Toole's Cerebrovascular Disorders, Sixth Edition

Toole's Cerebrovascular Disorders was the first modern book devoted to the care of stroke, originally published more than 40 years ago. Drs. E. Steve Roach, Kerstin Bettermann, and José Biller have completely revised and updated this sixth edition of the highly respected standard for stroke diagnosis and treatment, adding chapters on genetics, pregnancy-related stroke, and acute treatment. The practical focus of the book has not changed, retaining its emphasis on bedside diagnosis and treatment. Easily accessible for both stroke specialists and residents, this sixth edition has been modernized to keep pace with the rapid expansion of knowledge in stroke care and includes evidence-based recommendations, the latest technology and imaging, and risk factors. The text is supplemented with more than 200 images, many in color.

E. Steve Roach, MD, FAAN, FAHA, is Professor of Pediatrics and Neurology and Director of the Division of Child Neurology at The Ohio State University College of Medicine, Columbus, Ohio.

Kerstin Bettermann, MD, PhD, is Assistant Professor of Neurology at Penn State College of Medicine, Hershey, Pennsylvania.

José Biller, MD, FACP, FAAN, FAHA, is Professor of Neurology and Neurosurgery and Chairman of the Department of Neurology at Loyola University Chicago Stritch School of Medicine, Maywood, Illinois.

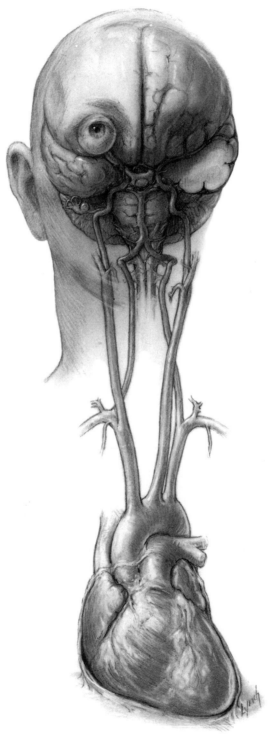

What is the hardest of all? What you as easiest would deem
To see with your eyes, what lies before your eyes.
Johann Wolfgang von Goethe

TOOLE'S
Cerebrovascular Disorders,
Sixth Edition

E. STEVE ROACH

The Ohio State University College of Medicine, Columbus, Ohio

KERSTIN BETTERMANN

Penn State College of Medicine, Hershey, Pennsylvania

JOSÉ BILLER

Loyola University Chicago Stritch School of Medicine, Maywood, Illinois

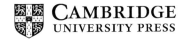

CAMBRIDGE UNIVERSITY PRESS
Cambridge, New York, Melbourne, Madrid, Cape Town, Singapore,
São Paulo, Delhi, Dubai, Tokyo

Cambridge University Press
32 Avenue of the Americas, New York, NY 10013-2473, USA

www.cambridge.org
Information on this title: www.cambridge.org/9780521866224

First published 2010

Printed in the United States of America

A catalog record for this publication is available from the British Library.

Library of Congress Cataloging in Publication Data

Roach, E. S. (Ewell Steve)
Toole's cerebrovascular disorders. – 6th ed. / E. Steve Roach, Kerstin Bettermann, José Biller.
p. ; cm.
Rev. ed. of: Cerebrovascular disorders / James F. Toole. 5th ed. c1999.
Includes bibliographical references and index.
ISBN 978-0-521-86622-4 (hardback)
1. Cerebrovascular disease. I. Bettermann, Kerstin. II. Biller, José. III. Toole, James F.,
1925– Cerebrovascular disorders. IV. Title. V. Title: Cerebrovascular disorders.
[DNLM: 1. Cerebrovascular Disorders. WL 355 R628t 2009]

RC388.5.T6 2009
616.8′1–dc22   2009013065

ISBN 978-0-521-86622-4 Hardback

We dedicate this book to
Lisa Hyde Roach
Wolfram, Katherine, and Sebastian Bettermann
Rhonda T. Biller

Contents

Contributor Affiliations

David C. Good, MD
Professor and Chair
Department of Neurology
Penn State University
College of Medicine
Hershey, Pennsylvania

Lumy Sawaki, MD, PhD
Associate Professor
Departments of Physical Medicine and Rehabilitation and
Neurology
University of Kentucky College of Medicine
Lexington, Kentucky

James F. Toole, MD
Walter C. Teagle Professor of Neurology
Wake Forest University School of Medicine
Winston-Salem, North Carolina

Foreword

I am honored that three such highly authoritative stroke neurologists have produced the sixth English edition of what began at Wake Forest in 1964 as a collaboration with my research Fellow, Aneel Patel. Our goal was to summarize the nascent field by writing the first textbook devoted solely to the prevention, diagnosis, management, and rehabilitation of stroke, emphasizing transient ischemic attacks – then a new concept. At that time there were no stroke journals or texts devoted solely to the topic even though stroke was already becoming recognized as a leading cause of disability and death worldwide.

We reviewed anatomy, physiology, patient presentation and examination, differential diagnosis, management, and rehabilitation. In those days our equipment was a detailed history, a reflex hammer, a tuning fork, a wisp of cotton, and a pin. We adopted the stethoscope as well as ophthalmoscope for neurologic use. There were few useful neurodiagnostic tests. Before ultrasound, computed tomography, computed tomography angiography, magnetic resonance imaging, and SPECT, we used skull X-rays to determine displacement of the calcified pineal gland because it was thought too daring to do an arteriogram. The prevailing attitude was "There is no treatment for stroke, so what purpose do dangerous studies serve?" I took the opposite view – that severe carotid stenosis, even if still asymptomatic, deserved medical and perhaps surgical intervention and that atherosclerosis could be stabilized and in some cases even reversed. At that time these were bold theories and actions. Gradually, of course, attitudes about stroke care have changed, and we have evolved from a largely intuitive approach to a more evidence-based mentality that is made possible by years of study and painstakingly completed multi-center clinical trials.

Dr. Richard L. Masland, previously at Wake Forest University and subsequently Director of the National Institute of Neurologic Diseases, along with Dr. Murray Goldstein designed and implemented the stroke portion of President Lyndon Johnson's so-called War on Heart Disease, Cancer, and Stroke. Our medical center subsequently became the third in the nation to be designated a stroke center. Over time we attracted a number of extraordinarily talented people,

including Dr. Lawrence McHenry, a medical historian who helped to develop cerebral blood flow measurement; Dr. William M. McKinney, who led the charge in developing and promoting ultrasound as a noninvasive neurovascular imaging tool; Dr. Richard Janeway, who rose to become dean of our medical college; and Dr. David Good, a neurorehabilitation specialist who has contributed to the last several editions of this book. Assisted by Diane C. Vernon and Ralph Hicks, we participated in the formation of national and international stroke societies and the editing of journals and texts, which have resulted in worldwide attention to this dread disorder – stroke.

We also attracted exceptional people for training, among them all three authors of this sixth edition of *Cerebrovascular Disorders*: E. Steve Roach, MD, a child neurologist specializing in stroke and genetics; Dr. José Biller, MD, a superb clinician and educator who focuses on stroke and cerebrovascular disorders; and most recently Kerstin Bettermann, MD, PhD, an expert in stroke and neurocirculatory physiology. I am proud to have influenced these and other outstanding colleagues, and as I leave the bedside for a more research-oriented life, I enthusiastically pass the baton to them as a team akin to that of Olympian Roger Bannister, neurocirculatory physiologist and neurologist, who electrified the world by doing the impossible – breaking the track barrier of the four-minute mile.[1] Of course, Bannister's hard-earned track record was quickly surpassed, as will be, one hopes, our current achievements in the study of stroke.

The six editions of *Cerebrovascular Disorders* mirror to a large extent the changes in our understanding of stroke and its diagnosis, prevention, management, and rehabilitation over the last four decades. Each succeeding edition incorporated an increasing array of new diagnostic techniques and reflected a progressively more sophisticated understanding of stroke in all its forms and presentations, increasingly supported by experimental models and patient-centered clinical trials. As evidenced by the numerous new pathological specimens that illustrate this sixth edition, it retains the firm grounding in neuroanatomy and pathology that characterized the previous editions. Like the earlier editions, this one strives to make the concepts that underlie stroke prevention, diagnosis, and management understandable to both clinicians and students. Moreover, this edition includes new developments in the prevention, diagnosis, and treatment of stroke, with new considerations of arterial dissection, genetic aspects, acute therapy, and vasculopathies as well as major updates of endovascular treatment, pathophysiology, technology, and primary and secondary stroke prevention. In the future, new concepts and methods will continue to accumulate, and so I applaud my author colleagues for providing a comprehensive, readable, and authoritative picture of what stroke care has become.

James F. Toole, MD
The Walter C. Teagle Professor of Neurology and Public Health Sciences
Wake Forest University Baptist Medical Center
Past President of the American Neurological Association
Past President of the World Federation of Neurology
Past President of the International Stroke Society

REFERENCE

1. Bascomb N. *The Perfect Mile: Three Athletes, One Goal, and Less than Four Minutes to Achieve It.* Boston: Houghton Mifflin; 2004.

Preface

Although Gregor Nymmann and Johann Jakob Wepfer wrote books on apoplexy as early as the seventeenth century, it was James F. Toole's first edition of *Cerebrovascular Disorders* in 1967 that defined stroke as a field for study. It summarized what was then known about the anatomy, pathophysiology, diagnosis, and treatment of stroke in a fashion that was so clear, logical, and positive that it sparked in many of us a lifetime interest in the study of cerebrovascular disease.

Despite centuries of observation, much of what we now deem useful knowledge about stroke has been discovered in the four decades since the 1967 appearance of *Cerebrovascular Disorders*. Stroke was then mostly a diagnosis based on bedside examination, knowledge of brain and vascular anatomy, clinical experience, and intuition. Therapeutic nihilism was the order of the day. Cerebral angiography could confirm certain diagnoses, and echoencephalography was used to detect displacement of the midline by a subdural hematoma or large intracerebral hemorrhage. Confirmation of a clinical diagnosis was difficult and awaited autopsy in the days before the now-ubiquitous imaging studies. The ensuing years have seen the development of multiple neuroimaging methods, new surgical and endovascular techniques, and new and more effective forms of therapy. But perhaps the most important long-term development in stroke care during the last few years has been the results of randomized clinical trials that increasingly augment clinical decisions.

The first five editions of *Cerebrovascular Disorders* chronicled the evolution of the field and, in many instances, included innovations that led to change. Our aim in writing this sixth edition is to maintain this tradition by creating a readily understandable and practical source of information about the prevention, diagnosis, and treatment of stroke to be a guide for experienced clinicians and trainees alike. It is our hope that ours as well as related books will continue to need updates, because, despite the extraordinary progress made, there is much still to discover and learn.

We thank some of the people who helped to create this book. Drs. David C. Good and Lumy Sawaki were kind enough to update their chapter on rehabilitation after stroke, and Dr. Toole contributed the first chapter on the history of the field. Artist George C. Lynch created numerous anatomical illustrations for the early editions, and some of these have been reused. We are particularly grateful for the unwavering editorial assistance provided by Lisa H. Roach, Ruth Vileikis, and Ralph Hicks with the help of Paula Griffin-Arnold, Linda Turner, and Gail White. Several colleagues provided illustrations or critiqued chapters, among them Nick Hogan, Louis Carragine, Dixon Moody, Geoffrey Heyer, and Sarkis Morales-Vidal.

In the interest of full disclosure, we should acknowledge that we three authors had the privilege of training with James F. Toole. As tempting as it might be to attribute any errors that may have crept into this book to gaps in our early training and subsequent mentoring, we alone are responsible for its content.

E. Steve Roach, MD
Kerstin Bettermann, MD, PhD
José Biller, MD

Toole's Cerebrovascular Disorders, Sixth Edition

A History of Cerebrovascular Disease since the Renaissance

James F. Toole, MD

Those who cannot remember the past are condemned to repeat it.

George Santayana

In the last three decades, there have been tremendous advances in technology and scientific knowledge that have revolutionized stroke prevention, diagnosis, and treatment. Noninvasive, painless, and safe imaging techniques now enable the clinician to pinpoint the size and location of brain lesions that in the not too distant past could be suspected but not easily or safely confirmed. Only 40 years ago, for example, the standard mode for differentiating brain hemorrhage from ischemic infarction was a lumbar puncture to examine for blood in the cerebrospinal fluid, and later a midline echogram might have been utilized to detect a shift of the midline structures caused by a unilateral cerebral lesion. Both of these techniques have been rendered obsolete by computed cranial tomography and magnetic resonance imaging studies. Similarly, therapeutics have improved dramatically. Clinical trials have better defined the usefulness of older drugs such as aspirin and anticoagulants, and tissue plasminogen activator (tPA) has emerged as a means to dissolve a clot and reestablish blood flow quickly enough to prevent brain tissue destruction.

In addition to these and other advances in diagnosis and treatment, infrastructural improvements in health care delivery, research collaboration and funding, and dissemination of information have spurred progress. Local, regional, national, and international health systems have been created for patients suffering with stroke. Responsibility for the care of individuals with stroke has shifted from individual physicians to specialized stroke treatment and rehabilitation teams that improve the outcome. Emergency therapies require knowledgeable health professionals to be available at all times. Large-scale public funding of biomedical research has enabled large multicenter clinical trials to provide data that increasingly dictate the treatment. Electronic editing and publishing have revolutionized medical research, communication, and clinical practice, in the process reducing costs and increasing the availability of information regarding effective therapy.

Knowledge of stroke rests on the generations of accumulated facts and observations that underpin our understanding of the pathophysiology of cerebrovascular disease. The threads of this long process are woven subtly into the fabric of our knowledge as eponymic names of signs and diseases and as long-accepted assumptions. But without a sense of the historical continuity of ideas, it is difficult to understand them. Therefore, we highlight some of the milestones in our understanding of cerebrovascular disease, concentrating on the post-Renaissance era.

OBSERVATIONAL STUDIES OF ANATOMY AND PATHOPHYSIOLOGY

Knowledge of human anatomy, and therefore understanding of function, were impeded during the Middle Ages when dissection of the human body was forbidden because resurrection of the body was an act of faith. Nevertheless, dissections were performed secretly in Bologna by Mondino di Luzi in the fourteenth century.[1] William Harvey, in England, is thought to have dissected the bodies of his own father and sister. Andreas Vesalius revolutionized the study of anatomy with the publication of his *De Humani Corporis Fabrica* (Figure 1-1), challenging the centuries-old teachings of Galen with new observations based on his human dissections.[2] Vesalius's pupil Fallopius illustrated the cerebral blood vessels in his *Observationes Anatomica* (1561) and included a description of the circle of Willis. However, it took many years for these early concepts of blood circulation to be reexamined and validated by Harvey[3] and accepted by others such as Wepfer, Lower, and Willis (Figure 1-2).[4–6]

Efforts toward prevention and therapy were scant because stroke was attributed to punishment by God, who "smote, or struck down" sinners, thus the origin of the term stroke. The first monographs on apoplexy were published by Gregor Nymmann from Wittenberg, Germany, in 1619 and Johann Jakob Wepfer working in Germany and Switzerland in 1658.[5,7] Wepfer was the first to record that stroke can be caused by hemorrhage as well as by clotting.

In 1658 Wepfer described "corpora fibrosa" in the wall of blood vessels as the cause for vascular stenosis and stroke

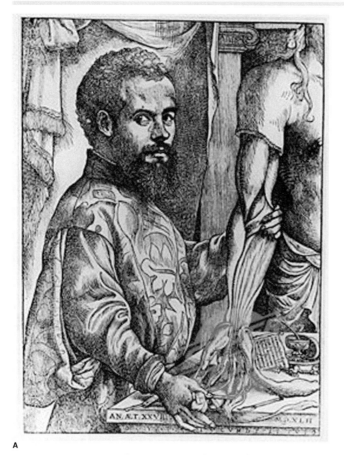

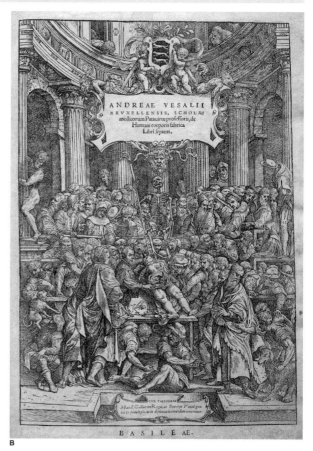

Figure 1-1. A: Andreas Vesalius. B: Illustration from Vesalius, *De Humani Corporis Fabrica* (1543).

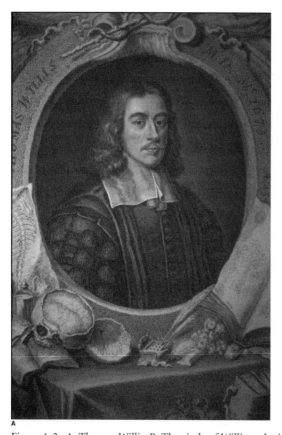

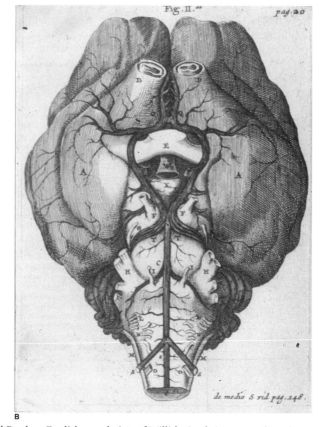

Figure 1-2. A: Thomas Willis. B: The circle of Willis as depicted in the Samuel Pordage English translation of Willis's *Cerebri Anatome* (1681).

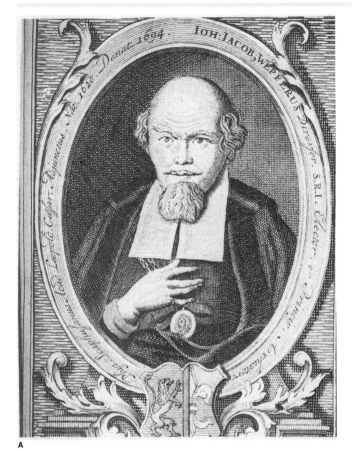

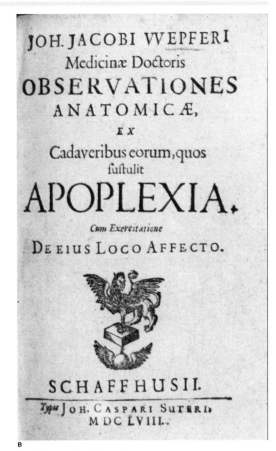

A B

Figure 1-3. A: Johann Jacobus Wepfer. B: Title page from Wepfer's *Apoplexia* (1658).

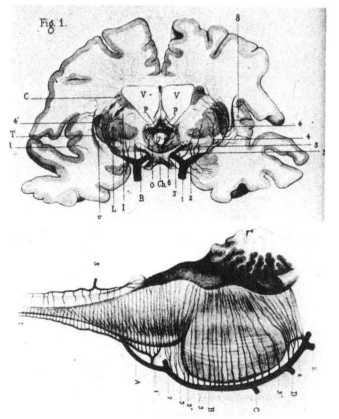

Figure 1-4. Duret's 1874 drawings of the distribution of the lenticulo-striate arteries and the penetrating branches of the basilar artery.

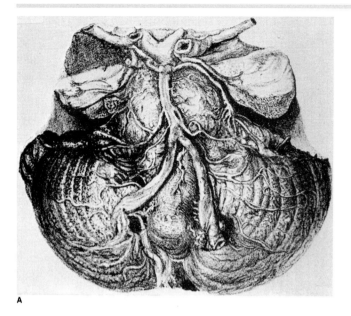
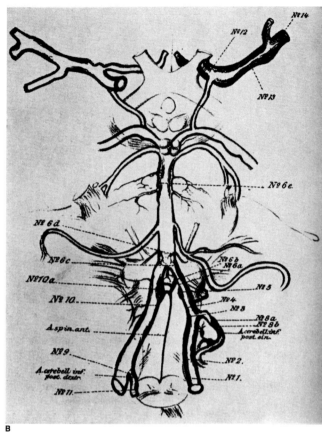

Figure 1-5. A: Autopsy drawing of Wallenberg's patient showing atherosclerosis of the major cerebral arteries. B: Another drawing illustrates the occlusion of the posterior inferior cerebral artery.

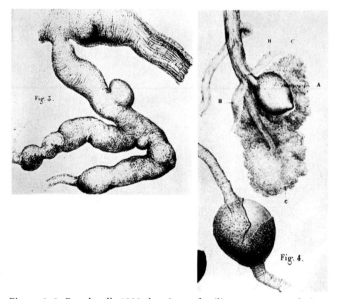

Figure 1-6. Bouchard's 1822 drawings of miliary aneurysms, lesions that he and Charcot believed to be the source of bleeding in intracranial hemorrhage.

(Figure 1-3).[5] Later, Bayle postulated that calcified carotid artery plaques could lead to stroke.[8] However, localization of cerebral function and the delineation of perfusion territories did not gain momentum until the eighteenth century. In 1754 von Swieten in his commentaries on Boerhaave's work stated that stroke could be caused by an embolism from the heart.[9] Morgagni of Padua correlated different clinical stroke types with postmortem studies in his monumental work *De Sebidus*.[10,11]

A MANUAL

OF

DISEASES OF THE NERVOUS SYSTEM

BY

W. R. GOWERS, M.D., F.R.C.P.,

ASSISTANT PROFESSOR OF CLINICAL MEDICINE IN UNIVERSITY COLLEGE, LONDON; PHYSICIAN TO
UNIVERSITY COLLEGE HOSPITAL AND TO THE NATIONAL HOSPITAL FOR
THE PARALYZED AND EPILEPTIC.

AMERICAN EDITION,

ISSUED UNDER THE SUPERVISION OF THE AUTHOR, AND CONTAINING ALL THE
MATERIAL OF THE TWO-VOLUME ENGLISH EDITION, WITH
SOME ADDITIONS AND REVISIONS.

WITH

THREE HUNDRED AND FORTY-ONE ILLUSTRATIONS.

PHILADELPHIA:
P. BLAKISTON, SON & CO.,
1012 WALNUT STREET.
1888.

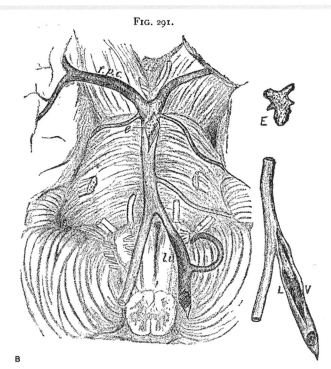

FIG. 291.

Figure 1-7. A: Title page of Gowers's *Manual of Diseases of the Nervous System*, the monograph that was sometimes called the "Bible of Neurology." B: Drawing of a vertebral artery embolism from Gowers's *Manual.*

The foundation for modern topography and classification of stroke was laid in the 1800s by the work of many individuals, including Abercrombie in Edinburgh, Carswell and Bright in London, and Heubner in Leipzig.[12–15] Additional contributions were made by Virchow and by Cohnheim[16,17] as well as by Charcot, Cruveilhier, Duret, and Foix in France.[16,18–21] Duret in 1873 was one of the first to delineate vascular territories (Figure 1-4), and numerous eponymic syndromes based on brainstem vascular occlusions (Figure 1-5) were described.[22–24] Charcot and others described anatomical variations, and Bouchard described dilations of the small penetrating arteries that they believed were responsible for brain hemorrhage (Figure 1-6).[21,25]

During the early to mid-nineteenth century, hemorrhagic and nonischemic stroke were differentiated by Carswell, Cruveilhier, Durand-Fardel, and many others.[14,19,26] Chiari in 1905 and Ramsay Hunt in 1914 established that cerebral vascular disease occurs at the carotid bifurcation in the neck.[27,28] They suggested that the carotid arteries should be examined clinically, an idea that was later made feasible by the introduction of cerebral angiography during the 1920s, ultrasound in the 1960s, and magnetic resonance angiography and cranial computed tomography (CT) angiography more recently.

Gowers in 1885 described cardiac embolism and thrombosis as an etiology of stroke (Figure 1-7).[29,30] This concept was later emphasized by Osler and McCrae in the neurological diseases portion of their influential *Modern Medicine – Its Theory and Practice.*[31] During the early twentieth century, it became obvious that atrial fibrillation could cause cerebral infarction, and in the 1990s warfarin was shown to reduce the risk of embolic stroke due to cardiac embolism. Warfarin was introduced for anticoagulation in humans in 1954.

In 1933 Wolkoff undertook the scientific study of cerebral arteriosclerosis, and Keele noted the effects of systemic hypertension on the carotid sinus region.[32,33] More recent contributions to stroke categorization were made by Zülch in Germany and C. Miller Fisher in the United States.[34–37] Until the 1950s the cause of carotid thrombosis was debated, with several authors suggesting syphilis or trauma as the etiology. In 1951, Fisher and Adams established that carotid artery atherosclerosis can cause cerebral infarction, often preceded by a transient ischemic attack due to embolic particles from an atherosclerotic plaque.[38] In 1961 Toole and colleagues presented two patients with stenosis of the left subclavian artery causing reversal of flow through the vertebral artery into the arm, introducing the concept of the subclavian steal syndrome.[39]

CEREBRAL PERFUSION, METABOLISM, AND NEUROIMAGING

In 1762 von Haller observed that the caliber of pial vessels changed during the cardiac cycle.[40] By 1783 Monro and Kellie in Scotland had formulated the doctrine named for them that the blood volume within the nonexpandable skull cavity tends to remain constant at all times.[41] However, Burrows showed in his 1846 monograph that the blood volume within the brain can vary somewhat with changing physiological states.[42] In 1850 Donders of Utrecht observed the response of pial vessels to asphyxia through a glass window in the skull.[43] Thereafter, Sherrington and Roy introduced the modern concept of cerebral vascular autoregulation.[44] Based partly on their demonstration of autoregulation of cerebral blood flow, Kety and Schmidt as well as McHenry developed methods to measure regional cerebral blood flow in patients using inert gases such as krypton and xenon.[45–49]

Imaging of arteries and veins using blood-borne radioopaque media and X-rays was introduced by Egas Moniz in Portugal.[50] He initially injected strontium bromide as an intraarterial contrast agent but later substituted iodinated contrast.[51] He was awarded the Nobel Prize – for his role in developing the now-discredited prefrontal leucotomy rather than his more long-lasting contribution to the diagnosis of vascular disease.[52] In 1961 Sokoloff initiated functional brain imaging by demonstrating the relation between regional cerebral blood flow and brain metabolism.[53,54] The use of single photon emission computed tomography (SPECT) for assessment of stroke patients today owes a debt to the first nuclide images by Kuhl and Edwards in 1963.[55]

The once critical bedside examination skills for localizing a brain lesion have been to some extent supplanted by the revolution in neuroimaging, especially computed cranial tomography in the 1970s and magnetic resonance imaging (MRI) in the 1980s. The construction of the first prototype camera based on the Compton effect, suggested in 1977, was performed by Singh and Doria in 1983.[56,57] The development of SPECT, xenon CT, positron emission tomography (PET), and functional MRI during the last three decades augment the ever-growing array of imaging techniques available for diagnosis and targeted treatment of stroke patients today.

Noninvasive visualization of anatomy of the brain became possible with the development of head CT by Oldendorf and then by Hounsfield and Cormack of Britain during the 1970s.[58–60] Subsequently, MRI was developed during the 1980s by Mansfield in Britain and by Lauterbur in the United States, who were awarded the Nobel Prize in 2003.[61,62] MRI was based on the magnetic resonance phenomenon independently characterized by the U.S. physicists Bloch and Purcell, both of whom received the Nobel Prize in physics in 1952.[63–65] Continued advances in computer technology and data analysis techniques have reduced the image acquisition time and created new avenues for acute stroke diagnosis and treatment. The development of CT angiography and MR angiography during the 1980s and the improvement of these techniques during subsequent years now allow rapid, precise visualization of the brain and its vasculature.

The subsequent initial application of Doppler techniques for blood vessel assessment by Olinger in 1969 and by Reid and Spencer in 1972 was quickly followed by the application of ultrasound to depict the brain's blood supply.[66,67] Olinger, based on previous work by Herz and Bliss, described the visualization of carotid arteries by B-mode ultrasound imaging.[66,68] In 1972 Blue and colleagues demonstrated the diagnostic validity of B-mode ultrasound images by comparing them to conventional carotid arteriography.[69] Miyazaki and Kato furthered transcranial Doppler as a diagnostic tool for stroke patients by recording changes in blood flow velocities through the intact human skull based on the Doppler effect.[70]

STROKE PREVENTION AND INTERVENTION

Identification of stroke risk factors provides a way to reduce the incidence of stroke by modifying the underlying condition or designing treatments based on specific pathophysiology. Recognition of the importance of tobacco use and systemic hypertension in the pathophysiology of cardiac disease and stroke led to more aggressive attempts to control them by education, diet, and medication, efforts that probably contributed to the decline in stroke incidence in recent years.[71]

The bark of the willow tree was used as a traditional herbal treatment for fever and pain in Europe long before its active ingredient acetylsalicylic acid (aspirin) was synthesized by chemists at the Bayer Company in Germany in 1887. In the 1960s the antithrombotic effect of aspirin was recognized, and the drug was introduced for the prevention of stroke in the 1970s.[72] Subsequent large-scale clinical trials showed that regular aspirin use reduced the risk of stroke due to atherosclerosis. Similarly, randomized clinical trials in the 1990s confirmed that warfarin, first introduced as an anticoagulant in humans in 1954, lowers the risk of ischemic stroke caused by cardiac embolism secondary to atrial fibrillation.

After 40 years of intense research, tPA (tissue plasminogen activator) was introduced in 1995 and became standard treatment for acute ischemic stroke for individuals presenting within 3 to 4.5 hours of symptom onset. However, the first randomized trial investigating the feasibility of a thrombolytic drug was published in 1963.[73] Further trials between 1963 and 1993 using tPA, urokinase, and streptokinase were inconclusive regarding the effectiveness and safety of thrombolytic drugs.[74–76] Neuroimaging techniques were incorporated into the multicenter acute stroke trial designs of the 1990s that demonstrated the feasibility of intravenous tPA administration in acute stroke patients, leading to the pivotal study of tPA by the National Institute of Neurological Disorders and Stroke (NINDS) in 1995 and FDA approval in 1996.[77,78]

SURGICAL AND INTRAVASCULAR THERAPIES

Before the use of carotid endarterectomy to prevent stroke from carotid atherosclerosis, carotid artery surgery was occasionally performed for other reasons, although often unsuccessfully.[79,80] Ligation of the common carotid artery without causing neurological deficit was documented in an aneurysm patient by Hebenstreit in 1793.[81] During the early twentieth century, carotid artery compression tests were explored and several initial carotid artery surgery efforts were recorded.[82,83] In 1916 Parczewski removed an arteriovenous aneurysm in the common carotid artery and performed a successful end-to-end anastomosis.[84] Carotid ligation was also an early means for controlling a distal carotid aneurysm.[85] In 1950 Gordon-Murray in Toronto restored the circulation to the common carotid artery of a 54-year-old man with syphilitic aortitis and occlusion of all four major cervicocephalic arteries.[83] The following year in

Table 1-1: Stroke Milestones

Discovery	Location	Person	Year
De Humani Corporis Fabrica, first drawings of cerebral circulation	Italy	Vesalius	1543
Depiction of circle of Willis	Italy	Fabricus	1561
Characterization of blood circulation and heart motion	UK	Harvey	1628
Description of physiological role of circle of Willis and described TIAs	UK	Willis	1621–1675
Syntagma Anatomicum, illustration of the complete circle of Willis	Germany	Vesling	1647
First monographs published on apoplexy	Germany, Switzerland	Wepfer	1619–1657
Description of atherosclerosis	Germany	Wepfer	1658
Arteries as etiology for stroke, describes calcified plaques	France	Bayle	1677
Apoplexy caused by cardiac embolism	Netherlands	von Swieten	1754
Four volumes on apoplexy	Italy	Morgagni	1761
Monro-Kellie doctrine	Scotland	Monro and Kellie	1783
Further description of TIAs	UK	Heberden	1802
Treatise on Apoplexy with first illustration of SAH, first to identify anemia as a cause of stroke	Ireland	Cheyne	1812
Pathological and Practical Researches on Disease of the Brain and Spinal Cord	UK	Abercrombie	1828
Observation of pial vessels via sealed glass window in closed skull; description of Takayasu arteritis case	Netherlands	Donders	1850
Description of carotid thrombosis causing blindness, studies on emboli, ICH	Germany	Virchow	1856
Mapping vascular territories	France	Duret and Charcot	1873–1874
Cerebral vascular autoregulation	UK	Sherrington and Roy	1890
Diseases of the Nervous System, ICH, aneurysms, cerebral emboli	Canada	Osler	1893
Discovery of X-rays	Germany	Roentgen	1895
Histopathology of arteriosclerosis, describes Alzheimer disease	Germany	Alzheimer	1897
Established that extracranial vascular disease leads to stroke	Italy	Chiari	1905
First description of carotid occlusion causing stroke	USA	Hunt	1914
Concept of hypertensive encephalopathy, chronic white matter disease	Germany	Binswanger	1917
Pneumo-encephalography	USA	Dandy	1918
Cerebral angiography description	Portugal	Moniz	1927
Catheter angiography, awarded 1956 Nobel Prize	Germany	Forssmann	1928
Scientific study of cerebral arteriosclerosis	Sweden	Wolkoff	1933
Plethysmography to measure CBF in humans	USA	Ferris	1941
Determination of human CBF and oxygen consumption	USA	Kety and Schmidt	1948
Cutaneous method for inserting arterial catheter	Sweden	Seldinger	1953
Carotid artery surgery	UK	Eastcott, Pickering, and Rob	1953
First Princeton Conference on cerebrovascular disease	USA	Wright	1954
Prospective Randomized Study of carotid endarterectomy	USA	DeBakey	1959

(continued)

Table 1-1 *(continued)*

Discovery	Location	Person	Year
Demonstration of increased rCBF with brain activity	USA	Sokoloff	1961
Quantitative measurement of rCBF in humans	Sweden	Ingvar and Lassen	1961
Reversal of flow in vertebral artery named subclavian steal	USA	Toole	1961
Tomographic brain images with SPECT	USA	Kuhl and Edwards	1963
Visualization of carotid arteries by B-mode ultrasound	USA	Olinger	1969
Ultrasound images of interior of blood vessels	USA	Reid and Spencer	1972
B-mode ultrasound scanning and results correlated with conventional arteriography	USA	Blue, McKinney, and Barnes	1972
Computerized cranial tomography	UK	Hounsfield, Ambrose, and Cormack	1973
SPECT	USA	Everett et al.	1977
Prototype of Compton camera built for SPECT	UK	Singh and Doria	1983
MRA imaging of arteries	USA	Dumoulin et al.	1987
Anticoagulation is proven effective for stroke prevention in atrial fibrillation, stroke centers introduced, tPA introduced, ACAS	USA		1970s–2000
NASCET and ACAS trials result in evidence-based indication for carotid endarterectomy	USA and Canada		1990s
fMRI developed for brain mapping	USA	Ogawa and Lee	1993
Nobel Prize for Medicine for MRI	USA	Mansfield and Lauterbur	2003
International Stroke Society, World Stroke Federation, and individual countries form societies for dissemination of knowledge through internet	Worldwide		2000–present

ACAS = Asymptomatic Carotid Atherosclerosis Study; CBF = cerebral blood flow; fMRI = functional magnetic resonance imaging; ICH = intracerebral hemorrhage; MRI = magnetic resonance imaging; NASCET = North American Symptomatic Carotid Endarterectomy Trial; rCBF = regional cerebral blood flow; SPECT = single photon emission computed tomography; TIA = transient ischemic attack; tPA = tissue plasminogen activator.

Argentina, Carrea and colleagues surgically reconstructed the carotid artery, joining the external carotid artery to the proximal internal carotid artery to reperfuse the brain.[86]

Strully and colleagues described one of the first endarterectomy procedures in 1953, and, in 1954 Eastcott and associates successfully reconstructed the carotid artery in an individual with intermittent hemiplegia.[87,88] In 1975 Michael DeBakey published the results of a cooperative study to determine the efficacy for stroke prevention by comparing endarterectomy to usual medical management and treatment. This was one of the first multicenter international trials in stroke treatment. DeBakey noted in that article that his first carotid endarterectomy patient had undergone an endarterectomy in 1953 and had lived for 19 years before death from coronary artery disease.[89,90] With the recent advancement of neuroimaging and the introduction of new microcatheters, endovascular interventions have now become state-of-the-art and may replace invasive surgical approaches for carotid disease.[91]

The development of microcatheters, thrombolytic agents, and intravascular devices have made acute stroke treatment feasible. In the early 1960s the concept of percutaneous luminal angioplasty was introduced, and Charles Dotter was one of the first to publish a technique for placing endovascular stents via a percutaneous approach.[92] As cerebral angiography improved, more intricate intravascular treatment techniques became feasible. Luessenhop and colleagues demonstrated the feasibility of intracranial artery catherization with flow-directed balloon-tipped catheters in 1964.[93,94] Gruentzig, a Swiss radiologist, was the first to perform transluminal coronary angioplasty in 1977.[95] The further development of new stents during the 1980s allowed stent applications starting with the work of Maass and colleagues.[96] He was one of the pioneers to use the earliest generation of newly developed self-expanding spring coils for stenting of the iliac and inferior cava vein and the aorta at the University of Zurich in Switzerland. In the early 1970s Serbinenko initiated endovascular therapy, reporting the first treatment of an intracranial aneurysm using a detachable balloon inserted via a newly developed microcatheter.[97,98] Stent development and catheter techniques evolved further during the 1970s and 1980s, first in the area of peripheral and coronary artery stenting and later in the treatment of cerebrovascular disease, allowing treatment of extra- and intracranial stenosis, vascular malformations, aneurysms, and the local injection of intra-arterial thrombolytics for acute ischemic stroke.

EVIDENCE-BASED MEDICINE AND STROKE ORGANIZATIONS

In reviewing the development of the field of stroke over the centuries it becomes apparent how much of our knowledge represents global interaction by physicians and scientists from many nations. The collaborative effort is demonstrated by the formation of national and international stroke societies, first in the United Kingdom in 1898, later in the United States, and now globally.

Research and care for patients with stroke and other neurologic illness in the United States was accelerated by the National Institutes of Health (NIH) and the National Institute of Neurologic Disease and Blindness (later the National Institute of Neurological Diseases and Stroke, or NINDS). At the end of World War II there were millions of veterans with neuropsychiatric disorders, accounting for an estimated 20% of patients in general hospitals. However, in 1950 there were relatively few neurologists, leading to a series of meetings and the identification of nervous system disorders as a national priority. The expansion of the NIH made possible the funding of the numerous large-scale, prospective multicenter clinical trials which have revolutionized our understanding of stroke in recent years. Many names are associated with this renaissance, but the most prominent are Drs. Richard L. Masland, Murray Goldstein, and Seymour Kety, who was appointed to oversee the internal research effort.[99] Ground-breaking clinical trials have studied the management of intracranial aneurysms, subarachnoid hemorrhage, carotid artery stenosis, transient ischemic attacks, hypertensive stroke, multiple infarct dementia, stroke due to sickle cell disease, and many other conditions.

Evidence-based medicine in neurology was introduced by the leadership of the Oxford Group with Sir Richard Doll and Richard Peto, who worked in synergy with new entrants to the neurosciences and neurology by designing, implementing, and reporting results of prospective randomized trials.

CEREBROVASCULAR DISEASE IN CHILDREN

Although stroke occurs in children much less often than in the elderly, incidence figures suggest that childhood stroke is more prevalent than cerebral tumors and many other neurological problems, making stroke in children a major public health issue. For many years, however, the occurrence of cerebrovascular disease among childhood went largely unrecognized and unstudied.

Willis described a newborn who had a cerebellar hemorrhage, and Morgagni recorded a cerebral hemorrhage in a 14-year-old boy.[100] Few additional developments occurred in childhood stroke until the nineteenth century, when several series of children with stroke appeared, including reports by Osler in 1889 and an 1891 series of 594 children by Sigmund Freud and Oscar Rie.[101,102] In 1890 Sachs and Peterson emphasized that children with acquired hemiplegia have vascular dysfunction.[103] Ford and Schaffer systematically studied etiology and outcome in a series of 70 children with acquired hemiplegia, foreshadowing the modern approach to the diagnosis and management of stroke during gestation, infancy, and childhood.[104] After this auspicious beginning, the study of childhood cerebrovascular disorders languished for several decades until the late 1960s, when moyamoya disease was described in Japan.[105,106]

The development of CT and then MRI and magnetic resonance angiography made noninvasive confirmation of a stroke diagnosis feasible. Then Roach, Biller, and others began to emphasize the importance of cerebrovascular dysfunction among children.[107,108] In Canada deVeber and colleagues used a large ischemic stroke registry to study the clinical features, risk factors, and outcome of ischemic stroke in children. Transcranial Doppler techniques were developed by Robert Adams and colleagues to predict stroke risk due to sickle cell disease, and these methods have now been used to select high-risk individuals with sickle cell disease for several randomized clinical trials.[109] The story is still unfolding.[110]

ADDITIONAL INFORMATION

Although our understanding of cerebrovascular disease has evolved at an uneven pace through the years, one can follow the threads of discovery through time, as concepts layer onto earlier ideas to form the foundation of what we now often take for granted. Knowing the pathway that we have followed adds depth and richness to of our understanding, but it is important to realize that our journey is far from finished. This brief overview is intended to highlight some of the major discoveries, hypotheses, and innovations (Table 1-1) that have stimulated the evolution of cerebrovascular disease as a discipline. For more details the reader is referred to the outstanding work on the history of neurology and stroke by McHenry, Garrison, Gurdjian, Fields, and Lemak.[111-114]

REFERENCES

1. Busacchi V. Mondino di' Liuzzi e i primordi della 'moderna' anatomia nell'antico Studio Bolognese. *Strenna Storica Bolognese.* 1987;**37**:101–112.
2. Vesalius A. *De humani corporus fabrica, libri VII.* Basel: Johannes Oporinus; 1543.
3. Harvey W. *Exercitatio anatomica de moru cordis et sanguinis in animalibus.* Francofurti: Fitzer; 1628.
4. Willis T. *Cerebri anatome: cui accessit nervorum descripto et usus.* London: J. Flesher; 1664.
5. Wepfer JJ. *Observations anatomicae, ex cadaveribus eorum, quos sustulit apoplexia, cum exercitatione de ejus loco affecto.* Schaffhausen: Joh. Caspari Suteri; 1658.
6. Lower R. *Tractus de corde, item de motu et colore sanguinis et chyli in eum transitu. Cui accessit dissertation de origine catarrhi, in qua oftenditur illum non provenire a cerebro.* 2nd ed. London: J. Redmayne; 1670.
7. Nymman G. *De apoplexia tractus.* 2nd ed. Witteberg: J.W. Fincelii; 1670.
8. Bayle F. *Tractatus de apoplexia.* Toulouse: B. Guillemette; 1677.
9. von Swieten G. *Of the Apoplexy, Palsy and Epilepsy. Commentaries upon the Aphorisms of Dr. Herman Boerhaave.* London: John & Paul Knapton; 1754.
10. Morgagni GB. *On the Seats and Causes of Diseases Investigated by Anatomy.* English translation in 3 volumes by B Alexander. London: Miller & Cadell, 1769.

11. Morgagni GB. *De sedibus, et causis morborum per anatomen indagatis libri quinque.* Vienna: ex typographica Remondiana; 1761.

12. Abercrombie J. *Pathological and Practical Researches on Diseases of the Brain and the Spinal Cord.* Edinburgh: Waugh and Innes; 1828.

13. Bright R. Cases illustrative of the effects produced when arteries and brain are diseased. *Guy's Hosp Rep.* 1836;**1**:9.

14. Carswell R. *Pathological Anatomy: Illustrations of the Elementary Forms of Disease.* London: Longman and Co.; 1838.

15. Heubner O. Topographie du Ernähiüngsgebiete einpelner Jormarteroem. *Zent Med Wiss.* 1872;**10**:817–821.

16. Virchow RLK. *Gesammelte Abhandlungen zur wissenschaftlichen Medizin.* Frankfurt: Meidinger; 1856.

17. Cohnheim J. *Vorlesungen über allgemeine Pathlogie.* Berlin: Hirschwald; 1882.

18. Foix C, Masson A. Le syndrome de "artère cérébrale postérieure." *Presse Méd.* 1923;**32**:361–365.

19. Cruveilhier J. *Anatomie pathologique du corps humain; descriptions avec figures lithographiees et coloriees; des diverses alterations morbides don't le corp humain est susceptible.* Paris: J.B. Bailliere; 1835.

20. Charcot JM. *Lectures on the Diseases of the Nervous System, delivered at the Salpêtrière, translated by G. Sigerson.* London: New Sydenham Society; 1877.

21. Charcot JM. *Leçons sur les localisations dans les maladies du cerveau.* Paris: Progrès Médical; 1876.

22. Duret H. Sur la distribution des artères nourricieres du bulbe rachidien. *Arch Physiol Norm Path.* 1873;**5**:97.

23. Duret H. Recherches anatomiques sur la circulation de l'encéphale. *Arch Phys Norm Path (2 sér).* 1874; **1**:60–69, 316–353, 664–693, 919–957.

24. Wallenberg A. Acute disease of the medulla. Embolus to the posterior inferior cerebellar artery? *Archiv Psychiatrie.* 1895;**24**:509–540.

25. Bouchard C. *A Study of Some Points in the Pathology of Cerebral Hemorrhage.* London: Simpkin, Marshall and Co.; 1872.

26. Durand-Fardel CLM. *Traitè du ramollissement du cerveau.* Paris: J.B. Baillière; 1843.

27. Chiari H. Über das Verhälten des Teilungswinkels der Carotis communis bei der Endasteritis chronic deformans. *Verh Deutsch Path Ges.* 1905;**9**:326.

28. Hunt JR. The role of the carotid arteries in the causation of vascular lesoins of the brain, with remarks on certain special features of the symptomatology. *Amer J Med Sci.* 1914;**147**:704.

29. Gowers WR. *A Manual of Diseases of the Nervous System.* Philadelphia: P. Blakiston, Son & Co.; 1888.

30. Gowers WR. *Lectures on the Diagnosis of Diseases of the Brain.* London: Churchill; 1885.

31. Osler W, McCrae T. *Modern Medicine: Its Theory and Practice.* Philadelphia: Lea & Febiger; 1910.

32. Wolkoff K. Über Atherosklerose der Gehirnarterien. *Bietr Z Path Anat Allg Path.* 1933;**91**:515.

33. Keele CA. Pathological changes in the carotid sinus and their relation to hypertension. *Quart J Med.* 1933;**2**:213–220.

34. Zulch KJ. Pathological aspects of cerebral accidents in arterial hypertension. *Acta Neurol Belg.* 1971;**71**:196–220.

35. Fisher CM. Lacunar strokes and infarcts: a review. *Neurology.* 1982;**32**:871–876.

36. Estol CJ. Dr C. Miller Fisher and the history of carotid artery disease. *Stroke.* 1996;**27**:559–566.

37. Fisher M. Occlusion of the carotid arteries: further experiences. *AMA Arch Neurol Psychiatry.* 1954;**72**:187–204.

38. Fisher M, Adams RD. Observations on brain embolism with special reference to the mechanism of hemorrhagic infarction. *J Neuropathol Exp Neurol.* 1951;**10**:92–94.

39. Reivich M, Holling HE, Roberts B, Toole JF. Reversal of blood flow through the vertebral artery and its effect on cerebral circulation. *N Engl J Med.* 1961; **265**:878–885.

40. von Haller A. *Elementa physiologiae corporis humani. Tomus quartus cerebrum nervi musculi.* Lausanne: Francisci Grasset; 1762.

41. Monro A. *Observations on the Structure and Functions of the Nervous System.* Edinburgh: W. Creech; 1783.

42. Burrows G. *On Disorders of the Cerebral Circulation and on the Connection between Affections of the Brain and Diseases of the Heart.* London: Longman, Brown, Green and Longmans; 1846.

43. Donders FC. De bevegingen der hersenen en de veranderingen der vaatvulling van de "Pia Mater," ook bij gesloten onuitzetberen schedel regtstreeks onderzocht. *Nederlandsche Lancet (Series 2).* 1850; **5**:521–553.

44. Roy CS, Sherrington CS. On the regulation of the blood-supply of the brain. *J Physiol.* 1890;**11**:85–158.

45. Kety SS, Schmidt CF. The nitrous oxide method for the quantitative determination of cerebral blood flow in man; theory, procedure and normal values. *J Clin Invest.* 1948;**27**:476–483.

46. Kety SS, Landau WM, Freygang WH Jr, Rowland LP, Sokoloff L. Estimation of regional circulation in the brain by the uptake of an inert gas. *Fed Proc.* 1955;**14**:85–86.

47. McHenry LC Jr. Measurement of cerebral blood flow. *N Engl J Med.* 1965;**273**:562–563.

48. McHenry LC Jr. Quantitative cerebral blood flow determination. Application of a krypton 85 desaturation technique in man. *Neurology.* 1964;**14**:785–793.

49. McHenry LC. Determination of cerebral blood flow by a krypton-85 desaturation method. *Nature.* 1963;**200**:1297–1299.

50. Moniz E. *L'angiographie cérébrale.* Paris: Masson; 1931.

51. Wolpert SM. Neuroradiology classics. *AJNR Am J Neuroradiol.* 1999;**20**:1752–1753.

52. Gorelick PB, Biller J. Egas Moniz: neurologist, statesman, and Nobel laureate. *J Lab Clin Med.* 1991;**118**:200–202.

53. Sokoloff L, Mangold R, Wechsler RL, Kenney C, Kety SS. The effects of mental arithmetic on cerebral circulation and metabolism. *J Clin Invest.* 1955;**34**:1101–1108.

54. Sokoloff L. Local cerebral circulation at rest and furing altered cerebral activity induced by anesthesia or visual stimulation. In: Kety SS, Elker G, eds. *Regional Neurochemistry.* Oxford: Pergamon Press; 1961:107–117.

55. Kuhl DE, Edwards RQ. Image separation radioisotope scanning. *Radiology.* 1963;**80**:653–662.

56. Everett DB, Fleming JS, Todd RW, Nightingale JM. Gamma-radiation imaging system based on the Compton effect. *Proc Inst Electr Eng.* 1977;**124**(11):995–1000.

57. Singh M, Doria D. An electronically collimated gamma camera for single photon emission computed tomography. Part II: Image reconstruction and preliminary experimental measurements. *Med Phys.* 1983;**10**:428–435.

58. Oldendorf WH. *The Quest for an Image of the Brain. Computerized Tomography in the Perspective of Past and Future Imaging Methods.* New York: Raven; 1980.

59. Hounsfield, GN. A method of and apparatus for examination of a body by radiation such as X-ray or gamma radiation. USPat#1, 283,915. 1972.

60. Cormack AM. Representation of a function by its line integrals, with some radiological applications. *J Appl Physiol.* 1963;**34**:2722.

61. Mansfield P. Muti-planar image-formation using NMR spin echoes. *J Phys C Solid State Phys.* 1977;**10**(3):L55–L58.

62. Lauterbur PC. Image formation by induced local interactions: examples employing nuclear magnetic resonance. *Nature.* 1973; **242**:190–191.

63. Bloch F. Nuclear induction. *Phys Rev.* 1946;**70**(7,8):460–474.

64. Purcell EM, Torry HC, Pound RV. Resonance absorption by nuclear magnetic moments in a solid. *Phys Rev*. 1946;**69**:37–38.

65. Carr HY, Purcell EM. Effects of diffusion on free precession in nuclear magnetic resonance experiments. *Phys Rev*. 1954;**94**:630–639.

66. Olinger CP. Ultrasonic carotid echoarteriography. *Am J Roentgenol Radium Ther Nucl Med*. 1969;**106**:282–295.

67. Reid JM, Spencer MP. Ultrasonic Doppler technique for imaging blood vessels. *Science*. 1972;**176**:1235–1236.

68. Hertz CH. Ultrasonic engineering in heart diagnosis. *Am J Cardiol*. 1967;**19**:6–17.

69. Blue SK, McKinney WM, Barnes R, Toole JF. Ultrasonic B-node scanning for study of extracranial vascular disease. *Neurology*. 1972;**22**:1079–1085.

70. Miyazaki M, Kato K. Measurement of cerebral blood flow by ultrasonic Doppler technique; hemodynamic comparison of right and left carotid artery in patients with hemiplegia. *Jpn Circ J*. 1965;**29**:383–386.

71. Whisnant JP. The decline of stroke. *Stroke*. 1984;**15**:160–168.

72. Craven LL. Acetylsalicylic acid, possible preventive of coronary thrombosis. *Ann West Med Surg*. 1950;**4**:95.

73. Meyer JS, Gilroy J, Barnhart MI, Johnson JF. Therapeutic thrombolysis in cerebral thromboembolism. Double-blind evaluation of intravenous plasmin therapy in carotid and middle cerebral arterial occlusion. *Neurology*. 1963;**13**:927–937.

74. Mori E, Yoneda Y, Tabuchi M, et al. Intravenous recombinant tissue plasminogen activator in acute carotid artery territory stroke. *Neurology*. 1992;**42**:976–982.

75. Yamagouchi T (for the Japanese Thrombolysis Study Group). Intravenous tissue plasminogen activator in acute thromboembolic stroke a placebo-controlled, double blind trial. In: del Zoppo GL, Mori E, Hacke W, eds. *Thrombolysis in Acute Ischemic Stroke*. New York: Springer-Verlag; 1993:59–65.

76. Haley EC Jr, Brott TG, Sheppard GL, et al. Pilot randomized trial of tissue plasminogen activator in acute ischemic stroke. The TPA Bridging Study Group. *Stroke*. 1993;**24**:1000–1004.

77. National Institute of Neurological Disorders and Stroke rt-PA Stroke Study Group. Tissue plasminogen activator for acute ischemic stroke. *N Engl J Med*. 1995;**333**:1581–1587.

78. The NINDS t-PA Stroke Study Group. Intracerebral hemorrhage after intravenous t-PA therapy for ischemic stroke. *Stroke*. 1997;**28**:2109–2118.

79. Thompson J. Carotid surgery: past is prologue? The John Homas Lecture. *J Vasc Surg*. 2003;**25**:131–140.

80. Robicsek F, Roush TS, Cook JW, Reames MK. From Hippocrates to Palmaz-Schatz, the history of carotid surgery. *Eur J Vasc Endovasc Surg*. 2004;**27**:389–397.

81. Hebenstreit EBG. *Zusatze zu Benj Bell's Abhandlung von den Geschwuren and deren Behandlung*. Germany; 1793.

82. Toole JF, Barrows LJ, Lambertsen CJ, Roberts B. Cerebral ischemia and infarction. *Am Pract Dig Treat*. 1961;**12**:147–154.

83. Fields WS, Lemak NA. *A History of Stroke, Its Recognition and Treatment*. New York: Oxford University Press; 1989.

84. von Parczewski S. Resektion und Naht der A carotis communis. *Munch Med Wochenschr*. 1916;**63**:1646–1647.

85. Walker AE. *A History of Neurological Surgery*. Baltimore: Williams & Wilkins; 1951.

86. Carrea R, Molins M, Murphy G. Surgical treatment of spontaneous thrombosis of the internal carotid artery in the neck. Carotid-carotideal anastomosis. *Acta Neurol Latinoamer*. 1955;**1**:71–78.

87. Strully KJ, Hurwitt ES, Blankenberg HW. Thrombo-endarterectomy for thrombosis of the internal carotid artery in the neck. *J Neurosurg*. 1953;**10**:474–482.

88. Eastcott HHG, Pickering GW, Robb CG. Reconstruction of internal carotid artery in a patient with intermittent attacks of hemiplegia. *Lancet*. 1954;**2**:994–996.

89. Debakey ME, Crawford ES, Cooley DA, Morris GC, Garret HE, Fields WS. Cerebral arterial insufficiency: one to 11-year results following arterial reconstructive operation. *Ann Surg*. 1965;**161**:921–945.

90. DeBakey ME. Successful carotid endarterectomy for cerebrovascular insufficiency. Nineteen-year follow-up. *JAMA*. 1975;**233**:1083–1085.

91. Thompson JE. The evolution of surgery for the treatment and prevention of stroke. The Willis Lecture. *Stroke*. 1996;**27**:1427–1434.

92. Dotter CT. Transluminally-placed coilspring endarterial tube grafts. Long-term patency in canine popliteal artery. *Invest Radiol*. 1969;**4**:329–332.

93. Luessenhop AJ, Velasquez AC. Observations on the tolerance of the intracranial arteries to catheterization. *J Neurosurg*. 1964;**21**:85–91.

94. Hopkins LN, Lanzino G, Guterman LR. Treating complex nervous system vascular disorders through a "needle stick": origins, evolution, and future of neuroendovascular therapy. *Neurosurgery*. 2001;**48**:463–475.

95. Gruntzig A. Transluminal dilatation of coronary-artery stenosis. *Lancet*. 1978;**1**:263.

96. Maass D, Kropf L, Egloff L, Demierre D, Turina M, Senning A. Transluminal implantation of intravascular "double helix" spiral prostheses: technical and biological considerations. *Esao Proc*. 1982;**9**:252–256.

97. Serbinenko FA. Catheterization and occlusion of major cerebral vessels and prospects for the development of vascular neurosurgery. *Vopr Neirokhir*. 1971; **35**:17–27.

98. Serbinenko FA. Balloon catheterization and occlusion of major cerebral vessels. *J Neurosurg*. 1974;**41**:125–145.

99. Rowland LR. *NINDs at 50. An Incomplete History Celebrating the Fiftieth Anniversary of the National Institute of Neurological Diseases and Stroke*. New York: Demos Medical Publications; 2003.

100. Schoenberg BS, Mellinger JF, Schoenberg DG. Cerebrovascular disease in infants and children: a study of incidence, clinical features, and survival. *Neurology*. 1978;**28**:763–768.

101. Osler W. *The Cerebral Palsies of Children: A Clinical Study from the Infirmary for Nervous Diseases*. Philadelphia: Blakiston; 1889.

102. Freud S. *Infantile Cerebral Paralysis*. Miami: University of Miami Press; 1968.

103. Sachs B, Peterson F. A study of cerebral palsies of early life, based upon an analysis of one hundred and forty cases. *J Nerv Ment Dis*. 1890;**17**:295–332.

104. Ford FR, Schaffer AJ. The etiology of infantile acquired hemiplegia. *Arch Neurol Psychiatry*. 1927;**18**:323–347.

105. Suzuki J, Takaku A. Cerebrovascular "moyamoya" disease. *Arch Neurol*. 1969;**20**:288–299.

106. Kudo T. Spontaneous occlusion of the circle of Willis. *Neurology*. 1968;**18**:485–496.

107. Roach ES, Riela AR. *Pediatric Cerebrovascular Disorders*. Mt. Kisco, NY: Futura; 1988.

108. Biller J, Mathews KD, Love BB, eds. *Stroke in Children and Young Adults*. Boston: Butterworth-Heinemann; 1994.

109. Adams RJ, McKie VC, Hsu L, et al. Stroke prevention trial in sickle cell anemia ("STOP"): study results. *N Engl J Med*. 1998;**339**:5–11.

110. Roach ES, Golomb MR, Adams RJ, et al. Management of stroke in infants and children. A scientific statement for healthcare professionals from a special writing group of the

Stroke Council, American Heart Association. *Stroke.* 2008;**39**: 2644–2691.

111. McHenry LC Jr. *Garrison's History of Neurology.* Springfield, IL: Charles C. Thomas; 1969.

112. McHenry LC Jr. *Cerebral Circulation and Stroke.* St. Louis, MO: Warren H. Green; 1978.

113. Gurdjian ES, Gurdjian ES. History of occlusive cerebrovascular disease I. from Wepfer to Moniz. *Arch Neurol.* 1979;**36**: 340–343.

114. Gurdjian ES, Gurdjian ES. History of occlusive cerebrovascular disease. II. After Moniz, with special reference to surgical treatment. *Arch Neurol.* 1979;**36**:427–432.

2

Interview and Examination

It is quite necessary to distinguish two different phenomena in the act of speech, namely, the power of creating words as signs of our ideas and that of articulating these same words. There is, so to speak, an internal speech and an external speech; the latter is only an expression of the former.

Jean-Baptiste Bouillaud

Diagnoses are missed not because of lack of knowledge on the part of the examiner, but rather because of lack of examination.

William Osler

Despite extraordinary advances in brain-imaging techniques in recent years, prompt recognition and accurate characterization of cerebrovascular disorders still depend on a detailed patient history and examination.[1-3] Interviewing a patient is a subtle and often neglected art designed to extract information that leads to an accurate diagnosis and to establish a relationship with the patient. The ability to do this effectively is the ultimate demonstration of the art of medicine in this age of accelerated science and technology.[4,5]

Recognition of the characteristic physical findings and typical clinical patterns of cerebrovascular disease (see Chapter 3) usually leads quickly to the correct diagnosis. Nevertheless, the individual with cerebrovascular disease can present special challenges. Defective memory, aphasia, and other stroke-related deficits of higher cortical function can make the task of information gathering difficult. The physician must in these instances take full advantage of the information available from the patient's family and other sources. Every effort must be made to ask straightforward questions that the patient can understand and to be aware of the ramifications of responses. Most importantly, the physician must always display a warm and sympathetic manner, even under the most trying circumstances.

INTERVIEWING THE PATIENT

As with any medical interview, the physician caring for a stroke patient should elicit and accurately record the sequence of events relating to the patient's illness. In addition, stroke-related cognitive and language deficits often become apparent during the initial interview. When done in the presence of a spouse or other family member, the interview provides an opportunity to gauge the reliability of the patient's memory and insight.

Often the most effective approach is to begin with the onset of symptoms or have the patient recall the first of several attacks. In the case of episodic dysfunction, it is often useful to review the most recent attack or an episode that was witnessed by another person who is present during the interview. Patients often recount their histories out of time sequence, ordering their symptoms in relationship to their emotional impact and perceived importance. Symptoms of lesser impact are often ignored. Even momentary loss of vision in an eye, for example, is usually frightening enough that it prompts the individual to seek medical attention, whereas nondominant hemisphere symptoms may be neglected altogether. Asking a family member for input or corroboration often generates vital information or insight. An equally important problem is amnesia for events occurring during a transitory neurologic episode. Only witnesses, such as family members or coworkers, can fill in accurate details in this situation.

Although the interview is usually conducted conversationally, nonverbal communication is also very important. Noting the affect, manner of sitting, facial expression, and eye movements sheds light on the patient's emotional reaction to the symptoms and facilitates communication. The physician should also be aware that his or her own verbal and nonverbal communication can either facilitate or inhibit effective communication.

The history should address the following questions:

1. What area of the nervous system is involved? Considering the patient's symptoms in light of his anatomy and function often allows us to accurately pinpoint the site of dysfunction even before examining the patient or performing diagnostic tests.

2. What was the patient doing when the difficulty began? The onset of symptoms during strenuous physical activity favors a hemorrhage, whereas onset during rest favors ischemia. Occurrence of symptoms only with certain body positions or during specific activities suggests a position-related vascular compromise such as subclavian steal syndrome.

3. Was the onset instantaneous, as often occurs with hemorrhage or embolus, or stepwise and perhaps preceded by short-lived but similar episodes, such as the transient ischemic attacks (TIAs) that often herald a cerebral thrombosis?

4. How severe did the symptom become before improvement began? Steady progression of symptoms suggests hemorrhage, whereas sudden onset of symptoms followed by rapid recovery suggests an embolus.

5. Are there residual deficits? A transient ischemic attack is an ischemic episode that resolves in less than 24 hours without causing an infarction (see Chapter 6). In fact, most TIAs last only a few minutes to an hour, and modern imaging techniques often demonstrate a small infarction even when the symptoms clear promptly. Often the patient thinks his arm or leg has simply "gone to sleep" because of the position in which the extremity has been maintained.

6. How many attacks has the patient had? If they have been numerous, he should at least be asked to describe, in detail, the first, the most recent, and the worst episode.

The patient and other observers should be questioned specifically about the following items if the information has not already been elicited:

1. Cognitive changes and memory
2. Loss of consciousness
3. Difficulties with speech, reading, or writing
4. Paralysis or sensory disturbance involving any part of the body
5. Depression
6. Visual symptoms
7. Seizures
8. Impairment of hearing or loss of balance
9. Headache
10. Trauma to the head or neck
11. Systemic disorders, such as diabetes mellitus, hypertension, or cardiac disease
12. Medications

Because information about these factors is so vital, they are considered individually here, even though their relationship to specific diseases will be discussed more fully in other chapters.

Cognitive Changes and Memory

The detail with which the patient describes his symptoms provides information about his insight, judgment, and recent and remote recall. Some people are unaware of their own higher cortical dysfunction and deny their cognitive impairment despite severe abnormality.[6,7] Up to a third of the patients with an ischemic stroke have cognitive impairment following the stroke (see Chapter 15).[8,9] This number is even higher in individuals who have had earlier strokes as well as in people with other risk factors for dementia.[10] For this reason it is a good idea to interview family members or friends to corroborate information about the patient's mental status, memory, and mood and to obtain details about the family history.

Loss of Consciousness

Loss of consciousness may occur without prodrome or after some seconds of lightheadedness or giddiness. Because unconsciousness is sometimes followed by amnesia for events surrounding the episode, some individuals are unable to remember precipitants.[11,12] It is essential, therefore, to have someone who observed the event describe its details. Important points to be noted are the following:

1. *Rapidity of onset:* An episode that is heralded by lightheadedness or other warning symptoms suggests syncope, cardiac dysrhythmia, partial-onset seizures, or hypoglycemia.

2. *Appearance of the patient during the attack:* Pallor and sweating are typical of syncope or hypoglycemia. Patients with cardiac dysrhythmias are often pale, whereas those with asystole are suffused or cyanotic (Stokes-Adams attacks).

3. *The rate and rhythm of the patient's heartbeat:* If a bystander has the presence of mind to take the patient's pulse during such an episode, this might provide the only clue to the diagnosis of an intermittent cardiac dysrhythmia.

4. *Repetitive body movements or urinary incontinence during the attack:* These findings suggest epileptic seizures because most patients who faint are limp and retain sphincter control. Occasional patients with syncope develop convulsive movements, especially toward the end of the episode.

Difficulties with Speech, Reading, or Writing

Language dysfunction commonly occurs with stroke. Temporary alterations in language function may go unrecognized by the patient. Hence, the physician must ask the family about lapses in conversation that could suggest temporary language difficulty, and the patient must be asked to read and write. Of course, the patient's educational level and baseline abilities must be taken into account when assessing for language deficits.

Individuals with aphasia may display change in fluency, loss of naming, expression, repetition, or comprehension (Table 2-1). Others have *paraphasias*, in which words are malformed or used in an inappropriate context. Nevertheless, the term *aphasia* is often applied to both complete and partial forms of acquired language dysfunction.[13]

Aphasia must be distinguished from dysarthria, in which the articulation is poor, but the form, content, and use of language is normal. Aphasia is important to recognize clinically because it localizes the lesion in the cerebral cortex, usually an area in the left hemisphere that is supplied by the middle cerebral artery.[14] There are exceptions: about 20% aphasic left-handers have right hemisphere lesions, anomic aphasias may result from diffuse cerebral lesions, and aphasia can occur with subcortical lesions. Language disturbance due to stroke is far more complicated than once imagined,[15–18] but the classic and common aphasia syndromes are described below.

Broca's aphasia results from a lesion of the third frontal gyrus. The speech output is diminished, often strikingly. Although there is relative preservation of comprehension of written and verbal speech, these too are usually abnormal when carefully tested. In its most severe form, there is complete absence of spoken language, and the individual is unable to read or repeat words.[19] Less severely affected patients and those who have partially recovered have some ability to speak, usually including some form of affirmative and negative response, but their verbal output remains sparse, grammatically inaccurate, and labored ("telegraphic"). The ability to say swear words and to use habitual expressions is often regained, as is the ability to sing or hum a melody. The patient is fully aware of his deficit

Table 2-1: Clinical Characterization of Commonly Encountered Aphasias

Syndrome	Fluency	Comprehension	Naming	Repetition	Hemiparesis
Broca	Nonfluent	Good	Poor	Poor	Common
Wernicke	Fluent	Poor	Variable	Poor	Rare
Anomic	Fluent	Good	Poor	Good	Rare
Conduction	Fluent	Good	Good	Poor	Rare
Global	Nonfluent	Poor	Poor	Poor	Common

and often becomes frustrated and depressed because of his inability to communicate.

Wernicke's aphasia results from a lesion in the area adjacent to the auditory cortex that is necessary for the understanding of auditory input, such as one's own or another person's speech.[20,21] With an abnormality in this area, speech is fluent and effortless but lacks normal content and is marked by paraphasic errors. The patient is unable to comprehend written or verbal communication and typically has little insight into the nature of his deficit.

Conduction aphasia occurs when a temporal or parietal lesion interrupts the arcuate fasciculus that connects Wernicke's and Broca's areas.[22,23] Speech is fluent but imperfect due to paraphasic and naming errors. Comprehension of spoken and written language is relatively preserved, but there is disproportionate difficulty with repeating sentences and with reading aloud.[24,25] Spelling, sentence structure, and punctuation are impaired, although penmanship is preserved.

Anomic aphasia is characterized by marked word-finding difficulty with relative preservation of fluency, repetition, and auditory comprehension. Some word-finding impairment occurs in all subtypes of aphasia, and, indeed, is a common end stage for most types of partially recovered aphasia.[26] Speech is normal except for difficulty naming and some paraphasic errors. Anomic aphasia has traditionally been attributed to a lesion of the angular gyrus, but lesions in various regions have been documented.[27–29]

Global aphasia is characterized by nonfluent verbal output and an inability to comprehend and to speak, usually resulting from large lesions of both Wernicke's and Broca's areas. Because the left motor cortex lies between these two regions, most patients with global aphasia also have right hemiparesis.[30] Occasionally two separate lesions destroy both Wernicke's and Broca's areas, producing global aphasia but sparing the motor cortex (Figure 2-1).[31] Global aphasia without hemiparesis may result from embolism, although it can also result from hemorrhage and other conditions.[32–34] Given that multiple or larger lesions are needed to cause global aphasia, it is not surprising that these individuals are less likely to recover than those with other types of aphasia.[26]

A few steps will identify the more common forms of aphasia. Listen to the patient's speech. Fluent but abnormal speech (Wernicke's aphasia) suggests a posterior lesion, whereas nonfluent speech (Broca's aphasia) usually occurs with an anterior lesion, and an inability to repeat spoken words suggests a disconnection of these two areas (conduction aphasia).[24,35] Table 2-1 presents a simple approach to the characterization of common aphasia syndromes. Many patients, however, have mixed forms of aphasia that are not easily categorized. Additional

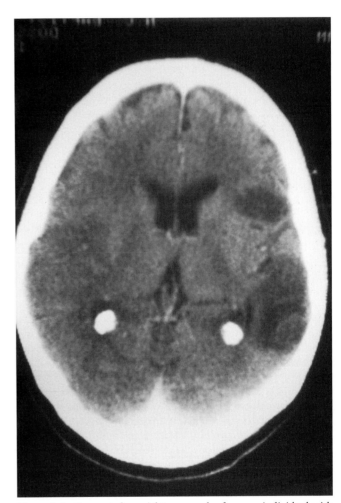

Figure 2-1. Computed cranial tomography from an individual with global aphasia without hemiparesis. Two infarctions correspond to Broca's and Wernicke's areas; the motor cortex between these lesions is spared.

information about the assessment of extra-Sylvian and subcortical aphasias is available elsewhere.[36]

Paralysis or Sensory Disturbances

Patients often use the terms *numbness* and *paralysis* interchangeably because many laymen do not realize that paralysis can occur without loss of sensation. Asking the patient to give specific examples of disturbed function (i.e., could he walk or eat

Table 2-2: Clinical Characteristics of Paroxysmal Events

	Syncope	Seizure	Functional
Onset age	Any age	Any age	Usually < 25 years
Posture at onset	Standing or sitting	Any position	Any position
Emotional issues	Not usually	Not usually	Usually
Premonitory features	Light-headedness, weakness, confusion	Automatisms or confusion with partial seizures	Dramatic gestures and staggering postures
Precipitating factors	Standing motionless, anemia, fright, hypoglycemia, drugs	Sleep loss, missed medications, drug withdrawal, menses, hypoglycemia	Emotional distress, sympathetic audience
Premonitory time	Few seconds	Variable (with partial seizures)	Often prolonged
Duration	Usually < 1 minute	< 2 minutes (unless status epilepticus)	Often > 15–20 minutes
Post-ictal state	Prompt recovery, with amnesia for period of unconsciousness	Confusion, amnesia, and somnolence (especially after longer seizures)	Total lack of recall
Incontinence	Rare	Common	Almost never
Involuntary movements	Motionless and limp; maybe mild clonic movements with prolonged attack	Tonic-clonic with generalized seizures, variable movements with partial seizures	Bizarre movements
Injury during attack	Rare	Common	Almost never
Autonomic function	Pallor, sweating, bradycardia	Cyanosis, flushing, tachycardia	None
Heart rate during attack	Slow or rapid	Rapid	Normal
EEG during attack	Background slowing	Spike discharge	Normal
EEG between attacks	Normal	Variable spikes	Normal

without assistance?) and briefly discussing the difference between weakness and numbness will usually help resolve the question. The pattern of weakness often points to a particular vascular territory. Weakness that is most pronounced in the arm, for example, suggests middle cerebral artery dysfunction, whereas leg weakness suggests anterior cerebral artery occlusion. In most instances a cortical lesion causes a mixture of motor, sensory, and cognitive deficits. Isolated loss of motor or sensory function more often occurs with interruption of the subcortical motor or sensory tracts, as occurs with a lacunar infarction.

In some instances paralysis due to psychological disturbance or malingering must be distinguished from neurogenic weakness. Abnormal neurologic signs help to confirm organic weakness, but transient ischemia can produce fleeting numbness or paralysis, leaving no residual neurological signs. Functional paralysis tends to have a dramatic onset in a public setting during a time of emotional stress.

Depression

Post-stroke depression is common and sometimes severe.[37,38] In some studies over half of the patients in a stroke unit exhibit overt sadness, crying, or subjective depression.[39] Other individuals develop emotional lability, either alone or in conjunction with depression.[40,41] Depression is more likely to occur with larger lesions and with very disabling lesions such as nonfluent aphasia, and it often persists for years following the stroke.[38,42] Although traditionally related to frontal lobe infarctions, recent studies have found little correlation between the anatomic loca-

tion of the stroke and the occurrence of depression.[41,43,44] It is important to recognize and treat post-stroke depression because it often impedes neurologic recovery. Not all depressed patients exhibit overt sadness; some develop alteration of sleep habits, poor appetite, or personality change.

Epileptic Seizures

A partial seizure followed by a post-ictal deficit can be difficult to distinguish from a TIA (Table 2-2), especially in a confused or unresponsive patient whose episode was not witnessed. Seizures can also result from cerebral ischemia, so even the occurrence of a well-described seizure does not fully exclude a vascular lesion. In one series of 535 consecutive stroke patients, for example, 33 individuals (6%) had one or more seizures during the week after their stroke, and 78% of these individuals had the seizure within 24 hours of the onset of the infarction.[45] Seizures can accompany any type of cerebrovascular lesion but occur more frequently in individuals with an embolism or intracranial venous thrombosis. Seizures are relatively uncommon in individuals with purely white matter lesions.[46] Seizures are more likely to develop after a hemorrhage than after an infarction, and seizures are particularly likely following a lobar hemorrhage.[47–49] The likelihood of developing delayed-onset seizures after an ischemic stroke is 7.4% at 5 years and 8.9% by 10 years.[45]

A history of epilepsy in an individual with a focal neurological deficit increases suspicions of a post-ictal deficit, but various congenital vascular lesions could be responsible for both long-standing epilepsy and a new-onset hemorrhagic or ischemic stroke in the same individual. Seizures are common, for example, in individuals with a cavernous malformation or an arteriovenous malformation (see Chapter 18).[50,51]

Visual Symptoms

The eyes may or may not be the mirror of the soul, but they do reflect cerebral vascular disease. Ophthalmologic symptoms are common with both carotid artery and vertebral-basilar system disease. For this reason it is particularly important to inquire about visual phenomena.

Amaurosis Fugax

One of the most common visual symptoms caused by cerebrovascular disease is amaurosis fugax, typically the result of retinal ischemia. However, there are many nonvascular causes of monocular vision loss (Table 2-3). Visual field defects caused by carotid distribution ischemia may result either from involvement of the visual pathways or the retina. Of the two, retinal ischemia is the more common, with symptoms and signs arising from the carotid artery homolateral to the symptomatic eye. The visual defect caused by retinal ischemia varies with the retinal vessel that is occluded. Concentric constriction of the field in the homolateral eye suggests hypotension in the ophthalmic artery, whereas an altitudinal or hemianopic progression, often described as a shade or veil being drawn across the visual field, indicates occlusion of a branch retinal artery (Figure 2-2).

Most individuals do not cover one eye during an attack and thus are unaware whether the visual loss involved just one eye or half of both visual fields. Some patients are so distraught by the abnormality that they believe both eyes to be blind when vision has become blurred or a scotoma has appeared in only one segment of the visual field. A cooperative patient can be taught to test his own visual fields during possible subsequent attacks. These patients report that vision is restored as abruptly as it fades.

Central Retinal Artery Occlusion

About half of the patients with retinal emboli have a branch retinal artery occlusion, and a third have a central retinal artery occlusion. Symptoms of central retinal artery occlusion can begin suddenly or in a stepwise fashion. Causes of central retinal artery occlusion include systemic hypertension, internal carotid artery occlusion, and cranial arteritis (see Chapter 10). Central retinal artery occlusion may result from arteritis from herpes zoster ophthalmicus. Injections near the maxilla during dental procedures may result in embolism of air, fat, or foreign substances to the central retinal artery via its anastomotic sites with the facial and internal maxillary arteries.[52] Retinal arteriolar spasm due to retinal migraine can cause transient monocular blindness, and retinal branch artery occlusion frequently occurs in individuals with Susac syndrome (see Chapter 13).[53]

Hemianopia

Whereas amaurosis fugax strongly suggests carotid artery disease, intermittent homonymous hemianopia is an unusual symptom of carotid ischemia. When infarction occurs, however, a dense hemianopia may develop if the posterior cerebral arterial territory has been affected, as occurs in cases of embryonal origin of the posterior cerebral artery (PCA) from the internal carotid.

Table 2-3: Causes of Transient Monocular Blindness

Embolism

- Carotid artery bifurcation stenosis
- Cardiac mural thrombus
- Intracardiac tumor
- Foreign body
- Air embolism

Hemodynamic

- Atheromatous disease
- Takayasu arteritis
- Cardiac failure, acute hypovolemia
- Microvascular (e.g., Susac syndrome)

Ocular

- Anterior ischemic optic neuropathy
- Central or branch retinal artery occlusion
- Central retinal vein occlusion
- Glaucoma
- Retinal detachment
- Vitreous hemorrhage

Neurologic

- Leber hereditary optic neuropathy
- Optic neuritis
- Optic nerve or chiasm compression
- Migraine

Psychiatric

- Somatoform disorder
- Malingering

Hematologic

- Hyperviscosity syndromes
- Thrombocytosis
- Polycythemia
- Coagulopathy
- Hemoglobinopathy (e.g. sickle cell disease)

Toxic

- Methanol

Diplopia

Transient horizontal or vertical diplopia is a frequent symptom of vertebrobasilar ischemia. Some patients describe double vision as "blurring," even though their vision is clear if one eye is kept closed. The attacks seldom last longer than 3 to 5 minutes and may be recurrent. Other conditions to be considered in the differential diagnosis of intermittent diplopia are palsies of cranial nerves III, IV, and VI and disorders of the extraocular

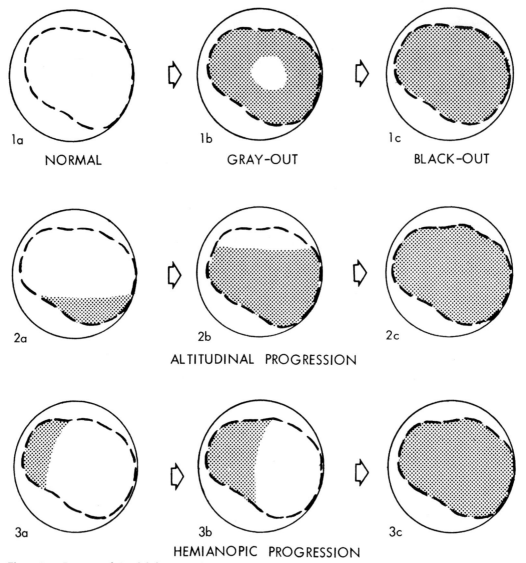

Figure 2-2. Patterns of visual defects in individuals with amaurosis fugax. *Top:* gradual concentric graying of the vision; *middle:* progressive altitudinal visual loss; *bottom:* hemianopic visual loss.

muscles themselves. These usually cause longer-lasting diplopia, which only rarely is intermittent in nature.

Homonymous Visual Field Defects

Homonymous visual field defects may result from dysfunction of the optic tract, lateral geniculate body, optic radiation (radiation of Gratiolet), or visual cortical areas of the occipital lobe. Sudden loss or impairment of vision that involves portions of both eyes suggests a homonymous field defect. Some patients first note a shadow or curtain obstructing their vision; others say that parts of objects suddenly disappear or that words or letters seem to be missing from a page of print. Because central vision is usually preserved, quadrantanopia or hemianopia may be undetected by the patient until it leads to an unusual number of mishaps, for example, stumbling into objects on the blind side or automobile accidents occasioned by the inability to see other cars from the "corner of the eye" on that side.

Some patients with attacks of vertebrobasilar artery ischemia have loss of their peripheral fields with preservation of macular vision. This constriction may be temporary as in ischemia, or permanent as in infarction of the occipital lobe. An acquired inability to read and failure to recognize objects, familiar surroundings, or the faces of people (visual agnosias) are due to an abnormality in the parieto-occipital association areas.

Cortical Blindness

Loss of vision despite normal fundi and unimpaired pupillary reaction to light is characteristic of cortical blindness. More often than not, such transient episodes presage serious sequelae. The condition can be distinguished from functional blindness by the absence of reflex blinking to visual threat or optokinetic nystagmus and by absent visual evoked potentials. The patient is often confused and disoriented, and he may deny blindness completely (Anton syndrome). Rarely, cortical blindness occurs when homonymous hemianopia is followed at a later time by a defect in the other half of the field of vision.

Oscillopsia

An illusion of either horizontal or vertical movement occurs when a patient with nystagmus or other eye movement abnormalities perceives the images in his visual field as they move across the retina. In the absence of drug intoxication, vertical nystagmus is usually a sign of a brainstem lesion, although such lesions are not always vascular in nature.

Deafness, Vertigo, and Ataxia

The auditory and vestibular apparatus encased in the petrous portion of the temporal bone is supplied by the vertebrobasilar arterial system. Episodes of vertigo, with or without an accompanying loss of hearing, may be due to vascular disease in the brainstem or in the vestibular apparatus itself. Some attacks are precipitated by changing the position of the head on the neck (as in looking up at a tall building) or by rotating the head to one side while backing an automobile or shaving. Sudden movement of the body or the head may precipitate violent vertigo, oscillopsia, nausea, and vomiting. At times it is difficult to distinguish between vertigo (usually associated with a feeling of spinning) and the unsteady feeling that precedes syncope.[54] Many patients with vertigo keep their eyes tightly closed during the attack and are therefore unable to say whether objects seem to be moving, but they hear and are acutely aware of their environment. In syncope the eyes are not always closed but vision dims and sounds grow more distant as consciousness fades. Vertiginous patients report that they or their environment moves, rotates, or spins. The movement of syncope is a sense of floating or drifting into weightlessness.

Some patients with vascular lesions have intermittent loss of hearing suggestive of Ménière disease, and others complain of noises in the head that are not tinnitus but bruits. The patient should always be asked for a description of sounds he may have in his head and should be questioned specifically about whether they are synchronous with the heartbeat. Occasionally a patient insists that he has an intracranial sound synchronous with his heartbeat, even though the physician cannot hear it. In such cases the examiner should ask the patient to imitate the sound and its rhythm while taking the patient's pulse.

Headache

Although headache is a nonspecific sign, it occurs in most patients with subarachnoid or intracerebral hemorrhage and frequently accompanies ischemic stroke. Headache is also reported by about a fourth of individuals with carotid insufficiency and a third of those with vertebrobasilar TIAs.[55] The site of the headache is not a reliable predictor of the lesion location.

Migraine (see Chapter 14) can lead to transient ischemic symptoms or even to cerebral infarction, although in many instances patients with complicated migraine attacks have additional underlying risk factors. Some individuals with chronic cerebrovascular compromise develop frequent intermittent pounding headaches that resemble migraine attacks, perhaps resulting from distention of collateral channels and vasodilatation to circumvent the obstruction. The important point is that headaches beginning anew in middle-aged or older individuals suggests a diagnosis other than migraine or tension headache, and the cause of these headaches must be pursued vigorously.

Individuals with occlusion of the transverse or other dural sinuses present with headache, papilledema, and other signs of increased intracranial pressure.[56–58] Similarly, carotid artery dissection or inflammation sometimes produces neck pain (carotidynia) that sometimes radiates into the head, and vertebral artery dissection often causes pain in the posterior neck and occipital region.[59]

Headache is also a common feature of many stroke risk factors. Patients with giant cell arteritis and other vasculitides, for example, frequently report headache. The same is true of systemic hypertension, polycythemia, thrombocytosis, and other stroke risk factors.

Trauma

In older patients, especially those who are receiving anticoagulant medication, even minor trauma may result in a subdural or intracranial hematoma (see Chapter 19). Likewise, relatively minor trauma may produce the intimal tears that lead to arterial dissections. Dissection occurs in the cervical or intracranial segments of the carotid arteries as well as in the vertebral arteries (see Chapter 12). Torsional wrenching movements of the neck are most likely to produce a dissection of the cervicocephalic vessels. Dissection following chiropractic manipulation has been reported.[60–63]

Systemic Diseases

Particularly important among the systemic diseases (see Chapters 10 and 11) are anemia, polycythemia, thrombocytosis, macroglobulinemia, monoclonal gammopathy, arteritis, hypertension, coronary artery disease with or without previous myocardial infarction, pulmonary disease, and diabetes mellitus, all of which can impair oxygenation or perfusion of the brain.

Medications and Substance Abuse

Medications that the patient has been taking, especially phenothiazine derivatives and hypotensive drugs, may cause or aggravate postural hypotension and transient attacks. An important, although unusual, complication of using monoamine oxidase inhibitors is a hypertensive crisis after consuming tyramine-rich food or drinks. This combination can cause cerebral vascular episodes. Alcohol, hypoglycemic drugs, phenytoin, and barbiturates are other medications that may affect the central nervous system and produce symptoms that simulate cerebral vascular disease.

Illicit drugs can lead to diffuse cerebral arteritis with multifocal cerebral infarctions or hemorrhage; intravenous use of drugs that are contaminated with inert substances can result in diffuse distribution of emboli to the vasculature of the brain.

OPHTHALMOLOGICAL EXAMINATION

Retinal Vascular Anatomy

The ophthalmic artery usually arises from of the internal carotid artery, and its direct continuation as the central retinal artery can be extremely important for the diagnosis of carotid artery disorder. The central artery of the retina runs adjacent to the nerve and pierces the meninges about 10 mm behind the eye, usually penetrating the papilla at the center of the optic nerve. It may branch immediately thereafter or deep within the substance of the nerve, so that it emerges as two or more divisions, usually including upper and lower branches. At times a cilioretinal artery supplies the macula independently of the central artery of the retina. It is of importance that the central retinal artery supplies the inner layers of the retina but does not supply the nerve itself. The central artery of the retina is, technically speaking, an arteriole that has a thick muscularis and some, but not much, adventitia. When one looks at the retinal circulation, one is looking at the blood column within its lumen and not at the media. With disease the "light streak" becomes apparent, and this is an index of the reflectivity of the diseased arteriole.

Ophthalmological Findings

The first maneuver is inspection of the conjunctiva for pallor and petechiae. At times congestion of the circumlimbal vessels (rubeosis oculi) suggests collateral circulation through the orbit due to carotid disease. Ptosis and pupillary abnormalities can be a clue to disease of the carotid artery; in particular, an oculo-sympathetic paresis or "incomplete" Horner syndrome can suggest ipsilateral internal carotid artery dissection. Occasionally the angular and/or anterior branch of the superficial temporal artery is hyperpulsatile, suggesting collateral circulation through the orbit caused by internal carotid stenosis or occlusion.

The optic disc and the central vessels are located and the veins are examined for characteristic pulsations. The diameters of the arteriole and vein are noted. Because the walls of the vessels themselves are not visible under physiological conditions, a change in the caliber of the bloodstream suggests an impingement on the lumen. If the streak of reflected light is wide and the column narrow, the walls have thickened. Lengthening of the arterioles is another part of the atherosclerotic process and distorts the relationship between the arteriole and the adjacent venule, causing "nicking." How closely retinal vascular changes parallel the neurovascular pathology is debated, but severely abnormal retinal vessels suggest significant atherosclerosis of the intracranial arterioles.

Atherosclerosis of any portion of the carotid artery proximal to the origin of the ophthalmic artery may be accompanied by reduction of pressure in the ophthalmic artery. When pressure is low enough, retinal ischemia produces attacks of loss of vision in that eye (amaurosis fugax) as well as hemorrhages and exudates secondary to endothelial hypoxia. If infarction of the optic nerve and retina occurs, the retina is pale, the disc white, the arteries difficult to see, and the veins attenuated.

Central Retinal Artery Occlusion

The signs and symptoms of central retinal artery occlusion include sudden, painless loss of vision in the affected eye; the globe is not usually tender. The pupil of the affected side is fixed or sluggish to direct light stimulation but usually responds consensually. Physical findings include a pale disc with attenuated arterioles and veins, a cloudy pale retina, and a "cherry-red" macula (Figure 2-3). If vision is not restored quickly, permanent blindness will result; later, there is atrophy of the inner retinal layers, and a pale disc heralds optic atrophy. Reduced pressure in the arterial supply to the globe is reflected in lower venous pressure. This leads to stagnation in out-flow with branch or central venous occlusion. However, retinal vein thrombosis in the absence of retinal artery occlusion features retinal edema and hemorrhage. This may be accompanied by reduced intraocular pressure as well.

Retinal Hemorrhage

An acute increase in intracranial pressure from any cause is transmitted to the retinal veins, resulting in an abrupt rise in

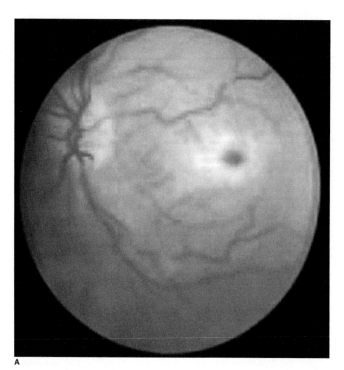

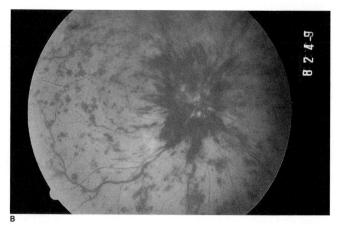

Figure 2-3.　A: Retinal appearance after a central retinal artery occlusion. Note the cloudy appearance of the retina, the indistinctness of the retinal arteries, and the cherry-red macular lesion. B: Retinal findings following thrombosis of the central retinal vein include retinal edema and perivenous hemorrhage.

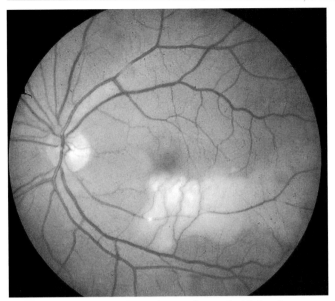

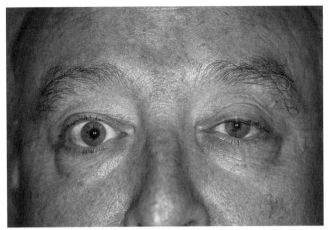

Figure 2-5. Left miosis and ptosis due to an oculosympathetic paresis, or partial Horner syndrome. Photograph courtesy of Dr. Carol Zimmerman.

Figure 2-4. Retinal embolus with secondary retinal infarction.

retinal venous pressure. In some individuals, a marked pressure change leads to hemorrhage into the optic nerve sheath or to retinal, preretinal (subhyaloid), subretinal, or vitreal hemorrhage (Terson syndrome).[64,65] The intraocular blood occupies the potential space between the retina and the vitreous body and can appear within minutes of a sudden rise in intracranial pressure. Retinal hemorrhages range in appearance from multiple small focal hemorrhages to large, crescent-shaped (Figure 17-2) or keel-shaped lesions (thus the term "boat" hemorrhage).

Retinal Emboli

Some patients with internal carotid artery atherosclerosis develop cholesterol-lipid emboli to the retinal arterioles (Hollenhorst plaques). There are three common types of retinal emboli: fibrin-platelet, cholesterol-lipid (Figure 2-4), and calcific or fibrinoid, each with specific characteristics. In rare instances retinal foreign body or air emboli are documented.

Horner Syndrome

An oculosympathetic paresis, or Horner syndrome (Figure 2-5), often accompanies either a carotid artery dissection or a brainstem lesion (e.g., Wallenberg syndrome). The ascending cervical sympathetic fibers within the carotid sheath are commonly affected by carotid artery dissection, leading to a homolateral oculosympathetic paresis.[66] Because the sudomotor fibers follow the path of the external carotid artery, they are spared with lesions of the internal carotid artery, and thus sweating remains normal over the ipsilateral face (thus a "partial" Horner syndrome). The descending sympathetic fibers course through the lateral brainstem, where they are vulnerable to lateral medullary infarction.[67–69]

NEUROVASCULAR EXAMINATION

The physical and neurologic examination of a patient with cerebral vascular disease should include specific observations for

the following: (a) systemic blood pressure along with postural hypotension or diminished cardiac output during a Valsalva maneuver, (b) abnormal pulsations of an artery or arterial branch supplying the head, (c) a cranial or cervical bruit, (d) unequal blood pressures or pulses in the arms, and (e) certain retinal abnormalities. Assessment of these special points constitutes the neurovascular examination. Although these observations are made as a part of the customary physical and neurologic examinations, they are considered separately in this chapter for emphasis.

Inspection

Inspection can suggest the presence of cerebrovascular disease as well as its etiology and pathogenesis. The examination should include the skin, which should be examined for color, visible pulsations in the external carotid system, and the vessels of the conjunctiva and retina. Pulsations of the superficial temporal arteries are seldom visible during youth but are commonly evident after middle age. Patients in the throes of migraine (see Chapter 14) sometimes display prominent hyperpulsatile arteries, as do many patients with stenosis or occlusion of the internal carotid artery because of the collateral network supplying the brain. Cranial arteritis (see Chapter 10) and encephalofacial angiomatosis (see Chapter 18) have stigmata of vascular disease.

Palpation

Palpation of the carotid artery in the neck occasionally reveals a thrill or diminished pulsations. Although the thrill is a clue to stenosis, the diminution or pulsations may mean nothing. Kinked or tortuous common carotid arteries can lie behind the trachea where they cannot be palpated. In these patients the superficial temporal arteries are usually found to be pulsating well, so that the examiner can be certain that the common and external carotid arteries are not occluded. When palpating the carotid artery, the examiner should remember that some patients have such a sensitive carotid sinus that even gentle massage or compression can cause bradycardia and hypotension and that vigorous palpation may dislodge an embolus.

Hyperpulsation of the superficial temporal artery suggests occlusion of the internal carotid with collateral circulation through the external carotid. Hypopulsation or the absence of pulsations in the superficial temporal artery, which is rare, suggests atherosclerotic involvement of the external carotid artery or cranial arteritis.

Pulsation of branches of the external carotid yields clues to the patency of the internal, as well as the external, carotid system. Comparison of one pulse with another may reveal an increase, a decrease, or even an absence of pulsations in one or more arteries. Most important for this purpose are the facial artery, which can be palpated beneath the angle of the jaw; the superficial temporal artery, which can be felt anterior to the tragus of the ear; and the posterior auricular and occipital arteries, which can be palpated in the occipital region. The common carotid arteries can be palpated at the bifurcation behind the angle of the jaw and low in the neck. The patency of the subclavian arteries can be verified by palpating above and below the clavicle as well as the radial and ulnar arteries. It is important to palpate the two radial arteries simultaneously to determine the possibility of delay in the arrival time of a pulse on one side, which, when found, suggests a steal syndrome (see Chapter 3).[70,71]

Diminution or absence of pulsations in one of the superficial temporal or occipital arteries suggests disease of that vessel or of the external or common carotid artery. If the artery is tender, cranial arteritis should be considered; if it is not, atherosclerotic occlusion is the probable cause. Increased pulsation of the superficial temporal or facial artery sometimes indicates stenosis or occlusion of the homolateral internal carotid artery with the development of collateral flow through the external system. Inability to palpate the common carotid, combined with the finding of good pulsations in the superficial temporal and occipital arteries, suggests a tortuous common carotid artery lying behind the trachea. If pulses in the subclavian artery are diminished or absent, the proximal portion of the vessel is diseased. In the absence of anemia or aortic stenosis, a thrill felt over any artery indicates disease at the site of the thrill. Absence of a radial, ulnar, or pedal pulse occurs in occlusive disease of the large vessels and suggests possibility of proximal stenosis of embolism. The absence of aortic, femoral, and pedal pulses is due to occlusion of the aorta by coarctation, embolus, or atherosclerosis. The reappearance of previously absent pulses suggests spasm, recanalization of arteries, or temporary diversion of blood flow.

Arterial Blood Pressure

Evaluation of arterial hypertension is considered in Chapter 9. Arterial blood pressures should be measured and compared in each arm and with the patient lying and standing. A difference exceeding 20 mm Hg in the systolic pressures between the two arms is strongly suggestive of subclavian artery disease. The blood pressure may fall precipitously in these individuals when the arm with the obstruction is exercised.

The blood pressure should be measured with the patient supine and then again after standing; several standing measurements may be needed because the pressure may be normally sustained for a minute or two, then fall to hypotensive levels. While standing, the patient should be asked to perform a Valsalva maneuver. The erect position may reduce pulse pressure,

Table 2-4: Causes of Cervical Bruits

Arterial stenosis

Atherosclerosis

Fibromuscular dysplasia

Neoplasm

Radiation vasculopathy

Arterial dissection

Arteritis

Occlusion with collateral channels

■ Padget disease of skull

Hemodynamic factors

■ Flow augmentation due to contralateral stenosis

■ Hyperthyroidism

■ Hemodialysis

■ Kinks and coils of arteries

■ Anemia

■ Arteriovenous (AV) shunts

■ AV malformation

■ AV fistula

Physiologically increased flow

■ Childhood

■ Pregnancy

■ Fever

Cardiac factors

■ Increased cardiac output

■ Transmitted murmur (especially for aortic valvular heart disease)

and the straining may cause a decreased cardiac output, which may precipitate symptoms of insufficiency.

Auscultation

Bruits at the carotid bifurcation occur in about 7% of patients over the age of 65 years. However, a bruit is but an indication of nonlaminar flow and can have many causes (Table 2-4). In isolation, a bruit over a cervicocephalic artery may or may not be significant.[72] But in an individual who is at risk for cerebrovascular disease, a cervical bruit suggests localized arterial stenosis, particularly when it occurs over the carotid bifurcation. Thus, a bruit is only one sign of vascular dysfunction, one to be evaluated in conjunction with the patient's other clinical and diagnostic findings.[73,74] A cervical bruit increases the likelihood of a cerebral infarction, but not necessarily in the arterial territory corresponding to the bruit.[75,76] One must undertake an orderly evaluation in each patient to determine the bruits' significance.

Any phenomenon that creates sufficient turbulence to disrupt the normally quiet laminar blood flow can cause a bruit. Thus, stenosis or vessel wall irregularity, if sufficiently severe, causes turbulent blood flow that creates an audible noise, the bruit. Similarly, thin individuals or children may have a bruit simply because it is easier to hear a normal amount of turbulence of blood flow. Not all bruits are hemodynamically consequential. Bruits can arise from turbulent flow due to anemia, arterial kinks, or conditions that increase blood flow through the vessel. Bruits are sometimes audible during pregnancy or in individuals with hyperthyroidism. A bruit that is heard only during a fever is likely due to transiently increased flow and not to vascular pathology. Occipital artery bruits are not usually associated with clinical phenomena and can be distinguished from the more important murmurs of the intracranial vessels by tracing the murmur along the distribution of the palpable vessel and obliterating it by digital compression.

After listening to the heart and lungs in the usual manner, attempt to detect murmurs caused by disease of the aortocranial arteries. One should listen for murmurs along the course of the vertebral and carotid arteries, particularly at the subclavian-vertebral junction, over the mastoids, along the common carotid artery, and at the carotid bifurcation just beneath the angle of the jaw. Because of its unique importance, the carotid bifurcation should be auscultated with particular care, with the patient's head first in the neutral position and then turned to one side and the other. Bruits that are not heard with the head in the neutral position may become evident when it is turned. The explanation may lie in the kinking or compressing of the artery by turning the head, but it is just as likely that the sternocleidomastoid muscle moving across the artery as the head is turned alters the audibility of bruits. At times the lateral mass of the first cervical vertebra (the atlas) can compress the artery from behind when the head is turned and, thus, produce turbulent flow.

Some bruits are audible only over the orbit, perhaps related to the conical megaphone-like configuration of the orbit. Thus the orbit has the potential to conduct sound from the depths of the head to the surface. Whatever the reason, cephalic murmurs are often audible over the orbits and nowhere else. The mastoid is another region to which murmurs are occasionally transmitted, perhaps because the dense petrous portion of the temporal bone conducts sound well. It will be recalled that the carotid artery passes through this bone and that the vertebral and basilar arteries lie close to it.

The importance of turning the head to different positions during auscultation has already been mentioned. The patient may also be examined while lying down with the head extended or sitting with the arms in various positions, particularly if no murmur is heard during the usual examination. The yield of such maneuvers may be better in patients who report hearing an intracranial sound than in unselected individuals. Because the subclavian artery runs behind the clavicle and can be compressed between the clavicle and the first rib when the arm is extended, the intensity of subclavian bruits varies with the position of the arm. Furthermore, a bruit emanating from the subclavian or vertebral artery can be heard by compressing the distal subclavian or axillary artery. If the murmur diminishes, it is subclavian; if it augments, it is vertebral.

Although no invariable rule can be made regarding the significance of a carotid murmur, a high-pitched systolic bruit heard at the carotid bifurcation often means stenosis in that location. If it persists into diastole, it is pathognomonic of tight stenosis of either the internal (90% of the time) or the external carotid (in 10%). Occlusion usually abolishes the murmur, but the diversion of blood into the external carotid may also cause a loud murmur. Similarly, a systolic bruit heard over one orbit suggests increased flow through a stenotic carotid siphon on that side or occlusion of the opposite carotid.

The significance of arterial murmurs can be summarized by the following generalities:

1. As a rule, murmurs become audible after the lumen has been reduced by about 50% of the cross-sectional area
2. With increasing stenosis, the pitch becomes higher
3. With increasing stenosis, the volume increases until the cross-sectional area of the lumen is reduced by more than two-thirds, at which point its intensity decreases and, finally, becomes inaudible when occlusion occurs
4. The loudness of the murmur correlates poorly with the severity of arterial stenosis and not at all with ulceration and/ or thrombus formation
5. As stenosis increases, so does the duration of the murmur produced by the constriction. Murmurs that continue into diastole suggest at least 90% reduction in the cross-sectional area. Therefore, the following general points can be made: (a) murmurs of low pitch or of high intensity or volume are generally associated with large orifices through which a large volume of blood is flowing under relatively high pressure; and (b) murmurs of high intensity, high pitch, and long duration suggest a high-velocity blood flow through a small orifice.

Even though some individuals with mild stenosis have loud bruits and others with a completely occluded vessel have none, listening for murmurs is the best bedside method for detecting atherosclerosis. The site of maximum bruit intensity usually overlies the vascular lesion, but this site does not always correlate with the lesion's severity because the volume, pitch, and transmission characteristics are unreliable predictors of the degree of lumen stenosis. The bruit's point of origin and maximum intensity, as well as its transmission characteristics, are the best means for determining the location of the lesion.

The common denominator of all bruits is turbulent flow, which may be the result of one or several of the following: abnormal blood viscosity, change in velocity of flow, irregularities in the lumen or in the intimal wall of the artery, and the relation of focal constriction to poststenotic dilatation of the artery.

Murmurs are classified according to their timing and duration in relationship to the cardiac cycle, as well as their intensity (volume), pitch, and transmission characteristics. Bruits are graded on a one to six scale; grade I is the faintest audible sound, and a grade VI murmur can still be heard with a stethoscope that has been just barely removed from contact with the skin surface.

Murmurs originating from the great vessels within the thorax may be audible over the upper portions of the chest wall but most often are loudest at the base of the neck over the common carotid or the subclavian arteries. Murmurs arising in the brachiocephalic trunk transmit into the right subclavian and the right common carotid artery. Those arising at the subclavian-vertebral junction may transmit out of the subclavian into the axilla, as well as up the vertebral artery into the neck. Bruits arising from the region of the carotid bifurcation, particularly on the internal carotid artery, transmit poorly into the cranial cavity.

When occlusion occurs, other vessels may develop sufficiently increased flow that murmurs may be heard over vessels other than the involved artery. A typical example of this occurs with occlusion of the internal carotid artery, in which murmurs may be heard over the homolateral external carotid or over the

Table 2-5: Examination Clues to Cerebrovascular Disorders

Finding	Possible Significance	Stroke Type	Suspected Pathogenesis
Skin			
Cyanosis	Cyanotic congenital heart disease	IS	Cardiac embolism, cerebral thrombosis (polycythemia)
Osler nodes, splinter hemorrhages	Infective endocarditis	IS, ICH, SAH	Cardiac embolism, infective aneurysm, vasculitis
Needle tracks	Drug addiction, infective endocarditis, HIV	IS, ICH, SAH	Cardiac embolism, infective aneurysm, vasculitis
Café-au-lait spots, axillary freckles, neurofibromas	Neurofibromatosis	IS, ICH, SAH	Arterial hypertension (renal artery stenosis, pheochromocytoma), moyamoya
Hypopigmented spots, ash-leaf spots, facial angiofibromas, ungual fibromas, shagreen patch	Tuberous sclerosis complex	IS, SAH	Cardiac embolism (rhabdomyomas), intracranial aneurysm
Excessive laxity	Ehlers-Danlos syndrome	IS, SAH	Aneurysm, dissection, CCF
Yellowish papules ("plucked chicken" appearance)	Pseudoxanthoma elasticum	IS, ICH, SAH	Aortic arch stenosis, aneurysm
Telangiectasias	Osler-Weber-Rendu	IS, ICH, SAH	Paradoxical embolism (pulmonary AVM), vascular malformations
Purpura	Henoch-Schönlein, cryoglobulinemia	IS, ICH	Vasculitis, hyperviscosity
Hemangiomas	Bannayan-Zonana syndrome	ICH	Brain hemangiomas (particularly cerebellum)
Upper facial nevus flammeus	Sturge-Weber syndrome	IS, CVT	Capillary venous angioma of leptomeninges, AVM
Malar skin rash	SLE, homocystinuria	IS, ICH, SAH, CVT	Prothrombotic state, vasculitis
Aphthous ulcers, oral and genital ulcers	Behçet disease	IS, CVT	Prothrombotic state, vasculitis
Angiokeratomas	Fabry disease	IS	Arterial hypertension, dolichoectasia, cardiac embolism (MI)
Livedo reticularis	Sneddon syndrome	IS	Prothrombotic state (APAS?)
Lentiginosi, blue nevi	Atrial myxoma	IS, ICH	Cardiac embolism, neoplastic aneurysm, arterial dissection
Xanthomas, xanthelasmas	Hyperlipidemia	IS	Atherosclerosis
Papules, atrophic lesions	Kohlmeier-Degos disease	IS, ICH	Prothrombotic state, vasculitis (?)
Adenopathy	Syphilis, HIV, sarcoidosis	IS, ICH	Vasculitis, vasculopathy, cardiac embolism
Hair			
Depigmented, brittle, twisted hair	Menkes kinky hair disease	IS, SAH	Tortuous and elongated cerebral arteries, angiodysplasia
Frontal baldness	Myotonic dystrophy	IS	Cardiac embolism
Eyes			
Horner syndrome	Cervico-cephalic arterial dissection	IS	Dissection
Pulsating exophthalmos	Carotid cavernous fistula	IS, ICH	Traumatic arteriovenous fistula
Lens subluxation	Marfan syndrome, homocystinuria	IS, ICH, CVT	Moyamoya, aortic dissection, MVP, intracranial aneurysm prothrombotic state

Table 2-5 *(continued)*

Finding	Possible Significance	Stroke Type	Suspected Pathogenesis
Retinal phlebitis	Eales disease	IS, ICH	Vasculopathy
Retinal angioma	Familial cavernous angiomatosis, Von Hippel Lindau disease	ICH, SCI	Vascular malformation, cerebellar hemangioblastoma, polycythemia, arterial hypertension
Retinal, subhyaloid, and vitreous hemorrhages	Terson syndrome	SAH	Intracranial aneurysm
Angioid streaks	Pseudoxanthoma elasticum	IS, ICH, SAH	Aortic arch stenosis, aneurysm
Corneal arcus	Hyperlipidemia	IS	Atherosclerosis
Corneal opacity	Fabry disease	IS	Arterial hypertension, cardiac embolism (MI)
Exudates (fundi)	Diabetes, hypertension, infective endocarditis, SLE	IS, ICH, SAH	Small and large vessel atherosclerotic disease, prothrombotic state, lipohyalinosis-fibrinoid arteriopathy, cardiac embolism, vasculitis, infective aneurysm
Hemorrhages (fundi)	Diabetes, hypertension, bleeding diathesis, ruptured aneurysm	IS, ICH, SAH	Small and large vessel atherosclerotic disease, lipohyalinosis-fibrinoid arteriopathy, hyperviscosity state, intracranial aneurysm
Fat globules	Fat embolism	ICH (petechial)	Fat embolism
Pharynx			
Tonsillar trauma	Carotid artery occlusion	IS	Dissection, thrombosis
Heart			
Murmur	Infective endocarditis, MVP, VSD, atrial myxoma, asymmetric septal hypertrophy	IS, ICH, SAH	Cardiac embolism, vasculitis, infective aneurysm
Atrial fibrillation	Nonvalvular, valvular, ischemic heart disease, cardiomyopathies, hyperthyroidism, etc.	IS	Cardiac embolism
Blood Vessels			
Diminished pulses	Premature atherosclerosis, aortic dissection, Takayasu	IS, ICH, SCI	Large vessel atherosclerosis, dissection, vasculitis
Diminished or absent femoral pulses compared with brachial pulse, upper extremity hypertension	Coarctation of the aorta	SAH	Intracranial aneurysm
Bruit	Premature atherosclerosis, fibromuscular dysplasia, arterial dissection	IS, ICH, SAH	Large vessel atherosclerosis, vasculopathy, dissection, prothrombotic state
Abdomen			
Flank mass, hematuria	ADPKD	SAH	Intracranial aneurysm
Extremities			
Xanthomas	Hyperlipidemia	IS	Atherosclerosis
Venous thrombosis	Primary or secondary prothrombotic states	IS, CVT	Prothrombotic state, paradoxical embolism
Clubbing	Cyanotic congenital heart disease	IS	Cardiac embolism

(continued)

Table 2-5 *(continued)*

Finding	Possible Significance	Stroke Type	Suspected Pathogenesis
Leg ulcers	Systemic vasculitis, Buerger disease, sickle cell disease	IS, ICH, SAH, SCI	Prothrombotic state, large vessel vasculopathy, moyamoya, aneurysm, vasculitis
Dactilytis	Sickle cell disease	IS, ICH, SAH, SCI	Prothrombotic state, large vessel vasculopathy, moyamoya, aneurysm
Short and broad hands, clinodactyly of the fifth finger, simian crease	Down syndrome	IS	Moyamoya
Limb hypertrophy	Klippel-Trenaunay-Weber syndrome	IS	Spinal cord AVM, cerebral arteriovenous fistula
Body Size			
Tall stature	Marfan syndrome, homocystinuria	IS, ICH, CVT	Moyamoya, dissection, prothrombotic state
Short stature	Progeria, mitochondrial encephalomyopathy, lactic acidosis, and stroke-like episodes (MELAS)	IS	Accelerated atherosclerosis, metabolic stroke
Neurological			
Mental retardation	Phakomatoses, homocystinuria, hereditary or chromosomal disorders leading to cognitive impairment and stroke, Down syndrome	IS, ICH, SAH, CVT	Cardiac embolism, aneurysm, prothrombotic state, moyamoya
Myotonia	Myotonic dystrophy	IS	Cardiac embolism
Progressive external ophthalmoplegia	Kearns-Sayre syndrome	IS	Cardiac embolism
Ataxia, lower extremity areflexia, high arches	Friedreich ataxia	IS	Cardiac embolism
Deficits in multiple vascular territories	Systemic disease, cardiac disorder	IS	Cardiac embolism, vasculitis, prothrombotic state

ADPKD = autosomal dominant polycystic kidney disease; APAS = Antiphospholipid Antibody Syndrome; AVM = arteriovenous malformation; CCF = carotid-cavernous fistula; CVST = cerebral venous sinus thrombosis; ICH = intracerebral hemorrhage; IS = ischemic stroke; MI = myocardial infarction; MVP = mitral valve prolapse; SAH = subarachnoid hemorrhage; SCI = spinal cord infarction; SLE = systemic lupus erythematosus; VSD = ventricular septal defect.

opposite internal carotid artery. The bruits in the former result from alternative collateral channels, whereas in the latter, the volume of flow through the opposite increases by about 40% to compensate for the obstruction in the opposite carotid. Often such murmurs are heard not only at the region of the carotid bifurcation but also in the orbit because of increased flow through the carotid siphon.

There are a variety of causes of internal carotid obstruction. The artery may be congenitally absent or atretic, conditions that are usually asymptomatic because of compensatory collateral circulation. Rarely, faucial tonsillitis or otitis media involves the adjacent segment of the internal carotid artery, leading to periarteritis and thrombosis, or an embolus from the heart occludes the artery. Other unusual causes include (a) external compression or invasion of the artery by neoplasm or cicatrix, (b) subintimal hematoma and dissection, (c) compression from behind by the lateral mass of the atlas, (d) fibromuscular dysplasia,

(e) inflammatory arteritis, and (f) radiation vasculopathy. By far the most frequent cause of carotid obstruction is atherosclerosis.

GENERAL EXAMINATION

Although attention must be focused on the neurological and ophthalmological examinations, the general physical examination offers many clues to the diagnosis of the patient with cerebrovascular disease. A thorough discussion of the general physical findings that are potentially relevant to the diagnosis of cerebrovascular disease is well beyond the scope of this text, but a system by system summary of some of the findings that could be relevant to the cerebrovascular system is provided in Table 2-5.

REFERENCES

1. Goldstein LB, Matchar DB. The rational clinical examination. Clinical assessment of stroke. *JAMA.* 1994;**271**:1114–1120.

2. Goldstein LB, Simel DL. Is this patient having a stroke? *JAMA*. 2005;**293**:2391–2402.

3. Ricci S. Clinical evaluation of patients with stroke is still worthwhile. *J Neurol Neurosurg Psychiatry*. 2000;**68**:547.

4. Laine C, Davidoff F. Patient-centered medicine. A professional evolution. *JAMA*. 1996;**275**:152–156.

5. Kimball CP. Techniques of interviewing. I. Interviewing and the meaning of the symptom. *Ann Intern Med*. 1969;**71**:147–153.

6. Ellis S, Small M. Localization of lesion in denial of hemiplegia after acute stroke. *Stroke*. 1997;**28**:67–71.

7. Santos CO, Caeiro L, Ferro JM, Albuquerque R, Figueira ML. Denial in the first days of acute stroke. *J Neurol*. 2006;**253**:1016–1023.

8. Leys D, Henon H, Kowiak-Cordoliani MA, Pasquier F. Poststroke dementia. *Lancet Neurol*. 2005;**4**:752–759.

9. Hoffmann M, Sacco R, Mohr JP, Tatemichi TK. Higher cortical function deficits among acute stroke patients: the stroke data bank experience. *J Stroke Cerebrovasc Dis*. 1997;**6**:114–120.

10. Pohjasvaara T, Erkinjuntti T, Ylikoski R, Hietanen M, Vataja R, Kaste M. Clinical determinants of poststroke dementia. *Stroke*. 1998;**29**:75–81.

11. Ott BR, Saver JL. Unilateral amnesic stroke. Six new cases and a review of the literature. *Stroke*. 1993;**24**:1033–1042.

12. Grewal RP. Severe amnesia following a unilateral temporal lobe stroke. *J Clin Neurosci*. 2003;**10**:102–104.

13. Darley FL. *Aphasia*. Philadelphia: W.B. Saunders Company; 1982.

14. Godefroy O, Dubois C, Debachy B, Leclerc M, Kreisler A. Vascular aphasias: main characteristics of patients hospitalized in acute stroke units. *Stroke*. 2002;**33**:702–705.

15. Willmes K, Poeck K. To what extent can aphasic syndromes be localized? *Brain*. 1993;**116**(Pt 6):1527–1540.

16. Blank SC, Scott SK, Murphy K, Warburton E, Wise RJ. Speech production: Wernicke, Broca and beyond. *Brain*. 2002;**125**:1829–1838.

17. Black PM, Black SE, Droge JA. Three models of human language. *Neurosurgery*. 1986;**19**:308–315.

18. Jordan LC, Hillis AE. Disorders of speech and language: aphasia, apraxia and dysarthria. *Curr Opin Neurol*. 2006;**19**:580–585.

19. Kerschensteiner M, Poeck K, Brunner E. The fluency-non fluency dimension in the classification of aphasic speech. *Cortex*. 1972;**8**:233–247.

20. Knepper LE, Biller J, Tranel D, Adams HP Jr, Marsh EE III. Etiology of stroke in patients with Wernicke's aphasia. *Stroke*. 1989;**20**:1730–1732.

21. Hillis AE, Wityk RJ, Tuffiash E, et al. Hypoperfusion of Wernicke's area predicts severity of semantic deficit in acute stroke. *Ann Neurol*. 2001;**50**:561–566.

22. Tanabe H, Sawada T, Inoue N, Ogawa M, Kuriyama Y, Shiraishi J. Conduction aphasia and arcuate fasciculus. *Acta Neurol Scand*. 1987;**76**:422–427.

23. Demeurisse G, Capon A. Brain activation during a linguistic task in conduction aphasia. *Cortex*. 1991;**27**:285–294.

24. Geschwind N. Disconnexion syndromes in animals and man. II. *Brain*. 1965;**88**:585–644.

25. Benson DF, Sheremata WA, Bouchard R, Segarra JM, Price D, Geschwind N. Conduction aphasia. A clinicopathological study. *Arch Neurol*. 1973;**28**:339–346.

26. Kertesz A, McCabe P. Recovery patterns and prognosis in aphasia. *Brain*. 1977;**100**(Pt 1):1–18.

27. Takeda M, Tachibana H, Shibuya N, et al. Pure anomic aphasia caused by a subcortical hemorrhage in the left temporo-parieto-occipital lobe. *Intern Med*. 1999;**38**:293–295.

28. Avila C, Lambon Ralph MA, Parcet MA, Geffner D, Gonzalez-Darder JM. Implicit word cues facilitate impaired naming performance: evidence from a case of anomia. *Brain Lang*. 2001;**79**:185–200.

29. Hadar U, Ticehurst S, Wade JP. Crossed anomic aphasia: mild naming deficits following right brain damage in a dextral patient. *Cortex*. 1991;**27**:459–468.

30. Heinsius T, Bogousslavsky J, Van Melle G. Large infarcts in the middle cerebral artery territory. Etiology and outcome patterns. *Neurology*. 1998;**50**:341–350.

31. Tranel D, Biller J, Damasio H, Adams HP Jr, Cornell SH. Global aphasia without hemiparesis. *Arch Neurol*. 1987;**44**:304–308.

32. Legatt AD, Brust JC. Global aphasia without hemiplegia. *N Engl J Med*. 1992;**327**:1244.

33. Legatt AD, Rubin MJ, Kaplan LR, Healton EB, Brust JC. Global aphasia without hemiparesis: multiple etiologies. *Neurology*. 1987;**37**:201–205.

34. Hanlon RE, Lux WE, Dromerick AW. Global aphasia without hemiparesis: language profiles and lesion distribution. *J Neurol Neurosurg Psychiatry*. 1999;**66**:365–369.

35. Naeser MA, Hayward RW. Lesion localization in aphasia with cranial computed tomography and the Boston Diagnostic Aphasia Exam. *Neurology*. 1978;**28**:545–551.

36. Biller J. *Practical Neurology*. 3rd ed. Philadelphia: Wolters-Kluwer/Lippincott Williams & Wilkins; 2009.

37. Ghika-Schmid F, Bogousslavsky J. Affective disorders following stroke. *Eur Neurol*. 1997;**38**:75–81.

38. Carota A, Rossetti AO, Karapanayiotides T, Bogousslavsky J. Catastrophic reaction in acute stroke: a reflex behavior in aphasic patients. *Neurology*. 2001;**57**:1902–1905.

39. Carota A, Berney A, Aybek S, et al. A prospective study of predictors of poststroke depression. *Neurology*. 2005;**64**:428–433.

40. Morris PL, Robinson RG, Raphael B. Emotional lability after stroke. *Aust NZ J Psychiatry*. 1993;**27**:601–605.

41. House A, Dennis M, Molyneux A, Warlow C, Hawton K. Emotionalism after stroke. *BMJ*. 1989;**298**:991–994.

42. Dam H. Depression in stroke patients 7 years following stroke. *Acta Psychiatr Scand*. 2001;**103**:287–293.

43. Nys GM, van Zandvoort MJ, van der Worp HB, de Haan EH, de Kort PL, Kappelle LJ. Early depressive symptoms after stroke: neuropsychological correlates and lesion characteristics. *J Neurol Sci*. 2005;**228**:27–33.

44. Kim JS, Choi-Kwon S. Poststroke depression and emotional incontinence: correlation with lesion location. *Neurology*. 2000;**54**:1805–1810.

45. So EL, Annegers JF, Hauser WA, O'Brien PC, Whisnant JP. Population-based study of seizure disorders after cerebral infarction. *Neurology*. 1996;**46**:350–355.

46. Bentes C, Pimentel J, Ferro JM. Epileptic seizures following subcortical infarcts. *Cerebrovasc Dis*. 2001;**12**:331–334.

47. Bladin CF, Alexandrov AV, Bellavance A, et al. Seizures after stroke: a prospective multicenter study. *Arch Neurol*. 2000;**57**:1617–1622.

48. De Reuck J, Hemelsoet D, Van Maele G. Seizures and epilepsy in patients with a spontaneous intracerebral haematoma. *Clin Neurol Neurosurg*. 2007;**109**:501–504.

49. Dennis MS. Outcome after brain haemorrhage. *Cerebrovasc Dis*. 2003;**16**(Suppl 1):9–13.

50. Yeh HS, Kashiwagi S, Tew JM Jr, Berger TS. Surgical management of epilepsy associated with cerebral arteriovenous malformations. *J Neurosurg*. 1990;**72**:216–223.

51. Regis J, Bartolomei F, Kida Y, et al. Radiosurgery for epilepsy associated with cavernous malformation: retrospective study in 49 patients. *Neurosurgery*. 2000;**47**:1091–1097.

52. Hall S, Carlin L, Roach ES, McLean WT. Herpes zoster and central retinal artery occlusion. *Ann Neurol*. 1983;**13**:217.

53. Aubar-Cohen F, Klein I, Alexandra JF, et al. Long-term outcome in Susac syndrome. *Medicine (Baltimore)*. 2007;**86**:93–102.

54. Sheehy JL. The dizzy patient. Eliciting his history. *Arch Otolaryngol*. 1967;**86**:18–20.

55. Ferro JM, Costa I, Melo TP, et al. Headache associated with transient ischemic attacks. *Headache*. 1995;**35**:544–548.

56. Symonds C. Otitic hydrocephalus. *Neurology*. 1956;**6**:681–685.

57. Bari L, Choksi R, Roach ES. Otitic hydrocephalus revisited. *Arch Neurol*. 2005;**62**:824–825.

58. Bousser MG, Russell RR. Cerebral venous thrombosis. In: Warlow CP, van Gijn J, eds. *Major Problems in Neurology*. London: W.B. Saunders Company; 1997:1–175.

59. Saeed AB, Shuaib A, Al-Sulaiti G, Emery D. Vertebral artery dissection: warning symptoms, clinical features and prognosis in 26 patients. *Can J Neurol Sci*. 2000;**27**:292–296.

60. Dziewas R, Konrad C, Drager B, et al. Cervical artery dissection – clinical features, risk factors, therapy and outcome in 126 patients. *J Neurol*. 2003;**250**:1179–1184.

61. Easton JD, Sherman DG. Cervical manipulation and stroke. *Stroke*. 1977;**8**:594–597.

62. Jeret JS, Bluth M. Stroke following chiropractic manipulation. Report of 3 cases and review of the literature. *Cerebrovasc Dis*. 2002;**13**:210–213.

63. Rothwell DM, Bondy SJ, Williams JI. Chiropractic manipulation and stroke: a population-based case-control study. *Stroke*. 2001;**32**:1054–1060.

64. Mills MD. Terson syndrome. *Ophthalmology*. 1998;**105**:2161–2163.

65. Kuhn F, Morris R, Witherspoon CD, Mester V. Terson syndrome. Results of vitrectomy and the significance of vitreous hemorrhage in patients with subarachnoid hemorrhage. *Ophthalmology*. 1998;**105**:472–477.

66. Biousse V, Touboul PJ, D'anglejan-Chatillon J, Levy C, Schaison M, Bousser MG. Ophthalmologic manifestations of internal carotid artery dissection. *Am J Ophthalmol*. 1998;**126**:565–577.

67. Lee H, Baik SK. Infarcts presenting with a combination of medial medullary and posterior inferior cerebellar artery syndromes. *J Neurol Sci*. 2004;**224**:89–91.

68. Kim JS, Lee JH, Suh DC, Lee MC. Spectrum of lateral medullary syndrome. Correlation between clinical findings and magnetic resonance imaging in 33 subjects. *Stroke*. 1994;**25**:1405–1410.

69. Sacco RL, Freddo L, Bello JA, Odel JG, Onesti ST, Mohr JP. Wallenberg's lateral medullary syndrome. Clinical-magnetic resonance imaging correlations. *Arch Neurol*. 1993;**50**:609–614.

70. Reivich M, Holling HE, Roberts B, Toole JF. Reversal of blood flow through the vertebral artery and its effect on cerebral circulation. *N Engl J Med*. 1961;**265**:878–885.

71. Toole JF. Reversed vertebral artery flow and cerebral vascular insufficiency. *Ann Intern Med*. 1964;**61**:159–162.

72. Shorr RI, Johnson KC, Wan JY, et al. The prognostic significance of asymptomatic carotid bruits in the elderly. *J Gen Intern Med*. 1998;**13**:86–90.

73. Cooperman M, Martin EW Jr, Evans WE. Significance of asymptomatic carotid bruits. *Arch Surg*. 1978;**113**:1339–1340.

74. Mackey AE, Abrahamowicz M, Langlois Y, et al. Outcome of asymptomatic patients with carotid disease. Asymptomatic Cervical Bruit Study Group. *Neurology*. 1997;**48**:896–903.

75. Ingall TJ, Homer D, Whisnant JP, Baker HL Jr, O'Fallon WM. Predictive value of carotid bruit for carotid atherosclerosis. *Arch Neurol*. 1989;**46**:418–422.

76. Howard VJ, Howard G, Harpold GJ, et al. Correlation of carotid bruits and carotid atherosclerosis detected by B-mode real-time ultrasonography. *Stroke*. 1989;**20**:1331–1335.

3

Syndromes of Vascular Dysfunction

The question of localization is only an application of the common physiology of the nervous system, of the facts that should be familiar to every student, and can be relearned, if necessary, with ease by every practitioner.

William R. Gowers

Disease is from of old and nothing about it has changed. It is we who change as we learn to recognize what was formerly imperceptible.

Jean-Martin Charcot

Cerebrovascular disease can produce a wide assortment of signs and symptoms, and the ability to recognize the clinical features of stroke is a valuable skill. Modern neuroimaging techniques (see Chapter 5) are essential for the proper diagnosis and management of individuals with cerebrovascular disease,[1] but a clinician who is able to recognize common patterns of vascular dysfunction and correlate the vascular and brain anatomy is sometimes able to accurately predict the nature and extent of the patient's disease based solely on the history and examination.

Although the size and location of a cerebrovascular lesion generally determine the patient's specific neurological signs, different forms of vascular dysfunction sometimes generate a characteristic clinical pattern. A cerebral embolism, for example, classically produces an almost immediate maximum deficit that sometimes resolves equally quickly (see Chapter 8), whereas this dramatic improvement occurs less often among individuals with cerebral thrombosis. Headache, signs of increased intracranial pressure, and impaired consciousness characterize intraparenchymal brain hemorrhage (see Chapter 16) and subarachnoid hemorrhage and occur less often with ischemic stroke. Individuals with dural sinus or cortical vein thrombosis (see Chapter 20) are more likely to develop seizures and signs of increased intracranial pressure than those with an arterial occlusion. Unfortunately the clinical manifestations of these conditions overlap sufficiently that it is not possible to precisely determine the nature of a patient's problem at the bedside.

The general approach to the evaluation of an individual with suspected cerebrovascular disease is described in Chapter 2.

In this chapter we outline the signs and symptoms associated with specific carotid and vertebrobasilar syndromes.

CAROTID ARTERY DYSFUNCTION

Applied Anatomy of the Carotid Artery

The brain receives blood from the heart via the aortic arch, which gives rise to the brachiocephalic (innominate), left common carotid, and left subclavian arteries. Arising behind the manubrium sterni, the brachiocephalic artery ascends to the level of the sternoclavicular notch, where it divides into the right common carotid and the right subclavian arteries (Figure 3-1). The left common carotid usually arises from the aortic arch just to the left of the brachiocephalic artery but may share a common origin with the brachiocephalic artery or spring from the brachiocephalic itself. A separate common trunk for the right and left common carotid artery is seen very rarely. The subclavian arteries give rise to the vertebral arteries. In some 5% of people, the left vertebral artery originates from the aortic arch proximal to the origin of the left subclavian artery. Paired vertebral and carotid arteries ascend through the neck and penetrate the skull to supply the brain.[2]

The two common carotid arteries with their adventitial sympathetic nerves lie adjacent to their respective jugular veins, the vagus nerves, and the cervical sympathetic chain. They ascend along either side of the trachea and behind the sternocleidomastoid muscle, approximately to the upper border of the thyroid cartilage just below the angle of the mandible, where each common carotid artery bifurcates into an external and an internal carotid artery. The external carotid artery supplies the neck, face, and scalp. The internal carotid artery and its branches supply the anterior two-thirds of the brain. About half of the time the common carotid bifurcation occurs at C4 just below the angle of the jaw. In another 30% it is above this level, and in the remainder it is below C4. These variations sometimes pose problems for the surgeon attempting reconstruction of the internal carotid artery. Just past its origin, the internal carotid has a bulbous expansion, the carotid sinus (Figure 3-2). This is richly supplied with receptors innervated by the glossopharyngeal

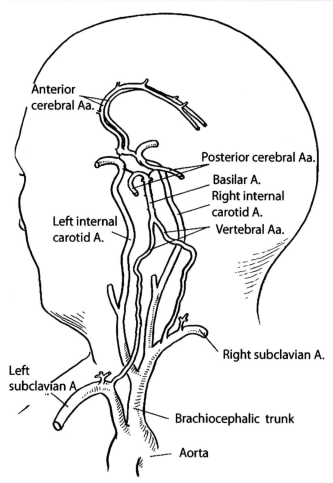

Figure 3-1. Origins of the cervicocephalic arteries.

nerve hand helps to regulate cardiac action. The carotid body is similarly innervated and lies adjacent to the sinus. The distinction between carotid bulb and sinus is important because confusion has arisen between anatomists and neurosonographers who use the above terminology and clinicians for whom the bulb is synonymous with sinus.

At its origin the external carotid artery lies anterior and medial to the internal carotid artery in the neck. The external carotid artery gives rise to the superior thyroid, facial, ascending pharyngeal, lingual, posterior auricular, and occipital arteries before terminating as the superficial temporal and maxillary arteries. The internal carotid artery ascends behind and lateral to the faucial tonsil. Just above the tonsil, the internal carotid artery lies anterior to the transverse processes of the upper three cervical vertebrae. The internal carotid artery penetrates the base of the skull through the carotid canal in the petrous portion of the temporal bone, where it is separated from the air cells in the middle ear by a bony wall that may be thin during youth and partially absorbed in later life.

The internal carotid enters the cranial cavity between the layers of the dura mater, where it lies just beneath the Gasserian ganglion, which it supplies with small branches. It then ascends abruptly along the posterolateral aspect of the sella turcica to enter the cavernous sinus. Within the venous plexus of the cavernous sinus, the carotid artery curves forward and then upward to a position medial to the anterior clinoid process, then doubles back to form the upper portion of the sinuous

curve known as the carotid siphon.[3,4] Hypophyseal arteries from this portion of the carotid perfuse the pituitary gland.[5] Branches in the siphon are (a) the meningohypophyseal trunk, which divides into the dorsal meningeal tentorial artery and the inferior hypophyseal artery, (b) the artery to the cavernous sinus, (c) the premamillary artery, and (d) the suprahypophyseal group. The paired superior and inferior hypophyseal arteries divide into capillary loops, which then form the pituitary and portal system.[6]

The internal carotid artery begins its subarachnoid course by perforating the dura mater medial to the anterior clinoid process and passing above the oculomotor nerve and below the optic nerve. At this level the clinically important branches of the internal carotid artery begin to arise in quick succession. These are, in their usual order of appearance, the ophthalmic, posterior communicating, anterior choroidal, and anterior and middle cerebral arteries.

Ethmoidal and lacrimal branches of the ophthalmic artery and the ascending pharyngeal, maxillary, and occipital arteries supply the dura mater.[7] The most important branch of the external carotid artery is the middle meningeal artery, which arises from the maxillary artery and provides the bulk of the meningeal circulation. It penetrates the base of the skull through the foramen spinosum of the sphenoid bone and runs forward and laterally in a groove or canal on the greater wing of the sphenoid, giving off branches to the dura mater.

Carotid Artery Anomalies

Hypoplasia or agenesis of the internal carotid artery can be confused with arterial stenosis or occlusion.[8] With hypoplasia, imaging studies of the skull base reveal a small or absent carotid canal.[9,10] Bilateral internal carotid artery agenesis is exceedingly rare.[11] Numerous anatomic variants have been described.[12–15]

Tortuosity, coiling, and kinking of the cervical arteries occur most frequently in the internal carotid artery and the first part of the vertebral artery.[16] Tortuosity and coiling are developmental conditions that ordinarily cause few symptoms, although stroke has been reported in individuals with an autosomal recessive disorder known as arterial tortuosity syndrome.[17–19] Kinking, on the other hand, is often acquired as a result of atherosclerosis in conjunction with a preexisting tortuous and dilated segment of the artery and may be symptomatic. In the absence of significant coexisting arterial stenosis, surgery is unlikely to be of use.

Common Carotid Artery Occlusion

Common carotid artery occlusion occurs in less than 1% of cases of carotid artery syndrome and is more frequent in the left common than in the right common carotid artery. Causes of common carotid occlusion include traumatic or spontaneous arterial dissection and deposition of an atheromatous plaque at the artery's origin at the aorta. One clinical clue to a carotid dissection is an oculosympathetic paralysis (partial Horner syndrome) that is ipsilateral to a carotid occlusion (Figure 2-5). If facial anhydrosis is present in addition to ptosis and miosis, the common or external carotid artery has likely been affected. Unusual causes for carotid occlusion include Takayasu arteritis, irradiation, coagulopathies, and cardiac embolism.[20,21]

Sometimes common carotid artery occlusion results from retrograde propagation of a clot from the internal carotid artery, an event with profound implications for the patient because it eliminates flow through the external carotid artery and with it a potential source of collateral blood flow. Robust collateral flow through an external carotid artery can maintain flow in the internal carotid artery despite occlusion of the common carotid artery.[20] If there is adequate collateral flow to prevent neurological dysfunction, an absent pulse lateral to the trachea may be the only physical finding. Similarly, in the face of a common carotid artery occlusion, flow of blood from the internal carotid into the external carotid artery can result in cerebral circulatory insufficiency. Hemisensory deficit is more commonly found with obstruction of the middle cerebral artery (MCA) than of the carotid artery because collateral circulation is not as great with the former.

Unilateral Internal Carotid Artery Stenosis and Occlusion

There are many causes for internal carotid artery dysfunction. Although in general the risk of stroke increases with increasing severity of carotid artery stenosis, the precise risk is difficult to reliably quantify in any given person.[22] Additionally, the likelihood of a stroke in one carotid territory depends to some extent on the severity of stenosis of the other cranial arteries.[23] The result of a sudden occlusion of the artery may be quite different from that caused by slowly progressive stenosis, which culminates finally in occlusion. Internal carotid artery occlusion occurs in the neck in 90% of cases and in the cavernous or terminal carotid in most of the remainder. Under either circumstance, eventually the thrombus extends upward or downward to fill the entire length of the artery.[24] Occlusion for more than a few hours may preclude a successful cervical carotid endarterectomy. From time to time the terminal intracranial portion of this long thrombus, while still friable and nonadherent, embolizes to the distal branches.

The presenting symptoms of internal carotid artery occlusion are influenced by the following factors:

1. The arterial segment involved – especially whether it is above or below the origin of the ophthalmic artery
2. The rapidity of development of the obstruction – whether gradually as with atherosclerosis or suddenly by dissection or embolus
3. The availability and adequacy of collateral circulation and the patency of the other major arteries
4. The area of brain affected – whether in the distribution of the anterior cerebral artery (ACA) or of the MCA or both.

About 25% of individuals with cerebral infarction due to carotid artery disease have carotid territory transient ischemic attacks (TIAs) before the infarction occurs. In most instances these TIAs result from microemboli in the form of cholesterol crystals, fibrin, or platelet aggregates cast off from atherosclerotic plaques. Obstruction of a small artery often produces a neurologic deficit, the duration of which depends on the adequacy of collaterals or on further distal movement of the embolus.[25]

Infarction related to atherosclerosis classically occurs during repose or sleep, often in the early morning hours, although there are, of course, many exceptions. It is not clear why this happens, but some researchers think it may be the result of physiological hypotension and hypoxemia due to circadian changes in blood constituents or mechanical compression of arteries due to prolonged rotation of the head. Cerebral emboli may occur at any time but may be more likely when the patient is awake and active. They may originate from the venous system, pulmonary veins, cardiac valves or chambers, or ulcerated plaques in the aortic arch or the arteries arising from it.

Visual symptoms sometimes herald the ictus and usually consist of a transient loss of vision in the homolateral eye, interpreted by some patients as "spots," a "blackout," or "blurred vision." Occasionally, retinal infarction develops, but, usually, the collateral arterial supply is so great that this does not occur. Some patients feel light-headed, but complete loss of consciousness is unusual. Similarly, presentation with focal seizures is unusual, and when seizures occur they are more likely to accompany an embolic than a thrombotic stroke.

Carotid territory dysfunction can result in many signs and symptoms, including paresthesias or numbness of the opposite fingers or face and weakness of an extremity. When the dominant hemisphere is affected, the patient may have difficulty with comprehension and communication. Subtle changes in personality may be detectable only by close associates. The manifestations of carotid artery stenosis can be divided into the following patterns:

1. Single or recurring TIAs: ipsilateral amaurosis fugax in combination with contralateral paresis or sensory deficit is virtually pathognomonic for carotid artery disease. Amaurosis fugax often results from emboli originating in the internal carotid artery, but the pathogenesis of cerebral TIAs in the carotid territory is more heterogeneous. As a generality, TIAs that result in hemiplegia are more likely to have resulted from relatively large cardiac emboli than from carotid sinus microemboli.
2. Unheralded ischemic stroke without a preceding TIA: Patients with large ischemic infarctions often worsen during the first few days after onset. Despite the different time course, the causes of ischemic stroke are basically similar to TIAs (see Chapter 6).
3. Some patients lack specific events that suggest a vascular etiology and may be misclassified as having a dementia or other conditions, particularly in the presence of bilateral carotid disease. There is some evidence that depression, irritability, drowsiness, confusion, emotional lability, and dementia may result from multiple cerebrovascular lesions.

Carotid Siphon Occlusion

Atheromatous changes and associated risk factors do not differ from those of age- and sex-matched controls with extracranial carotid disease. Nor is there a difference between matched groups with extracranial or intracranial internal carotid artery obstruction in numbers of strokes, TIAs, or death, which suggests that the prognosis of both is more related to age, sex, and disease severity than to the location of obstruction. Intracranial stenosis exceeding 80% has the worst prognosis for stroke, and the prognosis is better for individuals without tandem atheromatous lesions.

In younger adults and children, moyamoya disease is more likely to cause stenosis and occlusion of the intracranial carotid artery than atherosclerosis. Moyamoya is a radiographic syndrome of progressive carotid occlusion with dilated distal collateral vasculature that on catheter angiography resembles a puff of smoke (moyamoya is a Japanese term meaning "hazy," like a puff of smoke drifting through the air). By custom, individuals with idiopathic moyamoya are classified as having moyamoya *disease*, whereas those with known predisposing factors (e.g., cranial irradiation, neurofibromatosis type 1, or Down syndrome) are said to have moyamoya *syndrome*.[26] Moyamoya is presented in more detail in Chapter 13.

Rupture of the internal carotid artery within the cavernous sinus creates a carotid-cavernous fistula (see Chapter 18).

Bilateral Internal Carotid Artery Dysfunction

The effect of occlusion or stenosis of both carotids depends in part on collateral flow from the external carotid and vertebral-basilar systems. At one extreme bilateral occlusion may be asymptomatic, whereas other individuals have bilateral hemispheric infarction resulting in tetraplegia and coma. This devastating outcome typically occurs when one internal carotid has been occluded followed by the occlusion of the second carotid that had been providing blood flow to both hemispheres. In such patients symptoms suggestive of basilar artery insufficiency may be the result of simultaneous insufficiency of blood flow to both hemispheres, causing bilateral symptoms and signs. In other individuals a steal from the posterior to the carotid circulation may result in similar symptoms.

Because of the proximity of the internal carotid artery to the middle ear, carotid murmurs can sometimes be heard by the patient throughout his waking hours and may cause him great distress. Middle-ear infection affects the carotid canal, causing carotid periarteritis. Rarely, an aneurysm of the carotid artery in this location bulges into the middle ear and presents as a mass within it.

Mechanisms of Arterial Occlusion

When the occlusion is gradual and collateral blood flow is plentiful, occlusion of an internal carotid artery does not always cause a stroke.[27] When it does, the infarction tends to involve the cerebral cortex or a large subcortical region, similar to the pattern produced by an MCA occlusion or occlusion of both the MCA and ACA.[28] Small subcortical infarctions occur on the occluded side with the same frequency as in the opposite hemisphere, which suggests that these lesions may not be the direct result of the carotid occlusion.[29] The traditional teaching has been that TIAs stop once an artery becomes occluded (if a stroke does not occur at the time of occlusion, the patient is safe unless the collateral blood supply became occluded as well). However, there are many exceptions to this statement. For example, ischemia distal to an occluded carotid artery is common, probably because of thromboembolism in most instances. The common and external carotid arteries are typically diseased as well, providing a conduit for emboli to reach the brain or eye. Two-thirds of the patients retain a patent proximal stump of up to 10 mm in length that can be a source of emboli. The difficulty is knowing when the ischemic event in a given patient relates to an identified stump. This can be rarely done with absolute certainty, but it may be suspected if imaging demonstrates thrombus or if serial examinations reveal changing length of the stump.

Luminal stenosis of more than 60% of the cross-sectional area results in distal reduction of the arterial pulse pressure. Perfusion of brain requires pulsatile pressure for adequate flow, and flow is reduced when the luminal diameter has been reduced by 80% or more. At times, even occlusion of three or, rarely, four arteries does not result in cerebrovascular insufficiency, whereas, in other instances, carotid artery obstruction causes symptoms of

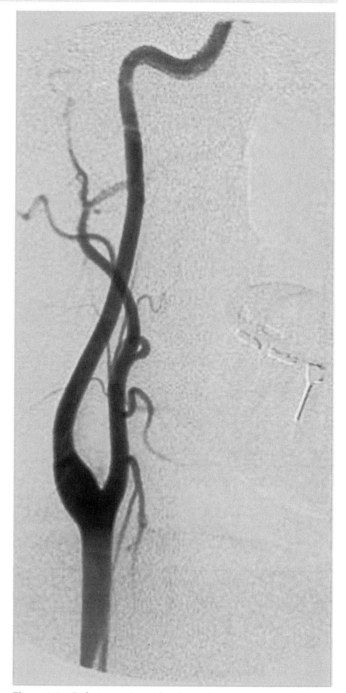

Figure 3-2. Catheter angiography shows the common carotid artery bifurcation to form the internal and external carotid arteries. Note the bulbous enlargement of the internal carotid artery just distal to the bifurcation.

vertebral-basilar territory ischemia by diverting blood to the carotid circulation through the posterior communicating arteries.

OPHTHALMIC ARTERY

Applied Anatomy

In most individuals the ophthalmic artery arises from the dorsal aspect of the first bend of the carotid siphon just above the diaphragma sellae and beneath the optic nerve (Figure 3-3). It enters the apex of the orbit through the optic foramen adjacent

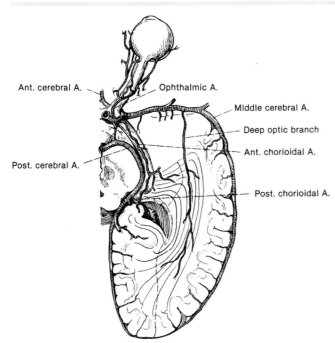

Ant. cerebral A.

Ophthalmic A.

Middle cerebral A.

Deep optic branch

Ant. chorioidal A.

Post. cerebral A.

Post. chorioidal A.

Figure 3-3. Vascular anatomy of the visual pathway relative to its blood supply.

to the optic nerve and then moves laterally and upwards to a supero-medial position relative to the optic nerve.[30] Rarely, it originates from the middle meningeal artery and enters the orbit through the superior orbital fissure.[31] There it divides into multiple branches that supply the orbital contents and anastomose with branches of the external carotid artery.[32] Its most important branch, the central artery of the retina, perforates the globe at the optic disk to divide into the branches that supply the retina. These are the arterioles seen when examining the optic fundus with an ophthalmoscope.

The central retinal artery enters the optic nerve about 10 mm behind the globe and supplies the inner two-thirds of the retina. It is an end-artery about 200 μm in diameter at the lamina cribrosa where it divides into superior and inferior branches, which subsequently redivide into nasal and temporal branches at the optic disc. Almost 50% of the population has a cilioretinal artery that may act as an independent blood supply to the peripapillary retina and to the macular region.

The retinal arterioles are about 100 μm in diameter. There are two main capillary networks: a superficial one in the ganglion cell layer and a deep one in the inner nuclear layer. In areas where the retina is thin (such as the parafoveal region and the peripheral retina), these two capillary networks anastomose. However, there is a capillary-free zone at the fovea. A separate set of capillaries, the radial peripapillary capillaries, carry blood to the retina, which lies in an arc around the macula. These relatively long, straight capillaries possibly are the source of hemorrhage that is sometimes associated with papilledema.

Usually the venules course alongside the arterioles, and the two are ensheathed in a common adventitia at crossing points. The diameter of the venules is approximately 100–120 μm and the central retinal vein is about 200 μm. The central retinal vein accompanies the central retinal artery along the optic nerve and is the main outflow channel. The superior ophthalmic vein is formed by the joining of the superior vortex veins. It exits the orbit through the superior orbital fissure. Two to four inferior

vortex veins join to form the inferior ophthalmic vein, which communicates with the superior ophthalmic vein after exiting through either the superior or the inferior orbital fissure. In 40% of the population, a medial ophthalmic vein is also present and drains into the cavernous sinus with the others.

Retinal Vascular Physiology

The retina has the greatest rate of oxygen consumption per gram of any tissue in the body and has two separate circulatory systems to meet this demand. The blood flow of the central retinal artery is about 28 μL/min. The choroidal circulation, with its much faster flow of 150 μL/min, has a more variable flow rate and a relatively lower arteriovenous oxygen gradient. The choroidal circulation supplies oxygen and nutrients to the macula lutea and the outer one-third of the retina and removes heat and waste products generated both by the conversion of light to chemical energy and by the metabolism of the rods and cones.

However, the retinal circulation is similar to that of the brain in that both autoregulate even though the retinal system is relatively less reactive to changes in partial pressure of CO_2 (PCO_2) and relatively more so to changes in partial pressure of oxygen (PO_2) compared to the cerebral circulation. Furthermore, there is a blood-retina barrier similar to the blood-brain barrier that restricts many molecules.

Amaurosis Fugax

Fleeting episodes of monocular blindness (*amaurosis fugax*) lasting from seconds to minutes, especially when recurrent, are very suggestive of retinal ischemia because of insufficiency of the homolateral ophthalmic or carotid artery (Table 3-1). There are numerous reasons for transient monocular visual loss in addition to circulatory compromise, but many of these can be eliminated solely on the basis of a detailed history and physical examination. Blindness due to cerebral vascular disease is most often sudden in onset, and the moment when it occurs is noted by the patient, who usually describes the attack as blurring of vision, blackout, or misty vision.[33] Sometimes a yellowish or greenish hue is noted as peripheral vision is lost. Occasionally vision is lost and regained in an altitudinal fashion, the common complaint being that of a "veil" or "shade" descending or ascending in front of one eye (Figure 2–2). The loss might involve the whole visual field or only a segment.

Parkin and associates followed 51 patients with amaurosis fugax for a mean of nearly 5 years.[34] Only three experienced minor permanent visual sequelae, but nearly half developed cerebral events. Eleven of 19 (58%) had no additional episodes after endarterectomy, but two (10%) had no change in the frequency or quality of their symptoms.

Because they do not cover one eye during an attack, most patients are unable to say whether just one eye or one-half of both visual fields was involved. Some patients mistake visual loss in one eye or one part of the visual field as complete blindness. Patients often report that vision is restored as abruptly as it fades.

The common denominator of all these is retinal ischemia secondary to a reduction of pressure or obstruction of flow on the arterial side of the retinal circulation. Obstruction of the carotid or the ophthalmic artery by thrombosis, embolus, or spasm can lower the pressure abruptly.[35–37] Individuals with a retinal Hollenhorst plaque (Figure 6-1) are more likely to have a stenotic carotid artery or an ulcerated arterial plaque, and

Table 3-1: Clinical Patterns of Amaurosis Fugax

Often Present	*Usually Absent*
Visual obscuration	Pain
Sudden onset	Simultaneous TIA
Rapid development	Prodrome
Brief duration	Scintillation
Vertical or altitudinal shade defect	Precipitating event

patients with a central retinal artery or branch artery occlusion are more likely to have risk factors than those with amaurosis fugax.[37] Individuals with amaurosis fugax have a lower risk of subsequent stroke than those with TIAs involving the brain.[38]

During the episode the involved retina is pale and the arterioles attenuated. Sometimes microemboli can be seen. At times phlebothrombosis develops as a result of the lowered venous pressure by arterial disease or phlebosclerosis. This results in prolonged impairment of vision because of retinal edema and hemorrhages, which are visible for days after the onset of the occlusion.

Anterior Ischemic Optic Neuropathy

The carotid arteries have long been implicated as a source of retinal arteriolar emboli, a cause of amaurosis fugax. The internal, common, and, rarely, external carotids have been found to be sources. There have been reports of amaurosis fugax caused by homolateral internal carotid occlusion due to emboli passing from the external carotid through various anastomotic connections to the ophthalmic artery and, finally, into the central retinal artery.

Ischemia of the optic nerve results in ischemic optic neuropathy (ION). The blood supply of the anterior segment of the optic nerve (optic nerve head) is mainly through the short posterior ciliary arteries that in turn arise from the ophthalmic artery, while the blood supply of the posterior segment of the optic nerve is through a centripetal vascular system formed by pial vessels arising from the first branches of the ophthalmic artery (but not from the short posterior ciliary arteries).

Ischemic optic neuropathy can be anterior or posterior. Anterior ION can be nonarteritic or arteritic, the latter being resulting primarily from giant cell arteritis (see Chapter 10). Acute anterior ischemic optic neuropathy is usually characterized by an acute onset of painless, monocular loss of vision, often noted on awakening. The optic nerve head is pale and edematous. The most commonly encountered visual field defect is an inferior altitudinal loss. An erythrocyte sedimentation rate (ESR) and C-reactive protein (CRP) test should be obtained in all patients with ION to rule out giant cell arteritis.

Venous stasis retinopathy consists of microaneurysms, punctate areas of capillary dilation, and small retinal hemorrhages; if it is severe, there is also dilation, darkening, and irregularity of the caliber of the major retinal veins in about 20% of patients with internal carotid occlusion. Preretinal neovascularization may occur in the chronic state. Visible improvement of neovascularization can occur within 48 hours of carotid endarterectomy.

Light-Sensitive Retinopathy

Although the majority of the ocular phenomena in patients with carotid artery disease consist of amaurosis fugax or ischemic optic neuropathy, another rare event is unilateral loss of vision caused by bright light. Because the retina has such a high metabolic rate, vascular compromise limits the rate at which the photo-pigment can recover. This may improve after carotid endarterectomy.[39]

MIDDLE CEREBRAL ARTERY

Applied Anatomy of the Middle Cerebral Artery

After giving off the anterior cerebral artery, the internal carotid becomes the middle cerebral artery. Numerous anatomical variants of the MCA have been documented.[40] The MCA supplies a much larger area than either the anterior or the posterior arteries and carries much of the blood received by the cerebral hemispheres. Although the area supplied by the MCA is relatively constant (Figure 3-4), considerable interindividual variation may be seen concerning the degree to which the MCA participates in the supply of the different structures.[41-45] It turns laterally into the Sylvian fissure, where it is encased by the base of the frontal lobe above and the superior surface of the temporal lobe below. The numerous paramedian or ganglionic

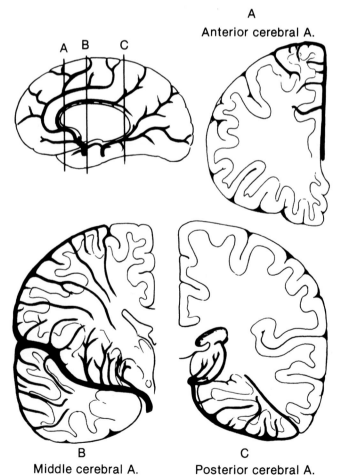

Figure 3-4. Distribution of the major cerebral arteries within the cerebral hemispheres.

branches, which it gives off into the anterior perforated substance, supply the putamen, the head of the caudate, the globus pallidus, and the genu and posterior limbs of the internal capsule.[46] The most prominent of these perforating end arteries are the lenticulostriates, which once were said to be the arteries of cerebral hemorrhage. These arteries are long and relatively unbranched in their course into the ganglia. They do not anastomose with one another as do the surface conducting arteries.[47]

In the Sylvian fissure on the lateral surface of the insula, the MCA divides into branches that travel in the sulci of the frontal and parietal lobes and the superior surfaces of the temporal lobe. The site of the main stem bifurcation and the course of its branches are variable. The anterior temporal artery, arising just distal to the origin of the lenticulostriate arteries, supplies the pole of the temporal lobe. The ascending frontal, or orbital frontal, artery is the largest and most complex branch of the MCA. Its branches pass deep in the sulci anteriorly and laterally, then ascend the convexity of the frontal lobe to anastomose terminally with branches of the callosomarginal artery over the lip of the hemisphere (Figure 3-5). The posterior temporal artery supplies the superior and lateral aspects of the temporal lobe. The posterior parietal artery proceeds laterally and posteriorly through the Sylvian fissure; in most persons it gives off a major branch, the angular artery, that helps to supply the lateral surface of the parietal lobe and superior portions of the temporal lobe of the brain. The terminal portions of these arteries anastomose with branches of the anterior and posterior cerebral arteries.

Middle Cerebral Artery Occlusion

The clinical syndromes produced by occlusion of the MCA or of one of its branches vary widely, depending on which branches are occluded and whether anastomotic channels are open.

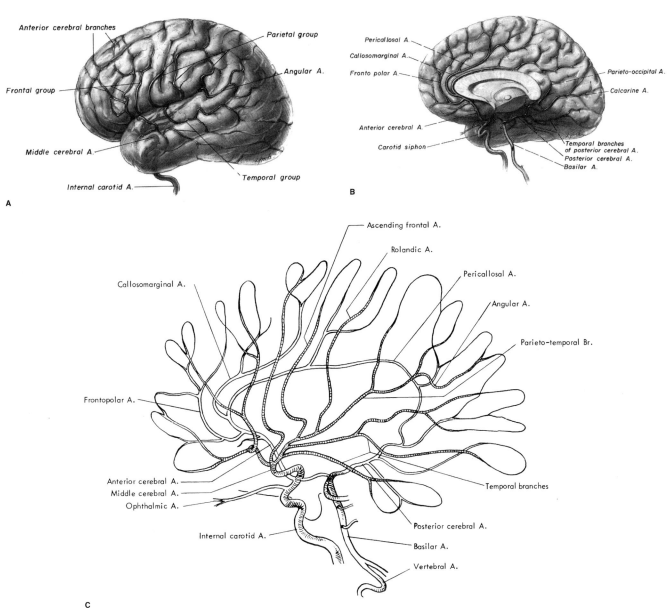

Figure 3-5. The branches of the internal carotid artery. A: Lateral view. B: Medial view. C: Schematic view.

When the MCA is occluded proximal to the lenticulostriate branches, extensive deep hemispheric infarction will include the anterior and posterior limbs of the internal capsule, and a cortical infarct surrounding the opercular region. The deficit will, therefore, include a dense hemiplegia, hemisensory loss, hemianopia, and a cortical deficit appropriate to the hemisphere.

The cortical deficits typically include global aphasia with the possibility of right-left confusion and graphic language disturbances if the dominant hemisphere is affected, and troublesome dyspraxias, lack of initiative, and failure to perceive the neurological deficit can occur with nondominant hemisphere lesions. Occlusion of the MCA distal to its lenticulostriate branches results in a variably sized infarction in the vicinity of the opercular cortex. In an individual with robust cortical collateral blood flow, occlusion of the MCA near the origin of the penetrating vessels results in subcortical infarction with relative preservation of the cortex.[48]

Because the MCA trifurcation is a frequent terminus of an embolism, recurrent major cerebral emboli may result in bilateral lesions of the opercular region. In the striking *bi-opercular syndrome*, paralysis of volitional movements of the tongue, jaw, pharynx, and facial musculature may suddenly be broken by a surprisingly full, emotionally induced movement (e.g., a smile or tongue protrusion). As both the upper and lower facial movements are impaired, the lesion could be mistaken for involvement of the lower motor neuron in the brainstem. However, jaw, facial, and gag reflexes are characteristically brisk, and limb movements are often normal.

Occlusion of the ascending frontal artery produces infarction of the third frontal convolution, which, on the dominant hemisphere, results in motor aphasia. Occlusion of the Rolandic artery produces sensory motor paralysis of the face and arm, and that of the angular artery produces infarction of the posterior limb of the Sylvian fissure and, if on the dominant hemisphere, receptive or global aphasia and apractognosia. When all of the cortical branches are obstructed, the infarction extends over the entire area, usually in varying degrees because of anastomoses in the distal distribution of these arteries. The usual effect is severe hemiplegia and sensory impairment.

Infarction in the middle cerebral distribution is often caused by embolism. Only in the minority is the occlusion due to atherosclerosis of the MCA itself. Artery-to-artery emboli arise from proximal atherosclerotic lesions or from an occluded internal carotid artery.[49] Thrombosis of the MCA due to atherosclerosis occurs only a tenth as often as internal carotid occlusion, but MCA atherosclerosis may occur more often in Asians.

Preceding homolateral amaurosis fugax is an important clue. As a rule, symptoms of MCA obstruction are more severe and abrupt than those of internal carotid artery because of the former's lack of collateral circulation. Additionally, headache is more common in individuals with carotid artery dysfunction than in those with MCA disease, and isolated aphasia without hemiparesis is more common in the MCA syndrome.

About a fourth of the individuals with an MCA occlusion experience TIAs before a major infarction. Clinical improvement or even complete clinical recovery following the ischemic event is possible. The embolus may disintegrate, the artery may recanalize, or leptomeningeal anastomotic circulation from branches of the posterior and anterior cerebral arteries may provide adequate collateral circulation. Any of these phenomena may allow some portion of the ischemic penumbra to survive, resulting in improved neurological function. Additionally, functional improvement is possible even after a completed infarction because of intrinsic brain plasticity. In contrast to internal carotid artery occlusion, a dramatic recovery after an occlusion of the MCA is less common.

The nature of the clinical dysfunction is determined by the specific area of the brain that is deprived of adequate blood flow (Figure 3-6). When the cortical branches are obstructed, the supply to the motor and sensory representation of the face and the upper limb are involved, and the leg is sometimes less severely affected. The signs may be localized, involving only weakness or numbness of a few fingers. Proximal movements are less involved than those distally. In the dominant hemisphere, speech functions are usually disrupted. Expressive aphasia from infarction of Broca's area, Wernicke's aphasia from an infarction in the posterior portion of the superior temporal gyrus, or global loss of speech may be present, as may transcortical aphasia or the disconnection syndromes (see Chapter 2). Confusion and agitated delirium sometimes occur after a right hemisphere infarction.[50]

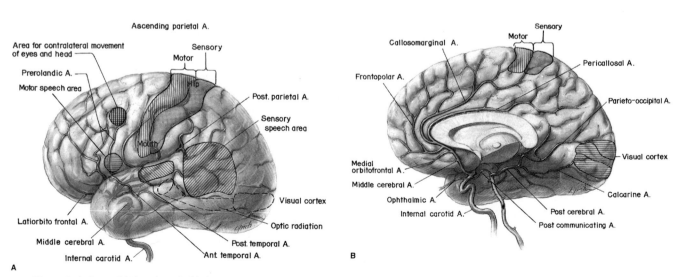

Figure 3-6. Lateral (A) and medial (B) views of a cerebral hemisphere showing areas of localized function relative to the blood supply.

Posterior parietal lesions may result in a lower visual quadrantanopia. The lateral lenticulostriate branches to the deeper structures supply the majority of the posterior limb of the internal capsule, and their obstruction gives rise to infarcts productive of severe hemiplegia with variable amounts of discriminative and crude sensory impairment and frequently an accompanying homonymous hemianopia contralateral to the lesion. This is one of the causes of hemiplegia, hemianesthesia, and hemianopia.

The cortical pursuit center lies within the distribution of the MCA in the parietal-occipital region. When the blood supply to this region is impaired, slow, smooth tracking movements in the direction toward the lesion are impaired. The frontal lobe gaze centers are also partially supplied by the MCA. The eyes tend to deviate toward the side with the lesion.

Posterior parietal lesions in the left hemisphere may lead to Gerstmann syndrome, which is characterized by bilateral finger agnosia, that is, inability to recognize, name, and select individual fingers when looking at the hands, disorientation for right and left, agraphia, and acalculia.[51] Bilateral cortical damage in the posterior parietal region may present as Balint syndrome with inability to perform visually guided operations (optic ataxia), hemispheric paralysis of visual fixation (inability to look in a particular direction or at a particular object although the head turns in the correct direction when a loud auditory signal is given), disturbance of visual attention (inability to respond to threatening visual stimuli), and simultanagnosia. Posterior temporal lesions may be associated with upper-quadrant anopia, Wernicke's aphasia (left hemisphere), or spatial delirium (right hemisphere). Bilateral lesions are rare but may result in cortical deafness. Occlusion of any of these vessels can result in homonymous hemianopsia. If only the fibers in the anterior-inferior bundle – Meyer's loop – are involved, the characteristic homonymous superior quadrantanopsia results.

Bilateral MCA Lesions

Bilateral MCA infarctions are more likely to occur as two separate events than at the same time. Typical findings include pseudobulbar palsy with swallowing difficulties, spastic attempts at speech, pathologic emotional lability, and spastic weakness of the upper limbs. Bilateral posterior parietal infarction may result in Balint syndrome.

Transient Global Amnesia

Transient global amnesia (TGA) is characterized by acute temporary loss of anterograde and recent retrograde memory.[52,53] One report estimated the incidence of TGA at 5.2 per 100,000 per year.[54] The reported TGA recurrence rate ranges from zero to 23.8%, but even individuals with recurrent TGA episodes are not at great risk for subsequent stroke.[54] The cause of TGA is still debated, and it appears that multiple triggers exist.[55,56]

Although there are well-documented individuals with both TGA and ischemic or even hemorrhagic stroke,[57–59] most people with TGA recover promptly, and individuals with TGA typically do not have more stroke risk factors than expected.[60–62] Migraine could cause some TGA episodes,[63–65] and individuals with TGA often complain of headache during or after an attack.[66] The incidence of migraine is higher in individuals with TGA in some series[60,67] but not in others.[54,68] TGA is occasionally documented after minor trauma,[69,70] brain tumor,[71] intracarotid amobarbital infusion,[72] with herpes encephalitis,[73] and with the use of drugs.[74] Recent reports suggest that TGA could also be triggered by abnormal cerebral venous outflow.[75,76]

Functional neuroimaging studies indicate that the amygdalae and hippocampi are the anatomic substrate of TGA.[77] Hippocampal lesions are documented more frequently with diffusion-weighted MRI that is done after 48 hours.[78–80] Positron emission tomography also suggests dysfunction in the amygdala,[81] and single photon emission computed tomography reveals transient focal hypoperfusion.[82]

Localizing the site of dysfunction to the amygdalae and hippocampi, however, does not fully explain the pathophysiology of TGA. Although there is no consensus on the pathophysiology of TGA, episodic loss of cerebral vasomotor control may be the common theme between migraine, minor trauma, various medications (these could alter autoregulation), the functional imaging results, and even the occasional patients with stroke.[83]

ANTERIOR CEREBRAL ARTERY

Applied Anatomy of the Anterior Cerebral Artery

The anterior cerebral artery branches from the internal carotid artery and proceeds anteromedially in a horizontal plane, crossing the optic nerve and the anterior perforated substance of the frontal lobe (Figure 3-4).[84,85] Numerous unnamed but highly important ganglionic branches penetrate the brain at this site. One vessel is of sufficient size to be named. The medial striate artery (recurrent artery of Heubner) arises from the midportion of the ACA and takes a recurrent course laterally, giving off a few branches to the orbital cortex, and then it dips into the anterior perforated substance to supply the anterior portion of the caudate nucleus and adjacent portions of the basal ganglia and anterior limb of the internal capsule.[84,86,87]

When the two ACAs reach the midline just above the optic chiasm at the base of the brain, they are joined by the short anterior communicating artery.[88] This highly important communication may be single, paired, trebled, or absent. In some individuals the proximal ACA is absent, and both distal ACAs fill from the same internal carotid artery via the anterior communicating artery.[86] Along with the two posterior communicating arteries and the basilar artery, the two ACAs and the anterior communicating artery complete the polygonal circle of Willis.[89]

Beyond their anastomosis via the anterior communicating artery, the two ACAs course around the genu of the corpus callosum into the interhemispheric fissure, where they become the pericallosal arteries. The two ACAs have branches to the corpus callosum and the medial surfaces of the two hemispheres. At the splenium they anastomose with distal branches of the posterior cerebral arteries, forming another connection between the carotid and vertebral-basilar systems.

The ACA gives off the frontopolar artery, which supplies the anterior portion of the frontal lobe on its medial side, and the callosomarginal artery, which runs in the cingulate sulcus to the paracentral lobule.[90,91] Consequently, the cingulum is bounded inferiorly by the ACA and superiorly by its callosomarginal branch. Branches of the callosomarginal artery ascend the medial aspect of the frontal lobe deep in the sulci, then loop over the superior margin of the hemisphere onto its lateral surface. They anastomose freely with the terminal branches of the MCA, which ascends on the lateral surface of the hemisphere from the Sylvian fissure. All these large named arteries branch and rebranch to form an extensive superficial network of surface vessels that ramify and anastomose with one another. From these surface vessels, perforating arteries that function as end arteries penetrate the brain.

Anterior Cerebral Artery Dysfunction

The clinical pattern resulting from occlusion of the ACA depends on the location of occlusion and the patency of anastomotic channels. Infarctions that are limited to the distribution of the ACA are relatively uncommon. Typical locations for infarction are the fronto-parietal cortex or the external capsule in the "watershed" or "border zone" between the MCA and ACA territories. This transitional zone ischemia may lead to a superficial fronto-parietal infarct or to a deep infarct involving the capsule.

The ACA is most often obstructed at its origin from the internal carotid artery. Because the ACA arises at a right angle from the internal carotid, emboli from the heart or the cervical carotid artery tend to bypass the origin of the ACA and continue instead in the MCA.[92] Even when the proximal ACA is completely occluded, distal flow is maintained if the anterior communicating artery is adequate. Occlusion of an ACA that normally supplies the contralateral ACA via the anterior communicating artery is likely to result in simultaneous bilateral ACA territory infarctions.

The ACA supplies the interhemispheric cortex matter and narrow parasagittal strips of cortex on the superior aspect of the cerebrum (Figures 3-4 and 3-5). The motor cortex in this region controls the leg muscles, and the classic clinical feature of an ACA distribution stroke is hemiparesis with greater involvement of the leg than the arm. However, Schneider and colleagues described a group of 63 stroke patients whose weakness predominantly involved the leg, and only 11 of the 63 individuals had an occlusion of the ACA.[93] Almost as many, nine patients, had an MCA distribution stroke, and the other individuals had a variety of lesions involving the internal capsule, thalamus, and brainstem.[93] Thus a predominance of leg weakness is not very specific. Rarely, infarction in the distribution of the left ACA results in aphasia as well as in diminished spontaneous speech.[94] Brodmann area 8, which lies within this vascular domain, is responsible for horizontal saccadic eye movements toward the contralateral field of vision. Disruption of this region often results in tonic eye deviation toward the ipsilateral side.

Occlusion proximal to the origin of the recurrent artery of Heubner may produce no deficit whatsoever if the anterior communicating artery allows ample collateral supply from the opposite ACA. However, if the anterior communicating artery is small, infarction of the anterior limb of the internal capsules may cause frontal dystaxia due to involvement of the fronto-pontocerebellar projections.

Infarction caused by pericallosal artery occlusion may cause disconnection in which the two hemispheres function independently, characterized by unilateral agraphia or inability to name objects felt by the disconnected hand. Obstruction of the ACA proximal to its callosomarginal branch may cause infarction of a large segment of the medial surface of the frontal lobe with resulting paralysis of the opposite lower limb, grasp reflex, incontinence, intellectual deterioration, sucking reflex, apraxia, and, sometimes, aphasia.

If the callosomarginal artery (Figure 3-5) is obstructed and if adequate anastomoses between it and the MCA do not exist, infarction of the paracentral lobule occurs, leading to paralysis of the contralateral leg with associated cortical sensory loss and incontinence due to lack of urinary and anal sphincter control. In such instances, the face, arm, and torso are spared because their cortical area of representation is supplied by the MCA.[93]

The junction of the ACAs and the anterior communicating artery is just rostral to the lamina terminalis, the thin anterior wall of the third ventricle. High pressure blood from a ruptured anterior communicating artery aneurysm often penetrates this thin membrane, explaining the high frequency of intraventricular hemorrhage with rupture of an aneurysm in this location.

Bilateral ACA Syndrome

Both ACAs can arise from a common stem, and in other individuals both ACAs become occluded. In such patients there may be urinary and bowel incontinence, abulia with decreased spontaneity, distractibility, and emotional lability. Signs include sucking and grasping reflexes, blepharospasm, and apraxia of gait. Abulia occurs with either dominant or nondominant hemisphere lesions. Some patients have reduced spontaneous speech, loss of emotional display of the face, and nearly complete akinesia of the contralateral limbs. The areas involved are usually the cingulate cortex and the supplementary motor area.

Combined ACA and MCA Occlusion

Occlusion of both these vessels is usually secondary to an internal carotid artery occlusion and typically leads to a devastating infarction. The patient is severely disabled at the onset by massive brain edema, which in some instances leads to life-threatening cerebral herniation. Patients who survive this acute phase are often left with severe and permanent disability due to loss of most of the hemisphere. The outlook is even bleaker if the dominant hemisphere is the one affected. Simultaneous infarction in two discrete territories of one hemisphere accounts for about 1% to 2% of first-time strokes. Hemispheric double infarctions usually occur in individuals with tight stenosis or occlusion of the internal carotid artery. Presenting symptoms include combinations of hemianopia, hemiparesis, and aphasia.

ANTERIOR CHOROIDAL ARTERY

Applied Anatomy of the Anterior Choroidal Artery

There is considerable variability in the configuration of the anterior choroidal artery.[95] At times originating from the posterior communicating or MCA, the anterior choroidal artery usually arises from the supraclinoid internal carotid artery just above the origin of the posterior communicating artery.[96] It typically measures about 1 mm in diameter and arises 2 mm to 4 mm distal to the origin of the posterior communicating artery, then runs posteriorly beneath the optic tract to the level of the anterior portion of the lateral geniculate body. Here it turns laterally and breaks into a number of branches, many of which enter the temporal horn of the lateral ventricle to supply the choroid plexus, to which it provides a generous amount of blood.[97] The anterior and posterior choroidal arteries join the carotid with the vertebrobasilar systems, and the anterior choroid arteries of each side interconnect the carotids. The anterior choroidal artery territory contains portions of the posterior limb of the internal capsule and auditory and optic projections. It also supplies the globus pallidus and gives off twigs that supply the optic tract, lateral geniculate body, posterior periventricular region, and medial temporal lobe.[98,99] Like the ganglionic branches of the posterior communicating artery and those of the anterior and middle cerebral arteries, the perforating branches of the anterior choroidal artery are end arteries that penetrate the brain and ramify into a capillary network.[96]

In its greatest ramification, it perfuses the optic tract, globus pallidus, the extreme posterior portion of the putamen, the uncus, pyriform cortex, amygdala, anterior hippocampus, and dentate gyrus of the temporal lobe. Medial branches penetrate the cerebral peduncle, substantia nigra, red nucleus, subthalamus, ventral anterior, ventral lateral, pulvinar, and reticular nuclei of the thalamus. Portions of the lateral geniculate body as well as the posterior limb and retrolenticular fibers of the internal capsule, including descending motor, ascending sensory, geniculocalcarine, auditory radiation, thalamo-parietal, denta-to-rubro-thalamic, and pallido-thalamic fibers, receive branches from the anterior choroidal artery. Portions of the caudate nucleus are supplied by the anterior choroidal artery as are parts of the corona radiata and the choroid plexus of the lateral ventricles.[100]

Anterior Choroidal Artery Syndrome

In its complete form, infarction in the territory of the anterior choroidal artery results in hemiplegia, hemisensory loss (usually transient loss of light touch and pin prick), and a hemideficit of the visual field.[101] However, the territory of the anterior choroidal artery varies greatly,[102] and incomplete forms of the syndrome are more frequent. Contralateral hemimotor or sensory loss and a superior homonymous quadrantanopia or hemianopia may result from involvement of the posterior limb of the internal capsule and retrocapsular sensory and visual radiations.

The optic tracts obtain much of their vascular supply from the anterior choroidal artery. Ischemic infarction of an optic tract results in incomplete, incongruous homonymous hemianopsia of variable density with sloping margins. With the proximity of the internal capsule and the thalamus, hemiparesis and hemihypesthesia contralateral to the occluded artery are common. Dysphasia, apraxia, and hemineglect may also occur, mimicking a MCA syndrome.

In one series the most common causes of anterior choroidal artery occlusion were cardiogenic embolism, large vessel atherosclerosis, and dissection of the internal carotid artery.[103] Anterior choroidal artery territory infarcts are commonly caused by small vessel occlusive disease, especially among patients with hypertension and diabetes mellitus (see Chapter 9).[104] Anterior choroidal artery territory infarcts have occurred after surgical treatment of internal carotid artery aneurysms, clipping or endovascular coiling of anterior choroidal artery aneurysms, temporal lobe resection for temporal lobe epilepsy, following thalamotomy, and after herpes zoster ophthalmicus.

Bilateral Anterior Choroidal Artery Syndrome

Bilateral anterior choroidal artery occlusion is uncommon but devastating.[105] Typically first one and then the other anterior choroidal arteries are occluded, resulting in a biphasic or stepwise clinical deterioration. It can produce acute pseudobulbar palsy with bilateral hemisensory and hemimotor deficit, bilateral upper quadrantanopsia, or bilateral pure motor hemiparesis and variable hemiataxic, hemisensory findings. A locked-in state may occur, and abulia may result from interruption of caudate-frontal lobe connections due to caudate ischemia. Dysarthria and severe pseudobulbar palsy resulting in a mute state have been reported.

POSTERIOR COMMUNICATING ARTERY

Anatomy of the Posterior Communicating Artery

The posterior communicating artery arises as the internal carotid artery sweeps backward above the sella turcica. It travels horizontally and slightly medially to join the posterior cerebral artery (PCA), which is the terminal branch of the basilar artery. From an embryologic standpoint, the posterior communicating and posterior cerebral arteries are branches of the carotid, but blood reaching the posterior cerebral arteries is usually derived from the vertebral-basilar system. The posterior communicating arteries vary greatly in caliber from person to person, and often one of the arteries is much smaller than the other or even altogether absent. Occasionally, both are threadlike, forming a tenuous link between the carotid and vertebral-basilar systems; rarely, both are vestigial.[106]

Perforating branches spring in great profusion from the side of the artery adjacent to the brain. The anterior group supplies the hypothalamus and ventral thalamus, the anterior third of the optic tract, and the posterior limb of the internal capsule. Those arising posteriorly penetrate the interpeduncular space to supply the subthalamic nucleus (body of Luys).[107] These paramedian (ganglionic) arteries do not anastomose with one another; hence, occlusion of any one of them produces infarction in the area deprived of its blood supply.

Dysfunction of the Posterior Communicating Artery

When sufficiently large, the posterior communicating arteries act as channels that equilibrate pressure between the carotid and the vertebral-basilar system. Blood in the two systems normally does not mix, but if pressure is reduced in one, blood from the other may compensate. In the face of rostral basilar artery or proximal posterior cerebral occlusion, for example, a well-developed posterior communicating artery can provide blood to the posterior cerebral cortex that would otherwise be infracted. Similarly, the posterior communicating artery can redirect blood from the anterior circulation to the brainstem after a vertebral artery occlusion.

Because of the proximity of the posterior communicating artery to CN III, an aneurysm of this artery often presents with a compressive oculomotor nerve palsy.[108–111]

DIFFERENTIAL DIAGNOSIS

Bedside differentiation of carotid and branch artery ischemic lesions from expanding lesions, such as neoplasm, intracerebral hemorrhage, chronic subdural hematoma, or abscess, can be difficult, especially in cases without an adequate history to establish the time course. With carotid disease, three major possibilities must be considered: (1) despite the presence of symptoms and signs of carotid artery syndrome, the patient has an unrelated intracranial lesion, for example, vascular dysfunction plus an unrelated neoplasm or subdural hematoma; (2) a nonvascular lesion is mimicking the typical signs of carotid artery dysfunction, for example, the sudden onset of symptoms from a neoplasm or demyelinating lesion; or (3) the lesion in one carotid artery is accompanied by preclinical or symptomatic disease in other extra- or intracranial arteries, for example, the opposite carotid or the coronary arteries. Having established that the patient suffers with carotid artery disease, the physician must then determine its etiology.

Headache of varying degrees of severity is a common symptom of internal carotid artery occlusion. Ipsilateral frontal and orbital pain is the most common occurrence. The pain varies in severity from mild to distressing and lasts hours to a few days subsequent to the occlusion. Occasionally it is contralateral to the occlusion, and, sometimes, it is occipital. The probable explanation is that there is painful distension of the collateral anastomotic arteries. It can perhaps be confused with cranial arteritis if, in addition to headache, the patient has jaw claudication resulting from external carotid artery stenosis or occlusion.

The symptoms and signs produced by obstruction of either carotid artery in the neck or the vertebral-basilar system depend, in part, on the interrelationship of the two carotid arteries through the circle of Willis. In many cases of atherosclerosis, stenosis of the carotid artery in the region of the carotid sinus occurs so slowly that there is ample time for collateral circulation to develop before obstruction of the carotid artery finally occurs. Such patients have no clinical signs until the opposite carotid artery or the vertebral-basilar system also becomes involved, at which time catastrophic bilateral cerebral damage or dysfunction of the opposite cerebral hemisphere occurs.

There are certain useful negative features for deciding that carotid artery disease is the basis of the patient's problem:

1. The absence of signs and symptoms suggesting brainstem involvement is a prerequisite for diagnosis of carotid artery disease. The most important brainstem phenomena of which to beware are the coincidental occurrence of bilateral motor and/or sensory symptoms and signs, oculomotor symptoms and signs, vertigo, incoordination out of proportion to spasticity or weakness, and loss of consciousness. Occasional exceptions are described below.
2. Binocular visual symptoms, particularly when the patient describes the simultaneous impairment or loss of all fields of vision, are not caused by carotid artery disease. An exception occurs when a patient who has already lost useful vision in one eye for any cause begins to experience amaurosis fugax in the remaining good eye. Many patients experiencing hemianopia, which could be of carotid or posterior circulation origin, believe they are experiencing a monocular phenomenon. Binocular involvement occurs as an uncommon event in patients with carotid artery disease. Furthermore, in 15% of individuals, the PCA originates from the internal carotid artery. Consequently the major supply of the PCA to the occipital (visual) cortex may come from an internal carotid artery lesion and explain a homonymous hemianopia. Homonymous visual involvement occurs with either carotid or vertebral-basilar disease and, by itself, cannot be used to distinguish which territory is involved.

3. Cardiac sources for emboli may coexist with symptomatic carotid artery disease. A patient with hemispheric symptoms who has myocardial infarction or atrial fibrillation is probably experiencing cerebral embolism rather than carotid artery disease per se.

Convulsions, syncope, vertigo, intellectual decline, and binocular involvement are relatively uncommon with carotid occlusion. When convulsions occur, they may begin before, during, or after other clinical evidence of stroke and may be focal or generalized. In some series up to 10% of the individuals with an ischemic infarction involving the cerebral cortex develop epileptic seizures. However, the incidence of seizures within 24 hours of presentation in one prospective of 6,044 stroke patients was 3.1%, although the seizure rate was higher for individuals with hemorrhagic stroke or subarachnoid hemorrhage (8.4%) and for those with ischemic stroke due to cardioembolic lesions.[112] In stroke patients who develop seizures, the lesion typically involves the cortex rather than the subcortical structures or brainstem.[113] About two-thirds of the individuals who had a seizure following a stroke did so within a month of having the stroke.[113]

Syncope is very common in older populations, and most patients do not have carotid artery disease. Even in the presence of overt disease of one or more carotid arteries, episodic cardiac dysrhythmia or hypotension is the usual primary cause. On rare occasions disease of the carotid sinus causes the baroreceptors to be hypersensitive with resultant syncope.

Vertigo and less specific "dizziness" are common at any age, but there is an increased incidence in the elderly. These phenomena have a variety of explanations, most of them involving the vestibular apparatus. They are frequent manifestations of disease in the vertebral-basilar territory and are not related to carotid artery disease.

Bilateral carotid artery territory infarction of a magnitude sufficient to reduce the total mass of functioning brain is attended by intellectual loss. From time to time, patients occlude one carotid artery without symptoms and then occlude the opposite internal carotid artery with results that vary from minor weakness to devastating bilateral infarction. In those patients who survive this second event, intellectual loss may be prominent. Vascular dementia occurs after repeated vascular insults (see Chapter 15).

VERTEBRAL ARTERY DYSFUNCTION

Vertebral Artery Anatomy

The vertebral arteries develop from longitudinal anastomoses between segmental arteries originating from the paired dorsal aortae and the hypoglossal arteries. The upper segmental arteries eventually disappear, leaving the seventh segmental artery to form the junction between the subclavian and vertebral arteries.

The right subclavian artery arises from the brachiocephalic artery behind the sterno-clavicular joint and lies wholly in the root of the neck. The left subclavian, arising from the aortic arch in the superior mediastinum, also has an intrathoracic course. In each case the vertebral artery is the first branch of the subclavian artery. The vertebral artery ascends for a short distance

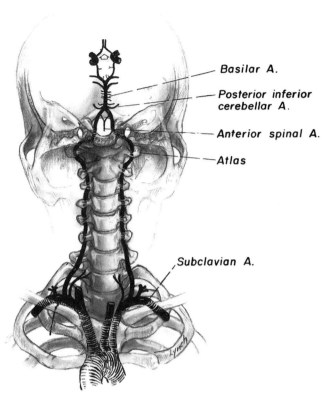

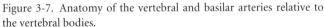

Figure 3-7. Anatomy of the vertebral and basilar arteries relative to the vertebral bodies.

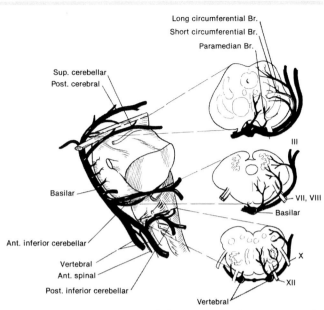

Figure 3-8. The relationship of the vertebrobasilar system to the brainstem.

through the neck just medial to the scalenus anterior muscle until it enters the osseous canal of the transverse processes of a cervical vertebra, usually that of the sixth cervical vertebra.[114] Less frequently it enters at C7 or C5, and, in rare instances, it travels to C4 before entering the canal. The two vertebral arteries join intracranially to form the basilar artery. The vertebral artery travels through the bony tunnel formed by the adjacent transverse processes and ligaments of the sixth cervical vertebra, up to the first cervical vertebra (Figure 3-7). In this tunnel it is accompanied by veins and a very dense plexus of sympathetic nerves that interconnect with cervical ganglia.

Abutting the artery on each level are cervical nerves and the joint spaces of the vertebrae. Twigs given off by the vertebral artery supply the cervical nerves, the vertebrae and their joints, and large muscular branches that exit through the vertebral foramina to supply the posterior muscles of the neck. Other branches of the vertebral artery enter the spinal canal along with the cervical nerves to supply portions of the upper spinal cord. Particularly important is a large, rather constant branch that enters the canal, usually at C5, to anastomose with the anterior spinal artery. This branch is a source of collateral circulation.

After going through C1, it travels in a groove around its posterior arch before entering the skull through the foramen magnum. In the suboccipital triangle, where it is covered only by soft tissues, it forms a loop akin to that of the carotid siphon and anastomoses freely with the occipital branch of the external carotid artery.

Entering the skull through the foramen magnum, the two vertebral arteries pierce the dura mater and ascend along the ventrolateral aspects of the medulla oblongata to which they give off numerous unnamed perforating arteries.[115,116] At the junction between the pons and the medulla, the vertebrals join to form the unique anastomosis that forms the basilar artery (Figure 3-8). Just after piercing the dura, each vertebral artery gives off its highly important anterior spinal ramus, which turns acutely downward on the lower medulla and angles toward the midline.[117,118] At the level of C2 to C3, it joins the anterior spinal ramus of the opposite side, and the two become a single artery that travels inferiorly in the medial fissure of the spinal cord (see Chapter 24).

The subclavian, vertebral, and basilar arteries form a unique system, for nowhere else in the body do two major arteries (the vertebrals) normally join to form a single one (the basilar). The posterior circulatory system is vital because it supplies all the ascending and descending tracts, most of the cranial nerves, and the nuclear aggregates that maintain consciousness, homeostasis, breathing, and deglutition.

Vertebral Artery Variations

Numerous variants of the vertebrobasilar anatomy have been documented. In most individuals such anomalies are harmless, but at times an aberrant vascular configuration affects the clinical presentation or the approach to therapy. One vertebral is typically larger than the other, and occasionally one vertebral artery is absent or so hypoplastic that it carries very little blood. In rare instances the vertebral arteries remain separate, each directly giving rise to a PCA. In 1% to 5% of individuals, the left vertebral artery arises directly from the arch of the aorta between the common carotid and the left subclavian arteries, and, in other instances, the left vertebral arises from one of the carotid arteries. Sometimes the right or left vertebral artery may have an anomalous duplicated origin.[119]

In other cases two vertebral arteries of normal size do not join in the usual fashion. In these instances one continues as the basilar and the other ends as the posterior inferior cerebellar artery. Such anomalies cause atypical clinical manifestations of the vertebral-basilar syndrome.

Mechanisms of Vertebral Artery Dysfunction

Normally the vertebral artery is about half the diameter of an internal carotid. Although the two carotid arteries are usually about equal in caliber, one vertebral artery is often much smaller than the other, so small in some instances that it contributes little to the brain's perfusion. In most such patients the opposite vertebral artery is unusually large, so that the total amount of blood flowing into the basilar artery is constant. At times the entire vertebrobasilar vascular system is hypoplastic, and the brainstem has marginal perfusion reserve aside from the flow it receives from the carotid circulation.

Unlike the internal carotid artery, which has few branches or anastomoses between its origin at the common carotid artery and its intracranial portion, the vertebral artery branches frequently as it ascends through the neck; it has many anastomoses with the thyrocervical trunk, the vertebral artery of the opposite side, and the occipital branch of the external carotid. These anastomoses may circumvent segmental occlusions, and so segmental occlusion is usually asymptomatic.

If pressures within the two vertebral arteries are equal, their bloodstreams remain somewhat segregated throughout the length of the basilar artery, the left vertebral supplying the left side of the cerebellum and brainstem and the right vertebral supplying the other. Pressure relations can be altered by anatomic variations, head turning, or pathologic situations, such as the subclavian steal syndrome, so that blood from one vertebral artery may fill the entire basilar artery and nourish all structures supplied by it.

Atheromatous plaques typically accumulate where the vertebral artery branches from the subclavian artery and along the course of the first part of the artery before it enters the foramen of the transverse process of the sixth cervical vertebra. Somewhat less commonly, the atheromatous process also affects the artery as it ascends through the vertebral canal; the regions between the transverse processes are particularly susceptible. It is surprising that atheromatous deposits are more common in the second straight portion of the artery than in the third portion, which bends around the transverse process of the atlas. The fourth portion, above the foramen magnum and below the junction of the two vertebral arteries, is usually involved only to a moderate degree, except at the ostium of the posterior inferior cerebellar artery.

The basilar artery, although it has no bends, is often affected by atherosclerotic plaques near its origin and termination and at branching points. Some physicians believe that the confluence of flow from the two vertebral arteries may set up injurious eddy currents that promote endothelial sheer stress and the development of atheromata.

The vertebral arteries are vulnerable to compression during extremes of extension of the skull on C1 or rotation at the atlanto-axial joint. Cervical spine injuries producing transient dislocation of one cervical vertebra to another ("whiplash" or hyperextension injuries) can traumatize the vertebral arteries within their canals. Hematoma or arterial dissection may occlude a vertebral artery. A similar mechanism may result from injudicious manipulation of the neck (as in chiropractic procedures), extreme extension of the neck during intubation of the trachea, or dental extraction and vigorous cervical traction.[120–124] Similarly, vertebral artery injuries are occasionally produced by gymnastics, wrestling, football, and swimming.[125–128] Arterial dissection from these activities is discussed in Chapter 12.

Atherosclerosis of the vertebral artery can be a nidus for thrombosis, which may occlude it or be cast off as an embolus to intracranial branches. Because the caliber of the vertebral artery is smaller than that of the basilar artery, any embolus that arises in the former will probably be propelled through it and lodge in the rostral end (top) of the basilar artery or in one of the basilar artery's branches.

Anomalies of the cranium and vertebral column may be associated with anomalies of the arterial tree. In both platybasia and occipitocervical synostosis, for example, there may be atresia of one vertebral artery or a failure of both vertebrals to join the basilar artery. In rare instances the vertebral artery arises from the common or the external carotid artery.

In an arthritic patient, a protruding osteophyte can impinge on a vertebral artery or narrow the space in which the vessel lies. Movement of one vertebra in relation to another, as in flexion and extension, lateral bending, or rotation of the head, may stretch or pinch an artery. Rotatory movements of the head and the neck occur, for the most part, at the C1 to C2 level. There the vertebral artery winds around the atlas and is subject to shearing force when the head is rotated. Under most circumstances, this is of no importance because increased flow through the other vertebral artery compensates for temporary reduction through its companion, but when one vessel is hypoplastic, stenosed, or occluded by atherosclerosis, such temporary occlusions are not as well tolerated. In addition, accompanying disease of the carotid arterial system or an anomaly of the posterior communicating artery of the circle of Willis increases the risk of infarction.

Similarly, rheumatoid arthritis can produce stenosis of the vertebral canal, and it can also result in rupture of the odontoid ligament with abnormal mobility of the atlantoaxial joint, causing bilateral compression of otherwise normal vertebral arteries. Also problematic are congenital anomalies of the cervical spine, such as craniocleidodysostosis and platybasia. In addition to their mechanical effects, these may coexist with anomalies of the vertebral arteries themselves. These osseous deformities, by limiting normal movement of the vertebral arteries within their canals, can lead to vascular insufficiency when the head is moved in relation to the neck. The same can occur with Paget disease of bone and basilar impression.

When the arm is extended, a cervical rib can compress or occlude the vertebral artery near its origin from the subclavian artery. Fibrous bands interconnecting such a cervical rib or even a normal rib to the vertebra may, under unusual circumstances, press on the artery and occlude it when the head, neck, and arm are in certain relationships to one another. Compression by muscle fascicles from the insertion of the longus colli and scalenus anticus at C6 can also produce temporary arterial obstruction during their contraction.

Table 3-2: Selected Brainstem Stroke Syndromes

Location	Eponym	Arterial Supply	Signs and Symptoms
Midbrain tegmentum, red nucleus, III, brachium conjunctivum corticospinal tract	Benedikt syndrome	Interpeduncular branches of basilar or posterior cerebral artery	Contralateral ataxia and weakness, ipsilateral CN III, variable movement disorder
Midbrain tegmentum, red nucleus, brachium conjunctivum, CN III	Claude syndrome	Posterior cerebral artery penetrating branches	Contralateral ataxia, ipsilateral CN III, tremor
Thalamus	Dejerine-Roussy syndrome	Penetrating thalamic branches of posterior cerebral artery	Contralateral sensory loss, contralateral pain
Lateral inferior pons	Raymond-Foville syndrome	Short circumferential branches of basilar artery or anterior inferior cerebellar artery	Ipsilateral facial weakness, ipsilateral lateral gaze palsy, contralateral weakness
Lateral pontine syndrome	Marie-Foix syndrome	Long circumferential branches of basilar, anterior inferior cerebellar artery	Contralateral weakness and sensory loss, ipsilateral ataxia
Unilateral ventral pons, fascicles of CN VI and VII	Millard-Gubler syndrome	Short circumferential and paramedian branches of basilar artery	Contralateral weakness sparing the face, ipsilateral lateral gaze paresis, ipsilateral face weakness
Midbrain tegmentum, superior cerebellar peduncles	Nothnagel syndrome	Basilar penetrating arteries, mesencephalic artery	Ipsilateral CN III palsy, contralateral ataxia
Lateral medullary	Wallenberg syndrome	Posterior inferior cerebellar artery (vertebral artery is primarily occluded)	Contralateral sensory loss, ipsilateral Horner, hoarseness, dysphagia, ipsilateral ataxia, facial sensory loss
Anterior cerebral peduncle	Weber syndrome	Midbrain penetrating branches of posterior cerebral artery	Ipsilateral CN III palsy, contralateral weakness

In some instances congenital anomalies or atherosclerosis may cause the vertebral artery to become unusually long, so that kinks or knuckles develop in it during movements of the arm or neck, obstructing flow through the artery. Loops tend to result from congenitally elongated arteries. Because the looped vessel is pliable and does not often impair flow, loops are generally less significant than a vessel kink.

Fibromuscular dysplasia is a noninflammatory arterial disorder characterized by hyperplasia of the vessel wall components with breakdown of normal elastic tissue. When found in vertebral arteries, the fibromuscular dysplasia is often bilateral. This disorder is presented in more detail in Chapter 13.

BASILAR ARTERY DYSFUNCTION

Blood carried through the vertebral-basilar system nourishes 10 of the 12 cranial nerves, all the ascending and descending tracts, the end organs for hearing and balance, and parts of the cerebral hemispheres. Hence, disease within this system can lead to many symptoms and signs, and numerous eponymic syndromes are named for lesions in different parts of the brainstem (Table 3-2).[129,130] The pattern in a given individual, however, usually clusters around one region of the brain. One person, for example, may have episodes of blindness with no vertigo, whereas another may have severe vertigo and loss of hearing without involvement of the occipital lobes. In the first case the symptoms are secondary to ischemia within the distribution of both posterior cerebral arteries and, in the second, to ischemia in the cochlea and semicircular canals or their neural connections in the brainstem. Despite the potentially devastating effects of an infarction within the posterior circulation, many patients do well.[131]

The typical TIA progresses swiftly from normal to maximum symptoms in less than 2 minutes. Common symptoms of vertebrobasilar TIAs include vertigo (with or without nausea and vomiting), diplopia, dysphagia, or dysarthria. If any occur alone, the attack may be due to a variety of etiologies, but, when they occur in combination with one another, the attack should then be considered a TIA.

The following clinical manifestations are suggestive of vertebrobasilar TIAs:

1. Vertigo with or without nausea and/or vomiting is the most common symptom. However, it is *not* usually indicative of a TIA when it occurs alone. When diplopia, dysphagia, or dysarthria occurs with the vertigo, the attack is most likely a TIA.
2. Motor deficit, such as weakness, clumsiness, or paralysis, in any combination of extremities up to tetraplegia. Motor deficits sometimes change from one side to another in different attacks.
3. Sensory deficits, such as numbness, including loss of sensation or paresthesias in any combination of extremities, including all four, or involving both sides of the face or mouth. This is frequently bilateral, but the distribution may change from side to side in different attacks.

4. Ataxia, imbalance, unsteadiness, or disequilibrium not associated with vertigo.
5. Loss of vision, complete or partial, in both homonymous fields (bilateral homonymous hemianopia).
6. Homonymous hemianopia.
7. Drop attacks.

It is estimated that about half of the individuals who eventually have an infarction in the distribution of the vertebral-basilar arterial system have one or many TIAs preceding it (see Chapter 6). These attacks, similar in etiology to those associated with the carotid artery syndrome, may be precipitated by one or more of the following factors: (a) changes in systemic blood pressure, (b) increased blood viscosity, (c) anemia, (d) erythrocytosis, (e) thrombocytosis, (f) hypoglycemia, (g) movements of the head on the neck, (h) trauma to the arteries, (i) cardiac disease including dysrhythmias, and (j) microembolism from a proximal atherothrombotic plaque.

Episodic vertigo and diplopia often accompanied by nystagmus, and, at times, nausea and vomiting are characteristic of vertebral-basilar territory ischemia. Such vertigo may wrongly be attributed to Ménière disease. The correct diagnosis can sometimes be made by differential caloric tests and by testing for positional nystagmus. Although vertigo is a common accompaniment of vertebral-basilar disease, vertigo alone is more characteristic of nonvascular disorders. If vertigo is the only symptom, vestibular neuronitis, benign paroxysmal postural vertigo (cupulolithiasis), and Ménière disease are more likely to be the explanation than impaired blood flow in the vertebral or basilar arteries.

Hemiparesis and hemiplegia with cranial nerve palsies are common, the clinical picture depending on the level of involvement of the brainstem. Cranial nerve involvement of the lower motor neuron type on one side, occurring simultaneously with hemiparesis on the other, is pathognomonic of brainstem abnormality (crossed neurologic signs).

Also strongly suggestive of vertebral-basilar territory ischemia is the "drop attack," in which the patient suddenly loses body tone and falls to the ground.[132] In this characteristic but uncommon syndrome, weakness usually subsides more slowly than it begins, and the patient evidently retains consciousness during the attack. The patient often attributes the fall to stumbling and looks for an obstruction in his path. Drop attacks are thought to be due to episodic ischemia of the lower brainstem or upper cervical cord with involvement of either the corticospinal tract or the reticular formation. Surprisingly enough, drop attacks have a relatively benign course and prognosis.[132]

A throbbing occipital headache, sometimes radiating down the neck along the course of the vertebral artery, may be the first symptom of impending posterior circulation ischemia. Although their genesis is uncertain, they are possibly related to hyperpulsation following sudden obstruction to flow within the vertebral artery. The increased pulsations may be within the vertebral artery itself, or within the anastomotic channels, particularly the occipital artery. Other possible causes are ischemia of the cervical muscles or dissection of a vertebral artery.

Examination of the Patient

Unless examined during a TIA or an evolving infarction, the patient's neurologic evaluation is typically normal. The neurovascular abnormalities that suggest vertebrobasilar disease are a

Table 3-3: Cerebellar Pressure Signs and Symptoms

Onset

- Infarction
- Dystaxia
- Dysmetria
- Dysarthria
- Awake but unable to walk or sit
- Vomiting

Intermediate stage

- Headache and perhaps nausea and vomiting
- Confusion
- Stupor
- VI nerve palsy, perhaps bilateral
- Horizontal gaze paresis
- Peripheral VII nerve palsy

Terminal state (herniation and brainstem compression)

- Coma
- Decorticate or decerebrate posturing
- Blood pressure, fluctuations, and lability
- Cardiac dysrhythmia
- Respiratory irregularities

bruit over the subclavian or mastoid region near the vertebral artery and unequal blood pressures in the two arms, which might occur with the subclavian steal syndrome. Even these clues are sometimes absent in patients with severe vertebrobasilar disease who have recurrent ischemic attacks. A murmur at the subclavian vertebral arterial junction is usually an incidental finding in asymptomatic persons.

In patients examined during a TIA or evolution of infarction, one of the following groups of abnormalities may be found: (a) homonymous hemianopia secondary to ischemia or infarction of the occipital lobes, (b) visual or auditory hallucinations related to a disturbance in the temporal lobe, (c) disturbances of consciousness with akinetic mutism, (d) hemi- or tetraparesis accompanied by cranial nerve deficit, dysmetria, dystaxia, dyssynergia, dysarthria, and/or dysphagia secondary to brainstem involvement, (e) positional nystagmus, (f) internuclear ophthalmoplegia, (g) various hemisensory deficits, (h) diplopia due to disturbances of brainstem pathways for conjugate gaze, and (i) Horner syndrome.

Cerebellar Infarction

Occlusion of any of the arteries supplying the cerebellum can lead to a cerebellar infarction, creating a lateralized deficit and, in some instances, clinically significant tissue swelling with brainstem compression or a herniation syndrome.[133] Such situations occur far less often after a cerebellar infarction than after a cerebellar hemorrhage (see Chapter 16), but the clinical progression (Table 3-3) and required management are similar.

Why some infarctions result in such massive swelling is not known, but the size of the stroke and the capacity for interstitial edema fluid to collect within the organ play a role. One suspects that bilateral lesions with boundary-zone infarction or anomalous vascular anatomy, as occurs when the posterior inferior cerebellar artery (PICA) and the anterior inferior cerebellar artery (AICA) arise from a single stem, are the most common progenitors. In other instances it is a component of brainstem infarction obscured in the constellation of signs of symptoms that occur during basilar artery thrombosis. Most commonly, cerebellar lesions are located in the distribution of the PICA or superior cerebellar artery (SCA). Less often, it occurs in the distribution of the AICA. Sometimes infarction may be bilateral without producing clinically significant edema.

The onset is characterized by homolateral signs if a hemisphere is involved or dystaxia if midline vermis is affected. Vertigo per se is not present in most cases. Signs of brainstem involvement occur if PICA, AICA, or basilar arteries are involved from its initiation. Development of such signs after some hours have elapsed should alert one to cerebellar edema with secondary brainstem compression.

Most cerebellar infarctions have a good prognosis, and recovery may be almost complete. However, occasional patients deteriorate rapidly because of intracranial hypertension resulting from obstructive hydrocephalus or herniation upward through the incisura of the tentorium cerebelli or downward through the foramen magnum (Table 3-3).[134,135] The prognosis for these individuals is poor. Hence deterioration of consciousness or the development of hydrocephalus or herniation on neuroimaging studies is an indication for emergency surgical intervention. Usually this consists initially of lateral ventricular drainage without decompression of the posterior fossa. However, lowering the supratentorial pressure may worsen any upward herniation, so that repeated imaging is very important. If deterioration continues, suboccipital craniectomy may be necessary. Thereafter, management is the same as that described for infarction in other locations (see Chapter 25). Corticosteroids have little effect on the edema caused by cerebellar infarction, but mannitol or hypertonic saline can be effective.

BASILAR ARTERY SYNDROMES

The basilar artery is formed at the junction of the medulla with the pons and runs along the ventral aspect of the pons (Figure 3-8). It ends where the pons joins the midbrain, forming the two posterior cerebral arteries. Although the posterior cerebral arteries are derived embryologically from the carotid system, blood flow through the posterior cerebral arteries comes from the vertebral-basilar system in about 90% of individuals. In some individuals both the anterior and the posterior circulations contribute to the blood supply of the posterior cerebral arteries.

Basilar Artery Occlusion

Fortunately, most infarctions within the basilar artery territory involve branch arteries or penetrating vessels rather than the entire basilar artery.[136] Complete occlusion of the basilar artery in an individual without adequate collateral blood flow leads to infarction of the pons, cerebellum, midbrain, and the two posterior cerebral arteries. The clinical correlate of this occurrence is

devastating and distinctive. The patient is comatose with preservation of some reflex responses, paralysis of the face and limbs, fixed eyes during head rotation, and ice-water caloric tests, unreactive or dilated pupils, decerebrate spasms, hyperthermia, and tachypnea.

Occlusion of the basilar artery occurs in its lower half three times as often as in the upper half, and embolism is the most common cause. Usually an atherosclerotic plaque narrows the lumen to less than 1 mm, and a superimposed thrombus completes the occlusion. Once occlusion has occurred, clotting takes place in the relatively stagnant, distal column. Large emboli entering the basilar artery after having traversed a vertebral artery may not stop until they reach the upper basilar near the posterior cerebral arteries, causing cortical blindness, coma, and bilateral CN III palsy. In most instances they are small enough to enter a normal PCA. Small emboli, however, may enter basilar branches (superior cerebellar artery, AICA, or PICA).

Parinaud Syndrome

Parinaud syndrome (which has several synonyms, including Sylvian aqueduct, peri-aqueductal, pretectal, or dorsal midbrain syndrome) includes supranuclear paresis of the conjugate vertical gaze (the patient cannot voluntarily look up but has intact Bell's phenomenon and oculocephalic reflexes) and paralysis of convergence. Other associated findings include large pupils with light-near dissociation, convergence retraction nystagmus on upward gaze, pathologic lid retraction (*Collier's sign*), lid lag, "pseudo-abducens palsy," and occasional paralysis of down gaze.

Locked-in Syndrome

Both sides of the lower pons simultaneously or separately can become the site of a lower basilar or branch infarct with the production of the "locked-in" syndrome, which consists of tetraplegia, loss of horizontal eye movements, and paralysis of face, mandible, and tongue.[137] Awareness is retained but may not be obvious because of the existence of total paralysis except for vertical eye movements.

Not all of the cases of locked-in syndrome are due to stroke, but the ones that are arise via occlusion of one or more penetrating basilar branches strategically supplying each side of the lower pons. Sometimes one basilar branch supplies both sides of the pons, and its occlusion alone can cause this disaster. The prognosis for locked-in syndrome due to stroke is generally poor,[138,139] but functional recovery is better for the individuals whose locked-in syndrome is nonvascular. A few individuals with stroke eventually show some improvement.[140]

Top of the Basilar Syndrome

Occlusion of the basilar artery occurs in its lower half more than in its upper half. Embolism is the most common cause of distal basilar artery occlusion, and basilar occlusion near its junction with the two posterior cerebral arteries generates a recognizable clinical pattern known as the *top of the basilar syndrome*.[141,142] The classic findings of top of the basilar syndrome include visual field deficits from occipital infarction and abnormal extraocular movements and pupillary dysfunction resulting from a midbrain infarction.[143,144] However,

Table 3-4: NIH Stroke Scale

1. Level of Consciousness (LOC)	[ ] 0 Alert	10. Right Arm Motor	[ ] 0 No drift
	[ ] 1 Drowsy		[ ] 1 Drift
	[ ] 2 Stuporous		[ ] 2 Some effort against gravity
	[ ] 3 Comatose		[ ] 3 No effort against gravity
			[ ] 4 No movement
2. LOC Questions	[ ] 0 Answers both correctly		[ ] X Untestable
	[ ] 1 Answers one correctly		
	[ ] 2 Both incorrect	11. Left Arm Motor	[ ] 0 No drift
			[ ] 1 Drift
3. LOC Commands	[ ] 0 Obeys both correctly		[ ] 2 Some effort against gravity
	[ ] 1 Obeys one correctly		[ ] 3 No effort against gravity
	[ ] 2 Both incorrect		[ ] 4 No movement
			[ ] X Untestable
4. Best Language	[ ] 0 No aphasia		
	[ ] 1 Mild–moderate aphasia	12. Right Leg Motor	[ ] 0 No drift
	[ ] 2 Severe aphasia		[ ] 1 Drift
	[ ] 3 Mute		[ ] 2 Some effort against gravity
			[ ] 3 No effort against gravity
5. Neglect	[ ] 0 No neglect		[ ] 4 No movement
	[ ] 1 Partial neglect		[ ] X Untestable
	[ ] 2 Complete neglect		
		13. Left Leg Motor	[ ] 0 No drift
6. Visual Fields	[ ] 0 No visual loss		[ ] 1 Drift
	[ ] 1 Partial hemianopsia		[ ] 2 Some effort against gravity
	[ ] 2 Complete hemianopsia		[ ] 3 No effort against gravity
	[ ] 3 Bilateral hemianopsia		[ ] 4 No movement
			[ ] X Untestable
7. Horizontal Gaze	[ ] 0 Normal		
	[ ] 1 Partial gaze palsy	14. Limb Ataxia	[ ] 0 Absent
	[ ] 2 Complete gaze palsy		[ ] 1 Present in 1 limb
			[ ] 2 Present in 2 or more limbs
8. Facial Strength	[ ] 0 Normal movement		[ ] X Untestable
	[ ] 1 Minor paresis		
	[ ] 2 Partial paresis	15. Sensory	[ ] 0 Normal
	[ ] 3 Complete palsy		[ ] 1 Partial loss
			[ ] 2 Dense loss
9. Dysarthria	[ ] 0 Normal articulation		
	[ ] 1 Mild–moderate		
	[ ] 2 Unintelligible or worse		
	[ ] X Untestable		

TOTAL NIHSS SCORE _____ (0–42)

Instructions for Scoring:
1. LOC: Score 0 for normal level of alertness. 1 if patient is drowsy, but can be easily aroused by minor stimulation. Score 2 if drowsy and requires repeated and strong stimulation, such as pain to elicit purposeful movements. Score 3 if no response or if only minimal reflex or autonomic responses are present.

(continued)

Table 3-4 *(continued)*

2. LOC Questions: Only score complete responses, score initial response only, do not prompt or give cues. Score 1 for patients who are unable to speak, such as intubated or severely dysarthric patients. Score 2 for aphasic or stuporous/comatose patients.
3. LOC Commands: Substitute with other one-step commands if necessary, such as when hand is paretic and cannot grip. Give credit for attempts to respond when limited by focal weakness. May use pantomime to communicate.
4. Language: Ask patients to name objects, read words and sentences, assess spontaneous speech. If patient has vision loss, place objects in his hand and ask the patient to identify them. Ask intubated to write. Score 1 if patient is able to communicate despite mild abnormalities in fluency, naming, repetition, or following commands. Score 2 for fragmented speech that requires much prompting and interpretation by the examiner. Score 3 for mute, global aphasic, or comatose patients.
5. Neglect: Score 0 for patients who pay attention to both sides of their body even if aphasic. Score 1 for patients with inattention to stimuli applied to one side of the body or for extinction to simultaneous stimulation of both sides. Test the following modalities: visual, spatial, tactile, auditory, neglect or presence of anosognosia. Score 2 for hemi-inattention to more than one modality, if patient does not recognize own hand or only orients to one side of space.
6. Visual Fields: Perform confrontational testing in all four quadrants and for each eye separately. Score 2 for quadrantanopsia, 3 for blindness, including cortical blindness.
7. Horizontal Gaze: Use voluntary or reflexive (oculocephalic response) responses. Score 1 for bilaterally abnormal gaze that improves with the oculophalic maneuver, or for abnormal gaze in only one eye. Score 2 for forced eye deviation or complete bilateral gaze paresis that does not improve with performing the oculophalic maneuver.
8. Facial Paresis: Score symmetry of grimace to painful supraorbital stimulation in patients who cannot follow commands. Score 1 for asymmetric face motions or a unilaterally flattened nasolabial fold. Score 2 for complete or near-complete paralysis of the lower face. Score 3 for paralysis involving the upper and lower face.
9. Dysarthria: Score 1 if the patient has slurred speech but can be understood. Score 2 if speech is unintelligible (in the absence of or out of proportion to any existing aphasia). Patients who are intubated or have other physical barrier to speak are untestable.
10./11. Arm Motor: Ask patient to elevate arms to 90 degrees palms up and to hold arms in this position for 10 seconds. Score 1 if the arm drifts before the end of the 10-second testing period, but does not hit the bed or other support. Score 2 if the patient lifts the arm, but cannot fully extend, or if the arm drifts all the way down.
12./13. Leg Motor: Ask patient to lift each leg separately to 30 degrees in the supine position and to hold for 5 seconds. Score 1 if the leg drifts before the end of the 5-second testing period, but does not hit the bed or other support. Score 2 if the patient lifts the leg, but cannot fully extend, or if the leg drifts all the way down.
14. Limb Ataxia: Test while patient has the eyes open. Ask the patient to perform the finger-nose-finger and knee-heel-shin maneuvers bilaterally. Score ataxia only if present out of proportion of any weakness. Do not score ataxia in patients who do not comprehend the command or whose limb is plegic. Score X if limb is amputated or joint is fused.
15. Sensory: Test sensation to pinprick or pain in stuporous patients. Only score sensory loss that is due to the acute stroke. Test arms and legs, trunk and face, not hands and feet. Score 2 if patient is not aware of being touched or does not respond to noxious stimulation (including comatose patients) or has acute bilateral sensory loss.

muscle weakness, incoordination, and alteration of consciousness are relatively common, particularly at the onset of symptoms.[142,145] Often thought to have a uniformly poor prognosis, some individuals with top of the basilar syndrome recover spontaneously, probably reflecting the duration and specific location of their underlying vascular lesion.[146]

VERTEBROBASILAR BRANCH ARTERIES

The branches of the vertebral-basilar system are customarily categorized as paramedian, short circumferential, and long circumferential arteries. This same classification was applied to the branches of the internal carotid artery, previously described. Although their size and the areas they supply vary widely from one individual to another, these arteries have reasonable anatomic predictability.[147] The anatomy and syndromes of the anterior inferior cerebellar artery and the superior cerebellar artery, both clinically important branches of the basilar artery, are discussed later in this chapter.

Posterior Inferior Cerebellar Artery

The posterior inferior cerebellar arteries originate from the vertebral arteries about 1 cm below their junction to form the basilar artery (Figure 3-8). They are the largest and most variable branches of the vertebral arteries. Each PICA travels down and around the lateral surface of the medulla to the level of the foramen magnum before looping back up to supply portions of the cerebellum.

These arteries supply a wedge-shaped area of the medulla, extending vertically from just above the level of the cuneate and gracile nuclei to the upper limit of the medulla. On the surface the area extends into an anteroposterior direction from just behind the inferior olivary nucleus to the inferior cerebellar peduncle. Centrally the apex of the wedge approaches the floor of the fourth ventricle. These arteries also supply part of the surface of the cerebellar hemispheres and, perhaps, part of the dentate nuclei.

Internal Auditory Artery

Particularly significant is the arterial supply of the inner ear, the semicircular canal, the saccule, the utricle, and the cochlea.[148,149] In more than 80% of persons coming to autopsy, the auditory artery stems from the anterior inferior cerebellar artery. In most of the remainder it originates directly from the basilar artery as the internal auditory artery. The auditory artery terminates in two branches, the cochlear and the vestibular. Each has a very tenuous anastomosis with the carotid circulation.

Just as the ophthalmic artery often affords a clue to disease of the carotid system, the internal auditory artery sometimes provides the first evidence of disease in the vertebral-basilar system. Because the auditory artery is, in effect, an end artery and because the semicircular canals are exquisitely sensitive, reduction of blood pressure and/or flow through this vessel may produce disturbances of equilibrium causing nausea, vomiting, and vertigo. Similar interruption of the cochlear supply causes sudden loss of hearing. If both occur together, the syndrome produced can mimic Ménière disease.

Anterior Inferior Cerebellar Artery

The anterior inferior cerebellar artery supplies the lateral portions of the tegmentum, the middle section of the brainstem, the inferior portion of the middle cerebellar peduncle, the inferior cerebellar peduncle, the flocculus, and the adjacent cerebellar hemisphere.[150–152] Isolated occlusion of the AICA is unusual, and in some instances it is secondarily occluded by atherosclerotic basilar artery occlusion.[153] The complete AICA syndrome results in cerebellar dysfunction, facial palsy, vertigo, deafness, and impairment of sensibility to light touch, pain, and temperature of the face on the side of this lesion; on the side opposite the lesion there is incomplete loss of pain and temperature sensibility over the torso and extremities.[154] However, most patients with an AICA occlusion do not develop this complete syndrome.[153]

Superior Cerebellar Artery

The superior cerebellar artery supplies the dorsolateral portion of the upper part of the brainstem, the superior cerebellar peduncle, the nuclei beneath the fourth ventricle, part of the dentate nucleus, part of the cortex of the superior part of the cerebellar hemisphere, and a variable part of the midbrain and pons. The three arteries that supply the cerebellum – the posterior and anterior inferior cerebellar arteries and the superior cerebellar artery – anastomose freely on the surface of the hemispheres.

Occlusion of the superior cerebellar artery causes signs of ipsilateral cerebellar dysfunction, abnormal movements of the upper and lower limbs on the same side, and contralateral loss of appreciation of pain and temperature over the entire body.[155–157] A cerebellar infarction caused by occlusion of the superior cerebellar artery tends to have more prominent gait disturbance and less prominent brainstem edema than did the individuals with a PICA occlusion.[158] It is not surprising, therefore, that the outcome after a superior cerebellar artery occlusion is a bit better than for individuals with a PICA occlusion.

Mesencephalic Artery

The length of artery between the bifurcation of the basilar artery into the posterior cerebral arteries and the junction of the posterior communicating arteries is considered to be a special artery. On embryologic and hemodynamic grounds, this arterial segment is distinct from the rest of the PCA and is called by some the mesencephalic artery. In the embryo two branches arising from the rostral end of the basilar artery constitute the mesencephalic artery. The PCA in the embryo arises from the carotid, and, during adult life, it retains this name even when it becomes the posterior communicating artery. The distal portion of the artery begins at the junction of the mesencephalic artery and ends at the occipital pole. The tip of the basilar artery and the mesencephalic artery give off perforating branches before forming the PCA. In the mesencephalic arterial syndrome, oculomotor disturbances, third nerve paralysis and, particularly, disturbance of vertical gaze can be observed. A loss of intellect resulting in dementia may be the result of rostral extension of the zone of infarction into the territory of the anterior branch of the mesencephalic artery.

Branch Artery Syndromes

An occluded artery is found in more than 75% of patients with infarcts in the vertebral-basilar system, and in the majority the occlusion is found intracranially in the distal portion of the vertebral or basilar artery or one of their branches. Moreover, infarction resulting from occlusion of the vertebral artery intracranially is three times more frequent than occlusion in the neck because of the extensive anatomic network in the cervical region. Such occlusions seldom extend beyond the C5–C6 level.

Distal occlusion often affects the origin of the posterior inferior cerebellar artery, resulting in infarction of the lateral medulla and/or inferior cerebellum. More than half of basilar thromboses result after occlusion of first one and then the other vertebral artery or occlusion of a single dominant vertebral artery. In addition, distal vertebral artery stenosis or thrombosis can be a source of embolism to the basilar and its branches.

Occlusion of both distal vertebral arteries where they join to form the basilar artery is usually associated with brainstem infarction due to posterior inferior cerebellar artery occlusions. From this location they may cause emboli to the posterior cerebral arteries with occipital lobe and central tegmental infarction.[159]

Posterior Inferior Cerebellar Artery

The blood supply to the lateral medulla consists of five or six branches spaced a few millimeters apart. Its lower one-third is supplied by branches from the vertebral artery, the middle third by the upper vertebral artery or PICA, and the upper third by the anterior inferior cerebellar artery and basilar arteries. Occlusion of the PICA leads to an infarction in the lateral medulla (Wallenberg syndrome). Infarction occurs more frequently in the distribution of the PICA (Figure 3-8) than in that of any other cerebellar artery. However, about three-fourths of the time, the lateral medullary syndrome results from an occluded intracranial vertebral artery.

Such lesions usually manifest by the sudden onset of vertigo, nystagmus, dysphagia, ataxia, nausea, and vomiting. Consciousness is not disturbed. There is a tendency to fall toward the involved side because of the cerebellar involvement, and spinothalamic function on the contralateral side of the body below the face is lost. Involvement of the descending root of the fifth cranial nerve causes homolateral loss of pain and temperature perception on the face.

Symptoms vary but include nausea, vomiting, loss of sensation in the ipsilateral side of the face, dysphagia, dysarthria, hoarseness, hiccoughs, dystaxia, diplopia, nystagmus, Horner syndrome, and/or oscillopsia. Headache in the occipital and ipsilateral mastoid region is often present initially, and headache may begin a week or two before the onset of neurological dysfunction.

There may be loss of pain and temperature sensation on the opposite side of the body, paralysis of the ipsilateral half of the soft palate, and, rarely, ipsilateral facial weakness, or facial pain. In the acute phase of lateral medullary infarction, respiratory, and cardiovascular complications presumably related to autonomic dysfunction are the most serious risk, accounting for 12% of mortality. The risk of recurrent stroke in the posterior circulation is about 2% per year. Most patients with a lateral medullary syndrome do well, but propagation of a vertebral artery thrombus into the basilar artery or preexisting occlusion of the contralateral vertebral artery can have devastating consequences.[160]

Medial Medullary Syndrome

Infarction of the medial medullary area, supplied by short penetrating branches of the anterior spinal artery, causes unilateral loss of hypoglossal nerve function with contralateral sensorimotor or pure motor hemiparesis.[161,162] Tingling sensation with decreased vibration and position sense is the most common sensory manifestation. Bilateral lesions may be occasionally present. The medial medullary syndrome is an uncommon stroke syndrome, with only a few dozen cases reported in the literature.[163] Occasionally lateral medullary involvement (see PICA syndrome) accompanies the medial involvement (Babinski-Nageotte syndrome). Bilateral ventral cervico-medullary infarction is seen very rarely. Dysarthria, tetraparesis, and respiratory arrests characterize its clinical picture.

Anterior Inferior Cerebellar Artery Syndrome

The AICA supplies the lateral pontomedullary structures, including the inferior part of the middle cerebellar peduncles, the inferior cerebellar peduncle, the anterior cerebellar hemisphere, vestibular and cochlear nuclei, including the exiting VII and VIII nerves, spinal trigeminal tract and nucleus, and medial lemniscus. In addition, the internal auditory artery supplying the inner ear usually arises from it.[149]

Occlusion of an AICA results in the lateral inferior pontine (Foville) syndrome. At the onset, vertigo may be severe. Unilateral deafness and vestibular disturbance are common, and some patients have additional facial numbness and weakness. The infarct lies in the infero-lateral pons, and the VIII nerve is involved, either within the brainstem or in its peripheral segment.

Vertical diplopia, dystaxia, dysarthria, and sensory loss of one side of the face occur ipsilateral to the lesion. On examination there is ipsilateral deafness, reduced or absent labyrinthine function, peripheral facial weakness, decreased sensation to pain and touch on the face, Horner syndrome, ipsilateral cerebellar signs, paresis of lateral gaze, nystagmus, and, occasionally, internuclear ophthalmoplegia. On the opposite side of the body, pain and temperature sensations are impaired, as are the corticospinal tract functions. Occlusion of an AICA is preceded by TIAs in about 50% of cases. Cerebellar infarction usually does not result from occlusion of the AICA because of abundant anastomoses with the superior and inferior cerebellar arteries. Because the AICA arises from the basilar artery at an angle of almost 90 degrees, emboli seldom lodge within it.

Pontine Paramedian Arteries

The pontine paramedian arteries (Figure 3-8) supply the antero-medial aspects of the pons. The abducens nerve, facial nerve, and corticospinal fibers course through their vascular domain. Occlusion of these arteries by emboli or atherosclerotic involvement of the basilar artery, from which these vessels take origin, can lead to peripheral nerve palsies. Lesions of the inferior ventral pons cause ipsilateral CN VI and CN VII paralysis and contralateral hemiparesis or hemiplegia.

The dorsal midpontine syndrome involves ipsilateral facial and gaze palsies, as well as contralateral hemiplegia of the body. Superior medial pontine syndrome consists of ipsilateral dystaxia, internuclear ophthalmoplegia (INO), and myoclonus (tremor) of the palate, pharynx, face, and/or eye, as well as contralateral hemiplegia.

Short Pontine Circumferential Arteries

Short circumferential branches from the basilar artery supply the antero-lateral aspects of the pons. Their involvement may result in ocular bobbing with abrupt, spontaneous, usually conjugate, downward jerks of both eyes, followed by a slow return to the midposition, suggestive of the movements of a fishing bob with a struggling fish hooked to the line.

Long Pontine Circumferential Arteries

The long pontine circumferential arteries arise not only from the basilar but also from the anterior inferior and the superior cerebellar arteries. The vascular supplies to the abducens nuclei, medial longitudinal fasciculi (MLF), and facial nuclei are derived from the basilar artery by way of the long circumferential arteries. A lesion in this region causes ipsilateral peripheral paralysis of CN VII and CN VI, paralysis of lateral gaze, and contralateral hypesthesia, ataxia, choreoathetoid movements, and tremor. Many cases are due to a neoplasm, but when vascular disease is the etiology, it is usually due to hemorrhage. The lateral tegmental syndrome includes anisocoria with the smaller pupil on the side of the lesion, INO, one-and-a-half syndrome (see below), paralysis of lateral gaze toward the side of the lesion, hemiparesis, hemihypesthesia, and cerebellar dysfunction.

The one-and-a-half syndrome consists of lateral conjugate gaze palsy with an ipsilateral INO.[164] The lesion involves the MLF and the parapontine reticular formation (PPRF) or the VI nerve nucleus and the adjacent interneurons. Involvement of the MLF causes INO, and involvement of either the PPRF or the VI nucleus and the surrounding interneurons causes lateral ipsilateral gaze palsy.

Arterial Supply to the Midbrain

The vascular supply to the midbrain consists of four groups of arteries, most of which derive their blood from the basilar artery. The paramedian, short circumferential, and long circumferential arteries supply most of the structures. The superior cerebellar arteries supply the caudal tegmentum in the region of the inferior colliculus and much of the lateral aspects of the midbrain. Because of the small diameter and significant variations of these vessels, the information presented under specific arteries is not necessarily proved by histologic pathology. The various findings presented, however, are consistent with disease within the distribution of the artery under which they are listed. Vascular disease of the midbrain is associated with nuclear palsies, nystagmus, INO, vertical gaze palsies, ptosis, hemiparesis, and tremors. Pupillary abnormalities are rare with midbrain lesions.

Midbrain Paramedian Arteries

Unnamed small arteries that take origin from the basilar, posterior cerebral, and posterior communicating arteries are collectively termed the paramedian arteries. The oculomotor nuclei, the red nuclei, and the MLF are supplied by paramedian branches originating from the basilar artery; the paramedian arteries that branch from the posterior cerebral and posterior communicating arteries supply the medial part of the crus cerebri, red nuclei, and substantia nigra. Pathologic correlations with clinical disease are very scant. These include a sudden onset of disturbance of the voluntary and reflex vertical gaze, hyperconvergence, convergence spasm, convergence nystagmus, failure of abduction not due to VI nerve dysfunction, elevation and retraction of the upper eyelids, and vertical nystagmus.

Oculomotor palsies due to nuclear damage occur commonly with infarction of the basilar and paramedian blood supplies. Because of the segmental arrangement of the subnuclei of the oculomotor nuclear complex, patients present occasionally with paresis of the inferior rectus and/or superior rectus with relative sparing of the median, inferior oblique, and levator palpebrae. Both the superior and inferior recti nuclei extend rostally like a peninsula beyond the bounds of the other subnuclei of the oculomotor nuclear complex. Infarction of this peninsula can cause isolated paresis of the superior and inferior recti, with sparing of other recti muscles. Complete nuclear oculomotor paralysis results in ptosis bilaterally and deviation of the eye outward and downward; the pupil is dilated and nonreactive because of the loss of parasympathetic input from the adjacent Edinger-Westphal nucleus. The Edinger-Westphal nucleus lies immediately rostral to the oculomotor complex and serves as the relay nucleus for parasympathetic pupillary constrictive fibers. If it is asymmetrically damaged, an eccentrically situated pupil may result, probably because of asymmetrical stimulation of pupillary constrictors.

A lesion within the inferomedial part of the cerebral peduncle may result in Benedikt syndrome, consisting of oculomotor palsy, contralateral hemiparesis, and contralateral involuntary movements and/or tremor. Paramedian midbrain lesion involving oculomotor fibers, red nucleus, and fibers exiting the superior cerebellar peduncle has been known to present with ipsilateral ophthalmoplegia, contralateral ataxia, and rubral tremor.

Midbrain Long Circumferential Arteries

The blood supply to the pretectal nuclear complex, which is responsible for pupillary reactivity and accommodation, is derived mainly from the long circumferential branches of the posterior cerebral arteries or from the quadrigeminal artery. Input to the superior colliculi comes from the contralateral visual field, and the output goes to both of the Edinger-Westphal nuclei after decussating through the posterior commissure. Unilateral injury to this structure has little effect but bilateral damage causes loss of accommodative and pupillary reactions.

POSTERIOR CEREBRAL ARTERY

Relevant Anatomy

In the majority of people, the two PCAs are the terminal branches of the basilar artery, but, in 5% to 30%, one of these arteries may originate from the internal carotid or be perfused mainly from the carotid via a posterior communicating artery. Each posterior communicating artery passes above the adjacent oculomotor nerve, then sweeps posteriorly and laterally around the midbrain, passing close to the free edge of the tentorium cerebelli. Soon after its origin from the basilar artery, the posterior communicating artery anastomoses with the

posterior communicating artery to complete the circle of Willis. Their branches eventually reach the medial aspect of the temporal and occipital lobes to terminate at the occipital pole (Figure 3-4).

Tiny circumferential branches supply the cerebral peduncle, the medial geniculate body, and the colliculi. Thalamogeniculate arteries supply the pulvinar and other structures of the posterior thalamus and the lateral geniculate body.[165] The posterior choroidal arteries arise near the origin of the posterior cerebral arteries and enter the transverse fissure to terminate in the choroid plexus of the third ventricle. They supply portions of the thalamus and the splenium, and anastomose with terminal branches of the anterior choroidal artery. The anterior and posterior temporal, the parieto-occipital, and the calcarine arteries supply the inferior surface of the temporal and occipital lobes of the brain. Their terminal branches anastomose with those of the anterior and middle cerebral arteries to form part of the leptomeningeal anastomotic circulation of the cerebral hemispheres.[166,167]

The calcarine artery, a branch of the internal occipital artery, supplies the primary visual cortex. The macular cortical region is at the extreme posterior pole and receives blood from both the calcarine and branches of the MCA, which explains the macular sparing with PCA occlusion.

In addition to its supply to the occipital lobes, several branches of the PCA supply the pineal gland, choroid plexus, thalamus, and parts of the basal ganglia, including the medial and lateral posterior choroidal arteries, the thalamo-perforating branches, and the thalamo-geniculate branches.[168] The inferior mesencephalic (paramedian) artery arises from the first few millimeters of the posterior cerebral stem. It travels to the inferior midbrain and supplies the trochlear nucleus, part of the third nerve nucleus, and the dentatothalamic projections.[169] The superior mesencephalic paramedian artery supplies a segment of the midbrain. The posterior thalamosubthalamic paramedian artery arises about 3 mm from the origin of the posterior cerebral and runs to the upper midbrain, subthalamus, and thalamus, supplying part of the III nerve, the vertical gaze centers, the subthalamic fibers serving the pupillary light reaction, the dentatothalamic radiation, and the posteromedial thalamic nuclei. The anterior thalamosubthalamic paramedian artery arises immediately distally and penetrates just posterior to the mammillary bodies, supplying the middle and anterior thalami. The mesencephalic arteries to the two sides may arise unilaterally from one posterior cerebral stem, sometimes by a common trunk that supplies bilateral symmetrical parts of the midline subthalamus and thalamus. A unilateral occlusion may produce a bilateral deficit, and in these cases an amnestic syndrome may occur suddenly.

Clinical Dysfunction of the PCA

The symptoms of PCA ischemia typically revolve around visual and sensory disturbances.[170] Infarction of both occipital lobes leads to cortical blindness, in which pupillary responses to light are preserved but vision is lost bilaterally.[171,172] The patient is sometimes unaware that he cannot see and denies being blind, sometimes confabulating imagined scenes and walking unconcernedly into objects.[173,174] Partial visual field defects are more common than complete cortical blindness, and several different patterns of visual disturbance have been described.[175] The visual defect resulting from the medial occipital lobe lesion is typically homonymous and congruous and involves only one sector of the visual field.

Occlusion of the PCA on the dominant side may cause infarction of the homolateral visual cortex and the splenium of the corpus callosum. In addition to contralateral homonymous hemianopia, splenial infarction causes disconnection of the right occipital lobe from the speech area, resulting in alexia without agraphia.

Visual hallucinations may assume many patterns, including flickering and colored lights or an after-image resulting from visual perseveration. Patients with paracentral scotomas may have hallucinations of flashing lights or colored lines that progress over time to form images of people moving about or to seeing half of a visitor's face melt like a Dali painting. Auditory hallucinations, in contrast, do not occur.

Individuals with PCA infarction may have disturbances of color perception (achromatopsia) or dyschromatopsia (in which colors seem too bright or the entire environment takes on a colored hue), especially after an infarction of the lower striate cortex. Patients with central achromatopsia usually complain that colors have lost their brightness or of difficulty distinguishing colors. Rarely, the individual can perceive colors but is unable to name or recognize them. The responsible lesion is in the white matter connections between the occipital lobe and the temporal-parietal cortex.

Various alterations of higher cortical function can follow a PCA occlusion, including the inability to recognize familiar faces (prosopagnosia) or acquired dyslexia. Infarction of the splenium of the corpus callosum may disconnect the right occipital lobe from the speech area, resulting in alexia without agraphia. Visual agnosia is common and usually associated with alexia. These patients may identify objects by touch, smell, or sound and may even draw and copy designs, but they cannot identify the item visually. Most of these individuals have bilateral association pathway lesions of the inferior longitudinal fasciculi of the cerebral hemispheres. Prosopagnosia is more commonly found with right-sided occipital lobe damage. Palinopsia is the persistence of a visual image after it has disappeared from the field of view. This visual perseveration and various other visual hallucinations have been reported with lesions of almost every part of the visual axis. Amnestic syndromes have also been documented.[176]

Despite the preponderance of visual and sensory symptoms in individuals with PCA occlusion, proximal PCA occlusion can mimic the findings of MCA occlusion, including hemiparesis and language dysfunction.[177,178] Other manifestations of PCA occlusion include aphasia, drowsiness, Parinaud syndrome, Balint syndrome (with characteristic apraxia of gaze, visual inattention and limb dystaxia, if performed under visual guidance), photophobia, cerebellar dystaxia, hemiballism, "rubral" tremor, thalamic pain, micropsia, anosognosia, confusion, and temporal lobe seizures.[107,179,180]

Pseudo-athetosis of the fingers, with frequent involuntary movements due to sensory loss, is a common accompaniment. Amnestic syndrome occurs due to damage to the hippocampal gyrus.

Any of the branch arteries of the PCA may be involved in infarctions. Most of the symptoms result from infarction in the distal superficial territory of the PCA or the posterior ventral nucleus of the thalamus (top of the basilar syndrome). The more proximal branches of the PCA supplying thalamus, subthalamus, peduncle, and upper mesencephalon may be involved in occlusion of the stem of the PCA. The penetrating branches

from the PCA stem may be blocked, causing stupor, paralysis of vertical gaze, cerebellar dystaxia, and hemiballism, if the nucleus of Luys is involved.

The superior cerebellar peduncle and the dentatothalamic radiation can be infarcted after it has crossed the midline in the lower midbrain. The contralateral limbs are dystaxic, and dysarthria may be severe.

In posterior paramedian lesions, there is stupor or coma due to involvement of the peri-aqueductal gray matter and posteromedial thalamus, impaired memory, paralysis of vertical gaze, small poorly reactive pupils, ptosis and blepharospasm, diplopia, partial III nerve paresis, cerebellar dystaxia, and dysarthria. This is caused by a V-shaped bilateral infarct extending anteriorly and superiorly from the ventral caudal part of the third ventricle to involve the medial rostral of the red nucleus, upper medial longitudinal fasciculus, medial dorsalis medialis, and medial third of the centrum medianum.

Many PCA territory infarctions are due to emboli, but a few result from atherosclerosis of the PCA. In general, emboli tend to cause a completed infarction within the PCA territory, whereas PCA atherosclerosis is more likely to result in TIAs.[170] Another cause of PCA distribution infarction is compression of the PCA against the tentorium during downward brain herniation.

Bilateral PCA Infarction

Bilateral PCA infarctions produce bilateral homonymous visual field loss that is manifest clinically as blindness with intact pupillary reactions to light. Many patients have confusion and an amnestic syndrome.[171] In some instances the patient is unconcerned or unaware of blindness and confabulates a description of his surroundings (Anton syndrome), so that the true state of affairs may not be recognized by casual observers. The denial includes concocted stories and excuses for not seeing, for example, "the light is too dim." These patients often have very small and varying amounts of retained vision, especially for pattern recognition.

Bilateral PCA occlusion or ischemia can arise from embolism to the top of the basilar artery or occlusion of one and then the other PCA. Infarction of one or both occipital lobes always suggests underlying vertebral-basilar artery disease.

THALAMIC SYNDROMES

The thalamogeniculate branches of the proximal PCA and the posterior choroidal arteries supply the lateral and posterior parts of the thalamus.[165] Pure sensory stroke is one manifestation of an infarction in the lateral part of the thalamus. The sensory hemisyndrome may be accompanied by hemiataxia or, sometimes, ataxic hemiparesis. However, thalamic lesions accounted for only 13 of the 100 patients with ataxic hemiparesis presented by Moulin and colleagues.[181] The other patients in this series had lesions in the internal capsule (39%), pons (19%), corona radiate (13%), lentiform nucleus (8%), frontal cortex (4%), and cerebellum (4%). Involuntary movements may be present when the projections from the striatum are interrupted. The thalamic pain (Dejerine-Roussy) syndrome consists of unilateral loss of sensation accompanied by intense pain, described as aching, burning, or "hot" (anesthesia dolorosa).[182,183]

Isolated occlusion of the posterior choroidal artery is uncommon. It leads to damage of the lateral geniculate body, the pulvinar, the posterior thalamus, and the hippocampus.[184]

Clinical manifestations of a posterior choroidal artery occlusion vary but include homonymous quadrantanopia, hemisensory loss, transcortical aphasia, and memory disturbance early in the course and pain and dystonia later.[184]

Occlusion of the thalamogeniculate branch of the PCA may result in the thalamic syndrome, in which pain and temperature perception is lost because of infarction in the portion of the thalamus that receives these impulses. Infarcts in the posterior thalamic nuclei may present with contralateral hemihypesthesia and a spectrum of contralateral motor phenomena, including ataxia, tremor, myoclonus, chorea, and akathisia (urge to move constantly and inner restlessness).

The paramedian territories of the thalamus are irrigated by the mesencephalic paramedian arteries (*vide supra*). The manifestations of paramedian territory infarcts include decreased consciousness, hemiparesis, hemiataxia, vertical gaze palsy, and neuropsychologic disturbance, such as dysphasia, memory loss, confusion, and hemi-neglect.[185,186] The arteries supplying the paramedian upper midbrain and the paramedian areas of the thalamus often arise together as a single pedicle from the proximal PCA; thus infarctions in these areas often occur in combination than in isolation. In addition, paramedian infarctions are often bilateral.

The anterolateral nuclei of the thalamus are supplied by the polar (or tuberothalamic) branches of the posterior communicating artery. With anterolateral infarctions, mild hemiparesis, abulia, aphasia (left-sided lesion), and hemi-neglect may be seen. Bilateral infarctions are rare. A significant amnestic state may be present when mamillothalamic tracts are involved.

ARTERIAL COMPRESSION SYNDROMES

Vascular compression of the trigeminal nerve by elongated and tortuous arteries at the nerve root entry zone suggest this to be a cause of some instances of trigeminal neuralgia.[187] Compression causing facial hemispasm, deafness, and glossopharyngeal neuralgia due to compression of the appropriate cranial nerve have all been reported.[188-190] In addition, a mega-dolico-basilar artery can impinge on the brainstem, causing cranial nerve compression or obstructive hydrocephalus by compression of the posterior third ventricle.[191-195] An aneurysm of the posterior communicating artery often presents with an oculomotor nerve compression syndrome.

DIFFERENTIAL DIAGNOSIS OF BRAINSTEM STROKE

The differential diagnosis of symptoms due to a vertebral-basilar TIA is more challenging than the differential diagnosis of symptoms caused by carotid artery disease. Because of the large number of structures supplied by the vertebral-basilar arterial system, disease of these arteries can mimic many nonvascular conditions. Particularly in younger individuals, acute demyelination due to multiple sclerosis can resemble stroke. Although brainstem tumors typically produce gradual clinical deterioration over several days or weeks, rapid deterioration due to hemorrhage within the tumor, obstruction of the cerebrospinal fluid flow, or herniation of brainstem tissue can cause acute deterioration that resembles that of a stroke. Vertigo can result from ischemia, but it occurs more often because of Ménière disease or labyrinthitis. Stupor or coma could result from stroke but could equally well be due to a metabolic disturbance or to

ingested drugs such as alcohol or barbiturates. Cardiac dysrhythmias can cause light-headedness, loss of consciousness, vertigo, and blurred vision – symptoms that also occur with intrinsic lesions of the posterior circulation.

Points in favor of a vascular etiology are older age, the presence of risk factors for cerebrovascular disease, recurrent episodic attacks that closely resemble one another (TIAs), a murmur along the course of the vertebral arteries, and inequality of brachial blood pressures. Even when these findings are all present, the underlying vascular disease may not be the cause of the patient's symptoms.

PERSISTENT PRIMITIVE ANASTOMOSES

There are numerous variations in the configuration of the circle of Willis. An atretic or absent anterior or posterior communicating artery may jeopardize the role of the circle of Willis as a potential collateral channel and increase the likelihood of brain infarction.[106,196-198] Additionally, the incidence of congenital saccular aneurysms is increased in individuals who have an unusual configuration of the circle of Willis.

During embryological development, several primitive arteries serve as anastomoses between different circulatory areas. Occasionally these arteries persist into adult life. The most common anomaly, a persistent trigeminal artery, is found in 0.2% of cerebral angiograms. In some instances only a remnant of the primitive trigeminal artery persist, causing an aneurysm or weakness in the vessel wall. Embryonic channels that can persist into adult life include the following:

1. The primitive trigeminal artery connecting internal carotid and basilar arterial systems. Trigeminal artery variants include cases with a direct anastomosis between the internal carotid artery and the cerebellar arteries.
2. The primitive otic artery connecting internal carotid and basilar arterial systems.
3. The primitive hypoglossal artery connecting internal carotid and basilar arterial systems.
4. The primitive proatlantal artery connecting internal and basilar arterial systems.
5. The primitive stapedial artery connecting internal carotid and middle meningeal arteries.
6. The primitive ophthalmic artery connecting the lacrimal branch of the ophthalmic artery with the middle meningeal artery.
7. The anastomotic channels between the two vertebral arteries.
8. The anastomotic channels between the ophthalmic and meningeal arteries.

STEAL SYNDROMES

Normally the arterial pressure is lower in the intracranial arteries than in the aortic arch or its branches. So long as this normal pressure gradient is maintained, arterial blood ascends through the carotid and vertebral arteries to supply the intracranial contents. However, an obstruction in a strategic location may alter the normal pressure gradient and cause blood flow to reverse course from the head toward the heart or arms (Figure 3-9). Symptomatic obstruction of the proximal subclavian artery with diversion of blood into the arm via the vertebral artery is known as the subclavian steal syndrome.[199-201]

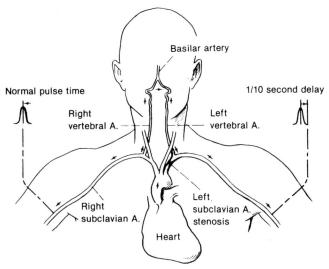

Figure 3-9. The hemodynamic pattern of subclavian steal syndrome also explains the left radial pulse delay that occurs with this syndrome. Stenosis of the proximal left subclavian artery results in lowered arterial pressure distally, allowing reversal of flow through the left vertebral artery into the distal subclavian artery, "stealing" blood from the brainstem.

Pathophysiology

Several other steal syndromes have now been described. Completely intracranial steal syndromes, for example, result from diversion of arterial blood into an arteriovenous malformation.[202–204] Obstruction in different locations produce different steal syndromes,[205,206] but in each case the volume and direction of abnormal flow depend on (a) the anatomy of the aortocranial arteries, which may be normal or anomalous, (b) the location of obstructions, and (c) the balance between demands of the limb and cerebral vascular beds for blood.

The anatomy and location of lesions remain the same, but the needs of the interconnected vascular beds are constantly changing. This causes the severity of flow reversal to fluctuate, explaining the intermittent nature of the patient's symptoms. For example, cutaneous vasodilatation and muscular exercise cause vasodilatation of limb vascular beds and augment the siphoning effect. Symptoms of vascular insufficiency in the brain or the upper extremity occur only if the needs of these tissues exceed the amount of blood available to them.

Etiology of Steal Syndromes

Atherosclerosis, usually involving the portion of the subclavian artery proximal to the origin of the left vertebral artery, is by far the most common form of obstructive lesion found in patients with reversed flow.[207] Congenital lesions include coarctation of the aorta and atresia of the proximal subclavian artery. Inflammatory angiopathy produced by such conditions as Takayasu disease (see Chapter 10) can also cause reversed flow.[208,209] The Blalock-Taussig operation (anastomosis of the proximal subclavian to the pulmonary artery) for the tetrology of Fallot also produces reversed flow, unless the left vertebral artery is also ligated.[210,211] In isolated instances subintimal dissection of the proximal subclavian artery (either spontaneous or after hyperextension or avulsing injuries to the left arm) has resulted in the subclavian steal.

Clinical Features

Catheter angiography and duplex ultrasound demonstrate an abnormal flow reversal in about 3% of patients studied for TIAs. In most of these individuals, however, no symptoms can be precipitated by limb exercise, nor does the steal adequately explain the patient's symptoms. Klemm and colleagues, for example, analyzed 324 patients with subclavian flow reversal and concluded that almost two-thirds of the patients were asymptomatic and that in others the symptoms were not explained by the mere presence of the steal.[212] Because it is often difficult to prove a cause and effect relationship between the occurrence of a steal and cerebrovascular insufficiency, it is probably wise to classify such instances as a *steal phenomenon* and to reserve the term *steal syndrome* for individuals whose symptoms can be reproduced by appropriate maneuvers. There are three main categories of steal symptoms:

1. Arm symptoms: Some patients complain of claudication, numbness, and tingling when the involved limb is exercised. Permanent weakness, wasting of the muscles, and vasomotor phenomena in the involved extremity are rare.
2. Symptoms of vertebral-basilar territory ischemia: Although syncope, dizziness, vertigo, unsteadiness, and occipital headache are the most frequent complaints, any of the other symptoms of vertebral-basilar insufficiency may occur.
3. Symptoms of carotid artery territory ischemia: These are rare but may occur in patients with stenosis of the brachiocephalic (innominate) artery or of both proximal subclavian arteries.

The most frequent signs and symptoms include the following:

1. Attacks of weakness (35%), or so-called drop attacks, involving all four extremities with or without loss of consciousness (18%), probably the result of ischemia of the upper spinal cord and lower brainstem.
2. Disequilibrium, tinnitus, vertigo, and nystagmus (52%), presumably resulting from vascular insufficiency of the inner ear.
3. Cerebellar dystaxia (25%).
4. Disturbances of ocular motility with diplopia (19%).
5. Hemianopia, graying of vision, or temporary blindness due to involvement of the posterior cerebral arteries with ischemia of the occipital lobes or lateral geniculate bodies (47%).
6. Occipital headaches precipitated by exercise (3%).
7. Transient global amnesia due to bitemporal ischemia (15%).
8. Limb claudication or finger gangrene (14%).

Diagnosis of Subclavian Steal Syndrome

The radial pulse on the affected side is diminished, and the arrival time of the pulse on the involved side is palpably delayed, a sign that is almost pathognomonic of subclavian steal. Systolic blood pressure readings in the two arms show a difference of at least 20 mm Hg, but diastolic pressures may remain equal. The disparity of blood pressure between the two may be accentuated, if measured with the patient standing erect and after exercise of the two arms. In equivocal instances, the pressure difference can be enhanced if both arms are exercised simultaneously; pressure in the involved

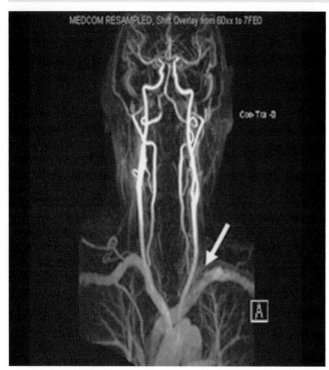

Figure 3-10. Magnetic resonance angiography from a 68-year-old man with disequilibrium and episodic binocular blurred vision. There is an abrupt loss of contrast opacification of the left subclavian artery (white arrow) 2 mm beyond its origin, most consistent with stenosis versus markedly reduced flow. Postcontrast MRA showed near-complete absence of flow-related enhancement in the left vertebral artery with complete opacification of this vessel, most consistent with subclavian steal.

arm is decreased, whereas that in the normal arm is maintained. Occasional patients have bilateral subclavian steal phenomenon.[213] Sudden deflation of the blood pressure cuff 3 minutes after inflation sometimes dramatically precipitates an attack of vascular insufficiency. Because neurological dysfunction is typically episodic, interictal examination reveals no abnormality of the central nervous system.

In some patients exercising the involved arm also induces claudication, causes the ipsilateral radial pulse to disappear, and accentuates the supraclavicular bruit, all signs of increased demand for blood by the exercising muscles. In an occasional patient this test precipitates vertigo, syncope, and headache, which suggests that some structures normally supplied by the vertebral-basilar system have been deprived of blood.

The easiest method for evaluating direction and velocity of flow through the great vessels of the upper thorax and the cervico-cranial regions is duplex ultrasound. Properly focused probes addressed to an artery, while compressing potential collaterals one at a time or adding physiological stress, such as limb exercise or change of head-neck or arm-shoulder relations, can detect changes in velocity, wave form, and direction in a most exquisite way. In some individuals, reversal of flow is intermittent and can be demonstrated only by having the patient exercise his arm during arteriography (Figure 3-9).

The diagnosis of the subclavian steal can sometimes be confirmed with magnetic resonance angiography (Figure 3-10). Catheter arteriography is justified when surgery or endovascular

therapy are contemplated. In such cases the abnormal flow patterns should be displayed, and the exact site and extent of the obstructive lesion must be demonstrated. To accomplish this, digital subtraction arteriography with serial exposures or cineradiography following injection of contrast material confirms the reversal of blood flow and pinpoints the location of the lesion.

Course and Prognosis

Symptoms do not occur in most individuals with reversed direction of flow. In some of the symptomatic cases, the development of collateral circulation eventually leads to a spontaneous remission.

Management of Subclavian Steal

Asymptomatic patients need no treatment. Patients with persistent arm claudication or symptoms of cerebral vascular insufficiency may benefit from intravascular angioplasty.[214] When the artery is completely occluded, bypass grafting of the subclavian artery to the carotid is best. The advantage of carotid-subclavian anastomosis is that it can be performed using the supraclavicular approach without performing a thoracotomy. In cases with reduced carotid flow, an axilloaxillary anastomosis can be considered. Surgical results are gratifying: postoperatively, the radial pulses and blood pressures are equal, and the patient is relieved of the symptoms of vertebral-basilar territory ischemia. Individuals with simultaneous visual symptoms and episodic paralysis may have coexistent carotid stenosis; these patients may benefit from carotid endarterectomy.[215]

ASSESSING SEVERITY

The NIH Stroke Scale (NIHSS) is a well-validated 15-item scale used to assess the severity of an acute stroke (Table 3-4).[216] The NIHSS yields a score between 0 (normal) and 42 (maximum score). The NIHSS score is a useful part of the decision tree when analyzing whether an individual might benefit from thrombolysis.[217] It provides an objective way to assess potential improvement or worsening of the patient's neurological status over time and allows comparison of neurological function before and after any type of intervention. However, it is not a diagnostic test and needs to be interpreted in conjunction with the history, results from diagnostic studies, and the clinical situation.

Table 3-4 outlines the application of the NIHSS. Below are general guidelines for the interpretation of the NIHSS score as it relates to the use of thrombolytic therapy:

NIHSS 1: Minor stroke or rapidly improving neurological symptoms. Consider not using tPA (except for isolated aphasia).
NIHSS 2–3: Mild stroke
NIHSS 4–10: Moderate stroke
NIHSS > 10: Severe stroke
NIHSS > 15: Typically indicates a large ischemic stroke
NIHSS > 25: May increase the possibility of hemorrhagic complications after the administration of intravenous thrombolytic therapy.

REFERENCES

1. Tatu L, Moulin T, Bogousslavsky J, Duvernoy H. Arterial territories of the human brain: cerebral hemispheres. *Neurology.* 1998;**50**:1699–1708.

2. Gillilan LA. Blood vessels, meninges, cerebrospinal fluid. In: Crosby EC, Humphrey T, Lauer EW, eds. *Correlative Anatomy of the Nervous System.* New York: Macmillan Company; 1962:550–579.

3. Tran-Dinh H. Cavernous branches of the internal carotid artery: anatomy and nomenclature. *Neurosurgery.* 1987;**20**:205–210.

4. Jimenez-Castellanos J, Carmona A, Catalina-Herrera CJ. Anatomical study of the branches emerging along the intracavernous course of the internal carotid artery in humans. *Acta Anat (Basel).* 1993;**148**:57–61.

5. Krisht AF, Barrow DL, Barnett DW, Bonner GD, Shengalaia G. The microsurgical anatomy of the superior hypophyseal artery. *Neurosurgery.* 1994;**35**:899–903.

6. Capo H, Kupersmith MJ, Berenstein A, Choi IS, Diamond GA. The clinical importance of the inferolateral trunk of the internal carotid artery. *Neurosurgery.* 1991;**28**:733–737.

7. Lasjaunias P, Moret J. The ascending pharyngeal artery: normal and pathological radioanatomy. *Neuroradiology.* 1976;**11**:77–82.

8. Lhermitte F, Gautier J-C, Poirier J, Tyrer JH. Hypoplasia of the internal carotid artery. *Neurology.* 1968;**18**:439–446.

9. Ide C, De CB, Mailleux P, Baudrez V, Ossemann M, Trigaux JP. Hypoplasia of the internal carotid artery: a noninvasive diagnosis. *Eur Radiol.* 2000;**10**:1865–1870.

10. Sachdev N, Laowattana S, Bonds LB, Thaver GH. Congenital carotid hypoplasia in ischemic stroke. *Neurology.* 2008;**70**:2086.

11. Cali RL, Berg R, Rama K. Bilateral internal carotid artery agenesis: a case study and review of the literature. *Surgery.* 1993;**113**:227–233.

12. Lie TA. *Congenital Anomalies of the Carotid Arteries.* Amsterdam: Excerpta Medica Foundation; 1968.

13. Bartels C, Horsch S. Classification of congenital arterial and venous vascular malformations. *Angiology.* 1995;**46**:191–200.

14. Borioni R, Garofalo M, Actis Dato GM, et al. Kinking of internal carotid artery: is it a risk factor for cerebro-vascular damage in patients undergoing cardiac surgery? *J Cardiovasc Surg (Torino).* 1994;**35**:325–326.

15. Teal JS, Rumbaugh CL, Segall HD, Bergeron RT. Anomalous branches of the internal cartoid artery. *Radiology.* 1973;**106**:567–573.

16. Koskas F, Bahnini A, Walden R, Kieffer E. Stenotic coiling and kinking of the internal carotid artery. *Ann Vasc Surg.* 1993;**7**:530–540.

17. Cartwright MS, Hickling WH, Roach ES. Ischemic stroke in an adolescent with arterial tortuosity syndrome. *Neurology.* 2006;**67**:360–361.

18. Callewaert BL, Willaert A, Kerstjens-Frederikse WS, et al. Arterial tortuosity syndrome: clinical and molecular findings in 12 newly identified families. *Hum Mutat.* 2008;**29**:150–158.

19. Coucke PJ, Willaert A, Wessels MW, et al. Mutations in the facilitative glucose transporter GLUT10 alter angiogenesis and cause arterial tortuosity syndrome. *Nat Genet.* 2006;**38**:452–457.

20. Belkin M, Mackey WC, Pessin MS, Caplan LR, O'Donnell TF. Common carotid artery occlusion with patent internal and external carotid arteries: diagnosis and surgical management. *J Vasc Surg.* 1993;**17**:1019–1027.

21. Chang YJ, Lin SK, Ryu SJ, Wai YY. Common carotid artery occlusion: evaluation with duplex sonography. *AJNR Am J Neuroradiol.* 1995;**16**:1099–1105.

22. Mansour MA, Mattos MA, Faught WE, et al. The natural history of moderate (50% to 79%) internal carotid artery stenosis in symptomatic, nonhemispheric, and asymptomatic patients. *J Vasc Surg.* 1995;**21**:346–356.

23. Faught WE, van Bemmelen PS, Mattos MA, et al. Presentation and natural history of internal carotid artery occlusion. *J Vasc Surg.* 1993;**18**:512–523.

24. Castaigne P, Lhermitte F, Gautier JC, Escourolle R, Derouesne C. Internal carotid artery occlusion. A study of 61 instances in 50 patients with post-mortem data. *Brain.* 1970;**93**:231–258.

25. Harrison MJ, Iansek R, Marshall J. Clinical identification of TIAs due to carotid stenosis. *Stroke.* 1986;**17**:391–392.

26. Roach ES, Golomb MR, Adams RJ, et al. Management of stroke in infants and children. A Scientific Statement for Healthcare Professionals from a Special Writing Group of the Stroke Council, American Heart Association. *Stroke.* 2008;**39**:2644–2691.

27. Cote R, Barnett HJ, Taylor DW. Internal carotid occlusion: a prospective study. *Stroke.* 1983;**14**:898–902.

28. Levine RL, Lagreze HL, Dobkin JA, Turski PA. Large subcortical hemispheric infarctions. Presentation and prognosis. *Arch Neurol.* 1988;**45**:1074–1077.

29. Mounier-Vehier F, Leys D, Pruvo JP. Stroke patterns in unilateral atherothrombotic occlusion of the internal carotid artery. *Stroke.* 1995;**26**:422–425.

30. Hayreh SS, Dass R. The ophthalmic artery: I. Origin and intracranial and intra-canalicular course. *Br J Ophthalmol.* 1962;**46**:65–98.

31. Gillilan LA. The collateral circulation of the human orbit. *Arch Ophthalmol.* 1961;**65**:684–694.

32. Macchi C, Catini C. The anatomy and clinical significance of the collateral circulation between the internal and external carotid arteries through the ophthalmic artery. *Ital J Anat Embryol.* 1993;**98**:23–29.

33. Gautier JC. Amaurosis fugax. *N Engl J Med.* 1993;**329**:426–428.

34. Parkin PJ, Kendall BE, Marshall J, McDonald WI. Amaurosis fugax: some aspects of management. *J Neurol Neurosurg Psychiatry.* 1982;**45**:1–6.

35. Winterkorn JMS, Kupersmith MJ, Wirtschafter JD, Forman S. Treatment of vasospastic amaurosis fugax with calcium-channel blockers. *N Engl J Med.* 1993;**329**:396–398.

36. Perez-Burkhardt JL, Gonzalez-Fajardo JA, Rodriguez E, Mateo AM. Amaurosis fugax as a symptom of carotid artery stenosis. Its relationship with ulcerated plaque. *J Cardiovasc Surg (Torino).* 1994;**35**:15–18.

37. Chawluk JB, Kushner MJ, Bank WJ, et al. Atherosclerotic carotid artery disease in patients with retinal ischemic syndromes. *Neurology.* 1988;**38**:858–863.

38. Poole CJ, Ross Russell RW. Mortality and stroke after amaurosis fugax. *J Neurol Neurosurg Psychiatry.* 1985;**48**:902–905.

39. Furlan AJ, Whisnant JP, Kearns TP. Unilateral visual loss in bright light. An unusual symptom of carotid artery occlusive disease. *Arch Neurol.* 1979;**36**:675–676.

40. Teal JS, Rumbaugh CL, Bergeron RT, Segall HD. Anomalies of the middle cerebral artery: accessory artery, duplication, and early bifurcation. *Am J Roentgenol Radium Ther Nucl Med.* 1973;**118**:567–575.

41. Gibo H, Carver CC, Rhoton AL Jr, Lenkey C, Mitchell RJ. Microsurgical anatomy of the middle cerebral artery. *J Neurosurg.* 1981;**54**:151–169.

42. van der Zwan A, Hillen B, Tulleken CA, Dujovny M, Dragovic L. Variability of the territories of the major cerebral arteries. *J Neurosurg.* 1992;**77**:927–940.

43. van der Zwan A, Hillen B. Review of the variability of the territories of the major cerebral arteries. *Stroke.* 1991;**22**:1078–1084.

44. van der Zwan A, Hillen B, Tulleken CA, Dujovny M, Dragovic L. Variability of the territories of the major cerebral arteries. *J Neurosurg.* 1992;**77**:927–940.

45. van der Zwan A. Hypertension encephalopathy after liquorice ingestion. *Clin Neurol Neurosurg.* 1993;**95**:35–37.

46. Marinkovic SV, Milisavljevic MM, Kovacevic MS, Stevic ZD. Perforating branches of the middle cerebral artery. Microanatomy and clinical significance of their intracerebral segments. *Stroke.* 1985;**16**:1022–1029.

47. Gillilan LA. Potential collateral circulation to the human cerebral cortex. *Neurology.* 1974;**24**:941–948.

48. Adams HP Jr, Damasio HC, Putman SF, Damasio AR. Middle cerebral artery occlusion as a cause of isolated subcortical infarction. *Stroke.* 1983;**14**:948–952.

49. Masuda J, Ogata J, Yutani C, Miyashita T, Yamaguchi T. Artery-to-artery embolism from a thrombus formed in stenotic middle cerebral artery. Report of an autopsy case. *Stroke.* 1987;**18**:680–684.

50. Mori E, Yamadori A. Acute confusional state and acute agitated delirium. Occurrence after infarction in the right middle cerebral artery territory. *Arch Neurol.* 1987;**44**:1139–1143.

51. Benton AL. Gerstmann's syndrome. *Arch Neurol.* 1992;**49**:445–447.

52. Quinette P, Guillery-Girard B, Dayan J, et al. What does transient global amnesia really mean? Review of the literature and thorough study of 142 cases. *Brain.* 2006;**129**:1640–1658.

53. Owen D, Paranandi B, Sivakumar R, Seevaratnam M. Classical diseases revisited: transient global amnesia. *Postgrad Med J.* 2007;**83**:236–239.

54. Miller JW, Petersen RC, Metter EJ, Millikan CH, Yanagihara T. Transient global amnesia: clinical characteristics and prognosis. *Neurology.* 1987;**37**:733–737.

55. Bettermann K. Transient global amnesia: the continuing quest for a source. *Arch Neurol.* 2006;**63**:1336–1338.

56. Menendez GM, Rivera MM. Transient global amnesia: increasing evidence of a venous etiology. *Arch Neurol.* 2006;**63**:1334–1336.

57. Grewal RP. Severe amnesia following a unilateral temporal lobe stroke. *J Clin Neurosci.* 2003;**10**:102–104.

58. Yoon B, Yoo JY, Shim YS, Lee KS, Kim JS. Transient global amnesia associated with acute intracerebral hemorrhage at the cingulate gyrus. *Eur Neurol.* 2006;**56**:54–56.

59. Bogousslavsky J, Regli F. Transient global amnesia and stroke. *Eur Neurol.* 1988;**28**:106–110.

60. Zorzon M, Antonutti L, Mase G, Biasutti E, Vitrani B, Cazzato G. Transient global amnesia and transient ischemic attack. Natural history, vascular risk factors, and associated conditions. *Stroke.* 1995;**26**:1536–1542.

61. Pantoni L, Bertini E, Lamassa M, Pracucci G, Inzitari D. Clinical features, risk factors, and prognosis in transient global amnesia: a follow-up study. *Eur J Neurol.* 2005;**12**:350–356.

62. Agosti C, Akkawi NM, Borroni B, Padovani A. Recurrency in transient global amnesia: a retrospective study. *Eur J Neurol.* 2006;**13**:986–989.

63. Olesen J, Jorgensen MB. Leao's spreading depression in the hippocampus explains transient global amnesia. A hypothesis. *Acta Neurol Scand.* 1986;**73**:219–220.

64. Teive HAG, Kowacs PA, Maranhao FP, Piovesan EJ, Werneck LC. Leao's cortical spreading depression: from experimental "artifact" to physiological principle. *Neurology.* 2005;**65**:1455–1459.

65. Tosi L, Righetti CA. Transient global amnesia and migraine in young people. *Clin Neurol Neurosurg.* 1997;**99**:63–65.

66. Caplan L, Chedru F, Lhermitte F, Mayman C. Transient global amnesia and migraine. *Neurology.* 1981;**31**:1167–1170.

67. Melo TP, Ferro JM, Ferro H. Transient global amnesia. A case control study. *Brain.* 1992;**115**(Pt 1):261–270.

68. Kushner MJ, Hauser WA. Transient global amnesia: a case-control study. *Ann Neurol.* 1985;**18**:684–691.

69. Vohanka S, Zouhar A. Transient global amnesia after mild head injury in childhood. *Act Nerv Super (Praha).* 1988;**30**:68–74.

70. Haas DC, Ross GS. Transient global amnesia triggered by mild head trauma. *Brain.* 1986;**109**(Pt 2):251–257.

71. Lisak RP, Zimmerman RA. Transient global amnesia due to a dominant hemisphere tumor. *Arch Neurol.* 1977;**34**:317–318.

72. Benke T, Chemelli A, Lottersberger C, Waldenberger P, Karner E, Trinka E. Transient global amnesia triggered by the intracarotid amobarbital procedure. *Epilepsy Behav.* 2005;**6**:274–278.

73. McCorry DJ, Crowley P. Transient global amnesia secondary to herpes simplex viral encephalitis. *QJM.* 2005;**98**:154–155.

74. Shukla PC, Moore UB. Marijuana-induced transient global amnesia. *South Med J.* 2004;**97**:782–784.

75. Akkawi NM, Agosti C, Borroni B, Padovani A. Detection of intracranial venous reflux in patients of transient global amnesia. *Neurology.* 2007;**68**:163.

76. Chung CP, Hsu HY, Chao AC, Chang FC, Sheng WY, Hu HH. Detection of intracranial venous reflux in patients of transient global amnesia. *Neurology.* 2006;**66**:1873–1877.

77. Di FM, Calabresi P. Ischemic bilateral hippocampal dysfunction during transient global amnesia. *Neurology.* 2007;**69**:493.

78. Matsui M, Imamura T, Sakamoto S, Ishii K, Kazui H, Mori E. Transient global amnesia: increased signal intensity in the right hippocampus on diffusion-weighted magnetic resonance imaging. *Neuroradiology.* 2002;**44**:235–238.

79. Sedlaczek O, Hirsch JG, Grips E, et al. Detection of delayed focal MR changes in the lateral hippocampus in transient global amnesia. *Neurology.* 2004;**62**:2165–2170.

80. Felix MM, Castro LH, Maia AC Jr, da Rocha AJ. Evidence of acute ischemic tissue change in transient global amnesia in magnetic resonance imaging: case report and literature review. *J Neuroimaging.* 2005;**15**:203–205.

81. Guillery B, Desgranges B, de la Sayette V, Landeau B, Eustache F, Baron JC. Transient global amnesia: concomitant episodic memory and positron emission tomography assessment in two additional patients. *Neurosci Lett.* 2002;**325**:62–66.

82. Lampl Y, Sadeh M, Lorberboym M. Transient global amnesia – not always a benign process. *Acta Neurol Scand.* 2004;**110**:75–79.

83. Kilian E, Oberhoffer M, Gulbins H, Uhlig A, Kreuzer E, Reichart B. Ten years' experience in aortic valve replacement with homografts in 389 cases. *J Heart Valve Dis.* 2004;**13**:554–559.

84. Ahmed DS, Ahmed RH. The recurrent branch of the anterior cerebral artery. *Anat Rec.* 1967;**157**:699–700.

85. Baptista AG. Studies on the arteries of the brain II. The anterior cerebral artery: some anatomic features and their clinical implications. *Neurology.* 1963;**13**:825–835.

86. Dunker RO, Harris AB. Surgical anatomy of the proximal anterior cerebral artery. *J Neurosurg.* 1976;**44**:359–367.

87. Aydin IH, Onder A, Takci E, Kadioglu HH, Kayaoglu CR, Tuzun Y. Heubner's artery variations in anterior communicating artery aneurysms. *Acta Neurochir (Wien).* 1994;**127**:17–20.

88. Crowell RM, Morawetz RB. The anterior communicating artery has significant branches. *Stroke.* 1977;**8**:272–273.

89. Perlmutter D, Rhoton AL Jr. Microsurgical anatomy of anterior cerebral anterior communicating recurrent artery complex. *Surg Forum.* 1976;**27**:464–465.

90. Perlmutter D, Rhoton AL Jr. Microsurgical anatomy of the distal anterior cerebral artery. *J Neurosurg.* 1978;**49**:204–228.

91. Marino R. The anterior cerebral artery: I. Anatomo-radiological study of its cortical territories. *Surg Neurol.* 1976;**5**:81–87.

92. Gacs G, Fox AJ, Barnett HJ, Vinuela F. Occurrence and mechanisms of occlusion of the anterior cerebral artery. *Stroke.* 1983;**14**:952–959.

93. Schneider R, Gautier JC. Leg weakness due to stroke. Site of lesions, weakness patterns and causes. *Brain*. 1994;**117**(Pt 2):347–354.

94. Alexander MP, Schmitt MA. The aphasia syndrome of stroke in the left anterior cerebral artery territory. *Arch Neurol*. 1980;**37**:97–100.

95. Takahashi S, Suga T, Kawata Y, Sakamoto K. Anterior choroidal artery: angiographic analysis of variations and anomalies. *AJNR Am J Neuroradiol*. 1990;**11**:719–729.

96. Rhoton AL Jr, Fujii K, Fradd B. Microsurgical anatomy of the anterior choroidal artery. *Surg Neurol*. 1979;**12**:171–187.

97. Fujii K, Lenkey C, Rhoton AL Jr. Microsurgical anatomy of the choroidal arteries: lateral and third ventricles. *J Neurosurg*. 1980;**52**:165–188.

98. Takahashi S, Fukasawa H, Ishii K, Sakamoto K. The anterior choroidal artery syndrome. I. Microangiography of the anterior choroidal artery. *Neurorad*. 1994;**36**:337–339.

99. Hupperts RM, Lodder J, Heuts-Van Raak EP, Kessels F. Infarcts in the anterior choroidal artery territory. Anatomical distribution, clinical syndromes, presumed pathogenesis and early outcome. *Brain*. 1994;**117**(Pt 4):825–834.

100. Helgason CM. A new view of anterior choroidal artery territory infarction. *J Neurol*. 1988;**235**:387–391.

101. Decroix JP, Graveleau P, Masson M, Cambier J. Infarction in the territory of the anterior choroidal artery. A clinical and computerized tomographic study of 16 cases. *Brain*. 1986;**109**(Pt 6):1071–1085.

102. Takahashi S, Ishii K, Matsumoto K, et al. The anterior choroidal artery syndrome. II. CT and/or MR in angiographically verified cases. *Neurorad*. 1994;**36**:340–345.

103. Leys D, Mounier-Vehier F, Lavenu I, Rondepierre P, Pruvo JP. Anterior choroidal artery territory infarcts. Study of presumed mechanisms. *Stroke*. 1994;**25**:837–842.

104. Palomeras E, Fossas P, Cano AT, Sanz P, Floriach M. Anterior choroidal artery infarction: a clinical, etiologic and prognostic study. *Acta Neurol Scand*. 2008;**118**:42–47.

105. Helgason C, Wilbur A, Weiss A, Redmond KJ, Kingsbury NA. Acute pseudobulbar mutism due to discrete bilateral capsular infarction in the territory of the anterior choroidal artery. *Brain*. 1988;**111**(Pt 3):507–524.

106. Fisher CM. The circle of Willis: anatomical variations. *Vasc Dis*. 1965;**2**:99–105.

107. Crozier S, Lehericy S, Verstichel P, Masson C, Masson M. Transient hemiballism/hemichorea due to an ipsilateral subthalamic nucleus infarction. *Neurology*. 1996;**46**:267–268.

108. Jacobson DM, Trobe JD. The emerging role of magnetic resonance angiography in the management of patients with third cranial nerve palsy. *Am J Ophthalmol*. 1999;**128**:94–96.

109. Kupersmith MJ, Heller G, Cox TA. Magnetic resonance angiography and clinical evaluation of third nerve palsies and posterior communicating artery aneurysms. *J Neurosurg*. 2006;**105**:228–234.

110. Nistri M, Perrini P, DiLorenzo N, Cellerini M, Villari N, Mascalchi M. Third-nerve palsy heralding dissecting aneurysm of posterior cerebral artery: digital subtraction angiography and magnetic resonance appearance. *J Neurol Neurosurg Psychiatry*. 2007;**78**:197–198.

111. Mansour N, Choudhari KA. Outcome of oculomotor nerve palsy from posterior communicating artery aneurysms: comparison of clipping and coiling. *Neurosurgery*. 2007;**60**:E582.

112. Szaflarski JP, Rackley AY, Kleindorfer DO, et al. Incidence of seizures in the acute phase of stroke: a population-based study. *Epilepsia*. 2008;**49**:974–981.

113. Teasell RW, McRae MP, Wiebe S. Poststroke seizures in stroke rehabilitation patients. *J Stroke Cerebrovasc Dis*. 1999;**8**:84–87.

114. Matula C, Trattnig S, Tschabitscher M, Day JD, Koos WT. The course of the prevertebral segment of the vertebral artery: anatomy and clinical significance. *Surg Neurol*. 1997;**48**:125–131.

115. Gillilan LA. Anatomy and embryology of the arterial system of the brainstem and cerebellum. In: Vinkin PJ, Bruyn GW, eds. *Handbook of Clinical Neurology*. Amsterdam: North-Holland Publishing Company; 1972:24–44.

116. Akar ZC, Dujovny M, Gomez-Tortosa E, Slavin KV, Ausman JI. Microvascular anatomy of the anterior surface of the medulla oblongata and olive. *J Neurosurg*. 1995;**82**:97–105.

117. Akar ZC, Dujovny M, Slavin KV, Gomez-Tortosa E, Ausman JI. Microsurgical anatomy of the intracranial part of the vertebral artery. *Neurol Res*. 1994;**16**:171–180.

118. Caruso G, Vincentelli F, Giudicelli G, Grisoli F, Xu T, Gouaze A. Perforating branches of the basilar bifurcation. *J Neurosurg*. 1990;**73**:259–265.

119. Takasato Y, Hayashi H, Kobayashi T, Hashimoto Y. Duplicated origin of right vertebral artery with rudimentary and accessory left vertebral arteries. *Neurorad*. 1992;**34**:287–289.

120. Di Duro JO. Stroke in a chiropractic patient population. *Cerebrovasc Dis*. 2003;**15**:156.

121. Dziewas R, Konrad C, Drager B, et al. Cervical artery dissection – clinical features, risk factors, therapy and outcome in 126 patients. *J Neurol*. 2003;**250**:1179–1184.

122. Easton JD, Sherman DG. Cervical manipulation and stroke. *Stroke*. 1977;**8**:594–597.

123. Frisoni GB, Anzola GP. Vertebrobasilar ischemia after neck motion. *Stroke*. 1991;**22**:1452–1460.

124. Rothwell DM, Bondy SJ, Williams JI. Chiropractic manipulation and stroke: a population-based case-control study. *Stroke*. 2001;**32**:1054–1060.

125. Rogers L, Sweeney PJ. Stroke: a neurologic complication of wrestling. A case of brainstem stroke in a 17-year-old athlete. *Am J Sports Med*. 1979;**7**:352–354.

126. Gosch HH, Gooding E, Schneider RC. Cervical spinal cord hemorrhages in experimental head injuries. *J Neurosurg*. 1970;**33**:640–645.

127. Schneider RC, Gosch HH, Norrell H, Jerva M, Combs LW, Smith RA. Vascular insufficiency and differential distortion of brain and cord caused by cervicomedullary football injuries. *J Neurosurg*. 1970;**33**:363–375.

128. Tramo MJ, Hainline B, Petito F, Lee B, Caronna J. Vertebral artery injury and cerebellar stroke while swimming: case report. *Stroke*. 1985;**16**:1039–1042.

129. Wolf JK. *The Classical Brain Stem Syndromes*. Springfield, IL: Charles C. Thomas; 1971.

130. Caplan LR, Wityk RJ, Glass TA, et al. New England Medical Center Posterior Circulation registry. *Ann Neurol*. 2004;**56**:389–398.

131. Glass TA, Hennessey PM, Pazdera L, et al. Outcome at 30 days in the New England Medical Center Posterior Circulation Registry. *Arch Neurol*. 2002;**59**:369–376.

132. Meissner I, Wiebers DO, Swanson JW, O'Fallon WM. The natural history of drop attacks. *Neurology*. 1986;**36**:1029–1034.

133. Chaves CJ, Caplan LR, Chung CS, et al. Cerebellar infarcts in the New England Medical Center Posterior Circulation Stroke Registry. *Neurology*. 1994;**44**:1385–1390.

134. Hornig CR, Rust DS, Busse O, Jauss M, Laun A. Space-occupying cerebellar infarction. Clinical course and prognosis. *Stroke*. 1994;**25**:372–374.

135. Laun A, Busse O, Calatayud V, Klug N. Cerebellar infarcts in the area of the supply of the PICA and their surgical treatment. *Acta Neurochir (Wien)*. 1984;**71**:295–306.

136. Liu GT, Crenner CW, Logigian EL, Charness ME, Samuels MA. Midbrain syndromes of Benedikt, Claude, and Nothnagel: setting the record straight. *Neurology*. 1992;**42**:1820–1822.

137. Chia LG. Locked-in syndrome with bilateral ventral midbrain infarcts. *Neurology.* 1991;**41**:445–446.

138. Katz RT, Haig AJ, Clark BB, DiPaola RJ. Long-term survival, prognosis, and life-care planning for 29 patients with chronic locked-in syndrome. *Arch Phys Med Rehabil.* 1992;**73**:403–408.

139. Haig AJ, Katz RT, Sahgal V. Mortality and complications of the locked-in syndrome. *Arch Phys Med Rehabil.* 1987;**68**:24–27.

140. Patterson JR, Grabois M. Locked-in syndrome: a review of 139 cases. *Stroke.* 1986;**17**:758–764.

141. Caplan LR. "Top of the basilar" syndrome. *Neurology.* 1980;**30**:72–79.

142. Mehler MF. The rostral basilar artery syndrome: diagnosis, etiology, prognosis. *Neurology.* 1989;**39**:9–16.

143. Baram TZ, Fishman MA. "Top of the basilar" artery stroke in an adolescent with Down's syndrome. *Arch Neurol.* 1985;**42**:296.

144. Mehler MF. The neuro-ophthalmologic spectrum of the rostral basilar artery syndrome. *Arch Neurol.* 1988;**45**:966–971.

145. Uson-Martin M, Gracia-Naya M. [Top of the basilar artery syndrome: clinico-radiological aspects of 25 patients]. *Rev Neurol.* 1999;**28**:698–701.

146. Mehler MF. Reversible rostral basilar artery syndrome. *Arch Intern Med.* 1988;**148**:166–169.

147. Torche M, Mahmood A, Araujo R, Dujovny M, Dragovic L, Ausman JI. Microsurgical anatomy of the lower basilar artery. *Neurol Res.* 1992;**14**:259–262.

148. Mazzoni A, Hansen CC. Surgical anatomy of the arteries of the internal auditory canal. *Arch Otolaryngol.* 1970;**91**:128–135.

149. Matsunaga T, Igarashi M, Kanzaki J. The course of the internal auditory artery and its branches. Computer-aided three-dimensional reconstructions. *Acta Otolaryngol Suppl.* 1991;**487**:54–60.

150. Naidich TP, Kricheff II, George AE, Lin JP. The normal anterior inferior cerebellar artery. Anatomic-radiographic correlation with emphasis on the lateral projection. *Radiology.* 1976;**119**:355–373.

151. Woischneck D, Hussein S. The anterior inferior cerebellar artery (AICA): clinical and radiological significance. *Neurosurg Rev.* 1991;**14**:293–295.

152. Martin RG, Grant JL, Peace D, Theiss C, Rhoton AL Jr. Microsurgical relationships of the anterior inferior cerebellar artery and the facial-vestibulocochlear nerve complex. *Neurosurgery.* 1980;**6**:483–507.

153. Amarenco P, Rosengart A, DeWitt LD, Pessin MS, Caplan LR. Anterior inferior cerebellar artery territory infarcts. Mechanisms and clinical features. *Arch Neurol.* 1993;**50**:154–161.

154. Oas JG, Baloh RW. Vertigo and the anterior inferior cerebellar artery syndrome. *Neurology.* 1992;**42**:2274–2279.

155. Kase CS, White JL, Joslyn JN, Williams JP, Mohr JP. Cerebellar infarction in the superior cerebellar artery distribution. *Neurology.* 1985;**35**:705–711.

156. Levine SR, Welch KM. Superior cerebellar artery infarction and vertebral artery dissection. *Stroke.* 1988;**19**:1431–1434.

157. Mani RL, Newton TH. The superior cerebellar artery: arteriographic changes in the diagnosis of posterior fossa lesions. *Radiology.* 1969;**92**:1281–1287.

158. Kase CS, Norrving B, Levine SR, et al. Cerebellar infarction. Clinical and anatomic observations in 66 cases. *Stroke.* 1993;**24**:76–83.

159. Caplan LR, Amarenco P, Rosengart A, et al. Embolism from vertebral artery origin occlusive disease. *Neurology.* 1992;**42**:1505–1512.

160. Caplan LR, Pessin MS, Scott RM, Yarnell P. Poor outcome after lateral medullary infarcts. *Neurology.* 1986;**36**:1510–1513.

161. Gan R, Noronha A. The medullary vascular syndromes revisited. *J Neurol.* 1995;**242**:195–202.

162. Ho KL, Meyer KR. The medial medullary syndrome. *Arch Neurol.* 1981;**38**:385–387.

163. Kim JS, Kim HG, Chung CS. Medial medullary syndrome. Report of 18 new patients and a review of the literature. *Stroke.* 1995;**26**:1548–1552.

164. Pierrot-Deseilligny C, Chain F, Serdaru M, Gray F, Lhermitte F. The 'one-and-a-half' syndrome. Electro-oculographic analyses of five cases with deductions about the physiological mechanisms of lateral gaze. *Brain.* 1981;**104**:665–699.

165. Milisavljevic MM, Marinkovic SV, Gibo H, Puskas LF. The thalamogeniculate perforators of the posterior cerebral artery: the microsurgical anatomy. *Neurosurgery.* 1991;**28**:523–529.

166. Vander Eeken HCM. *The Anastomoses between the Leptomeningeal Arteries of the Brain.* Springfield, IL: Charles C. Thomas; 1959.

167. Weidner W, Hanafee W, Markham CH. Intracranial collateral circulation via leptomeningeal and rete mirabile anastomoses. *Neurology.* 1965;**15**:39–48.

168. Marinkovic SV, Milisavljevic MM, Kovacevic MS. Anastomoses among the thalamoperforating branches of the posterior cerebral artery. *Arch Neurol.* 1986;**43**:811–814.

169. Milisavljevic M, Marinkovic S, Lolic-Draganic V, Kovacevic M. Oculomotor, trochlear, and abducens nerves penetrated by cerebral vessels. Microanatomy and possible clinical significance. *Arch Neurol.* 1986;**43**:58–61.

170. Pessin MS, Kwan ES, DeWitt LD, Hedges TR III, Gale D, Caplan LR. Posterior cerebral artery stenosis. *Ann Neurol.* 1987;**21**:85–89.

171. Castillo M, Falcone S, Naidich TP, Bowen B, Quencer RM. Imaging in acute basilar artery thrombosis. *Neuroradiology.* 1994;**36**:426–429.

172. Brandt T, Steinke W, Thie A, Pessin MS, Caplan LR. Posterior cerebral artery territory infarcts: clinical features, infarct topography, causes and outcome. Multicenter results and a review of the literature. *Cerebrovasc Dis.* 2000;**10**:170–182.

173. Argenta PA, Morgan MA. Cortical blindness and Anton syndrome in a patient with obstetric hemorrhage. *Obstet Gynecol.* 1998;**91**:810–812.

174. Misra M, Rath S, Mohanty AB. Anton syndrome and cortical blindness due to bilateral occipital infarction. *Indian J Ophthalmol.* 1989;**37**:196.

175. Aldrich MS, Alessi AG, Beck RW, Gilman S. Cortical blindness: etiology, diagnosis, and prognosis. *Ann Neurol.* 1987;**21**:149–158.

176. Servan J, Verstichel P, Catala M, Rancurel G. [Amnestic syndromes and confabulation in infarction of the posterior cerebral artery area]. *Rev Neurol (Paris).* 1994;**150**:201–208.

177. Chambers BR, Brooder RJ, Donnan GA. Proximal posterior cerebral artery occlusion simulating middle cerebral artery occlusion. *Neurology.* 1991;**41**:385–390.

178. North K, Kan A, de Silva M, Ouvrier R. Hemiplegia due to posterior cerebral artery occlusion. *Stroke.* 1993;**24**:1757–1760.

179. Devinsky O, Bear D, Volpe BT. Confusional states following posterior cerebral artery infarction. *Arch Neurol.* 1988;**45**:160–163.

180. Servan J, Verstichel P, Catala M, Yakovleff A, Rancurel G. Aphasia and infarction of the posterior cerebral artery territory. *J Neurol.* 1995;**242**:87–92.

181. Moulin T, Bogousslavsky J, Chopard JL, et al. Vascular ataxic hemiparesis: a re-evaluation. *J Neurol Neurosurg Psychiatry.* 1995;**58**:422–427.

182. Wessel K, Vieregge P, Kessler C, Kompf D. Thalamic stroke: correlation of clinical symptoms, somatosensory evoked potentials, and CT findings. *Acta Neurol Scand.* 1994;**90**:167–173.

183. Bogousslavsky J, Regli F, Uske A. Thalamic infarcts: clinical syndromes, etiology, and prognosis. *Neurology.* 1988;**38**:837–848.

184. Neau JP, Bogousslavsky J. The syndrome of posterior choroidal artery territory infarction. *Ann Neurol*. 1996;**39**:779–788.
185. Guberman A, Stuss D. The syndrome of bilateral paramedian thalamic infarction. *Neurology*. 1983;**33**:540–546.
186. Clark JM, Albers GW. Vertical gaze palsies from medial thalamic infarctions without midbrain involvement. *Stroke*. 1995;**26**:1467–1470.
187. Lye RH. Basilar artery ectasia: an unusual cause of trigeminal neuralgia. *J Neurol Neurosurg Psychiatry*. 1986;**49**:22–28.
188. Ueda S, Kohyama Y, Takase K. Peripheral hypoglossal nerve palsy caused by lateral position of the external carotid artery and an abnormally high position of bifurcation of the external and internal carotid arteries – a case report. *Stroke*. 1984;**15**: 736–739.
189. Adler CH, Zimmerman RA, Savino PJ, Bernardi B, Bosley TM, Sergott RC. Hemifacial spasm: evaluation by magnetic resonance imaging and magnetic resonance tomographic angiography. *Ann Neurol*. 1992;**32**:502–506.
190. Eidelman BH, Nielsen VK, Moller M, Janetta PJ. Vascular compression, hemifacial spasm, and multiple cranial neuropathy. *Neurology*. 1985;**35**:712–716.
191. Besson G, Bogousslavsky J, Moulin T, Hommel M. Vertebrobasilar infarcts in patients with dolichoectatic basilar artery. *Acta Neurol Scand*. 1995;**91**:37–42.
192. Buttner U, Ott M, Helmchen C, Yousry T. Bilateral loss of eighth nerve function as the only clinical sign of vertebrobasilar dolichoectasia. *J Vestib Res*. 1995;**5**:47–51.
193. Kim P, Ishijima B, Takahashi H, Shimizu H, Yokochi M. Hemiparesis caused by vertebral artery compression of the medulla oblongata. Case report. *J Neurosurg*. 1985;**62**:425–429.
194. Levine RL, Turski PA, Grist TM. Basilar artery dolichoectasia. Review of the literature and six patients studied with magnetic resonance angiography. *J Neuroimaging*. 1995;**5**:164–170.
195. Passero SG, Rossi S. Natural history of vertebrobasilar dolichoectasia. *Neurology*. 2008;**70**:66–72.
196. Riggs HE, Rupp C. Variation in form of circle of Willis. *Arch Neurol*. 1963;**8**:8–14.
197. Battacharji SK, Hutchinson EC, McCall AJ. The circle of Willis – the incidence of developmental abnormalities in normal and infarcted brains. *Brain*. 1967;**90**:747–758.
198. Lehrer HZ. Relative calibre of the cervical internal carotid artery. Normal variation with the circle of Willis. *Brain*. 1968;**91**: 339–348.
199. Reivich M, Holling HE, Roberts B, Toole JF. Reversal of blood flow through the vertebral artery and its effect on cerebral circulation. *N Engl J Med*. 1961;**265**:878–885.
200. Toole JF. Reversed vertebral-artery flow – subclavian-steal syndrome. *Lancet*. 1964;**1**:872–873.
201. Toole JF. Interarterial shunts in the cerebral circulation. *Circulation*. 1966;**33**:474–483.
202. Sheth RD, Bodensteiner JB. Progressive neurologic impairment from an arteriovenous malformation vascular steal. *Pediatr Neurol*. 1995;**13**:352–354.
203. Nencini P, Inzitari D, Gibbs J, Mangiafico S. Dementia with leucoaraiosis and dural arteriovenous malformation: clinical and PET case study. *J Neurol Neurosurg Psychiatry*. 1993;**56**:929–931.
204. Norbash AM, Marks MP, Lane B. Correlation of pressure measurements with angiographic characteristics predisposing to hemorrhage and steal in cerebral arteriovenous malformations. *AJNR Am J Neuroradiol*. 1994;**15**:809–813.
205. Kendall BE, Andrew J. Neurogenic intermittent claudication associated with aortic steal from the anterior spinal artery complicating coarctation of the aorta. *J Neurosurg*. 1972;**37**: 89–94.
206. Hirano T, Uyama E, Tashima K, Mita S, Uchino M. An atypical case of adult moyamoya disease with initial onset of brain stem ischemia. *J Neurol Sci*. 1998;**157**:100–104.
207. Thomassen L, Aarli JA. Subclavian steal phenomenon. Clinical and hemodynamic aspects. *Acta Neurol Scand*. 1994;**90**: 241–244.
208. Grosset DG, Patterson J, Bone I. Intracranial haemodynamics in Takayasu's arteritis. *Acta Neurochir (Wien)*. 1992;**119**:161–165.
209. Ringleb PA, Strittmatter EI, Loewer M, et al. Cerebrovascular manifestations of Takayasu arteritis in Europe. *Rheumatology (Oxford)*. 2005;**44**:1012–1015.
210. Folger GM, Shar KD. Subclavian steal in patients with Blalock-Taussig anastomosis. *Circulation*. 1965;**31**:241–248.
211. Kurlan R, Krall RL, DeWeese JA. Vertebrobasilar ischemia after total repair of tetralogy of Fallot: significance of subclavian steal created by Blalock-Taussig anastomosis. Vertebrobasilar ischemia after correction of tetralogy of Fallot. *Stroke*. 1984;**15**:359–362.
212. Hennerici M, Klemm C, Rautenberg W. The subclavian steal phenomenon: a common vascular disorder with rare neurologic deficits. *Neurology*. 1988;**38**:669–673.
213. Giles KA, Poirier VC. Bilateral subclavian steal: a review of an unusual twist in a common disorder. *AJNR Am J Neuroradiol*. 1993;**14**:485–488.
214. Sueoka BL. Percutaneous transluminal stent placement to treat subclavian steal syndrome. *J Vasc Interv Radiol*. 1996;**7**: 351–356.
215. Smith JM, Koury HI, Hafner CD, Welling RE. Subclavian steal syndrome. A review of 59 consecutive cases. *J Cardiovasc Surg (Torino)*. 1994;**35**:11–14.
216. Brott T, Adams HP Jr, Olinger CP, et al. Measurements of acute cerebral infarction: a clinical examination scale. *Stroke*. 1989;**20**:864–870.
217. Lyden P, Lu M, Jackson C, et al. Underlying structure of the National Institutes of Health Stroke Scale: results of a factor analysis. NINDS tPA Stroke Trial Investigators. *Stroke*. 1999;**30**:2347–2354.

4

Pathophysiology of Ischemic Stroke

In some respects at least, myths and science fulfill a similar function: they both provide human beings with a representation of the world and of the forces that are supposed to govern it. They both fix the limits of what is considered as possible. … Whether mythic or scientific, the view of the world that man builds is always largely a product of his imagination. For, in contrast to what is frequently believed, the scientific process does not consist merely in observing, in collecting data and deducing a theory from them. One can watch an object for years without ever producing any observation of scientific interest. Before making a valuable observation, it is necessary to have some idea of what to observe, a preconception of what is possible.

François Jacob

Cerebral ischemia causes a complex chain of events altering blood flow, metabolism, and cellular function throughout multiple areas of the brain. Current concepts of stroke pathophysiology are broadly based on experimental studies involving cell cultures or animal models of permanent or transient global and focal ischemia. Animal experiments demonstrate a significant species variability in susceptibility to hypoperfusion and hypoxia as well as in brain viability following recanalization and reperfusion after thrombolysis of an acute arterial occlusion. It is sometimes difficult to extrapolate data from these studies to humans for clinical applications. Our understanding of stroke pathophysiology in humans is based partly on pathological examinations and the use of neurodiagnostic techniques. However, these studies allow only a momentary glimpse into a continuous pathophysiological process that unfolds over time. The following section will describe the molecular, pathophysiological, and pathological sequelae of an acute interruption of cerebral blood flow. Modern imaging techniques that help to understand the evolving dynamics of brain ischemia and guide management are discussed in more detail in Chapter 5. The clinical findings depend largely on the specific vascular territory affected and are discussed in Chapter 3.

PHYSIOLOGY OF CEREBRAL PERFUSION AND METABOLISM

Although the brain accounts for only 1% to 2% of the total body mass, it receives approximately 20% of the resting cardiac output. Cellular function, integrity, and survival depend on adequate tissue perfusion and oxygenation. This is especially crucial for the brain with its tremendous energy demand, which is required not only to maintain cerebral metabolism but also to fuel neuronal signaling and information processing. At rest, the human brain is responsible for about 20% of the body's entire oxygen utilization. About half of this amount is used to operate the sodium/potassium ion channel pumps of neuronal membranes, maintaining the ionic concentration gradients that provide the basis for synaptic electrical signaling.

The brain's metabolic rate can influence neural coding profoundly. The cellular activity that supports complex brain functions such as maintenance of consciousness and cognition is metabolically expensive.[1] Its high metabolic rate makes the brain susceptible to ischemic-hypoxic injury, and some portions of the brain are more vulnerable to such injury than others.[2] In global cerebral ischemia, consciousness and higher cognitive functions are lost a few seconds after cerebral blood flow (CBF) ceases. Brain areas with less neuronal complexity and energy demand fail in successive order. Prolonged interruption of perfusion results in cerebral ischemia and hypoxia, and the ensuing energy failure and cell death affects all major constituents of the functional brain unit: neurons, endothelial cells, and neuroglia.

The brain needs a constant supply of blood to maintain the exchange of gases, fluids, solutes, nutrients, and metabolic waste products. The normal cerebral perfusion rate in humans is about 50 ml/100 mg/minute and is tightly controlled by autoregulation of cerebral blood flow.[3] The brain derives its energy predominantly from oxidative phosphorylation of glucose. Under resting conditions cerebral oxygen consumption is about 4 ml/100 g/min, and its glucose utilization is about 30 μmol/100 g/min. With normally functioning brain blood flow, the blood volume and energy metabolism (measured as cerebral metabolic rate of oxygen and glucose) are coupled and are higher in gray matter than in white matter. Brain volume is approximately 1500 ml, of which the neuroglia constitute 700–900 ml, neurons 500–700 ml, blood volume 100–150 ml, and extracellular fluid and cerebrospinal fluid (CSF) 100–150 ml each. Of the cells, neurons are the most vulnerable to ischemia.

Cerebral blood flow depends on cerebral perfusion pressure and cerebrovascular resistance. Cerebrovascular resistance is determined by vascular tone and blood viscosity. The perfusion pressure is determined by the difference between the systemic arterial pressure and the venous pressure at the point of the subarachnoid space, where the perfusion pressure is approximated by the intracranial pressure (ICP). A high-flow, low-pressure system allows cerebral perfusion throughout the entire cardiac cycle with relatively pronounced flow even during diastole. Hemodynamics are controlled by vascular autoregulation, allowing the brain to adjust to changes in systemic blood pressure to maintain steady perfusion. Alteration of vascular tone in arterioles and capillaries leads to adaptation of cerebrovascular resistance and may take several seconds to occur.

In normal individuals CBF remains constant when the mean arterial systemic pressure ranges between 60 and 160 mm Hg. These upper and lower limits can vary in different diseases and with changing physiological conditions. For example, activation of the sympathetic nervous system can shift the autoregulatory plateau toward higher upper limits.[4] Autoregulation is achieved by a complex system of local and global mechanisms acting in concert to adjust the resistance of cerebral vascular beds. Although the precise mechanisms are not fully understood, vascular resistance is probably controlled by the interaction of multiple neurogenic, myogenic, metabolic, and endothelial factors.

Cerebral autoregulation also allows the brain to regulate regional cerebral perfusion in response to the varying functional and metabolic demands. Activation and inactivation of neuronal networks for information processing are circumscribed spatiotemporal events that require precise control of regional cerebral perfusion. The regional flow changes caused by mental activity, however, have no measurable effect on overall cerebral perfusion. Cerebral perfusion and vascular reactivity can be measured by transcranial Doppler (TCD) examination, perfusion cranial computed tomography (CT), perfusion magnetic resonance imaging (MRI), positron emission tomography (PET), or single-proton-emission-computed-tomography (SPECT) following the administration of acetazolamide, inhalation of CO_2, hyperventilation, or breath holding. These methods provide an estimate of the cerebrovascular reserve, that is, the ability to increase or decrease cerebral blood flow following various stimuli.

PATHOPHYSIOLOGY

Hypoxia

The brain can survive anoxia for a time if the tissue is well perfused and metabolites do not accumulate, because infarction results in part from tissue acidosis and endothelial injury that, if reversed quickly, allows restitution of brain function. However, it is unusual for severe anoxia to occur without simultaneous reduction in the mean arterial blood pressure, such as occurs during cardiovascular collapse.

Encephalopathy may occur as an immediate or delayed response to anoxia. Some patients recover near-normal neural function only to suffer a progressively evolving neurologic disorder thought to be the delayed consequence of anaerobic metabolism, particularly lactic acidosis and the presence of free radicals.

Anoxia affects all brain tissues, but anoxic damage can be localized or multifocal, perhaps because of variations in local metabolic needs. Especially vulnerable are the cerebral cortex, basal ganglia, and Purkinje cells of the cerebellum. In other cases the border zone areas are most affected, particularly if systemic hypotension is a concomitant feature. At other times local

stenosis or impairment of arterial flow and pressure promotes hypoxic-ischemic changes confined to that vascular territory. The continued availability of glucose permits continuing glycolysis and lactic acidosis, leading in some settings to further tissue destruction. Therefore, elevated blood glucose caused by diabetes mellitus or the administration of intravenous fluids should be avoided.

Several categories of hypoxia have been described: anemic, stagnant, cellular, or anoxic. Anoxia is the result of decreased blood oxygen due to respiratory insufficiency, whereas anemic anoxia is the result of reduced oxygen-carrying capacity of the blood, such as occurs in carbon monoxide poisoning or severe blood loss anemia. Stagnant anoxia results from reduction of blood flow, as in severe hypotension or cardiac arrest, whereas cellular (histotoxic) anoxia is caused by interference with the utilization of oxygen by the cells (e.g., cyanide poisoning).

Ischemia

Ischemia is caused by a decrease in CBF sufficient to interfere with cerebral function. Although ischemia results in hypoxia, the two terms are not interchangeable. Hypoxia means low blood oxygen with normal flow to remove metabolites, whereas ischemia implies not only impaired delivery of oxygen and glucose but also failure to remove carbon dioxide, lactic acid, and other metabolites. Cerebral oxygen consumption averages 50 ml/min for the whole brain. When the arterial oxygen tension (PaO_2) drops from its normal level of about 100 mm Hg to as low as 50 mm Hg, the CBF increases slightly. At a PaO_2 of 40 mm Hg, patients develop confusion and, at 20 mm Hg, coma. The effects of hypoxia are aggravated in the presence of concomitant hypotension or ischemia.[5–7]

Global ischemia is usually produced by a sudden and severe reduction in arterial pressure, as may occur during shock. If it persists for more than a few minutes, cerebral damage occurs, particularly in the gray matter. Areas in the boundary zone between the vascular territories (*watershed areas*) are particularly vulnerable to ischemia (see below). Different regions of the brain vary in their ability to withstand hypoxia and ischemia.[8] Even within the territory of a single occluded cerebral artery the response to hypoxia differs between the core of the lesion, where the cells are quickly killed by the absence of oxygen, and the peripheral portion of the lesion (the *ischemic penumbra*), where the cells are damaged by secondary metabolic changes that occur in response to low levels of oxygen and ischemic injury.[9] The word *penumbra* is derived from Latin, meaning "half shade" (from *paenes* "almost" and *umbra* "shadow") and is primarily used in astronomy to describe the portion of a shadow that receives direct light from only a part of the light source.

After cardiac arrest, both CBF and metabolism are reduced by half. Continuing coma and failure of recovery reflect the underlying brain injury and not the persistence of global ischemia. Reduction of flow to 20 ml/100 g/min produces electroencephalographic changes. Levels of about 15 ml/100 g/min will cause somatosensory-evoked responses to disappear, and when CBF drops to 10 ml/100 g/min, a massive afflux of potassium ensues, resulting in neuronal death if it is not immediately reversed.

Cerebral ischemia triggers a complex cascade of hemodynamic, cellular, and metabolic events during which cell death occurs as a dynamic process starting almost immediately with the occlusion of an artery and continuing to evolve over many days (Figure 4-1). At the same time mechanisms of cell repair

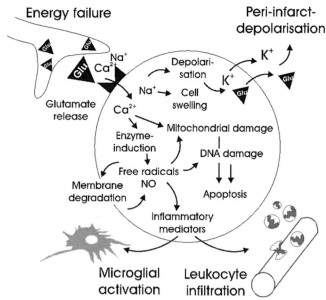

Figure 4-1. The ischemic cascade: Multiple pathophysiological mechanisms are induced by acute cerebral ischemia, resulting in inflammation, apoptosis, peri-infarct depolarizations lipolysis of cell membranes, and cell damage that may cause secondary cellular injury. Reprinted with permission from Dirnagl et al.[65]

and neuroplasticity are initiated. Ischemia-induced signaling cascades decide about cell survival, neurological deficit, and stroke mortality. The effects of cerebral ischemia can extend well beyond a specific vascular territory to influence metabolism and function of neuronal networks in remote areas of the brain by transneural deactivation. Basal ganglia infarctions, for example, can reduce cerebral blood flow and glucose metabolism in ipsilateral and contralateral cortical areas. Cerebral ischemia also has systemic effects on the organism as a whole. Stroke can cause changes in cardiac function, blood pressure, and body temperature or induce immunosuppression by overactivation of the sympathetic nervous system.[10–13]

The sympatho-adrenal and adrenocortical systems are activated during an acute stroke. Changes in cardiac function, blood pressure, blood glucose, serum cortisol, serum lipids, the renninangiotensin system, and body temperature may result from this activation. The cardiac effects are primarily dysrhythmias following subfrontal, hypothalamic, or brainstem infarctions. At times, there are pronounced changes in the S-T segments and T-waves, possibly the result of vasomotor responses within the neural network of the myocardium, resulting from circulating catecholamines released from the adrenal medulla and the postganglionic nerve terminals controlled by the brain at the highest level. Neurogenic pulmonary edema is associated with overactivation of the sympatho-adrenal system.

Cerebral Autoregulation

In the critically hypoperfused brain, autoregulatory hemodynamics are impaired or abolished. Brain arteries in ischemic areas are already maximally dilated in an attempt to maintain perfusion and do not respond to normal physiological stimuli. In this situation CBF is determined only by systemic perfusion pressure. Regional cerebral flow cannot be controlled by alteration of vasomotor tone, resulting in the uncoupling of cerebral perfusion and energy metabolism. If vascular autoregulation is impaired, regional blood flow may not meet increasing metabolic needs in areas with high electric synaptic activity and low perfusion. In these brain regions the energy crisis leads quickly to cellular injury.[14,15] Additionally, impaired autoregulation can induce an intracerebral steal phenomenon in which blood is shunted from the poorly perfused peri-infarct zone to well-perfused healthy tissue, amplifying ischemia in the penumbral zone. This may be one of several mechanisms by which the infarct core grows over time.[16]

After a few hours of recirculation, delayed postischemic circulatory disturbance may cause dissociation between maintained autoregulation and absent CO_2 reactivity (postischemic hypoperfusion syndrome). Systemic vasoactive drugs are ineffective, but they may have more effect if applied locally. The role of spasm and various other complications of postischemic resuscitation will be discussed later in this chapter.

The degree to which the adventitial neurons contribute to homeostatic control of brain circulation is still debated. There are a number of substances that can modulate responsivity, particularly in the endothelial cells, which appear able to recognize the presence of vasoactive substances and generate signals that alter the tone of muscle cells.

Autoregulation is mediated by a neural network, as evidenced by the fact that in some brainstem diseases autoregulatory responses of the two cerebral hemispheres may be lost. In addition to localized loss of regulation caused by cerebral infarction, there is often loss of autoregulation in a similar position on the opposite hemisphere.[17] The mechanism underlying this phenomenon is unknown, but it is thought that the entire arteriolar system is controlled by a network involving the intrinsic dopaminergic system, probably in conjunction with local myogenic responses in the arteriolar walls.

Oxygen Extraction Fraction

The brain has developed protective mechanisms to ensure adequate perfusion and oxygenation if CBF decreases but remains above a critical threshold. This is accomplished by collateralization of blood flow, vascular autoregulation, and increase of the oxygen extraction fraction. The oxygen extraction fraction is the amount of oxygen consumed by the brain and equals the arterial-to-venous difference of oxygen content in blood. If CBF decreases to rates between 25 and 40 ml/100 g/min, the oxygen extraction fraction can increase by about 50% to 60%.[18,19] This response is found in the ischemic penumbra. An increased oxygen extraction fraction can temporarily maintain cellular metabolism and function but indicates marginal perfusion during which the brain is at risk for permanent damage and cell death. In the irreversible damaged core of an ischemic stroke, CBF has fallen below the critical perfusion threshold, and the protective mechanism of an increased oxygen extraction fraction has failed.

Usually within 24 hours the affected area becomes reperfused at a rate that is more than adequate for the residual oxygen demand of the previously ischemic tissue. At this stage oxygen extraction is considerably reduced, often to levels as low as 10% to 30%. These two patterns – raised and lowered oxygen extraction – appear to represent true ischemia and established infarction, respectively.

BRAIN INFARCTION

Cerebral infarction – the death of neurons, glia, and blood vessels – is caused either by insufficient blood carrying oxygen and nutrients or by reduced removal of metabolic products. Each of the causes, such as anoxia, ischemia, or hypoglycemia, has its own characteristic features, zones of vulnerability, and histopathology. For example, hypoxic infarction caused by lack of oxygen, despite normal circulation, affects basal ganglia and cortex, whereas hypoglycemia with normal flow and oxygenation results in characteristic subcortical laminar necrosis. Ischemic infarction may be caused by oligemia, despite normal glucose and oxygenation, with secondary hypoxia, impaired cellular nutrition, and accumulation of metabolites and heat with resulting cell death. It is by far the most common cause for brain infarction.

Regional CBF studies often show a local area of ischemia, sometimes surrounded by an area of hyperemia.[20] Hyperemic foci are most likely to be present during the first few days and after an occluded artery has recanalized, as happens with cerebral embolism. Increased flow around the ischemic area is the equivalent of the "red veins" seen at surgery through an ischemic area. This relative excess of blood supply that exceeds metabolic needs has been termed "luxury perfusion syndrome."

Positron emission tomography (PET) demonstrates that acute cerebral ischemia disrupts the normally close relation between CBF and metabolism.[21,22] During the first 24 to 48 hours, the decrease in CBF is relatively greater than that of oxygen consumption, implying that a true state of ischemia exists ("misery perfusion"). After 72 hours the depression of metabolism is relatively more profound than that of CBF, leading to perfusion greater than is required by the depressed metabolism ("luxury perfusion").

Studies with PET have confirmed previous observations that an acute cerebral infarct in one hemisphere can lead to diffuse depression of blood flow and metabolism in the opposite hemisphere that is at a maximum in the area that represents the mirror image of the infarct.[23] Interruption of connecting neural pathways provides a plausible but incomplete explanation of these phenomena.

PATHOLOGIC FINDINGS

At autopsy the arteries may have advanced atherosclerosis without there being any infarctions in the brain. Although new infarctions do not become visible for about 72 hours, they are palpable as circumscribed areas of softening within the substance of the brain within a day of occurrence. Within minutes of arterial occlusion, multiple foci of cortical pallor begin to coalesce, evolving within hours into a large pale region where red arterial blood becomes dark blue because of stagnation.

In most cases infarction is the result of arterial obstruction and follows the outline of the arterial bed distal to the point of occlusion.[24,25] Infarction due to venous occlusion affects the area it normally drains (Chapter 20). Infarct dimensions generally depend on the size of the vessel obstructed. In addition, the shape and size of the zone of infarction depend on the efficiency of collateral channels. When these are inadequate, obliteration of a main artery results in infarction of its entire territory. If collaterals exist, the infarct may be a wedge in the center of its field of distribution. On the other hand, if a major artery is occluded in association with stenosis of an adjacent main artery, the infarct may be massive because the occluded artery now diverts flow through anastomotic channels, so that flow and pressure are inadequate for either.

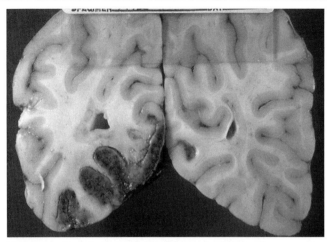

Figure 4-2. Occipital lobe gyriform hemorrhagic infarction secondary to uncal herniation causing compression of the posterior cerebral artery.

Infarcts caused by obstruction of a penetrating artery (lacunes) may barely be visible; those resulting from interruption of the carotid arterial supply may almost destroy an entire hemisphere. Infarction is always sharply delineated from the surrounding normal brain and can be identified by its grayish white appearance and mushy consistency. Multiple tiny infarctions visible in the internal capsule, putamen, thalamus, pons, and, sometimes, the cerebellum constitute the lacunar state (see Chapter 9). They are fluid-filled vacuoles surrounding arteries that may contain small thrombi. Sometimes they collapse and become nearly invisible slits.

In the early stages of infarction, there may be enough edema to displace and distort surrounding structures. When an entire hemisphere is edematous, the gyri are flattened and the sulci obliterated. The cingulate gyrus of the frontal lobe may be displaced beneath the falx cerebri, and herniation of the hippocampal gyrus through the tentorium may compress the posterior cerebral artery against the sharp edge of the tentorium cerebelli, causing ischemic infarction in the occipital lobe. If blood flow is reestablished, the infarction may become hemorrhagic (Figure 4-2).The midline structures may shift to such a degree that the midbrain is compressed against the sharp edge of the tentorium on the opposite side, resulting in homolateral upper motor neuron signs. In severe cases an indentation of the peduncle by the incisura (Kernohan's notch) can be seen at autopsy (Figure 4-3).

In cases of massive infarction of the cerebellum (see Figure 25-8), the structures in the posterior fossa are compressed, and the cerebellum may herniate up through the incisura and/or down through the foramen magnum. In such instances hydrocephalus secondary to obstruction of the aqueduct often occurs.

No change is seen microscopically for up to 6 hours after an ictus. Neurons swell thereafter, yet by 24 hours they are shrunken, hyperchromatic, and pyknotic. Chromatolysis and nuclear eccentricity may be seen. Astrocytes swell and fragment, and myelin sheaths degenerate. The axis cylinders are particularly sensitive and soon fragment, while the oligodendrocytes swell and disappear. Capillaries are relatively resistant, although their endothelium swells. Polymorphonuclear cells may be abundant during the first 24 to 36 hours. At 48 hours microglia proliferate and enter the infarcted tissue to ingest the fatty products of

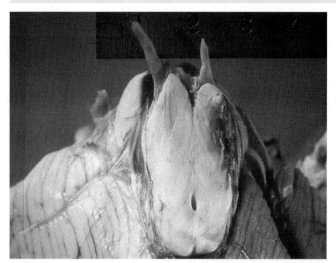

Figure 4-3. Coronal specimen shows necrosis of the contralateral cerebral peduncle due to uncal herniation (Kernohan's notch syndrome) caused by a large hemorrhagic infarction with uncal herniation.

myelin breakdown, forming fatty macrophages. After 3 weeks these begin to decrease in number, gradually diminishing for many months.[26]

After several days the surviving capillaries become more prominent, and new capillaries appear. In the surrounding undamaged tissue, astrocytes begin to proliferate, forming large cells with abundant pale cytoplasm. Astroglial fibers are laid down on the borders of the infarct. A fine collagenous fibroglial deposition covers the persisting capillaries within the infarct, forming the basis of a trabecular framework. As necrotic material is phagocytosed and macrophages decrease in number, the interstices of the meshwork fill with fluid.[26]

After about 2 to 3 months, the necrotic material is resorbed, and a cavity is left. At the periphery there is proliferation of capillaries and swollen astrocytes, and the cavity itself is traversed by glial and fibrovascular elements. The overlying leptomeninges are thickened, and in the later stages the cortex may be depressed and the adjoining ventricle dilated.

Microscopically, three distinct zones can be discerned in a large brain infarction:

1. An inner area of coagulative necrosis where all cells (including those in the capillaries) have unstainable nuclei
2. A central zone containing prominently vacuolated neuropil, leukocytic infiltrates, swollen axons, and thickened capillaries
3. An outer marginal zone containing hyperplastic astrocytes mixed with occasional neurons.

HEMORRHAGIC INFARCTION

Autopsy studies find that 50% to 70% of strokes resulting from emboli are hemorrhagic, compared with only 2% to 20% of the lesions without a source for embolism. Furthermore, they are evident in only about 5% of cranial CT performed within 48 hours of onset. The cumulative incidence of hemorrhagic transformation by CT reaches 40% during the first 2 weeks after infarction. Apart from hemorrhagic infarctions, parenchymal hematomas may develop in the territory of primary infarction. The most reliable predictors of hemorrhagic transformation are

large infarct size, use of anticoagulants, and treatment with thrombolytic agents. Surprisingly, hypertension, either acute or chronic, does not increase the likelihood of hemorrhagic transformation. Well-developed collateral supply to the ischemic area probably increases the risk of hemorrhagic transformation. Another mechanism is the reperfusion of the occluded artery due to spontaneous thrombolysis and distal clot migration.

At autopsy there is a combination of ischemic infarction and blotchy hemorrhages on the brain surface. Microscopically, hemorrhages are seen predominantly in the gray matter, distributed around the necrotic blood vessels, and in association with phagocytes containing hemosiderin. In the late stages the leptomeninges acquire a rusty brown color, and the hemorrhage is seen as a cavity enclosed by a golden brown wall.[26]

Unlike cerebral hemorrhage, which dissects between nerve fibers and along tracts, a hemorrhagic infarct destroys all of the tissues in the distribution of the involved artery or vein. After a cerebral hemorrhage heals, its walls are in close apposition, whereas those of a hemorrhagic infarct tend to be widely separated with the cavity spanned by fibroglial tissue.

Occlusion of cerebral veins or venous sinuses frequently cause hemorrhagic infarction (see Chapter 20), and these venous lesions are usually more edematous than an arterial infarction. Because a venous occlusion impedes venous outflow, it causes hemorrhage within its venous territory and involves both white and gray matter equally.

BOUNDARY ZONE (HEMODYNAMIC) INFARCTION

Reduced arterial blood pressure can be systemic or localized. In either case as perfusion pressure falls, cerebral arterioles dilate. When this vasodilatation is maximal, autoregulation ceases, and, if blood pressure is further reduced, CBF decreases in parallel. In such cases the boundary or watershed zones between arterial territories are the first regions to become oligemic. Thereafter, the distribution of brain damage caused by prolonged and profound hypotension is determined by the balance between the selective vulnerability of the regional brain tissues and the blood flow it receives. Watershed infarctions constitute about 10% of ischemic brain infarcts and as many as 40% of those in patients with documented carotid stenosis or occlusion (Figure 4-4). The locations of infarction conform to one of three patterns:

1. Watershed infarction – Damage is greatest at the edges between the territories of the major cerebral and cerebellar arteries. In the cerebral cortex it is most severe in the parietal-temporal-occipital triangle at the junction of the anterior, middle, and posterior cerebral arteries. A typical example is the combination of extracranial arterial stenosis or occlusion with subsequent systemic hypotension. This situation is particularly common following an apparently asymptomatic internal carotid occlusion, after which the patient may develop leukoaraiosis in the distribution of the border zones between anterior, middle, and posterior cerebral arterial distributions.[27,28] Hypotensive ischemia in an individual with these marginally perfused areas can lead to border zone infarctions. In some cases these events are preceded or accompanied by syncope or "limb-shaking" transient ischemic attacks (TIAs), and many occur during acute cardiac events that may overshadow this serious complication.

The border zone between the anterior and middle cerebral arteries extends over the frontoparietal area and crosses the

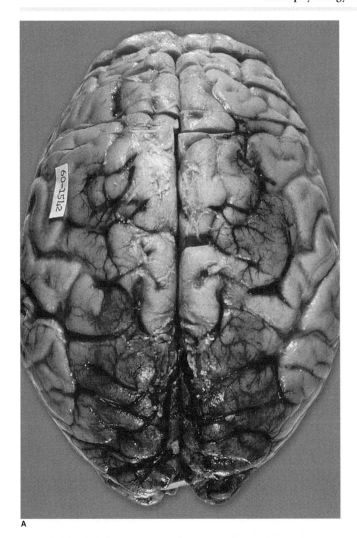

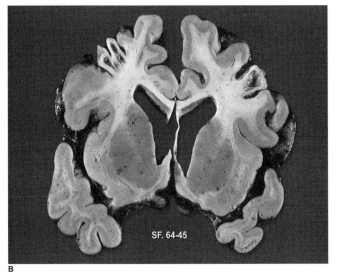

SF. 64-45

Figure 4-4. A: Pathological specimen demonstrates a watershed infarct of both cerebral hemispheres. B: Coronal brain section demonstrates selective parasagittal necrosis.

sensory and motor homunculi at approximately the level of the cortical representation of the arm. Therefore, involvement of this watershed zone causes a characteristic clinical syndrome consisting of paralysis and sensory loss, predominantly involving

the arm. The face is spared, and there is no dysphasia. Bilateral infarction of these border zone areas produces the "man in the barrel" syndrome with bibrachial paresis and relative sparing of the legs.

The three-vessel border zone of the anterior, middle, and posterior cerebral arteries occurs in the parieto-occipital area (Figure 4-4). The clinical manifestations of lesions in this location are homonymous hemianopia with visual agnosia, disorientation in space, apraxia, dyslexia, dysgraphia, and dyscalculia. The neurological deficits of patients with bilateral infarctions in the middle-posterior or triple-vessel watershed areas include cortical blindness, sometimes accompanied by formed visual hallucinations, replaced by disturbances of visual localization, such as estimation of distance and length, visual attention and fixation, convergence, pursuit, and reflex blinking to threat. All of these in combination can be expressed as dementia. Other watershed areas are those between the posterior inferior cerebellar artery (PICA), the anterior inferior cerebellar artery (AICA), and the superior cerebellar artery (SCA), between the recurrent artery of Heubner and the lenticulostriate arteries or the lenticulostriate and pial branches of the middle cerebral artery in the basal ganglia, and the internal border zone between the circumferential penetrating branches of the basilar artery in the brainstem. Bilateral hemispheric border zone infarctions may be confused, at times, with brainstem lesions.

2. Generalized – Ischemic lesions can encompass the cortex, basal ganglia, thalami, and cerebellar nuclei but spare the hippocampi. This unusual pattern results when hypotension is gradual in onset but profound and prolonged as occurs in shock.

3. Combination of boundary zone and generalized patterns – Most typically, combinations occur after hypotension, as might occur with a cardiac arrest.

BIOCHEMICAL MECHANISMS

The Ischemic Cascade

Reduced or absent cerebral perfusion causes an almost immediate decrease in neuronal and glial metabolism. Protein synthesis is highly susceptible to cerebral hypoperfusion and decreases rapidly if perfusion decreases by 50% or more. If it decreases further, anaerobic utilization of substrate replaces oxidative phosphorylation of glucose yielding only about 5% of the amount of adenosine triphosphate (ATP) produced by aerobic glycolysis. Although anaerobic production of ATP increases, it does not keep pace with cellular demands because the brain does not store glycogen or glucose. ATP levels fall and cellular failure ensues.

Because of energy failure, membrane-bound ion channel pumps cease to work, and extracellular cytotoxic ions such as calcium leak into the cytoplasm.[29,30] Calcium activates catabolic enzymes such as kinases, calmodulin, proteinases, lipases, and free radicals and can damage mitochondrial and cellular membranes. The production of reactive oxygen species is upregulated. These species can react with NO synthase (NOS) leading to the creation of peroxynitrite and free radicals and activation of inflammatory mediators such as prostaglandins and leukotrienes. Inflammatory mediators in turn activate microglia and leukocyte adhesion, causing inflammatory tissue injury.[31]

Free radicals damage membranes of the cells and cell organelles by peroxidation and induce programmed cell death by

DNA fragmentation. In transient ischemia and in the penumbra of a permanent ischemic focus, mitochondria play a key role in causing apoptosis.[32] Intracellular calcium and free radicals can disrupt the inner mitochondrial membrane, increasing ion permeability and leading to swelling of the mitochondria. The external membrane of the swollen mitochondria is damaged, and apoptotic factors such as cytochrome c and caspase 9 are activated, signaling the beginning of the molecular cascade of apoptotic cell death.[33–35]

Metabolism of neurons and glia served by the arteriole has a profound effect on local blood flow. Neuronal activity, for example, causes carbon dioxide, heat, and metabolites to accumulate. These products find their way to the venous capillaries and are eventually carried off, but, first, they cause arteriolar dilatation and increase of blood flow. This phenomenon is dramatically demonstrated in focal seizures that sometimes occur in the setting of ischemic or hemorrhagic stroke. When groups of neurons become active, metabolism in brain tissue increases, as does blood flow, to satisfy increased requirements for oxygen and glucose and to carry away heat, CO_2, and metabolites, such as lactic acid, histamine, and water, that accumulate in the area.[36]

Because the brain does not store glucose in significant quantities and cannot shift to an effective anaerobic cycle if blood flow is cut off even for 10 seconds, neuron activity is impaired, lactic acid is produced, and soon the tissue ceases to function. Neurons and supporting glia remain alive but functionless for as long as 30 minutes before cellular death occurs. If blood flow is impaired but not completely cut off, neurons may be functionless but viable for 6 to 8 hours – rarely up to 48 hours.[37,16]

Arterioles dilate in response to an increase in adenosine and hydrogen ions, including lactic acid. This effect occurs whether blood flowing through surrounding extracellular fluid is altered or not. As a consequence, one can imagine that blood flow through the millions of arterioles that serve the billions of cellular groups is constantly in a state of flux. When a finger moves or the iris changes caliber, flow to the neurons controlling them must alter. During seizures this response to lactic acid and hydrogen ions is carried to dangerous extremes because acid metabolites overwhelm the arterioles, producing maximal dilatation and hyperemia of the brain, destroying the normal autoregulatory response, so that tissue perfusion fluctuates directly with changes in arterial pressure. Cortical hyperemia is so pronounced that oxygenated venous blood can be seen flowing from the site. When arterial or tissue PCO_2 or lactic acid is increased, CBF increases, even if arterial pressure remains constant. Any increase in arterial pressure will be transmitted directly into the arteriolar-capillary network to create a dangerous increase in perfusion pressure. Then, if arterial pressure falls, perfusion does also and the damage is compounded.

The possibility that restoration of flow during the interval between loss of neuron activity and tissue death might restore function is the basis for therapy of the evolving cerebral infarction. The clinical state of the patient during this time depends on the area of the brain involved. For example, a large area in the nondominant hemisphere may become ischemic without causing any detectable abnormality but, if blood supply to a *small* area of mesencephalic gray matter in the upper brainstem is interrupted, coma ensues rapidly. One might argue that, throughout our lives, we maintain only a tenuous link with consciousness.

It is important to recognize that focal ischemia differs from global ischemia. For example, there is collateral flow in focal ischemia that results in a penumbra of viable tissue – a situation not present in generalized ischemia. This gradation in degree of flow impairment results in a complex situation with delivery of glucose under anaerobic conditions, causing lactic acidosis in some tissue. Whether ischemia is focal or general, at a CBF less than 10 ml/100 g/min the following changes begin to occur:

1. Depletion of ATP
2. Failure of the Na^+/K^+ ion pump causes the neuronal membrane to depolarize, increase of glutamate release from presynaptic nerve terminals
3. This allows penetration of extracellular calcium ion into the cell
4. This, in turn, activates phospholipase, which attacks membrane and liberates free fatty acids, including prostaglandins, leukotrienes, and free acid radicals
5. Profound intracellular (mostly lactic) acidosis due to disruption of oxidative phosphorylation
6. Redistribution of H_2O between the extra- and intracellular compartments.

Within an area of ischemic infarction there is graded metabolic abnormality from a small degree through total energy failure. There may be anaerobic utilization of substrate in the border zone, causing acidosis without energy failure.

After irreversible damage to brain cells their membranes burst, releasing their contents of lipids, long-chain fatty acids, calcium, and potassium, as well as polypeptides, prostaglandins, and free radicals. These can magnify damage in surrounding cell systems and may further extend the zone of injury. Regardless of which compound is responsible, the end result is a derangement of cellular metabolism, which, in the presence of ischemia, intensifies the damage.[38]

During hypoxia, energy requirements are served by glycolytic degradation of glucose to lactic acid, but this falls short of providing even resting requirements. Furthermore, the accumulation of lactic acid is harmful. Normal aerobic glucose utilization yields approximately 20 times more energy than glycolysis, so that even under maximum stimulation of the glycolytic pathway only 30% to 40% of the energy requirement of tissue can be served. In addition, glycolysis can be continued only so long as glucose or glycogen is available, and, as a rule, local supplies are quickly exhausted. Maximum glucose transport from blood to brain cell can only be doubled, which is another rate-limiting factor.[39,40]

Most of the energy required for biosynthesis of neurotransmitters must be reconstituted during and after nerve transmission across synaptic junctions. In hyperthermic states this process is accelerated, increasing the metabolic demand for oxygen that must be met to prevent tissue breakdown. Expenditure of electrical activity requires increased metabolism and oxygen consumption, which is supplied by an increase in CBF to the affected region. Anesthesia, hypothermia, and repose reduce oxygen needs.[41,42] Sleep, on the other hand, requires a maintenance of oxygen consumption with continuation of energy, metabolism, and, consequently, increased CBF.[43]

NEUROGENIC MECHANISMS

Sympathetic nerve fibers from the stellate ganglia surround the carotid and vertebral arteries and their intracranial branches.

Their terminal fibers follow the penetrating arteries into the substance of the brain to end within the arterioles. There is evidence that neural fibers assist with regional redistribution of blood in response to local metabolic changes, and some investigators hypothesize that they also play a major role in overall regulation.[44] Parasympathetic dilator fibers from the facial nerve join the plexus surrounding the internal carotid artery via the greater superficial petrosal nerve. The stellate, middle, and upper cervical sympathetic plexuses evidently contribute only a weak constrictor effect. Blocking the cervical sympathetics in normal people has no effect on brain blood flow; yet the diffuse vasospasm that may occur in some clinical states – for example, embolism – may conceivably be mediated by overreaction of the sympathetic plexus to a foreign body in the arterial system.

The area postrema plays a major role in the neurohumoral control of the peripheral circulation. Because the blood brain barrier (BBB) is absent in the area postrema, circulating substances can modulate its activity. Electrical stimulation of the area postrema decreases blood flow to the choroid plexus, but the CBF increases, particularly in the frontal regions.

Although the major cerebral arteries are enmeshed in a rich noradrenergic, dopaminergic, and cholinergic network, their precise roles remain obscure. Some evidence suggests that they protect the brain during sudden and marked rises in blood pressure.[45] For example, hypertensive encephalopathy can be induced in animals at a low arterial pressure if the arteries have been denervated. The function of the intraparenchymal adrenergic system arising from the locus ceruleus remains unknown, although changes in capillary surface area and capillary permeability have been attributed to it. Similarly the role of acetylcholine in vasodilation remains to be clarified. It has been tradition that cerebral blood vessels are innervated by sympathetic, norepinephrine-secreting vasoconstrictor fibers and parasympathetic acetylcholine vasodilator fibers.

Up to 15 peptides have been identified in cerebral vessels, but their role, if any, in the regulation of the cerebral circulation remains unclear.[46] Vasoactive intestinal peptide (VIP) is one of the most important transmitters in the resistance vessels of the brain.

NITRIC OXIDE

Another mode for arterial dilatation may be dependent on intact endothelium, which can release endothelium-derived nitric oxide (NO). NO is synthesized from L-arginine by several isoforms of NO synthase.[47] When the rate of blood flow increases, the lateral force or shear stress on the endothelium increases. Endothelial cells sense and release relaxing factors, resulting in "flow-dependent" vasodilation. NO dilates both large arteries and resistance vessels,[48] and it has a strong platelet antiaggregant effect.

CARBON DIOXIDE AND OXYGEN

Cerebral arterioles respond with exquisite sensitivity to variations in CO_2 tension in the arterial blood ($PaCO_2$). This tension is maintained normally at a pressure of about 40 mm Hg. In the range of 20 to 55 mm Hg, each unit of change alters CBF by about 1 to 2 ml/100 g/min. When a person exhales excessive quantities of CO_2, his $PaCO_2$ may fall as low as 15 to 20 mm Hg; cerebral vasoconstriction then results and may reduce blood flow by 75%. The effect of this reactive constriction can be seen in the electroencephalogram as diffuse slowing of brain rhythms. In the anxious individual who hyperventilates, severe respiratory alkalosis can develop, leading to loss of consciousness and, in some cases, convulsions. Labored breathing after exercise does not produce cerebral vasoconstriction because muscle contraction results in the accumulation of lactate and CO_2, which counteracts the respiratory reduction of CO_2.

When a person inhales CO_2 mixed with air or when pulmonary disease prevents exhalation of the CO_2 normally produced by body metabolism, cerebral vasodilation results and may increase blood flow by as much as 50% in the acute situation. Respiratory acidosis may overcome the intrinsic autoregulatory capacity of the cerebral vessels, causing intensive vasodilation and sometimes transudation of fluid. This leads to cerebral edema and ICP with headache. Clinically, this condition is seen in patients whose respiratory mechanics are impaired by obesity (Pickwickian syndrome), musculoskeletal diseases, and pulmonary diseases, such as emphysema and alveolar capillary block. Chronic CO_2 retention, however, leads to a compensatory adaptation and normalization of the CBF.

Generally speaking, the effects of too much or too little oxygen on autoregulation are the opposite of those described for CO_2. Arterial Po_2 is normally about 80 mm Hg, whereas jugular venous Po_2 is about 34 mm Hg. Oxygen tension in tissue is somewhat less than that in the capillaries because oxygen must diffuse from the blood through the capillary wall into the tissue surrounding it. Although hypoxia results in some vasodilation, this is seldom enough to maintain constant oxygenation. Vasodilation begins when the PaO_2 drops below 80 mm Hg and becomes maximal at an arterial Po_2 of about 25 mm Hg. Consciousness is lost when the PaO_2 falls to 18 mm Hg.[49]

Following interruption of blood flow oxygen levels fall rapidly within the area of hypoperfusion. The brain can survive brief periods of anoxia provided that cerebral perfusion remains intact, but oxidative phosphorylation is impaired and metabolism will depend on shifting to anaerobic glycolysis. However, compared to aerobic conditions ATP production in anaerobic metabolism remains significantly decreased with subsequent danger of permanent brain damage and neurological deficit. Different areas of the brain exhibit different susceptibility to hypoxic injury. This selective hypoxic susceptibility may be determined by vascular supply, genetic factors, design of local neuronal circuits, regional characteristics of receptors, or other unknown variables. Hypoxia-susceptible regions include parts of the hippocampus, the basal ganglia, the Purkinje cells in the cerebellum, or certain cortical cell layers, to name a few. The effect of increased oxygen levels in the setting of acute cerebral infarction remains currently investigational.

When supplementary oxygen is given to patients with deficient pulmonary gas exchange, the effect may be to depress respiration, thereby causing a decrease in the exchange of oxygen and CO_2. The resultant accumulation of CO_2 in the bloodstream may lead to CO_2 narcosis. The administration of oxygen to people with normal pulmonary exchange causes a slight increase in the volume of oxygen dissolved in the plasma. If oxygen pressure is increased as much as three atmospheres, a much larger volume of oxygen is carried to the brain, but hyperoxia can be toxic to the neurons and interfere with function. Moderate elevations of ambient atmospheric pressure, in contrast, may improve brain oxygenation and exert a neuroprotective effect without undue toxicity. However, the use of hyperbaric and normobaric oxygen treatment for ischemic stroke remains controversial.

INTRACRANIAL PRESSURE

Encased within its bony cavity, the brain has a specific gravity somewhat greater than that of the CSF that surrounds it. In the erect position, it lies semisuspended from the veins that connect it to the dura, delicately poised on the arteries and the bony structures below.

With each systole a pulse of blood courses through the cerebral arteries, transmitting an impulse to the brain and possibly increasing its volume somewhat. Under normal conditions the brain itself probably distends little, if at all, because venous blood leaves the parenchyma as rapidly as arterial blood enters. The volume of blood within the intracranial arteries and veins at any one time is normally about 100 ml. If this changes for any reason, a concomitant readjustment in the volume of the CSF takes place; otherwise, pressure within the skull would be altered because the brain is not compressible (Monro-Kellie doctrine). Nevertheless, normal or slightly raised ICP bears no consistent relationship to CBF. However, in the presence of ICP exceeding 30 mm Hg, increased CBF raises ICP and results in a further decrease in flow.[50]

BRAIN-BLOOD BARRIER

Except for the area postrema, choroid plexus, pineal, and posterior pituitary gland, all of the brain is protected by an endothelial and a biochemical barrier. The tight junctions between the vascular endothelial cells and the relative paucity of pinocytic vesicles effectively exclude most blood macromolecules from the brain. By the same token, the BBB prevents brain chemicals, such as neurotransmitters, from leaking into the blood. However, areas of the brain that produce hormones or function as chemoreceptors are supplied by capillaries with a porous endothelium that facilitates easy exchange of materials between the brain and the blood.

In general, lipid-soluble substances can diffuse easily through the BBB, while water soluble molecules require a carrier system to reach brain cells. Large and charged molecules also have difficulty traversing the blood-brain barrier. Moreover, after an injury the endothelium itself can secrete substances that have a profound effect on local flow.

The blood-brain interface has multiple barrier systems that regulate the passage of substances between blood and brain to preserve homeostasis. In pathological states these endothelial-astrocytic regulatory systems may be unequally affected, resulting in differences in rapidity of both transfer of various metabolites. Either or both may be disturbed and result in neural dysfunction.

About 90% of the energy needed for transmission of neural impulses and for maintenance of membrane gradients is obtained by glucose metabolism. Temporary occlusion of an artery with subsequent restitution of pressure and flow is accompanied by marked reactive hyperemia followed by leakage of fluid from the capillaries until there is a secondary breakdown of the BBB, associated permanent ischemia, and closure of the capillary bed.[51] The endothelial and glial cells swell during or immediately after the ischemic insult, resulting in marked reduction of the lumens of the cerebral capillaries. To a certain degree this depends on the pathogenesis, that is, hypotension, microembolus, or anoxia.

Complete interruption of CBF in the normothermic brain causes suppression of the electrical activity within 12 to 15 seconds, inhibition of transsynaptic excitation after 2 to 4 minutes, and abolition of electrical excitability after 4 to 6 minutes. Metabolism and all anabolic processes break down shortly later. Catabolic processes during the first hour of ischemia are minor, but severe disturbances of ion homeostasis occur. Extracellular potassium rises from 3 meq/l to more than 50 meq/l, and extracellular sodium decreases to about the same level. The cells imbibe as much as 50% of the extracellular fluid volume and swell proportionately, causing ion shifts. Brain osmolality during this time increases by more than 50 milliosmols.

After blood flow is restored, equilibration of the osmotic and ionic concentration gradients causes severe brain swelling. Brain volume may increase more than 10 volume percent, causing a remarkable increase in intracranial pressure of up to 75 mm Hg. In addition, endothelial swelling and changes in blood viscosity prevent recirculation (no-reflow phenomenon). However, restoration of sufficient perfusion pressure can keep damaged tissue alive, sometimes as long as 1 hour, presumably by keeping the capillaries patent, while washing away products of cellular metabolism, such as heat, lactic acid, and hydrogen ions.

Ischemic stroke results in failure of ion channel pumps with subsequent loss of ion concentration gradients. Sodium then diffuses into the cells, increasing the osmotic pressure. Water follows the increased osmotic pressure, and the cells start to swell. Cytotoxic brain edema develops, affecting mainly the gray matter. Initially functional endothelial cells can control the sodium influx into the extracellular compartment. Subsequent disruption of the BBB induced by impaired cerebral autoregulation, acute reperfusion injury, or decreased cerebral perfusion leads to leakage of sodium into the extracellular space. This increase in extracellular fluid characterizes vascular edema. Cells continue to swell, increasing cerebral edema. This affects mainly the white matter, and ICP can increase dramatically.[52] Following large territory strokes such as an acute middle cerebral artery infarction, both forms of edema develop simultaneously, leading to malignant cerebral edema. Especially in young people who have nonatrophic brains with tightly packed neurons, volume expansion in the limited room of the skull is not tolerated, and lethal edema can develop rapidly. In this situation emergent hemi-craniectomy can be life saving.

MICROCIRCULATORY COMPROMISE

During circulatory arrest or episodes of severely decreased cerebral perfusion pressure blood viscosity increases, and endothelial cells and microglia are damaged and swell, compromising blood flow in the microcirculation.[53] Despite reinstitution of perfusion pressure and systemic blood flow within adequate time limits for cerebral resuscitation, CBF does not reestablish sufficiently to avoid brain injury under these circumstances. Similarly, recanalization of blood flow by thrombolysis of a temporarily occluded artery may not lead to adequate cerebral blood flow in the supplied vascular territory on postinterventional imaging studies. Recanalization does not necessarily equal adequate cerebral perfusion because focal ischemic stroke can cause significant impairment of flow in the microvasculature as well. Potential mechanisms involved in this process include leukocyte endothelial adhesion, disruption of the BBB, integrin-matrix interactions, and activation of platelets and deposition of fibrin in small vessels.

In addition to the effects of ischemia on the brain and vasomotor tone, stagnant blood within the vascular bed is also affected. Stasis initiates platelet adhesion and aggregation followed by formation of a fibrin gel. After ischemic infarction, there is platelet aggregation that can be quantitated by elevated levels of platelet factor 4, a protein stored in dense bodies within the platelet and released during the irreversible phase of platelet aggregation. This antiheparin protein is located in the alpha granules bound to the glycosaminoglycan carrier chondroitin sulfate. This phenomenon is common to all the platelets in the systemic circulation as well as the affected brain circulation.

Microcirculatory changes include vasodilatation, segmental spasm, and paralysis. The column of blood stagnates and darkens due to O_2 extraction. Arterial spasm may develop. With restoration of flow, the chain of events reverses. Venous blood becomes red. Flow becomes laminar and the cortex resumes it normal color. There ensues a hyperemic state caused by vasoparalysis. Then endothelial blebs may obstruct microcirculation and limit reperfusion.

REPERFUSION INJURY

Following cerebral hypoperfusion in acute stroke, postischemic hyperperfusion or luxury perfusion can develop. Although hyperperfusion in the penumbral zone can help to recanalize flow in temporarily closed blood vessels and can limit infarct growth, it can lead to reperfusion injury in the core of the infarction. In the ischemic core endothelial cells are damaged, causing disruption of the blood brain area. If hyperemia occurs, it can lead to increased edema and hemorrhagic transformation.

THE ISCHEMIC PENUMBRA

Acute ischemic stroke causes an area of dying tissue surrounded by hypoperfused, nonfunctional, but still potentially viable brain surrounding the ischemic core. The core of an ischemic infarction has been shown to grow in a centrifugal fashion over time (Figure 4-5). PET studies in humans have demonstrated infarct

extension up to 48 hours following cerebral infarction and possibly longer. Within the core cerebral perfusion has decreased below the critical threshold necessary to maintain cellular energy metabolism. Affected cells have lost structural integrity and become irreversibly damaged by ischemia. Cells in the ischemic core die and necrosis develops. Surrounding this epicenter cerebral blood flow has diminished but can temporarily sustain brain metabolism, function, and structural integrity. This zone, characterized by oligemia and by an increased oxygen extraction fraction, is called the penumbra. Depending on the severity and duration of ischemia and the efficiency of reperfusion, penumbral tissue may fully recover or die. In the penumbra cellular death involves a combination of both necrosis and apoptosis. In contrast to necrosis, apoptosis is characterized by condensation of the nucleus and breakdown of cellular components without induction of an inflammatory response.

The evolution of cerebral infarction is a highly dynamic process. PET studies suggest that regions with rCBF below 12 ml/100 g/min do not retain their viability and undergo infarction, whereas regions with rCBF between 12 and 22 ml/100 g/min are in an unstable state where infarction will occur if perfusion disturbance persists. Neural depolarizations, transmitter release, oxygen and substrate demand, depletion of ATP, and influx of calcium are all increased in the penumbra tissue. In this unstable ("to be or not") state, evidently lasting only a few hours, ischemic penumbra may preserve its vitality given that early restoration of perfusion has occurred, either spontaneously or through interventional thrombolysis.

Normally CBF in the resting state is greater through the frontal areas of the brain than that in the parietal and temporal regions – the "hyperfrontal" pattern. If a person becomes anxious or excited, this baseline flow becomes exaggerated. Furthermore, the resting pattern changes in response to various activities. For example, if a subject opens and closes his right hand repeatedly, flow increases in the left motor strip and, to a lesser degree, in the right as well. Similarly, tracking eye movements produce a focal blood flow increase in the frontal eye areas and in the occipital regions. In contrast, a motionless stimulus, for instance, a stationary light, increases CBF only in the inferior occipital area. On the other hand, a complex act, such as speaking, increases flow in the mouth and tongue motor and supplementary motor areas and in the auditory cortices,

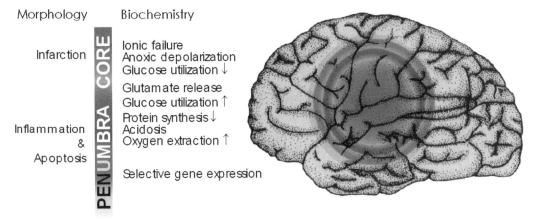

Figure 4-5. The ischemic penumbra can enlarge over time. Early intervention aims at restoring function of this area of viable tissue. Reprinted with permission from Dirnagl et al.[66]

with changes being more pronounced in the left supplementary motor and mouth regions. Listening to speech induces an increase in CBF in the left and, to a lesser extent, to the right temporal auditory cortices and Wernicke's area. Listening to music, calculating, and stereo perception produce their own characteristic alterations in rCBF. Metabolic mapping shows patterns of local brain increases similar to those of rCBF, suggesting that there is a close coupling between blood flow and metabolism and that increases in rCBF are mediated by increased metabolic requirements of activated neurons.

In contrast to the sequence of events caused by focal or global ischemia, anoxia is always generalized and affects all bodily tissues. The extreme and generalized vasodilatation that results from hypoxia creates an enormous blood flow through the oxygen-starved tissue. All cells, including capillary endothelium, are affected, so that they swell and later occlude their lumens. Endothelial cells are relatively resistant to hypoxic injury and are more susceptible to injury from lactic acidosis seen in stenotic arteries. However, with mild hypoxia, flow remains increased, so there is neither formation of clot nor accumulation of metabolites. Increasing concentrations of lactic acid and carbon dioxide cause extracellular acidosis with relaxation of smooth muscle cells and an increase in regional blood flow.

In the acute phase of arterial occlusion, there is a reduction in CBF, perhaps accompanied by a hyperemic flow in adjacent zones. The initial hyperemia occurs in response to metabolic needs and represents luxury perfusion. The delayed hyperemia occurs in the chronic stage and is probably the result of the growth of new capillaries. Therefore, the stages of evolution of ischemia can be divided into one of hypoperfusion with normal metabolism, a second one with hyperperfusion and impaired metabolism, and a final stage of infarction.[54]

Imaging studies indicate multiple penumbral layers of brain tissue showing different degrees of impaired neuronal and metabolic function. PET studies in patients with acute stroke show the infarcted core characterized by decreased CBF and oxygen metabolism, surrounded by areas of hypoperfusion but increased oxygen extraction fraction and normal glucose metabolism, surrounded by regions with normal to increased glucose metabolism, but decreased CBF and oxygen consumption. Animal experiments have shown the existence of multiple penumbral layers, characterized by different molecular events such as expression of genes or the presence of proteins triggered by thresholds of perfusion.[38,55] Electrical activity and ionic and transmitter homeostasis all have their own thresholds of CBF reduction before they become disrupted.

The mechanisms underlying the extension of the infarcted core over time are not completely understood. Continued artery-to-artery embolic events and thrombus propagation can be important for infarct progression. In addition, postischemic hyperexcitability may significantly contribute to the delayed progression of brain damage. Following cerebral hypoperfusion, excitatory transmitters are released from synapses and damaged cell membranes. They induce depolarization of cellular membranes, causing a wave of spreading electrical depression that originates in the penumbra and travels across the

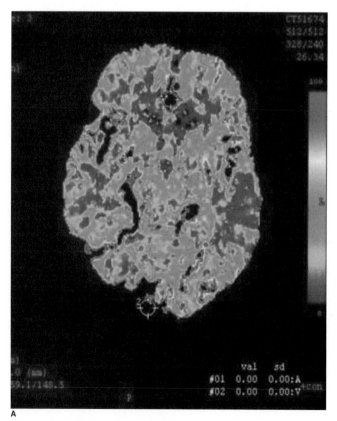
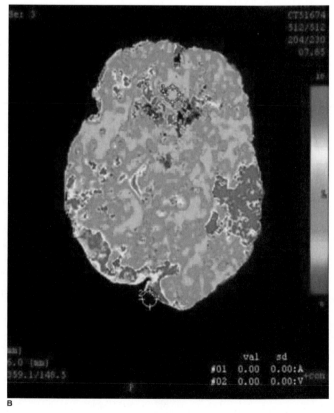

Figure 4-6.   Imaging of the penumbra by perfusion cranial CT in an individual with left posterior MCA territory ischemia: (A) an area of decreased CBF (*dark blue*), (B) increased MTT of the contrast agent (*red*). The noncontrast cranial CT was within normal limits before and following the administration of tPA.

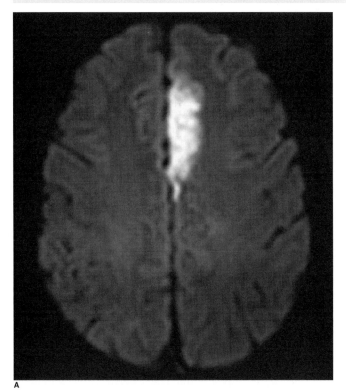
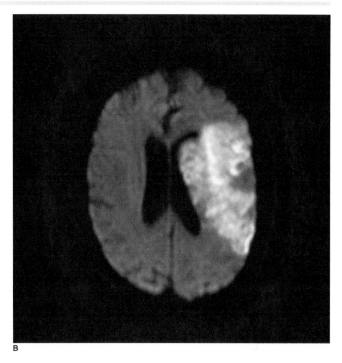

Figure 4-7. Brain MRIs illustrating acute infarctions visible by restricted diffusion that appears bright on diffusion-weighted sequences. A: Diffusion-weighted axial MRI showing an acute left anterior cerebral artery infarction in a man who was subsequently found to have infectious endocarditis and cardioembolic stroke. B: Diffusion-weighted axial MRI showing an acute infarction in the left middle cerebral artery territory. The patient presented with acute aphasia and right hemiparesis and numbness.

entire hemisphere. These postischemic depolarizations activate rather large groups of neuronal networks, which requires energy and oxygen. In the penumbral zone, which is characterized by neuronal uncoupling, this may enhance energy depletion, causing cellular damage and death. Cortical spreading depression has also been identified as the main mechanism underlying gene induction in the remote nonischemic cortex. This dynamic spatiotemporal pattern of gene induction may cause remote cell damage or, alternatively, mediate neuroprotection, tissue remodeling, and functional recovery.

Imaging the Ischemic Penumbra

To identify stroke patients who might benefit from thrombolysis and to better understand the brain's pathophysiological mechanisms, functional imaging is essential. Chapter 5 considers the clinical diagnostic evaluation in more detail.

Imaging modalities include, among others, positron emission tomography, SPECT, stable-xenon computed tomography, diffusion/perfusion weighted (DW/PW)–based MRI mismatch, magnetic resonance spectroscopy (MRS), or most recently dynamic cerebral perfusion computer tomography.[56] Dynamic perfusion CT is readily available in most institutions treating acute ischemic stroke patients and allows assessment of rCBF and blood volume (rCBV). Pixel-by-pixel calculation of rCBF, rCBV, and contrast mean transit time (MTT) results in construction of brain maps representing normal brain tissue, infracted areas, and the penumbra.[57] The methods provide information on infarct size, extent of the penumbra, and assessment of clinical prognosis for acute stroke patients, although it

has been argued that quantification of physiological flow parameters is problematic (Figure 4-6).

MRI is used to differentiate between the ischemic core, visible within minutes on DW-MRI (Figure 4-7), and the potentially salvageable ischemic penumbra, visible on PW-MRI. However, the magnetic resonance concept of the diffusion-perfusion mismatch has some shortcomings in identifying the penumbra reliably.[58] The addition of MR-spectroscopy allows metabolic imaging of lactate as a marker of ischemia and evaluation of energy metabolism by measurement of phosphorus and its chemical compounds, and can estimate neuronal loss and damage to cellular membranes. Currently it remains controversial which of the imaging studies, CT-based techniques, SPECT, or MRI, is more feasible to use in identifying salvageable tissue.

PET is able to measure physiological flow parameters such as rCBF, rCBV, and metabolic rates of glucose, oxygen, and other metabolites quantitatively, but its wide application is limited by relatively high costs and complex logistics.[59,60]

Combination of different imaging modality promises more precise construction of probability maps predicting which part of the penumbral tissue becomes infracted and which can be preserved by an acute intervention. However, these combined investigational methods are time consuming and technically complex.

PHYSIOLOGIC VARIABLES

CBF and the brain's response to hypoxia and ischemia are influenced by a variety of normal and abnormal physiologic factors. Younger individuals, for example, may have greater tolerance to periods of hypoxia and ischemia. The body temperature can increase or decrease the brain's metabolic demands, rendering it more or less susceptible to the effects of hypoxia. Maintenance of blood flow during hypoxia results in lengthened tissue survival, perhaps because blood flow carries away toxic metabolites and heat of metabolism.

Metabolic requirements, as expressed by blood glucose and the availability of other nutrients, also have an effect, and hypoglycemia combined with hypoxia and ischemia is a worse combination than any of the three alone. Similarly, by increasing the brain's metabolic demands, a seizure can exacerbate an already dire situation during a period of hypoxia or ischemia.

Temperature

Clinical and experimental studies demonstrate a hyperthermia-dependent exacerbation of ischemic injury and neurological outcome.[61,62] Metabolic processes can be accelerated by an increase in temperature, resulting in increased utilization of cellular energy and additional metabolic stress to the hypoperfused brain tissue. Consequently hyperthermia accentuates the metabolic energy depletion within the penumbra. In addition, hyperthermia accelerates all biochemical reactions involved in the pathophysiology of the ischemic cascade contributing to the conversion of the penumbra into an irreversible lesion. Recent work suggests a neuroprotective effect of hypothermia with improved neurological outcome following global hypoxia/ischemia after cardiac arrest and potentially after focal brain ischemia.

Blood Pressure

Ischemic stroke results in regional loss of autoregulation. Therefore blood flow in these areas parallels the systemic perfusion pressure. If systemic blood pressure rises too high, the BBB can be disrupted, which can result in cerebral edema or hemorrhagic transformation. Stroke patients with chronic hypertension and sustained high blood pressure are especially predisposed to develop cerebral edema and hemorrhagic transformation. On the other hand, in patients with chronic hypertension the autoregulatory plateau is shifted to higher values. If systemic blood pressure is reduced dramatically, these individuals can develop ischemic infarctions at relatively high blood pressures. In the acute phase of an infarction the blood pressure must be monitored continuously and needs to be adjusted to relatively higher values to maintain cerebral perfusion.

Glucose

Hypoperfusion and ischemia cause acute substrate deficiency, depleting cells of necessary energy. Furthermore there is evidence that hypoglycemia can activate excitatory amino acids such as aspartate and glutamate, which are potent cytotoxic agents involved in the ischemic cascade. Yet in acute ischemic stroke hyperglycemia increases mortality and infarct size and has a detrimental effect on neurological outcome.[63–65] This is especially seen in patients receiving thrombolytics. The effect of glucose levels on stroke outcome may depend on residual brain perfusion in the penumbra and the status of vascular collaterals. In small infarctions with good collateralization of blood flow hyperglycemia may even improve neurological outcome by facilitation of energy metabolism. Below a critical perfusion threshold elevated glucose may have the opposite effect. Glucose levels should be normalized to 120–150 mg/dl in nondiabetic patients and to 120–200 in diabetic patients with acute ischemic stroke.

Sleep

Frequent changes in regional flow occur not only in the awake but also in the sleeping brain. The average CBF increases mildly during slow-wave sleep and more markedly during rapid eye movement (REM) sleep. On the other hand, CBF and metabolism are depressed during coma, from any cause, with the extent of the metabolic change generally paralleling the depth of coma.

Seizures

Seizures, either spontaneous or those induced by electroconvulsive therapy, are accompanied by greatly increased CBF and metabolism. Within a seizure focus, local CBF and glucose metabolism almost double, whereas the overall flow increases are more modest. If seizures occur as complication of a stroke, they should be treated appropriately, especially because they can increase the metabolic demand on the brain in the acute phase.

CONCLUSION

Advances in basic sciences and neuroimaging technology allow us to better understand the basic pathophysiology of brain hypoxia, ischemia, and the metabolic effects of stroke. Despite the complexity of the accumulating data, this improved understanding will ultimately help improve patient management and clinical outcome. Unraveling the pathophysiological mechanisms involved in primary and secondary ischemic injury might lead the way to new stroke treatments such as novel drugs, tissue engineering, or stem cell therapy.

REFERENCES

1. Laughlin SB, de Ruyter van Stevenick RR, Anderson JC. The metabolic cost of neuronal information. *Nature Neurosci.* 1998;**1**: 36–41.
2. Shulman RG, Rothman DL, Behar KL, Hyder F. Energetic basis of brain activity: implications for neuroimaging. *Trends Neurosci.* 2004;**27**(8):489–495.
3. Aaslid R, Lindegaard KF, Sorteberg W, et al. Cerebral autoregulation dynamics in humans. *Stroke.* 1989;**20**:45–52.
4. Strandgaard S, Paulson OB. Cerebral autoregulation. *Stroke.* 1984;**15**:413–416.
5. Ernsting J. The effects of hypoxia upon human performance and the electroencephalogram. *Int Anesthesiol Clin.* 1966;**4**:245–259.
6. Smith AL. Effect of anesthetics and oxygen deprivation on brain blood flow and metabolism. *Surg Clin North Am.* 1975;**55**:819–836.
7. Michael JA. Neurophysiological effects of hypoxia. *Monogr Neural Sci.* 1973;**1**:65–121.
8. Astrup J, Siesjö BK, Symon L, et al. Thresholds in cerebral ischemia – the ischemic penumbra. *Stroke.* 1981;**12**:723–725.
9. Heiss WD. Flow thresholds of functional and morphological damage of tissue. *Stroke.* 1983;**14**:329–331.
10. Klehmet J, Harms H, Richter M, et al. Stroke-induced immunodepression and post-stroke infections: Lessons from the Preventive Antibacterial Therapy in Stroke trial. *Neuroscience.* 2009; **158**:1184–1193.
11. Chamorro A, Amaro S, Vargas M, et al. Catecholamines, infection, and death in acute ischemic stroke. *J Neurol Sci.* 2007;**252**:29–35.

12. Prass K, Meisel C, Höflich C, et al. Stroke-induced immunodeficiency promotes spontaneous bacterial infections and is mediated by sympathetic activation reversal by poststroke T helper cell type1-like immunostimulation. *J Exp Med*. 2003;**198**:725–736.

13. Yrjanheikki J, Tikka T, Keinanan R, et al. A tetracycline derivative, minocycline, reduces inflammation and protects against focal cerebral ischemia with a wide therapeutic window. *Proc Natl Acad Sci USA*. 1999;**96**:13496–13500.

14. Novak V, Chowdhary A, Farrar B, et al. Altered cerebral vasoregulation in hypertension and stroke. *Neurology*. 2003;**60**:1657–1663.

15. Markus HS. Cerebral perfusion and stroke. *J Neurol Neurosurg Psychiatry*. 2004;**75**:353–361.

16. Wise RJS, Bernardi S, Frackowiak RSJ, et al. Serial observations on the pathophysiology of acute stroke. The transition from ischemia to infarction as reflected in regional oxygen extraction. *Brain*. 1983;**106**:197–222.

17. Masdeu JC, Brass LM. SPECT imaging of stroke. *J Neuroimaging*. 1995;**5**(Suppl 1):14–22.

18. Ackerman RH, Alpert NM, Correia JA, et al. Positron imaging in ischemic stroke disease. *Ann Neurol*. 1984;**15**(Suppl):S126–130.

19. Ibaraki M, Shimosegawa E, Miura S, et al. PET measurements of CBF, OEF, and CMRO2 without arterial sampling in hyperacute ischemic stroke: method and error analysis. *Ann Nucl Med*. 2004;**18**:35–44.

20. Heiss W-D, Kracht LW, Thiel A, et al. Penumbral probability thresholds of cortical flumazenil binding and blood flow predicting tissue outcome in patients with cerebral ischaemia. *Brain*. 2001;**124**:20–29.

21. Ebinger M, De Silva DA, Christensen S, et al. Imaging the penumbra – strategies to detect tissue at risk after ischemic stroke. *J Clin Neurosci*. 2009;**16**:178–187.

22. Baron JC. Mapping the ischemic penumbra with PET: implications for acute stroke treatment. *Cerebrovasc Dis*. 1999;**9**:193–201.

23. Powers WJ, Zazulia AR. The use of positron emission tomography in cerebrovascular disease. *Neuroimaging Clin N Am*. 2003;**13**:741–758.

24. Friedman M, Byers SO. Experimantal thromboatherosclerosis. *J Clin Invest*. 1961;**40**:1139–1152.

25. Zugibe FT, Brown KD. Histochemical studies in atherogenesis. *Circulat Res*. 1961;**9**:897–905.

26. Feigin I, Budzilovich GN. The general pathology of cerebrovascualr disease. In: Vinken PJ, Bruyn GW, eds. *Handbook of Clinical Neurology. Vascular Diseases of the Nervous System*. Part I. Amsterdam: North-Holland Publishing Company; 1972:118–127.

27. Fisher CM. Occlusion of the carotid arteries: further experiences. *Arch Neurol Psych*. 1954;**72**:187–204.

28. Zülch KJ. Die Pathogenese von Massenblutung und Erweichung unter besonderer Berücksichtigung klinischer Gesichtspunkte. *Acat Neurochir*. 1961;**7**(Suppl):51–117.

29. Xiong ZG, Zhu XM, Chu XP, et al. Neuroprotection in ischemia: blocking calcium-permeable acid sensing ion channels. *Cell*. 2004;**118**:687–698.

30. Paschen W. Role of calcium in neuronal injury. *Brain Res Bull*. 2000;**53**:409–413.

31. Endres M, Dirnagl U. Ischemia and stroke. *Adv Exp Med Biol*. 2002;**513**:455–473.

32. Zjemg Z, Zjap J, Steomberg GL, et al. Cellular and molecular events underlying ischemia-induced neuronal apoptosis. *Drug News Perspect*. 2003;**16**:497–503.

33. Mergenthaler P, Dirnagl U, Meisel A. Pathophysiology of stroke: lessons from animal models. *Metab Brain Dis*. 2004;**19**:151–167.

34. Majno G, Joris I. Apoptosis, oncosis, and necrosis. An overview of cell death. *Am J Pathol*. 1995;**146**:3–15.

35. Yuan J, Yanker B. Apoptosis in the nervous system. *Nature*. 2000;**407**:802–809.

36. Clarkson AN, Sutherland BA, Appleton I. The biology and pathology of hypoxia-ischemia: an update. *Arch Immunol Ther Exp*. 2005;**53**(3):213–225.

37. Hossmann YA. Viability thresholds and the penumbra of focal ischemia. *Ann Neurol*. 1994;**36**:557–565.

38. Ginsberg MD. Adventures in the pathophysiology of brain ischemia: penumbra, gene expression, neuroprotection. The 2002 Thomas Willis Lecture. *Stroke*. 2003;**34**:214–223.

39. Shi H, Liu KJ. Cerebral tissue oxygenation and oxidative brain injury during ischemia and reperfusion. *Front Biosci*. 2007;**12**:1318–1328.

40. Lust WD, Taylor C, Pundik S, et al. Ischemic cell death: dynamics of delayed secondary energy failure during reperfusion following focal ischemia. *Metab Brain Dis*. 2002;**17**:113–121.

41. Nagel S, Papadakis M, Hoyte L, et al. Therapeutic hypothermia in experimental models of focal and global cerebral ischemia and intracerebral hemorrhage. *Expert Rev Neurother*. 2008;**8**:1255–1268.

42. Lazzaro MA, Prabhakaran S. Induced hypothermia in acute ischemic stroke. *Expert Opin Investig Drugs*. 2008;**17**:1161–1174.

43. Yenari M, Kitagawa K, Lyden P, et al. Metabolic downregulation: a key to successful neuroprotection? *Stroke*. 2008;**39**:2910–2917.

44. Baumbach GL, Heistad DD, Siems JE. Effects of sympathetic nerves on composition and distensibility of cerebral arterioles in rats. *J Physiol*. 1989;**416**:123–140.

45. Mayhan WG, Werber AH, Heistad DD. Protection of cerebral vessels by sympathetic nerves and vascular hypertrophy. *Circulation*. 1987;**75**:107–112.

46. Asahi M, Wang X, Mori T, et al. Effects of matrix metalloproteinase 9 gene knockout on the proteolysis of blood-brain barrier and white matter components after cerebral ischemia. *J Neurosci*. **2201**;21:7724–7732.

47. Samdani AF, Dawson TM, Dawson WL Nitric oxide synthase in models of focal ischemia. *Stroke*. 1997;**28**:1283–1288.

48. Dalkara T, Yoshida T, Irikura K, et al. Dual role of nitric oxide in focal cerebral ischemia. *Neuropharmacology*. 1994;**33**:1447–1452.

49. Kety SS. The physiology of the cerebral circulation. In: Vinken PJ, Bruyn GW, eds. *Handbook of Clinical Neurology. Vascular Diseases of the Nervous System*. Part I. Amsterdam: North-Holland Publishing Company; 1972:118–127.

50. Dietrich WD. Morphological manifestations of reperfusion injury in brain. *Ann NY Acad Sci*. 1994;**723**:15–24.

51. Klotzo I. Neuropathological aspects of barin edema. *J Neuropathol Exp Neurol*. 1967;**26**:1–14.

52. Ayata C, Ropper AH. Ischaemic brain oedema. *J Clin Neurosci*. 2002;**9**:113–124.

53. del Zoppo GJ, Mabuchi T. Cerebral microvessel responses to focal ischemia. *J Cereb Blood Flow Metab*. 2003;**23**:879–894.

54. Fieschi C, et al. Therapeutic window for pharmacological treatment in acute focal cerebral ischemia. *Ann NY Acad Sci*. 1988;**522**:662–666.

55. Weinstein PR, Hong S, Sharp FR. Molecular identification of the ischemic pneumbra. *Stroke*. 2004;**35**(Suppl 1):2666–2670.

56. Guadagno JV, Donnan GA, Markus R, et al. Imaging the ischemic penumbra. *Curr Opin Neurol*. 2004;**17**:61–67.

57. Schramm P, Schellinger PD, Klotz E, et al. Comparison of perfusion computed tomography and computed tomography angiography source images with perfusion-weighted imaging and diffusion-weighted imaging in patients with acute stroke of less than 6 hours' duration. *Stroke*. 2004;**35**:1657–1658.

58. Guadagno JV, Warburton EA, Aigbirhio FI, et al. Does the acute diffusion-weighted imaging lesion represent penumbra as well

as core? A combined quantitative PET/MRI voxel-based study. *J Cereb Blood Flow Metab.* 2004;**24**:1249–1254.

59. Heiss W-D, Sobesky J, v. Smekal U, et al. Probability of cortical infarction predicted by Flumazenil binding and diffusion-weighted imaging signal intensity. *Stroke.* 2004;**35**:1892–1898.

60. Heiss WD. Imaging the ischemic penumbra and treatment effects by PET. *Keio J Med.* 2001;**50**:249–256.

61. Zaremba J. Hyperthermia in ischemic stroke. *Med Sci Monit.* 2004;**10**:RA148–153.

62. Kagansky N, Levy S, Knobler H. The role of hyperglycemia in acute stroke. *Arch Neurol.* 2001;**58**:1209–1212.

63. Alvarez-Sabin J, Molina CA, Ribo M, et al. Impact of admission hyperglycemia on stroke outcome after thrombolysis: risk stratification in relation to time to reperfusion. *Stroke.* 2004;**35**:2493–2498.

64. Nagi M, Pfefferkorn T, Haberl RL. Blutzucker und Schlaganfall. *Nervenarzt.* 1999;**70**:944–949.

65. Dirnagl U, Simon RP, Hallenbeck JM. Ischemic tolerance and endogenous neuroprotection. *Trends Neurosci.* 2003;**26**;248–254.

66. Dirnagl U, Iadecola C, Moskowitz MA. Pathobiology of ischaemic stroke: an integrated view. *Trends Neurosci.* 1999;**22**:391–397.

5

Diagnostic Evaluation of Stroke

The misuse of diagnostic techniques begins when the physician fails to have the proper medical question in mind. The technique is often asked to answer the wrong question.

J. Willis Hurst

Stroke and transient ischemic attacks (TIAs) are medical emergencies, just as are their cardiac equivalents, acute myocardial infarction and unstable angina. A TIA is a warning sign of an impending stroke, and its acute management provides a window of opportunity for primary stroke prevention. The stroke risk following a TIA is estimated to be 3% to 18% during the first month.[1–5] Acute stroke patients must be evaluated urgently if they are to benefit from thrombolysis or other types of acute therapy and to prevent stroke extension and treat medical complications. Similarly, intracranial hemorrhage is an emergency, and timely assessment can lead to more rapid therapy and an improved outcome. Therefore any type of cerebrovascular event requires immediate diagnostic evaluation and intervention.

Techniques for obtaining a focused neurological history and comprehensive examination are presented in Chapter 2. This chapter reviews the diagnostic studies that are useful in the assessment of cerebrovascular dysfunction.

GENERAL APPROACH TO PATIENT EVALUATION

Although an array of neuroimaging methods is available to assess patients with acute ischemic or hemorrhagic stroke, the studies need to be individualized and tailored to the clinical situation. The diagnostic evaluation is likely to be substantially different for a young patient versus an old one or for an individual with an infarction as opposed to one with a hemorrhagic stroke. Whenever possible the initial evaluation should be minimally invasive, then progress to more invasive methods when necessary.

Cranial computed tomography (CT) or brain magnetic resonance imaging (MRI) are usually performed emergently to rule out intracranial hemorrhage, identify the location and extent of a cerebral infarction, and exclude other conditions such as a brain tumor or central nervous system (CNS) infection. Most medical centers still focus initially on structural brain imaging with cranial CT, but the increasing availability and rapid advancement of new generations of ultra-fast CT scanners and more sophisticated software allow simultaneous assessment of the brain vasculature and tissue perfusion status even during the initial scan.

Neuroimaging plays an important role in the early identification of patients who may benefit from thrombolysis or other acute vascular intervention and allows clinicians to monitor therapeutic results and observe for complications such as hemorrhagic transformation or cerebral edema. It is also the basis for endovascular treatment of vascular lesions or diagnosis of the vascular abnormalities underlying intracranial hemorrhages. The patient's neuroimaging studies must be interpreted in light of information gleaned earlier from the history and neurological examination. Generally this is best accomplished at a site with a stroke team experienced in the planning and interpretation of diagnostic studies along with experience in acute therapeutic intervention and clinical management.[6–8]

Determination of the exact onset time of stroke symptoms, preferably verified by a third party, is essential if thrombolytic agents are to be considered. Time is of the essence in these individuals, so a cranial CT or brain MRI with diffusion-weighted imaging (DWI) and perfusion-weighted imaging (PWI) sequences to differentiate ischemic and hemorrhagic infarction and to detect early signs of brain ischemia and arterial occlusion should be initiated quickly after the patient arrives.

LABORATORY STUDIES

After a complete history and general physical and neurological examinations (see Chapter 2), a complete blood count, coagulation studies, serum glucose and electrolyte values, and a pregnancy test for women of childbearing age are appropriate. Further laboratory studies depend on individual history and clinical circumstances. In patients older than 60 years, basic studies include a complete blood count with differential, fibrinogen, coagulation studies, basic metabolic panel, fasting lipid profile, sedimentation rate, HbA1c, thyroid stimulating hormone, and homocysteine level. A baseline chest X-ray is usually appropriate. Stroke in younger individuals or an unusual clinical presentation usually triggers a more extensive evaluation for less common causes of cerebrovascular lesions. Additional laboratory studies include a urine drug screen, tests for rheumatologic disorders, evaluation for thrombophilia and a hypercoagulable state with a thrombophilia screen, and measurement of antiphospholipid antibodies.

The majority of stroke patients undergo a swallowing evaluation by a speech therapist after initial bedside screening to avoid aspiration pneumonia secondary to dysphagia. However, swallowing function should be reassessed after several days in initially obtunded patients, who often perform better after their level of awareness has improved. Reevaluation frequently shows relatively rapid recovery from dysphagia, and the placement of a percutaneous endogastric feeding tube can sometimes be avoided in these individuals.[9–11]

Patients with suspected cardiac embolism should undergo a transthoracic echocardiogram with intravenous injection of agitated saline to screen for an intracardiac shunt, calculate the ejection fraction, and assess myocardial and valvular function and morphology. Especially if the visual quality of the images is poor, as in very obese patients, or if a more precise view of the left atrium or the aortic arch is needed, a transesophageal echocardiogram is preferable.

CRANIAL COMPUTED TOMOGRAPHY

Noncontrast cranial CT is useful for initial evaluation of patients with suspected cerebral ischemia or hemorrhage because it is quick, widely available, relatively inexpensive, and easy to perform. Intracerebral hemorrhage (ICH) or subarachnoid hemorrhage (SAH) is quickly confirmed with CT (Figure 5-1) and secondary complications such as hydrocephalus or impending herniation are easily identified. Similarly, most subarachnoid hemorrhages are evident on CT, and the pattern of the subarachnoid bleeding often offers the first clue about the site of the bleeding. Subdural and epidural hematomas are readily apparent with CT (see Chapter 19).

Cranial CT shows ischemic cerebral infarction (Figure 5-2), but the early signs of an infarction on CT are often subtle or absent, and small lesions are easily missed. Early CT findings include a discrete hypo-attenuation in the lentiform nucleus or the lateral margins of the insula, termed insular ribbon sign, volume reduction of the cortical sulci, or loss of the gray-white matter differentiation due to early edema. A hyperdensity within an artery indicates the presence of a thrombus (Figure 5-2). The prognostic value of early CT findings increases with the number of abnormalities present and can help to identify candidates for thrombolysis.[12] However, even in the presence of an extensive ischemic stroke, the cranial CT may be initially normal or show only subtle findings. Malignancies or microhemorrhages may be overlooked with CT, and it is harder to determine the age of an infarct with CT than with MRI. These factors are important when evaluating the safety of tissue plasminogen activator (tPA) administration because there is an increased risk for intraparenchymal hemorrhage in patients with large infarctions, in those with small and unrecognized hemorrhages, such as from cerebral amyloid angiopathy, and in patients presenting long after symptom onset.[13–17]

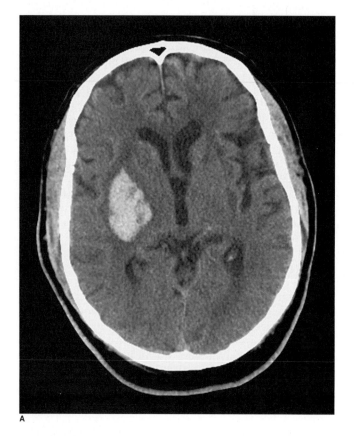
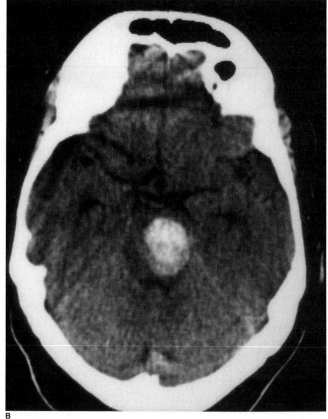

Figure 5-1. A: Cranial CT of a hypertensive patient with a left putaminal hemorrhage. B: Acute pontine hemorrhage in a comatose patient.

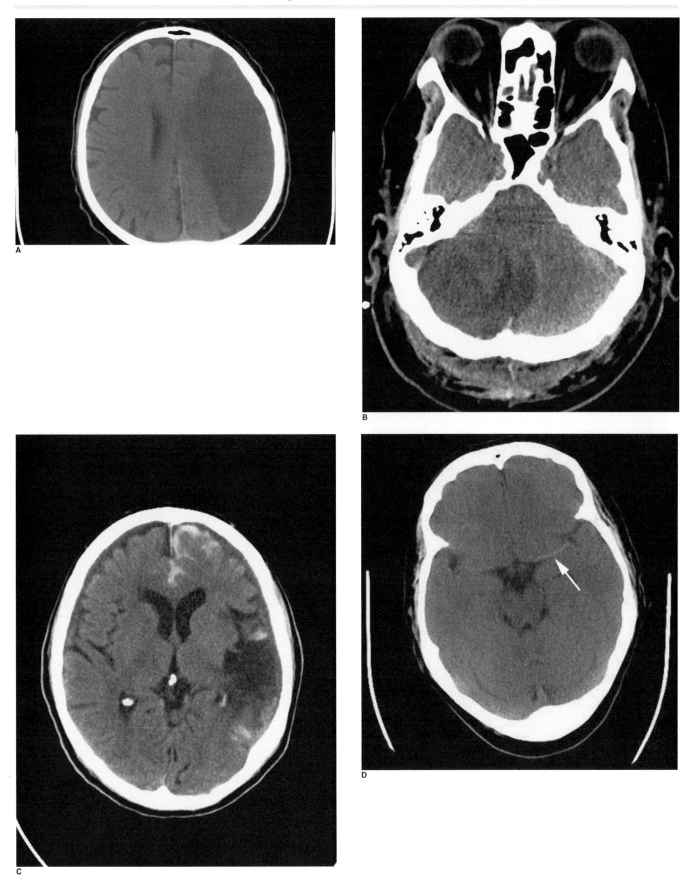

Figure 5-2. A: Cranial CT in shows a large hypodense lesion in the left middle cerebral artery territory. B: Large right cerebellar lesion with mass effect consistent with infarction in the distribution of the posterior inferior cerebellar artery. C: Noncontrast CT shows a subacute infarction in the left perisylvian region in a man taking warfarin for atrial fibrillation but with a subtherapeutic INR. Note the hyperdense areas at the anterior and posterior margins of the infarction (representing hemorrhagic conversion of the infarction) along with the subarachnoid hemorrhage along the left frontal convexity and in the anterior interhemispheric fissure. D: Hyperdensity of the left middle cerebral artery (*arrow*) represents thrombus within the vessel.

Dynamic perfusion CT of the brain with contrast, when performed during the initial scan, can add important information for the management of acute stroke patients, guiding the decision for thrombolysis. Following intravenous administration of a contrast agent, brain perfusion is measured by parenchymal density changes resulting from passage of the contrast bolus over time. Software processing of these images takes less than 10 minutes and generates perfusion maps that identify normal tissue, the irreversible damaged ischemic core, and the potentially salvageable ischemic penumbra (Figure 5-3). From these data the probability for conversion of ischemic brain tissue to infarction can be determined. The risk-benefit ratio of thrombolysis for a specific patient and the final size of the infarction can be estimated.

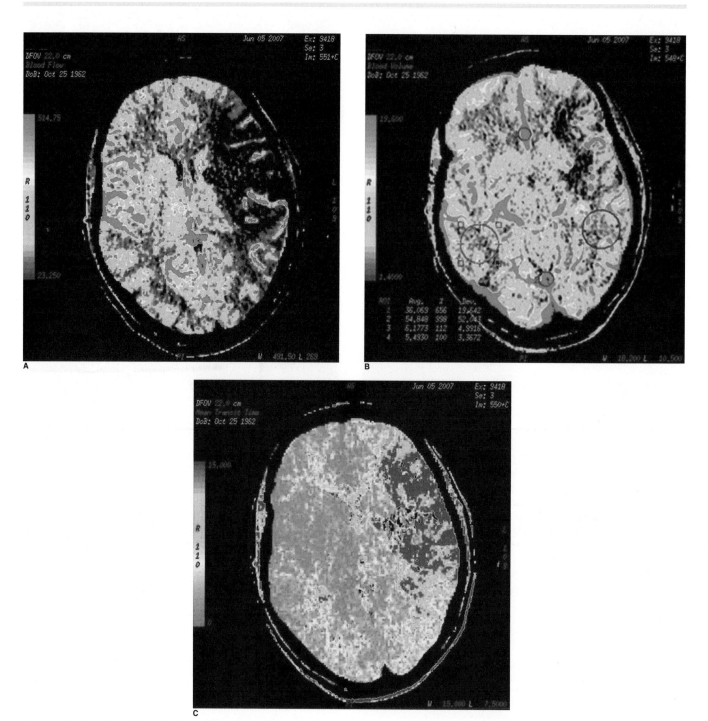

Figure 5-3. Perfusion CT studies from a patient who presented at the end of the three-hour time limit for thrombolysis and instead underwent mechanical thrombectomy and intra-arterial thrombolysis. Her studies show matching areas of significantly decreased cerebral blood flow (A), cerebral blood volume (B), and decreased mean transit time (C) within the left middle cerebral artery territory, findings that collectively suggest a completed infarct without evidence of an ischemic penumbra.

Perfusion CT provides information about the flow of the contrast agent (mean transit time or MTT), time to maximum peak of the contrast agent, bolus passage time, cerebral blood volume (CBV), and cerebral blood flow (CBF), which are presented in parametric maps. Perfusion status in these different maps can be compared to derive characteristic patterns that correlate with residual collateralization of blood flow, final infarct size, and clinical outcome. The ischemic core is characterized by reduced CBF and CBV. In the hyperacute phase of cerebral ischemia, CBF is reduced within the infarcted core. Surrounding capillaries become maximally dilated in an attempt to maintain perfusion, and CBV remains temporarily stable or even increases. With progressive failure of cerebral autoregulation and decrease in perfusion, CBV starts to fall. Analogous to the perfusion/diffusion mismatch in MRI, a CBF/CBV mismatch can indicate the presence of tissue at risk that may respond to acute intervention.[18,19]

Perfusion deficits in other parametric maps, for example, the TPP map, also have been analyzed to assess the evolution of ischemia and clinical outcome in stroke patients receiving thrombolysis compared to those not undergoing any acute intervention. The clinical application of these techniques is beyond the scope of this text, and the interested reader is referred to the rapidly evolving literature.[19–21]

CT ANGIOGRAPHY

Cranial CT without contrast infusion for the assessment of stroke patients may soon be replaced by multimodal CT, which includes not only structural imaging and dynamic perfusion studies of the brain, but also CT angiography (CTA) of the intracranial and extracranial arteries. CTA takes an additional 5–10 minutes of scan time and allows three-dimensional reconstructions of blood vessels. It yields important information about stroke etiology and vascular status and is highly sensitive and specific in detecting arterial occlusion or stenosis. The degree of arterial stenosis can be reliably estimated, and, in contrast to MR angiography, the method is not susceptible to low-flow artifacts. Cortical veins, venous sinuses, and vascular malformation can be easily visualized.[22–27] The extent of atherosclerotic disease in the brain-supplying arteries can be determined, and the residual arterial lumen in an area of atherothrombosis and the plaque size can be measured. The appearance and stability of a plaque correlates with future stroke risk. CTA can facilitate decision making between medical treatment or carotid endarterectomy, angioplasty, and endovascular stenting.

Cranial CT is still the preferred imaging modality for rapid diagnosis of intracranial hemorrhage, and CTA often can help to pinpoint the underlying vascular lesion responsible for the hemorrhage with minimal additional processing time. It can detect high- and low-flow arteriovenous malformations and aneurysms as small as 2–3 mm in diameter.[28–31] Three-dimensional reconstruction of CT angiographic images allows for more exact anatomical characterization of vessel abnormalities in different projection planes and assessment of the anatomical relation between vessels and bony structures (Figure 5-4). CTA is increasingly used for preoperative diagnosis and intervention planning. Being noninvasive, CTA is also ideal for postintervention follow-up, monitoring of patients with unruptured aneurysms, and screening of high-risk populations for intracranial hemorrhage.[32]

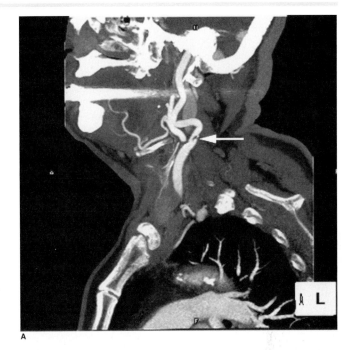

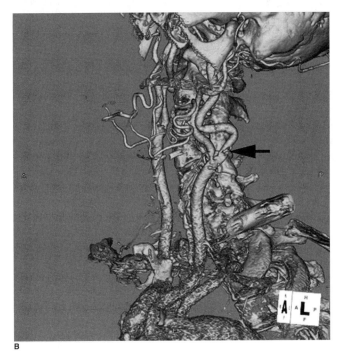

Figure 5-4. A: CT angiography demonstrates focal stenosis of the proximal left internal carotid artery (*arrow*) due to a suspected dissection in a 60-year-old man presenting with neck pain and a left Horner syndrome. B: A three-dimensional reconstruction of the cervical arteries shows this same lesion more clearly (*arrow*) and better demonstrates an out-pouching of contrast along the posterior aspect of the proximal left internal carotid artery consistent with a small dissection.

BRAIN MRI

Brain MRI (Figure 5-5) is a rapidly evolving imaging modality that is essential for the diagnosis of acute brain ischemia and clinical management of stroke patients. It is usually more sensitive and specific than cranial CT and thus more likely to identify small infarctions, detect hyperacute stroke, and depict infarctions

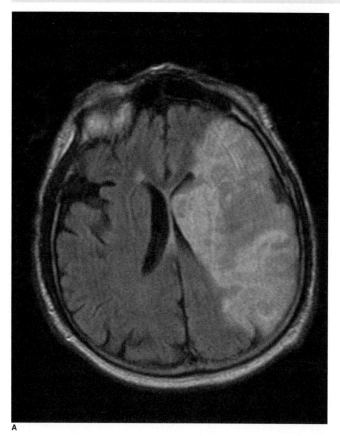

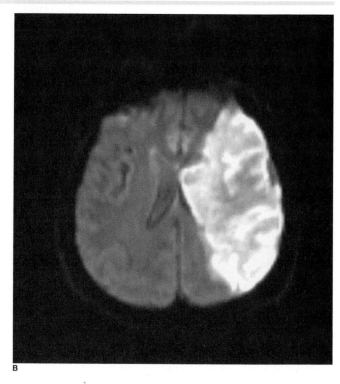

Figure 5-5. A and B: Cranial MRI shows a T_2 hyperintense signal abnormality with restricted diffusion present throughout most of the left middle cerebral artery territory consistent with acute infarct. The patient had a left internal carotid artery occlusion.

within the brainstem (Figure 5-6). With the recent development of susceptibility weighted imaging, intracranial hemorrhage can be more reliably identified. MRI provides information about location and extension of infarction and hemorrhage and the underlying stroke pathophysiology by assessing vessel anatomy, hemodynamics, and vascular function. Additionally it allows imaging of the arterial and venous systems, characterization of an atherosclerotic plaque, assessment of collateral circulation, and measurement of cerebral tissue perfusion, metabolism, and brain function.

MRI is essential for establishing the time course of cerebral infarction. DWI and PWI sequences can identify even subtle brain injury soon after the onset of ischemia and correlate well with event duration.[32,33] Brain injury is visible on DWI-MRI in about 50% of patients with clinical symptoms lasting longer than 1 hour and in 70% of patients with events lasting 12 to 24 hours.[33] Mosely and colleagues noted that changes in water diffusion associated with the development of brain edema can be used for acute stroke imaging.[34,35] Tissue with cytotoxic edema is characterized by restricted water diffusion, which is visible within minutes following symptom onset. Areas of restricted water diffusion appear bright on DWI-MRI and dark on the corresponding apparent diffusion coefficient (ADC) map. With normalization of water movement during the course of ischemia, the DWI signal intensity diminishes, and the infarcted area becomes detectable on T_2-weighted and fluid-attenuated inversion recovery (FLAIR) sequences. Signal abnormalities on ADC maps corresponding to the areas of restricted diffusion on DWI can help to distinguish

infarction from T_2 shine-through artifact. Reversibility of diffusion-weighted imaging abnormalities in humans during the acute stroke phase correlates with clinical improvement.[36]

Using DWI and PWI in combination with standard T_1 and T_2 sequences allows imaging of the ischemic penumbra, the target of acute stroke therapy. The penumbra is the area surrounding the infarcted core that is characterized by misery perfusion and impaired function in the face of preserved cell structure. Areas of restricted diffusion on DWI are presumed to represent the irreversibly damaged ischemic epicenter surrounded by the penumbra, which appears dark on PWI sequences. The penumbra is represented by the resulting perfusion/diffusion mismatch.[37] However, the use of a diffusion-perfusion mismatch to identify an ischemic penumbra has shortcomings. Normalization of disturbed water diffusion and disappearance of signal brightness in some instances after treatment up to 6 hours after symptom onset suggests that DWI-MRI abnormalities may not always represent irreversibly damaged ischemic tissue.[38–40]

New MRI sequences might overcome these limitations and help identify additional parameters for thrombectomy and thrombolysis beyond those currently in use. PWI-MRI allows the assessment of hemodynamics and brain tissue perfusion using gadolinium contrast, or noninvasively by arterial spin labeling echo sequences using blood as an innate contrast agent. Perfusion deficits following acute ischemic stroke can be visualized within 5 minutes by these techniques.[41,42] During PWI data acquisition, bolus arrival time, MTT, CBF, and CBV can be calculated following administration of an intravenous contrast agent.

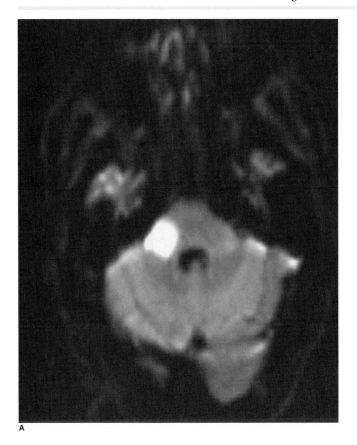 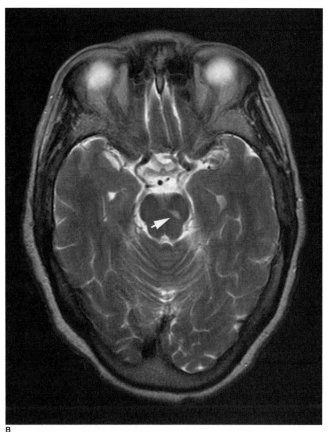

Figure 5-6. A: Cranial MRI demonstrates an acute infarction (restricted diffusion) involving the right brachium pontis in an elderly woman with hypertension, diabetes, dyslipidemia, and a recent coronary artery bypass procedure. B: Another patient with arterial hypertension and diffuse atherosclerosis has a chronic lacunar infarction (*arrow*) in the midbrain.

Functional MRI utilizing blood oxygen level-dependent (BOLD) contrast analysis can sometimes identify the penumbra more reliably than a PWI/DWI mismatch.[43] BOLD MRI analyzes the oxyhemoglobin to deoxyhemoglobin ratio measured in capillaries and venous vessels, which reflects the oxygen extraction fraction and cerebral metabolic rate comparable to PET imaging. Tissue at risk for infarct extension is characterized by an increased oxygen extraction fraction and decreased oxygen consumption. Susceptibility weighted imaging with T_2^*-weighted MRI sequences also has been shown to be useful in the setting of acute brain ischemia because the susceptibility rate of signal changes on T_2^*-weighted MRI directly relates to the degree of misery perfusion within the penumbra.[44] The addition of MR spectroscopy allows metabolic imaging of lactate as a marker of anaerobic glycolysis in areas of ischemia and the evaluation of energy metabolism by measurement of phosphorus and its chemical compounds to estimate neuronal loss and damage to cellular membranes following infarction.[45,46] Many of these techniques are still investigational, and it remains uncertain whether CT, PET, SPECT, or MRI-based techniques or a combination are more reliable in identifying salvageable tissue.

MAGNETIC RESONANCE ANGIOGRAPHY

In addition to imaging the penumbra and the infarction, it is important to collect information on the cerebral vascular status. MRI with and without contrast allows structural imaging of the carotid arteries, the aortic arch, the intracranial vessels, the vertebral-basilar system, and smaller intracranial vasculature. MR angiography (MRA) and CTA are excellent methods for noninvasive evaluation of the intracranial and extracranial vessels. Areas of stenosis, vascular malformations, arterial dissection, or other vascular pathologies can be rapidly identified. Two-dimensional contrast angiography and three-dimensional time-of-flight MR techniques can demonstrate embolic occlusion of the carotid arteries and their branches, arterial dissection, fibromuscular dysplasia, and other vascular abnormalities and also estimate the degree of arterial stenosis (Figure 5-7).

An MRA of the carotid artery allows accurate measurement of carotid artery stenosis when compared to carotid ultrasound, CTA, and catheter angiogram. However, MRA tends to overestimate the degree of stenosis in low-flow states or in areas of vascular tortuosity, resulting in signal drop-out or the production of flow artifacts. Gadolinium-enhanced three-dimensional MRA techniques allow better assessment of carotid artery stenosis, but at times it can be impossible to distinguish between high-grade stenosis and occlusion based on MRA alone.[47–49] Further, MRA can provide information about collateral flow, assessment of vascular function, and the quality of autoregulation and vascular reserve. It sometimes demonstrates arteriovenous malformations and aneurysms.[31] Intracranial MRA allows imaging of the circle of Willis and its variations as well as assessment of collateral blood flow and intracranial artery stenosis. With more advanced techniques MRI-based velocity

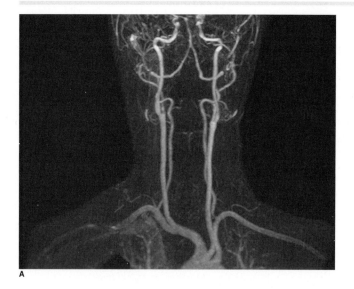
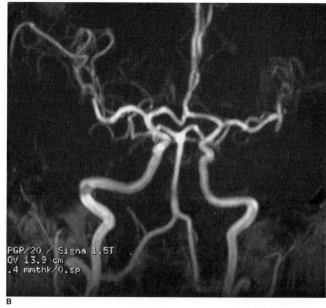

Figure 5-7. A: MRA study of the cervicocephalic vessels. B: MRA of the intracranial arteries. Note the poor filling of the left middle cerebral artery in this woman with vasculopathy of pregnancy.

measurements and determination of flow direction will become possible.[50]

MRA can directly visualize a blood clot before and after intra-arterial thrombolysis. Susceptibility-weighted imaging (SWI) can help detect dislocated clots that may be missed by MRA. However, susceptibility artifact can be problematic with this technique. $T_2{}^*$-weighted gradient echo sequences have also shown promise in the detection of isolated thrombus within cerebral sinuses and veins, which can be visualized by alterations in blood flow and by measuring hemoglobin degradation products.

SWI techniques are based on magnetic susceptibility artifacts produced by local inhomogeneities in the magnetic field and are highly sensitive for the detection of blood products. Recently SWI has been used to identify microhemorrhages, and the technique is highly sensitive for the detection of intracranial hemorrhage within 6 hours of symptom onset. $T_2{}^*$-weighted imaging can help to identify spontaneous hemorrhagic transformation in ischemic stroke earlier than conventional cranial CT and can help identify stroke patients at risk to develop hemorrhagic transformation following intravenous thrombolysis.

Assessment of carotid plaque burden by MRA helps to estimate the severity of atherosclerotic disease for prognostic purposes. Serial imaging of the carotid arteries depicts the atherosclerosis over time and allows one to analyze the response to therapy. Plaque compensation can be measured noninvasively based on unique MRI characteristics of different atheroma components.[51] Plaque imaging can be improved by the use of gadolinium or other paramagnetic contrast agents to differentiate between the fibrous cap and the necrotic lipid core. Areas of neovascularization into the plaque can also be detected by these methods.[52] In symptomatic patients, plaque characteristics such as a ruptured fibrous cap, intraplaque hemorrhage, large lipid-rich core, or a larger maximum wall thickness are associated with a higher risk of stroke. High-resolution MRI will be able to detect unstable carotid artery plaques that feature plaque erosion, ulceration, thrombosis,

intraplaque hemorrhage, thin fibrous cap, large lipid core, and associated inflammatory response. It allows measurement of cap thickness, detects areas of plaque rupture, and identifies deposits of calcium, fibrous tissue, hemorrhage, lipid accumulation, and necrosis.[53,54]

In the future molecular MRI utilizing targeted contrast agents may provide new insights into the development of atherosclerosis by measuring the degree of inflammation and neovascularization based on the application of enzymatic conversion of paramagnetic plaque compounds or assembly-disassembly of paramagnetic nanoparticles.[55–58] Targeted MRI agents may directly visualize molecular pathways and cellular processes of arthrosclerosis. Surface thrombus, indicating unstable plaque, can already be measured by fibrin-targeted nanoparticles. These new MRI techniques may prove able to directly visualize arterial wall modeling and remodeling, to identify unstable plaque, to monitor therapeutic responses, and to identify early subclinical stages of atherosclerosis.[59]

EMISSION TOMOGRAPHY

Building on the development of the cranial CT in the 1980s, emission tomography techniques including positron emission tomography (PET) and single proton emission computed tomography (SPECT) emerged. These imaging modalities allow functional brain imaging by measuring cerebral perfusion and metabolism. PET and SPECT are nuclear medicine–based approaches and use static radiotracers or specific receptor-binding radiopharmaceuticals to analyze brain metabolism and blood flow as indirect measures of neuronal function. Disadvantages include the utilization of radioactive substances, the relatively high imaging costs, and the relative poor spatial resolution of the images. However, PET remains the most accurate method for quantitative measurement of regional cerebral perfusion and for metabolism of glucose and oxygen, the key energy resources for brain function and cellular integrity.[60]

Positron Emission Tomography

PET imaging is based on the natural decay of positron-emitting isotopes in brain tissue, which are either injected intravenously or inhaled in form of radioactive gases, usually oxygen or nitrogen. The method is commonly used to measure the regional cerebral blood flow (rCBF), and the metabolic rate of oxygen (CMRO2) and glucose (rCMG), and the cerebral blood volume (rCBV).

PET has been extensively used in animal models of permanent and temporary arterial occlusion as well as in humans to document changes in those parameters associated with stroke and TIAs.[61-64] Following an arterial occlusion, brain perfusion declines rapidly below a critical threshold required to maintain cellular function. Regions with cerebral blood flow between 12 and 22 ml/100 g/min that lie within the penumbra are characterized by diminished perfusion and an increased oxygen extraction fraction. Within the penumbra, the oxygen extraction fraction increases from about 40% under normal conditions to about 90% during hypoperfusion. If reperfusion and reconstitution of blood flow occurs at the time of an increased oxygen extraction fraction, brain tissue may completely recover. Within the center of the ischemic core regional cerebral blood flow has fallen below 12 ml/100 g/min and CMRO2 to below 65 ml/100 g/min. Potential viable tissue within the penumbra shows rCBF values around 12 to 20 ml/100 g/min and CMRO2 values of more than 65 ml/100 g/min. However, these values vary significantly between individuals and within different regions of the brain.[65]

PET studies have shown that the ischemic core extends over time unless the occluded vessel recanalized within the therapeutic time window.[61] In rare cases the penumbra can exist up to 48 hours following onset of brain ischemia.[66] Early recanalization, either spontaneously or after therapeutic intervention, can be visualized by PET showing increased rCBF and near-to-normal CMRO2 values associated with rapid clinical improvement and subsequently relatively small infarcts on brain MRI or cranial CT.

During brain ischemia, the regional oxygen extraction fraction by itself is not a reliable predictor of tissue viability, and multitracer receptor imaging, such as with [18]-F-fluoromisonidazol and [11]-C flumezenil, allows differentiation between irreversible damaged tissue and the penumbra[67,68] and thus helps to identify individuals who might benefit from thrombolysis and intra-arterial intervention beyond the conventional treatment windows.

In patients with atherosclerotic disease PET can be used to assess the vasomotor reserve and the risk of hemodynamic compromise. High-grade carotid or intracranial arterial stenosis or occlusion causes maximal vasodilatation and is often associated with impaired cerebral autoregulation. This is demonstrated by an increase in rCBV on [15]-oxygen PET.[69-71] Cerebral perfusion pressure in vascular occlusive disease can be estimated by the CBF/CBV quotient. If the CBF/CBV quotient falls below a critical value, the brain can compensate by increasing the oxygen extraction fraction. However, a high-grade arterial stenosis associated with a low CBF/CBV quotient and maximal increase in regional oxygen extraction fraction suggests a marginal cerebral vascular reserve. Although these patients are at higher risk for hemodynamic compromise and subsequent infarction, the relationship between rCBF, rCBV, and the regional oxygen extraction fraction is complex, and assessment of hemodynamic impairment by PET often does not correlate precisely with the risk of cerebral infarction.[72] Assessment of the vasomotor reserve by SPECT may therefore be a preferable alternative.

Single Proton Emission Computed Tomography

SPECT analyzes the emission of protons from radioisotopes during their natural decay in brain tissue detected by gamma-ray cameras. Because the spatial resolution of SPECT is limited, its images tend to be blurred. The method is mainly utilized to assess cerebral blood flow. Commonly used isotopes to measure regional cerebral blood flow include 133-xenon, which is inhaled, or 123-I-labeled radiopharmaceuticals and 99-Tc-labeled isotopes, which are injected intravenously. SPECT measures rCBF and rCBV quantitatively, and the estimated regional oxygen extraction fraction is derived from rCBF and rCBV ratios (Figure 5-8).

Comparable to PET, receptor imaging is possible with SPECT using dopaminergic, serotonergic, GABAergic, or cholinergic radioligands or alternative transmitter systems. These technologies are used mainly for research and are infrequently utilized as clinical imaging studies for acute cerebral ischemia.[73] Receptor imaging techniques based on SPECT compounds such as 123-I-iomazenil show neuronal integrity following cerebral ischemia and may prove helpful to manage stroke patients clinically.[74,75]

SPECT furthermore is a useful diagnostic tool for the assessment of cerebral vasoreactivity and the hemodynamic reserve in patients with atherosclerotic carotid disease.[76] Inhalation of CO_2 or injection of acetazolamide causes vasodilatation of cerebral arterioles, and the degree of vasodilatation reflects the cerebral vascular reserve. The CBF/CBV quotient estimates the perfusion reserve. Misery perfusion is characterized by an increase in rCBV and a decrease in rCBF. Diminished vessel dilation following

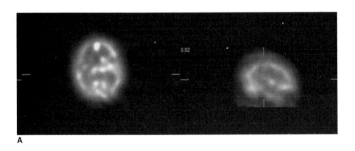

A

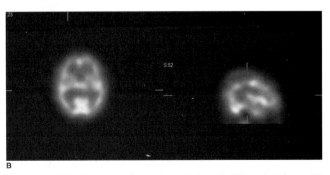

B

Figure 5-8. Single photon emission tomography (SPECT) scan images in the transaxial and sagittal planes done both with (A) and without (B) intravenous acetazolamide infusion. After intravenous acetazolamide, there is decreased perfusion in the right hemisphere primarily in a watershed region. A repeat study a few days later without acetazolamide (B) shows an improved, although not yet normal, perfusion pattern.

CO_2 inhalation or acetazolamide challenge indicates poor vascular hemodynamic reserve and helps to identify patients with carotid artery disease who may benefit from carotid artery stenting, endarterectomy, or possibly extracranial-intracranial-(EC-IC) carotid artery bypass surgery.[77–79]

CATHETER ANGIOGRAPHY

With the development of cerebral angiography by Moniz, it became apparent that extracranial occlusive disease is a major cause for ischemic stroke.[80] Despite the advent of less invasive imaging techniques, catheter angiography remains the most accurate means of assessing the cervicocerebral vasculature. Catheter angiography allows visualization of the extracranial and intracranial vasculature, including the medium-sized and small arteries that are not accurately depicted by MRA or CTA. It is still the most reliable way to identify an arterial dissection, demonstrate structural vessel abnormalities such as an arteriovenous malformation or aneurysm, or differentiate high-grade stenosis from vessel occlusion. Selective catheter angiography can be used to analyze the adequacy and source of intracranial or extracranial collateral flow, often critical information when planning surgical or endovascular procedures.

Not only is catheter angiography used for diagnosis, but it is also the basis for planning and performing endovascular therapeutic procedures.[81] Intravascular treatment techniques have been developed for arteriovenous malformations, arterial aneurysms, and cerebral venous sinus thrombosis. The development of new catheter techniques and new contrast agents has made angiography-based interventions the method of choice to treat many intracranial vascular abnormalities. In acute stroke patients who present beyond the 3- to 4.5-hour interval for intravenous tPA administration, angiography provides access for intra-arterial pharmacological or mechanical thrombolysis, thrombectomy, and angioplasty and stenting of stenotic lesions.

The complete angiographic evaluation of the cerebrovascular system should encompass views of the aortic arch, the cervical arteries including common carotid and internal and external carotid arteries, the vertebrobasilar circulation, and the major intracranial branches of these vessels. A nonselective aortogram can serve as preliminary road map, but selective catheterization of both common carotid and the vertebral arteries is needed to completely assess the entire cerebral vasculature and the status of the collateral circulation (Figure 5-9). Projections should include anterior-posterior, lateral as well as oblique views to allow optimal delineation of vascular pathology. Visualization of all major cranial arteries is desirable, but it is wise to study the artery of primary clinical interest first in case the study has to be aborted.

Most catheter angiography studies now utilize high-resolution image-intensified fluoroscopy with rapid-sequence X-ray generators. Three-dimensional rotational angiography allows reconstructions of three-dimensional images similar to those acquired during CTA and MRA. After transfemoral injection of a contrast agent via a small catheter, imaging data are sampled by moving the imaging system through an arch around the patient. Rapid data acquisition and display with digital road mapping capability is essential for the safe performance of diagnostic and therapeutic angiography. Newer high-contrast resolution digital subtraction angiography requires application of relatively small amounts of contrast, reducing the likelihood of contrast-induced nephropathy in patients with coexisting chronic renal insufficiency.[82]

Even in experienced hands, catheter angiography carries some risk, and the risk may be slightly higher in individuals with atherosclerosis. Consequently, in many medical centers vascular interventions are now based on MRA, CTA, or carotid duplex studies alone. The reported risk of permanent neurological deficit from diagnostic angiography is 0.3% to 5.7%, and the risk for transient neurological deficits is 0.3% to 6.8%.[83–87] The overall stroke risk is about 1% but is 2-to-3-fold higher in patients with symptomatic atherosclerotic disease than in those with asymptomatic lesions.[88–90] However, clinically silent infarctions after a diagnostic angiography can be demonstrated with cranial MRI in some patients.[91–93] The risk for ischemic injury is significantly lower when experienced interventionalists perform the procedure avoiding the use of multiple catheters, prolonged procedure time, and misdiagnosis from poor technique and limited experience in interpretation of imaging data.[94,95]

LUMBAR PUNCTURE

Analysis of the cerebrospinal fluid (CSF) is useful in specific situations, although lumbar puncture is unnecessary in most individuals with suspected cerebrovascular dysfunction. Lumbar puncture should probably be avoided in patients with brain lesions that are large enough to cause concern about brain herniation, but most other patients tolerate lumbar puncture well.

CSF analysis is important in stroke patients who have an unexplained fever or signs of CNS infection. Ischemic stroke is sometimes the first indication of chronic meningitis or early tuberculous meningitis. Bacterial meningitis can also cause vasculitis and stroke, but not usually as its initial manifestation. Syphilis serology should be done in patients with unexplained ischemic stroke. Evidence of inflammation (typically an excessive number of white blood cells and increased protein content) is present in some individuals with noninfectious vasculitis of the cerebral vessels.

Occasionally a mild subarachnoid hemorrhage that is not apparent on CT can be demonstrated via lumbar puncture (see Chapter 17). However, there is usually little need to do a lumbar puncture solely to confirm subarachnoid bleeding that is already obvious radiographically.

ULTRASOUND

Ultrasonography of the brain-supplying vessels is completely noninvasive and provides information about both the hemodynamics and the anatomy of the vessels. The hemodynamic evaluation typically includes Doppler ultrasonography, whereas structural imaging is done with B-mode ultrasonography. Their combination in duplex sonography forms the foundation for diagnostic testing in individuals with suspected cerebrovascular disease. The technique is operator dependent, so it must be performed and interpreted by trained, experienced individuals to yield accurate results. The clinical usefulness of carotid duplex ultrasonology is limited by a higher than normal carotid bifurcation, a short neck, deeply situated vessels, and extensive acoustic shadowing that prevents adequate visualization of the vessels. In these cases CTA and MRA are the preferred noninvasive imaging modalities.

Carotid Duplex Ultrasound

Blood cells move at a variety of speeds and directions within the vessel at any point in time, causing an array of Doppler

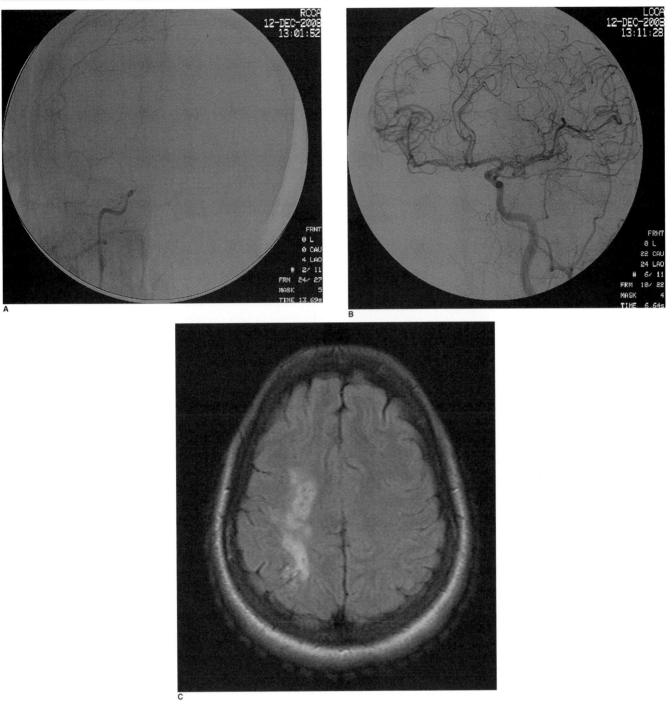

Figure 5-9. A: Catheter angiography demonstrates occlusion of the right internal carotid artery just distal to the origin of the right ophthalmic artery. B: There is rapid cross-filling of the right anterior cerebral artery and the right middle cerebral artery via the anterior communicating artery. C: Nevertheless, a cranial MRI shows a watershed distribution infarction in the right parietal lobe.

frequency shift values in any acquired sample volume. Specific characteristics of the spectral waveform depend not only on flow hemodynamics at the point of interrogation but also on flow hemodynamics proximally and distally.[96]

The internal carotid and vertebral arteries are low-resistance vascular beds with low pulsatility, generating a spectral waveform pattern that is quite distinct from that of the vessels with higher peripheral resistance such as the external carotid artery.

In normal vessels with laminar flow, the Doppler spectrum is usually narrow with a relatively smooth acoustic envelope. Narrowing of a vessel leads to a predictable series of hemodynamic changes. Those changes manifest in alteration of peak systolic and end diastolic velocities, spectral bandwidth, and shape of the envelope.

Controlled clinical trials have shown that carotid endarterectomy is beneficial for symptomatic patients with 70% to

99% stenosis of the internal carotid artery (see the North American Symptomatic Carotid Endarterectomy Trial or NASCET) and for asymptomatic patients with 60% to 99% ICA stenosis (see the Asymptomatic Carotid Artery Stenosis or ACAS study).[97,98] These and related studies demonstrate a beneficial effect from readily available therapy, creating a clear clinical mandate to accurately measure the degree of carotid stenosis. Carotid duplex ultrasonography provides a hemodynamic assessment of carotid stenosis rather than merely a linear measurement of stenosis. When performed by trained sonographers using a standard imaging protocol and ongoing quality assurance, this technique can reach 90% specificity.[99,100]

In the presence of 95% to 99% stenosis, flow velocity values are variable. Color flow imaging and power Doppler can help to differentiate between subtotal and total occlusion by demonstrating trickle flow or a "string sign." A residual lumen diameter of less than 2 mm, which is considered as a B-mode imaging threshold for tight stenosis, as well as the use of common carotid artery volume flow rate are also helpful as adjunctive data for interpretation.

The vertebral artery should be included as a routine part of a complete vascular duplex examination. Compared to catheter angiography, vertebral duplex ultrasonography has a sensitivity of 80% and specificity of 83% to 90% for detection of 50% or greater stenosis at the vertebral artery origin.[101] Although the ultrasound findings are not specific, a vertebral artery dissection can be detected and monitored noninvasively by Doppler, CTA, or MRA in a suggestive clinical setting.[102] The pattern of flow velocity changes in the vertebral artery may help localize the site of occlusion in the subclavian, vertebral, and basilar arteries.

B-mode or brightness mode imaging provides a two-dimensional display of the grayscale image of soft tissue and vessels and allows real-time interrogation of the thickness and appearance of the vessel wall.[103] It is safe, noninvasive, readily available, and relatively inexpensive. It has the ability to identify mobile thrombus on the surface of a complex plaque that may require urgent treatment. The composition and thickness, and thus the elasticity, of the vessel wall may change over time. Early changes due to atherosclerosis include thickening of the arterial intima and media layers and increased vessel stiffness. High-resolution B-mode ultrasonography provides visualization of the vessel wall in detail (Figure 5-10). Thickening of the intima and media can be accurately assessed up to 0.1 to 0.3 mm[104–106] and is now widely used to study subclinical atherosclerosis and

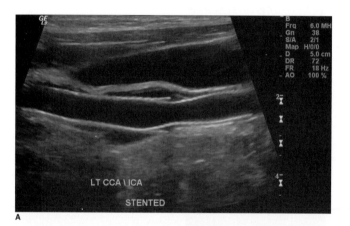

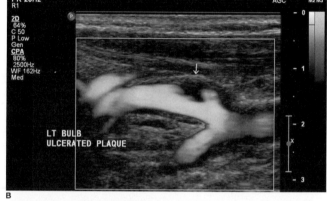

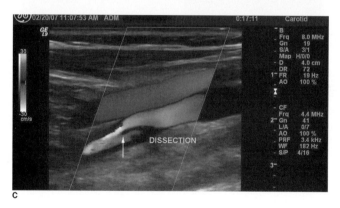

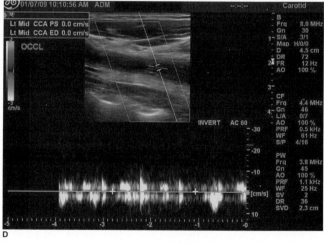

Figure 5-10. Ultrasound depiction of the cervicocephalic arteries. A: B-mode ultrasound demonstrates a stent in the left common carotid artery extending into the proximal internal carotid artery. B: Large ulcerated plaque (*arrow*) of the left carotid artery bifurcation. C: Dissection of the right internal carotid artery (*red*). A flap (*arrow*) divides the true and false lumen. D: With occlusion of the left common carotid artery there is no detectable color flow within the vascular lumen, and the spectral analysis shows absent arterial flow. Ultrasound images are courtesy of the Vascular Laboratory at Penn State College of Medicine, Hershey, Pennsylvania.

regression and progression of atherosclerotic lesions in association with risk factor modification.[107–110]

A unique strength of B-mode imaging is its ability to assess atherosclerotic plaque characteristics (Figure 5-10). Plaques that are primarily homogeneous and echogenic or calcified are usually found to have substantial fibrous components and are probably more stable.[111] Plaques that are heterogeneous, with marked surface ulceration or intraplaque hemorrhage, are often referred to as complex plaques, which are less stable and have a greater risk of causing cerebral ischemia.[112–115]

Color-flow imaging provides real-time two-dimensional flow velocity information and better visualization of vessel walls, hypoechoic plaques, differentiation between ulcerated plaque and intraplaque hemorrhage, recognition of carotid dissection, reconstitution of the vessel distal to an occlusion, or vessel tortuosity. It accurately differentiates between subtotal and total occlusion of the ICA with a sensitivity of 87% to 100% and a specificity of 84% compared to conventional angiographic findings.[116–119]

Transcranial Doppler

Transcranial Doppler sonography (TCD) is a real-time noninvasive method to evaluate intracranial hemodynamics in the circle of Willis. Established clinical TCD indications include detection of intracranial stenosis or occlusion of the major basal cerebral arteries, assessment of collateral flow in patients with intracranial or extracranial arterial stenosis or occlusion, evaluation of vasospasm, screening vascular status in sickle cell disease, and assessment of potential cerebral circulatory arrest (brain death). In experienced hands, TCD data are reproducible because there is normally little significant variation between two sides or between studies on different days, making it an ideal noninvasive test for repeated measurements.[120–125]

Increased flow velocities can be observed in many pathological conditions that decrease the vessel lumen, such as intracranial stenosis, intracranial dissection, vasospasm, arteriovenous malformation, or cerebral embolism. Decreased velocity may be due to an inadequate acoustic window, poor angle of insonation, cardiac dysfunction, more proximal stenosis, distal hypoperfusion in that territory, or markedly increased intracranial pressure. Absence of Doppler signals from an artery suggests occlusion of that arterial segment. Highly pulsatility waveforms with low diastolic flow velocity suggest high resistance distally as with increased intracranial pressure or multifocal, diffuse cerebral atherosclerosis, but can also occur with cardiac dysfunction, such as aortic insufficiency. Asymmetrical increases in pulsatility of the waveform may indicate mass effect as with intracerebral hemorrhage. Reversed flow direction in certain arterial segments may indicate collateral flow distal to proximal occlusive lesion, as with reversed anterior cerebral artery flow direction distal to an internal carotid artery occlusion.

Transcranial color-flow duplex ultrasonography allows direct visualization of the course of intracranial vessels, brain parenchyma, and bony structures. It can image multiple vessels simultaneously. Flow in veins, aneurysms, and arteriovenous malformation can be identified.[126–129] It can be rapidly performed at the bedside to provide data regarding stroke subtype and mechanism. This may be especially helpful in the setting of acute stroke. The evolution of ultrasound contrast may help the clinician to make decisions on treatment or additional evaluation in acute stroke. Serial follow-up studies are useful to monitor the result of thrombolytic therapy.

TCD can also be used to evaluate the cerebrovascular reserve by different physiological challenges, including breath holding, hyperventilation, inhalation of 5% CO_2, or the administration of intravenous acetazolamide.[130–138] When compared with SPECT or PET, TCD is noninvasive, nonradioactive, and less expensive, and it has excellent correlation with results obtained by acetazolamide SPECT.[139]

Cerebral microembolism can be reliably detected by TCD in numerous clinical settings, including for patients with prosthetic cardiac valves, cardiac conditions, extracranial carotid stenosis, vertebrobasilar ischemia, and during carotid endarterectomy, cerebral contrast angiography, carotid angioplasty, and cardiopulmonary bypass.[140–144] Sequential TCD monitoring for cerebral microembolism may play an important role in the patients with acute stroke to assist with the classification of stroke subtype, understanding the prognosis of stroke, and making decisions on the best preventive therapy.[145,146]

Patients with a patent foramen ovale (PFO) can be assessed by TCD monitoring. Agitated saline or commercial ultrasound contrast agents are injected intravenously while the MCA signal is monitored. Such agents are too large to cross the pulmonary capillary bed, but if there is a patent foramen ovale or a right-to-left intracardiac shunt, bubbles cross to the left side of the heart to enter systemic circulation. When they pass the TCD beam, these small bubbles act as emboli and cause distinct embolic signals. The use of Valsalva increases the diagnostic yield. Such TCD evaluation for intracardiac shunts is reported to have 77% to 100% sensitivity and 94% to 100% specificity compared to contrast transesophageal echocardiography. In fact, some researchers feel that contrast TCD may be better able to identify pulmonary A-V fistulae, which transesophageal echocardiography may miss.[147–149]

Newer ultrasound approaches have recently been developed. Three-dimensional ultrasound images, which are reconstructed from a series of conventional two-dimensional ultrasound images, have been used for carotid atheromatous plaque visualization and imaging of intracranial vessels. Plaque morphology is more precisely differentiated, and the plaque volume quantification is typically less affected by echo shadowing after three-dimensional reconstruction.[150–154]

BIOMARKERS IN CEREBROVASCULAR DISEASE

There is growing interest in biomarkers that may help to identify individuals at risk for cerebral ischemic events and to provide prognostic clinical outcome data in stroke patients. Most biomarkers are measured in plasma, serum, or, less commonly, cerebrospinal fluid or urine. The presence of these compounds may indicate a specific underlying pathophysiological process, that is, cerebral ischemia or a vulnerable plaque formation with altered patterns in circulating vasculature derived proteins. Several proteins involved in the modulation of the coagulation system, inflammatory responses, lipid transport, vascular matrix formation, or platelet function have been studied, but thus far no single marker has proved effective to predict the risk of ischemic cerebral events.

The future development of biomarker panels may help to detect unstable atherosclerotic plaque, predict vascular ischemic events, and assess stroke severity and treatment responses. More than a thousand candidate proteins have been studied for use in screening, diagnosis, and clinical management of ischemic stroke and cardiovascular disease to date. These potential markers include a variety of brain-derived proteins (e.g., neuron-specific enolase, protein S100B, glial fibrillary acidic protein), indicators of vascular inflammation such as high-sensitivity C-reactive protein (hsCRP), cell adhesion molecules (CAMs, selectins, beta 2 integrins), interleukins, tumor necrosis factor, interferons, and markers of oxidative stress and atherosclerosis, lipoprotein-associated phospholipase A2, and extracellular matrix markers (metalloproteinases, procollagen peptides, tissue inhibitors of metalloproteinases), to name just a few. The list of currently available biomarkers is extensive, and a detailed description is beyond the scope of this chapter. The interested reader is referred to the extensive literature for further details.[155–161]

Atherosclerosis is a major cause for ischemic stroke, and therefore biomarkers of chronic inflammation associated with atheroma formation, plaque rupture, and subsequent embolization may predict future ischemic vascular events and therapeutic response.[161] In particular, high-sensitivity C-reactive protein (CRP) has been promising as an independent predictor of ischemic stroke in several studies.[162–164] Even modest elevation of plasma CRP in the absence of traditional vascular risk factors appears to be associated with an increased risk of cerebrovascular and cardiovascular events. Patients with ischemic stroke and elevated CRP levels have a higher risk of myocardial infarction. However, it remains unclear whether therapeutic reduction of CRP levels, for instance, by statins or anti-inflammatory agents, would lower the risk of ischemic stroke.[165,166] There is insufficient evidence to routinely use CRP as marker of therapy effectiveness or as independent predictor for vascular events in primary and secondary stroke prevention.

Vascular risk factors such as arterial hypertension, tobacco use, hyperlipidemia, and diabetes upregulate leukocytes, CRP, and fibrinogen levels, with subsequent cytokine activation and release of adhesion molecules such as sICAM-1, cVCAM, or sE-selectin that mediate chronic inflammation, platelet activation, and coagulation. Modulation of the vessel wall with positive or negative remodeling during the process of atheroma formation is mediated by extracellular matrix proteins that determine collagen content and the structure of the vascular matrix. Atherosclerotic plaque formation is associated with increase in collagen content, often with altered structure and higher smooth muscle cell content.[167] Circulating proteins involved in this process include procollagen peptides (PINP, PCP, ICTP) and matrix metalloproteinases (MMPs) as well as their tissue inhibitors of MMPs (TIMPs). Several studies suggest that the process of atherosclerosis can be monitored by assaying circulating levels of these factors.[168–170] MMP-9 in particular has been shown to be elevated in individuals with hypertension, diabetes, and coronary artery disease and in tobacco users. It is a predictor of cardiovascular events, can be lowered by statins, and is associated with worse neurological outcome and increased risk of hemorrhagic transformation in ischemic stroke[171–174] Tissue inhibitor of MMP is positively correlated with traditional vascular risk factors and carotid atherosclerosis.[175] However, circulating extracellular matrix proteins are not tissue specific, and their relation with cerebral ischemic events needs to be established in future longitudinal prospective studies.

Although multiple risk factors of ischemic stroke and biomarkers of atherosclerosis have been identified, no single test yet has sufficient sensitivity or specificity to be used in the routine management of patients with ischemic cerebrovascular disease. Currently available biomarkers have a relative high rate of diagnostic errors leading to misclassification of patients. Composites biomarker panels developed by proteomic techniques designed to simultaneously identify specific proteins that may be associated with stroke and atherosclerosis may soon provide new tools for risk factor screening and clinical management of stroke.

GENETIC TESTING IN CEREBROVASCULAR DISEASE

There is growing clinical interest in the genetic causes of cerebrovascular disease, and several specific gene disorders are known to promote it (see Chapter 21). Many other genes collectively control the function of the physiologic parameters that determine an individual's propensity to develop a stroke – control of coagulation, platelet function, lipid metabolism, arterial blood pressure, response to injury, and others. Relatively few of these genes yield a specific and predictable stroke risk, and fewer still can currently be tested in a clinical setting. However, the number of commercially available genetic screening tests is increasing and no doubt will continue to do so.

Among the most established genetic tests is screening for a *Notch3* gene mutation on chromosome 19p13 that causes cerebral autosomal dominant arteriopathy with subcortical infarcts and leukoencephalopathy (CADASIL). CADASIL is an inherited cerebrovascular disease that can cause extensive ischemic white matter changes on neuroimaging studies, stroke, vascular dementia, migraine-like headache, seizures, and psychiatric disorders (see also Chapter 21). Testing of all 23 exons carrying known mutations for CADASIL is currently available.[176]

Mitochondrial myopathy, encephalopathy, lactic acidosis, and stroke (MELAS), a progressive neurodegenerative disorder causing lactate acidosis, seizures, ophthalmoplegia, ragged red fiber myopathy, and stroke-like episodes, can be diagnosed by genetic testing. Polymerase chain reaction and restriction fragment length polymorphism can now detect mDNA point mutations that are associated with MELAS.[177] The test is done on whole blood.

Genetic testing for inherited forms of cerebral amyloid angiopathy (CAA) is discussed in Chapter 15. Recently additional genes have been identified that are associated with malformation of arteries, capillaries, and venous structures.[178] There is an ongoing search for genes that would facilitate screening of patients at risk for intracranial aneurysms; so far only a few mutations have been well characterized.[179]

Multiple cerebral cavernous malformations (see Chapter 18) result from a dominantly inherited mutation of any of three genes. These include the *CCM1* and *CCM2* genes on chromosome 7 and the *CCM3* gene on chromosome 3. *CCM1* is caused by a mutation in the *KRIT1* gene that causes disturbances in cell adhesion, migration, and angiogenesis. The functions of *CCM2* mutations that are found in 20% of families with cavernous malformations and of *CCM3*, found in 40% of all inherited cases, remain to be identified.[180]

Other available genetic tests with relevance to the cerebrovascular system include those for hereditary hemorrhagic telangiectasia, familial hemiplegic migraine, factor V Leiden, the prothrombin G20210A mutation, Williams syndrome, hemophilia A and B, pseudoxanthoma elasticum, and neurofibromatosis type 1. In addition, genetic screening is possible for some metabolic conditions and lipid metabolism disorders that promote stroke. Over the next few years, the array of genetic tests available for cerebrovascular risk factors is likely to increase dramatically. In addition, increasing recognition of genetic factors that alter one's response to therapy or one's response to an injury are likely to have a major impact on our approach to the care of individuals with stroke.

REFERENCES

1. Johnston SC, Nguyen-Huynh MN, Schwarz ME, et al. National stroke association guidelines for the management of transient ischemic attacks. *Ann Neurol.* 2006;**60**:301–313.

2. Johnson SC, Gress DR, Browner WS, Sidney S. Short-term prognosis after emergency-department diagnosis of transient ischemic attack. *JAMA.* 2000;**284**:2901–2906.

3. Coull AJ, Lovett JK, Rothwell PM. Population based study of early risk of stroke after transient ischaemic attack or minor stroke: implications for public education and organization of services. *BMJ.* 2004;**328**:326–328.

4. Hill MD, Yiannakoulias N, Keerakathil T, et al. The high risk of stroke immediately after transient ischemic attack: *a population-based study. Neurology.* 2004;**62**:2015–2020.

5. Kleindorfer D, Panagos P, Pancioli A, et al. Incidence and short-term prognosis of transient ischemic attack in a population-based study. *Stroke.* 2005;**36**:720–723.

6. Fjaersetoft H, Indredavik B, Lydersen S. Stroke unit care combined with early supported discharge: long-term follow-up of a randomized controlled trial. *Stroke.* 2003;**34**(11):2691–2692.

7. Cadilhac DA, Ibrahim J, Pearce DC, et al. Multicenter comparison of processes of care between Stroke Units and conventional care wards in Australia. *Stroke.* 2004;**35**(5):1035–1040.

8. Mohammad YM, Divani AA, Jradi H, et al. Primary stroke center: basic components and recommendations. *South Med J.* 2006;**99**(7):749–752.

9. Hamdy S, Rothewell JC, Aziz Q, Thompson DG. Organization and reorganization of human swallowing motor cortex: implications for recovery after stroke. *Clin Sci (Lond).* 2000;**99**(2): 151–157.

10. Smithard DG. Swallowing and stroke. Neurological effects and recovery. *Cerebrovasc Dis.* 2002;**14**(1):1–8.

11. Singh S, Hamdy S. Dysphagia in stroke patients. *Postgrad Med J.* 2006;**82**(968):383–391.

12. Moulin T, Cattin F, Crepin-Leblond T, et al. Early CT signs in acute middle cerebral artery infarction: predictive value for subsequent infarct locations and outcome. *Neurology.* 1996;**47**(2): 366–375.

13. Brott TG, Haley EC Jr, Levy DE, et al. Urgent therapy for stroke. Part I. Pilot study of tissue plasminogen activator administered within 90 minutes. *Stroke.* 1992;**23**(5):632–640.

14. Haley EC Jr, Levy DE, Brott TG, et al. Urgent therapy for stroke. Part II. Pilot study of tissue plasminogen activator administered 91–180 minutes from onset. *Stroke.* 1992;**23**(5):641–645.

15. Okada Y, Sadoshima S, Nakane H, Utsunomiya H, Fujishima M. Early computed tomographic findings for thrombolytic therapy in patients with acute brain embolism. *Stroke.* 1992;**23**(1):20–23.

16. Bozzao L, Angeloni U, Bastianello S, et al. Early angiographic and CT findings in patients with hemorrhagic infarction in the distribution of the middle cerebral artery. *AJNR Am J Neuroradiol.* 1991;**12**(6):1115–1121.

17. Horowitz SH, Zito JL, Donnarumma R, Patel M, Alvir J. Computed tomographic-angiographic findings within the first first five hours of cerebral infarction. *Stroke.* 1991;**22**(10):1245–1253.

18. Harrigan MR, Leonardo J, Gibbons KJ, Guterman LR, Hopkins LN. CT perfusion cerebral blood flow imaging in neurological critical care. *Neurocrit Care.* 2005;**2**(3):352–366.

19. Wintermark M. Brain perfusion-CT in acute stroke patients. *Eur Radiol.* 2005; **15**(Suppl 4):D28–31.

20. Pepper EM, Parsons MW, Bateman GA, Levi CR. CT perfusion source images improve identification of early ischaemic change in hyperacute stroke. *J Clin Neurosci.* 2006;**13**(2):199–205.

21. Murphy BD, Fox AJ, Lee DH, et al. Identification of pneumbra and infarct in acute ischemic stroke using computed tomography perfusion-derived blood flow and blood volume measurements. *Stroke.* 2006;**37**(7):1771–1777.

22. Shrier DA, Tnaka H, Numaguchi Y, et al. CT angiography in the evaluation of acute stroke. *AJNR Am J Neuroradiol.* 1997;**18**:1011–1020.

23. Josephson SA, Bryant SO, Mak HK, Johnston SC, Dillon WP, Smith WS. Evaluation of carotid stenosis using CT angiography in the initial evaluation of stroke and TIA. *Neurology.* 2004; **63**(3):412–413.

24. Barlett ES, Walters TD, Symons SP, Fox AJ. Diagnosing carotid stenosis near-occlusion by using CT angiography. *AJNR Am J Neuroradiol.* 2006;**27**(3):632–637.

25. Kaufmann TJ, Kallmes DF. Utility of MRA and CTA in the evaluation of carotid occlusive disease. *Semin Vasc Surg.* 2005;**18**(2): 75–82.

26. Dross P, Fisher B. Clinical applications of computed tomography angiography in neuroimaging. *Del Med J.* 2005;**77**(6): 211–217.

27. Forsting M. CTA of the ICA bifurcation and intracranial vessels. *Eur Radiol.* 2005; **15**(Suppl l4):D25–27.

28. Chen Y, Manness W, Kattner K. Application of CT angiography of complex cerebrovascular lesions during surgical decision making. *Skull Base.* 2004;**14**(4):185–93; discussion 193.

29. van Gelder JM. Computed tomographic angiography for detecting cerebral aneurysms: implications of aneurysm size distribution for the sensitivity, specificity, and likelihood ratios. *Neurosurgery.* 2003;**53**(3):597–605; discussion 605–606.

30. Goddard AJ, Tan G, Becker J. Computed tomography angiography for the detection and characterization of intra-cranial aneurysms: current status. *Clin Radiol.* 2005;**60**(12):1221–1236.

31. Anzalone N, Scomazzoni F, Strada L, Patay Z, Scotti G. Intracranial vascular malformations. *Eur Radiol.* 1998;**8**(5):685–690.

32. Kamal AK, Segal AZ, Ulug AM. Quantitative diffusion-weighted MR imaging in ischemic attacks. *AJNR Am J Neuroradiol.* 2002; **23**(9):1533–1538.

33. Kidwell CS, Alger JR, Di Salle F, et al. Diffusion MRI in patients with transient ischemic attacks. *Stroke.* 1999;**1174**:2762–2763.

34. Moseley ME, Cohen Y, Kucharczyk J, et al. Diffusion-weighted MR imaging of anisotropic water diffusion in cat central nervous system. *Radiology.* 1990;**176**(2):439–445.

35. Moseley ME, Cohen Y, Mintorovitch J, et al. Early detection of regional cerebral ischemia in cats: comparison of diffusion- and T2-weighted MRI and spectroscopy. *Magn Reson Med.* 1990; **14**(2):330–346.

36. Kidwell CS, Saver JL, Mattiello J, et al. Thrombolytic reversal of acute human cerebral ischemic injury shown by diffusion/ perfusion magnetic resonance imaging. *Ann Neurol.* 2000;**47**(4): 462–469.

37. Warach S. Measurement of the ischemic pneumbra with MRI: it's about time. *Stroke.* 2003;**34**(10):2533–2534.

38. Rivers CS, Wardlaw JM, Armitage PA, et al. Do acute diffusion- and perfusion-weighted MRI lesions identify final infarct volume in ischemic stroke? *Stroke.* 2006;**37**(1):98–104.

39. Butcher KS, Parsons M, MacGregor L, et al. Refining the perfusion-diffusion mismatch hypothesis. *Stroke.* 2005;**36**(6):1153–1159.

40. Sobesky J, Zaro W, Lehnhardt FG, et al. Does the mismatch match the pneumbra? Magnetic resonance imaging and positron emission tomography in early ischemic stroke. *Stroke.* 2005;**36**(5):980–985.

41. Moseley ME, Mintorovitch J, Cohen Y, et al. Early detection of ischemic injury: comparison of spectroscopy, diffusion-, T2-, and magnetic susceptibility-weighted MRI in cats. *Acta Neurochri Suppl (Wien)*. 1990;**51**:207–209.

42. Moseley ME, Kucharczyk J, Mintorovitch J, et al. Diffusion-weighted MR imaging of acute stroke: correlation with T2-weighted and magnetic susceptibility-enhanced MR imaging in cats. *AJNR Am J Neuroradiol*. 1990;**11**(3):423–429.

43. Geisler BS, Brandhoff F, Fiehler J, et al. Blood oxygen level-dependent MRI allows metabolic description of tissue ar risk in acute stroke patients. *Stroke*. 2006;**37**:1778–1784.

44. Hermier M, Nighoghossian N. Contribution of susceptibility-weighted imaging to acute stroke assessment. *Stroke*. 2004;**35**:1989–1994.

45. Wardlaw JM, Marshall I, Wild J, et al. Studies of acute ischemic stroke with proton magnetic resonance spectroscopy: relation between time from onset, neurological deficit, metabolite abnormalities in the infarct, blood flow, and clinical outcome. *Stroke*. 1998;**29**(8):1618–1624.

46. Graham GD, Kalvach P, Blamire AM, et al. Clinical correlates of proton magnetic resonance spectroscopy findings after acute cerebral infarction. *Stroke*. 1995;**26**(2):225–229.

47. Jewells V, Castillo M. MR angiography of the extracranial circulation. *Magn Reson Imaging Clin N Am*. 2003;**11**(44):585–597.

48. Mitra D, Connolly D, Jenkins S, et al. Comparison of image quality, diagnostic confidence and interobserver variability in contrast enhanced MR angiography and 2D time of flight angiography in evaluation of carotid stenosis. *Br J Radiol*. 2006;**79**(939):201–207.

49. Fellner C, Lang W, Janka R, Wutke R, Bautz W, Fellner FA. Magnetic resonance angiography of the carotid arteries using three different techniques: accuracy compared with intraarterial X-ray angiography and endarterectomy specimens. *J Magn Reson Imaging*. 2005;**21**(4):424–431.

50. Bammer R, Skare S, Newbould R, et al. Foundations of advanced magnetic resonance imaging. *NeuroRx*. 2005;**2**:167–196.

51. Morasch MD. New diagnostic imaging techniques. *Perspec Vasc Surg Endovasc Ther*. 2005;**17**(4):341–350.

52. Crouse, JR III. Imaging atherosclerosis: state of the art. *J Lipid Res*. 2006;**47**:1677–1699.

53. Yuan C, Kerwin WS. MRI of atherosclerosis. *J Magn Reson Imaging*. 2004;**19**(6):710–719.

54. Saam T, Ferguson MS, Yarnykh VL, et al. Quantitative evaluation of carotid plaque composition by in vivo MRI. *Arterioscler Thromb Vasc Biol*. 2005;**25**(1):234–239.

55. Kooi ME. Cappendijk VC, Cleutjens KB, et al. Accumulation of ultrasmall superparamagnetic particles of iron oxide in human atherosclerotic plaques can be detected by in vivo magnetic resonance imaging. *Circulation*. 2003;**107**(19):2453–2458.

56. Trivedi RA, U-King-Im JM, Graves MJ, et al. In vivo detection of macrophages in human carotid atheroma: temporal dependence of ultrasmall superparamagnetic particles of iron oxide-enhanced MRI. *Stroke*. 2004;**35**(7):1631–1635.

57. Winter PM, Morawski AM, Caruthers SD, et al. Molecular imaging of angiogenesis in early-stage atherosclerosis with alpha(v) beta3-integrin-targeted nanoparticles. *Circulation*. 2003;**18**:2270–2274.

58. Linder JR. Microbubblers in medical imaging: current applications and future directions. *Nat Rev Drug Discov*. 2004;**3**(6)527–532.

59. Nighoghossian N, Derex L, Douek P. The vulnerable carotid artery plaque. Current imaging methods and new perspectives. *Stroke*. 2005;**36**:2764–2772.

60. Powers WJ, Zazulia AR. The use of positron emission tomography in cerebrovascular disease. *Neuroimaging Clin N Am*. 2003;**13**(4):741–758.

61. Heiss WD, Herholz K. Assessment of pathophysiology of stroke by positron emission tomography. *Eur J Nucl Med*. 1994;**21**(5):455–465.

62. Heiss WD, Podreka I. Role of PET and SPECT in the assessment of ischemic cerebrovascular disease. *Cerebrovasc Brain Metab Rev*. 1993;**5**(4):235–263.

63. Heiss WD. Imaging the ischemic penumbra and treatment effects by PET. *Keio J Med*. 2001;**50**(4):249–256.

64. Wise RJ, Bernardi S, Frackowiak RS, Jones T, Legg NJ, Lenzi GL. Measurement of regional cerebral blood flow, oxygen extraction ratio and oxygen utilization in stroke patients using ositron emission tomography. *Exp Brain Res*. 1982;Suppl. **5**:182–186.

65. Lenzi GL, Frackowiak RS, Jones T. Cerebral oxygen metabolism and blood flow in human cerebral ischemic infarction. *J Cereb Blood Flow Metab*. 1982;**2**(3):321–335.

66. Fieschi C. Cerebral blood flow land energy metabolism in vascular insufficiency. *Stroke*. 1980;**11**(5):431–432.

67. Heiss W-D, Sobesky J, v Smekal U, et al. Probability of cortical infarction predicted by flumazenil binding and diffusion-weighted imaging signal intensity. A comparative Positron Emisssion Tomography/Magnetic Resonance Imaging study in early ischemic stroke. *Stroke*. 2004;**35**:1892–1898.

68. Hatazawa J, Shimosegawa E. Imaging neurochemistry of cerebrovascular disease with PET and SPECT. *Q J Nucl Med*. 1998;**42**(3):193–198.

69. Gibbs JM, Wise RJ, Leenders KL, Jones T. Evaluation of cerebral perfusion reserve in patients with carotid-artery occlusion. *Lancet*. 1984;**1**(8372):310–314.

70. Sette G, Baron JC, Mazoyer B, Levasseur M, Pappata S, Crouzel C. Local brain haemodynamics and oxygen metabolism in cerebrovascular disease. Positron emission tomography. *Brain*. 1989;**112**(Pt. 4):931–951.

71. Yamauchi H, Fukuyama H, Kimura J, Konishi J, Kameyama M. Hemodynamics in internal carotid artery occlusion examined by positron emission tomography. *Stroke*. 1990;**21**(10):1400–1406.

72. Itoh M, Hatazawa J, Pozzilli C, et al. Haemodynamics and oxygen metabolism in patients after reversible ischaemic attack or minor ischaemic stroke assessed with positron emission tomography. *Neuroradiology*. 1987;**29**(5):416–421.

73. Masdeu JC, ed. Single-photon emission computed tomography in the practice of neurology. *J Neuroimaging*. 1995;**5**(Suppl 1):S14–22.

74. Saur D, Buchert R, Knab R, Weiller C, Rother J. Iomazenil-single-photon emission computed tomography reveals selective neuronal loss in magnetic resonance-defined mismatch areas. *Stroke*. 2006;**37**(11):2713–2719.

75. Nakagawara J, Sperling B, Lassen NA. Incomplete brain infarction of reperfused cortex may be quantitated with iomazenil. *Stroke*. 1997;**28**(1):124–132.

76. Hirano T, Minematsu K, Hasegawa Y, Tanaka Y, Hayashida K, Yamaguchi T. Acetazolamide reactivity on 123I-IMP single photon emission computed tomography in patients with major cerebral artery occlusive disease: correlation with positron emission tomography parameters. *J Cereb Blood Flow Metab*. 1994;**14**(5):763–770.

77. Imaizumi M, Kitagawa K, Hashikawa K, et al. Detection of misery perfusion with split-dose 123I-iodoamphetamine single-photon emission computed tomography in patients with carotid occlusive diseases. *Stroke*. 2002;**33**(9):2217–2223.

78. Ogasawara K, Ogawa A, Terasaki K, Shimizu H, Tominaga T, Yoshimoto T. Use of cerebrovascular reactivity in patients with symptomatic major cerebral artery occlusion to predict 5-year outcome: comparison of xenon-133 and iodine-123 single-photon emission computed tomography. *J Cereb Blood Flow Metab*. 2002;**22**(9):1142–1148.

79. Kuroda S, Shiga T, Ishikawa T, et al. Reduced blood flow and preserved vasoreactivity characterize oxygen hypometabolism due to incomplete infarction in occlusive carotid artery diseases. *J Nucl Med*. 2004;**45**(6):943–949.

80. Moniz E. *L'angiographie Cérébrale*. Paris: Masson; 1931.

81. Hopkins LN, Ecker RD. Cerebral endovascular neurosurgery. *Neurosurgery*. 2008;**62**:1483–1501.

82. Barr JD. Cerebral angiography in the assessment of acute cerebral ischemia: guidelines and recommendations. *J Vasc Interv Radiol*. 2004;**15**:S57–S66.

83. Qureshi AI, Luft AR, Sharma M, Guterman LR, Hopkins LN. Prevention and treatment of thromboembolic and ischemic complications associated with endovascular procedures: part II – clinical aspects and recommendations. *Neurosurgery*. 2000;**46**: 1360–1375.

84. Earnest RL, Forbes G, Sandok BA, et al. Complications of cerebral angiography: prospective assessment of risk. *Am J Roentgenol*. 1984;**142**:247–253.

85. Dion JE, Gates PC, Fox AJ, et al. Clinical events following neuroangiography: a prospective study. *Stroke*. 1987;**18**:997–1004.

86. Grzyska U, Freitag J, Zeumer H. Selective cerebral intraarterial DSA. Coplication rate and control of risk factors. *Neuroradiology*. 1990;**32**:296–299.

87. Willinsky RA, Taylor SM, terBrugge K, et al. Neurologic complications of cerebral angiography: prospective analysis of 2,899 procedures and review of the literature. *Neuroradiology*. 2003; **227**:522–528.

88. Kerber CW, Cromwell LD, Drayer BP, et al. Cerebral ischemia. I. Current angiographic techniques, complications, and safety. *Am J Roentgenol*. 1987;**130**:1097–1103.

89. Executive committee for the Asymptomatic Carotid Atherosclerosis Study. Endarterectomy for asymptomatic carotid artery stenosis. *JAMA*. 1995;**273**:1421–1428.

90. Mani RL, Eisenberg RL, McDonald EJ Jr, et al. Complications of catheter cerebral angiography: analysis of 5000 procedures. I. Criteria and incidence. *Am J Roentgenol*. 1978;**131**:861–865.

91. Bendszus M, Koltzenberg M, Burger R, et al. Silent embolism in diagnostic cerebral angiography and neurointerventional procedures: a prospective study. *Lancet*. 1999;**354**:1594–1597.

92. Britt PM, Heiserman JE, Snider RM, et al. Incidence of pastangiographic abnormalities revealed by diffusion-weighted MR imaging. *AJNR Am J Neuroradiol*. 2000;**31**:1329–1334.

93. Crawley F, Stygall J, Lunn S, et al. Comparison of microembolism detected by transcranial Doppler and neuropsychological sequelae of carotid surgery and percutaneous transluminal angioplasty. *Stroke*. 2000;**31**:1329–1334.

94. Horowitz MB, Dutton K, Purdy PD. Assessment of complication types and rates related to diagnostic angiography and interventional neuroradiologic procedures. *Interventional Neuroradiol*. 1998;**4**:27–37.

95. Johnston DC, Chapman KM, Goldstein LB. Low rate of complications of cerebral angiography in routine clinical practice. *Neurology*. 2001;**57**:2012–2014.

96. Kremkua FW. *Doppler Ultrasound: Principle and Instruments*. Philadelphia: W. B. Saunders Co.; 1995.

97. Barnett HJ, Taylor DW, Eliasziw M, et al. Benefit of carotid endarterectomy in patients with symptomatic moderate or severe stenosis. North American Symptomatic Carotid Endarterectomy Trial Collaborators. *N Engl J Med*. 1998;**339**:1415–1425.

98. Endarterectomy for asymptomatic carotid artery stenosis. Executive Committee for the Asymptomatic Carotid Atherosclerosis Study. *JAMA*. 1995;**273**:1421–1428.

99. Alexandrov AV, Brodie DS, McLean A, et al. Correlation of peak systolic velocity and angiographic measurement of carotid stenosis revisted. *Stroke*. **28**:343–347.

100. Schwartz SW, Chambless LE, Baker WH, et al. Consistency of Doppler parameters I predicting arteriographically confirmed carotid stenosis. *Stroke*. 1997;**28**:343–347.

101. Bartels E, Fuchs H-H, Flugel KA. Duplex ultrasonography of vertebral artery in cerebral atherosclerosis. *Angiology*. 1992;**43**: 169–180.

102. Hoffman M, Sacco RL, Chan S, Mohr JP. Noinvasive detection of vertebral artery dissection. *Stroke*. 1993;**24**:815–819.

103. Kremkau FW. Doppler principles. *Semin. Roentgenol*. 1992;**27**: 6–16.

104. Kanters SDJM, Algra A, van Leeuwen MS, Banga JD. Reproducibility of in vivo carotid intima-media thickness measurements: a review. *Stroke*. 1997;**28**:665–671.

105. Howard G, Burke GL, Evans GW, et al. Relations of intimal-medial thickness among sites within the carotid artery as evaluated by B-mode ultrasound. *Stroke*. 1994;**25**:1581–1587.

106. Howard G, Sharrett AR, Heiss G, et al. Carotid artery intimal-medial thickness distribution in general populations as evaluated by B-mode ultrasound. *Stroke*. 1993;**24**:1297–1304.

107. Bae JH, Kim WS, Riohal CS, Lerman A. Individual measurement and significance of carotid intima, media, and intima-media thickness by B-mode ultrasonographic image processing. *Arterioscler Thromb Vasc Biol*. 2006;**2**(10):2380–2385.

108. Poredos P. Intima-media thickness: indicator of cardiovascular risk and measure of the extent of atherosclerosis. *Vasc Med*. 2004;**9**(1):46–54.

109. Bonithon-Kopp C. Prevalence of and risk factors for intima-media thickening: a literature review. In: Touboul PJ, Crouse JR II, eds. *Intima-media Thickness and Atherosclerosis. Predicting the Risk?* New York: Parthenon Publishing Group; 1997:27–44.

110. O'Leary DH, Polak JF, Kronmal RA, Manolio TA, Burke GL, Wolfson SK Jr. Carotid-artery intima and media thickness as a risk factor for myocardial infarction and stroke in older adults. *N Engl J Med*. 1999;**340**:14.

111. Hatsukami TS, Ferguson MS, Beach W, et al. Carotid plaque morphology and clinical events. *Stroke*. 1997;**28**:95–100.

112. Perez-Burkhardt JL, Gonzalez-Fajardo JA, Rodriguez E, Mateo AM. Amaurosis fugax as a symptom of carotid artery stenosis. Its relationship with ulcerated plaque. *J Cardiovasc Surg*. 1944; **35**:15–18.

113. Sterpetti AV, Schultz RD, Feldhaus RJ, et al. Ultrasonographic features of carotid plaque and the risk of subsequent neurologic deficits. *Surgery*. 1988;**104**:652–660.

114. Reilly LM, Lusby RJ, Hughes L, et al. Carotid plaque histology using real-time ultrasonography: clinical and therapeutic implication. *Am J Surg*. **146**:188–193.

115. Baroncini LA, Pazin FA, Murta LO Jr, et al. Ultrasonic tissue characterization of vulnerable carotid plaque: correlation between videodensitometric method and histological examination. *Cardiovasc Ultrasound*. 2006;**4**:32.

116. Lee DH, Gao FQ, Rankin R, et al. Duplex and color Doppler flow sonography of occlusion and near occlusion of the carotid artery. *AJNR Am J Neuroradiol*. 1996;**17**:1267–1274.

117. Mansour MA, Mattos MA, Hood DB, et al. Detection of total occlusion, string sign, and preocclusive stenosis of the internal carotid artery by color-flow duplex scanning. *Am J Surg*. 1995;**170**:154–158.

118. Colquhoun I, Oates CP, Martin K, et al. The assessment of carotid and vertebral arteries: a comparison of CFM duplex ultrasound with intravenous digital subtraction angiography. *Br J Radiol*. 1992;**65**:1069–1074.

119. Griewing B, Morgenstern C, Driesner F, et al. Cerebrovascular disease assessed by color-flor and power Doppler ultrasonography. Comparison with digital subtraction angiography in internal carotid artery stenosis. *Stroke*. 1996;**27**:9–100.

120. Newell DW. Transcranial Doppler ultrasonography. *Neurosurg Clin N Am*. 1994;**5**:619–631.

121. Babikian VL, Wechsler LR. *Transcranial Doppler Ultrasonography*. St Louis: Mosby Year Book; 1993.

122. Ringelstein EB, Kahlscheuer B, Niggemeyer E, Otis SM. Transcranial Doppler sonography: anatomical landmarks and normal velocity values. *Ultrasound Med Biol*. 1990;**16**:745–761.

123. Hennerici M, Rautenberg W, Sitzer G, Schwartz A. Transcranial Doppler ultrasound for the assessment of intracranial arterial flow velocity. Part I. Examination technique and normal values. *Surg Neurol*. 1987;**27**:439–448.

124. Asaslid R, Markwalder T-M, Nornes H. Noinvasive transcranial Doppler ultrasound recording of flow velocity in basal cerebral arteries. *J Neursurg*. 1982;**57**:769–774.

125. Sloan MA, Alexandrov AV, Tegeler CH, et al. Assessment: transcranial Doppler ultrasonography: report of the Therapeutics and Technology Assessment Subcommittee of the American Academy of Neurology. *Neurology*. 2004;**62**(9):1468–1481.

126. Seidel G, Kaps M, Gerriets T. Potential and limitations of transcranial color-coded sonography in stroke patients. *Stroke*. 1995;**26**:2061–2066.

127. Baumgartner RW, Mattle HP, Aaslid R. Transcranial color-coded duplex sonography, magnetic resonance angiography, and computed tomography angiography; methods, applications, advantages, and limitations. *J Clin Ultrasound*. 1995;**23**:89–111.

128. Kaps M, Seidel G, Bauer T, Behrmann B. Imaging of the intracranial vertebrobasilar system using color-coded ultrasound. *Stroke*. 1992;**23**:1577–1582.

129. Becker GM, Winkler J, Hoffmann E, Bogdahn U. Imaging of cerebral arteriovenous malformations by transcranial color-coded real-time sonography. *Neuroradiology*. 1990;**32**:280–288.

130. Silvestrini M, Troisi E, Matteis M, et al. Transcranial Doppler assessment of cerebrovascular reactivity in symptomatic and asymptomatic severe carotid stenosis. *Stroke*. 1996;**27**:1970–1973.

131. Hilgertner L, Majchrowski A. Breath holding and carotid compression test. A comparison of two methods for cerebrovascular reactivity assessment. *Cerebrovasc Dis*. 1966;**6**(Suppl 3):18 (Abstract).

132. Stoll M, Hamann G, Jost V, et al. Time course of the acetazolamide effect in patients with extracranial carotid artery disease. *J Neuroimag*. 1996;**6**:144–149.

133. Dahl A, Russell D, Nyberg-Hansen R, et al. Simultaneous assessment of vasoreactivity using transcranial Doppler ultrasound and cerebral blood flow in healthy subjects. *J Cereb Blood Flow Metab*. 1994;**14**:974–981.

134. Dahl A, Russell D, Nyberg-Hansen R, Rootwelt K, Blakke SJ. Cerebral vasoreactivity in unilateral carotid artery disease. A comparison of blood flow and regional cerebral blood flow measurements. *Stroke*. 1994;**25**:621–626.

135. Karnik R, Valentin A, Ammerer H-P, et al. Evaluation of vasomotor reactivity by transcranial Doppler and acetazolamide test before and after extracranial-intracranial bypass in patients with internal carotid artery occlusion. *Stroke*. 1992;**23**:812–817.

136. Klingelhofer J, Sander D. Doppler CO_2 test as an indicator of cerebral vasoreactivity and prognosis in severe intracranial hemorrhage. *Stroke*. 1992;**23**:962–966.

137. Markus HS, Harrison MJG. Estimation of cerebrovascular reactivity using transcranial Doppler, including the use of breath-holding as the vasodilatory stimulus. *Stroke*. 1992;**23**:668–673.

138. Ringelstein EB, Eyck SV, Mertens I. Evaluation of cerebral vasomotor reactivity by various vasodilating stimuli: comparison of CO_2 to acetazolamide. *J Cereb Blood Flow Metab*. 1992;**12**:162–168.

139. Dahl A, Lindegaard KF, Russel D, et al. A comparison of transcranial Doppler and cerebral blood flow studies to assess cerebral vasoreactivity. *Stroke*. 1992;**23**:15–19.

140. Koennecke HC, Mast H, Trocio SS, et al. Microembolic in patients with vertebrobasilar ischemia. Association with vertebrobasilar and cardiac lesions. *Stroke*. 1997;**28**:593–596.

141. Droste DW, Hagedorn G, Notzold A, et al. Bigated transcranial Doppler for the detection of clinically silent circulating emboli in normal persons and patients with prosthetic cardiac valves. *Stroke*. 1997;**28**:588–592.

142. Molloy J, Markus HS. Multigated Doppler ultrasound in the detection of emboli in a flow model and embolic signals in patients. *Stroke*. 1996;**27**:1548–1552.

143. Daffertshofer M, Ries S, Schminke U, Hennerici M. High-intensity transient signals in patients with cerebral ischemia. *Stroke*. 1996; **27**:1844–1849.

144. Barbut D, Yao FS, Hager DN, et al. Comparison of transcranial Doppler ultrasonography to monitor emboli during cardiac bypass surgery. *Stroke*. 1996;**27**:87–90.

145. Sliwka U, Lingnau A, Stohlmann W-D, et al. Prevalence and time course of microembolic signals in patients with acute stroke. A prospective study. *Stroke*. 1997;**28**:593–596.

146. Eicke BM, von Lorentz J, Paulus W, Tegeler CH. Serial transcranial Doppler monitoring after transient ischemic attack. *J Neuroimag*. 1996;**6**:174–176.

147. Keegan BM, Yeung M, Shuaib A. Transcranial Doppler ultrasonography is more sensitive than transeophageal echocardiography in the detection of right to left shut. *Neurology*. 1996; **46**:A301 (Abstract).

148. Nuzzaci G, Right D, Borgioli F, et al. The use of transcranial Doppler and echocardiography to detect interartrial shunting. *Cerebrovasc Dis*. 1996;**6**(Suppl 3):14 (Abstract).

149. Chimowitz MI, Nemec JJ, et al. Transcranial Doppler ultrasound identifies patients with right-to-left cardiac or pulmonary shunts. *Neurology*. 1991;**41**:1902–1904.

150. Griewing B, Schminke U, Morgenstern C, Walker ML, Kessler C. Three-dimensional ultrasound angiography (power mode) for the quantification of carotid artery atherosclerosis. *J Neuroimag*. 1997;**7**:40–45.

151. Downey DB, Fenster A. Vascular imaging with a three-dimensional power Doppler system. *Am J Roentgenol*. 1995;**165**:665–668.

152. Picot PA, Rickey DW, Mitchell R, et al. Three-dimensional colour Doppler imaging. *Ultrasound Med Biol*. 1994;**19**:95–104.

153. Rankin RN, Fenster A, Downey DB, et al. Three dimensional sonographic reconstruction: techniques and diagnostic applications. *Am J Roentgenol*. 1993;**161**:696–702.

154. Bainbridge D. 3-D imaging for aortic plaque assessment. *Semin Cardiothorac Vasc Anesth*. 2005;**9**(2):163–165.

155. Anderson L. Candidate-based proteomics in the search for biomarkers of cardiovascular disease. *J Physiol*. 2005;**563**:23–60.

156. Adkins JN, Varnum SM, Auberry KJ, et al. Toward a human blood serum proteome: analysis by multidimensional separation coupled with mass spectrometry. *Mol Cell Proteomics*. 2002; **1**:947–955.

157. Anderson NL, Anderson NG. The human plasma proteome: history, character, and diagnostic prospects. *Mol Cell Proteomics*. 2002;**1**:845–867.

158. Braeckman L, De Bacquer D, Delanghe J, Claeys L, De Backer G. Associations between hjaptoglobin polymorphism, lipids, lipoproteins and inflammatory variables. *Atherosclerosis*. 1999;**143**: 383–388.

159. Esmon CT. Coagulation and inflammation. *J Endotoxin Res*. 2003;**9**:192–198.

160. Johansson L, Jansson JH, Boman K, Nilsson TK, Stegmayr B, Hallmans G. Tissue-plasminogen activator, plasminogen activator

inhibitor-1 complex as risk factors for the development of a first stroke. *Stroke.* 2000;**31**:26–32.

161. Lindsberg PJ, Grau AJ. Inflammation and infections as risk fctors for ischemic stroke. *Stroke.* 2003;**34**:2518–2532.

162. Elkind MS. Inflammation, atherosclerosis, and stroke. *Neurologist.* 2006;**12**(3):140–148.

163. Di Napoli M, Schwaninger M, Cappelli R, et al. Evaluation of C-reactive protein measurement for assessing the risk and prognosis in ischemic stroke: a statement for health care professionals from the CRP Pooling Project members. *Stroke.* 2005;**36**(6): 1316–1329.

164. Vivanco F, Martin-Ventura JL, Duran MC, et al. Quest for novel cardiovascular biomarkers by proteomic analysis. *J Proteome Res.* 2005;**4**(4):1181–1191.

165. Castillo J, Rodriguez I. Biochemical changes and inflammatory response as markers for brain ischaemia: molecular markers of diagnostic utility and prognosis in human clinical practice. *Cerebrovasc Dis.* 2004;**17**(Suppl 1):7–18.

166. Schwartz RS, Bayes-Genis A, Lesser JR, Sangiorgi M, Henry TD, Conover CA. Detecting vulnerable plaque using peripheral blood: inflammatory and cellular markers. *J Interv Cardiol.* 2003;**16**(3):231–242.

167. Stary HC, Chandler AB, Dinsmore RE, et al. A definition of advanced types of atherosclerotic lesions and a histological classification of atherosclerosis: a report from the Committee on Vascular Lesions of the Council on Arteriosclerosis, American Heart Association. *Artheriosler Thromb Vasc Biol.* 1995;**15**:1512–1531.

168. Sundström J, Vasan RS. Circulating biomarkers of extracellular matrix remodeling and risk of atherosclerotic events. *Curr Opin Lipidol.* 2006;**17**:45–53.

169. Galis ZS, Sukhova GK, Lark MW, Libby P. Increased expression of matrix metalloproterinases and matrix degrading activating in vulnerable regions of human atherosclerotic plaques. *J Clin Invest.* 1994;**94**:2493–2503.

170. Fabunmi RP, Sukhova GK, Sugiyama S, Libby P. Expression of tissue inhibitor of metalloproteinases-3 in human atheroma and regulation in lesion-associated cells: a potential protective mechanism in plaque stability. *Circ Res.* 1998;**83**:270–278.

171. Montaner J, Alvarez-Sabin J, Molina C, et al. Matrix metalloproteinase expression after human cardioembolic stroke: temporal profile and relation to neurological impairment. *Stroke.* 2001; **32**:1759–1766.

172. Montaner J, Fernandez-Cadenas I, Molina CA, et al. Matrix metalloproteinase-9 pretreatment level predicts intracranial hemorrhagic complications after thrombolysis in human stroke. *Circulation.* 2003;**107**:598–603.

173. Montaner J, Fernandez-Cadenas I, Molina CA, et al. Safety profile of tissue plasminogen activator treatment among stroke patients carrying a common polymorphism (C-1562T) in the promoter region of the matrix metalloproteinase-9 gene. *Stroke.* 2003;**34**:2951–2955.

174. Castellanos M, Leira R, Serena J, et al. Plasma metalloproteinase-9 concentration predicts hemorrhagic transformation in acute ischemic stroke. *Stroke.* 2003;**34**:40–66.

175. Beaudeux JLL, Giral P, Bruckert E, et al. Serum matrix metalloproteinase-3 and tissue inhibitor of metalloproteinases-1 as potential markers of carotid atherosclerosis in infranclinical hyperlipidemia. *Atherosclerosis.* 2003;**169**:139–146.

176. Federico A, Bianchi S, Dotti MT. The spectrum of mutations for CADASIL diagnosis. *Neurol Sci.* 2005;**26**(2):117–124.

177. Fan H, Civalier C, Booker JK, Gulley ML, Prior TW, Farber RA. Detection of common disease-causing mutations in mitochondrial DNA (mitochondrial encephalomyopathy, lactic acidosis with stroke-like episodes MTTL1 3243 A>G and myoclonic epilepsy associated with ragged-red fibers MTTK 8344A>G) by real-time polymerase chain reaction. *J Mol Diagn.* 2006;**8**(2): 277–281.

178. Wang QK. Update on the molecular genetics of vascular anomalies. *Lymphat Res Biol.* 2005;**3**(4):226–233.

179. Dichgans M, Hegele RA. Update on the genetics of stroke and cerebrovascular disease 2006. *Stroke.* 2007;**38**(2):216–218.

180. Labauge P, Denier C, Bergametti F, Tournier-Lasserve E. Genetics of cavernous angiomas. *Lancet Neurol.* 2007;**6**(3):237–244.

6

Transient Ischemic Attacks

Unaccustomed attacks of numbness and anesthesia are signs of impending apoplexy.

Hippocrates

Since before the time of Thomas Willis, physicians have been aware that recurrent, short-lived episodes of focal neurologic deficits can precede cerebral infarction; yet, until about 1951, these warnings were ignored because there was no specific therapy to offer.[1] An estimated 400,000 individuals experience a transient ischemic attack (TIA) per year compared to 750,000 strokes per year. Having a TIA increases risk of stroke or ischemic events in other vascular beds. Following a TIA, the risk of recurrent event may be as high as 10.5% within the first 90 days, with the greatest risk apparent during the first week.[2–3]

DEFINITION

A TIA is a rapidly developing temporary focal neurologic deficit related to ischemia of the brain or retina that lasts less than 24 hours and is not accompanied by evidence of cerebral infarction. Yet, most TIAs last only a few minutes. Their importance lies in the fact that they may be harbingers of impending infarction. TIAs involving the carotid circulation should be distinguished from those involving the vertebrobasilar circulation.

Typical of TIAs in the carotid circulation include ipsilateral amaurosis fugax, contralateral sensory or motor dysfunction, aphasia, contralateral homonymous hemianopia, or any combination thereof (Table 6-1). Carotid TIAs may also present as transient episodes of monocular blindness on exposure to bright light or orthostatic limb-shaking events.[4]

The following symptoms represent typical TIAs in the vertebrobasilar system: bilateral or shifting motor or sensory dysfunction, complete or partial loss of vision in both homonymous fields, or any combination of these symptoms. Isolated diplopia, vertigo, dysarthria, and dysphagia are unlikely to represent TIAs, but in combination with one another or with any of the symptoms just listed, any of these symptoms could result from a vertebrobasilar TIA (Table 6-2).

Table 6-1: Carotid Distribution TIA Presentations

Contralateral weakness, clumsiness, or paralysis

Contralateral numbness or paresthesias

Dysphasia or dysarthria

Transient blurring of vision or blindness in ipsilateral eye (amaurosis fugax)

Contralateral homonymous hemianopia

Combinations of the above

Table 6-2: Vertebrobasilar TIA Presentations

Bilateral or shifting weakness or clumsiness

Ataxia, imbalance, or disequilibrium not associated with vertigo

Bilateral or shifting numbness or paresthesias

Dysarthria

Diplopia

Partial or complete blindness in both homonymous visual fields

Combinations of the above

Transient vertigo, diplopia, dysarthria, or dysphagia by themselves are insufficient to establish a definite diagnosis of VB TIA.

Approximately 10% of patients with a TIA have a stroke in the 90 days following the TIA, with half of these having a stroke within 2 days of the TIA. With the advent of diffusion-weighted imaging (DWI) magnetic resonance sequences, the time-based definition of TIAs proved inadequate, because infarctions are sometimes evident radiographically in patients whose clinical manifestations resolved completely within a few hours. Thus, a new "tissue-based" definition (versus the traditional time-based definition) of TIAs has been proposed: brief episodes of neurological dysfunction caused by focal retinal or brain ischemia with symptoms typically lasting less than 60 minutes, and without evidence of acute infarction.[5]

EPIDEMIOLOGY AND NATURAL HISTORY

TIAs have an age- and gender-adjusted incidence rate of 68.2 to 83 per 100,000.[6] The ominous implication of a TIA is underscored by the fact that, in the Caucasian population of the United States, the likelihood of stroke occurring in persons 65 to 74 years of age is about 1% per year, but, in a matched TIA population, the probability increases to 5% to 8% per year. Furthermore, as many as 60% of TIA sufferers die from cardiovascular disease within the ensuing 5 years. A TIA forewarns of infarction in 30% to 50% of patients who suffer atherothrombotic infarction, in 15% to 25% of lacunar infarctions, and in perhaps 10% of cardioembolic infarctions.

TIAs are more common in whites than in other races, probably because of the greater prevalence of atherosclerosis in whites. Men are affected twice as frequently as women, and the onset occurs most often in 50-to-70-year-old individuals. About 40% are hypertensive, 50% have ischemic heart disease, and 20% have diabetes mellitus.

About 90% of TIAs occur in the carotid distribution, 7% in the vertebrobasilar, and 3% in both. These percentages vary with the populations surveyed and are probably skewed by referral patterns that preselect patients with carotid disease referred for surgical evaluation.

PATHOGENESIS OF TIAS

TIAs are most often caused by thromboembolism associated with large artery atherosclerosis (25% to 50%), cardioembolism (10% to 30%), or small vessel (lacunar) disease (10% to 15%).

Microembolism

Of the many causes of TIAs, atherothromboembolism (see Chapter 7) is by far the most common. A thrombus is formed when platelets adhere to vessel walls at lesion-prone sites and undergo activation and aggregation via various inflammatory processes and coagulation cascades.[7] Atherosclerotic plaques shed aggregations of fibrin, platelets, or cholesterol crystals that are carried in the bloodstream to the brain and in the optic fundus (Figure 6-1) during TIAs. Other causes include cardioembolism, most often related to nonvalvular atrial fibrillation, acute myocardial infarction, valvular heart disease (e.g., rheumatic mitral stenosis, prosthetic heart valves), or dilated cardiomyopathies. Embolism from aortic atherosclerosis, thrombophilic conditions, coagulopathies, and hyperviscosity can also cause ischemic attacks. It is likely that most TIAs are initiated by an embolism lodging in the proximal portion of a microcirculatory arterial bed that obstructs the lumen and irritates the wall, causing vasoconstriction of the distal arterioles. However, many individuals with TIAs clearly have multiple contributing factors. Ultimately, a temporary discrepancy between the metabolic needs of neurons and the available supply of blood containing oxygen and other nutrients is the final common pathway.

The pathophysiology of short episodes may differ from those of longer duration, with episodes lasting less than 30 minutes

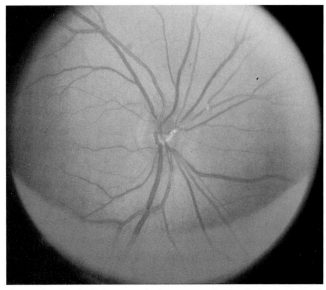

Figure 6-1. Retinal photograph shows an embolism lodged at branch point of a retinal artery. Photograph courtesy of Dr. Nick Hogan.

due to artery-to-artery fibrin/platelet emboli and those of longer duration due to blood clots from the valves or chambers of the left heart. In one study only 8% of patients with TIAs lasting longer than an hour had an abnormal extracranial arteriogram, suggesting a cardiac origin in such cases. On the other hand, 37% of those with TIAs of lesser duration had carotid stenosis. This difference may be related to the size of the embolic particle or clot. The heart may be the source for larger clots that impact larger arteries, whereas microemboli speed easily through the large and lodge only in the small arteries.

Vasospasm

Vasospastic disorders are rarely reported as a cause of this clinical problem.[8] Vasospasm can impede flow through the internal carotid and vertebral arteries as well as the circle of Willis. A remarkable reduction in the caliber of the arteries has been seen by neurosurgeons when the large arteries at the base of the brain are manipulated during surgery. This vasospasm occurs in response to (a) abnormalities such as emboli within the lumen of the artery, (b) subarachnoid bleeding, (c) manipulation of the artery, (d) vasoconstrictor substances in the blood, or (e) cranial trauma. In individuals with subarachnoid hemorrhage, vasospasm is segmental and may be protective by helping to limit the extent of bleeding; however, if spasm is severe or persistent, it can cause brain infarction.

Spasm of the penetrating arteries and arterioles has been likened to the beaded, sausage-shaped segmental spasm that can be seen in the retinal arterioles of patients who have grade II hypertensive retinopathy. When it is more intense and prolonged, it involves the entire circumference and length, reduces blood flow, and is associated with ischemia leading to transudates and then exudates similar to those found in grades III and IV hypertensive retinopathy. Spasm of this degree is always secondary to some other primary process, for instance, sustained severe hypertension, subarachnoid hemorrhage, vasoconstrictor agents, or irritation of the arteriolar bed by local trauma, such as embolus.

Hypotension

Episodic hypotension with or without stenosis in the appropriate arterial distribution seldom results in a TIA. For example, surgical repair of severely stenotic carotid arteries requires the artery to be clamped for about 20 minutes. During this time, over 90% of patients develop no symptoms or signs. Furthermore, restoration of the arterial lumen does not necessarily increase hemispheric blood flow, even though the attacks cease. Last, it has been a common experience that TIAs cease after carotid occlusion occurs, emphasizing that TIAs generally result from emboli – not a reduced perfusion pressure. However, regional hypoperfusion caused by strategically distributed atherosclerotic plaques coupled with anomalies of the circle of Willis can promote boundary zone (watershed) ischemia. This concept, as well as that of leukoariosis resulting from hypoperfusion in the penetrating arterial system, is discussed in Chapters 3 and 5.

Hematologic Causes

Even when the arteries, arterioles, capillaries, and veins are apparently normal, abnormalities in the blood constituents can cause TIAs. These can be divided into as many groups as there are blood constituents. For details, the reader is referred to Chapter 11.

Head and Body Positions

Rapid, extreme degrees of rotation or extension of the head on the neck that (e.g., when working overhead or backing up a car) may cause a feeling of giddiness, imbalance, or light-headedness. This phenomenon is usually caused by angular acceleration of the head that triggers a vestibular response. However, TIAs may stem from mechanical alterations of flow through the arteries in the neck, especially in individuals with basilar impression, platybasia, arterial anomalies, or cervical spondylosis. When turning the head to the opposite side, the vertebral artery is compressed. With cervical osteoarthritis, especially if one vertebral artery is hypoplastic, rotation of the head may lead to symptomatic vertebrobasilar ischemia. Extreme and prolonged rotation, as might occur during sleep, coma, or anesthesia, can result in a TIA or infarction. There have been reports of temporary worsening or precipitation of neurologic deficit when a recumbent person sits or stands. In patients with severe carotid stenosis, cerebral perfusion can be so marginal that a reduction in hydrostatic pressure in the erect position results in limb-shaking TIAs.

Reversal of Cephalic Blood Flow

Lesions of the subclavian or brachiocephalic trunk, the aortic arch, or even the common carotid artery may cause a steal syndrome – inversion of the normal pressure gradients that leads to blood flow away from the brain. Subclavian steal syndrome is discussed in Chapter 3.

Other Abnormalities of the Vessel Wall

Although atherosclerosis is the most frequent cause of TIAs, other nonatherosclerotic cerebral vasculopathies including kinking, cervicocephalic arterial dissections, cervicocephalic fibromuscular dysplasia, vasculitis, or radiation-induced accelerated atherosclerosis may lead to TIAs (see Chapters 12 and 13).

CLINICAL FEATURES

Theoretically, there are as many varieties of TIAs as there are brain functions. As a consequence of the arterial anatomy, certain syndrome patterns are, however, more frequent. Perhaps there is a loss of power in hand or foot, which rapidly progresses to involve an extremity and then, perhaps, the entire side of the body, including the face. Others describe numbness or abnormal sensation, such as lack of feeling that occurs during local anesthesia. It is neither painful nor tingling. Although not common, weakness or numbness of several fingers or the hand may be the sole manifestation of a TIA because of their extensive cortical representation.

A careful history is crucial for the recognition and management of TIAs, because the patient's examination is usually normal by the time they present. Even with a careful history, recognition of TIAs is sometimes difficult, and experienced observers do not always agree. The symptoms of transient ischemic attacks are protean and depend on the vascular territory involved.

When the carotid artery territory is involved, the symptoms reflect ischemia to the ipsilateral retina or brain. Amaurosis fugax (fleeting blindness) is typically characterized by a sudden, painless, and temporary monocular visual loss due to retinal hypoperfusion (see Chapter 2). The visual disturbance is often described as a transient (lasting seconds or minutes) graying, fogging, or blurring of vision, sometimes as if a shade descended over the eye. Pain and scintillations are usually absent. Rarely, similar episodes may be precipitated by a change in posture, exercise, or exposure to bright light; the last is often associated with severe ipsilateral carotid artery occlusive disease. Hemispheral ischemia usually causes weakness and/or numbness of the contralateral face or limbs. Language difficulties and cognitive and behavioral changes may also occur. Rarely, transient episodes of anosognosia may be the presenting feature of a hemispheric TIA.

Vertebrobasilar territory TIAs include symptoms such as dystaxia; vertigo, dizziness or light-headedness; dysarthria; diplopia; dysphagia; partial or complete blindness in both homonymous visual fields; cortical blindness; unilateral, bilateral, or shifting weakness; clumsiness or paralysis; weakness or paralysis of the legs or all four extremities (drop attacks) with preservation of consciousness; bilateral or shifting numbness or paresthesias; or combinations of the above. Vertebrobasilar TIAs may also be associated with episodes of visual inversion, impaired visual accommodation, tinnitus, hearing loss, occipital headaches, or trigeminal autonomic symptoms.[4,9]

The abrupt inability to record memories – a disorder of sudden onset and characteristic of short duration – has been recognized as a distinct entity since first described by Bender in 1956[10] and is now called transient global amnesia (see Chapter 3). Affected individuals are most often middle-aged men. The episodes rarely last longer than 24 hours. Headache before or during the attack is rather common. In many instances the ictus is precipitated by strenuous physical activity, for instance, sports, excitement, heavy exertion, such as sexual intercourse or exposure to thermal extremes, such as a sauna bath or desert heat. The patients who have been examined during an attack have neither physical nor neurologic abnormalities other than memory deficits. Both recent and remote memories are affected during the episode, but, after its termination, the permanent amnesia encompasses only the period between onset and cessation of the attack.

Some attacks are characterized by partial or complete blindness of one or both eyes. This dramatic event, which one imagines would frighten the patient, generally subsides too rapidly for panic, but it is usually sufficient to make the patient seek medical attention.

A well-known, albeit rare, feature of severe carotid stenosis is the presence of "limb-shaking" TIAs, which are often confused with either focal seizures or tremors. Limb-shaking TIAs consist of brief (typically 1 or 2 minutes) involuntary, rhythmic jerking movements of the contralateral arm and hand, or arm, hand, and leg, often precipitated by standing and resolving while sitting. Limb-shaking TIAs may also be precipitated by hyperventilation in patients with moyamoya and result from transient hypoperfusion of the contralateral frontal-parietal cortex.

Patients with isolated confusion or amnesia seldom have vertebrobasilar TIAs.[11] However, episodic behavioral abnormality or amnesia may be a rare manifestation of TIAs, if the limbic system is involved. There may even be no recognized clinical symptoms or signs of recurrent focal dysfunction if the patient denies illness because of emotional response or inattention associated with nondominant hemisphere lesions. A particularly troublesome problem is the possibility of such attacks occurring during sleep (one-third of one's life), during which no awareness of abnormality is possible.

Many patients with seemingly asymptomatic extracranial atherosclerosis have nonfocal neurologic symptoms that may, nevertheless, be related to ischemic brain disease. Some patients are referred because of failing memory, others with behavioral change, and still others with such evanescent phenomena as wooziness, light-headedness, giddiness, and a subjective feeling of not being able to think quickly. Another common complaint is the change in ability to recall stored information at will, such as the names of acquaintances one has not seen for a while, leading to embarrassing situations. Although such symptoms are nonspecific and difficult to interpret, some of these transitory phenomena may represent symptomatic cerebrovascular disease.

If a patient is seen during an episode, the symptoms and signs are indistinguishable from those of an evolving cerebral infarction. In a series of patients examined during an attack, it was observed that many patients were unaware of their deficit, especially visual field deficits.

Symptom Onset

Almost invariably TIAs develop from their first manifestation to full expression within 60 seconds. This extraordinary rapidity is a hallmark that is very useful for differentiating TIAs from migraines or partial seizures. Brevity is one of the major arguments for the pathogenesis of most TIAs being embolic in nature.

Duration of Symptoms

The time boundaries for TIAs were arbitrarily devised to eliminate phenomena that persist for less than 30 seconds or more than 24 hours. Surprisingly, all definitions stipulate the maximum duration, but none define their brevity. Most TIAs resolve within 30 minutes. Almost half of TIAs persist less than 5 minutes, another quarter subside within an hour, and the remainder are gone within 24 hours. Those lasting less than 1 hour are more likely to be caused by a microembolism from an artery, whereas those persisting longer tend to originate from the heart. Generally speaking, the time taken from the moment the attack is first noted until its height is less than the time taken for recovery to occur after symptoms begin to diminish.

Headache

Headache may be associated with TIAs in 15% to 25% of cases of stroke and TIA. Distinguishing the individuals with headache associated with a TIA from those with a deficit due to complicated migraine can be difficult, and some would argue that complicated migraine is merely a type of TIA (see Chapter 14). A diagnosis of complicated migraine is readily apparent in patients with the classic pattern of focal neurological deficit followed immediately by severe unilateral headache and vomiting, but even these individuals can be a diagnostic challenge when seen during the initial phase of an attack before the headache begins. Migraine is so common that a personal or family history of migraine provides little diagnostic help, except perhaps when there is a strong family history of complicated migraine. Additionally, some cerebrovascular conditions feature intermittent headaches that are indistinguishable from those of migraine that begin well before a neurological deficit appears. Thus, one must be cautious about attributing an acute neurological deficit to migraine.

Bickerstaff described a syndrome involving headache, along with symptoms consistent with brainstem ischemia, which he felt was due to a migrainous disturbance in the basilar artery system. Young women are affected most commonly. A family history of migraine is common. The onset is usually visual, with either total loss of vision or strong positive visual phenomenon. Following this, vertigo, dysarthria, bilateral acroparesthesia, perioral numbness, and ataxia may occur. These symptoms last several minutes, then resolve quickly, and, in contrast to TIAs, the patient is often left with a severe, throbbing occipital headache, nausea, and vomiting.

Patients with ischemic oculopathy (ocular ischemic syndrome), a manifestation of carotid artery occlusive disease, may complain of ipsilateral orbital or ocular pain often relieved by lying down. Loss of consciousness is seldom seen with carotid TIAs, but patients may report a transient confusion or a daze. Vague symptoms such as giddiness, dizziness, or forgetfulness by themselves are not typical of TIAs (Table 6-3).

Frequency of Attacks

Some patients suffer only one episode in a lifetime, while others report 20 or more brief attacks in one day. Closely approximated episodes, especially with increasing frequency, are an ominous sign that usually portends infarction. These crescendo TIAs are an alerting mechanism for urgent evaluation and appropriate management. In most instances, however, there are fewer than one or two attacks a month.

The probability that an embolic TIA is caused by atherosclerosis depends on the age and sex of the patient. Those occurring in youth suggest the possibility of another source, such as rheumatic heart disease, congenital anomaly, or collagen vascular diseases. Above age 50 atherosclerosis becomes the probable explanation, and above age 70, perhaps the only consideration.

Neurovascular Examination

The neurovascular examination (see Chapter 2) often signals extracranial carotid disease. Most important is auscultation for

Table 6-3: Symptoms Not Usually Attributed to TIA unless Accompanied by Other Phenomena

Unconsciousness, including syncope

Dizziness or wooziness

Sensory symptoms

Tonic and/or clonic activity

Bowel or bladder incontinence

Impaired vision associated with alteration of consciousness

Symptoms associated with migraine

Scintillating scotomata

Vertigo

Dysarthria

Dysphagia

Diplopia

Confusion

Amnesia

Table 6-4: ABCD2 Score

Age 60 or older	1 point
Blood pressure ≥ 140/90	1 point
Clinical	
▪ Unilateral weakness	2 points
▪ Speech impairment	1 point
Duration	
▪ 60 minutes or more	2 points
▪ Less than 60 minutes	1 point
Diabetes	1 point

Table 6-5: Physical Findings Associated with TIAs

Carotid Circulation

- Abnormal pulsation of the external carotid branches or common carotid arteries on either side
- Arterial bruit localized over either carotid bifurcation and/or the contralateral orbit
- Microemboli, confined to the ipsilateral retina
  - Bright plaques (Hollenhorst)
    - Cholesterol crystals
  - White plugs
    - Platelet fibrin
  - Calcific emboli
    - Calcium
- Diminished pressure in the ipsilateral ophthalmic artery
- Venous stasis (hypotensive) retinopathy
  - Dilated and tortuous retinal veins
  - Midperipheral retinal microaneurysms
  - Blossom-shaped hemorrhages in midperipheral retina
  - Retinal nerve fiber layer splinter hemorrhages
- Diminished temperature over the medial aspect of the ipsilateral forehead

Vertebrobasilar Circulation

- Bruits at the subclavian-vertebral junction and along the course of the vertebral artery to the mastoid
- Unequal blood pressures in the two arms (subclavian steal)

bruits, which are likely to be absent in patients with a complete occlusion and present in those with stenosis.[12] If a patient is seen during an episode, symptoms and signs are indistinguishable from those of an evolving cerebral infarction, and, during an attack, many patients were unaware of their own deficit, especially of visual field deficits.

The atheroma itself is not usually the cause of TIAs or cerebral infarction. Rather, it is the process of ulceration that can cause clinical phenomena due to platelet or other emboli. These may result in crystals visualized in the retina (Hollenhorst plaques) and evanescent neural deficits. Careful funduscopic examination in patients with carotid artery disease may demonstrate retinal microemboli or changes suggestive of venous stasis retinopathy (hypotensive retinopathy).

Risk Stratification and Prognosis

Johnston et al.[13] introduced a new unified score for risk stratification in patients with TIAs, known as the ABCD2 score. The ABCD2 score is based on age (60 or older), blood pressure (≥ 140/90), clinical features, TIA duration (60 minutes or more vs. < 60 minutes), and diabetes (Table 6-4).

Although clinicians must be careful when applying numerical rating scales to individual patients, the ABCD2 score is one of the best predictors of stroke risk during the two-day window, during which approximately half of subsequent strokes occur. Scores of 3 or greater indicate a moderate to high stroke risk and justify prompt hospital admission.

As long as neurologic deficit is present, the TIA cannot be identified as such (differential diagnosis: stroke). If the patient has an acute neurologic deficit and is apparently in the throes of a TIA, he or she must be hospitalized immediately for an immediate diagnostic evaluation and management appropriate to the etiology of the TIA (Table 6-5).

DIFFERENTIAL DIAGNOSIS

A TIA should be diagnosed only if the following criteria are met:

1. The neural dysfunction must be localized to a specific vascular distribution

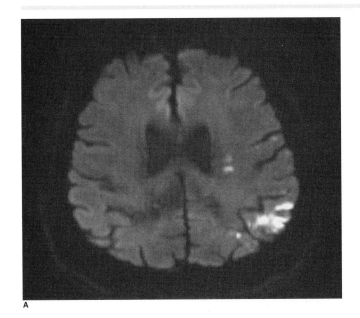

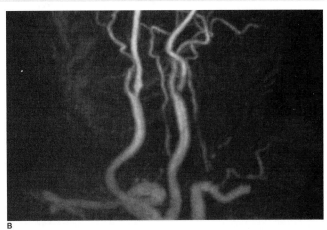

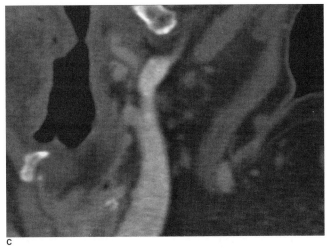

Figure 6-2. A 76-year-old man with hypertension and diabetes presented with transient nonsensical speech. A carotid ultrasound demonstrated 80% to 99% diameter stenosis of the left ICA and a calcified plaque in the left proximal ICA; the right ICA showed 1% to 49% diameter stenosis. A: MRI shows scattered foci of restricted diffusion in the distribution of the posterior division of the left middle cerebral artery. B: MRA shows a focal moderate to severe stenosis at the origin of the left ICA, best seen on the postcontrast sequences. C: CT angiogram shows a severe critical stenosis at the origin of left ICA.

2. The duration of the attack is usually less than 15 minutes but must not exceed 24 hours
3. The patient must have no abnormal neurologic signs between attacks, unless there has been previous infarction or other brain lesion.

Even if these criteria are met, it is not always possible to differentiate TIAs from other disorders, such as Ménière disease, epilepsy, syncope, benign paroxysmal vertigo, psychophysiological reactions, and complicated migraine. Several ophthalmological disorders can mimic TIAs, including angle-closure glaucoma, retinal tears or detachments, lightning streaks of Moore (vertically oriented flashes perceived by the patient in the temporal fields after eye movements), flick phosphenes, optic neuropathies, transient visual obscurations associated

with increased intracranial pressure. Metabolic abnormalities, particularly hypoglycemia, hyperglycemia, and hyponatremia, may occasionally cause transient focal neurologic deficits.

Recurrent short-lived episodes without lasting deficit sometimes occur in patients with intracranial arterial occlusions and, occasionally, in those with brain neoplasms. In such cases cranial computed tomography (CT), magnetic resonance imaging (MRI), and/or CT angiography or catheter cerebral arteriographic examination is indispensable (Figure 6-2).

One may encounter patients with TIAs in whom a full evaluation fails to identify any abnormality. Indeed, 28% to 40% of all aortocervical cranial arteriograms demonstrate no pathoanatomic cause for TIAs. In such cases it may be that the lesion lies in the microcirculation that comprises 80% to 90% of the vascular bed. Alternatively, the cause of such TIAs may be emboli from pulmonary veins, the left atrium or ventricle, or the aortic arch where lesions or clots are notoriously difficult to diagnose, although transesophageal echocardiography is superior to arteriography in this situation and cardiac MRI may prove useful.

When the history and clinical findings suggest a transient vascular disorder, the physician must determine its pathogenesis and triggering mechanisms before concluding that the patient is suffering with atherothrombotic disease. Even if atherosclerosis is the probable cause, the physician must still ascertain what precipitated the attack and whether an unrelated systemic or intracranial disorder contributed to the symptoms. The following are some of the possibilities.

Systemic Disease

1. Hypotension, such as that resulting from acute blood loss, myocardial infarction, antihypertensive medications, hypersensitivity of the carotid sinus reflex, or cardiac dysrhythmias
2. Intracranial embolism from paradoxical embolization of heart valves or mural thrombus of the endocardium should be considered in patients with potential right-to-left shunts, such as patent foramen ovale (PFO) or pulmonary arteriovenous fistulas (see Chapter 8)
3. Hematologic disease, such as polycythemia, sickle cell anemia, and thrombocytosis (see Chapter 11)
4. Substance abuse from barbiturates, alcohol, narcotics, or other drugs of misuse
5. Endocrine disorders such as diabetes mellitus or thyroid disease.

Intracranial Disease

Intracranial disease sometimes causes transient dysfunction:

1. *Cerebral hemorrhage* – About 10% of hemorrhages remain "encapsulated" and cause no bleeding into the cerebrospinal fluid (CSF) (Chapter 16).
2. *Subdural hematoma* – A head injury that appears trivial to the patient and his family may produce a subdural hematoma. Such a sequel to trauma is most likely to occur in the elderly and in patients who have been given anticoagulants.
3. *Neoplasm* – Both benign and malignant neoplasms occasionally cause sudden loss of neurologic function and simulate vascular episodes.
4. *Epilepsy* – Partial seizures are sometimes accompanied by short-lived focal neurologic deficits (post-ictal paralysis or sensory march) that can simulate TIAs. Limb-shaking TIAs could be confused with partial seizures.
5. *Ménière disease* – This may simulate vertebrobasilar ischemia (see Chapters 2 and 3).
6. *Migraine* – The differential diagnosis includes migrainous aura or TIAs with cephalgia such as occurs in 15% to 25% of the individuals with TIAs (see Chapter 14).
7. *Aneurysm* – Rarely clots form within the aneurysmal sac, then embolize distally and cause TIAs.
8. *Familial paroxysmal ataxia* – This syndrome is characterized by sudden onset of frequently recurrent gait dystaxia, dysarthria, and nystagmus lasting up to 3 hours per episode. It is responsive to acetazolamide could be confused with a TIA.

A central issue in the evaluation of patients with TIAs is the degree to which the TIA signals the need for emergency inter-

Table 6-6: Diagnostic Evaluation of Patients with TIAs

MRI including diffusion-weighted MRI

CT (if MR not available or contraindicated)

Carotid duplex ultrasound

Transcranial Doppler, MRA or CTA

ECG

Transthoracic echocardiography

TEE (selected patients)

Holter monitoring (selected patients)

CBC, CMP, PT (INR), aPTT, fasting lipid profile

Hemoglobin A1C (optional)

Erythrocyte sedimentation rate (selected patients)

CRP-HS (optional)

Hypercoagulable evaluation (selected patients)[a]

[a] See Chapters 11 and 20.

vention to prevent what might be a disastrous cerebral infarction. Differing pathogenesis may explain why some patients have a higher risk than others. Therefore, it is our practice to evaluate all TIA patients as emergencies. The carotid system may well be one in which arterial ulcerations and microembolism are the underlying causes, whereas in the vertebrobasilar system, the situation may be one of stenosis and compromise of pressure and flow. Whichever the mechanism, the two situations are considered separately here because diagnostic modalities and therapeutic options differ for the two.

DIAGNOSTIC EVALUATION

Certain procedures should be done on most patients who suffer a TIA. In addition to the general physical, neurological, and neurovascular examinations (see Chapter 2), these tests help to pinpoint the underlying mechanism of ischemia: large vessel atherothrombotic, small vessel lacunar, cardioembolic, nonatherosclerotic vasculopathies, hypercoagulable states, etc. (Table 6-6). In addition to the studies designed to identify common etiologies of TIAs, physicians must be alert to unusual causes if the customary studies are unrevealing. Herein lies the art of medicine and judgment that only extensive clinical experience can provide.

When a carotid distribution TIA occurs, ultrasound examination of the carotid bifurcation must be performed according to standardized laboratory protocols.[14] If ultrasound examination (see Chapter 5) of the internal carotid artery demonstrates the artery to be patent and the lumen compromised less than 60%, we treat the patient medically. The AHA/ASA 2006 guidelines advocate the use of antiplatelet therapy, specifically aspirin, clopidogrel, or extended-release dipyridamole/aspirin for the prevention of stroke.[15] Management of risk factors is also integral to prevention strategies.

The arteriographic image must be projected in such a way that one has an impression, first, of the degree of stenosis and, second, whether ulceration is present. It is surprising to realize that in arteriographic, pathologic, or surgical correlations, the accuracy of radiologic diagnosis of ulceration is only about 80%. The reasons for this include the possibility that the pathology has changed between arteriography and surgery and that the arteriogram is limited by the fact that one can visualize only the contour abnormalities of the arterial tube. This requires three or four projections, which are sometimes overlain by either bone or adjacent arteries, which cannot be subtracted. Another possibility is that ulcerations can be filled with a clot, so that the column of dye is not distorted.

Four criteria, sonographic or arteriographic, have been established for the diagnosis of ulceration: (a) penetrating niche, (b) irregularity of the silhouette of the artery, (c) delayed washout of contrast material in a segment of artery between areas of stenosis, and (d) a wall of circumscribed double density of contrast medium superimposed on the artery.

MEDICAL MANAGEMENT

A recent TIA is an urgent situation necessitating rapid assessment designed to identify and correct underlying stroke risk factors as well as to initiate appropriate therapy. Each patient with recurrent neurologic deficit must be individualized. The key to therapy is, whenever possible, the removal or treatment of any triggering mechanisms.

Modification of risk factors such as arterial hypertension, diabetes, hyperlipidemia, cigarette smoking, and obesity is fundamental in the management of these patients. Antiplatelet therapy is highly effective in reducing the risk of recurrent vascular events and is recommended over warfarin for noncardioembolic TIAs.

Platelet Antiaggregant Therapy

Antiplatelet agents such as aspirin, clopidogrel, and the combination of extended-release dipyridamole plus aspirin, play a critical role in the secondary prevention of atherothrombotic events.[15–17]

Aspirin is the best prophylaxis for prevention of late-stage atherosclerotic complications such as stroke and myocardial infarction (MI). Meta-analyses have shown that aspirin reduces the combined risk of stroke, MI, and vascular death by approximately 25%. The utility of aspirin is based on its irreversible acetylation of platelet cyclo-oxygenase, which decreases platelet aggregation and prevents release of vasoactive substances. However, it does not inhibit the degradation of prothrombin to thrombin, so that hemostasis is only moderately impaired, and severe bleeding is unusual. Furthermore, aspirin does not inhibit adhesion of platelets to damaged endothelium, nor does it prevent the release of smooth muscle growth factors that allow the process to continue.

The acetyl moiety of aspirin combines with the platelet membrane and permanently inhibits platelet cyclo-oxygenase because platelets do not synthesize proteins. Thus, aspirin prevents thromboxane A_2 production for the 7-to-10-day life of the platelet, and as little as 30–60 mg daily may be sufficient to inhibit aggregation. Aspirin also inhibits prostacyclin (PGI_2) production by the endothelium. However, small intermittent doses of aspirin do not have a lasting effect on the production of PGI_2 in blood vessels because normal endothelial cells have an excellent capacity for protein synthesis, allowing cyclo-oxygenase and PGI_2 to be restored to normal within a few hours. Whether atherosclerotic blood vessels resynthesize cyclo-oxygenase after aspirin inhibition is unknown; theoretically, restoration of PGI_2 in atherosclerotic plaque could be inhibited by therapy aimed at controlling platelet aggregation.

The characteristics of plaques and their effects on blood flow add still another dimension to the interaction between aspirin, platelets, and the arterial wall. For example, in slow-flow, low-pressure systems, the spontaneous initiation of the coagulation cascade is of more importance than is platelet-initiated thrombogenesis, whereas the reverse is true in arterial fast-flowing systems. Moreover, debris cast into the bloodstream by degenerated plaque can serve as the nidus for platelet-initiated thrombi.

Drugs that interfere with platelet function have been evaluated by randomized prospective trials that have tested primary prevention of myocardial infarction as well as secondary prevention in patients with myocardial infarction, TIAs, or nondisabling cerebral infarction. These studies do not mean that platelet antiaggregants are the definitive stroke preventives because some patients have break-through strokes despite taking aspirin. Furthermore, in two trials there was a disturbing increase in the incidence of intracerebral hemorrhage in the aspirin arm, which can be a complication of its chronic use.

Recommendations regarding dose of aspirin range from 50 to 325 mg a day; however, for patients suffering an acute ischemic stroke, the lowest effective dose is 160 mg.[18–19]

One of the major dilemmas of therapy is individual variation in medication responsivity. Most individuals have a stable, reproducible dose- or concentration-response relationships for many drugs, allowing doses to be adjusted individually. However, others differ substantially in their response because of genetic makeup, concurrent diseases, gastrointestinal absorption, metabolic factors, and interaction with other drugs.[20]

The other antiplatelet agents that have proven efficacy in stroke prevention are clopidogrel, ticlopidine, and aspirin plus extended-release dipyridamole. Clopidogrel is a platelet adenosine diphosphate receptor antagonist. Clopidogrel is given as a single dose 75 mg daily. In a study of more than 19,000 patients with atherosclerotic vascular disease (manifested as either recent ischemic stroke, recent MI, or symptomatic peripheral arterial disease), 75 mg of clopidogrel was modestly more effective (8.7% relative risk reduction) than 325 mg of aspirin in reducing the combined risk of ischemic stroke, MI, or vascular death. Ticlopidine acts primarily by irreversible inhibition of the adenosine diphosphate pathways of the platelet membrane. Ticlopidine at a dose of 250 mg twice daily reduces the relative risk for death and nonfatal stroke by 12% in comparison to aspirin. Individuals taking ticlopidine sometimes develop neutropenia and thrombotic thrombocytopenia purpura. Consequently, since the advent of clopidogrel, ticlopidine is now seldom used except in Japan, where physicians still use it (but at a reduced dose of only 200 mg/day).

Dipyridamole is a cyclic nucleotide phosphodiesterase inhibitor. The combination of low-dose aspirin and extended-release dipyridamole has been shown to be effective in reducing the rate of nonfatal stroke and offers a potential alternative to aspirin alone for stroke prevention. The PRoFESS trial examined the safety and efficacy of aspirin and extended-release dipyridamole versus clopidogrel for recurrent stroke in more than 20,000 patients. This trial enrolled 20,322 patients (from 695 centers in 35 countries) with recent noncardioembolic ischemic stroke. Almost a third of patients (32%) were from Asia. Randomization guaranteed an equal balance of demographic factors and medical history between the two groups. Mean follow-up was 2.5 years. PRoFESS compared 10,181 patients treated with aspirin plus extended-release dipyridamole (25 mg ASA + 200 mg ER-DIP bid) with 10,151 patients treated with clopidogrel (75 mg/d CLO) alone. PRoFESS was originally designed to test the superiority of ASA + ER-DIP over CLO in 15,500 patients. This was modified to 20,000 patients after six protocol amendments because of lower-than-expected outcome events. Sequential statistical testing of noninferiority followed by superiority testing was planned. Using data from CAPRIE and from the meta-analysis of the ATC, and following the method of Fisher, the prestated margin of noninferiority was 1.075, and it involved the prespecification of a hazard ratio. The primary endpoint (recurrent stroke of any type) occurred among 916 patients (9.0%) receiving ASA + ER-DIP, and in 898 patients (8.8%) receiving CLO (hazard ratio 1.01; 95% CI: 0.92–1.11). Ischemic stroke accounted for 87.4% (1,585 of 1,814) of the recurrent strokes. The composite endpoint of vascular death, nonfatal myocardial infarction, and nonfatal stroke was identical in the two groups: 1,333 patients (13.1%) (hazard ratio for ASA + ER-DIP versus CLO was 0.99; 95% CI: 0.92–1.07.) The rates of most tertiary (efficacy) outcomes were also equal in both groups. Hemorrhagic events occurred in 4.1% of ASA + ER-DIP recipients and among 3.6% of CLO recipients (hazard ratio 1.15; 95% CI: 1.00–1.32; p = +0.06). PRoFESS failed to meet the prespecified noninferiority margin of 1.075.[21]

Currently there is no evidence regarding the efficacy of combining clopidogrel and aspirin in ischemic stroke patients unless patients have a history of acute coronary syndrome or have an endovascular stent deployed.

Dietary changes which increase prostacyclin and alter platelet aggregability may develop into worthwhile therapeutic strategies. Those who eat fish as a major component of diet may have elevated levels of eicosopentanoic acid that reduces platelet aggregability. Consequently, some add fish oil supplements to diets designed to reduce atherogenesis.

Anticoagulant Therapy

Warfarin is indicated for primary and secondary prevention of stroke among patients with nonvalvular atrial fibrillation. Warfarin is also indicated for prevention of stroke in patients with rheumatic atrial fibrillation, mechanical prosthetic heart valves, or other selected subgroups of patients with high-risk cardiac sources of embolism. Other potential indications for warfarin include TIAs associated with extracranial cervicocephalic arterial dissections or TIAs associated with selected hypercoagulable states.

Regimen for Warfarin Therapy

Coumarin and warfarin sodium are synthetic oral anticoagulants that inhibit hepatic synthesis of vitamin K–dependent clotting factors II, VII, IX, and X. Patients should be treated to an international normalized ratio (INR) range of 2.0 to 3.0.

A major problem in long-term administration is compliance with the routine of daily medication and frequent blood sampling for medication adjustments. Some patients who are sensitive to a particular drug may manifest toxicity at concentrations considered in the therapeutic range, whereas others may require concentrations above the therapeutic range before efficacy occurs. Therefore, neither efficacy nor toxicity can be quantified by measuring drug concentrations, although such

measurements may be used, along with other laboratory data and clinical signs and symptoms, as evidence of lack of efficacy or toxicity.

Patients with cerebral embolism from high-risk cardiac disorders (see Chapter 8) may require one of these drugs indefinitely. If it seems advisable to discontinue anticoagulants after a patient has been taking them for any length of time, the dose should be reduced gradually to avoid hypercoagulability – the so-called rebound effect. Even if the prothrombin time (PT) is found to be unduly prolonged as the result of an overdose, it is usually wise to administer, at most, a very small dose of vitamin K_1 oxide, to return the prothrombin time *toward* normal rather than *to* normal.

Furthermore, drug interactions that alter the bioavailability of vitamin K, such as antibiotics, mineral oil, or cholestyramine, must be considered when treating patients with oral anticoagulants. Other interactions are those that alter hepatic metabolism and change the dose requirements. The amount of anticoagulant medication required by a given patient varies according to the climate – the warmer the weather, the larger the dose required to achieve the same effect. Other factors that may affect the prothrombin time and the required dosage of anticoagulants are certain medications, for example, salicylates, barbiturates, phenylbutazone, and antibiotics; vitamin K ingested in food and multiple-vitamin mixtures; consumption of alcohol; intercurrent illnesses (especially gastroenteritis); and the use of organic solvents in the patient's hobby or occupation. In the rare pregnant patient who requires anticoagulants, heparin rather than coumarin should be used.

The most common complication of anticoagulant therapy is bleeding from any one of a number of sites, even though the PT may be within the therapeutic range. If bleeding from the gastrointestinal or urinary tract occurs when the PT is within the targeted range, one should consider an underlying lesion, such as carcinoma, ulcer, renal stone, or cystitis. Hemoptysis or epistaxis is rarely a problem, and hemarthrosis or bleeding into the muscles after minor trauma is even more infrequent. Patients with ischemic brain disease who are maintained on anticoagulants may develop subdural or epidural hematomas within the calvaria or in the spinal canal, sometimes after lumbar puncture or minor trauma to the back. These may be insidious, and the symptoms and signs may be mistakenly attributed to progression of the cerebrovascular process, rather than to the hematoma.

Blood Pressure Medications

Blood pressure treatment resulting in a decrease in mean diastolic blood pressure of 5 mm Hg over 2 to 3 years is associated with a 40% reduction in risk of stroke. Available evidence from large randomized trials appears to support the use of a diuretic with or without an angiotensin-converting enzyme (ACE) inhibitor.

SURGICAL-ENDOVASCULAR MANAGEMENT

Data from large randomized clinical trials have established carotid endarterectomy (CEA) as the standard treatment for severe symptomatic carotid artery stenosis. Timely surgical intervention in selected patients with hemispheric TIAs, amaurosis fugax, or nondisabling carotid territory ischemic strokes within the previous 6 months, and with 70% to 99% diameter reducing carotid stenosis, can significantly reduce the risk for recurrent cerebral ischemia or death. In centers with a low surgical risk, CEA also provides modest benefit in symptomatic patients with carotid artery stenosis of 50% to 69%.[22-29] The indications for urgent or emergent CEA remain controversial.[30]

Data from SPACE and EVA-3S failed to show a benefit for carotid artery angioplasty and stenting (CAS) in recently symptomatic patients who were randomized to CEA or CAS. Two additional trials (ICSS and CREST) continue to actively randomize patients.[31]

COURSE AND PROGNOSIS

Reports of the frequency with which TIA patients suffer cerebral infarction range from 2% to 62% with the consensus being that about 25% eventually suffer infarction in the location of the TIA within 3 years of the onset. When assessed retrospectively, the range is from 9% to 74%. Therefore, both retrospective and prospective studies affirm the serious nature of TIAs, and they must be treated accordingly. Of TIA patients who eventually develop infarction, the short time often elapsing between the two determines that these patients be evaluated urgently and treated as emergencies. About 36% of subsequent infarctions occur within a month and 50% within 12 months of onset of TIAs.

Following a TIA, the risk of cerebral infarction is increased up to 10 times within 5 years and is greatest in the first few months. However, only about 20% of infarctions are preceded by TIAs. It is estimated that about one-third of those who suffer recurrent transient neurologic deficit continue to have attacks without developing permanent disability; another third eventually have cerebral infarction; and, in the remainder, the attacks cease spontaneously. Unfortunately, we have no way to predict the group into which an individual will fall, but there is some indication that the natural history of attacks secondary to vertebral-basilar territory ischemia is more benign than that associated with carotid artery syndrome. Five-year mortality rates in TIA patients average about 20% to 25%. However, the majority of these fatalities are secondary to myocardial rather than cerebral infarction.

The incidence and prevalence of TIAs varies with race, sex, age, and, surprisingly, by geographic location. The causes for some of this variation are known but for others constitute the raison d'être for ongoing clinical research. Note how incidence and prevalence increase with age in all groups and how women are "protected" until after menopause. Furthermore, TIA varies among racial groups residing in one geographic area.

Hospital-based reports reflect referral patterns and selection bias, particularly the time elapsed between TIA and admission to hospital. However, most reports emanate from this source, resulting in bias. Using proportional hazards analyses, the impact of TIA increases with age, cigarette use, previous stroke or myocardial infarction, and diabetes mellitus.

To a large degree, prognosis of TIA depends on its etiology and concomitant diseases. In younger populations in whom excess risk is generally less, etiologies such as valvular and congenital heart disease and hypotension are major contributors to TIA. In the elderly hypertension and atherosclerosis become major contributors to risk, and the course and prognosis is poorest.

A hitherto poorly investigated potential contributor to risk is family clustering of stroke. Whether this is a genetic predisposition or an environmental factor, such as dietary habits or attitudes toward medical intervention, is unknown.

REFERENCES

1. Fisher CM. Transient monocular blindness associated with hemiplegia. *Trans Am Neurol Assoc.* 1951;**76**:154–158.
2. Johnston SC, Gress DR, Browner WS, Sidney S. Short-term prognosis after emergency department diagnosis of TIA. *JAMA.* 2000;**284**:2901–2906.
3. Rothwell PM, Giles MF, Flossmann E, et al. A simple score (abcd) to identify individuals at high early risk of stroke after transient ischaemic attack. *Lancet.* 2005;**366**:29–36.
4. Feldman E, Wilterdink JL. The symptoms of transient cerebral ischemic attacks. *Sem Neurol.* 1991;**11**:135–145.
5. Albers GW, Caplan LR, Easton JD, et al. Transient ischemic attack: proposal for a new definition. *N Engl J Med.* 2002;**347**:1713–1716.
6. Rosamond W, Flegal K, Friday G, et al. Heart disease and stroke statistics – 2007 update. A report from the American Heart Association statistics committee and stroke statistics subcommittee. *Circulation.* 2006;**16**:762–772.
7. Steinhubl SR, Moliterno DJ. The role of the platelet in the pathogenesis of atherothrombosis. *Am J Cardiovasc Drugs.* 2005;**5**:399–408.
8. Libman RB, Masters SR, de Paola A, Mohr JP. Transient monocular blindness associated with cocaine abuse. *Neurology.* 1993;**43**: 228–229.
9. Maramattom BV. Transient ischemic attack with trigeminal autonomic symptoms. *J Neurol Neurosurg Psychiatry.* 2005;**76**:104.
10. Bender MB. Syndrome of isolated episode of confusion with amnesia. *J Hillside Hospital.* 1956;**5**:212–215.
11. Albucher JF, Martel P, Mas JL. Clinical practice guidelines: diagnosis and immediate management of transient ischemic attacks in adults. *Cerebrovasc Dis.* 2005;**20**:220–225.
12. Caplan LR. The frontal artery sign – a bedside indicator of carotid occlusive disease. *N Engl J Med.* 1973;**288**:1008.
13. Johnston SC, Rothwell PM, Nguyen-Huyn MN, et al. Validation and refinement of scores to predict very early stroke risk after transient ischemic attack. *Lancet.* 2007;**369**:283–292.
14. Grant E, Benson CB, Moneta GL, et al. Carotid artery stenosis: gray scale and Doppler US Diagnosis Society of Radiologists in Ultrasound Consensus Conference. *Radiology.* 2003;**229**:340–346.
15. Sacco RL, Adams R, Albers G, et al. Guidelines for prevention of stroke in patients with ischemic stroke or transient ischemic attack: a statement for healthcare professionals from the American Heart Association/American Stroke Association Council on Stroke: cosponsored by the Council on Cardiovascular Radiology and Intervention: The American Academy of Neurology affirms the value of this guideline. *Stroke.* 2006;**37**:577–617.
16. Goldstein LB, Adams R, Alberts MJ, et al. Primary prevention of ischemic stroke: A guideline from the American Heart Association/American Stroke Association Stroke Council: cosponsored by the Atherosclerotic Peripheral Vascular Disease Interdisciplinary Working Group; Cardiovascular Nursing Council; Clinical Cardiology Council; Nutrition, Physical Activity, and Metabolism Council; and the Quality of Care and Outcomes Research Interdisciplinary Working Group: the American Academy of Neurology affirms the value of this guidelines. *Circulation.* 2006;**113**(24):e873–923.
17. Biller J. The role of antiplatelet therapy in the management of ischemic stroke: implementation of guidelines in current practice. *Neurolog Res.* 2008;**30**(7):669–677.
18. Weisman SM, Graham DY. Evaluation of the benefits and risks of low-dose aspirin in the secondary prevention of cardiovascular and cerebrovascular events. *Arch Intern Med.* 2002;**162**:2197–2202.
19. Smith SC, Allen J, Blair SN, et al. AHA/ACC Guidelines for secondary prevention for patients with coronary and other atherosclerotic vascular disease. 2006 update. *Circulation.* 2006;**113**: 2363–2372.

20. Biller J. Aspirin nonresponse in patients with arterial causes of ischemic stroke: Considerations in detection and management. *J Neurol Sci.* 2008;**272**:1–7.

21. Sacco RL, Diener HC, Yusuf S, et al. PRoFESS Study Group. Aspirin and extended-release dipyridamole versus clopidogrel for recurrent stroke. *N Engl J Med.* 2008;**359**(12):1238–1251.

22. Mayberg MR, Wilson SE, Yatsu F. VA Symptomatic Carotid Stenosis Group. Carotid endarterectomy and prevention of cerebral ischemia in symptomatic carotid stenosis. *JAMA.* 1991;**266**:3289–3294.

23. European Carotid Surgery Trialists' Collaborative Group. Randomised trial of endarterectomy for recently symptomatic carotid stenosis: final results of the MRC European Carotid Surgery Trial (ECST). *Lancet.* 1998;**351**:1379–1387.

24. North American Symptomatic Carotid Endarterectomy Trial Collaborators. Benefit of carotid endarterectomy in patients with symptomatic moderate or severe stenosis. *N Engl J Med.* 1998;**339**: 1415–1425.

25. Executive Committee for the Asymptomatic Carotid Atherosclerosis Study. Endarterectomy for asymptomatic carotid artery stenosis. *JAMA.* 1995;**273**:1421–1428.

26. Halliday A, Mansfield A, Marro J, et al. MRC Asymptomatic Carotid Surgery Trial (ACST) Collaborative Group. Prevention of disabling and fatal strokes by successful carotid endarterectomy in patients without recent neurological symptoms: randomized controlled trial. *Lancet.* 2004;**363**:1491–1502.

27. North American Symptomatic Carotid Endarterectomy Trial Collaborators. Beneficial effect of carotid endarterectomy in symptomatic patients with high-grade carotid stenosis. *N Engl J Med.* 1991;**325**:445–453.

28. MRC European Carotid Surgery Trial. Interim results for symptomatic patients with severe (70–99%) or with mild (0–29%) carotid stenosis: European Carotid Surgery Trialists' Collaborative Group. *Lancet.* 1991;**337**:1235–1243.

29. Biller J, Feinberg W, Castaldo JE, et al. Guidelines for carotid endarterectomy: a statement for healthcare professionals from a special writing group of the Stroke Council, American Heart Association. *Stroke.* 1998;**29**:554–562.

30. Van der Mierem G, Duchateau J, De Vleeschauwer P, et al. The case for urgent carotid endarterectomy. *Acta Clin Belg.* 2005;**105**: 403–406.

31. Barrett KM, Brott TG. Carotid artery stenting versus carotid endarterectomy: current status. Neurology Clinics. *Preoperative Perioperative Issues Cerebrovas Dis.* 2006;**24**(4):681–691.

7

Atherosclerosis of the Cervicocranial Arteries

It is very common in examining the brain of persons who are considerably advanced in life, to find the trunks of the internal carotid artery upon the side of the sella turcica very much diseased, and this disease extends frequently more or less into the small branches. The disease consists in a bony or earthy matter being deposited in the coats of the arteries, by which they loose a part of their contractile and distensile powers, as well as of their tenacity. The same sort of diseased structure is likewise found in the basilar and its branches.

Mathew Baillie

Atherosclerosis affects millions of people worldwide, and by the end of the next decade, it is likely to become the leading cause of death worldwide.[1–3] Atherosclerosis of the arteries supplying the brain has been found in mummified Egyptians preserved from 4000 B.C.E., so this disease has probably afflicted mankind ever since he indulged his gastronomic urges by eating the forbidden fruit.[4] Although atherosclerosis does not always result from the rise of various cardiometabolic risk factors including the greater problem of rising obesity and its associated pathologies, it has been known for decades that people with a low prevalence of atherosclerosis may migrate around the world, change their eating habits and environment, and acquire increased prevalence of the disease.

Atherosclerosis is a diffuse systemic vascular disorder affecting large and medium-sized arteries causing patchy intimal plaques known as atheromas. Atherosclerosis is known to begin early in life with pathological studies showing that fatty streaks start as early as 2 years of age. However, it usually does not become symptomatic until middle age or thereafter.[5] Because of the systemic nature of atherosclerosis, having a transient ischemic attack (TIA) or stroke increases the likelihood of a recurrent stroke or ischemic events in other vascular beds.

CLINICAL MANIFESTATIONS OF ATHEROSCLEROSIS

Two of the three leading causes of death in the United States of America, namely, cardiovascular disease and stroke, often result from atherosclerosis.[6] Because of the diffuse nature of atherosclerosis, individuals with a history of stroke or TIAs are also at

risk for ischemic events in the coronary vascular bed. The pathologic process begins with superficial erosion or rupture of an atherosclerotic lesion that initiates hemostasis, including platelet aggregation and fibrin deposition, leading to thrombus formation at the site of the vascular lesion. Atherosclerosis affects predominantly large and medium-size arteries, and atheromas are made up of various lipids, blood cells, and blood products, leading to focal thickening and fibrosis (the plaque). These arterial lesions cause one or more of the following complications, namely, stenosis of the lumen, progressive weakening of the vessel wall (aneurysm formation), calcification, ulceration, thrombosis, and thromboembolism.[7–9] However, there are frequent exceptions to the above pattern; for example, small meningeal arterial branches may be affected by atherosclerosis in patients with diabetes, or the media and adventitia can be secondarily affected during the formation of atherosclerotic aneurysm.

Atherosclerosis can cause both TIAs (see Chapter 6) and ischemic stroke. Specific neurological findings depend on location and duration of ischemia distal to the atherosclerotic vessel and are not unique to atherosclerosis. Whether or not a brain infarction occurs in a given individual with atherosclerosis is influenced by the availability of collateral blood supply, the presence of other risk factors, the existence of other comorbidities, and the effectiveness of earlier treatment. Common syndromes of vascular dysfunction are reviewed in Chapter 3.

The distinction between symptomatic and asymptomatic cerebrovascular atherosclerotic steno-occlusive disease may depend on the patient's recognition of sometimes subjective and evanescent events and on whether the patient's physician recognizes the implications of subtle complaints. Some nonspecific symptoms, such as giddiness and forgetfulness, are difficult to interpret. Nondisabling symptoms are often ignored by the patient. In other individuals, strokes occur in a so-called silent brain area, causing neuroimaging lesions but no symptoms and no detectable neurologic deficits.[10] Patients may be unaware of nondominant hemispheric TIAs and even of small infarctions, illustrating anew the value of observations by family and skilled observers, particularly regarding behavioral changes and memory.

The identification of underlying atherosclerosis before it becomes symptomatic has therapeutic implications. Although the history and neurovascular examination are valuable screening methods, they must be augmented by more objective information, especially in asymptomatic individuals. The widespread availability of accurate, noninvasive imaging techniques that can be repeated over time to assess a lesion's longitudinal change makes it feasible to begin therapy before the onset of symptoms in some individuals. Ultrasound techniques such as color-coded high-definition power duplex and three-dimensional imaging provide precise categorization of flow disturbance, wall characteristics, size, type, and frequency of microemboli (see Chapter 5).

Superficial wedge-shaped infarctions have a predilection for the anterior, middle, and posterior cerebral arteries, where the smaller branches of one artery form anastomoses with those of another. Local arterial pressures in these watershed areas are normally the lowest in the system, so that any generalized reduction first reaches critical levels in these terminal branches, especially those of the parietal region. The more deeply situated infarctions of the cerebrum are most commonly found in the region of the internal capsule.

Compression of a cranial nerve or brainstem structure by a dilated, tortuous, atherosclerotic artery can cause cranial nerve dysfunction, a cerebellopontine angle syndrome, trigeminal neuralgia, or hemifacial spasm. Binasal hemianopsia sometimes results when a dilated and calcified internal carotid artery compresses the lateral margins of the optic nerves and chiasm. Elongation of the terminal portion of the basilar artery may invaginate into the third ventricle, sometimes resulting in cognitive impairment due to obstructive hydrocephalus.

Atherosclerosis per se does not cause Parkinsonism, but the two conditions frequently occur together in elderly individuals, and they can have overlapping clinical manifestations. Individuals with cerebrovascular disease whose findings resemble those of "lower body Parkinsonism" typically have associated upper motor neuron dysfunction, dementia, and/or pseudobulbar signs in addition to their extrapyramidal signs. In patients with widespread disease, lacunar state is often found at postmortem examination.

Even though the clinical signs associated with pseudobulbar palsy (involuntary emotional expression) are superficially suggestive of primary medullary (bulbar) dysfunction, most individuals have bilateral lesions in the corticobulbar tracts with supranuclear paralysis of the lower cranial nerves, characterized by dysarthria, dysphagia, and an immobile facies. The typical location of lesions is in the posterior limb of the internal capsules, often the result of multiple lacunes (see Chapter 9). Because one side is usually involved before the other, most patients have a history of focal deficit followed by more recent paralysis on the opposite side and superimposed pseudobulbar signs. The patient has difficulty speaking and protruding his tongue. The jaw jerk and muscle stretch reflexes are hyperactive, and Hoffmann's and Babinski's signs may occur bilaterally. Bilateral corticospinal tract lesions cause the gait to be slow, clumsy, unsteady, and shuffling (*marche-a-petit-pas*). Diffuse cerebral involvement may cause lability of affect and other personality changes, with inappropriate and uncontrolled laughter or crying in response to minor emotional stimuli.

RISK FACTORS FOR ATHEROSCLEROSIS

For atherosclerosis in general, advanced age, male gender, arterial hypertension, dyslipidemia, diabetes mellitus, tobacco use, and a diet high in saturated fats are the main risk factors. In addition, obesity, lack of exercise, prolonged use of oral contraceptives, and high-carbohydrate diets are contributory factors. The most studied risk factors are elevated levels of low-density lipoprotein (LDL) and very low-density lipoprotein (VLDL) in blood. It appears that in any given individual more than one factor can act synergistically and contribute to the development of atherosclerotic lesions.[11–13]

Fewer risk factors are known to specifically increase the risk for craniocervical atherosclerosis and stroke, with advancing age, arterial hypertension, diabetes mellitus, and dyslipidemias leading the list. It is generally accepted that factors that contribute to atherosclerosis in general are also likely to contribute to the development of carotid artery and intracranial atherosclerosis, but the association may be less than statistically significant or less thoroughly studied.

Arterial Hypertension

There are approximately 1 billion people with arterial hypertension worldwide, with an estimated 65 million (ages 65–75 years) in the United States alone.[14] Hypertension occurs earlier and more frequently among African American men and women. Hypertension is a well-known risk factor for ischemic stroke and intracerebral hemorrhage. Hypertension also increases the risk for atherosclerosis fourfold, probably because it accelerates atherogenesis. Atherosclerosis in individuals with systemic hypertension does not differ qualitatively from that in normotensive individuals but, instead, is worse at the usual sites of predilection and involves segments of the arterial tree that are generally spared. This accelerated process is even more rapid when serum cholesterol levels exceed 220 mg/dl.

Current theories of atherogenesis suggest different explanations for the vascular effects of arterial hypertension. An early aspect of atherogenesis is thought to involve altered endothelial permeability.[15] Similarly, arterial hypertension itself induces some thickening of the intima and increased endothelial permeability. Thus, if we regard atherosclerosis as a disease of accretion, hypertension will enhance it – the more lipid in the plasma, the more lipid in the intima. The brain of an adult receives approximately 55 ml of blood flow per 100 grams of tissue per minute, and, at heightened systolic and diastolic blood pressures, the regions prone to hemodynamic variation, such as the carotid artery bifurcation, will suffer more severely in hypertensives than in normotensives. The carotid bulb is the first segment of the internal carotid artery after its origin. The bulbous enlargement of the carotid bulb is predisposed to the formation of atheromatous plaques.

Cholesterol and Lipoproteins

Cholesterol is a lipid component of cell membranes and a precursor of bile acids and steroid hormones that travels in the blood as spherical particles of lipoprotein. The cholesterol level in blood plasma is determined partly by the fat and cholesterol content of the diet. Other factors, such as obesity and physical inactivity, may also play a role.

Three major classes of lipoproteins can be measured in the serum: very low-density lipoproteins (VLDLs), low-density lipoproteins (LDLs), and high-density lipoproteins (HDLs). The LDL is the major atherogenic class and typically contains 60% to 70% of the total serum cholesterol, whereas HDL usually contains 20% to 30%. HDL is inversely and LDL directly correlated with risk for coronary heart disease and stroke. The VLDL, which is composed mainly of triglycerides, contains 10% to 15% of the total serum cholesterol. Because most of the cholesterol in the serum is found in the LDL, the concentration of total cholesterol is closely correlated with the concentration of LDL cholesterol. Thus, although LDL cholesterol is the actual target of cholesterol-lowering efforts, total serum cholesterol can be used as a marker during the initial evaluation of serum lipids because testing is more readily available and less expensive. However, LDL cholesterol offers more precision and is, therefore, preferred for clinical decisions about interventions to lower blood cholesterol.

HDLs are intimately involved in the metabolic pathways of chylomicrons and VLDLs. They appear to facilitate the clearance of triglycerides from human plasma. HDLs may also have an important function facilitating the egress of cellular cholesterol and, hence, in controlling its accumulation in arterial smooth muscle cells. HDLs participate in the catabolism of chylomicrons and VLDLs by making available their apoC proteins.

The origin of HDL is enigmatic; both the intestine and the liver appear to participate in its production. The intestine is evidently a source of apoA proteins, which enter the bloodstream bound to lymph chylomicrons. Many believe that apoproteins are transferred to HDLs during chylomicron degradation. HDL is catabolized in the liver and peripheral tissues; the catabolism is enhanced in people who have decreased concentrations of HDL in their plasma.[16–19]

Homocysteine

Homocysteine is an amino acid formed by the conversion of methionine to cysteine. Homocysteine is metabolized by either transsulfuration or remethylation. About a quarter of individuals with symptomatic atherosclerosis may have elevated plasma homocysteine levels due to various factors. High levels of homocysteine are associated with increased susceptibility to heart attacks, stroke, carotid artery stenosis, and adverse outcomes after angioplasty. High levels of homocysteine have been associated with genetic defects in the enzymes involved in homocysteine metabolism, cigarette smoking, vitamin/nutritional deficiencies, and a variety of medical conditions. Homozygosity for methylene-tetrahydrofolate reductase (MTHFR) C677I is associated with hyperhomocysteinemia, a genetic variant present in approximately 10% of Western Europeans. Elevated levels of homocysteine have a toxic effect on the endothelium and in this fashion accelerate atherosclerosis.[20–26]

PATHOLOGY OF ATHEROSCLEROSIS

Site of Predilection and Age of Occurrence

The highest prevalence of stenosis exceeding 50% of the original lumen size in men and women occurs between the ages of 60 and 79 years. Most stenotic lesions in the cervical arteries are situated at the level of the carotid bifurcation. Next in frequency is the origin of the vertebral arteries followed by subclavian artery stenosis, with a predominance of lesions in the left subclavian artery. The least frequent site is the origin of the common carotid artery, with the left side dominating.

The pattern of extracranial and intracranial artery occlusive lesions depends on age, gender, and race/ethnicity of the population selected.[27–29] Lesions in the extracranial arteries are mul-

tiple in two-thirds of the cases. In the intracranial arteries, the atherosclerotic changes are most often located in the larger vessels: (a) terminal internal carotid artery, (b) basilar artery, (c) petrous portion of the internal carotid artery, (d) middle cerebral artery, (e) anterior cerebral and pericallosal arteries, and (f) posterior cerebral artery. Occlusions occur most often in the internal carotid artery and are less common in the basilar artery.

Atherosclerosis is of greatest clinical importance when it occurs in the coronary arteries, the arch of the aorta and its aortocranial branches, the renal arterial tree, and the aortoiliac vessels. Persons with extensive atherosclerosis in any of these locations remain asymptomatic until perfusion distal to the stenosis is compromised, as occurs with sudden reduction of flow through a stenotic artery below a critical level, thrombosis superimposed on an atherosclerotic plaque, or emboli from an ulcerated plaque to the distal arterial bed. Although atherosclerosis of the aortocranial arteries is the subject of this chapter, the clinician must consider it in relation to the more generalized disease, particularly of the coronary, peripheral arterial, and renal arterial trees. For purposes of classification, the intracranial branches of the carotid and vertebral arteries have customarily been considered separately from their extracranial arterial trunks. This artificial division has no sound basis in anatomy or physiology because the aortocranial system functions almost as a unit, from thoracic origin to intracranial capillary bed.

Visual Appearance

Over time the arteries become thickened (Figure 7-1) and less pliable, whereas the lumen is typically eccentric and narrowed but may enlarge. Beneath the intima, which may be ulcerated, friable, or covered with thrombus, are found atheromatous plaques containing gummous material. Beneath the plaques there may be fresh or old hemorrhage resulting from rupture of the vasa vasorum or from a newly formed vascular network. Concomitant weakening of the arterial wall may lead to dilation, fusiform aneurysm, or subintimal dissection; ulceration of the endothelium may allow the contents of the plaque to be discharged into the bloodstream as emboli.

When an artery is occluded by thrombus or embolus, blood flow in the distal segment is arrested, and clot forms as far as the next branch where flow is maintained by collateral channels. For example, when the internal carotid artery becomes occluded at its sinus, thrombus usually extends up to the caroticotympanic or ophthalmic artery, where collateral flow develops and prevents clotting. At times, however, it may continue past these branches into the ophthalmic, anterior, and middle cerebral branches of the carotid artery. Later, fibroblastic proliferation causes the clot to adhere firmly to the wall of the vessel with resultant organization of the clot and, in about 3 weeks, beginning fibrosis of the artery.

The most serious consequence of atherosclerosis is thrombosis, which is often facilitated by ulceration and fibrin deposition on the surface of the plaque (Figure 7-2). The thrombus becomes organized, a process that increases the thickness of the plaque and progressively reduces the remaining lumen. Concomitantly, the underlying arterial wall atrophies, which results in bulging of a segment of the artery (ectasia) leading to a localized saccular dilatation called atherosclerotic aneurysm (Figure 7-3).

Thrombi adherent to fibrous plaques and their subsequent organization are likely to be a means by which plaques progress

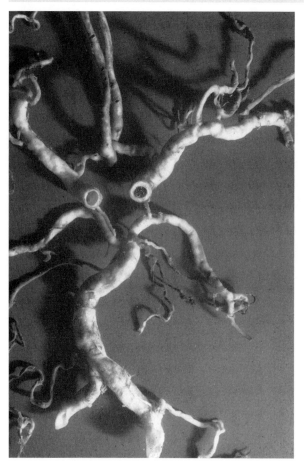

Figure 7-1. Thickening and tortuosity of the major arteries due to atherosclerosis.

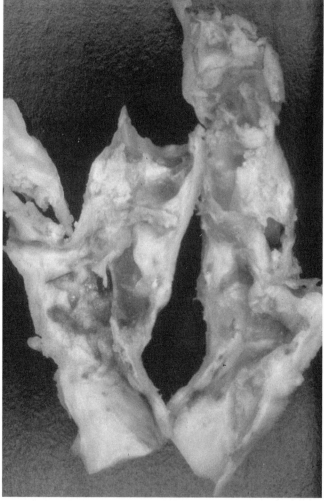

Figure 7-2. A carotid artery plaque removed at endarterectomy reveals an irregular, fibrin-coated luminal surface. Photograph courtesy of Dr. David Lefkowitz.

to severe stenotic lesions. Thromboembolism is the major complication that interrupts downstream perfusion, leading as a consequence to ischemic necrosis in the myocardium, the brain, or an extremity.

Among people within any group, the severity of atherosclerotic lesions varies widely. There is also a difference in the severity of atherosclerosis among a given patient's different arterial beds. Although systemic factors, such as dyslipidemia, seem to influence the severity of atherosclerosis, local tissue factors also modify the rate of progression within the same individual. Focal characteristics of the lesions, even within the same arterial segment, point to the existence of local tissue factors in atherogenesis.

Bifurcations and angulations of arteries or irregularities on the surface of the endothelium disturb laminar flow and create turbulence and eddy currents in the bloodstream, resulting in further injury, after which high-density chylomicrons and lipoproteins can collect in these roughened areas. There is progressive involvement of such important sites as the origins of the aortocranial arteries, the origin of the vertebrals from the subclavian artery, and the bifurcation of the common carotid artery (Figure 7-4), the proximal one to two centimeters of the internal

carotid artery including the carotid sinus and angulations, such as the carotid siphon. Despite severe involvement in these regions, areas in between may remain free of disease. When atherosclerosis causes these arteries to become elongated, dilated, and tortuous, their angles are changed, so that laminar flow is further distorted and the resulting eddy currents further damage the arteries and accelerate the process.

In the vertebral arteries and basilar artery, however, the distribution of atherosclerotic plaques is more general. Some authorities believe that the lipid deposits in the vertebral arteries that occur in the segments between the transverse processes of the cervical vertebrae are possibly related to greater pulsation of these segments. In the first two centimeters after their origin, plaques can form in the vertebral arteries where the artery lies close to the transverse process and the dorsal root ganglion. Perhaps these plaques are related to direct pressure of these structures against the arterial wall.

It has been impossible to confirm a cause-and-effect relationship between atherosclerosis and diffuse brain atrophy; on the other hand, the cervical portions of the brain arteries have not been examined in a large enough series to allow for valid correlations to be made. When such an atrophic brain is sectioned, the

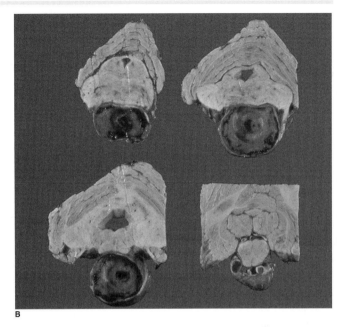

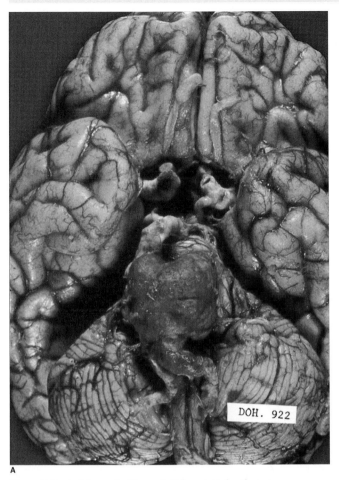

Figure 7-3. A: A large, fusiform, dolichoectatic basilar artery aneurysm resulting from atherosclerosis. B: In cross section, there is thrombus within the lesion with preservation of the lumen within the center of the clot. Note the indentation of the brainstem.

cortical ribbon is seen to be narrowed, and the bulk of the white matter beneath is decreased. The ventricles are dilated symmetrically. The cut ends of the sclerotic penetrating arteries may protrude above the cut surface, and old infarctions of varying ages may be seen irregularly scattered throughout the substance of the brain. Such individuals may have had vascular dementia (vascular cognitive impairment) or Binswanger disease.

Microscopic Pathology

With light microscopy, plaques characteristically contain foam cells swollen with fat. In addition, cholesterol crystals that may initiate a giant-cell reaction are found in the subintimal layers. In advanced cases the internal elastic membrane is ruptured, and the medial coat of the artery shows degenerative changes.

Calcification often occurs in the carotid bulb or in the cavernous and petrous segments of the internal carotid arteries and in the proximal and distal parts of the vertebral arteries. Nevertheless, plaques are rare in the petrous and cavernous segments of the internal carotid artery. There is little correlation between the occurrence of calcification and the development of atherosclerotic intimal changes. However, the presence of lipids and macrophages within the plaque predict a lower likelihood of restenosis following endarterectomy (Figure 7-5).[30]

PATHOGENESIS OF ATHEROSCLEROSIS

The development of moderate to severe atherosclerosis in intracranial arteries often lags behind that in the aorta and coronary arteries by one or two decades, although in high risk individuals the cervical and intracranial arteries may be affected first.

Thrombogenesis

Atherosclerosis is an important stimulus for thrombogenesis.[31–32] Platelets react to the exposed intima and become adherent, release their contents, aggregate, and, sometimes, embolize. Furthermore, they may release vasoactive substances, one of which is the vasoconstrictor prostaglandin thromboxane A_2, which promotes further platelet aggregation. Endothelial cells and platelets oxidize arachidonic acid, an 18-carbon unsaturated fatty acid, to prostaglandins, which have major effects on vasomotor tone and responsiveness. The rate-limiting enzyme of arachidonic acid oxidation is cyclo-oxygenase, which is irreversibly inhibited by acetyl radicals, such as those in aspirin. The metabolites of arachidonate differ according to cell type. Platelets convert arachidonate into thromboxane A_2, whereas endothelial cells convert it into prostacyclin (PGI_2), a potent vasodilator and inhibitor of platelet aggregation. Thus, the same

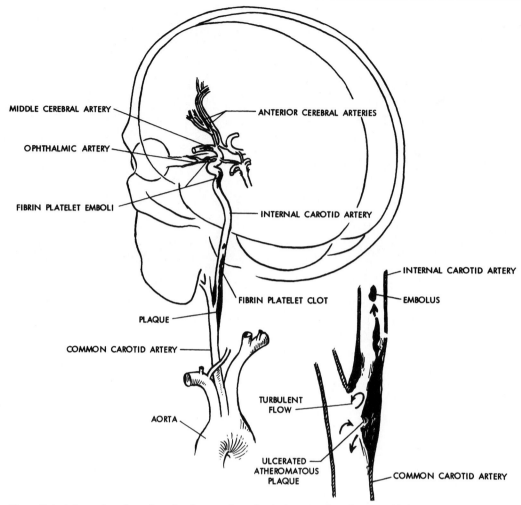

Figure 7-4. Atherosclerosis tends to develop at points of turbulence, such as the carotid bifurcation and the siphon of the internal carotid artery. The inset illustrates the tendency for emboli to arise from the stenotic areas.

precursor may be oxidized by platelets or by normal vascular walls into products with opposite actions. Both act on adenylate cyclase and are rapidly inactivated in the blood.

The dynamic equilibrium between prostacyclin produced by endothelium and thromboxane A_2 produced by platelets serves to maintain normal blood flow without deposition of platelets on vascular surfaces and to permit normal localized hemostasis when vascular damage occurs. When a vessel is injured, endothelial damage exposes the flowing blood to collagen, initiating platelet adhesion and aggregation causing platelet plug formation, which stabilizes when thrombin forms and produces fibrin. Thrombin augments local platelet aggregation, promotes clot formation, and stimulates synthesis of PGI_2, which helps to modulate the clot size. Therefore, both thromboxane and prostacyclin levels are transiently increased by vascular injury, but their relationship may be governed by a number of factors. Furthermore, damaged vascular surface and stasis promote thrombin generation, and turbulent flow favors platelet activation. Moreover, atherosclerosis may inhibit both prostacyclin production and its action because atherosclerotic arteries produce less prostacyclin than normal vascular tissue, possibly because more prostacyclin synthetase is inactivated by the lipid peroxides in atheromas. Free radicals can also destroy

the biologic activity of PGI_2. Last, mild hypoxia stimulates PGI_2 production, but severe ischemic hypoxia inhibits PGI_2 formation, and accompanying local tissue acidosis promotes inactivation of PGI_2. The ability of the vascular endothelium to synthesize PGI_2 in response to thrombin is limited, because thrombin receptors on the endothelial surface are rapidly inactivated and fail to respond to repeated exposure to thrombin. Thus, in the setting of atherosclerotic or ischemic blood vessels, hyperactive platelets may shift the balance between antithrombotic and prothrombotic prostaglandins to favor thrombosis.

Hemodynamic Implications

Although a number of factors contribute to the hemodynamic significance of a carotid artery atherosclerotic lesion, the principal element is the relationship between the cross-sectional area of the residual lumen at the level of the lesion and the cross-sectional area of the normal artery distal to the abnormality. A 75% reduction in cross-sectional area stenosis is pressure-significant, and a 90% cross-sectional area stenosis reduces flow. Although the flow through an artery is not reduced until the constriction exceeds 70% of its cross-sectional area, less profound changes can profoundly alter the pulse-wave contour and flow

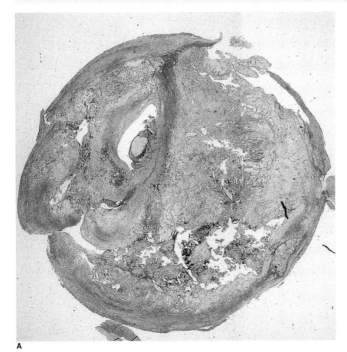
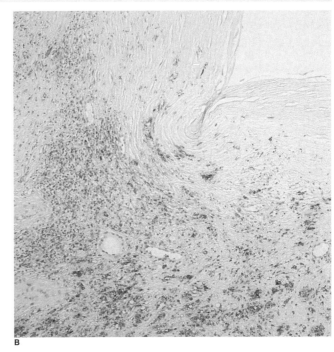

Figure 7-5. A: The carotid artery lumen is almost occluded by extensive lipid-laden plaque-containing cholesterol crystals (Picro-Serius red collagen stain with × 20 magnification). B: CD-68 stained carotid plaque demonstrates heavy macrophage infiltration (× 100). These findings predict a lower likelihood of carotid artery restenosis after endarterectomy. Reprinted with permission from Hellings et al.[30]

velocities. These alterations in flow velocities may damage the vessel wall, the blood elements, and, eventually, the brain itself, which depends to a certain extent on pulsatile flow for propulsion through its microcirculation. As the constriction increases further, the flow disturbance becomes more pronounced.

Perfusion of the brain requires pulsatile pressure for optimal flow, so that stenosis of about 60% to 70% begins to reduce tissue perfusion pressure distal to the stenosis. Therefore, if the patient's symptoms are in the same distribution as a surgically accessible carotid stenosis, then removal of constrictions exceeding 70% should prevent further episodes. There are times, however, when even occlusion of three or, rarely, four arteries does not result in symptoms of brain ischemia. As a consequence, sophisticated medical judgment based on understanding of flow dynamics and the likelihood for embolism must be made before recommending a specific surgical procedure.

The normal column of blood streaming into the carotid bifurcation develops a helical flow pattern in the carotid sinus. Therefore, the outer wall of the sinus experiences oscillations in wall shear, both in magnitude and direction, induced by transitory flow separation phenomena that are induced by the helical pattern. Wall shear stress is generally low in this region, but, in the neighborhood of the flow divider, the wall has relatively high shear with essentially unidirectional flow. This may be the reason why atherosclerotic plaques tend to remain well demarcated at their peripheral aspects. Indeed, atherosclerosis tends to localize along the outer wall of the bifurcation where mean and maximum shear are low and oscillate greatly with the cardiac cycle. Furthermore, the length of time particles in blood remain against the wall is much greater along the outer wall of the bifurcation than along the flow divider.

It is important to realize that blood flow in different regions can differ markedly because of (a) congenital variations, such as hypoplasia or agenesis of a segment of the circle of Willis, which occur in perhaps 60% of individuals, (b) the vagaries of atherosclerosis, which may destroy different segments of this anastomotic system, and (c) brain work, which increases metabolism and blood flow requirements. These three factors affect the potential for collateral circulation to any given region of the brain and may produce local deficiencies in blood flow while elsewhere cerebral blood flow is normal. Superimposed on these local factors, systemic stresses (e.g., reduction in systemic blood pressure, alterations in blood and plasma viscosity, anemia, hypoxia, and hypoglycemia) can act as triggering mechanisms, which result in temporary or even permanent deficits in the brain areas most compromised by atherosclerosis.

Atherosclerotic lesions are sometimes the site of thrombosis, but often the infarction occurs via a distal artery-to-artery embolism from the stenotic site. These emboli tend to be smaller than those from the heart, and thus the ischemic lesions they produce tend to be smaller and more often transient than cardiac emboli. However, it has been extremely difficult to correlate atherosclerotic ulcers with TIAs or cerebral infarction because the means for their identification and characterization remain inexact.

Formation of Atherosclerosis

Current theories of atherogenesis include the inflammatory response-to-injury paradigm, monoclonal proliferation, the lipid-lipoprotein hypotheses, and combinations of the above. The initial events stem from the endothelial cell responses to a variety of injuries at the cellular and subcellular level. Adhesion of blood monocytes and platelets is believed to be mediated by vascular cell adhesion molecules (VCAMs) and intercellular adhesion molecules (ICAMs). Increased endothelial cell permeability and replication lead to inward migration of the adherent mononuclear cells. Powerful chemotactants, such as oxidized LDLs, monocyte chemotactic protein-1 (MCP-1), and macrophage colony-stimulating factor (MCSF) cause the migration of the mononuclear cells through gaps between endothelial cells. In the intima the monocytes become macrophages and accumulate oxidized LDLs to become foam cells. Further enlargement of the lesion may depend on factors produced by the macrophages, such as interleukin (IL), tissue necrosis factor (TNF), MCSF, and growth factors. One result may be the recruitment of smooth muscle cells into the lesion from the medial smooth muscle cells or myointimal cells, which, in turn, become lipid-laden foam cells. T-lymphocytes are identifiable, but their precise role is not known. Growth factors derived from platelets, monocytes, smooth muscle cells, and serum thus contribute to the growth of the atherosclerotic plaque.

The monoclonal theory suggests that plaques begin as the result of mutation or cloning, induced perhaps as a response to stress injury or even a chronic viral infestation of the media of the artery, which continues until mitoses form a mound of tissue that elevates the endothelium. Lipids, mostly cholesterol and cholesteryl oleate, are then deposited in the smooth muscle cells and macrophages of the arterial intima.

Increased plasma levels of lipids, especially LDL, induced by high-fat diet or one of the well-characterized, genetically transmitted hyperlipoproteinemias, may lead to increased lipid in the atherosclerotic lesions. Once in the intima, LDL oxidation may play a key role in chemotaxis, cell adhesion, cell motility, and cell necrosis. Lipoprotein (a) is an atherogenic lipoprotein that could interfere with plasminogen turnover and stimulate smooth muscle cell division.[33]

In response to vascular injury or vasospasm, the arterial vasa vasorum initiate neovascularization, forming new vessels that deposit material to the injury zone that eventually become plaques. The vasa vasorum may play a key role in the enlargement of atherosclerotic lesions by hemorrhage into the lesion.

Boundary Layer Separation

Plaques build up preferentially at bifurcations, curvatures, and branching points of an artery, distorting laminar flow. Two fluid dynamic factors that may cause this and increase atherogenesis are the mechanical damage of high-shear stress with turbulence and the mass transfer of blood-borne substances into the arterial wall in regions of eddy currents. Carotid atherosclerosis develops in areas of low vessel-wall shear stress, most commonly the carotid bulb.

Stress Proteins

These relate to the major components of the advanced plaque, one of which is a necrotic center that includes cell debris, cholesterol crystals, cholesterol esters, calcium, and thromboplastic substances. Necrosis can occur in relation to fully developed fibrolipid plaques and is a common event in the depths of severely affected areas. It may be partially ischemic in origin because intimal thickening disturbs the nutritional state of tissue that cannot be reached by the vasa vasorum.

Stress proteins (SPs) synthesized during homeostatic disturbances have been strongly conserved through evolution,

clearly indicating that they play a vital role in survival of the organism. Their presence enhances the cells' ability to recover from stress, but precisely how they do this is not known. SPs have ATP-binding sites and also bind fatty acids. Thiol oxidants and heavy metals appear to induce SPs, and certain SPs may even form a complex with steroid receptors. SPs may have a major effect on the denaturation of proteins, and they may stabilize other proteins. In the context of advanced atheroma, oxygen deprivation may be assumed and the synthesis of SPs induced. Potentially the lack of an SP response at the site of oxygen deprivation could initiate arterial cell death and generate a necrotic plaque.[34]

EVALUATION FOR ATHEROSCLEROSIS

Ultrasonic determinations utilize Doppler for flow velocity and B-mode for wall imaging. Combined as duplex, and now with three-dimensional imaging, ultrasonic examinations can be used to delineate flow, the thickness of the arterial wall and the arterial lumen, and whether plaques in the wall contain calcium and presence of embolic debris in the bloodstream. At times, blood clots, ulcerations, or a static column of blood distal to obstruction can be detected.[35]

Transfemoral catheter cerebral arteriography (Figure 7-6) remains the most precise method for demonstrating lesions of the cervicocephalic vessels, but whenever possible, noninvasive studies using ultrasound and verification with magnetic resonance angiography (MRA) or multidetector computed tomography angiography (CTA) are preferred. More information on the diagnostic studies that are commonly used to evaluate atherosclerosis is provided in Chapter 5.

MANAGEMENT OF ATHEROSCLEROSIS

By the time aortocervical atherosclerosis has developed to such a degree that the patient has symptoms or signs caused by it, there is seldom much to be done that can reverse the process. Conversely, progression may be slowed or stopped by proper management of arterial hypertension, diabetes mellitus, and other cerebrovascular risk factors. Treatment of atherosclerosis can be divided into (1) risk factor reduction, (2) medical therapy with antiplatelet agents and cholesterol-lowering agents, and (3) endarterectomy and other procedures designed to reopen obstructed vessels.

Risk Factor Reduction

Dietary Changes

Because low-fat, low-carbohydrate diets may reduce serum lipids, individuals with atherosclerosis should restrict their intake of these foods. Such a regimen may retard atherogenesis. Adipose tissue is active metabolically and is the major site for lipid fuel storage, which it supplies as fatty acids during fasting. Excess lipid deposition in adipose tissue (obesity) is a risk factor for atherosclerosis. The obese patient should have the caloric intake restricted until his weight has reached the minimum recommended for the height and body build. For many patients, the goals of cholesterol reduction can be achieved by diet alone, and lifestyle changes are important even in individuals who are prescribed medication.

The purpose of decreasing total fat intake is to facilitate reduction of saturated fatty acid intake and to promote weight reduction. Total fat in the current American diet averages 35%

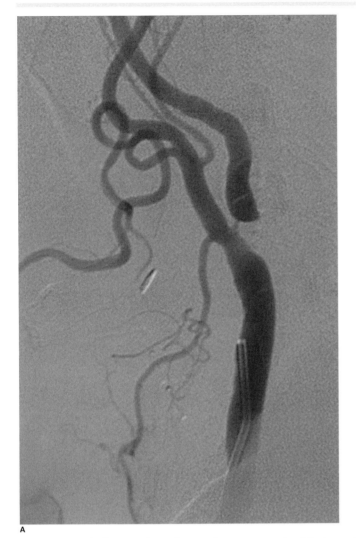 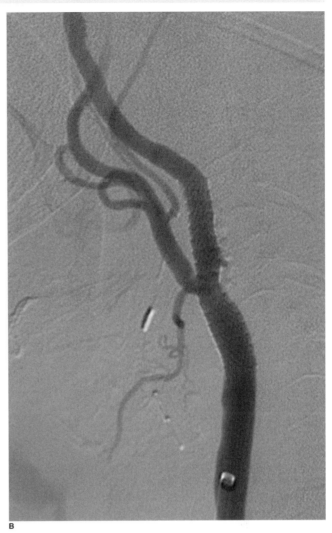

Figure 7-6. A: Catheter angiography reveals severe stenosis of the internal carotid artery just past its bifurcation from the common carotid artery. B: This same artery is widely patent after a stent was placed.

to 40% of calories, but should be no more than 30%. Saturated fatty acids should be decreased to less than 10% of calories. For most patients saturated fatty acid intake will have to be reduced by about one-third.

When dietary saturated fatty acids are decreased, polyunsaturated fatty acids can be increased to 10% of calories. The usual American diet contains about 7% of calories as polyunsaturated fatty acids, which should be a minimum value for the therapeutic diets. There are two major categories of polyunsaturated fatty acids, commonly referred to as omega-6 and omega-3. The major omega-6 fatty acid is linoleic acid, which has 18 carbon atoms and two double bonds. Substitution of linoleic acid for dietary saturated fatty acids results in a fall in plasma cholesterol. Although very high intakes of linoleic acid were once advocated for cholesterol lowering, lack of information about the consequences of long-term ingestion of large amounts of linoleic acid has led most investigators to recommend a ceiling of 10% of total calories. Several vegetable oils are rich in linoleic acid, including safflower oil, sunflower seed oil, soybean oil, and corn oil.

The best source of omega-3 fatty acids are the fish oils, which have very elongated carbon chains and are highly polyunsaturated. The major acids in this class are eicosapentaenoic acid and docosahexaenoic acid. Intake of omega-3 fatty acids should be differentiated from consumption of fish, only some of which are rich in omega-3 acids. Epidemiological data suggest that frequent consumption of fish of any type, seemingly independent of omega-3 fatty acid content, is associated with reduced coronary heart disease (CHD) risk.

Monounsaturated fatty acids, mainly oleic acid, should comprise 10% to 15% of total calories. Oleic acid is the major fatty acid found in olive oil, canola oil, and high-oleic forms of sunflower and safflower oils. Recent evidence indicates that oleic acid may cause as much of a decrease in LDL-cholesterol levels as linoleic acid when either is substituted for saturated fatty acids in the diet.

Most diets specify an intake of carbohydrates of 50% to 60% of calories. When dietary fat is reduced, it should be replaced by simple sugars (monosaccharides and disaccharides), complex digestible carbohydrates (starches), and complex indigestible carbohydrates (fiber). Complex carbohydrates should make up more than half of digestible carbohydrates; this will help ensure ingestion of desirable quantities of vegetable products that contain vitamins, minerals, and fiber. In most people, when digestible carbohydrates are substituted for cholesterol-raising saturated fatty acids, the LDL-cholesterol level will fall to about the same extent as when oleic acid and linoleic acid are substituted in this manner. Very high-carbohydrate diets can raise plasma triglycerides, but when fat intakes are in the vicinity of 30% of calories, this triglyceride response is minimal.

Obesity is not only associated with elevated serum LDL-cholesterol levels but is an independent risk factor for cardiovascular disease. Abdominal obesity, rather than general, may be more related to stroke risk. It is important, therefore, to reduce caloric intake or increase energy expenditure to achieve weight reduction in the obese. Weight reduction will lower the LDL-cholesterol level in many people as well as reduce plasma triglycerides and raise HDL-cholesterol levels. Some patients with high-risk LDL-cholesterol levels are extremely sensitive to caloric intake and weight reduction, and establishment of desirable body weight will completely correct their elevated LDL-cholesterol concentrations. The importance of caloric restriction in overweight, high-risk individuals cannot be overemphasized. Weight reduction and maintenance of ideal weight should be considered for all overweight patients who have had either a TIA or stroke.

Cholesterol

High total cholesterol and high LDL concentrations are correlated with atherosclerosis. Newly absorbed cholesterol enters the circulation with chylomicrons, which are degraded to cholesterol-rich chylomicron remnants; the latter may be atherogenic. Cholesterol in the diet comes from animal products. The flesh of all animals contains cholesterol; it is present in both muscle and fat, and both have approximately the same concentrations on a wet-weight basis. Particularly rich sources are egg yolk and organ meats (liver, sweetbreads, and brain). Some shellfish (e.g., shrimp) also are moderately high in cholesterol. Dairy products containing butterfat also contribute cholesterol to the diet. Increased blood cholesterol levels, more specifically increased levels of LDL cholesterol, are casually related to an increased risk of CHD. Coronary risk rises progressively with cholesterol level, particularly when cholesterol levels rise above 200 mg/dl. There is also substantial evidence that lowering total and LDL-cholesterol levels will reduce the incidence of CHD.

Both nonpharmacologic and pharmacologic methods are used to lower blood cholesterol levels. These two approaches are complementary, and, together, they represent a coordinated strategy aimed at reducing cholesterol levels and coronary risk. Lifestyle modifications involve dietary intervention and increased physical activity. Lipid-modifying therapy with statins has definitively established that reduction of LDL cholesterol reduces cardiovascular risk. Statins appear likely to benefit stroke survivors as well. Lipid-lowering agents may slow progression of atherosclerotic plaque growth and may possibly cause a regression in plaque formation.

Hyperhomocysteinemia

High levels of homocysteine damages the vascular endothelium and accelerates atherosclerosis in both large and small arteries. Homocysteine levels above 10.5 uM/L are elevated and can be reduced by alteration of diet or by supplementation with folic acid, along with pyridoxine (vitamin B_6) and vitamin B_{12}. One clinical trial, however, failed to demonstrate a reduction in recurrent stroke or myocardial infarction in individuals who received these vitamins even though the homocysteine levels dropped in the individuals who received vitamins.[26] The U.S. food industry has been ordered to fortify all grains and cereals with folate to reduce the incidence of neural tube defects and secondarily to reduce homocysteine levels.

Alcohol Consumption

The average intake of alcohol among Americans is approximately 5% of total calories, but this value varies widely among individuals. Alcohol affects lipoprotein metabolism in several ways. It does not affect LDL-cholesterol concentrations, but it does increase triglyceride concentrations and HDL-cholesterol levels in many individuals. Elimination or reduction of alcohol consumption is recommended in heavy drinkers and restriction of alcohol consumption to not more than two drinks per day is recommended for moderate drinkers and nonpregnant women.

Exercise

Whether exercise specifically prevents cerebral atherosclerosis is still uncertain, but daily exercise of at least 30 minutes is recommended as a good measure of health for all patients who are capable of participating in a moderate-intensity regime.

Medical Management of Atherosclerosis

Control of Cholesterol

Secondary causes of hyperlipidemia (e.g., diabetes, hypothyroidism, nephrotic syndrome, and alcohol dependence) should be identified and treated. The discovery of specific competitive inhibitors of 3-hydroxy-3-methylglutaryl-coenzyme-A reductase (HMG CoA reductase) opened up a new avenue of therapy for patients with primary hypercholesterolemia. Just as oil and water cannot mix without a detergent, cholesterol cannot enter the bloodstream unless it is transported within an LDL. LDL ferries cholesterol to LDL receptors. Low cholesterol levels in the liver trigger the production of more receptors that extract LDL from the blood. But, if the liver does not make enough receptors, the LDL levels in the blood will rise.

Patients with ischemic stroke or TIA with elevated cholesterol, comorbid coronary artery disease, or evidence of an atherosclerotic lesion are best managed with statins. Likewise, the Stroke Prevention by Aggressive Reduction in Cholesterol Levels (SPARCL) study demonstrated that treatment with atorvastatin 80 mg daily significantly reduced the risk of nonfatal or fatal stroke and the risk of stroke or TIA among patients without prior history of CAD. Although atorvastatin was associated with fewer ischemic strokes than placebo, hemorrhagic strokes were more frequent in the atorvastatin group.[36] Currently six statins are available: atorvastatin (Lipitor®), simvastatin (Zocor®), pravastatin (Pravachol®), fluvastatin (Lescol®), lovastatin (Mevacor®), and rosuvastatin (Crestor®). Therapy is best initiated at the lowest dose, once daily, preferably at bedtime.

Reported side effects (often transient) of statins include changes in bowel function, headaches, nausea, fatigue, insomnia, and skin rash. Although statin-induced myositis is often emphasized, there have been relatively few cases of true inflammatory myopathy associated with the use of statins. Statin myotoxicity occurs in about 5% of patients, with manifestations ranging from asymptomatic elevations of the serum creatine kinase (CK), to diffuse myalgias, to a myopathy with possible muscle necrosis and rhabdomyolysis. Peripheral neuropathy is another potential complication. Biochemical changes have included increases in transaminases and CK. Approximately 1.9% of patients have developed persistent increases in transaminase levels of greater than three times normal after 3 to 16 months of therapy requiring discontinuance of therapy. Careful monitoring of liver function studies is essential.[36–39]

Other cholesterol-lowering agents include cholesterol absorption inhibitors (ezetimibe), bile acid suppressants, fibrates, and nicotinic acid. Nicotinic acid has been shown to lower CHD risk in clinical trials, and its long-term safety has been established. Nicotinic acid is the preferred drug in patients with concurrent hypertriglyceridemia (triglycerides ≥ 250 mg/dl) because bile acid sequestrants tend to increase them.[13,36–39]

Control of Hypertension

Hypertension is the most important preventable and treatable cause for symptomatic cerebrovascular disease. The goal of therapy is to provide safe optimal protection against cardiovascular and target organ (e.g., heart, brain, and kidney) complications. Sustained systolic and diastolic hypertension accelerates atherogenesis. The target blood pressure may be individualized according to age, ethnicity, and coexisting co-morbidities.[13] The optimal antihypertensive regimen has not been determined, but it should include targeted lifestyle modifications as well as antihypertensive agents. Available antihypertensive medications, used alone or in combination, include diuretics, beta blockers, angiotensin-converting enzyme inhibitors, angiotensin receptor blockers, calcium channel blockers, and alpha-blocking drugs. However, recent studies suggest that among patients with uncomplicated hypertension, first-line therapy with beta blockers may offer less protection against stroke, especially among elderly individuals with hypertension.[12]

Platelet Antiaggregant Therapy

Platelet antiaggregants are a mainstay of stroke prevention therapy (Chapter 25). Antiplatelet therapy is recommended over oral anticoagulants for patients with noncardio-embolic ischemic stroke or TIA. A meta-analysis of patients with prior stroke or TIA demonstrated a 28% relative risk reduction in nonfatal stroke, and a 16% reduction in fatal stroke with the use of antiplatelet therapy.[13]

Of these agents, three are viable options in the United States according to evidence-based guidelines to prevent stroke: aspirin (50–325 mg/day), clopidogrel, and aspirin plus extended-release dipyridamole. Of these antiplatelet agents, aspirin is the most thoroughly studied and well established. A meta-analysis by the antiplatelet trialists showed that aspirin is the best prophylaxis for prevention of end-stage atherosclerotic complications such as stroke and myocardial infarction.

One of the major dilemmas of therapy is individual variation in response to medications. Most patients show stable, reproducible dose- or concentration-response relationships for many drugs, allowing doses to be titrated individually. However, others differ substantially in their dose- or concentration-response relationships because of genetic makeup, concurrent diseases, gastrointestinal absorption, metabolic factors, or use of other drugs.[13,40–41]

Carotid Endarterectomy

Results from a number of major prospective studies provide compelling evidence of the benefit of carotid endarterectomy (CEA) performed by experienced surgeons in improving the chance of stroke-free survival in high-risk symptomatic patients.

The number of patients needed to treat to prevent one stroke among symptomatic individuals with carotid stenosis of 50% to 69% is 15, whereas for the symptomatic patients with 70% to 99% stenosis, the number needed to treat is only six.

Data from a number of randomized clinical trials concerning the efficacy of CEA in patients with asymptomatic carotid artery stenosis are now available. Given the low risk for ipsilateral cerebral infarction among patients with asymptomatic carotid artery stenosis, some experts recommend surgery only when the degree of stenosis is greater than 80%, provided that the operation is performed by an experienced surgeon with a complication rate (combined arteriographic and surgical) of < 3%. For best results, there must be a team approach for the appropriate evaluation, selection, and management. Meticulous anesthesia, surgery, and postoperative care are the essential components of what must be a seamless team approach.[42–49]

Even though there may be a valid indication for CEA, primary considerations must include the patient's physiological age, the presence of potentially life-limiting diseases, the combined angiographic, anesthetic, and surgical morbidity and mortality at the institution where the procedure would be performed, and the facilities available for complete management of any complications that might arise.

Factors that greatly increase risk are angina pectoris, previous myocardial infarction, cardiac decompensation, sustained hypertension, chronic obstructive pulmonary disease, severe obesity, and physiological age exceeding 75 years. Occlusion of the opposite internal carotid, intracranial carotid artery disease, extensive length of plaque in the artery to be operated, high bifurcation, and soft thrombus adhering to an ulcerative lesion all add to the inherent risk.

Stenting of the Cervicocerebral Vessels

There is increasing interest in arterial angioplasty and stenting, an approach that has proved successful for coronary and aorto-femoral atherosclerosis and for some patients with carotid or vertebral artery stenoses. It is technically feasible and minimally invasive and can be performed with local anesthesia. When positioned, the balloon on the catheter tip is inflated, fracturing the plaque and dilating the artery, after which a specially constructed stent can be placed to prevent recurrent stenosis. Although this procedure avoids surgery, the danger of emboli or arterial dissection is approximately 6% for symptomatic and 3% for asymptomatic carotid stenosis patients and is more dangerous for women than men. However, it is useful for subclavian stenosis because the initial, reversal of vertebral flow by subclavian steal prevents emboli to the brain. In the case of smooth stenosis without ulceration, such as that which occurs in fibromuscular dysplasia, some practitioners have had encouraging success without sequelae in both carotid and vertebrobasilar stenosis. If they prove to be safer than endarterectomy, catheter techniques may become another therapeutic option.

At present, the use of carotid angioplasty and stenting is supported only by a series of observational studies.[50–53] In contrast, there is strong evidence for the clinical efficacy of CEA, at least in carefully selected patients, in the form of multiple controlled clinical trials. Although preliminary reports of prospective multicenter studies of safety and angiographic effectiveness are encouraging, it will be years before adequately controlled carotid angioplasty studies with acceptable statistical power emerge. Carotid angioplasty and stenting has the potential to provide safer, cheaper management. However, it also could carry the risk of increased stroke, death, or disability (see Chapters 6 and 25).

REFERENCES

1. Baker AB, Flora GC, Resch JA, Loewwenson R. The geographic pathology of atherosclerosis: a review of the literature with some personal observations on cerebral atherosclerosis. *J Chronic Dis.* 1967;**20**:685–706.
2. Bhatt DL, Steg PG, Ohman EM, et al. International prevalence, recognition and treatment of cardiovascular risk factors in outpatients with atherothrombosis. *JAMA.* 2006;**295**:180–189.
3. Nichols FT, Shaltoni HM, Yatsu FM. A cerebrovascular perspective of atherosclerosis. In: Fisher IM, ed. *Handbook of Clinical Neurology.* Vol. 92 (3rd Series). *Stroke,* Part I. Amsterdam: Elsevier; 2009;**11**:215–238.
4. Shattock S. A report on the pathological condition of the aorta of King Memephthah, traditionally regarded as the Pharaoh of the Exodus. *Proc R Soc Med Pathol Sect.* 1909;**2**:122–127.
5. Rigal RD, Lovell FW, Townsend FM. Pathologic findings in the cardiovascular systems of military flying personnel. *Am J Cardiol.* 1960;**6**:19–25.
6. Strong JP. Atherosclerotic lesions. Natural history, risk factors and topography. *Arch Pathol Lab Med.* 1992;**116**:1268–1275.
7. Stary HC, Chandler AB, Glavov S, et al. A definition of initial fatty streak, and intermediate lesions of atherosclerosis. A report from the Committee on Vascular Lesions of the Council on Arteriosclerosis, American Heart Association. *Circulation.* 1994;**89**:2462–2478.
8. Stary HC, Chandler AB, Dinsmore RE, et al. A definition of advanced types of atherosclerotic lestions and a histological classification of atherosclerosis. A report from the Committee on Vascular Lesions of the Council on Arteriosclerosis, American Heart Association. *Circulation.* 1995;**92**:1355–1379.
9. Stehbens WE. *Pathology of the Cerebral Blood Vessels.* St. Louis: Mosby; 1972.
10. Witterdink JL, Easton JD. Vascular event rates in patients with atherosclerotic cerebrovascular disease. *Arch Neurol.* 1992;**49**(8):857–863.
11. Ross R. The pathogenesis of atherosclerosis: a perspective for the 1990's. *Nature.* 1993;**362**:801–809.
12. Bangalore S, Messerli FH, Kostis JB, Pepine CJ. Cardiovascular protection using beta-blockers: a critical review of the evidence. *J Am Coll Cardiol.* 2007;**50**:563–572.
13. Sacco RL, Adams R, Albers G, et al. Guidelines for prevention of stroke in patients with ischemic stroke or transient ischemic attack: a statement for healthcare professionals from the American Heart Association/American Stroke Association Council on Stroke: co-sponsored by the Council on Cardiovascular Radiology and Intervention: the American Academy of Neurology affirms the value of this guideline. *Stroke.* 2006;**37**:577–617.
14. Wolf-Maier K, Cooper RS, Banefas Jr, et al. Hypertension prevalence and blood pressure levels in 6 European countries, Canada, and the United States. *JAMA.* 2003;**289**:2363–2369.
15. Fajardo LF. The complexity of endothelial cells. A review. *Am J Clin Pathol.* 1989;**92**:241–250.
16. Crouse JR III. Gender, lipoproteins, diet and cardiovascular risk. Sauce for the goose may not be sauce for the gander. *Lancet.* 1989;**1**(8633):318–320.
17. Garcia JH, Khang-Loon H. Carotid atherosclerosis: definition, pathogenesis and clinical significance. *Neuroimaging Clin N Am.* 1996;**6**(4):801–810.
18. Steinberg D, Witztum JL. Lipoproteins and atherogenesis. Current concepts. *JAMA.* 1990;**264**:3047–3052.
19. Lewis JC, Taylor RG. Localization of lipoprotein in pre- and post-transition atherosclerotic lesions following short-term incubation with [^{125}I] LDL. *Histochem J.* 1994;**26**(11):833–843.
20. Boysen G, Brander T, Christensen H, et al. Homocysteine and risk of recurrent stroke. *Stroke.* 2003;**34**(5):1258–1261.
21. Iso H, Moriyama Y, Sato S, et al. Serum total homocysteine concentrations and risk of stroke and its subtypes in Japanese. *Circulation.* 2004;**109**(22):2766–2772.
22. Kelly PJ, Rosand J, Kistler JP, et al. Homocysteine, MTHFR 677CT polymorphism, and risk of ischemic stroke: results of a meta-analysis. *Neurology.* 2002;**59**(4):529–536.
23. Kim NK, Choi BO, Jung WS, et al. Hyperhomocystinemia as an independent risk factor for silent brain infarction. *Neurology.* 2003;**61**(11):1595–1596.
24. Li Z, Sun L, Zhang H. Elevated plasma homocysteine was associated with hemorrhagic and ischemic stroke, but methylenetetrahydrofolate reductase gene C677T polymorphism was a risk factor for thrombotic stroke: a Multicenter Case-Control Study in China. *Stroke.* 2003;**34**(9):2085–2090.
25. McIlroy SP, Dynan KB, Lawson JT, et al. Moderately elevated plasma homocysteine, methylenetetrahydrofolate reductase genotype, and risk for stroke, vascular dementia, and Alzheimer disease in Northern Ireland. *Stroke.* 2002;**33**(10):2351–2356.
26. Toole JF, Malinow MR, Chambless LE, et al. Lowering homocysteine in patients with ischemic stroke to prevent recurrent stroke, myocardial infarction, and death: the Vitamin Intervention for Stroke Prevention (VISP) randomized controlled trial. *JAMA.* 2004;**291**(5):565–567.
27. Moossy J. Cerebral infarcts and the lesions of intracranial and extracranial atherosclerosis. *Arch Neurol.* 1966;**14**(2):124–128.
28. Heart Disease and Stroke Statistics – 2007 Update. A report from the American Heart Association Statistics Committee and Stroke Statistics Subcommittee. *Circulation.* 2007;**115**:e69–e171.
29. Strong JP, Eggen DA, Tracy RE. *The Geographic Pathology and Topography of Atherosclerosis and Risk Factors for Atherosclerotic Lesions.* New York: Plenum; 1978.
30. Hellings WE, Moll FL, de Vries JP, et al. Atherosclerotic plaque composition and occurrence of restenosis after carotid endarterectomy. *JAMA.* 2008;**299**:547–554.
31. Chandler A. *An Overview of Thrombosis and Platelet Involvement in the Development of the Human Atherosclerotic Plaque.* New York: Springer; 1990:359–377.
32. Davies MJ, Woolf N. Atherosclerosis: what is it and why does it occur? *Br Heart J.* 1993;**69**:53–511.
33. Gordon DJ, Rifkind BM. High density lipoprotein – the clinical implications of recent studies. *N Engl J Med.* 1989;**321**:1311–1316.
34. Landers SC, Gupta M, Lewis JC. Ultrastructural localization of tissue factor on monocyte-derived macrophages and macrophage foam cells associated with atherosclerotic lesions. *Virchows Arch.* 1994;**425**(1):49–54.
35. Bond N, Barnes RW, Riley WA, et al. High resolution B-mode ultrasound scanning methods in the atherosclerosis risk in communities (ARIC) cohort. *J Neuroimaging.* 1991;**1**:68–73.
36. Amarenco P, Bogousslavsky J, Callahan A III, et al. High-dose atorvastatin after stroke or transient ischemic attack. *N Engl J Med.* 2006;**355**:549–559.
37. Expert Panel on Detection and Treatment of High Blood Cholesterol in Adults (Adult Treatment Panel III). Executive summary of the Third Report of the National Cholesterol Education Program (NCEP). *JAMA.* 2001;**285**:2486–2497.
38. Reamy BV, ed. *Hyperlipidemia Management for Primary Care. An Evidence-Based Approach.* New York: Springer; 2008.
39. Switzer JA, Hess DL. Statins in stroke: prevention, protection and recovery. *Expect Rev Neurother.* 2006;**6**:195–202.

40. Gorelick PB. Use of antiplatelet agents for the prevention of first and recurrent stroke. Stroke prevention in American Academy of Neurology. *Continuum*. 2005;**11**(4):77–96.

41. Biller J. Aspirin nonresponse in patients with arterial causes of ischemic stroke: considerations in detection and management. *J Neurolog Sci*. 2008;**272**:1–7.

42. Barnett, HJM, Taylor, DW, Eliasziw M, et al. Benefit of carotid endarterectomy in patients with symptomatic moderate or severe stenosis. North American Symptomatic Carotid Endarterectomy Trial Collaborators. *N Engl J Med*. 1998;**39**:1415–1425.

43. Chaturvedi, S, Bruno A, Feasby F, et al. Carotid endarterectomy. An evidence based review: report of the Therapeutics and Technology Assessment Subcommittee of the American Academy of Neurology, *Neurology*. 2005;**65**:794–801.

44. European Carotid Surgery Trialists' Collaborative Group. Risk of stroke in the distribution of an asymptomatic carotid artery. *Lancet*. 1995;**345**:209–212.

45. European Carotid Surgery Trialists' Collaborative Group. Endarterectomy for moderate symptomatic carotid stenosis: interim results from the MRC European Carotid Surgery Trial. *Lancet*. 1996;**347**:1591–1593.

46. Hacke W, Brown MD, MasJ-L. Carotid endarterectomy versus stenting: an international perspective. *Stroke*. 2006;**37**:344.

47. Halliday A, Mansfield A, Marco J, et al. Prevention of disabling and fatal strokes by successful carotid endarterectomy in patients without recent neurological symptoms. *Lancet*. 2004;**363**:1491–1502.

48. Pullicino P, Halperin J. Combining carotid endarterectomy with coronary bypass surgery: is it worth the risk? *Neurology*. 2005;**64**:1332–1333.

49. Rothwell PM, Eliasziw M, Gutnikov SA, et al. For the Carotid Endarterectomy Trialists Collaboration. Effect of endarterectomy for symptomatic carotid stenosis in relation to clinical subgroups and to the timing of surgery. *Lancet*. 2004;**363**:915–924.

50. Dominick JH, McCabe AC, Pereira AC, et al. Restenosis after carotid angioplasty, stenting, or endarterectomy in the Carotid and Vertebral Artery Transluminal Angioplasty Study (CAVATAS). *Stroke*. 2005;**356**:281–286.

51. Higishida RT, Meyers PM, Connors JJ III, et al. Intracranial angioplasty and stenting for cerebral atherosclerosis. *Am J Neurodiol*. 2005;**26**:2323–2327.

52. Qureshi AL, Kirmani JF, Divani AA, et al. Carotid angioplasty with or without stent placement versus carotid endarterectomy for treatment of carotid stenosis: a meta-analysis. *Neurosurgery*. 2005;**56**:1171–1181.

53. Yadav JS, Wholey MH, Kuntz R, et al. Protected carotid artery stenting versus endarterectomy in high risk patients. *N Engl J Med*. 2004;**351**:1493–1501.

8

Embolism and Stroke

Premonitory symptoms are rare in embolism. When present they are not true prodromata, but consist of lighter attacks of the same character, due to the obstruction of small vessels by small emboli, or else they are really the first symptoms of the onset, when the obstruction is incomplete and the occlusion is gradual. There is no persistent preceding headache or other indication of encephalic disease. Until the plug obstructs the vessel, the brain is in a normal state. In thrombosis from atheroma, on the other hand, premonitory symptoms are frequent, being present in the majority of cases.

William R. Gowers

About one-third of all ischemic cerebrovascular events are due to embolism.[1] In the pre-antibiotic era, many cerebral emboli resulted from infective endocarditis and valvular heart disease resulting from rheumatic fever, a condition that has become uncommon in developed countries. In 1885 Osler described chronic heart disease, endocarditis, aortic atheroma, clot originating from aneurysms or the pulmonary veins, pregnancy-related hypercoagulability, and mitral valve abnormalities in rheumatic fever as common causative entities.[2,3] An aging population, widespread use of antibiotics, and rapid advancement of medical technology have resulted in a shift of common etiologies. Procedure-related embolic events and cerebral embolism from mechanical heart valves or atrial fibrillation have become major causes for cerebral embolism.

Sources for brain embolism vary with the age of the patient. Congenital heart disease or substance abuse-related infective endocarditis more commonly occur in younger adults, whereas emboli secondary to atherosclerosis, atrial fibrillation, or cardiac valvular lesions are seen most often in older patients. Causes of cerebral embolism are listed in Table 8-1, and we consider the common and a few of the uncommon risk factors individually below.

CARDIOGENIC CEREBRAL EMBOLISM

About 15% to 20% of all ischemic strokes are due to intracardiac thrombus formation followed by systemic embolism.[1] Cardiogenic emboli arise from the left ventricle or left atrium, commonly in individuals with atrial fibrillation or cardiac valvular disease. Intracardiac thrombus formation also occurs in some individuals after a myocardial infarction or in response to congestive heart failure, and individuals with multiple risk factors are at even greater risk of embolism. Less common causes of cardiogenic embolism include valvular vegetations and intracardiac tumors.

Rhythm Disorders

Stroke has been reported in individuals with most types of cardiac arrhythmias, although atrial fibrillation is by far the arrhythmia that is most likely to cause cerebral embolus. Stroke, in turn, can induce arrhythmia. Intracranial hemorrhage is more likely to cause an arrhythmia than an ischemic stroke. Lesions involving the hypothalamus, limbic system, and orbitofrontal cortex have all been associated with reflex effects on the heart and lungs.

Prolonged electrocardiographic monitoring for ambulatory patients allows one to test the clinical suspicion that cardiac dysrhythmias can result in episodic cerebral vascular insufficiency and/or cerebral infarction. More than half of patients with cardiac dysrhythmia are unaware of it. They may present with diffuse symptoms such as light-headedness, dizziness, and, sometimes, visual disturbances, syncope, or seizure-like episodes.

Significant slowing or rapidity of the heart rate causes decreased cardiac output and can cause global cerebral ischemia. Dysrhythmia per se causes abnormality in flow and irregularities of pulse pressure with secondary peaks and valleys in flow. If, in addition, narrowing of arteries supplying the brain is also present, perfusion of border zones within the brain can fail, resulting in a transient ischemic attack (TIA) or infarction.

Sick Sinus Syndrome

The sick sinus syndrome, which is diagnosed by prolonged electrocardiographic monitoring, is a sinoatrial conduction disorder resulting in bradyarrhythmia, sometimes interspersed with bouts of tachycardia. It usually occurs in individuals with

Table 8-1: Risk Factors for Cerebral Embolism

Cardiac arrhythmia

- Atrial fibrillation
- Supraventricular tachycardia
- Sick sinus syndrome

Impaired left ventricular function

Myocardial infarct

Congestive heart failure

Cardiomyopathy

Congenital heart disease

- Transposition of the great vessels
- Tetralogy of Fallot
- Eisenmenger complex
- Truncus arteriosus
- Ebstein anomaly
- Septal defects
- Patent foramen ovale
- Atrial septal defect
- Atrial septal aneurysm with and without patent foramen ovale

Valvular heart disease

- Rheumatic fever
- Prosthetic heart valves
- Infective endocarditis
- Nonbacterial thrombotic endocarditis
- Libman-Sacks endocarditis

Cardiac tumors

- Atrial myxoma
- Rhabdomyoma
- Papillary fibroelastoma

Artery-to-artery embolism (e.g., atherosclerosis)

Dissection of extra- and intracranial arteries

Aortic atheroma

Procedure related

- Extracorporeal membrane oxygenation (ECMO)
- Cardiac surgery and catheterization
- Endovascular procedures

Foreign body

Gas embolism

Fat embolism

Paradoxical embolism with left to right shunts

Neoplasm

atherosclerosis but may develop earlier in patients with Friedreich ataxia or muscular dystrophy. Emboli occur more commonly in the patients who have the rhythm disruption fluctuating between abnormally slow and very rapid rates.

Atrial Fibrillation

Atrial fibrillation is one of the most prevalent causes of stroke, TIA, and silent ischemic brain injury, becoming increasingly common with age.[4,5] It occurs in more than 10% of people older than 80 years of age and is associated with more severe stroke, poorer clinical outcome, and a higher mortality rate than embolic stroke without atrial fibrillation.[6,7] Stroke typically results from systemic embolization of a thrombus from the left atrium or the left atrial appendage. Embolism can occur spontaneously or during cardioversion. Many individuals with atrial fibrillation have coexisting stroke risk factors such as arterial hypertension and atherosclerosis, so not all strokes in these patients can be attributed to the atrial fibrillation.

Atrial fibrillation frequently develops in the setting of cardiac disease, for example, with rheumatic mitral valve damage or following prosthetic mitral valve replacement.[8] Atrial fibrillation can occur with or without underlying structural heart disease. The abnormal rhythm can be permanent, paroxysmal, or persistent (i.e., terminating spontaneously in less than a week). Cerebral embolization can occur with all types of atrial fibrillation and can develop as early as within 72 hours following acute onset.[9] Paroxysmal atrial fibrillation often goes unnoticed by the patient but is frequently associated with recurrent episodes of embolization and high risk for ischemic stroke without anticoagulation. Traditional teaching notwithstanding, patients who have been cardioverted and rhythm controlled to normal sinus rhythm remain at considerable risk for recurrent embolism.[10,11]

Most emboli develop in the left atrial appendage. Patients at highest risk for cerebral embolization are those with previous cerebral ischemic events or a history of previous systemic embolization, valvular disease, history of hypertension or diabetes, impaired left ventricular function, or those who are older than 75 years. In contrast, patients with atrial fibrillation who are younger than 60 years are at lower risk.[12,13] Transesophageal echocardiogram (TEE) is the method of choice to detect atrial thrombi, spontaneous echocontrast, and aortic plaque.

Stratification of the stroke risk in individuals with nonvalvular atrial fibrillation allows physicians to individualize therapy based on a patient's estimated stroke risk. The CHADS$_2$ index categorizes the stroke risk based on a patient's age, arterial hypertension, diabetes mellitus, cardiac failure, or prior stroke or TIA (Table 8-2).[14] In patients with none of these factors (i.e., a CHADS$_2$ score of 0), the risk of warfarin is greater than the stroke risk, so aspirin is recommended. Individuals with a CHADS$_2$ score of greater than one should receive warfarin unless it is contraindicated. Anticoagulation with warfarin, with a target international normalized ratio (INR) of 2.0 to 3.0, reduces the stroke risk in high-risk individuals with atrial fibrillation by about 68%.[9,15,16]

The targeted INR needs to be at the higher end of the therapeutic range in high-risk atrial fibrillation patients with mechanical prosthetic heart valves. Despite a significant reduction in stroke risk, only about 50% to 60% of all eligible atrial fibrillation patients receive warfarin therapy. Of these, a significant number remain suboptimally anticoagulated because of the narrow therapeutic

Table 8-2: Stroke Risk Stratification in Patients with Nonvalvular Atrial Fibrillation

CHADS$_2$ Risk Criteria	Score
Prior stroke or TIA	2
Age > 75 years	1
Arterial hypertension	1
Diabetes mellitus	1
Heart failure	1

Patients (N = 1733)	Adjusted Stroke Rate (%/ year) (95% CI)	CHADS$_2$ Score
120	1.9 (1.2–3.0)	0
463	2.8 (2.0–3.8)	1
523	4.0 (3.1–5.1)	2
337	5.9 (4.6–7.3)	3
220	8.5 (6.3–11.1)	4
65	12.5 (8.2–17.5)	5
5	18.2 (10.5–27.4)	6

The adjusted stroke risk was derived from a multivariate analysis assuming no aspirin usage. Treatment recommendations based on the above stratification scoring are provided in the text. CHADS$_2$ = Cardiac failure, hypertension, age, diabetes mellitus, and prior stroke or TIA (doubled). CI = confidence interval. Data were drawn from van Walraven et al.[125] and from Gage et al.[126] Table was modified with permission from Fuster.[14]

window of warfarin, medical noncompliance, and multiple drug interactions. Patients with INRs below 2.0 are at increased risk for more severe stroke and have a higher mortality.[17] The potential benefits of anticoagulation must be weighted against the risk of hemorrhage. Elderly patients, those in whom the INR is difficult to maintain within the goal range, and patients on concomitant antiplatelet therapy are at increased bleeding risk.

Patients who cannot tolerate anticoagulation or those who have a contraindication to oral anticoagulation therapy should receive aspirin. However, aspirin is inferior to warfarin for prevention of ischemic stroke in high risk patients with nonvalvular atrial fibrillation.[18] Aspirin is more effective in younger patients with nonstructural heart disease and for the prevention of minor strokes, but overall it provides only modest effects for stroke prevention in patients with atrial fibrillation. Combined antiplatelet therapy with aspirin and clopidogrel does not improve stroke prevention, but combined therapy has an increased risk of hemorrhage.

Patients with atrial fibrillation often have associated small vessel ischemic cerebrovascular disease or coronary artery disease requiring concomitant use of aspirin together with warfarin. Aspirin and warfarin combination therapy compared to warfarin monotherapy does not result in decreased stroke risk in patients who have only atrial fibrillation, but combination therapy is associated with an increased risk of hemorrhagic complications. This combination should therefore not be used for stroke prevention in atrial fibrillation unless other indications for antiplatelet therapy are present. Cardioversion and

rhythm control do not eliminate the need for anticoagulation because of the associated risk of recurrent episodes of atrial fibrillation that may lead to cerebral embolization. Long-term anticoagulation is presented in more detail in Chapter 25.

Myocardial Infarction

About 2% of patients with myocardial infarct develop embolic cerebral infarction within a month after an index cardiac event, particularly if it involves the endocardium, causing a pedunculated and mobile left ventricular thrombus. The likelihood increases even more when the left ventricle and/or septum is involved. Observational studies using serial TEEs in myocardial infarction patients indicate that most left ventricular thrombi develop within the first 2 weeks, but clots have been observed in as early as 24 hours following a myocardial infarction.[19–21] Based on echocardiographic data, it has been estimated that at least 5% of patients with anterior wall myocardial infarct develop a left ventricular thrombus, but recent cardiac magnetic resonance imaging (MRI) studies suggest that formation of small thrombi may occur even more frequently.[22,23]

Patients with a large anterior wall myocardial infarct, atrial fibrillation, cardiac decompensation, left ventricular dysfunction, ventricular aneurysm, or an akinetic segment following a myocardial infarction are at high risk for ischemic stroke. Other predictors include older age, previous stroke, and size of the infarction. Rarely embolic cerebral infarcts occur as a complication of percutaneous coronary intervention for acute cardiac infarction. Overall the incidence of left ventricular thrombus formation has decreased with acute thrombolysis and endovascular therapy.[24]

Echocardiography is routinely used in myocardial infarction patients to monitor cardiac function, detect potential complications, and monitor thrombus resolution. Due to its high resolution, ECG-gated cardiac MRI is more sensitive but is currently not routinely utilized.

Early endovascular reperfusion therapy and thrombolysis combined with improved high-acuity clinical care of individuals with myocardial infarction have lowered the rate of ventricular thrombus formation and subsequent cerebral embolization.[25] Use of unfractionated or low-molecular-weight heparin for 10 days and heparin followed by systemic anticoagulation with warfarin reduces the risk of left ventricular thrombus formation in patients with anterior wall ST-elevation MI in the acute phase.[26–28] Most emboli occur during the first 3 to 4 months, but delayed embolization has been observed, especially in high-risk patients with severe structural cardiac damage and dysrhythmias following infarction. Patients with severe left ventricular dysfunction, left ventricular thrombus, and severe regional wall motion abnormalities, especially apical hypo- and akinesia, should receive warfarin therapy.[29] The need for lifelong anticoagulation beyond the first 3 to 12 months is somewhat controversial.[30] The decision should be made on individual basis estimating embolization risk and monitoring cardiac function by serial echocardiograms. The target INR typically is 2.0 to 3.0. All patients should also receive concomitant aspirin for secondary prevention of myocardial infarction. Patients with coronary artery stents require clopidogrel for 4 to 12 months depending on stent type. The risks and benefits of various thrombotic combination therapies need to be carefully considered, and interdisciplinary care is mandated to avoid intracranial or systemic hemorrhage.

Cardiac Failure

Cardiomyopathy causes generalized ventricular dilatation, decreases cardiac output, and promotes pulmonary venous stasis. Thrombi accumulate in the trabeculae carneae cordis of the apices of the right and left ventricles, and emboli may dislodge into the lungs or the brain. These patients are predisposed to cardiac decompensation and atrial fibrillation, which increases the risk even further. One study of patients who died as a result of cardiomyopathy demonstrated platelet-fibrin thrombi in the heart chambers in 50% of these cases.

The classification of the cardiomyopathies into the hypertrophic, restrictive, and dilated types is based on anatomic and physiologic features. Patients with idiopathic cardiomyopathy show both dilatation and hypertrophy. Hypertrophic cardiomyopathy, defined as idiopathic hypertrophy of the left ventricle with normal chamber size, probably represents several disease entities. Dilated cardiomyopathy is characterized by dilatation and impaired systolic function of the left ventricle without evident cause, usually associated with cardiac decompensation. Dilated cardiomyopathy also occurs in patients with a history of heavy alcohol intake, cocaine, or organic solvent abuse. Nutritional abnormalities, such as beriberi due to thiamine deficiency, account for some cases.

Patients with impaired left ventricular function and severely decreased ejection fraction of < 30% are at increased risk for left ventricular thrombus formation and cerebral embolization. There seems to be a linear relation between decreased ejection fraction and risk for ischemic stroke, which is more pronounced in women than men.[31,32]

Patients with heart failure and previous ischemic stroke should receive warfarin therapy. Anticoagulation is also indicated in MI patients who develop a mural thrombus, severe left ventricular dysfunction, or severe regional wall motion abnormalities. Although not validated by well-designed trials, warfarin therapy should be considered in patients with symptomatic heart failure, independent of the underlying etiology, when it is associated with an ejection fraction less than 30% or with ventricular thrombus formation.[33] The optimal INR range has not been established, but a goal INR between 2.0 to 3.0 is generally accepted to represent standard of medical care. Aspirin may be beneficial in patients with heart failure who cannot tolerate anticoagulation.[32] The use of ACE inhibitors, which are commonly used to treat patients with heart failure, may also help to reduce the hypercoagulable tendency that is frequently associated with this condition.[9,34]

Congenital Heart Disease

Cerebral infarctions occur in up to 17% of patients with congenital heart disease. Congenital heart lesions that allow mixing of arterial and venous blood and promote cyanosis are the defects most likely to cause stroke (see Chapter 22). Tetralogy of Fallot, hypoplastic ventricle syndrome, and transposition of great vessels are the lesions most likely to cause stroke, but most congenital heart lesions carry some risk.

Increasingly, individuals with congenital heart disease are surviving into late adulthood. It is estimated that there are about one million adult survivors of congenital heart disease in the United States. Some of these patients whose congenital lesion has been repaired still have residually altered hemodynamic function and thus an increased risk of stroke. Older patients with congenital heart disease may also develop accelerated atherosclerosis with secondary thrombotic and lacunar infarcts.

Cardiac disease may cause stroke in a variety of ways. A diseased heart valve or endocardium can be the locus for thrombus, which may embolize to the brain. Impaired cardiac output caused by insufficient perfusion, hypokinesis of the muscle wall, or outflow obstruction may reduce cerebral perfusion to critical levels. Furthermore, medications or interventions designed for the management of circulatory disorders may impair normal brain function. It is likely that individuals with an underlying coagulation abnormality in addition to their congenital heart disease have a greater risk of thromboembolism than with only the cardiac disease. The stroke risk goes up during catheterization and operative procedures. Finally, there is some evidence that individuals with congenital heart disease have a higher incidence of intracranial aneurysms and major vessel dissection.[35]

Cardiogenic stroke or TIA can result from an embolism from the left side of the heart or from paradoxical embolism from the venous circulation via an atrial septal defect or pulmonary right to left shunt. Patients with congenital heart disease are predisposed to ischemic events from prostatic heart valves, abnormalities of the left atrium and appendage, endocarditis, or atrial fibrillation. Paradoxical emboli can originate in the leg or pelvic veins or after thrombus formation at the site of an atrial septal aneurysm or patent foramen ovale (PFO).

Atrial Septal Lesions

In the fetal circulation oxygenated blood from the umbilical veins enters the right atrium and is shunted to the left atrium via a patent foramen ovale, bypassing the lung circulation. After birth the lungs inflate, and the associated sudden increase in left atrial pressure typically seals the flaplike connection. However, in 25% to 30% of the general population the PFO persists and can be demonstrated by echocardiography following intravenous injection of agitated saline during a Valsalva maneuver. Bubbles of saline that cross paradoxically from the right to the left side of the heart during transient episodes of increased right atrial pressure are visible by ultrasound.

Less often a congenital atrial septal defect (ASD) results from incomplete septation during fetal development. Like a PFO, an ASD can cause paradoxical embolism during episodes of transiently elevated right atrial pressure, which may result in ischemic stroke, TIA, or systemic atrial embolization to other organs or the extremities.

Atrial septal aneurysms have been found in 1% of autopsies, in 2% of all patients, and 6% to 15% of patients with possible embolic stroke referred for a TEE.[36–38] These lesions consist of redundant hypermobile septal tissue causing turbulent flow predisposing to aggregation of fibrin and platelets on the left atrial side, which may cause arterial embolization. Atrial septal aneurysm can occur in isolation, but is more commonly associated with a PFO or ASD.[39] If an atrial septal aneurysm is perforated, it presents functionally like an ASD, causing shunting of blood and potentially paradoxical embolic events.

In patients with cryptogenic stroke, which in some series constitutes 20% to 30% of all strokes in patients younger than 65 years, ASDs are relatively common. However, PFOs occur in 25% to 30% of the general population and usually remain asymptomatic. Results from prospective studies that explored the association of atrial septal aneurysm and PFO with cryptogenic stroke and recurrent stroke risk are controversial.[40–44]

Based on the currently available studies, it remains difficult to assess the risk of index stroke or a recurrent cerebral ischemic event associated with the presence of a PFO or septal aneurysm.[45–47] The American Academy of Neurology 2004 practice parameter concluded that an isolated PFO is not associated with a meaningful risk of recurrent stroke or death in patients who already had a cryptogenic stroke, that the data on atrial septal aneurysm and recurrent stroke risk are insufficient, and that a combination of an atrial septal aneurysm and PFO possibly increases the risk for recurrent stroke in patients younger than 55 years of age.[48]

The majority of people with PFO remain asymptomatic throughout life. However, there appears to be a higher incidence of cryptogenic stroke, vascular headaches, and paradoxical embolism, including gas embolism occurring during scuba diving or fat embolism after trauma in these individuals. Clinical presentation depends on the vascular territory involved, but smaller emboli may be clinically silent.

Neuroimaging studies often show infarcts in multiple vascular territories (Figure 8-1) or a cortical wedge-shaped stroke extending into the white matter. The diagnosis of an atrial shunt is best confirmed by TEE with agitated saline injection. TEE allows high-resolution imaging of the left atrium and left appendage where most thrombi are located, but offers limited visualization of the left ventricle. It is superior to transthoracic echocardiography (TTE) but is invasive and should therefore not be used routinely as the imaging study of first choice. Frequently an atrial septal defect can be detected by TTE. Transcranial Doppler studies with agitated contrast solution can also detect a right-to-left shunt but cannot differentiate between a cardiac or pulmonary source. Imaging studies of the lower extremities and pelvic veins are frequently negative.

The best management for these individuals is uncertain. Treatment options for atrial septal defects include endovascular or surgical closure, anticoagulation, and antiplatelet therapy. It is unclear whether device closure for PFO is superior to medical therapy, because recurrent ischemic strokes after PFO closure have been observed.[49–51] In cryptogenic stroke the causal relationship between an atrial septal defect and ischemic stroke remains difficult to establish because of the high frequency of PFOs among otherwise normal individuals. Furthermore the natural history of patients with atrial septal aneurysm or PFO who had a TIA or ischemic stroke but who do receive treatment is unknown.

Until results from ongoing studies on percutaneous closure of isolated PFO become available, antiplatelet therapy with aspirin or an alternative antiplatelet agent is the first line of therapy for most patients who have had an ischemic cerebral event and who do not wish to participate in any of the ongoing trials comparing device closure with medical treatment.[41,43] It has been suggested that patients with recurrent strokes or TIAs despite antiplatelet therapy should undergo a percutaneous device

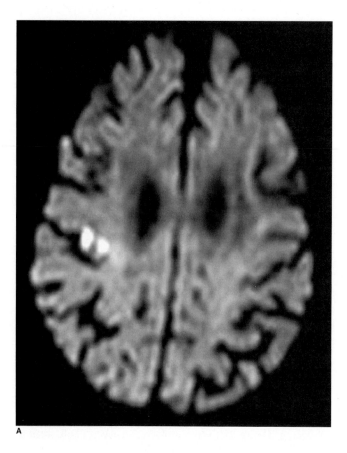
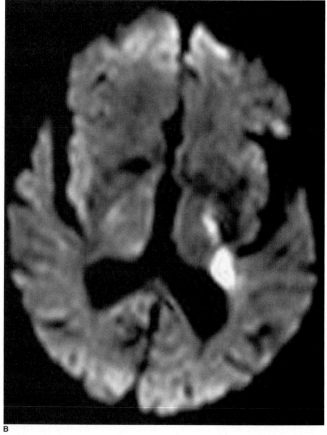

Figure 8-1. A and B: Diffusion-weighted MRI from a man with multiple ischemic infarctions due to cardiogenic emboli (he had atrial fibrillation and cardiomyopathy, and his echocardiogram showed a left atrial thrombus). Note several different ischemic lesions in different vascular territories, a pattern suggestive of multiple emboli.

closure, but evidence-based data are currently limited.[52] Patients with PFO and concurrent hypercoagulable state or other indication for anticoagulation should receive warfarin.[30]

A similar approach seems reasonable in individuals who have both a PFO and an atrial septal aneurysm because evidence-based data are limited. There are no clear recommendations regarding the use of medical treatment or device closure in this setting. As isolated ASA are relatively uncommon, no guidelines are in place to comment on treatment for stroke patients with isolated septal aneurysm. However, because of the risk of thrombus formation, treatment with an antiplatelet agent such as aspirin and risk factor modification seems indicated. Patients with ASD should probably undergo device closure because of the presence of a relatively high-volume shunt, which increases the chance of paradoxical embolism and right heart failure.

Valvular Heart Disease

Valvular heart disease and prosthetic heart valves provide a nidus for clot formation (Figure 8-2) and thus are risk factors for cardioembolic stroke. Systemic emboli can originate from valve thrombosis, vegetations, or left atrial or ventricular thrombus.

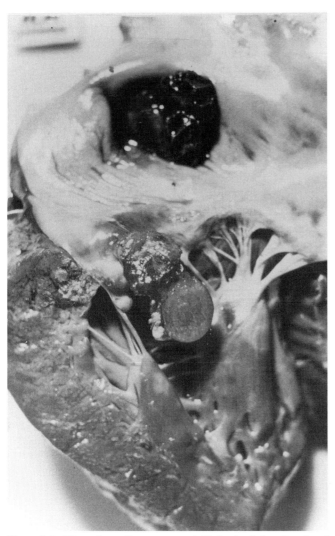

Figure 8-2. Thrombus adherent to a calcified mitral ring. Reprinted with permission from Pomerance.[127]

Infective Embolism

Compared to the pre-antibiotic era, infective endocarditis has become much less common. About 10,000 to 15,000 new cases of infectious endocarditis are diagnosed each year,[53] and many of those occur in elderly patients who are at increased risk to develop valvular heart disease requiring valve replacement, which is associated with an increased risk of endocarditis. Emboli originate mainly from the left side of the heart but can also occur with tricuspid valve vegetations in the setting of paradoxical emboli through a PFO or an arteriovenous lung shunt.

Many cases of infective endocarditis are due to infections with *Staphylococcus aureus* (about 32%) or *Streptococcus viridans* (about 18%), which cause more valvular damage and have a higher rate of complications and embolization than *Enteroccocus endocarditis* (about 11% of all cases).[54] Organisms with low virulence produce localized arteritis or focal arterial wall damage with aneurysm formation, whereas more virulent organisms cause meningitis or an abscess. Multiple types of brain lesions may occur in the same patient, but arteritis and stroke are more common than abscess or septic aneurysm.[55,56]

Systemic symptoms and cardiac signs predominate initially in individuals with infective endocarditis. Patients often have fever but can be nonfebrile and may or may not have a heart murmur. Headache is usually present, and mental status change is common. The nature of the neurological deficits depends on the location, number, and size of the lesions. Ischemic stroke can be the first presenting symptom of infectious embolism, or it can occur later from infectious arteritis.[57] Rupture of an infectious aneurysm is followed immediately by signs of subarachnoid or intraparenchymal hemorrhage. Because of their more peripheral location, septic aneurysms are more likely to cause intraparenchymal hemorrhage than saccular aneurysms (see Chapter 17).[58]

Branches of the middle cerebral artery are the most common location for infective emboli (Figure 8-3), but any portion of the cerebral circulation can be affected.[59] Septic aneurysms can be distinguished from saccular or fusiform aneurysms

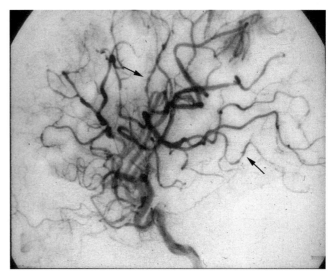

Figure 8-3. Cerebral catheter angiogram from a patient with infective endocarditis demonstrates multiple areas of arterial stenosis and beading (arrows) resulting from arteritis due to septic emboli.

microscopically by intense acute inflammation. The arterial media and elastica are damaged, but the acute nature of this process is usually apparent. An abscess may form about the aneurysm, and the offending organism can sometimes be seen or cultured.[60]

Anticoagulation is discouraged in individuals with native valve infective endocarditis, but there are high-risk subgroups in which the embolism risk may be high enough to justify anticoagulation. Patients with prosthetic valve endocarditis have an embolism risk approaching 50% without warfarin treatment, and anticoagulation or valve replacement should be strongly considered. Retrospective studies suggest a potential protective effect of antiplatelet agents to prevent embolism, but only when initiated at least 6 months before infectious embolism.[61] If antiplatelet therapy is initiated after the diagnosis of infectious embolism has been established, there is an increased risk of hemorrhagic complications and no benefit to prevent cerebral emboli.[62]

A 4- to 8-week course of antibiotics that is adequate to cure infective endocarditis should also be sufficient to eliminate septic intracranial arteritis in the early stages before an aneurysm or abscess has formed. Despite some risk of additional emboli, anticoagulation is best avoided because of the risk of aneurysm formation and rupture. Some aneurysms resolve with antibiotics, but persistence of an aneurysm after 2 months of appropriate antibiotic therapy, radiographic enlargement of an aneurysm, or the development of symptoms related to an aneurysm all are indications for surgery or endovascular treatment. Thin slice magnetic resonance imaging (MRI) or computed tomography angiography (CTA) are less invasive means of following the aneurysm than catheter angiography, although arguably less reliable as well. Selected aneurysms may lend themselves to endovascular treatment.[63,64]

Various parasites including *Trichinella spiralis, Entamoeba histolytica*, cysticercus, and schistosoma may embolize and encyst in the small arteries of the brain.

Rheumatic Valvular Heart Disease

Rheumatic valvular heart disease used to be the most frequent cause of mitral valve dysfunction and cerebral embolism in the United States and remains so in many parts of the developing world. Systemic emboli occur in about 20% of patients, with an estimated 40% of those lodging in the brain arteries. The annual risk of recurrent embolism is about 10%. Atrial fibrillation caused by rheumatic or ischemic heart disease increases the risk of cerebral embolism. It contributes a 17-fold increase. Emboli to the middle cerebral artery are the most common.

Mitral valve stenosis results from rheumatic fever but has become quite rare. In patients with mitral valve stenosis cerebral emboli can develop. Observational studies before mitral valve replacement and use of anticoagulation showed that up to 30% of patients with mitral valve stenosis have evidence of systemic embolization. The risk of embolization increases with the presence of left atrial thrombus.[65]

Mitral Valve Prolapse

The association of mitral valve prolapse (MVP) and cerebral ischemic events is uncertain. Observational studies and community surveys have found conflicting results.[66–76] Based on the conflicting data available, it is difficult to establish an association between MVP and the risk of ischemic stroke and TIA. In young patients ischemic cerebral events are rare, whereas MVP is a relatively common echocardiographic finding, and an association might be coincidental. However, in patients with MVP who are older than 50 years of age and have other vascular risk factors, there might be an increased risk for stroke.[71] There is no consensus for antiplatelet or warfarin therapy. The current guideline by the 2008 Eighth ACCP Consensus Conference on Antithrombotic Therapy[77] and the 2006 American College of Cardiology/American Heart Association guidelines[78] agreed that antithrombotic therapy is not recommended in patients without a history of systemic embolism, unexplained transient ischemic attacks, ischemic stroke, or atrial fibrillation. In contrast, the 2006 ACC/AHA guidelines suggest that aspirin therapy (75 to 325 mg) may be considered for individuals in sinus rhythm with echocardiographic evidence of high-risk MVP. Aspirin (up to 325 mg daily) is recommended in patients with unexplained transient ischemic attacks who are in sinus rhythm and have no associated atrial thrombi. Warfarin therapy with a target INR of 2 to 3 is recommended for patients with documented systemic embolism or recurrent transient ischemic attacks who have failed aspirin therapy.

Nonbacterial (Marantic) Thrombotic Endocarditis

Formerly known as marantic endocarditis, nonbacterial thrombotic endocarditis (NBTE) complicates cancer (often mucin-producing carcinomas) and other disorders with "hypercoagulable states" and a variety of other systemic conditions, including intravascular coagulation (DIC) and systemic lupus erythematosus (SLE).[79] Episodes of arterial thromboembolism are most frequently due to NBTE.[80] Nonbacterial thrombotic endocarditis is characterized by valvular lesions, mostly found in patients with advanced stages of adenocarcinoma. The lesions can consist of small platelet aggregates or large vegetations and are frequently found on the aortic or the mitral valve. Most vegetations are associated with lung cancer, but can also be found in prostate, ovarian, or gastrointestinal cancer, among other cancers. Cerebral embolization is relatively common because fragments of vegetations get easily dislodged into the cerebrovascular circulation. There is minimal inflammatory reaction of the endocardium.

Fewer than half of the patients have a heart murmur, and small lesions can easily be missed by echocardiography so that the diagnosis can be difficult. Hypercoagulable state associated with malignancy is an important differential diagnosis in these patients. Some cases of acute ischemic stroke in patients with malignancy may be due to paradoxical brain embolism arising from deep vein thrombosis and a right-to-left shunt.[81] Thrombophlebitis elsewhere in the body should arouse suspicion of NBTE. The occurrence of multiple emboli and its association with malignancies and with a variety of cardiovascular, pulmonary, renal, and gastrointestinal disorders should provide clues for recognition of this disorder.

The 2008 ACCP Guidelines recommend that patients with NBTE and systemic or pulmonary emboli should receive treatment with full-dose intravenous unfractionated heparin or subcutaneous low-molecular-weight heparin.[77] Full-dose intravenous unfractionated heparin or subcutaneous low-molecular-weight heparin should be initiated in patients with disseminated cancer or debilitating disease who are found to have aseptic vegetations. Anticoagulation should be continued lifelong.[82] If possible, the underlying malignancy should be treated.

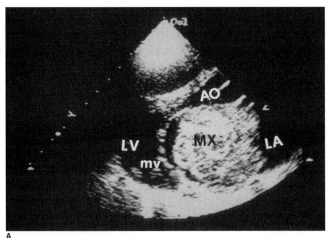
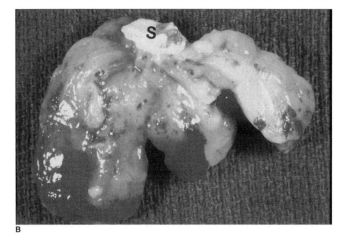

Figure 8-4. A: Echardiogram showing an atrial myxoma in an individual with a large embolic left middle cerebral artery territory infarction. B: Surgically removed atrial myxoma specimen. Note the pedunculated nature of the tumor and the associated thrombus. AO = aorta, LA = left atrium, LV = left ventricle, MX = myxoma, S = stalk. Reprinted with permission from Bayir et al.[128]

Libman-Sacks Endocarditis

Libman-Sacks (verrucous) endocarditis occurs in about 10% to 40% of patients with SLE and may be associated with the antiphospholipid antibody syndrome.[83] Verrucae are most commonly localized on the aortic and mitral valves. They consist of accumulations of immune complexes, mononuclear cells, fibrin, and platelet thrombi that can be best visualized by TEE. When these lesions heal, fibrosis, scars, and calcifications develop that can damage the heart valve. Typically verrucous endocarditis is asymptomatic, but when verroucous fragments break off, they can produce systemic emboli.

Prosthetic Heart Valves

Mechanical prosthetic heart valves have a considerable risk of systemic embolization and cerebral ischemic events. Patients with a mechanical mitral valve are especially at high risk for thrombus formation and systemic embolization. In patients on warfarin therapy the risk for cerebral embolism is 1% per patient-year.[84,85] Patients with mechanical heart valves require lifelong anticoagulation with warfarin and close monitoring of their INR, which often is targeted to stay at the upper ranges of the therapeutic window. If patients need to discontinue warfarin to undergo a procedure, bridging with low-molecular-weight heparin, such as subcutaneous enoxaparin, may not be sufficient for prevention of thromboembolic events.[86] In these situations intravenous heparin should be used instead. Patients with bioprosthetic valves do not require systemic anticoagulation.

Cardiac Tumors

With an incidence of less than 1%, primary cardiac tumors are rare. More frequently the heart is involved in metastatic disease, where masses have been found in up to 20% of patients dying of cancer.[87] The vast majority of primary cardiac tumors are benign. In adults most intracardiac tumors are myxomas followed by papillary fibroelastomas and lipomas.

Rhabdomyomas, which occur in two-thirds of individuals with tuberous sclerosis complex, are the most common intracardiac tumors in children. Based on the paucity of clinical reports, however, it appears that cardiac rhabdomyomas do not create nearly as great a risk of embolic stroke as do atrial myxomas, so rhabdomyomas do not always need to be electively removed.[88–90]

Benign myxomas occur predominantly in the left atrium at the border of the fossa ovalis (Figure 8-4), but they can arise in the right atrium or, less frequently, in the ventricles. They are prone to cause cerebral tumor emboli because of protrusion of the friable tumor into the left atrium or ventricle. Emboli may be either from tumor fragments or from thrombus attached to the neoplasm.[91] The motility of the tumor within the heart, rather than its size, tends to determine the risk of embolism.[92] Neurologic manifestations are common and include focal deficits, cognitive disturbances, syncope, seizures, and headaches. Rare presentations of left atrial myxoma are mental status change, spinal cord ischemia, and subarachnoid hemorrhage.[93] Myxomas can cause multiple cerebral aneurysms, at times years after the cardiac lesion has been removed.[94] Like other aneurysms, myxoma-related aneurysms result in subarachnoid or intraparenchymal hemorrhage (see Chapter 17).

Approximately 25% of patients have no cardiac symptoms to alert the neurologist to the underlying cause of ischemic or hemorrhagic strokes. Some patients, however, present with fever, weight loss, and laboratory results suggesting the presence of a connective tissue disease. Although the etiology of these symptoms is not known, the production of various cytokines and growth factors by the tumor may play a role. The main differential diagnosis of cardiac myxoma is infective endocarditis. Soft, systolic murmurs may be present, and a characteristic tumor "plop" sometimes results when a pedunculated tumor strikes the endocardial wall.

Cranial CT and brain MRI may show single or multiple infarctions or space-occupying lesions. Depending on its size the tumor can be detected by TTE, TEE, cardiac ultra-fast CT imaging, or cardiac magnetic resonance. Transvenous biopsy may be helpful, but is only rarely indicated. Generally noninvasive imaging is sufficient to make the decision for surgery until a definitive histological diagnosis is made following resection.

Prompt resection is indicated to avoid the risk of systemic embolization or cardiovascular complications, including sudden death.[95–97] The results of surgical resection are generally excellent. In rare instances with multiple recurrent atrial myxomas cardiac transplantation may be indicated. Atrial myxomas recur in about 2% to 5% of cases.

Papillary fibroelastomas are the second most common primary cardiac tumor in adults. Symptoms usually are caused by embolization, either of the tumor fragments or due to thromboembolism. The most common clinical presentation is that of cerebral embolization, followed by angina, myocardial infarction, sudden death, heart failure, syncope, and systemic or pulmonary embolic events. Patients with evidence of embolization should undergo surgical resection, which generally has excellent results.

ARTERY-TO-ARTERY EMBOLISM

Emboli composed of cholesterol crystals dislodged from atheromatous plaques situated on the carotid and vertebral-basilar arteries and the aorta are common. These plaques form over years, and, if they become ulcerated, they can release a plaque fragment or clot, which obstructs small distal arteries to produce infarction. In other cases the plaques may accumulate platelets, cells, and thrombi, which can cause local obstruction of larger arteries or travel to distal arteries and cause embolic occlusion. Embolism from arterial dissection or an aneurysmal sac is rare but should be considered as a possible etiology, especially in patients with familial tendency for aneurysms.

Carotid artery atherosclerosis can cause artery-to-artery embolism and is discussed in detail in Chapter 7. Carotid bifurcation plaques are a frequent source of emboli to the brain and retina (see Figure 6-1), resulting in TIAs, amaurosis fugax, retinal ischemia, or ischemic strokes.

AORTIC ATHEROSCLEROTIC PLAQUE

Aortic atherosclerotic plaques, especially when complex and unstable, are a common source of cerebral emboli.[98,99] Thromboemboli tend to be single and lodge in medium or large arteries of the brain. Cholesterol embolism, less common in this setting, is due to dislodgement of small pieces of aortic atheromatous material, typically causing multiple small artery occlusions resulting in retinal ischemia, livedo reticularis, or multiple small cerebral infarcts. Emboli occur only with lesions of the ascending aorta and the aortic arch.

The risk of embolization increases with ulcerated or mobile plaques and plaque size of > 4 mm. Atherosclerotic plaque formation is related to classical vascular risk factors including, but not limited to, hypertension, diabetes mellitus, dyslipidemia, age, tobacco use, or elevated C-reactive protein. Complex aortic plaques have a high rate of embolization.[100,101] The risk of embolism varies with plaque's characteristics on TEE and location. Cerebral embolization due to dislodging of debris from the aorta can occur during catheterization, percutaneous coronary intervention, intra-aortic balloon pump, and cardiac surgery.

The neurological manifestations depend on the vascular territory affected by embolism. Mortality associated with severe aortic plaque may be as high as 20% within 3 years of diagnosis.[102] Almost 20% of the deaths are attributed to complications of stroke. Furthermore, patients with complex or large aortic plaque are also at higher risk of intraoperative stroke during cardiopulmonary bypass surgery, which has been reported to be as high as 39%.[103]

Aortic plaques can be identified and characterized by magnetic resonance angiography, TEE, and CTA. TEE is the diagnostic method of choice for the detection and measurement of thoracic aortic plaques. Conscious sedation is required in approximately half of the patients, but the method is relatively minimally invasive and has a low risk of complication.

Patients with cerebral thromboembolism due to atherosclerotic plaque should be aggressively treated to prevent recurrent stroke. Vascular risk factors need to be appropriately modified. The patient should receive aspirin or an alternative antiplatelet regimen, statins, blood pressure control, counseling about tobacco use, and glycemic control. The goal is to reduce thrombus size and to induce plaque stabilization.

The optimal treatment of complex aortic arch plaque is uncertain, given the limited data and absence of randomized trials. For eligible patients with history of ischemic stroke and complex atheroma, some authors suggest chronic warfarin therapy with a goal INR of 2.0 to 3.0,[104] whereas others suggest chronic aspirin therapy. For patients without stroke who have atheroma with a mobile component, expert opinions are also divided. Some suggest chronic therapy with warfarin (INR goal 2.0 to 3.0); others prefer chronic aspirin or alternative antiplatelet therapy. There are no guidelines to help make decisions regarding the target INR. The efficacy of aspirin or alternative antiplatelet agents in this setting is also unknown.

Statin therapy for stroke risk reduction in patients with severe thoracic aortic atherosclerosis has been evaluated only in observational studies.[102] Statins may induce aortic plaque stabilization and potentially plaque regression.[105–108] The SPARCL trial showed a reduction of recurrent stroke and TIA following daily administration of 80 mg of atorvastatin.[109] LDL levels recommended by the American Heart Association probably should be achieved (LDL < 100 mg/dl for the general population and < 70 mg/dl in patients with cerebral ischemic events or at high risk for atherosclerosis in other vascular beds).

The role of surgical therapy is not clearly defined. Newer surgical techniques for replacing the aortic arch or aortic filters designed to prevent cerebral embolism are being studied.

EMBOLISM DURING CARDIAC PROCEDURES

Cerebral embolism due to dislodging of debris from atherosclerotic lesions occurs as a complication of invasive cardiovascular and cerebrovascular procedures, including catheterization, percutaneous coronary intervention, intraaortic balloon pump, cardiac surgery, carotid endarterectomy, and endovascular procedures within the extra- and intracranial cerebral circulation.

The reported incidence of stroke related to cardiac operations ranges from 0.4% to 14%.[110–112] Perioperative stroke rates associated with coronary artery bypass graft surgery (CABG) range between 0.8% and 5%.[113,114] Intraprocedural cerebral emboli can be thromboembolic, atheroembolic, or related to air entering the circulation. Thrombi or atheromatous debris can be released from complex plaques during clamping and unclamping, construction of coronary artery bypass graft anastomoses, from severely calcified and diseased cardiac valves, or by turbulent blood flow. Gaseous emboli enter the arterial circulation via open cardiac chambers, vascular instrumentation sites, or at arterial anastomoses. Stroke after an uncomplicated procedure is frequently due to cardiogenic emboli. Atrial fibrillation is a common postoperative complication that seems to play a major role in this setting.

Whenever possible patients should undergo brain MRI to confirm the diagnosis of stroke and to treat the underlying cause, although treatment is mainly supportive. There is an increased incidence of neuropsychological deficits in patients undergoing cardiac surgery, which are thought to be related to the intraoperative occurrence of cerebral microemboli.[115]

Improved intraoperative monitoring and improved technology such as new filter systems or endovascular protective devices may help to prevent some of these cerebral ischemic events.

FOREIGN BODY EMBOLISM

Trauma to systemic veins, the heart, lungs, or aortocranial arteries can introduce air or solid foreign material into the bloodstream, which may travel to the brain. Among the agents that have been inadvertently or maliciously introduced into the arterial tree are bullets, air, calcium from the heart valves or aortic arch, antifoaming agents, talcum crystals, cotton, catheters, device fragments, and other items (Figure 8-5).

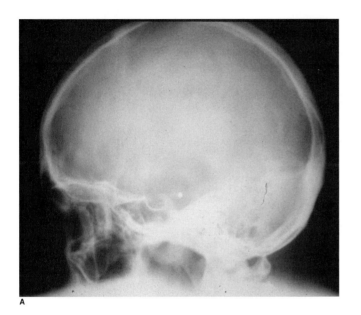

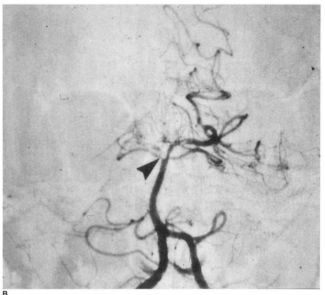

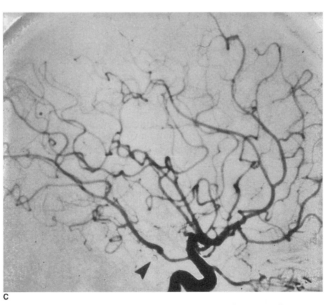

Figure 8-5. A: Lateral skull X-ray following a self-inflicted shotgun wound to the chest shows a pellet posterior to the sella turcica. B and C: Catheter cerebral angiogram shows that the pellet (*arrowheads*) is occluding the proximal posterior cerebral artery, which continues to be perfused via the posterior communicating artery. The patient recovered completely. Reprinted with permission from Roach and Riela.[129]

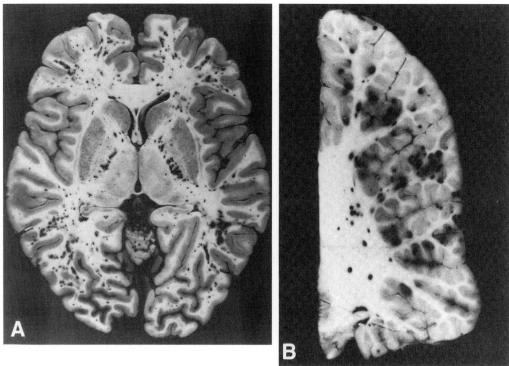

Figure 8-6. The characteristic appearance of fat embolism in the cerebral hemispheres (A) and cerebellum (B). Note the extensive white matter petechiae with sparing of the cortex. Part A reprinted with permission from Kamenar and Kozachuk.[130]

FAT EMBOLISM

Fat embolism is an occasional complication of trauma to the long bones, especially those that contain marrow, and due to pelvic fractures. Closed fractures and multiple fractures are associated with an increased risk. Several days after a crushing injury or fracture, the patient develops signs secondary to obstruction of pulmonary, cerebral, and renal capillaries by fat globules sized 10 to 40 µm. There are two theories regarding the source of these globules: (1) the crushed adipose cells of the marrow release fat into the marrow veins and (2) the normally emulsified chylomicrons of the bloodstream aggregate into large globules that cannot pass through capillary beds. As fat globules become coated with platelets, thrombocytopenia develops. Platelet aggregates have been proposed to contribute to the focal lesions caused by capillary obstruction. Patent foramen ovale may be an important contributing factor in pathogenesis. As right-heart pressure increases in response to Valsalva maneuvers or pulmonary embolization, fat droplets may paradoxically embolize through a patent foramen ovale.

The clinical presentation is highly variable, and at times the diagnosis is difficult. Dyspnea, tachypnea, and hypoxemia are typically the first symptoms, followed by encephalopathy, seizures, stupor, or coma and multifocal neurological deficits. A characteristic petechial rash may develop on the head, neck, anterior thorax, maxillae, and subconjunctiva. In surviving patients the neurological deficits are usually transient with a good chance of complete recovery. If the patient dies, the brain shows widespread petechiae (Figure 8-6). Microscopically, fat emboli are widely distributed throughout the central nervous system, being most numerous in the white matter of the cerebrum. Reported mortality rates vary between 5% to 15%.[116] A similar syndrome can develop following silicone embolism syn-drome. In those patients neurological deficits are often associated with rapid clinical deterioration and mortality.[117] Brain MRI may demonstrate high T_2 signal hyperintensities.

Treatment is supportive. The use of corticosteroids is controversial. Early fracture immobilization may help to prevent fat embolism after trauma, and correction of hypoxemia and hypo-volemic shock is of proven benefit.

AIR EMBOLISM

The most common causes of air embolism are interventional procedures involving the dural sinuses or veins of the head, neck, and chest as well as cardiac interventions. Patients in the intensive care setting are at increased risk for air embolism because of the instrumentation of the central venous system and use of positive pressure mechanical ventilation, which may induce venous or arterial gas emboli. Upright position under these conditions is a particular risk.

The clinical picture depends on the rate and amount of air introduced into the circulation. Introduction of large volumes of 300–500 ml of air at a rate of 100 ml/sec is typically a fatal event. In the microcirculation bubbles cause endothelial dysfunction and damage, accumulation of platelets, fibrin, and neutrophils. Complements and mediators of inflammation and free radicals are released, causing breakdown of the blood-brain barrier and cerebral edema. Bubbles also directly occlude the microcirculation, causing ischemic brain damage.[118,119]

The diagnosis should be considered in patients with acute onset of cardiopulmonary and neurological deterioration occurring in a plausible clinical setting. Patients typically present with dyspnea, wheezing, rales, respiratory failure, signs of shock, acute right-sided heart failure, change in mental status,

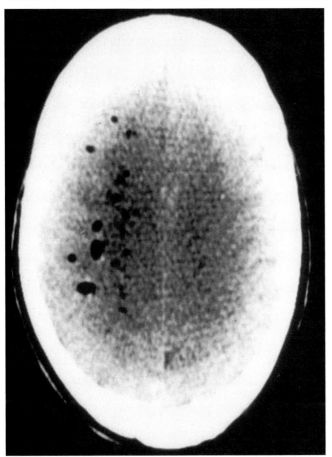

Figure 8-7. Multiple right hemisphere air emboli are evident on a CT scan.

and focal neurological deficits. The differential diagnosis includes acute diseases of the heart and lung, stroke of other etiology, or hypoxic brain injury. There is no single confirmatory diagnostic test. Frequently chest X-ray and laboratory findings are normal or nonspecific. Neuroimaging studies may demonstrate multiple small strokes, intraparenchymal gas (Figure 8-7), and diffuse cerebral edema.

Identification of the source of air emboli to prevent recurrence and supportive care are the cornerstones of therapy. Patients with "air lock" from large volumes of air obstructing right ventricular outflow should be placed in the left lateral decubitus or the Trendelenburg position. Hyperbaric oxygen treatment can reduce bubble size so that air bubbles redissolve in the bloodstream. Furthermore, it increases nitrogen absorption and the amount of oxygen dissolved in blood, reducing the risk of hypoxemic damage.[120]

Nitrogen Bubbles (Bends)

Embolism caused by bubbles of nitrogen is the most frequent cause of neurologic abnormality in persons who are subjected to rapid reduction in atmospheric pressure, particularly scuba divers or miners. During rapid decompression, microbubbles can form from inert nitrogen, which is usually dissolved in the blood. Microbubbles coalesce to act as a vapor lock, plugging arterioles and capillaries and producing tissue hypoxia. Seizures, joint pain, mental status changes, focal neurological deficits,

stupor, or coma can develop. Treatment consists of immediate restoration of increased ambient atmospheric pressure in a hyperbaric chamber, followed by slow decompression ranging over hours to days. If detected and treated immediately, full recovery is the rule.

Neoplasm-Related Embolism

In addition to embolism from atrial myxoma, dislodged tumor fragments from carcinoma of the lung, breast, stomach, kidney, or thyroid or from choriocarcinoma or malignant melanoma can deposit in the brain vasculature.[121–124] They are carried in the bloodstream, usually as aggregates, until they seed into the brain. Atrial myxomas and certain lung neoplasms occasionally send off emboli that are large enough to obstruct and even grow in the wall of an artery, producing immediate or delayed neurologic deficit. They cause a variety of abnormalities, including aneurysms, because of implantation of invasive cells in the arterial wall, which weaken it.

PATHOPHYSIOLOGY OF CEREBRAL EMBOLISM

Although blood clot is by far the most common, any solid, liquid, gaseous, or foreign material can embolize through an artery and produce ischemia. In addition to causing obstruction, the embolic material may act as an irritant, causing vasospasm, endothelial damage, or inflammatory changes in the segment where it lodges or affecting the entire distal arterial bed. Therefore, not only the artery it obstructs but also the effect it has on the vascular tree and especially the microcirculatory bed determine the neurologic abnormalities that occur. Symptoms depend on the vessel obstructed. An embolus large enough to lodge in the internal carotid artery and to obliterate all distal blood flow produces vastly different symptoms from one that lodges in a terminal branch of the middle cerebral artery. This interplay between the branch occluded and the response of the vascular tree varies from person to person. Some patients respond with intense vasospasm to a small embolus, whereas others may tolerate a large one with little or no consequence. Spasm seems to occur more frequently in younger patients, perhaps because their arteries are less sclerotic.

An embolus entering the aortocranial circulation may enter an artery supplying blood to the eye or the brain. The flow through the internal carotid artery is about three times that of the external carotid, and, although fragments more often tend to travel into the internal carotid, some foreign material in the common carotid may be swept into the external carotid system and then to the mucous membranes and skin, rather than traversing through the internal carotid to the brain.

The initial obstruction generally occurs at a bifurcation site because the lumens of the branches are smaller than those of the parent artery. In this location an embolus may obstruct one or both of the branches, producing ischemia of distal tissues. Stasis of the blood column leads to platelet rolling, leukocyte adhesion, and thrombus formation, both proximally and distally in the stagnant column. As tissue metabolism continues, carbon dioxide accumulates locally, causing maximal dilatation of regional arteries, capillaries, and veins. Neuronal function ceases within seconds, and, if collateral channels do not take over immediately, capillary diapedesis and edema develop. If the embolus moves on into distal branches before irreversible changes begin, neuronal function is promptly restored.

When an embolus that had initially lodged at a bifurcation breaks apart, the fragments move into distal branches that had been too small for the whole embolus to traverse. As they proceed distally into the necrosing area, the restoration of blood flow through the now-weakened arterial system is reestablished, sometimes changing what had been a bloodless area into a hemorrhagic one. In addition, good collateral supply from the leptomeningeal network increases the risk of hemorrhagic transformation. Consequently, in patients with cerebral embolism, hemorrhagic infarctions frequently exist side by side with ischemic ones.

In contrast to the local dilatation produced by carbon dioxide and accumulating metabolites, spasm may occur in a large portion of the regional arterial bed as soon as the foreign material has entered it. The result is ischemia and, perhaps, infarction in areas remote from the embolus itself.

PATHOLOGICAL FINDINGS

In many cases with a clinical picture typical of cerebral embolism, emboli may not be found at autopsy, even when the vessels are examined in detail. Many explanations for this apparent lack of clinicopathologic correlation have been offered:

1. Massive vasospasm may occur in response to a very small embolus, so that a large deficit is produced by a small foreign body
2. The original large embolus may divide into smaller and smaller fragments that lodge in distal arterioles and, thus, are visible only using microscopy
3. Fixatives used to prepare the specimen may dissolve or dislodge emboli, such as cholesterol crystals or a blood clot
4. Intrinsic thrombolysis may have dissolved blood clots that were temporarily obstructing an artery.

Hemorrhagic cerebral infarction is the typical lesion of embolism. Approximately 50% to 60% of embolic cerebral infarctions are at least microscopically hemorrhagic, and frankly hemorrhagic arterial infarcts are more common with embolism than thrombosis. In such cases the uncut brain usually shows edema over a large area, which is often stippled with multiple petechial hemorrhages in gray, but not white, matter. The gyri are swollen and red-brown. A section made through the lesion shows it primarily to involve the cortex and subcortical white matter. Microscopic analysis shows varying amounts of disintegration of neurons, myelin sheaths, and neuroglia, together with perivascular hemorrhages.

Septic emboli have a similar distribution, but frequently lead to suppuration and abscess formation. At times, metastatic emboli also result in acute infarction. Parasites blocking the cerebral capillaries may produce ischemia, hemorrhage, and a fibroglial or granulomatous reaction, often with calcification. In patients dying of a fat embolism, the lungs and kidneys, as well as the brain, are typically involved (Figure 8-6). The brain is edematous, and numerous petechial hemorrhages are found in the white matter with little, if any, involvement of the gray matter. Microscopic examination shows sudanophilic granules distributed throughout the gray and white matter, but the rich capillary anastomotic arrangement of the gray matter causes it to be free of hemorrhage and microinfarction.

In contrast to the above picture, there are no characteristic changes in the brain of a patient dying from an air embolism. The arteries supplying it may show bubbles of air, and there may be large quantities of air in the right atrium and ventricle.

Even when the embolus itself cannot be found, its source can usually be demonstrated. This is most often the pulmonary veins, the left atrium or its auricular appendage, the mitral valve, or the endocardium of the left ventricle; the aortic valve is an unusual source of emboli. In the presence of chronic pulmonary infection, the possibility of septic embolus as the cause of neurologic deficit should be considered.

Occasionally a thrombus is dislodged so completely that no remaining clot can be found at the primary site. When this occurs, the massive embolus from the pulmonary veins, the left atrium, or the atrial appendage may produce acute obstruction of the orifice of the mitral valve, with resulting sudden generalized ischemic anoxia, or it may pass through the left ventricle to lodge in the ostium of one of the great vessels coming off the arch.

Emboli that originate or lodge in the cervical arteries are seldom discovered because standard autopsy technique does not include examination of the length of the carotid, the subclavian, and the vertebral arteries. Whenever the heart and lungs do not reveal the source of an embolus to the brain, the cervical segments of the aortocranial arteries should be dissected.

DIAGNOSIS OF CEREBRAL EMBOLISM

There is no laboratory test that provides absolute proof of a thromboembolism. Except with infectious embolism, the initial blood count and CSF examination are usually normal, but hemorrhagic infarction may later cause blood to appear in the CSF. Chest X-rays are frequently normal or show nonspecific changes.

Cranial CT is usually normal at the onset but, depending on the course of the illness, later shows some combination of infarction or hemorrhagic infarction. The early cranial CT finding of hyperdensity of the proximal middle cerebral artery often indicates an embolic occlusion. Other early CT findings include sulcal effacement and effacement of basal ganglia/white matter frontiers on the infarct side. Identification of these early cranial CT signs is important during the evaluation for thrombolytic therapy.

Prolonged electrocardiographic monitoring may reveal cardiac dysrhythmias that have not been diagnosed clinically and may show an unsuspected myocardial infarction or paroxysmal atrial fibrillation as the source of embolism. TEE may show valvular lesions, wall motion abnormalities, thrombi, and positive echocontrast. The accuracy of echocardiography for the detection of shunts can be increased using a solution containing air microbubbles injected intravenously. In a person with an apparent cerebral embolus for which no source can be found, more infrequent causes such as atrial myxoma should be considered. Ultrasonography is often helpful in detecting and localizing embolic sources in stroke patients and in detecting intracardiac shunts. An EEG may show a focal disturbance corresponding to the ischemia area.

Magnetic resonance imaging is superior to CT when assessing lesion topography and the extent of infarction, but it is equally unable to distinguish embolic from nonembolic infarction. Multiple infarctions in different vascular territories, a pattern that suggests embolic disease, are better detected by MRI than cranial CT. Therefore, MRIs should be used when possible.

Magnetic resonance angiography is helpful for defining stenosis or occlusion of arteries or veins. Diffusion/perfusion MRI is highly sensitive to detect cerebral ischemia and penumbral tissue. Gradient-echo MRI can reliably detect microhemorrhage. Arteriography can be diagnostic when an intraluminal clot is demonstrated, and an occlusion at the branch point of an artery is suggestive of an embolism.

Later in the course of the illness, results of tests that had initially been normal may change. Because some emboli produce tissue hypoxia and infarction that may eventually become hemorrhagic, repeat examination of the cerebrospinal fluid may show red blood cells, xanthochromia, or an elevated protein level. Cranial CT may also show hemorrhage or an abnormal uptake of contrast material in the region of the infarction. Diagnostic evaluation for stroke is presented in more detail in Chapter 5.

PROGNOSIS AND CLINICAL COURSE

Not surprisingly, the prognosis is largely dependent on the size and number of emboli as well as the location of the resulting infarctions. Most patients survive the initial cerebral embolism; some recover completely, but others have major neurologic deficits. Death is most often due to the effects of secondary cerebral edema. A remarkable return of neurologic function may begin within hours of onset, perhaps because of the disappearance of vasospasm and restoration of flow. In some patients an embolus initially lodged in a large artery may move into smaller distal branches as the arterial spasm diminishes. In other cases, collateral circulation may account for the rapid return of function. Whatever the cause, this rapid improvement may closely simulate a TIA, and overall the prognosis is generally good.

REFERENCES

1. Cardiogenic brain embolism. The second report of the Cerebral Embolism Task Force. *Arch Neurol.* 1989;**46**:727–743.
2. Osler W. *The Principles and Practice of Medicine.* New York: D. Appleton and Company; 1892.
3. Osler W. On malignant endocarditis. *Br Med J.* 1885;**1**:467–470.
4. Ferro JM. Atrial fibrillation and cardioembolic stroke. *Minerva Cardioangiol.* 2004;**52**:111–124.
5. Kempster PA, Gerraty RP, Gates PC. Asymptomatic cerebral infarction in patients with chronic atrial fibrillation. *Stroke.* 1988;**19**:955–957.
6. Lin HJ, Wolf PA, Kelly-Hayes M, et al. Stroke severity in atrial fibrillation. The Framingham Study. *Stroke.* 1996;**27**:1760–1764.
7. Lloyd-Jones DM, Wang TJ, Leip EP, et al. Lifetime risk for development of atrial fibrillation: the Framingham Heart Study. *Circulation.* 2004;**110**:1042–1046.
8. Kannel WB, Abbott RD, Savage DD, McNamara PM. Epidemiologic features of chronic atrial fibrillation: the Framingham study. *N Engl J Med.* 1982;**306**:1018–1022.
9. Hart RG, Pearce LA, Aguilar MI. Meta-analysis: antithrombotic therapy to prevent stroke in patients who have nonvalvular atrial fibrillation. *Ann Intern Med.* 2007;**146**:857–867.
10. Wyse DG, Waldo AL, DiMarco JP, et al. A comparison of rate control and rhythm control in patients with atrial fibrillation. *N Engl J Med.* 2002;**347**:1825–1833.
11. Van Gelder I, Hagens VE, Bosker HA, et al. A comparison of rate control and rhythm control in patients with recurrent persistent atrial fibrillation. *N Engl J Med.* 2002;**347**:1834–1840.
12. Gage BF, Boechler M, Doggette AL, et al. Adverse outcomes and predictors of underuse of antithrombotic therapy in medicare beneficiaries with chronic atrial fibrillation. *Stroke.* 2000;**31**:822–827.
13. Go AS, Hylek EM, Borowsky LH, Phillips KA, Selby JV, Singer DE. Warfarin use among ambulatory patients with nonvalvular atrial fibrillation: the anticoagulation and risk factors in atrial fibrillation (ATRIA) study. *Ann Intern Med.* 1999;**131**:927–934.
14. Fuster V, Ryden LE, Cannom DS, et al. ACC/AHA/ESC 2006 guidelines for the management of patients with atrial fibrillation – executive summary: a report of the American College of Cardiology/American Heart Association Task Force on Practice Guidelines and the European Society of Cardiology Committee for Practice Guidelines (Writing Committee to Revise the 2001 Guidelines for the Management of Patients with Atrial Fibrillation). *J Am Coll Cardiol.* 2006;**48**:854–906.
15. Rockson SG, Albers GW. Comparing the guidelines: anticoagulation therapy to optimize stroke prevention in patients with atrial fibrillation. *J Am Coll Cardiol.* 2004;**43**:929–935.
16. Cooper NJ, Sutton AJ, Lu G, Khunti K. Mixed comparison of stroke prevention treatments in individuals with nonrheumatic atrial fibrillation. *Arch Intern Med.* 2006;**166**:1269–1275.
17. Hylek EM, Evans-Molina C, Shea C, Henault LE, Regan S. Major hemorrhage and tolerability of warfarin in the first year of therapy among elderly patients with atrial fibrillation. *Circulation.* 2007;**115**:2689–2696.
18. van Walraven C, Hart RG, Singer DE, et al. Oral anticoagulants vs aspirin in nonvalvular atrial fibrillation: an individual patient meta-analysis. *JAMA.* 2002;**288**:2441–2448.
19. Asinger RW, Mikell FL, Elsperger J, Hodges M. Incidence of left-ventricular thrombosis after acute transmural myocardial infarction. Serial evaluation by two-dimensional echocardiography. *N Engl J Med.* 1981;**305**:297–302.
20. Weinreich DJ, Burke JF, Pauletto FJ. Left ventricular mural thrombi complicating acute myocardial infarction. Long-term follow-up with serial echocardiography. *Ann Intern Med.* 1984;**100**:789–794.
21. Greaves SC, Zhi G, Lee RT, et al. Incidence and natural history of left ventricular thrombus following anterior wall acute myocardial infarction. *Am J Cardiol.* 1997;**80**:442–448.
22. Srichai MB, Junor C, Rodriguez LL, et al. Clinical, imaging, and pathological characteristics of left ventricular thrombus: a comparison of contrast-enhanced magnetic resonance imaging, transthoracic echocardiography, and transesophageal echocardiography with surgical or pathological validation. *Am Heart J.* 2006;**152**:75–84.
23. Mollet NR, Dymarkowski S, Volders W, et al. Visualization of ventricular thrombi with contrast-enhanced magnetic resonance imaging in patients with ischemic heart disease. *Circulation.* 2002;**106**:2873–2876.
24. Chiarella F, Santoro E, Domenicucci S, Maggioni A, Vecchio C. Predischarge two-dimensional echocardiographic evaluation of left ventricular thrombosis after acute myocardial infarction in the GISSI-3 study. *Am J Cardiol.* 1998;**81**:822–827.
25. Vaitkus PT, Barnathan ES. Embolic potential, prevention and management of mural thrombus complicating anterior myocardial infarction: a meta-analysis. *J Am Coll Cardiol.* 1993;**22**:1004–1009.
26. Turpie AG, Robinson JG, Doyle DJ, et al. Comparison of high-dose with low-dose subcutaneous heparin to prevent left ventricular mural thrombosis in patients with acute transmural anterior myocardial infarction. *N Engl J Med.* 1989;**320**:352–357.
27. Kontny F, Dale J, Abildgaard U, Pedersen TR. Randomized trial of low molecular weight heparin (dalteparin) in prevention of left ventricular thrombus formation and arterial embolism after

acute anterior myocardial infarction: the Fragmin in Acute Myocardial Infarction (FRAMI) Study. *J Am Coll Cardiol.* 1997;**30**:962–969.

28. Nordrehaug JE, Johannessen KA, von der Lippe G. Usefulness of high-dose anticoagulants in preventing left ventricular thrombus in acute myocardial infarction. *Am J Cardiol.* 1985;**55**:1491–1493.

29. Antman EM, Hand M, Armstrong PW, et al. 2007 focused update of the ACC/AHA 2004 guidelines for the management of patients with ST-elevation myocardial infarction: a report of the American College of Cardiology/American Heart Association Task Force on Practice Guidelines. *J Am Coll Cardiol.* 2008;**51**:210–247.

30. Sacco RL, Adams R, Albers G, et al. Guidelines for prevention of stroke in patients with ischemic stroke or transient ischemic attack: a statement for healthcare professionals from the American Heart Association/American Stroke Association Council on Stroke: co-sponsored by the Council on Cardiovascular Radiology and Intervention: the American Academy of Neurology affirms the value of this guideline. *Stroke.* 2006;**37**: 577–617.

31. Dries DL, Rosenberg YD, Waclawiw MA, Domanski MJ. Ejection fraction and risk of thromboembolic events in patients with systolic dysfunction and sinus rhythm: evidence for gender differences in the studies of left ventricular dysfunction trials. *J Am Coll Cardiol.* 1997;**29**:1074–1080.

32. Loh E, Sutton MS, Wun CC, et al. Ventricular dysfunction and the risk of stroke after myocardial infarction. *N Engl J Med.* 1997;**336**:251–257.

33. Hunt SA, Abraham WT, Chin MH, et al. ACC/AHA 2005 Guideline Update for the Diagnosis and Management of Chronic Heart Failure in the Adult: a report of the American College of Cardiology/American Heart Association Task Force on Practice Guidelines (Writing Committee to Update the 2001 Guidelines for the Evaluation and Management of Heart Failure): developed in collaboration with the American College of Chest Physicians and the International Society for Heart and Lung Transplantation: endorsed by the Heart Rhythm Society. *Circulation.* 2005;**112**:e154–e235.

34. Jafri SM, Mammen EF, Masura J, Goldstein S. Effects of warfarin on markers of hypercoagulability in patients with heart failure. *Am Heart J.* 1997;**134**:27–36.

35. Schievink WI, Mokri B, Piepgras DG, Gittenberger-de Groot AC. Intracranial aneurysms and cervicocephalic arterial dissections associated with congenital heart disease. *Neurosurgery.* 1996;**39**:685–690.

36. Silver MD, Dorsey JS. Aneurysms of the septum primum in adults. *Arch Pathol Lab Med.* 1978;**102**:62–65.

37. Agmon Y, Khandheria BK, Meissner I, et al. Frequency of atrial septal aneurysms in patients with cerebral ischemic events. *Circulation.* 1999;**99**:1942–1944.

38. Pearson AC, Nagelhout D, Castello R, Gomez CR, Labovitz AJ. Atrial septal aneurysm and stroke: a transesophageal echocardiographic study. *J Am Coll Cardiol.* 1991;**18**:1223–1229.

39. Mugge A, Daniel WG, Angermann C, et al. Atrial septal aneurysm in adult patients. A multicenter study using transthoracic and transesophageal echocardiography. *Circulation.* 1995;**91**: 2785–2792.

40. Lamy C, Giannesini C, Zuber M, et al. Clinical and imaging findings in cryptogenic stroke patients with and without patent foramen ovale: the PFO-ASA Study. Atrial Septal Aneurysm. *Stroke.* 2002;**33**:706–711.

41. Mas JL, Arquizan C, Lamy C, et al. Recurrent cerebrovascular events associated with patent foramen ovale, atrial septal aneurysm, or both. *N Engl J Med.* 2001;**345**:1740–1746.

42. Burger AJ, Sherman HB, Charlamb MJ. Low incidence of embolic strokes with atrial septal aneurysms: a prospective, long-term study. *Am Heart J.* 2000;**139**:149–152.

43. Homma S, Sacco RL, Di Tullio MR, Sciacca RR, Mohr JP. Effect of medical treatment in stroke patients with patent foramen ovale: patent foramen ovale in Cryptogenic Stroke Study. *Circulation.* 2002;**105**:2625–2631.

44. Handke M, Harloff A, Olschewski M, Hetzel A, Geibel A. Patent foramen ovale and cryptogenic stroke in older patients. *N Engl J Med.* 2007;**357**:2262–2268.

45. Di Tullio MR, Sacco RL, Sciacca RR, Jin Z, Homma S. Patent foramen ovale and the risk of ischemic stroke in a multiethnic population. *J Am Coll Cardiol.* 2007;**49**:797–802.

46. Meissner I, Khandheria BK, Heit JA, et al. Patent foramen ovale: innocent or guilty? Evidence from a prospective population-based study. *J Am Coll Cardiol.* 2006;**47**:440–445.

47. Petty GW, Khandheria BK, Meissner I, et al. Population-based study of the relationship between patent foramen ovale and cerebrovascular ischemic events. *Mayo Clin Proc.* 2006;**81**: 602–608.

48. Messe SR, Silverman IE, Kizer JR, et al. Practice parameter: recurrent stroke with patent foramen ovale and atrial septal aneurysm: report of the Quality Standards Subcommittee of the American Academy of Neurology. *Neurology.* 2004;**62**:1042–1050.

49. Windecker S, Wahl A, Chatterjee T, et al. Percutaneous closure of patent foramen ovale in patients with paradoxical embolism: long-term risk of recurrent thromboembolic events. *Circulation.* 2000;**101**:893–898.

50. Anzola GP, Morandi E, Casilli F, Onorato E. Does transcatheter closure of patent foramen ovale really "shut the door"? A prospective study with transcranial Doppler. *Stroke.* 2004; **35**:2140–2144.

51. Berthet K, Lavergne T, Cohen A, et al. Significant association of atrial vulnerability with atrial septal abnormalities in young patients with ischemic stroke of unknown cause. *Stroke.* 2000;**31**:398–403.

52. Wu LA, Malouf JF, Dearani JA, et al. Patent foramen ovale in cryptogenic stroke: current understanding and management options. *Arch Intern Med.* 2004;**164**:950–956.

53. Bayer AS. Infective endocarditis. *Clin Infect Dis.* 1993;**17**: 313–320.

54. McDonald JR, Olaison L, Anderson DJ, et al. Enterococcal endocarditis: 107 cases from the international collaboration on endocarditis merged database. *Am J Med.* 2005;**118**:759–766.

55. Weeks SG, Silva C, Auer RN, Doig CJ, Gill MJ, Power C. Encephalopathy with staphylococcal endocarditis: multiple neuropathological findings. *Can J Neurol Sci.* 2001;**28**:260–264.

56. Masuda J, Yutani C, Waki R, Ogata J, Kuriyama Y, Yamaguchi T. Histopathological analysis of the mechanisms of intracranial hemorrhage complicating infective endocarditis. *Stroke.* 1992; **23**:843–850.

57. Davenport J, Hart RG. Prosthetic valve endocarditis 1976–1987. Antibiotics, anticoagulation, and stroke. *Stroke.* 1990;**21**: 993–999.

58. Barrow DL, Prats AR. Infectious intracranial aneurysms: comparison of groups with and without endocarditis. *Neurosurgery.* 1990;**27**:562–573.

59. Roach MR, Drake CG. Ruptured cerebral aneurysms caused by micro-organisms. *N Engl J Med.* 1965;**273**:240–244.

60. Ahuja GH, Jain N, Vijayaraghavan M, Roy S. Cerebral mycotic aneurysm of fungal origin. *J Neurosurg.* 1978;**49**:107–110.

61. Anavekar NS, Tleyjeh IM, Anavekar NS, et al. Impact of prior antiplatelet therapy on risk of embolism in infective endocarditis. *Clin Infect Dis.* 2007;**44**:1180–1186.

62. Chan KL, Dumesnil JG, Cujec B, et al. A randomized trial of aspirin on the risk of embolic events in patients with infective endocarditis. *J Am Coll Cardiol*. 2003;**42**:775–780.

63. Chapot R, Houdart E, Saint-Maurice JP, et al. Endovascular treatment of cerebral mycotic aneurysms. *Radiology*. 2002; **222**:389–396.

64. Chun JY, Smith W, Halbach VV, Higashida RT, Wilson CB, Lawton MT. Current multimodality management of infectious intracranial aneurysms. *Neurosurgery*. 2001;**48**:1203–1213.

65. Goswami KC, Yadav R, Bahl VK. Predictors of left atrial appendage clot: a transesophageal echocardiographic study of left atrial appendage function in patients with severe mitral stenosis. *Indian Heart J*. 2004;**56**:628–635.

66. Barnett HJM, Jones MW, Boughner DR, Kostuk WJ. Cerebral ischemic events associated with prolapsing mitral valve. *Arch Neurol*. 1976;**33**:777–782.

67. Kostuk WJ, Boughner DR, Barnett HJ, Silver MD. Strokes: a complication of mitral-leaflet prolapse? *Lancet*. 1977;**2**: 313–316.

68. Barnett HJ, Boughner DR, Taylor DW, Cooper PE, Kostuk WJ, Nichol PM. Further evidence relating mitral-valve prolapse to cerebral ischemic events. *N Engl J Med*. 1980;**302**:139–144.

69. Tharakan J, Ahuja GK, Manchanda SC, Khanna A. Mitral valve prolapse and cerebrovascular accidents in the young. *Acta Neurol Scand*. 1982;**66**:295–302.

70. Drory Y, Shahar A. Mitral valve prolapse and thromboembolic brain disease. *Isr J Med Sci*. 1991;**27**:44–48.

71. Avierinos JF, Brown RD, Foley DA, et al. Cerebral ischemic events after diagnosis of mitral valve prolapse: a community-based study of incidence and predictive factors. *Stroke*. 2003;**34**:1339–1344.

72. Carolei A, Marini C, Ferranti E, Frontoni M, Prencipe M, Fieschi C. A prospective study of cerebral ischemia in the young. Analysis of pathogenic determinants. The National Research Council Study Group. *Stroke*. 1993;**24**:362–367.

73. Wolf PA, Sila CA. Cerebral ischemia with mitral valve prolapse. *Am Heart J*. 1987;**113**:1308–1315.

74. Nishimura RA, McGoon MD, Shub C, Miller FA, Jr, Ilstrup DM, Tajik AJ. Echocardiographically documented mitral-valve prolapse. Long-term follow-up of 237 patients. *N Engl J Med*. 1985;**313**:1305–1309.

75. Jones HR Jr, Naggar CZ, Seljan MP, Downing LL. Mitral valve prolapse and cerebral ischemic events. A comparison between a neurology population with stroke and a cardiology population with mitral valve prolapse observed for five years. *Stroke*. 1982;**13**:451–453.

76. Gilon D, Buonanno FS, Joffe MM, et al. Lack of evidence of an association between mitral-valve prolapse and stroke in young patients. *N Engl J Med*. 1999;**341**:8–13.

77. Salem DN, O'Gara PT, Madias C, Pauker SG. Valvular and structural heart disease: American College of Chest Physicians Evidence-Based Clinical Practice Guidelines (8th edition). *Chest*. 2008;**133**:593S–629S.

78. Bonow RO, Carabello BA, Chatterjee K, et al. ACC/AHA 2006 guidelines for the management of patients with valvular heart disease: a report of the American College of Cardiology/American Heart Association Task Force on Practice Guidelines (Writing Committee to Revise the 1998 guidelines for the management of patients with valvular heart disease) developed in collaboration with the Society of Cardiovascular Anesthesiologists endorsed by the Society for Cardiovascular Angiography and Interventions and the Society of Thoracic Surgeons. *J Am Coll Cardiol*. 2006;**48**:e1–e148.

79. Biller J, Challa VR, Toole JF, Howard VJ. Nonbacterial thrombotic endocarditis. *Arch Neurol*. 1982;**39**:95–98.

80. Khorana AA, Francis CW, Culakova E, Fisher RI, Kuderer NM, Lyman GH. Thromboembolism in hospitalized neutropenic cancer patients. *J Clin Oncol*. 2006;**24**:484–490.

81. Iguchi Y, Kimura K, Kobayashi K, Ueno Y, Inoue T. Ischaemic stroke with malignancy may often be caused by paradoxical embolism. *J Neurol Neurosurg Psychiatry*. 2006;**77**:1336–1339.

82. Rogers LR, Cho ES, Kempin S, Posner JB. Cerebral infarction from non-bacterial thrombotic endocarditis. Clinical and pathological study including the effects of anticoagulation. *Am J Med*. 1987;**83**:746–756.

83. Mandell BF. Cardiovascular involvement in systemic lupus erythematosus. *Semin Arthritis Rheum*. 1987;**17**:126–141.

84. Cannegieter SC, Rosendaal FR, Briet E. Thromboembolic and bleeding complications in patients with mechanical heart valve prostheses. *Circulation*. 1994;**89**:635–641.

85. Cannegieter SC, Rosendaal FR, Wintzen AR, van der Meer FJ, Vandenbroucke JP, Briet E. Optimal oral anticoagulant therapy in patients with mechanical heart valves. *N Engl J Med*. 1995;**333**:11–17.

86. Stamou SC, Lefrak EE. Delayed presentation of low molecular weight heparin treatment failure in a patient with mitral valve prosthesis. *J Card Surg*. 2007;**22**:61–62.

87. Lam KY, Dickens P, Chan AC. Tumors of the heart. A 20-year experience with a review of 12,485 consecutive autopsies. *Arch Pathol Lab Med*. 1993;**117**:1027–1031.

88. Konkol RJ, Walsh EP, Power T, Bresnan MJ. Cerebral embolism resulting from an intracardiac tumor in tuberous sclerosis. *Pediatr Neurol*. 1986;**2**:108–110.

89. Kandt RS, Gebarski SS, Goetting MG. Tuberous sclerosis with cardiogenic cerebral embolism: magnetic resonance imaging. *Neurology*. 1985;**35**:1223–1225.

90. Roach ES, Golomb MR, Adams RJ, et al. Management of stroke in infants and children. A scientific statement for healthcare professionals from a special writing group of the Stroke Council, American Heart Association. *Stroke*. 2008;**39**:2644–2691.

91. Savino JS, Weiss SJ. Images in clinical medicine. Right atrial tumor. *N Engl J Med*. 1995;**333**:1608.

92. Lee VH, Connolly HM, Brown RD Jr. Central nervous system manifestations of cardiac myxoma. *Arch Neurol*. 2007;**64**:1115–1120.

93. Knepper LE, Biller J, Adams HP, Bruno A. Neurologic manifestations of atrial myxoma. A 12-year experience and review. *Stroke*. 1988;**19**:1435–1440.

94. Jean WC, Walski-Easton SM, Nussbaum ES. Multiple intracranial aneurysms as delayed complications of an atrial myxoma: case report. *Neurosurgery*. 2001;**49**:200–202.

95. Keeling IM, Oberwalder P, Anelli-Monti M, et al. Cardiac myxomas: 24 years of experience in 49 patients. *Eur J Cardiothorac Surg*. 2002;**22**:971–977.

96. Bhan A, Mehrotra R, Choudhary SK, et al. Surgical experience with intracardiac myxomas: long-term follow-up. *Ann Thorac Surg*. 1998;**66**:810–813.

97. Bakaeen FG, Reardon MJ, Coselli JS, et al. Surgical outcome in 85 patients with primary cardiac tumors. *Am J Surg*. 2003; **186**:641–647.

98. Amarenco P, Cohen A, Tzourio C, et al. Atherosclerotic disease of the aortic arch and the risk of ischemic stroke. *N Engl J Med*. 1994;**331**:1474–1479.

99. Atherosclerotic disease of the aortic arch as a risk factor for recurrent ischemic stroke. The French Study of Aortic Plaques in Stroke Group. *N Engl J Med*. 1996;**334**:1216–1221.

100. Tunick PA, Rosenzweig BP, Katz ES, Freedberg RS, Perez JL, Kronzon I. High risk for vascular events in patients with protruding aortic atheromas: a prospective study. *J Am Coll Cardiol*. 1994;**23**:1085–1090.

101. Cohen A, Tzourio C, Bertrand B, Chauvel C, Bousser MG, Amarenco P. Aortic plaque morphology and vascular events: a follow-up study in patients with ischemic stroke. FAPS Investigators. French Study of Aortic Plaques in Stroke. *Circulation.* 1997;**96**:3838–3841.

102. Tunick PA, Nayar AC, Goodkin GM, et al. Effect of treatment on the incidence of stroke and other emboli in 519 patients with severe thoracic aortic plaque. *Am J Cardiol.* 2002;**90**:1320–1325.

103. Stern A, Tunick PA, Culliford AT, et al. Protruding aortic arch atheromas: risk of stroke during heart surgery with and without aortic arch endarterectomy. *Am Heart J.* 1999;**138**:746–752.

104. Ferrari E, Vidal R, Chevallier T, Baudouy M. Atherosclerosis of the thoracic aorta and aortic debris as a marker of poor prognosis: benefit of oral anticoagulants. *J Am Coll Cardiol.* 1999; **33**:1317–1322.

105. Lima JA, Desai MY, Steen H, Warren WP, Gautam S, Lai S. Statin-induced cholesterol lowering and plaque regression after 6 months of magnetic resonance imaging-monitored therapy. *Circulation.* 2004;**110**:2336–2341.

106. Yonemura A, Momiyama Y, Fayad ZA, et al. Effect of lipid-lowering therapy with atorvastatin on atherosclerotic aortic plaques detected by noninvasive magnetic resonance imaging. *J Am Coll Cardiol.* 2005;**45**:733–742.

107. Pitsavos CE, Aggeli KI, Barbetseas JD, et al. Effects of pravastatin on thoracic aortic atherosclerosis in patients with heterozygous familial hypercholesterolemia. *Am J Cardiol.* 1998;**82**:1484–1488.

108. Corti R, Fuster V, Fayad ZA, et al. Effects of aggressive versus conventional lipid-lowering therapy by simvastatin on human atherosclerotic lesions: a prospective, randomized, double-blind trial with high-resolution magnetic resonance imaging. *J Am Coll Cardiol.* 2005;**46**:106–112.

109. Amarenco P, Bogousslavsky J, Callahan A III, et al. High-dose atorvastatin after stroke or transient ischemic attack. *N Engl J Med.* 2006;**355**:549–559.

110. Roach GW, Kanchuger M, Mangano CM, et al. Adverse cerebral outcomes after coronary bypass surgery. Multicenter Study of Perioperative Ischemia Research Group and the Ischemia Research and Education Foundation Investigators. *N Engl J Med.* 1996;**335**:1857–1863.

111. Stamou SC, Hill PC, Dangas G, et al. Stroke after coronary artery bypass: incidence, predictors, and clinical outcome. *Stroke.* 2001;**32**:1508–1513.

112. Anyanwu AC, Filsoufi F, Salzberg SP, Bronster DJ, Adams DH. Epidemiology of stroke after cardiac surgery in the current era. *J Thorac Cardiovasc Surg.* 2007;**134**:1121–1127.

113. Ascione R, Reeves BC, Chamberlain MH, Ghosh AK, Lim KH, Angelini GD. Predictors of stroke in the modern era of coronary artery bypass grafting: a case control study. *Ann Thorac Surg.* 2002;**74**:474–480.

114. McKhann GM, Goldsborough MA, Borowicz LM Jr, et al. Predictors of stroke risk in coronary artery bypass patients. *Ann Thorac Surg.* 1997;**63**:516–521.

115. Clark RE, Brillman J, Davis DA, Lovell MR, Price TR, Magovern GJ. Microemboli during coronary artery bypass grafting. Genesis and effect on outcome. *J Thorac Cardiovasc Surg.* 1995; **109**:249–257.

116. Mellor A, Soni N. Fat embolism. *Anaesthesia.* 2001;**56**:145–154.

117. Schmid A, Tzur A, Leshko L, Krieger BP. Silicone embolism syndrome: a case report, review of the literature, and comparison with fat embolism syndrome. *Chest.* 2005;**127**:2276–2281.

118. Heckmann JG, Lang CJ, Kindler K, Huk W, Erbguth FJ, Neundorfer B. Neurologic manifestations of cerebral air embolism as a complication of central venous catheterization. *Crit Care Med.* 2000;**28**:1621–1625.

119. Dutka AJ, Kochanek PM, Hallenbeck JM. Influence of granulocytopenia on canine cerebral ischemia induced by air embolism. *Stroke.* 1989;**20**:390–395.

120. Murphy BP, Harford FJ, Cramer FS. Cerebral air embolism resulting from invasive medical procedures. *Ann Surg.* 1985; **201**:242–245.

121. Dickens WN, Sayre GP, Clagett OT, Goldstein NP. Tumor embolism of the basilar artery: case report. *Arch Neurol.* 1961;**5**:655–658.

122. Umemura S, Kishino D, Tabata M, et al. Systemic tumor embolism mimicking gefitinib ('IRESSA')-induced interstitial lung disease in a patient with lung cancer. *Intern Med.* 2005;**44**:979–982.

123. Ho KL. Neoplastic aneurysm and intracranial hemorrhage. *Cancer.* 1982;**50**:2935–2940.

124. Olmsted WW, McGee TP. The pathogenesis of peripheral aneurysms of the central nervous system: a subject review from the AFIP. *Radiology.* 1977;**123**:661–666.

125. van Walraven C, Hart RG, Wells GA, et al. A clinical prediction rule to identify patients with atrial fibrillation and a low risk for stroke while taking aspirin. *Arch Intern Med.* 2003;**163**:936–943.

126. Gage BF, Waterman AD, Shannon W, Boechler M, Rich MW, Radford MJ. Validation of clinical classification schemes for predicting stroke: results from the National Registry of Atrial Fibrillation. *JAMA.* 2001;**285**:2864–2870.

127. Pomerance A. Pathological and clinical study of calcification of the mitral valve ring. *J Clin Pathol.* 1970;**23**:354–361.

128. Bayir H, Morelli PJ, Smith TH, Biancaniello TA. A left atrial myxoma presenting as a cerebrovascular accident. *Pediatr Neurol.* 1999;**21**:569–572.

129. Roach ES, Riela AR. *Pediatric Cerebrovascular Disorders.* 2nd ed. New York: Futura; 1995.

130. Kamenar E, Kozachuk A. Non-cardiac sources of cerebral embolism: fat and air emboli. *Handbook of Clinical Neurology*, part III, volume 55. Amsterdam: Elsevier Science Publishers; 1989: 177–201.

9

Lacunar Strokes and Hypertensive Encephalopathy

Remember, as a working rule, that symptoms of sudden onset, due to an organic cause, indicate a vascular lesion. They indicate the rupture of a vessel or the obstruction of a vessel; the former, as we have seen, causing hemorrhage, the latter softening.

William R. Gowers

Arterial hypertension is a serious public health problem that affects millions of individuals worldwide. Hypertension's effects are particularly insidious because its lack of consistent early signs and symptoms make early diagnosis less likely, an unfortunate occurrence because hypertension is readily treatable. The effects of chronic arterial hypertension on the cardiovascular system can be devastating, all the more so when it occurs in tandem with other cardiovascular risk factors. Chronic arterial hypertension increases the rate of atherosclerosis formation, promotes both ischemic stroke and symptomatic coronary artery disease, and causes intracerebral hemorrhage (see Chapter 16). In this chapter we review the effects of arterial hypertension on the cerebrovascular system and the clinical manifestations of lacunar infarction.

ARTERIAL HYPERTENSION

Arterial hypertension is an enormous worldwide public health problem. As many as 65 million people in the United States and 1 billion worldwide have arterial hypertension.[1-8] Arterial hypertension, defined as systolic blood pressure (SBP) greater than 140 mm Hg or diastolic blood pressure (DBP) greater than 90 mm Hg, is a dominant risk factor of the more than 750,000 new or recurrent strokes that occur each year in the United States. Likewise, arterial hypertension is the most powerful risk factor for all forms of vascular dementia (vascular cognitive impairment).

The importance of lowering blood pressure in reducing cardiovascular death and total mortality as well as renal morbidity and mortality has been demonstrated in numerous clinical trials.[5-12] Overall, blood pressure reduction trials have shown a reduction in stroke by 38%. The JNC7 report emphasizes that patients at risk, including those with diabetes mellitus or a history of stroke, should be treated with medications.[5-6]

Prehypertension is defined as SBP between 120 and 139 mm Hg, or DBP between 80 and 89 mm Hg; optimal blood pressure is defined as SBP less than 120 mm Hg and diastolic blood pressure less than 80 mm Hg. Table 9-1 shows the classification of blood pressure for adults as detailed in the JNC7 report.[5-6] The incidence and prevalence of arterial hypertension increases steadily with age. Arterial hypertension occurs more often in African Americans.[13] Epidemiologic data suggest that elevated SBP is a stronger risk factor than elevated DBP for the development of cardiovascular disease in all but the youngest ages.

Isolated systolic hypertension, defined as SBP greater than 140 and DBP less than 90 mm Hg, is frequently associated with coronary artery disease, thrombotic and hemorrhagic stroke, dementia, peripheral arterial disease, and slowly progressive heart and kidney failure. Overall, isolated systolic hypertension in the elderly increases the risk of cardiovascular disease twofold compared with younger subjects with systolic-diastolic hypertension.[1-3] A reasonable target blood pressure for adults is less than 140/90 mm Hg. However, among individuals with diabetes mellitus, renal insufficiency, or heart failure, the target blood pressure should be less than 130/80 mm Hg.

Pathophysiology

Arterial blood pressure fluctuates in a diurnal rhythm, with the nadir occurring during sleep and the zenith during daytime activities. Superimposed on this circadian cycle are abrupt, short-lived elevations and reductions that result from vasomotor readjustments to stress, such as emotion, dreaming during sleep, exertion (particularly coitus), and changes in posture. With each passing year, blood pressure tends to increase gradually from the normal childhood range to adult levels.

Despite continual changes in systemic blood pressure, the pressure in the arteriolar-capillary network of the brain remains constant. When arterial blood pressure increases, the cerebral arterioles constrict, the degree depending on the pressure elevation. If this is of short duration and the pressure is not too high, there is no apparent harm, but, if pressure is sustained at even moderate elevations for months or years, hyalinization of the muscularis occurs, and the wall of the lumen loses its capacity to

Table 9-1: Classification of Blood Pressure for Adults (Aged 18 or Older, According to JNC 7)[a]

Category	SBP (mm Hg)	DBP (mm Hg)
Normal[b]	< 120 and	< 80
Prehypertension	120–139 and	81–89
Hypertension[c]		
Stage 1	140–159 or	90–99
Stage 2	≥ 160 or	≥ 100

Adapted with permission from Chobanian et al.[6]

[a] Not taking antihypertensive drugs and not acutely ill. When systolic and diastolic pressures fall into different categories, the higher category should be selected to classify the individual's blood pressure status. Isolated systolic hypertension is defined as systolic blood pressure of 140 mm Hg or greater and diastolic blood pressure below 90 mm Hg and staged appropriately.

[b] Normal blood pressure with respect to cardiovascular disease risk is below 120/80 mm Hg. However, unusually low readings should be evaluated for clinical significance.

[c] Based on the average of two or more readings taken at each of two or more visits after an initial screening. JNC VII, Seventh report of the U.S. Joint National Committee for Detection, Evaluation, and Treatment of High Blood Pressure.

adapt to change in arterial pressure. This is a dangerous situation because it means that the cerebral arterioles can no longer dilate or constrict appropriately to compensate for fluctuations in systemic pressure or needs of brain tissues. Reduction in arterial pressure can then lead to inadequate perfusion and brain ischemia, whereas an increase in systemic arterial pressure can result in excessive perfusion pressure in the capillary bed with resultant hyperemia, edema, and, possibly, hemorrhage.

Among normotensive subjects, cerebral blood flow remains the same between mean arterial blood pressures (MABPs) of approximately 60 to 160 mm Hg; this is known as cerebral pressure autoregulation. Patients with chronic hypertension have their autoregulation curves shifted to the right: that is, their breakdown and breakthrough points are higher than those of normotensives. If the systemic MABP is raised above 160 mm Hg, cerebral blood flow (CBF) suddenly increases. Such observations suggest that the first stage of hypertensive encephalopathy results from a sudden increase in blood flow with overdistention of the arteriolar tree, disruption of the blood-brain barrier, and consequent edema and local damage. Damaged tissue requires less blood flow, which may explain why decreased CBF has been observed in the later stages of hypertensive encephalopathy. Cerebral edema may also increase the intracranial pressure and result in diminished CBF. Because the breakthrough point of autoregulation occurs more readily during hypercapnia, optimizing cardiorespiratory function is an important part of treating hypertensive encephalopathy.

Diagnosis of Presymptomatic Hypertension

Arterial hypertension goes undiagnosed in a substantial number of individuals.[1–3] Hypertension accelerates atherogenesis. Blood pressure is a continuous physiologic trait. The disease is not the blood pressure values but rather the cardiovascular

abnormalities that result. Hypertension is typically a silent disease that produces no symptoms until arteries in target organs, such as the heart (clinical, electrocardiographic, or radiologic evidence of coronary artery disease; left ventricular hypertrophy or "strain" by electrocardiography; or left ventricular hypertrophy by echocardiography), kidneys (serum creatinine > 1.5 mg/dl, proteinuria of 1+ or greater, microalbuminuria), retina (hemorrhages or exudates, with or without papilledema); and/or brain (transient ischemic attacks or strokes), become affected.

Hypertension should not be diagnosed on the basis of a single blood pressure measurement. Initially elevated readings must be confirmed on at least two subsequent occasions, with average levels of DBP of 90 mm Hg or greater or SBP of 140 mm Hg or greater sustained after rest. Therefore, blood pressure must be determined at each patient visit.

The SBP is defined as the first appearance of a Korotkoff sound and the DBP by the disappearance of the Korotkoff sound (phase 5). Because blood pressure is variable and can be affected by multiple extraneous factors, it should be measured with an appropriately sized cuff to the arm circumference and in such a manner that the values obtained are representative of the patients' usual level. The following techniques are strongly recommended.[1–3,14] Patients should be seated with the arm bared, supported, and positioned at heart level. They should not have smoked or ingested caffeine within 30 minutes before measurement, which should begin after 5 minutes of quiet rest. Two or more readings should be averaged. If the first two readings differ by more than 5 mm Hg, additional readings should be obtained.

Repeated blood pressure measurements will determine whether initial elevations persist and require close observation or prompt attention, or whether they have returned to normal and need only periodic repeated measurements. Initial blood pressure readings that are markedly elevated or associated with evidence of target organ damage may require immediate drug therapy. The timing of subsequent readings should be based on the baseline level.

As an adjunct to repeated office readings, blood pressure may be measured at the work site or at home by the patient himself or a family member. Twenty-four-hour ambulatory blood pressure devices are available but not recommended for diagnosis and follow-up except for those in whom therapeutic decisions are difficult because of marked lability in blood pressure.

Clinical evaluation of patients with suspected arterial hypertension should be directed to answer the following questions: (a) Does the patient have primary or secondary (possibly reversible) hypertension? (b) Is target-organ involvement present? (c) Are other cardiovascular risk factors other than high blood pressure present?

Each patient requires a complete physical examination. Physical examination should always include blood pressure measurements at least in both arms (preferably both arms and one leg in the initial evaluation), weight and height measurements, funduscopic examination (with pupil dilation if needed), palpation of the thyroid gland, detailed cardiac, lung, abdominal, and cervical auscultation, and extremity examination with palpation of peripheral pulses, especially the femoral arteries.

Management of Presymptomatic Hypertension

Treatment of mild hypertension requires conviction and patience. Physicians are often reluctant to prescribe long-term pharmacologic therapy for asymptomatic patients. Low-salt diets have been shown to effectively decrease blood pressure. Some hypertensive patients benefit from an increase in potassium intake. The hyperinsulinemia and hypoleptinemia associated with obesity may increase sympathetic nervous system activity, and weight loss in patients who are obese will bring about a reduction in blood pressure. The value of regular exercise and lifestyle changes needs to be emphasized.[1–3]

The benefits of blood-pressure-lowering therapy for the prevention of fatal and nonfatal stroke in middle-aged subjects has been well established. Blood pressure targets should be individualized according to age, ethnicity, and co-morbidities, although treatment benefit seems to occur with an as little as 10 mm Hg systolic pressure reduction and 5 mm Hg diastolic pressure reduction. The optimal antihypertensive regimen has not been determined, but available evidence from large randomized trials appears to support the use of a diuretic with or without an angiotensin-converting enzyme (ACE) inhibitor, a recommendation that is now included in the guidelines for the prevention of secondary stroke. Potential contraindications to specific drugs should be assessed.

In the Heart Outcomes Prevention Evaluation (HOPE) Study, ramipril was associated with a 22% relative risk reduction (RRR) in the composite endpoint of stroke, myocardial infarction (MI), and vascular death, compared with placebo in high-risk individuals with a history of stroke or transient ischemic attack (TIA; relative risk: 0/78; 95% CI: 0.70–0.86; $p < 0.001$).[15]

The Perindopril Protection against Recurrent Stroke Study evaluated the effects of the ACE inhibitor perindopril alone or with the diuretic indapamide (prescribed at the discretion of the treating physician) versus placebo in over 6,100 patients with previous stroke or TIA within the last 5 years. Treatment with perindopril, with or without indapamide, resulted in an RRR of 28% (95% CI: 17–38%) for recurrent stroke and 26% (95% CI: 16–34%) for major vascular events (vascular death or nonfatal MI or stroke) compared with placebo.[16]

Evidence from the Losartan Intervention for Endpoint Reduction in Hypertension (LIFE) Study, a double-blind, prospective parallel group study designed to compare the effects of losartan with those of atenolol on the reduction of cardiovascular morbidity and mortality among hypertensive patients, suggests that losartan may reduce the risk of recurrent stroke. In this study of 9,193 hypertensive patients, use of the angiotensin receptor blocker losartan was associated with a significant RRR of 25% ($p = 0.001$) in fatal or nonfatal stroke compared with the beta-blocker atenolol after 4 or more years.[17]

Rigorous blood pressure control is particularly recommended for diabetic patients. Primary prevention guidelines emphasize blood pressure targets of ≤ 130/80 mm Hg in patients with type 1 or 2 diabetes. More than one class of antihypertensive agents will be required in many patients to achieve optimal blood pressure control. In the United Kingdom Prospective Diabetes Study, a 44% reduction (95% CI: 11% to 65%; $p = 0.013$) in risk of stroke was observed in diabetic patients with blood pressure that was well controlled with an intensive treatment regimen.[18]

The American Diabetes Association recommends that all patients with diabetes who have concomitant hypertension should be treated with a regimen that includes an ACE inhibitor or an angiotensin receptor blocker.[19]

The results of the Anglo-Scandinavian Cardiac Outcomes Trial (ASCOT) suggest that beta blockers are less effective than alternate therapies in preventing strokes, especially in elderly patients.[12]

The tangible results of hypertension control have been repeatedly demonstrated. The benefits of antihypertensive therapy include a 12% reduction in all-cause mortality, a 20% reduction in coronary artery disease, and a 36% reduction in stroke.[1–3] Despite these numbers, underdiagnosis and suboptimal treatment of arterial hypertension remain common. The "rule of halves" still applies: half of the patients with arterial hypertension have not been diagnosed, half of those who have been diagnosed are not on treatment, and half of those receiving treatment lack adequate control. Treatment of mild hypertension requires conviction and patience.

LACUNAR INFARCTION

Small vessel or penetrating artery disease (lacunes) typically occurs in patients with long-standing arterial hypertension. Available evidence suggests that structural changes of the cerebral vasculature due to arterial hypertension are characterized by fibrinoid angiopathy, lipohyalinosis, and microaneurysm formation. Accelerated hypertensive arteriolar damage of the small-diameter penetrating arteries is operative in a large number of patients with lacunar infarction. Micro-atheroma of the ostium of a penetrating artery, embolism, or changes in hemorrheology are pathophysiologically operative in the remainder of cases.[12,19–35]

Lacunes are small ischemic infarcts in the deep regions of the brain or brainstem resulting from occlusion of a single perforating vessel. The most frequent sites of lacunes are the putamen, basis pontis, thalamus, posterior limb of the internal capsule, and caudate nucleus, in that order. Lacunes may also occur in the anterior limb of the internal capsule, subcortical cerebral white matter, cerebellar white matter, and corpus callosum. Most lacunes are asymptomatic, and although they generally carry a relatively favorable prognosis, multiple lacunes may lead to pseudobulbar palsy or dementing states. In general, most patients with lacunar infarcts have a good functional recovery with a lower recurrence rate and higher survival rate than other ischemic stroke subtypes. Shortly before onset of a lacunar stroke, TIAs may occur. Associated headaches are infrequent. However, the mere occurrence of a "lacunar" syndrome in a patient with arterial hypertension or diabetes mellitus is not sufficient for a diagnosis of a lacunar infarct, and other causes of ischemic stroke must be excluded (Table 9-2).[19–35]

Patients may have but one lacune, but the majority have two or three; in other patients there are lacunes concomitant with microhemorrhages and even large infarctions. The differentiation between a lacune and what might be called a small infarction is arbitrary. It lies in whether penetrating or surface conducting arteries are involved, which determines the size and location of the resultant infarction.

The size of a lacune depends on the location of the occlusion along the length of the penetrator: those distal are as small as 3 mm in diameter; those at the origin of the penetrating artery can be as large as 15 mm. After phagocytosis of the infarcted tissues, the residual cavity is a lacune (hole). A multiplicity is called the lacunar state. They are the most common cerebrovascular lesions in elderly hypertensive patients.

Among the Japanese the frequency of lacunar infarcts far exceeds infarctions in the middle cerebral artery (MCA)

Table 9-2: Small Vessel Disease, Lacunes, and Subcortical Infarcts

Not all subcortical ischemic lesions are lacunar infarctions

Not all subcortical "lesions" are lacunes (i.e., enlarged perivascular spaces, etc.)

Not all "small vessel disease" results in lacunes

Not all lacunar syndromes are caused by lacunar infarctions

Not all lacunar infarctions are associated with arterial hypertension

Not all anterior choroidal artery infarcts are caused by small vessel disease

Not all striato-capsular infarctions are lacunes

Not all pure motor hemiparesis and sensorimotor stroke predict lacunar infarcts

Not all progression of paresis is associated with poor prognosis

Not all lacunes carry a good prognosis (dementia, pseudobulbar state, greater recurrence rate if associated with leukoaraiosis)

---

distribution. Why does this apparent racial predisposition exist, and why does atherosclerotic plaque repeatedly occur in certain positions along the course of these specific arteries? Some suggested reasons are hypertension, flow dynamics, or tethering of the artery that anchors certain segments. In youth, the artery changes caliber as much as 20% during the cardiac cycle, reducing to 8% during adult life and usually becoming a rigid pipe during senescence. There is no evidence to suggest that hypertension per se results in MCA stenosis, but it stands to reason that in such patients hypertension will result in better perfusion of the distal vascular bed. The correlative is that reduction to normotension may result in cerebrovascular insufficiency, a point that in the future will undoubtedly be addressed using transcranial Doppler interrogation of the MCA before and after treatment of hypertension.[36–37]

Clinical Features of Lacunes

Lacunar infarcts account for up to 20% of strokes. Ten to 15% of patients have preceding TIAs before developing lacunar infarction. Not all lacunes result in clinically recognized symptoms. In some instances they are discovered as incidental findings by cranial computed tomography (CT) or magnetic resonance imaging (MRI), or at autopsy. Such patients may have a trivial clinical impairment, such as transient weakness or sensory change in a limb; sometimes the deficit evolves over hours and occasionally days.

At least 20 lacunar syndromes have been recognized. The best recognized clinical syndromes include pure motor stroke, pure sensory stroke, dysarthria–clumsy hand syndrome, ataxic hemiparesis syndrome, and sensorimotor stroke.[20–29]

Pure Motor Stroke

Pure motor signs are the most common expression of lacunar stroke (about 60% of cases). Hemiparesis or hemiplegia results from infarction in the anterior limb of the internal capsule, corona radiata, or basis pontis. In either case the lesion is opposite the paralysis and is not accompanied by aphasia,

apraxia, agnosia, sensory, or visual field defects. Patients may have a series of preceding TIAs (capsular warning signs). Clinical findings usually do not distinguish between capsular of pontine pure motor hemiparesis, but the combination of dysarthria and a history of previous transient gait abnormality or vertigo would favor a pontine location. Ischemic cortical lesions may also cause pure motor hemiparesis. A pure motor monoparesis is seldom caused by a lacunar infarct.[21,24,32,34,38]

Pure Sensory Stroke

Accounting for approximately 10% to 20% of lacunar infarction cases, pure sensory stroke is manifested by isolated hemisensory loss or unilateral paresthesias involving the face, arm, and leg. Paresthesias are typically described as numbness, sleeping sensations, tingling, stiffness, or a dead feeling and sometimes gnawing and continuous pain, at times without signs to corroborate its organicity. The affected side may feel distorted in size or compressed. This condition is usually the result of a lacune in the postero-ventral nucleus of the thalamus. Small ischemic strokes in the internal capsule/corona radiata, subthalamus, midbrain, or the parietal cortex may also cause a pure sensory stroke, as may pontine lacunes localized to the medial lemniscus or paramedian dorsal pons.[30,32–35,39–42]

Dysarthria–Clumsy Hand Syndrome

The dysarthria–clumsy hand syndrome occurs in about 10% of lacunar infarctions; it manifests as a sudden onset of moderate to severe dysarthria, central facial weakness, deviation of the tongue on protrusion, slight dysphagia, clumsiness and slowness in fine manipulations of the affected hand, some weakness and ataxia on the finger-to-nose test, and an extensor plantar response. The patient experiences mild imbalance on walking, and some corticospinal tract signs are present. The lesion responsible is often in the contralateral pons between its upper third and lower two-thirds. Lacunar infarcts in the internal capsule and cerebral peduncle may also cause this syndrome. Lacunar infarctions or small hemorrhages involving the putamen and genu of the internal capsule may also cause the dysarthria–clumsy hand syndrome, often associated with micrographia.[21,25,32,34,35,43]

Ataxic Hemiparesis

In ataxic hemiparesis syndrome, the ataxia and weakness involve the leg more than the arm. The responsible lesion often lies where the corona radiata funnels into the internal capsule or in the ventral pons. In spite of its name, the ataxia is probably not due to involvement of the cerebellum but rather to damage to the corticopontine pathways. This syndrome has also been described with contralateral thalamocapsular lesions, lesions of the contralateral red nucleus, lesions of the corona radiata, lentiform nucleus, with superior cerebellar artery territory infarcts, and with superficial anterior cerebral artery (ACA) territory infarcts in the paracentral area.[21,23,29,32,34,35,44]

Sensorimotor Stroke

Usually the lenticulostriate branches of the middle cerebral artery supply the internal capsule, whereas most of the thalamus is supplied by the perforating branches from the posterior cerebral artery. Presumably in some individuals, the boundary between these two supply areas are variable because, in rare cases, a single small end-arterial infarct can involve both the ventral thalamus and the internal capsule and cause a sensorimotor hemisyndrome.[32,34,35]

Diagnostic Evaluation

Cranial computed tomography and magnetic resonance imaging are the essential neuroimaging tests. However, despite their phenomenal capabilities, these studies may not demonstrate lacunar lesions if images are made too early following onset, if the lesion is less than 3 mm in size and lies between tomographic slices, or if artifact from bone or other structures obscures the area of interest. CT or MRI may show characteristic small cavities if the cuts are made in the appropriate locations using a high-resolution scanner, but, in most cases they demonstrate only the atrophic changes seen with brain aging, even though lacunes are present. Correlations using CT or MRI as the standard show that most lacunes are asymptomatic and one-third occur in normotensive patients.[45–47] Gradient-echo MRI studies of cerebral microbleeds, considered evidence of advanced microangiopathy, suggest that patients with lacunar infarcts and associated white matter changes (leukoaraiosis) may be more prone to bleeding.[48–50] Additional evidence suggests that such microbleeds are more frequently observed in patients with recurrent stroke of either hemorrhagic or ischemic infarcts.[51]

Catheter cerebral angiography is typically normal or shows only the patient's coexisting atherosclerosis, and similarly the cerebrospinal fluid is normal. When lacunar syndrome is diagnosed by clinical findings and neuroimaging studies, catheter angiography is not needed for confirmation of the diagnosis.[34–35]

Management of Lacunar Infarction

Patients with lacunar infarcts demonstrate the best survival and functional recovery of any stroke subtype, regardless of the treatment strategy employed.[52–53] Although treatment of hypertension plays a central role in management, it should be remembered that lacunar infarctions are not caused solely by a combination of hypertension and small vessel disease. Artery-to-artery embolism, cardiogenic embolism, and hematologic disorders may be the etiology in some cases. Similar therapeutic approaches should be considered for patients with lacunar infarction as for patients with cerebral infarction in general (see Chapter 25). The American Heart Association/American Stroke Association (AHA/ASA) and the American College of Chest Physicians have outlined evidence-based recommendations for antiplatelet therapy in patients with ischemic stroke or TIA (see Chapters 6 and 25).[54–55] Anticoagulants are of no proven value in this setting and may be potentially harmful given the large number of lacunar stroke patients who are hypertensive.

Lacunar infarction may be associated with nonreversible hypertensive vascular changes, carrying a risk of cerebral ischemia when the pressure is lowered too aggressively. After the neurologic deficit has stabilized, the goal is to prevent further morbidity and mortality associated with high blood pressure by targeting blood pressure values of 140/90 mm Hg. The decision to initiate treatment in individual patients requires physicians to consider at least two factors: the severity of blood pressure elevation and the presence of other complications. Recent evidence suggests that nonpharmacologic approaches – particularly weight reduction, salt restriction, and moderation of alcohol consumption – may lower elevated pressure and also improve the efficacy of pharmacologic agents. Therefore, nonpharmacologic approaches are used both as definitive intervention and as an adjunct to pharmacologic therapy and should be an integral part of antihypertensive therapy. Because of the clear relationship between obesity and blood pressure, all obese hypertensive adults should begin a weight reduction program.

Excess alcohol intake may lead to elevated blood pressure, poor adherence to antihypertensive therapy, and, occasionally, refractory hypertension. Therefore, for controlling hypertension, those who drink should consume no more than 1 ounce of ethanol daily.

Course and Prognosis of Lacunae

Partial recovery is the rule, and maintenance of blood pressure near normotensive levels is the goal of management. Unfortunately many patients have concomitant atherosclerosis, which may become symptomatic if hypertension is corrected too far or too abruptly. The pseudobulbar palsy sometimes seen in association with the lacunar state is described in Chapter 3.

In the Oxfordshire series, the annual incidence of lacunar infarction was 0.33/1000 without excess risk for men. Case fatality rate was 9.8% at one year, and the rate of recurrence was 12% in the first year. Of the survivors, two-thirds are able to live independently.[52,53,56–59]

HYPERTENSIVE ENCEPHALOPATHY

Of the many millions of Americans with arterial hypertension, fewer than 1% develop a hypertensive emergency. Encephalopathy may be secondary to severe essential hypertension or to uncontrolled hypertension resulting from primary hyperaldosteronism, glomerulonephritis, pheochromocytoma, Cushing syndrome, eclampsia, or autonomic dysreflexia in patients with spinal cord injuries above T6. Of these, acute nephritis and toxemia of pregnancy are the most frequent offenders. Some features of hypertensive encephalopathy have been noted in patients receiving monoamine oxidase (MAO) inhibitors as antidepressants. In these patients the hypertensive crises are sometimes precipitated by the ingestion of foods rich in tyramine. Amphetamines and cocaine use as well as abrupt clonidine withdrawal can also cause findings suggestive of hypertensive encephalopathy.[1–3,60–62]

Hypertensive crises are differentiated into hypertensive urgencies and hypertensive emergencies, the latter defined by whether there is evidence of target organ damage. The presence of a hypertensive emergency (such as hypertensive encephalopathy) implies the need for rapid blood pressure reduction by the use of intravenous antihypertensive medications, with a target reduction of the mean arterial blood pressure by 20% to 25% within a few hours.

Hypertensive encephalopathy describes a group of life-threatening acute and usually transient neurologic phenomena in patients with extremely elevated arterial blood pressure. Oppenheimer and Fishberg found the brains of patients who died with the syndrome to be pale and swollen.[63] Because no histopathologic studies were made, they attributed the abnormality to intense arterial spasm with resultant cerebral edema and coined the term *hypertensive encephalopathy*. The term quickly became a catch-all for a variety of intracranial catastrophes in patients with persistent arterial hypertension, making it difficult to define a clear-cut syndrome that excludes the possibility of multifocal cerebral hemorrhages and microinfarctions. If the diagnosis is restricted to reversible cerebral disorders associated with a marked or sudden rise in blood pressure in the absence of any evidence of uremia, cerebral infarction, or cerebral hemorrhage, it is found that hypertensive encephalopathy occurs very infrequently, and, when it does, it may be suspected by characteristic MR findings.

Etiology and Pathogenesis

Arteriolar spasm in response to extreme elevation of the blood pressure leads to breakdown of the blood-brain barrier, cerebral edema and reduced blood flow. It is suspected that the key factors are the mean arterial blood pressure (diastolic pressure plus one-third of the pulse pressure) and the rate of increase in pressure. Sustained arterial hypertension can be tolerated, but rapid elevation of the mean pressure to 150 mm Hg or above may result in an elevation of the cerebral perfusion pressure (breakthrough hyperperfusion) beyond the limits of the autoregulatory response. The diffuse vasospasm leads to reduced flow into the microcirculation and causes increased capillary permeability and cerebral edema. The end result is transudation of fluid into the extracellular space (cerebral edema), rupture of capillaries (petechial hemorrhages), and, sometimes, tissue necrosis (ischemic microinfarction). Even though the process is diffuse, the sequence of events listed above is multifocal, and a constellation of focal neurologic deficits may develop. On MRI there is a predominance of lesions in the parieto-occipital white matter, primarily a result of vasogenic rather than cytotoxic edema.[64–67]

Pathologic Findings

Neuropathologic changes consist of severe vascular alterations with fibrinoid necrosis of the arterioles and thrombosis within both arterioles and the capillary bed. The results include microinfarction, petechial hemorrhages, and edema. The pathology in patients who succumb to acute hypertensive encephalopathy depends on the stage of evolution of the disorder and the phase of management at the time of death. In the acute phase the brain is usually swollen and pale, with flattening of the gyri and obliteration of the sulci. Signs of increased intracranial pressure (incisural and transforaminal herniation) are apparent. Petechiae may be noted over the surface and on cut section minute slit hemorrhages and lacunae may be visible. Large infarcts and hemorrhages are not part of the syndrome of hypertensive encephalopathy but may complicate it. In addition to neuronal swelling and degeneration secondary to ischemia, necrotizing arteriolitis and microinfarcts with glial scars often occur.

Signs and Symptoms

The constellation of symptoms and signs that signal the onset of hypertensive encephalopathy are (a) altered state of consciousness, (b) severe headache, (c) nausea and vomiting, (d) visual disturbances, (e) focal or generalized seizures, and (f) focal neurologic deficits, in the setting of severe systemic hypertension that is relatively acute in onset. The initial symptom of encephalopathy is frequently the subacute onset of generalized or suboccipital headache, which increases gradually in intensity. The pain is usually aggravated by coughing and straining, commonly exaggerated in the early morning hours and accompanied by vomiting. Transient attacks of blindness, paresis, and generalized or focal convulsions are common. After a variable interval, somnolence, disorientation, confusion, delirium, stupor, and coma occur, culminating in the triad of headaches, convulsions, and altered consciousness.

The severity of hypertension varies, but in general the diastolic pressure is usually above 120 mm Hg and may be as high as 160 mm Hg; the mean arterial pressure is often 150 to 200 mm Hg. In women with toxemia of pregnancy and children with acute glomerulonephritis, however, encephalopathy may occur when arterial pressure is no higher than 180 mm Hg systolic and 110 mm Hg diastolic. Furthermore, patients with other abnormalities that can result in diffuse cerebral dysfunction (e.g., uremia) have a lower threshold for hypertensive encephalopathy. Patients with long-standing hypertension show evidence of left ventricular enlargement and often have a diastolic gallop rhythm that suggests incipient cardiac decompensation.

In the early stages the patient is commonly confused and often hyperirritable, with focal twitching and myoclonic movements of the extremities. Mental obtundation with lethargy and impaired memory may be an initial manifestation. Hemiparesis, aphasia, or some other evidence of focal neurologic dysfunction is often present. Unilateral blindness and hemianopia occasionally occur. Funduscopic examination usually shows grades III to IV hypertensive retinopathy. There have been cases in which the fundus showed only severe retinal arteriolar spasm without hemorrhages, exudates, or papilledema.[68]

Differential Diagnosis

The differential diagnosis includes (a) acute anxiety with extreme but temporary elevations of blood pressure, (b) the use of combinations of MAO inhibitor antidepressants with tyramine-rich foods, and (c) primary intracranial pathology, which results in hypertension. Amphetamines and other drugs have been associated with acute hypertension and arteritis. Elevated systolic and diastolic pressure and grades III (narrowing, nicking, and retinal hemorrhages or exudates) to IV (papilledema) hypertensive retinopathy, especially when accompanied by severe headache, vomiting, drowsiness, and focal or generalized seizures, suggest the possibility of hypertensive encephalopathy. Although the absence of signs of meningeal irritation helps exclude subarachnoid hemorrhage, a cerebral infarct or encapsulated cerebral hemorrhage must still be considered, and a CT or MRI scan should be done.[1–3,60–62] At times systemic lupus erythematosus (SLE) can mimic hypertensive encephalopathy by causing cerebral angiitis.[69]

Laboratory Findings

In an emergency situation when a patient's condition is rapidly deteriorating, reduction of blood pressure should precede time-consuming laboratory tests. Emergency CT or MRI may be normal in early stages but show brain edema with small ventricles and all structures in their normal position in more advanced cases. MRI shows generally symmetric multifocal areas of increased signal density in both gray and white matter. Resolution of the clinical features of encephalopathy is accompanied by return of the MRI image to normal. If imaging is normal, one should proceed with antihypertensive therapy. A lumbar puncture need not be performed as a routine test.[70]

Course of Hypertensive Encephalopathy

Recurring, self-limited episodes of confusion, lethargy, and seizures are sometimes seen in patients with uncontrolled severe hypertension. Unless hemorrhage or extensive brain swelling occurs, the prognosis depends on the extent to which the blood pressure can be controlled and on the severity of the concomitant cardiac and renal disease.

Management of Hypertensive Encephalopathy

Adequate reduction in blood pressure results in a sometimes dramatic recovery with disappearance of headache, vomiting, somnolence, and neurologic deficits. If prompt recovery does not occur, the physician must conclude that either his diagnosis is in error or there is an associated complicating process, such as cerebral hemorrhage, uremia, or drug intoxication.

Many different agents (e.g., nitroprusside, nicardipine, labetalol, esmolol, hydralazine, or enalapril) are available for the treatment of hypertensive encephalopathy.[70,71] In general, intravenous antihypertensive therapy, with readily titratable agents, should aim at lowering the mean arterial blood pressure by 20% to 25% over the initial 2 to 4 hours. Patients with hypertensive encephalopathy should be treated in an intensive care unit. The increased intracranial pressure is reduced when the blood pressure is lowered and usually does not require specific treatment. Repeated lumbar punctures to reduce cerebrospinal fluid pressure may precipitate herniation of the brain and hence should not be done. Seizures should be controlled by the usual antiepileptic drugs. Cardiac decompensation, when present, should be managed by the usual methods. Once the crisis has been controlled, the underlying cause of the patient's hypertension should be sought. If a remediable cause is not found, well-controlled long-term management with antihypertensive medications is necessary.

REFERENCES

1. Lip GYH, Hall JE. *Comprehensive Hypertension*. Philadelphia: Mosby Elsevier; 2007.
2. Willerson JT, Cohn JN, Hein J, Wellens J, Holmes DR Jr. *Cardiovascular Medicine*. 3rd ed. New York: Springer; 2007.
3. Kaplan NM. *Kaplan's Clinical Hypertension*. 9th ed. Philadelphia: Lippincott Williams & Wilkins; 2006.
4. Fields LE, Burt VL, Culter JA, et al. The burden of adult hypertension in the United States 199–2000. A rising tide. *Hypertension*. 2004;**44**:498–504.
5. Chobanian AV, Bakris GL, Black HR, et al. National High Blood Pressure Education Program Coordinating Committee: Seventh report of the Joint National Committee on Prevention, Detection, Evaluation, and Treatment of High Blood Pressure: JNC 7. Complete Version. *Hypertension*. 2003;**42**:1206–1252.
6. Chobanian AV, Bakris GL, Black HR, et al. The Sevent Report of the Joint National Ccommittee on Prevention, Detection, Evaluation, and Treatment of High Blood Pressure. The JNC 7 Report. *JAMA*. 2003;**289**:2560–2572.
7. Guidelines Committee: 2003 European Society of Hypertension – European Society of Cardiology guidelines for the management of arterial hypertension. *J Hypertens*. 2003;**21**:1011–1015.
8. Whitworth JA. World Health Organization (WHO) International Society of Hypertension (ISH) statement on management of hypertension. *J Hypertens*. 2003;**21**:1983–1992.
9. ALLHAT Officers and Coordinators for the ALLHAT Collaborative Research Group: Major outcomes in high-risk hypertensive patients randomized to angiotensin converting enzyme inhibitor or calcium channel blocker vs. diuretic: the Antihypertensive and Lipid-Lowering Treatment to Prevent Heart Attack Trial (ALLHAT). *JAMA*. 2002;**288**:2981–2997.
10. Blood Pressure Lowering Treatment Trialists; Collaboration: effects of different blood-pressure lowering regimens on major cardiovascular events. Results of prospectively-designed overviews of randomized trials. *Lancet*. 2003;**362**:1527–1535.
11. Williams B, Poulter NR, Brown MJ, et al. Gyidelines for management of hypertension: report of the Fourth Working Party of the British Hypertension Society – BHS IV: British Hypertension Society Guidelines. *J Hum Hypertens*. 2004;**18**:139–184.
12. Dahlof B. Sever PS, Poulter NR, et al. The ASCOT Investigators. Prevention of cardiovascular events with an antihypertensive regimen of amlodipine adding perindopril as required versus atenolol adding bendroflumethiazide as required, in the Angio-Scandinavian Cardiac Outcome Trial-Blood Pressure Lowering Arm (ASCOT-BPLA): a multicentre randomized controlled trial. *Lancet*. 2005;**366**:895–906.
13. Ong GL, Cheung BMY, Man YB, et al. Prevalence, awareness treatment and control of hypertension among United States adults 1999–2004. *Hypertension*. 2007;**49**:69–75.
14. Pickering TG, Hall JE, Appel LJ, et al. Recommendations for blood pressure measurement in humans and experimental animals. Part I: blood pressure measurement in humans. *Hypertension*. 2005; **45**:142–161.
15. Yusuf S, Sleight P, Pogue J, et al. Heart Outcomes Prevention Evaluation Study Investigators. Effects of an angiotensin-converting-enzyme inhibitor, ramipril on cardio vascular events in high-risk patients. *N Engl J Med*. 2000;**342**:145–153.
16. Progress Collaborative Group. Randomized trial of a perindopril-based blood pressure lowering regimen among 6105 individuals with previous stroke or transient ischemic attack. *Lancet*. 2001;**358**:1033–1041.
17. Dahlof R, Devereux R, Kjeldsen S, et al. Cardiovascular morbidity and mortality in the Losartan Intervention for Endpoint Reduction in Hypertension study (LIFE): a randomized trial against atenolol. *Lancet*. 2002;**359**:995–1003.
18. UK Prospective Diabetes Study Group. Efficacy of atenolol and captopril in reducing risk of both macrovascular and microvascular complications in type 2 diabetes. (UKPDS 39). *BMJ*. 1998;**317**:713–720.
19. Implications of the United Kingdom Prospective Diabetes Study American Diabetes Association. Position statement. *Diabetes Care*. 2003;**26**:528–532.
20. Marie P. Des foyers lacumaires de disintegration et de differentes autres états cavitaires dev cerveau. *Rev Med (Paris)*. 1901;**21**:281–298.
21. Fisher CM. Lacunar: small, deep cerebral infarcts. *Neurology*. 1965;**15**:774–784.
22. Fisher CM. Pure sensory stroke involving face, arm, and leg. *Neurology*.1965;**15**:76–80.
23. Fisher CM, Cole H. Homolateral ataxia and crural paresis: a vascular syndrome. *J Neurol Neurosurg Psychiatry*. 1965;**28**:48–55.
24. Fisher CM, Curry HB. Pure motor hemiplegia of vascular origin. *Arch Neurol*. 1965;**13**:30–44.
25. Fisher CM. A lacunar stroke. The dysarthria-clumsy hand syndrome. *Neurology*. 1967;**17**:614–617.
26. Fisher CM. The arterial lesions underlying lacunes. *Acta Neuropathol (Berl)*. 1968;**12**:1–15.
27. Fisher CM, Caplan LR. Basilar branch occlusion. A cause of pontine infarction. *Neurology*. 1971;**21**:900–905.
28. Fisher CM. Bilateral occlusion of basilar artery branches. *J Neurol Neurosurg Psychiatry*. 1977;**40**:1182–1189.
29. Fisher CM. Ataxic hemiparesis. A pathologic study. *Arch Neurol*. 1978;**35**:126–128.
30. Fisher CM. Thalamic pure sensory stroke. A pathologic study. *Neurology*. 1978;**28**:1141–1144.
31. Fisher CM. Capsular infarcts: the underlying vascular lesions. *Arch Neurol*. 1979;**36**:65–73.

32. Fisher CN. Lacunar strokes and infarcts: a review. *Neurology.* 1982;**32**:871–876.

33. Fisher CM. Pure sensory stroke and allied conditions. *Stroke.* 1982;**13**:434–437.

34. Mohr JP. Lacunes. *Stroke.* 1982;**13**:3–11.

35. Kappelle LJ, vanGijin J. Lacunar infarcts. *Clin Neurol Neurosurg.*1986;**88**:3–17.

36. Donnan GA, Norrving B. Lacunes and lacunar syndrome. In: *Handbok of Clinical Neurology.* Vol. 93 (3rd series). *Stroke.* Part II. Fisher M, ed. Edinburgh: Elsevier. 2009;**27**:559–575.

37. Yamaguchi T, Nishimaru K, Minematsu K. Benefits and hazards of antiplatelet therapy in ischemic cerebrovascular diseases. *J Jpn Coll Angiol.* 1994;**39**:279–285.

38. Nighoghossian N, Ryvlin P, Trouillas P, et al. Pontine versus capsular pure motor hemiparesis. *Neurology.* 1993;**43**:2197–2201.

39. Kim JS. Pure sensory stroke: clinical-radiological correlates of 21 cases. *Stroke.* 1992;**23**:983–987.

40. Kim JS. Restricted nonsacral sensory syndrome. *Stroke.* 1996;**27**:988–990.

41. Kim JS. Sensory symptoms restricted to proximal body parts in small cortical infarction. *Neurology.* 1999;**53**:889–890.

42. Shintani S. Clinical-radiologic correlations in pure sensory stroke. *Neurology.* 1998;**51**:297–302.

43. Urban PP, Hopf HC, Zorowka PG, et al. Dysarthria and lacunar stroke: pathophysiologic aspects. *Neurology.* 1996;**47**:1135–1141.

44. Sakai T, Murakami S, Ito K. Ataxic hemiparesis with trigeminal weakness. *Neurology.* 1981;**31**:635–636.

45. Donnan GA, Gress BM, Bladin PF. A prospective study of lacunar infarctions using computerized tomography. *Neurology.* 1982;**32**:49–56.

46. Ay H, Oliveira-Filho J, Buonanno FS, et al. Diffusion-weighted imaging identifies an onset of lacunar infarction associated with embolic source. *Stroke.* 1999;**30**:2644–2650.

47. Doefe CA, Kerskens CM, Romero BL, et al. Assessment of diffusion and perfusion deficits in patients with small subcortical ischemia. *AJNR Am J Neuroradiol.* 2003;**24**:1355–1363.

48. Fan YH, Mok VC, Lam WW, et al. Cerebral microbleeds and white matter changes in patients hospitalized with lacunar infarcts. *J Neurol.* 2004;**251**:537–541.

49. Fan YH, Zanf L, Lam WW, et al. Cerebral microbleeds as a risk factor for subsequent intracerebral hemorrhages among patients with acute ischemic stroke. *Stroke.* 2003;**34**:2459–2462.

50. Kato H, Izumiyama M, Izumiyama K, et al. Silent cerebral microbleeds on T2-weighted MRI: correlation with stroke subtype, stroke recurrence, and leukoaraiosis. *Stroke.* 2002;**33**:1536–1540.

51. Naka H, Nomura E, Wakabayashi S, et al. Frequency of asymptomatic microbleeds on T2-weighted MR images of patients with recurrent stroke: association with consideration of stroke subtypes and leukoaraiosis. *AJNR Am J Neuroradiol.* 2004;**25**:714–715.

52. Petty GN, Porown RD Jr, Whisuant JP, et al. Ischemic stroke subtypes: a population-based study of functional outcome, survival, and recurrence. *Stroke.* 2000;**31**:1062–1068.

53. deJong G, van Raak L, Kessels F, Lodder J. Stroke subtype and mortality. A follow-up study in 998 patients with a first cerebral infarct. *J Clin Epidemiol.* 2003;**56**:262–268.

54. Adams RJ, Alber G, Alberts MJ, et al. Update to the AHA/ASA recommendations for the prevention of stroke in patients with stroke and transient ischemic attack. *Stroke.* 2008;**39**:1647–1652.

55. Albers GW, Amarenco P, Easton JD, et al. Antithrombotic and thrombolytic therapy for ischemic stroke: American College of Chest Physicians Evidence-Based Clinical Practice Guidelines (8th ed). *Chest.* 2008;**133**:630S–669S.

56. Bamford J, Sandercock P, Jones L, et al. The natural history of lacunar infarction: the Oxfordshire Community Stroke Project. *Stroke.* 1987;**18**:545–551.

57. Gandolfo C, Moretti C, Dall-Agata D, et al. Long term prognosis of patients with lacunar syndromes. *Vascular Diseases of CNS.* London: Churchill; 1976.

58. Gandolfo C, Moretti C, Dall-Agaia D, et al. Long-term prognosis of patients with lacunar syndromes. *Acta Neurol Scand.* 1986;**74**:224–229.

59. Loeb C, Gandolfo C, Croce R, Conti M. Dementia associated with lacunar infarction. *Stroke.* 1992;**23**:1225–1229.

60. Dinsdale HB. Hypertensive encephalopathy. *Stroke.* 1982;**13**:717–719.

61. Phillips S, Whisnant J. Hypertension and the brain. The National High Blood Pressure Education Program. *Arch Int Med.* 1992;**152**(5):938–645.

62. Chow W-H, Messing RD. Hypertensive encephalopathy and the blood-brain barrier: is 8 PKC a gatekeeper? *J Clin Invest.* 2007;**118**(1):17–20.

63. Oppenheimer BS, Fishberg AM. Hypertensive encephalopathy. *Arch Intern Med.* 1928;**41**(2):264–278.

64. Schwartz T, Jones K, Kalina P, et al. Hypertensive encephalopathy: findings of CT, MR imaging, and SPECT imaging in 14 cases. *Am J Roentgenol.*1992;**159**:379–383.

65. Sheth RD, Riggs JE, Bodensteiner JB, et al. Parietal occipital edema in hypertensive encephalopathy: a pathogenic mechanism. *Eur Neurol.* 1996;**36**:25–28.

66. Pavlakis SG. Topical review: hypertensive encephalopathy reversible occipitoparietal encephalopathy, or reversible posterior leukoencephalopathy: three names for an old syndrome. *J Child Neurol.* 1999;**14**(5):277–281.

67. Hinchey J, Chaves C, Appignani B, et al. A reversible posterior leukoencephalopathy syndrome. *N Engl J Med.* 1996;**334**:494–500.

68. Hayreh S, Servais G, Virdi P. Fundus lesions in malignant hypertension versus hypertensive optic neuropathy. *Opthalmology.* 1986;**93**:74–87.

69. Jones BV, Egelhoff JC, Patterson RJ. Hypertensive encephalopathy in children. *AJNR Am J Neuroradiol.* 1997;**18**(1):101–106.

70. Bonovich DC. Hypertension and hypertensive encephalopathy. In: Biller J, ed. *The Interface of Neurology and Internal Medicine.* Kluwer: Wolters/Lippincott Williams and Williams; 2008;**9**:67–71.

71. Suarez JI, ed. *Critical Care Neurology and Neurosurgery.* New York: Humana Press; 2004.

10

Inflammatory Angiopathies and Stroke

Though we name the things we know, we do not necessarily know them because we name them.

Homer W. Smith

Inflammation of the cranial vessels can occur either in the setting of a widespread systemic vasculitis or as a localized process limited to the arteries of the head and neck. Giant cell arteritis and Takayasu arteritis affect medium and large arteries, whereas other forms of arteritis, such as polyarteritis nodosa, affect smaller ones, and still others, such as systemic lupus erythematosus (SLE) and noninfectious granulomatous angiitis, attack arterioles, capillaries, and venules (Table 10-1). Some of these conditions arise from an abnormal immune response; others result from a normal inflammatory response to an infection (Table 10-2). Despite the diverse nature of the arteritides, they are linked by their common tendency to disrupt the cerebral circulation, resulting in brain infarction or less commonly in intracranial hemorrhage.

In this chapter we first consider the primary arteritides, conditions that often affect the brain but are generally not tied to a specific underlying infection or systemic autoimmune disorder; we then discuss vasculitis arising from infections and systemic disorders.

GIANT CELL ARTERITIS

Hutchinson first thoroughly described giant cell arteritis in 1890, although the disorder was probably known well before this time.[1,2] Early descriptions of giant cell arteritis emphasized abnormalities of the superficial temporal artery (thus the term *temporal arteritis*), but when individuals with intracranial and systemic arteritis began to appear, *giant cell arteritis* better reflected its initial histopathologic features. The more limiting terms *temporal* and *cranial arteritis* continue to be used on occasion. The clinical and pathologic manifestations of giant cell arteritis overlap those of other forms of vasculitis, and many individuals with giant cell arteritis also exhibit systemic signs of polymyalgia rheumatica.

Giant cell arteritis is the most common form of systemic vasculitis among individuals of European descent over 50 years of age.[3] The mean age of individuals with giant cell arteritis in one study was 69 years, but it rarely occurs in younger adults and even children.[4-6] There is a strong predilection for women, and giant cell arteritis occurs more often in Caucasians, especially those of Scandinavian or northern European descent. The HLA-DR4 haplotype occurs more often in individuals with either giant cell arteritis or polymyalgia rheumatica.[7]

Clinical Features

The clinical features of giant cell arteritis and polymyalgia rheumatica often overlap: general fatigue and weakness, abdominal discomfort, anorexia with loss of weight, and sometimes low-grade recurrent fever with nocturnal diaphoresis. The patient is often ill-appearing and complains of headache and myalgia. Individuals who present with headache tend to be diagnosed earlier than those with other complaints.[3] Over half of the individuals with polymyalgia rheumatica have muscle pain in the neck or in the shoulder or pelvic girdle, and the insertions of tendons sometimes become painful. Some individuals develop joint pain and synovitis, causing stiffness of the knee, wrist, and metacarpal joints, which is particularly evident on awakening. In one study individuals with giant cell arteritis were more likely to develop cardiac disease.[8]

Most patients with giant cell arteritis develop headache sooner or later; in one study, for example, 203 of 240 (86.4%) patients complained of headache.[3] With the inflammation in the large branches of the external carotid artery, the pain initially emanates from the scalp, but over time headache tends to become more generalized and more severe. Pain can also result from ischemia of the temporal muscles during mastication. Occasional patients have isolated neck pain or cluster-like headache.[9]

The superficial temporal artery is often exquisitely tender.[3] It can become visibly enlarged (Figure 10-1), difficult to compress, and, in advanced cases, pulseless. The overlying skin may become erythematous, hot, and edematous. Rarely, ischemia of the scalp results in areas of necrosis.

Visual loss due to optic nerve ischemia is the most frequent and most dramatic neurological complication of giant cell arteritis.[10] Visual loss is most often due to decreased blood flow

Table 10-1: Classification of the Vasculitides

Vasculitis due to infections

- Infective arteritis
- Meningitis
- Human immunodeficiency virus
- Syphilis
- Fungal
- Neuroborreliosis
- Herpes zoster

Necrotizing vasculitis

- Churg-Strauss syndrome
- Kawasaki disease
- Microscopic polyangiitis
- Polyarteritis nodosa
- Wegener granulomatosis

Primary angiitis of the CNS

Giant cell vasculitides

- Takayasu arteritis
- Giant cell arteritis

Hypersensitivity vasculitis

- Henoch-Schönlein purpura
- Cryoglobulinemia
- Hypocomplementemic vasculitis
- Drug induced

Vasculitis due to systemic diseases

- Behçet disease
- Mixed connective tissue disease
- Paraneoplastic vasculitis
- Rheumatoid arthritis
- Systemic lupus erythematosus
- Scleroderma
- Sjögren syndrome
- Thromboangiitis obliterans

to the posterior ciliary arteries, causing infarction of the optic nerve head (anterior ischemic optic neuropathy). Less commonly, visual loss results from retinal infarction due to central retinal artery occlusion. Typically the patient develops complete or partial monocular visual loss within a 12- to 24-hour span. The retinal arterioles exhibit decreased caliber and blood flow, and secondary central retinal artery occlusion sometimes occurs. Optic disc edema evolves to optic nerve pallor and optic atrophy in individuals with significant visual loss (Figure 10-1).

In a prospective study of 174 individuals, 48 people (27.5%) suffered visual loss, including 23 individuals (13.2%) with permanent visual loss.[11] Undoubtedly the risk of eventual blindness due to untreated giant cell arteritis would be even higher in untreated patients. Episodic visual loss is common initially, but once optic nerve infarction occurs, vision does not usually recover, even with corticosteroid treatment. An elevated platelet count increases the likelihood of visual loss, whereas the coexistence of polymyalgia rheumatica or other systemic signs lessens it.

Cerebral infarction occurs less often than optic nerve ischemia and is more likely to occur in the posterior than the anterior circulation, resulting at times in cortical blindness. Rarely there is double vision due to a cranial nerve VI palsy or even a more severe ophthalmoplegia. Cerebellar infarction, diabetes insipidus, or spinal cord ischemia have been reported. Vascular cognitive impairment is rare.

Fatal complications result from giant cell arteritis in about 10% of patients. Causes of death include ruptured aortic aneurysm, arterial dissection, stroke, and myocardial infarction.[6] Because most of the affected individuals are elderly, it can be difficult to be certain whether a stroke or myocardial infarction resulted from arteritis.

Laboratory Findings

About half of the patients have mild leukocytosis and a normocytic, normochromic anemia. The platelet count is often elevated. In untreated patients, the erythrocyte sedimentation rate (ESR) is typically above 50 mm in the first hour (Westergren method), but it can be normal even at the time of diagnosis.[12,13] A normal ESR becomes more likely over time but does not predict a milder clinical course. Elevation of the C-reactive protein (CRP) may be a more dependable indicator of giant cell arteritis than the ESR, and combining these two studies could be the most reliable approach.[14] Although patients with an ESR of greater than 100 mm/hour develop more constitutional

Table 10-2: Anatomic Distribution of Vasculitides Affecting the Brain

	Aorta	Large Artery	Medium Artery	Small Artery	Arteriole	Capillary	Veins/Venule
Giant cell arteritis	+	++	++	−	−	−	−
Takayasu arteritis	++	++	−	−	−	−	−
Polyarteritis nodosa	−	−	++	++	+	−	−
Primary angiitis	−	−	++	++	++	++	+
Wegener arteritis	−	−	+	++	++	++	+
Hypersensitivity angiitis	−	−	−	−	+	++	++

Legend: ++ = typically affected; + = variably affected; − = not affected.

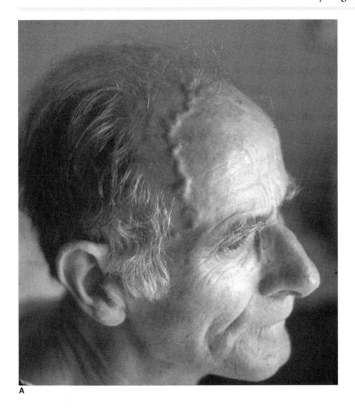

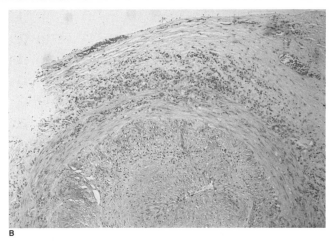

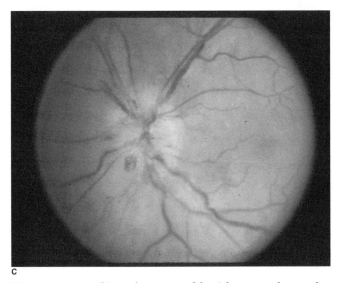

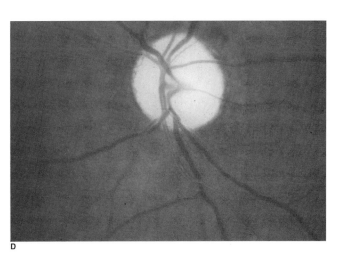

Figure 10-1. A: Striking enlargement of the right temporal artery due to giant cell arteritis in a 70-year-old man with a 6-month history of frontal headache and weight loss. B: Temporal artery biopsy from a patient with giant cell arteritis showing lymphocytic infiltration and lumen occlusion. C: Optic nerve edema and infarction due to giant cell arteritis. D: Chronic optic atrophy following acute visual loss due to giant cell arteritis. Parts C and D courtesy of Dr. Carol F. Zimmerman.

symptoms, markedly abnormal laboratory markers of inflammation do not correlate precisely with an increased likelihood of ischemic complications.[15]

Angiography is not usually necessary for the diagnosis of giant cell arteritis, but Doppler ultrasonography can help to identify abnormal segments of the temporal artery before biopsy. When the intracranial arteries are affected, angiography reveals multifocal arterial stenosis.[16] Segmental narrowing of larger vessels can mimic arterial dissection.[17] Magnetic resonance imaging sometimes shows localized or patchy areas of dural contrast enhancement[18] as well as cerebral infarction and other complications.[16]

Pathologic Findings

Temporal arteritis preferentially affects the superficial temporal, ophthalmic, posterior ciliary, and vertebral arteries. Aortic involvement tends to be a late complication, occurring in about

10% of the patients. The characteristic histological changes usually include transmural inflammation of the medium-sized and large arteries. The typical features of giant cell arteritis are granulomatous pan-arteritis with inflammation and thickening of the vessel walls, disruption of the internal elastic lamina, giant cell infiltration, and arterial occlusion or stenosis (Figure 10-1). Early in the course there is more intense lymphocytic infiltrate and more numerous giant cells, whereas in the chronic phase the inflammation is less intense and there are fewer giant cells.[6] The lumen is eventually occluded by intimal hyperplasia, and the media is partially replaced by connective tissue.

A definite pathological diagnosis of giant cell arteritis requires histological verification of inflammatory cells in the arterial wall. The arterial inflammation can be multifocal, however, and so histological examination of several different areas of the biopsy specimen is usually recommended. One study identified three patients with "skip lesions" in the temporal artery biopsy among 35 individuals (8.5%) with giant cell arteritis;[19] another found only one additional example of giant cell arteritis among 132 initially normal temporal artery biopsy specimens by reexamining the biopsy specimens at multiple levels.[20]

Some studies suggest a role for the herpes simplex virus in the pathogenesis of giant cell arteritis. Powers and colleagues used a polymerase chain reaction technique to identify herpes simplex DNA in 21 of 24 (88%) temporal artery biopsy specimens that were histologically positive for giant cell arteritis. No herpes simplex DNA was identified in 10 renal artery specimens from their age-matched control group.[21] An earlier study of 10 biopsy-confirmed cases of giant cell arteritis found no evidence of varicella zoster viral infection.[22]

Diagnosis and Management

Because of the risk of sudden and generally irreversible visual loss, corticosteroids should be started immediately when giant cell arteritis is suspected, even before the diagnosis has been confirmed. Thus, corticosteroids should be considered in an elderly individual with increasingly severe unexplained headache and an elevated ESR rate and one or more physical signs compatible with giant cell arteritis.

A long segment (2.5 to 4.0 cm in length) temporal artery biopsy should be done as soon as possible after presentation; several days of corticosteroid therapy does not typically eliminate the histological evidence of arteritis. Examination of several different areas of the biopsy specimen is usually done because of the segmental nature of the inflammation, and some authors advocate sampling both temporal arteries to increase the diagnostic yield. However, the likelihood of missing the diagnosis by examining a single area is relatively small.[20]

Prednisone at 1 mg/kg/day should be given for 1 to 3 months or 1.5 mg/kg/day in individuals with transient ischemic attacks, stroke, or visual loss. Maintenance therapy for 1 to 2 years is typically recommended, reducing the daily steroid dose by 2.5 mg to 5 mg every month provided the patient remains asymptomatic and the ESR remains low.[23] In patients with acute visual loss, stroke, or transient ischemic attacks, high dose (1–2 mg/kg) of intravenous methylprednisolone for several days is often prescribed. Dramatic resolution of pain within 72 hours of starting corticosteroids can have diagnostic and prognostic importance. The patient's general condition also improves rapidly, and the ESR normalizes within 3 weeks in half of the cases. Alternate day corticosteroid therapy is ineffective. Adding methotrexate to corticosteroids does not lower the risk of initial treatment failure, but combined treatment may reduce the rate of relapse once a patient is in remission.[24,25] Unfortunately, both optic nerve infarction and ischemic stroke sometimes occur, even in individuals taking corticosteroids.[26,27]

TAKAYASU ARTERITIS

Named for the Japanese ophthalmologist who so vividly described its ocular changes in 1906, Takayasu arteritis is also known as pulseless disease or obliterative brachiocephalic arteritis. Although any portion of the aorta or its major branches can be involved, it most often affects the aortic arch and its branches. Oddly, it is frequently identified in Asia and Mexico but rarely in Europe and North America (where the annual incidence is estimated to be 2.6 per million).[28–31] Affected individuals typically present between the ages of 12 and 40 years, and there is a strong predilection for women.

Clinical Features

In the early stages Takayasu arteritis often causes constitutional symptoms rather than vascular insufficiency. Common early symptoms include fever, asthenia, fatigue, vague musculoskeletal pain, arthralgia, anorexia, anemia, and weight loss. These nonspecific symptoms can persist for months before the onset of vascular signs. Takayasu arteritis most often affects the aortic arch and its branches, including the carotid, vertebral, and subclavian arteries (Figure 10-2 A).[32] Recurring headaches are common, as are syncope and vertigo. Unilateral, and occasionally bilateral, amaurosis fugax can arise from carotid artery involvement. Transient ischemic attacks are more common than brain infarction. Coronary artery disease leads to angina in some individuals.[33]

When Takayasu arteritis affects the mid-aorta (Figure 10-2 B), compromise of the renal, celiac, and superior mesenteric arteries can result in abdominal angina, intestinal malabsorption, and renovascular hypertension. The aortic bifurcation syndrome (Leriche syndrome), involving the terminal aorta and the iliac arteries, produces intermittent claudication of the hips and legs and, in males, impotence secondary to failure of tumescence. Involvement of the renal, coronary, or pulmonary arteries superimpose the symptoms of hypertension and cardiopulmonary disease on those caused by ischemia of the brain, eye, and arms. Individuals with rapid progression to vascular compromise have less time to develop collateral circulation and tend to develop more signs of distal ischemia.

The subclavian, brachial, and radial pulses are often absent in the later stages. Thus, although about half of the patients develop systemic hypertension, many of them have a spuriously normal or low blood pressure reading because of stenosis or occlusion of the proximal arteries of the arms. The carotid pulses are often diminished, and the carotid sinuses may be hypersensitive. Pulsations, thrills, and bruits in the collateral vessels of the head, neck, or chest suggest an obstructive lesion of the aortic arch and its major branches, but they are not specific for this syndrome. Trophic changes, such as perforation of the nasal septum, alopecia, and ulceration of the oral mucous membranes, sometimes develop when cranial blood flow is severely compromised.

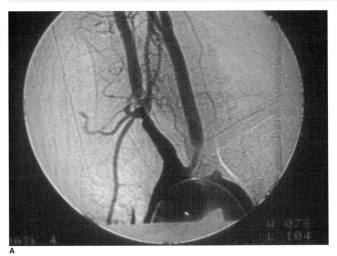 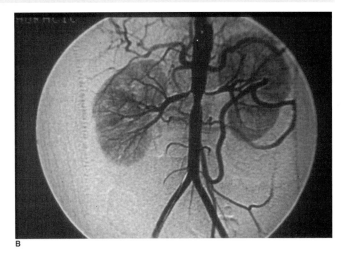

Figure 10-2. Digital subtraction angiogram from an individual with Takayasu arteritis. A: Both subclavian arteries are occluded, and the carotid arteries are stenotic. The left common carotid arises atypically from the brachiocephalic trunk. B: The abdominal aorta is stenotic just beneath its junction with the renal arteries, which are also narrowed.

Ophthalmoscopic examination may reveal stasis with segmentation of the retinal arterioles and veins. Occasional patients have such reduced blood pressure and flow in the retinal and cerebral arteries that they assume a head-low posture in an effort to increase blood flow and improve vision. Characteristic peripapillary neovascularization and arteriovenous anastomoses may also be present; cataracts and conjunctival injection are relatively common.

In the face of carotid artery occlusion, the vertebrobasilar system may provide collateral circulation to the entire brain. Because vertebral artery flow may rarely be compromised by different head postures, the vascular symptoms sometimes become more prominent with extension of the neck or head turning. Standing may decrease cerebral perfusion in this already compromised circulation and cause the symptoms of cerebrovascular insufficiency. During limb exercise, claudication and brainstem ischemia manifested by diplopia, dysphagia, blurring of vision, and incoordination may be prominent symptoms (subclavian steal syndrome). Brain infarction is common in untreated individuals with Takayasu arteritis.[34]

Laboratory Findings

Although the majority of patients have an elevated ESR, it is normal in about a quarter of the patients with active disease.[31] About half the patients have a normocytic, normochromic anemia with leukocytosis. The results of serologic studies for syphilis are negative.

Various degrees of stenosis or occlusion of the subclavian, brachiocephalic, carotid, and vertebral arteries are evident on catheter cerebral angiography (Figure 10-2), magnetic resonance angiography, and cranial computed tomography (CT) angiography.[34] In a few individuals, obstruction of the proximal subclavian or brachiocephalic artery allows reversal of blood flow through the vertebral artery and causes vertebral-basilar territory ischemia (subclavian steal).[34] Rare patients develop arterial dissection.[35] Ultrasound demonstrates the arterial lesion as well as the direction and velocity of flow,[36] and transcranial Doppler sometimes shows microemboli distal to the stenotic arteries.[36,37]

Pathologic Findings

Most commonly involved are the aortic arch and the brachiocephalic, common carotid, and subclavian arteries, with sparing of their intracranial segments. Affected arteries have patchy intimal thickening, longitudinal scarring, and segmental changes that narrow the lumen or lead to aneurysmal dilatation. Thrombosis of the vessel is common, although eventual recanalization often follows. Microscopically, active granulomas display edema, fragmentation of the elastica, and focal or diffuse collections of lymphocytes, plasma cells, macrophages, and giant cells. The inflammation involves predominantly the adventitia and outer media, and over time endothelial proliferation leads to obliteration of the lumen. The endarteritis and perivascular cuffing of syphilis are not present, and no caseation is evident. Chronically, the affected segments develop medial fibrosis, and the inflammation often wanes. Long-term, atherosclerotic lesions sometimes develop at the site where the artery was inflamed.[38]

Course and Prognosis

Takayasu arteritis has protean manifestations and a somewhat unpredictable course. Systemic hypertension caused by coarctation of the aorta and renal artery stenosis is another complication. Untreated, there is slowly progressive compromise of cerebral and peripheral blood flow. Nevertheless, many treated patients have a relatively benign neurological course despite the persistence of severe arterial compromise. In a recent series of 20 patients followed for 20 years, for example, two had suffered a stroke before diagnosis and another had persistent transient ischemic attacks.[30]

Management

High-dose corticosteroids often halt the inflammatory process and prevent arterial stenosis if started early. If remission is not achieved with corticosteroids alone, cytotoxic agents should be added. In one series, almost two-thirds of the patients achieved remission, although relapse was common.[31] Platelet inhibitors or anticoagulants may benefit individuals with symptomatic arterial stenosis. Angioplasty may relieve symptomatic chronic arterial stenosis, but restenosis is common.[39]

POLYARTERITIS NODOSA

Polyarteritis nodosa (PAN) may result from an infection that triggers an autoimmune reaction to the medium-sized and small arteries that contain a well-developed muscularis. The transmural necrotizing vasculitis of PAN preferentially affects the skin, joints, gastrointestinal tract, kidneys, and peripheral nerves. Some individuals are infected with hepatitis B virus (HBV),[40] and other infections may play a role in the remaining patients. The classic descriptions of PAN note the systemic nature of the arteritis but stress that the pulmonary circulation is usually spared. The peripheral nervous system is more often affected than the central nervous system, and peripheral neuropathy may be the only neurologic manifestation of the disease.

Clinical Features

Polyarteritis nodosa is four times more common in men than women and typically begins between 20 and 40 years of age. The initial signs and symptoms usually reflect systemic disease: myalgia, fever, malaise, anorexia with weight loss, postprandial abdominal pain (from mesenteric ischemia), arthralgias, and subcutaneous nodules may precede the neurological symptoms by months or years. Variable skin changes include livedo reticularis, ulcerations, ecchymoses, and, least commonly, palpable nodules.[40] At times, inflamed arteries are visible on the dorsum of the hand or foot and may be tender to palpation. Renal involvement occurs early and is characterized by flank pain, hematuria, proteinuria, azotemia, and hypertension.

The neurological symptoms vary, but headache is the most common complaint.[41] The severity, location, and duration of the headache varies, and, in some instances, the headache stems from systemic hypertension rather than arteritis. Focal or generalized seizures are frequent, and chorea has been reported. Confusion, delirium, disorientation, and behavior change are particularly common features of brain involvement. About half the patients develop either generalized symmetrical polyneuropathy or mononeuritis multiplex. Facial palsy, deafness, oculomotor palsy, or other cranial neuropathies may be selectively involved and can be the initial neurological manifestation.

Polyarteritis nodosa can produce several neurovascular syndromes, although brain vascular lesions rarely occur early in its course.[41–43] Occlusion of a superficial or the penetrating arterial branch results in a variety of infarction syndromes.[44] Obstruction of a major artery, such as the basilar, results in disastrous neurologic deficits. If the wall of a surface conducting artery is weakened, aneurysmal dilatation and rupture results in subarachnoid hemorrhage. Penetrating arteries may also rupture to produce intracerebral or intracerebellar hemorrhage.[42,45]

Changes in the optic fundus are common. Some of these abnormalities (e.g., arteriolar spasm, hemorrhages, and exudates) are secondary to systemic hypertension; papilledema is the result of increased intracranial pressure. Occlusion of the central retinal artery or its branches may result in sudden monocular visual loss.[41]

Laboratory Findings

Anemia, leukocytosis with eosinophilia, and elevation of the ESR occur in about half the cases. The urine frequently contains protein, red blood cells, and very characteristic red blood cell casts. Antinuclear antibodies and rheumatoid factor are sometimes weakly positive but of no practical value in this setting. The same is true for ANCA positivity. The cerebrospinal fluid (CSF) pressure is typically normal, but in a few patients the protein is increased and increased numbers of lymphocytes and polymorphonuclear cells occur. The rare patient with subarachnoid hemorrhage has blood-stained CSF.[41]

Cranial computed tomography (CT) or magnetic resonance imaging (MRI) may show one or more infarctions.[46,47] Arterial beading, occlusion, or aneurysm formation are apparent with catheter angiography and sometimes with magnetic resonance angiography (MRA) or CT angiography. The definitive diagnosis is established by a biopsy of involved tissue.

Pathologic Findings

There is a widespread misconception that PAN seldom affects the central nervous system (CNS), but 8% to 46% of cases examined by autopsy show involvement of the arteries of the brain. Typically polyarteritis nodosa affects the medium-sized and small arteries.[41] In one autopsy study, five of 19 patients had one or more cerebral infarctions, and one had a brain hemorrhage. The intracranial arterial lesions may cause subarachnoid hemorrhage, intracerebral hemorrhage, hemorrhagic infarction, or multiple small hemorrhages distributed throughout the hemispheres. The brain is swollen, and, on cut sections, multiple infarctions of various sizes and in various distributions may be seen.

There is inflammation of the adventitia and muscularis of the arteries, which are infiltrated with polymorphonuclear cells, lymphocytes, eosinophils, and reactive proliferation. The arterioles are thickened, and the lumen of the vessel is small and eccentric and may be occluded with thrombus. The pathology of PAN closely resembles that of Kawasaki syndrome in children.[48] In others the clinical and pathological manifestations overlap those of giant cell arteritis and other forms of vasculitis.[49,50]

Management and Prognosis

The treatment of PAN hinges on whether it is idiopathic or associated with HBV.[51] About half of the patients with isolated PAN achieve at least a temporary remission with only high-dose corticosteroids,[40] and the remission may persist for several years. In refractory cases or those with major organ involvement, a combination of cyclophosphamide (2 mg/kg/day orally provided the renal function is normal) and corticosteroids is preferable.[40] Because immunosuppression can hasten hepatic dysfunction in individuals with HBV,[52] their regimen should be modified to include an antiviral agent.[40] Medications that could aggravate the disorder (e.g., hydralazine, the sulfonamides, and certain antibiotics) should be avoided.

Renal impairment develops early and is often accompanied by intractable hypertension. Causes of death include renal decompensation with hypertension, stroke, and myocardial infarction. Only about half of the individuals with multiple organ involvement that includes the central nervous system survive for 5 years.

PRIMARY ANGIITIS OF THE CNS

Isolated angiitis of the CNS may not be nearly as rare as once believed. It is distinguished from most other forms of arteritis that affect the nervous system by the paucity of the usual systemic signs of inflammation. The pathogenesis of isolated CNS angiitis remains obscure, but some investigators suspect a hypersensitivity reaction or an autoimmune process.

Clinical Features

The disease affects both sexes equally. It typically occurs in middle-aged adults, but a few patients have been children and elderly adults.[53–55] Common early symptoms include headache, vomiting, and altered mental function. In contrast to other forms of arteritis that affect the nervous system, fever, arthralgia, myalgia, and elevation of the ESR are conspicuously uncommon in individuals with primary angiitis.[56] As the disease worsens, various focal neurological deficits occur, and some individuals develop convulsions. The clinical course is variable; some patients have a relentlessly downhill course, whereas others achieve long-term remission or develop a relapsing and remitting pattern in response to therapy.[56,57]

Laboratory Findings

The ESR and the white blood cell count are typically normal or only mildly elevated. Likewise, assays for antinuclear antibodies and rheumatoid factor are normal.[56] The CSF is most often normal, although a few patients have slightly elevated pressure and some an elevated protein level or modestly increased lymphocyte count.[56]

MRI or CT may show multifocal brain infarctions (Figure 10-3) and, on occasion, hemorrhage.[58] Arteriography shows multifocal segmental narrowing, dilatation, beading, and/or occlusions of small cortical arteries.[59]

Pathologic Findings

The brain parenchyma has small areas of infarction with loss of neurons distributed throughout the cerebrum, brainstem, and cerebellum. The vessels of the leptomeninges are sometimes more extensively affected than those in the brain (Figure 10-3). The lumen is narrowed and the intima thickened. Inflammation affects the entire vessel wall and is made up of lymphocytes, large mononuclear cells, and multinucleated giant cells.[54,60]

Diagnosis and Management

Brain and meningeal biopsy should be performed in selected patients, and, if inflammatory angiitis is confirmed, corticosteroids and cyclophosphamide should be administered.[60] Isolated CNS angiitis was once thought to have a uniformly poor outcome, but with aggressive treatment, many patients achieve a sustained remission. However, the prognosis is unpredictable.

WEGENER GRANULOMATOSIS

Wegener granulomatosis is characterized by granulomatous inflammation of the respiratory tract, focal glomerulonephritis, and necrotizing vasculitis.[61] Men are affected slightly more often than women, and the disease usually affects individuals in middle age although children and the elderly are sometimes affected. Antineutrophilic cytoplasmic antibodies (ANCAs), possibly in conjunction with an intercurrent infection, evidently play a key role in the pathogenesis of Wegener granulomatosis.[61]

Clinical Features

Wegener granulomatosis is distinguished clinically from other forms of arteritis by its consistent involvement of the upper and lower respiratory tract, frequent sinusitis, and ulceration of the mucous membranes. These and other systemic symptoms generally precede the neurologic signs, but stroke is occasionally the initial complication.[62]

The nervous system is involved in about a third of the individuals with Wegener granulomatosis, and some patients develop more than one type of neurologic complication.[63,64] Individuals with polyneuropathy or mononeuropathy multiplex far outnumber those with cerebrovascular complications.[64] Wegener granulomatosis can lead to brain infarction, intraparenchymal hemorrhage, subarachnoid hemorrhage, or venous thrombosis.[62,65,66] In addition, localized leptomeningeal inflammation can impair the function of cranial nerves or cause diabetes insipidus.

Churg-Strauss syndrome is similar to Wegener granulomatosis, and the two conditions are considered by some to be variants of the same condition.[67] Affected individuals tend to have eosinophilia and asthma, and they are less likely to develop renal disease.[68] Both conditions involve small blood vessels, feature necrotizing granulomas, and have positive c-ANCA assays.[68]

Pathologic Findings

Necrotizing granulomatosis of the upper and lower respiratory tract is followed by granulomas of the brain and/or by more generalized vasculitis. Only two of 12 autopsied cases in one series had evidence of active vasculitis.[64] The inflammation involves small arteries and veins. All layers are infiltrated by histiocytes, polymorphonuclear cells, and fibrinoid necrosis.

Laboratory Findings

Acutely, the ESR is increased and the CRP is elevated. In individuals with systemic manifestations of Wegener granulomatosis, testing for c-ANCA and related antibodies has better than a 96% sensitivity, but the sensitivity is lower in people with localized disease.[61,69] Cranial CT or MRI demonstrate cerebral atrophy, strokes, or isolated granulomas.[70] Additionally, MRI may depict high-signal lesions of the white matter and thickened areas in the leptomeninges with striking contrast enhancement.[67,71]

Management

Cyclophosphamide, the drug of choice, is given orally, 1 to 2 mg/kg/day in a single dose and, in severe cases, up to 3 mg/kg/day. Prednisone at 1 mg/kg/day may be necessary in the beginning because the effect of cyclophosphamide may be delayed for several weeks. Intravenous immunoglobulin (IVIG) may be useful.[72]

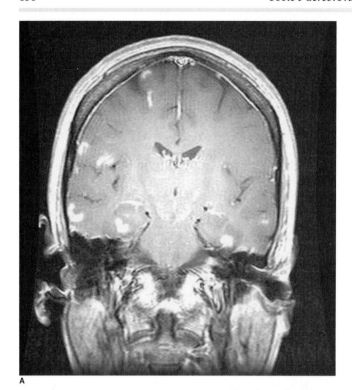

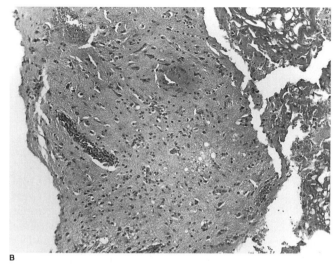

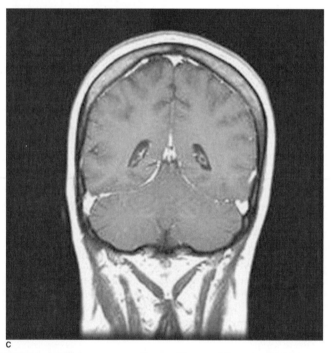

Figure 10-3. A: T$_2$-weighted cranial MRI with gadolinium contrast (from a 38-year-old woman with increased migraine frequency and new-onset paresthesias, aphasia, and cognitive deterioration) shows multiple small enhancing lesions consistent with infarctions. B: Biopsy of this patient's right temporal lobe showed perivascular mononuclear lymphocytic and plasma cell infiltrates suggestive of primary cerebral arteritis. Although not well shown in this picture, the brain tissue around some of these vessels contained reactive astrocytes and degenerating neurons (hematoxylin-eosin, original magnification × 400). C: Repeat T$_2$-weighted MRI after 6 months of clophosphamide and dexamethasone shows resolution of the lesions.

HYPERSENSITIVITY VASCULITIS

Hypersensitivity vasculitis includes Henoch-Schönlein (anaphylactoid) purpura, vasculitic drug reactions, hypocomplementemic vasculitis, and cryoglobulinemia. These entities tend to involve the skin more than other sites, typically with purpura or urticaria.[73] Henoch-Schönlein purpura is a hypersensitivity vasculitis that affects children more often than adults.[74] It characteristically causes purpura, glomerulonephritis, arthralgia, and gastrointestinal lesions. The disorder has been documented after a variety of infections. Relatively few Henoch-Schönlein purpura patients with neurovascular complications have been described, starting with Osler's description in 1914 of a patient who developed hemiparesis. Common neurological symptoms are headache, altered mental status, and epileptic seizures, but various focal neurological deficits have been described.[75,76] Rare patients develop subarachnoid or intraparenchymal hemorrhage.[77–79]

Deposits of IgA complexes and nonsegmental inflammation have been demonstrated within the small vessels (arterioles, capillaries, and venules).[80] Fibrinoid necrosis and microinfarctions occur adjacent to these vascular lesions.[81] The levels of circulating immune complexes correlate with the clinical severity in some individuals, although not in the population as a whole.[82]

Many patients with anaphylactoid purpura respond to oral corticosteroids or pulse methylprednisolone. Plasmapheresis and oral cyclophosphamide are effective in others.[83]

Allergic drug reactions with immune complex deposition result from sulfonamides and other medications, and usually clear once the medication is removed. Initial symptoms are typically fever and headache, followed by a rash and cough. Neurologic complaints include generally nonspecific symptoms such as mental status alteration or seizures, but cranial neuropathy and stroke are occasionally documented.[81]

Vasculitis associated with cryoglobulinemia typically involves the skin and glomeruli, and only occasionally the brain. This syndrome often accompanies hepatitis C infection or lymphoproliferative disorders. The vasculitis affects the arterioles, capillaries, and venules.[68] Cryoglobulins contain IgG, IgM, complement, and lipoprotein. These precipitate below 37°C, ultimately leading to vessel wall damage and occlusion of small vessels.[68,81]

ARTERITIS CAUSED BY INFECTION

Infectious Embolism

Emboli resulting from infective endocarditis or from a pulmonary arteriovenous fistula can cause cranial arteritis. Infective endocarditis typically occurs in children with congenital heart disease or in adults with rheumatic valvular heart disease, prosthetic heart valves, or a history of intravenous drug use. Pulmonary arteriovenous fistulas occur in disorders such as hereditary hemorrhagic telangiectasia (see Chapter 18). Infectious cardiac emboli generally result from various strains of *Streptococcus* or *Staphylococcus*,[84] but other bacterial and fungal infections occur especially in debilitated or immunocompromised individuals.[85,86] Although infective endocarditis has become less common because of the lower incidence of rheumatic heart disease and the availability of antibiotics, cerebrovascular complications remain common among individuals with infective endocarditis. Hart and colleagues, for example, noted that stroke occurred in 21% of 212 episodes of infective endocarditis.[87] Infective embolism is considered in more detail in Chapter 8.

Meningitis

The cerebral vessels lie in proximity to the meninges and traverse the subarachnoid space, so it is not surprising that vascular inflammation and occlusion should occur in individuals with meningitis. Bacterial infections account for most instances of stroke, but there are occasional reports of stroke due to viral or even amoebic meningitis.[88] Stroke can occur even before the other signs of meningitis develop, especially with partially treated meningitis or with organisms that produce a less fulminant initial clinical course.[89] Delayed or inappropriate treatment probably increases the likelihood of stroke. Individuals with meningitis complicated by stroke tend to have a lower initial CSF glucose and a higher leukocyte count. In extremely ill patients, it can be difficult to distinguish the effects of the infection itself from those of secondary vascular occlusion.

In one series about a third of 86 consecutive adults with bacterial meningitis developed cerebrovascular complications.[90] Angiography, performed in 27 of these 86 patients, documented frequent cerebrovascular lesions, including occlusion of both large and medium-sized arteries, focal arterial stenosis, and sinovenous occlusion.[90] The reported stroke risk in children with bacterial meningitis ranges from 5% to 27%.[91]

Stroke is common in individuals with tuberculous meningitis. One study found cerebral arteritis or phlebitis in 22 of 23 autopsied cases, and in this cohort there were five infarctions and eight hemorrhagic infarctions.[92] Stroke is more common in children with tuberculous meningitis than in adults.[93] Ischemic infarction occurred in 25 of 65 (38%) children with tuberculous meningitis in one series and in about half of the 198 children in another series.[94,95] Because of its propensity for basilar meningitis, tuberculous meningitis tends to cause basal ganglia infarction.[96]

Prompt and appropriate antibiotic therapy should theoretically reduce the risk of stroke due to meningitis, although a full discussion of specific therapeutic agents is beyond the scope of this book. If administered early, corticosteroids seem to improve the overall outcome of patients with bacterial meningitis, but there is little evidence that these agents reduce the risk of stroke from meningitis.

Herpes Infections

Individuals with herpes zoster ophthalmicus sometimes develop an ipsilateral cerebral infarction several days or weeks after the zoster eruption.[97] Most of the lesions are infarctions within the anterior circulation, but one patient suffered an intracranial hemorrhage and another developed a central retinal artery occlusion.[98,99] Another patient suffered multiple infarctions due to a varicella zoster vasculitis without cutaneous signs of the virus.[100]

Intracranial herpetic angiitis may result from transmission of the virions to the intracranial vessel wall from the trigeminal ganglion via the intracranial branches of the ophthalmic nerve, resulting in arterial inflammation and occlusion. Necrotizing arteritis of the large and small cerebral arteries was demonstrated at autopsy of one 69-year-old woman, along with herpes-like virus particles in the middle cerebral artery.[101]

Although the mechanism is not well understood, some children develop a cerebral infarction following systemic chicken pox.[102,103] A case-control study found a statistically significant link between stroke and recent chicken pox. Seven of 11 (64%) children with an idiopathic ischemic stroke had varicella within the preceding 9 months, versus only four of the 44 (9%)

children in the control group.[104] Another study found a three-fold increase in recent varicella infections among children with unexplained ischemic stroke.[105] Most individuals have a single infarction within the anterior circulation, although there are exceptions.[106,107] The interval from the varicella infection until the stroke varies from days to several months. Segmental narrowing of the intracranial arteries has been demonstrated with both MRA and standard angiography, and these lesions are presumed to represent arteritis.

Human Immunodeficiency Virus

Cerebrovascular disease occurs with increased frequency in individuals infected with the human immunodeficiency virus (HIV).[108] The prevalence of stroke increases in individuals with more advanced disease.[109] One study[109] of 772 individuals estimated a combined prevalence for infarction and transient ischemic attacks to be 1.9%, but many individuals with vascular lesions do not have overt symptoms. Before the availability of effective therapy for HIV, Park and colleagues estimated that 1.3% of individuals per year had stroke symptoms, but they found cerebrovascular lesions in 24% of the patients who were autopsied.[110]

Both infarction and hemorrhage occur, and any part of the brain may be affected. Patients with HIV can develop cerebrovascular lesions via more than one mechanism. Infection of the cerebral vascular endothelium by the human immunodeficiency virus is evidently a major factor. One man had recurrent strokes due to vasculitis that pathologically resembled primary cerebral angiitis.[111] Several HIV-infected patients have developed intracranial or carotid aneurysms.[112,113] Some have additional vascular risk factors from coexisting infective endocarditis, thrombocytopenia, or other infections (such as hepatitis B virus or syphilis).[113,114] The clinical picture may be confusing when signs of a stroke are superimposed on those of progressive encephalopathy from the infection or on nonvascular complications of HIV.

Pathological findings include one or multiple brain infarctions and, in some patients, brain hemorrhage. Calcium deposits within vessel walls and in the adjacent brain produce characteristic calcified lesions on CT. There is progressive intimal fibroplasia as well as disruption of the elastic lamina and the media.[110,115] Some patients develop frank vasculitis characterized by giant multinucleated cells, lymphocyte and plasmocyte infiltration, and intimal fibrosis.[111]

Syphilis

Syphilis was once the most prevalent worldwide risk factor for cerebrovascular disease, and given the surge in neurosyphilis cases in recent years, it remains a significant stroke risk factor. In the Western countries at least, most patients with syphilis are treated early enough that CNS involvement is relatively uncommon except in high-risk individuals (such as those with HIV or intravenous drug abusers who use contaminated needles). Additionally, individuals with syphilis tend to contract HIV and other infections, further increasing the stroke risk and perhaps promoting a more fulminant clinical course.[116]

In one large series the majority of the patients presented with neuropsychiatric signs, but about a quarter of the patients developed a stroke.[117] Stroke occurs in some individuals after the onset of mental status changes or frank dementia. Infarctions due to syphilis can occur in any portion of the brain or spinal cord, but the middle cerebral artery territory is the vessel most often affected.[118–120] The lesions are often multiple and bilateral.[121] Affected vessels may be entirely intracranial or both the intracranial and extracranial, and stroke sometimes results from syphilitic changes of the aorta.[118]

The diagnosis of neurosyphilis is confirmed by a reactive CSF Venereal Disease Research Laboratory (VDRL) or a positive fluorescent treponemal antibody absorption (FTA-ABS) assay in an individual with typical clinical findings.[117] The CSF protein is often elevated and the white blood cells too numerous.[122] Given the potential co-infection with HIV, it is advisable to test each person with syphilis for HIV. Computed tomography and MRI reveal one or more ischemic infarctions, sometimes superimposed on diffuse cortical atrophy. Catheter cerebral angiography shows segmental narrowing or occlusion of both large and medium-sized arteries.[119,123]

Treatment with antibiotics quickly reduces the risk of stroke due to syphilis, but a complete discussion of the treatment of neurosyphilis is beyond the scope of this text. Individuals infected with HIV should begin appropriate antiviral agents.

Fungal Infection

Although uncommon, fungal meningitis and/or vasculitis should be suspected in individuals at high risk because of altered immunity.[124] Vasculitis and stroke can result from fungal meningitis, direct extension from nearby paranasal sinuses or the orbits, or fungal septicemia. Ischemic stroke and increased intracranial pressure result from thrombosis of the intracranial arteries or a dural venous sinus, whereas subarachnoid or intraparenchymal hemorrhage results from arterial destruction or mycotic aneurysm rupture.[124–127] In some instances the stroke risk is compounded by HIV or other infections.[128] Aspergillosis and mucormycosis invade the vessel locally, whereas *Candida* and *Coccidiomycosis* tend to produce a chronic meningitis that in turn produces vascular inflammation.[81,129]

Neuroborreliosis (Lyme Disease)

Isolated reports suggest that neuroborreliosis incites cerebral arteritis that in turn leads to brain infarction as well as subarachnoid or intraparenchymal hemorrhage.[130–132] Although it seems intuitive that neuroborreliosis, like other chronic infections of the CNS, could produce vascular inflammation and stroke, given the frequency of the infection and the paucity of such reports, Lyme disease does not appear to be a huge risk factor. Only one of 281 consecutive patients with noncardioembolic stroke, for example, had serologic evidence of *Borrelia burgdorferi*.[133] Clinical suspicion should increase in a younger individual living in an endemic area for the infection who has few other risk factors.

The CSF has a lymphocytic pleocytosis and an increased protein level. Elevated *B. burgdorferi* antibodies are found in the serum and CSF.[130,131] The vascular lesion is best demonstrated by MRI. Treatment with antibiotics normalizes the CSF abnormalities and should reduce the inflammation and thus the stroke risk.[131]

SYSTEMIC LUPUS ERYTHEMATOSUS

Systemic lupus erythematosus has protean manifestations, but the tissues most often affected are the skin, joints, and kidneys. Peripheral neuropathy is the most common neurologic complication, but involvement of the CNS is relatively common.

SLE promotes stroke in several ways: vasculitis, antiphospholipid antibodies, verrucous (Libman-Sacks) endocarditis, and enhanced atherosclerosis can all occur in individuals with SLE, and each of these increases the risk of stroke.[134]

Clinical Features

Women develop SLE four times more often than men. The disorder typically manifests between the ages of 15 and 40 years, but both childhood onset and late adult onset is common. Malar eruption (butterfly rash), arthralgias, and eventually renal disease are its hallmarks, but the array of general signs and symptoms is highly variable and cannot be discussed here in detail.

The most frequent neurologic complication is peripheral neuropathy, ranging from a nonspecific symmetrical sensory-motor neuropathy to mononeuritis multiplex. In one study 60 of 519 (11.6%) patients with SLE developed epileptic seizures.[135] Cognitive dysfunction and mental status changes are even more common and range from confusion to delirium to frank psychosis. SLE increases the risk of both ischemic and hemorrhagic stroke but not of subarachnoid hemorrhage.[136] Cerebrovascular complications tend to occur later in the course of the disease, but they can occur at any time. Brain dysfunction due to SLE can result from cerebritis as well as stroke, and distinguishing these two at the bedside can be challenging.

Untreated, the course of SLE disease is variable, with about three-fourths of the patients surviving more than 1 year but only one-fifth being alive beyond 5 years. Spontaneous, although often temporary, remission occurs in up to 40% of the patients, and the course is intermittent in about 20%. The most common mode of death is renal failure.

Laboratory Findings

Fever, anemia (normochromic, hypochromic, or hemolytic), an increased ESR, a false-positive serum reaction for syphilis, and, at times, thrombocytopenia are nonspecific findings of SLE. The diagnosis is supported by the presence of fluorescent antinuclear anti-dsDNA antibodies in the blood.

Antiphospholipid antibodies occur with increased frequency in individuals with SLE and have been implicated as a cause of stroke.[137] Only a third of patients with SLE have the lupus anticoagulant, and most individuals who have it do not have SLE. Patients with vasculitis plus antiphospholipid antibodies or endocarditis compound their risk of vascular complications; individuals with traditional stroke risk factors such as smoking, increased age, and elevated serum levels of C-reactive protein also have greater risk.[138] The diagnosis and treatment of antiphospholipid antibodies are discussed more completely in Chapter 11.

Computed tomography may show one or more infarctions, and MRI, in addition, may show areas of cerebritis. Differentiating cerebritis from a vascular lesion can be difficult unless the lesion corresponds to an obvious vascular territory, and a diffusion-weighted MRI sequence may be useful in this setting.[139] The electroencephalogram is often abnormal but nonspecific, with focal or generalized slowing and, less commonly, epileptiform activity.[135,140]

The CSF is usually normal, but individuals with neuropathy often have an elevated CSF protein, and those with either cerebritis or CNS vasculitis may, in addition, have pleocytosis. Renal biopsy may reveal characteristic vascular changes that offer both diagnostic and prognostic information because the usual life-threatening complication of this disorder is renal failure.

Pathologic Findings

In severe cases the peritoneal, pleural, and pericardial surfaces are involved with inflammatory reaction, adhesions, and effusions. The heart may be enlarged, and verrucous vegetations (Libman-Sachs endocarditis) may occur on the mitral or aortic valves. The large arteries are not usually affected.

The brain or spinal cord may be edematous with thickened meninges, and either ischemic infarction or petechial hemorrhage may be seen scattered in the hemispheres and brainstem. The arterioles, capillaries, and venules may be diffusely inflamed and sometimes occluded by blood clot, fibrinoid material, or platelet aggregations, resulting in adjacent microinfarctions of the brain parenchyma.

Management

Corticosteroid therapy slows progression of the illness and, in some patients, may keep it under control for years. During the acute phase of cerebral lupus, cyclophosphamide has been advocated as an adjunctive treatment.

BEHÇET DISEASE

Behçet disease is a chronic multisystem vasculitis that is most prevalent in the Middle East, the Mediterranean region, and the Far East. It occurs most frequently in young and middle-aged adults but has been diagnosed in the elderly, in children, and even in a neonate whose mother was affected.[141] A familial pattern occurs in about 10% of the cases.[142,143] Individuals whose disease begins before 25 years of age do poorly compared to those who develop symptoms later.[144] The clinical course also tends to be more severe in males.[143,145]

The clinical hallmarks of Behçet disease are recurrent oral and genital ulcerations, arthritis, chronic iridocyclitis, and erythema nodosum or other skin lesions. Occasionally neurological symptoms develop first.[143,145] Cardiac, pulmonary, or gastrointestinal dysfunction occurs less often.[145] The frequency of neurological involvement is 13.0% in men and 5.6% among women,[146] including individuals with nonvascular complications such as meningeal inflammation and neuropathy. Headache is the most common neurological symptom, especially during acute phases of the illness, and memory loss is common.[146] Ischemic stroke can affect either the brainstem or the cerebral hemispheres.[147,148] Subarachnoid hemorrhage can result from either a ruptured aneurysm or from arterial dissection.[149,150] There have been a few reports of dural sinus thrombosis.[151,152]

Pathology

The brainstem and basal ganglia are the brain sites most likely to be affected, with relative sparing of the cerebellum and cerebral cortex.[143] Typical brain findings include multifocal demyelination or gliosis. There may be inflammation of the leptomeninges. Affected vessels contain perivascular infiltration with lymphocytes and neutrophils. Thrombosis is seen infrequently.[145]

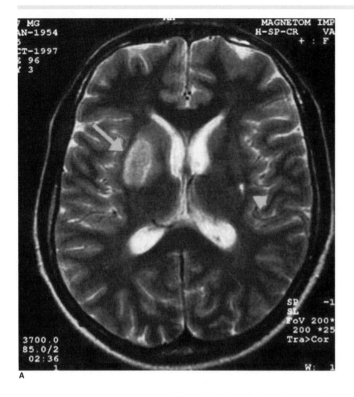
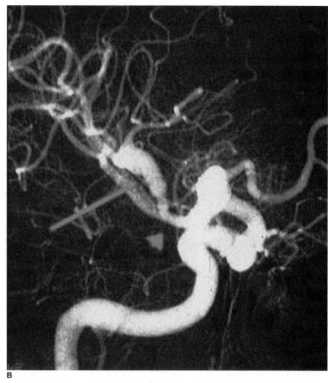

Figure 10-4. A: An MRI reveals bilateral basal ganglia infarctions (*arrows*) due to Behçet disease. B: An angiogram of an individual with Behçet disease shows subtle stenosis (*arrowhead*) of the proximal right middle cerebral artery and aneurysmal dilatation of a middle cerebral branch (*arrow*). Reprinted with permission from Krepsi et al.[147] Photographs courtesy of Professor Gulsen Akman-Demir.

Diagnosis

There is no specific laboratory test for Behçet disease, so the diagnosis rests largely on clinical observations.[153] The ESR is inconsistently elevated during acute phases of the disease. The pathergy test is often abnormal but is nonspecific. Affected individuals are more likely to be HLA-B51 positive.[143] The CSF may be normal or display pleocytosis (variable numbers of neutrophils and lymphocytes) and an elevated protein level.[143] The CSF glucose is usually normal. Thrombin generation and fibrinolysis are increased, but these do not predict thrombotic complications.[154]

The MRI typically shows high signal white matter lesions with relative sparing of the cerebellum and the cerebral cortex.[152,155,156] Segmental irregularity of the arteries and aneurysmal dilatation (Figure 10-4) can be seen with MRA in individuals with frank vasculitis.[147] Brain lesions are evident on MRI even in many individuals without neurological signs and symptoms.

Treatment

No treatment is uniformly effective, but corticosteroids may be helpful early in the course and for acute exacerbations. Immunosuppressive agents may help some individuals stabilize or achieve a long-term remission.[143,153] Some authors favor the use of cyclosporine and colchicine. Sakane and colleagues have reviewed the treatment options for Behçet disease in more detail.[153] A chronic relapsing and remitting course is typical, but over time the disease tends to become less active and may extinguish itself.[143]

OTHER CNS VASCULITIDES

Vasculitis is seen so infrequently in a few disorders that the connection could be coincidental. Some of these are referenced here but not discussed in detail.

Paraneoplastic vasculitis more often affects the peripheral than the central nervous system. Some individuals with a neoplasm are hypercoagulable, and others develop paraneoplastic encephalomyelitis, making it harder to recognize a vasculitis-mediated stroke.

Individuals with rheumatoid arthritis rarely develop cranial arteritis and brain infarction; those who do have a necrotizing vasculitis that is similar to that of polyarteritis nodosa.[157,158] About 10% of the patients with mixed connective tissue disease develop neurologic issues, but only a few of these individuals have cerebrovascular disease.[81,159] Sjögren syndrome may cause systemic vasculitis and, on rare occasions, brain infarction or subarachnoid hemorrhage.[160,161] Occasional individuals with dermatomyositis develop cerebral arteritis.[162]

A few individuals with scleroderma have developed an ischemic stroke.[163,164] Whether the vascular lesions in these patients result from vasculitis or from a noninflammatory vasculopathy is debated.[163] There is scant evidence of inflammation, but some of the patients respond to corticosteroids.

Several reports implicated neurocysticercosis as a stroke risk factor.[165,166] Stroke in these patients has been attributed to chronic meningitis, to inflammation of vessels adjacent to the brain cysts, and to endarteritis,[167] and some reports describe focal arterial stenosis suggestive of arteritis.[166] However, neurocysticercosis is common in many parts of the world; it is the most common parasitic infection among immunocompetent individuals. Recent studies suggest that the occurrence of stroke in individuals with cysticercosis may be coincidental.[168]

THROMBOANGIITIS OBLITERANS (BUERGER DISEASE)

First described in 1908 by Leo Buerger, thromboangiitis obliterans (Buerger disease) is an obliterative vascular disease that typically leads to ischemia of the extremities and often culminates in limb amputation.[169] Although claudication of the extremities is characteristic, ischemia of the gut, renal artery stenosis, and cerebrovascular dysfunction have all been described.[170,171] Thromboangiitis obliterans classically occurs in young to middle-aged men who are heavy smokers, although in recent reports the male predominance has become less striking.

Stroke due to thromboangiitis obliterans is relatively uncommon. In one series of 46 patients who were followed for a cumulative 883 patient years, for example, only one individual, a 59-year-old man, developed a focal neurological deficit.[172] The clinical pattern of cerebral Buerger disease may include transient ischemic attacks, an isolated fixed focal neurologic deficit, or recurrent infarctions in the same vascular distribution.[173,174]

Confirmation of cerebral thromboangiitis obliterans can be difficult, but it should be considered in young individuals with typical peripheral arterial occlusive disease, especially when they are heavy smokers.[175] Cerebral catheter angiography reveals multiple arterial occlusions with formation of collateral channels around the occlusion, similar to the pattern in the peripheral vasculature in these individuals.[173] Transcranial Doppler studies reveal decreased blood flow velocity of the cerebral arteries in some individuals with Buerger disease.[176]

The pathogenesis of thromboangiitis obliterans is still debated, but it appears to be a segmental inflammatory non-atherosclerotic process affecting the small to medium-sized arteries and sometimes the veins. Acutely there is vessel wall inflammation and foci of giant cells.[177] The internal elastic lamina remains intact. Adventitial fibrosis occurs, and there is swelling of the endothelium of the vasa vasorum.[178] The suspected pathogenesis is an immune-mediated endarteritis, and anti-endothelial cell antibodies have been demonstrated.[177,179]

Cessation of tobacco use is the mainstay of therapy and usually halts the progression of the disease.[177,180] Lumbar sympathectomy, infusion of prostacyclin analogues, and surgical bypass procedures or angioplasty have been used to relieve severe claudication.[181–183]

REFERENCES

1. Hutchinson L. On a peculiar form of thrombotic arteritis of the aged which is sometimes productive of gangrene. *Arch Surg (London)*. 1890;**1**:323–329.
2. Appelbloom T, Van Eigem A. How ancient is temporal arteritis? *J Rheum*. 1990;**17**:929–931.
3. Gonzalez-Gay MA, Barros S, Lopez-Diaz MJ, Garcia-Porrua C, Sanchez-Andrade A, Llorca J. Giant cell arteritis: disease patterns of clinical presentation in a series of 240 patients. *Medicine (Baltimore)*. 2005;**84**:269–276.
4. Lie JT, Gordon LP, Titus JL. Juvenile temporal arteritis – biopsy study of four cases. *JAMA*. 1975;**234**:496–499.
5. Tomlinson FH, Lie JT, Nienhuis BJ, Konzen KM, Groover RV. Juvenile temporal arteritis revisited. *Mayo Clin Proc*. 1994;**69**:445–447.
6. Lie JT. Aortic and extracranial large vessel giant cell arteritis: a review of 72 cases with histopathologic documentation. *Semin Arthritis Rheum*. 1995;**24**:422–431.
7. Weyand CM, Ma-Krupa W, Goronzy JJ. Immunopathways in giant cell arteritis and polymyalgia rheumatica. *Autoimmun Rev*. 2004;**3**:46–53.
8. Ray JG, Mamdani MM, Geerts WH. Giant cell arteritis and cardiovascular disease in older adults. *Heart*. 2005;**91**:324–328.
9. Jimenez-Jimenez FJ, Garcia-Alba E, Zurdo M, Martinez-Onsurbe P, Ruiz de Villaespesa A. Giant cell arteritis presenting as cluster headache. *Neurology*. 1998;**51**:1768–1769.
10. Kattah JC, Mejico L, Chrousos GA, Zimmerman LE, Manz HJ. Pathologic findings in a steroid-responsive optic nerve infarct in giant-cell arteritis. *Neurology*. 1999;**53**:177–180.
11. Liozon E, Herrmann F, Ly K, et al. Risk factors for visual loss in giant cell (temporal) arteritis: a prospective study of 174 patients. *Am J Med*. 2001;**111**:211–217.
12. Kansu T, Corbett JJ, Savino P, Schatz NJ. Giant cell arteritis with normal sedimentation rate. *Arch Neurol*. 1977;**34**:624–625.
13. Neish PR, Sergent JS. Giant cell arteritis. A case with unusual neurologic manifestations and a normal sedimentation rate. *Arch Intern Med*. 1991;**151**:378–380.
14. Hayreh SS, Podhajsky PA, Zimmerman B. Occult giant cell arteritis: ocular manifestations. *Am J Ophthalmol*. 1998;**125**:521–526.
15. Gonzalez-Gay MA, Lopez-Diaz MJ, Barros S, et al. Giant cell arteritis: laboratory tests at the time of diagnosis in a series of 240 patients. *Medicine (Baltimore)*. 2005;**84**:277–290.
16. Moritani T, Hiwatashi A, Shrier DA, Wang HZ, Numaguchi Y, Westesson PL. CNS vasculitis and vasculopathy: efficacy and usefulness of diffusion-weighted echoplanar MR imaging. *Clin Imaging*. 2004;**28**:261–270.
17. Reinhard M, Schmidt D, Schumacher M, Hetzel A. Involvement of the vertebral arteries in giant cell arteritis mimicking vertebral dissection. *J Neurol*. 2003;**250**:1006–1009.
18. Joelson E, Ruthrauff B, Ali F, Lindeman N, Sharp FR. Multifocal dural enhancement associated with temporal arteritis. *Arch Neurol*. 2000;**57**:119–122.
19. Poller DN, van Wik Q, Jeffrey MJ. The importance of skip lesions in temporal arteritis. *J Clin Pathol*. 2000;**53**:137–139.
20. Chakrabarty A, Franks AJ. Temporal artery biopsy: is there any value in examining biopsies at multiple levels? *J Clin Pathol*. 2000;**53**:131–136.
21. Powers JF, Bedri S, Hussein S, Salomon RN, Tischler AS. High prevalence of herpes simplex virus DNA in temporal arteritis biopsy specimens. *Am J Clin Pathol*. 2005;**123**:261–264.
22. Nordborg C, Nordborg E, Petursdottir V, et al. Search for varicella zoster virus in giant cell arteritis. *Ann Neurol*. 1998;**44**:413–414.
23. Ferro JM. Vasculitis of the central nervous system. *J Neurol*. 1998;**245**:766–776.
24. Jover JA, Hernandez-Garcia C, Morado IC, Vargas E, Banares A, Fernandez-Gutierrez B. Combined treatment of giant-cell arteritis with methotrexate and prednisone. A randomized, double-blind, placebo-controlled trial. *Ann Intern Med*. 2001;**134**:106–114.
25. Hoffman GS, Cid MC, Hellmann DB, Guillevin L, Stone JH, Schousboe J. A multicenter, randomized, double-blind, placebo-controlled trial of adjuvant methotrexate treatment for giant cell arteritis. *Arthritis Rheum*. 2002;**46**:1309–1318.
26. Staunton H, Stafford F, Leader M, O'Riordan D. Deterioration of giant cell arteritis with corticosteroid therapy. *Arch Neurol*. 2000;**57**:581–584.

27. Collazos J, Garcia-Monco C, Martin A, Rodriguez J, Gomez MA. Multiple strokes after initiation of steroid therapy in giant cell arteritis. *Postgrad Med J*. 1994;**70**:228–230.

28. Lupi-Herrera E, Sanchez-Torres G, Marcushamer J, Mispireta J, Horwitz S, Vela JE. Takayasu's arteritis. Clinical study of 107 cases. *Am Heart J*. 1977;**93**:94–103.

29. Hall S, Barr W, Lie JT, Stanson AW, Kazmier FJ, Hunder GG. Takayasu arteritis. A study of 32 North American patients. *Medicine*. 1985;**64**:89–99.

30. Ringleb PA, Strittmatter EI, Loewer M, et al. Cerebrovascular manifestations of Takayasu arteritis in Europe. *Rheumatology (Oxford)*. 2005;**44**:1012–1015.

31. Kerr GS, Hallahan CW, Giordano J, et al. Takayasu arteritis. *Ann Intern Med*. 1994;**120**:919–929.

32. Nakao K, Ikeda M, Kimata S, et al. Takayasu's arteritis – clinical report of eighty-four cases and immunological studies of seven cases. *Circulation*. 1967;**35**:1141–1155.

33. Takei M, Sasaki Y, Suyama K, et al. Surgically treated case of complete obstruction of the left main coronary artery caused by Takayasu's arteritis. *Am Heart J*. 1993;**126**:458–459.

34. Kim HJ, Suh DC, Kim JK, et al. Correlation of neurological manifestations of Takayasu's arteritis with cerebral angiographic findings. *Clin Imaging*. 2005;**29**:79–85.

35. Yamato M, Lecky JW, Hiramatsu K, Kohda E. Takayasu arteritis: radiographic and angiographic findings in 59 patients. *Radiology*. 1986;**161**:329–334.

36. Hoffmann M, Corr P, Robbs J. Cerebrovascular findings in Takayasu disease. *J Neuroimaging*. 2000;**10**:84–90.

37. Kumral E, Evyapan D, Aksu K, Keser G, Kabasakal Y, Balkir K. Microembolus detection in patients with Takayasu's arteritis. *Stroke*. 2002;**33**:712–716.

38. Filer A, Nicholls D, Corston R, Carey P, Bacon P. Takayasu arteritis and atherosclerosis: illustrating the consequences of endothelial damage. *J Rheumatol*. 2001;**28**:2752–2753.

39. Giordano JM. Surgical treatment of Takayasu's arteritis. *Int J Cardiol*. 2000;**75**(Suppl 1):S123–S128.

40. Stone JH. Polyarteritis nodosa. *JAMA*. 2002;**288**:1632–16339.

41. Ford RG, Siekert RG. Central nervous system manifestations of periarteritis nodosa. *Neurology*. 1965;**15**:114–122.

42. Iaconetta G, Benvenuti D, Lamaida E, Gallicchio B, Signorelli F, Maiuri F. Cerebral hemorrhagic complication in polyarteritis nodosa. Case report and review of the literature. *Acta Neurol (Napoli)*. 1994;**16**:64–69.

43. Semmo AN, Baumert TF, Kreisel W. Severe cerebral vasculitis as primary manifestation of hepatitis B-associated polyarteritis nodosa. *J Hepatol*. 2002;**37**:414–416.

44. Reichart MD, Bogousslavsky J, Janzer RC. Early lacunar strokes complicating polyarteritis nodosa: thrombotic microangiopathy. *Neurology*. 2000;**54**:883–889.

45. De Reuck J. Dorsal thalamic haemorrhage complicating polyarteritis nodosa: a clinico-pathologic case report. *Acta Neurol Belg*. 2003;**103**:40–42.

46. Kasantikul V, Suwanwela N, Pongsabutr S. Magnetic resonance images of brain stem infarct in periarteritis nodosa. *Surg Neurol*. 1991;**36**:133–136.

47. Provenzale JM, Allen NB. Neuroradiologic findings in polyarteritis nodosa. *AJNR Am J Neuroradiol*. 1996;**17**:1119–1126.

48. Scully RE, Mark EJ, McNeely BU. Case records of the Massachusetts General Hospital: Case 43–1986. *N Engl J Med*. 1986;**315**:1143–1154.

49. Bert RJ, Antonacci VP, Berman L, Melhem ER. Polyarteritis nodosa presenting as temporal arteritis in a 9-year-old child. *AJNR Am J Neuroradiol*. 1999;**20**:167–171.

50. Picard O, Brunereau L, Pelosse B, Kerob D, Cabane J, Imbert JC. Cerebral infarction associated with vasculitis due to varicella zoster virus in patients infected with the human immunodeficiency virus. *Biomed Pharmacother*. 1997;**51**:449–454.

51. Guillevin L, Lhote F. Treatment of polyarteritis nodosa and microscopic polyangiitis. *Arthrit Rheumat*. 1998;**41**:2100–2105.

52. Lam KC, Lai CL, Trepo C, Wu PC. Deleterious effects of prednisolone in hepatitis B surface antigen-positive chronic active hepatitis. *N Engl J Med*. 1981;**304**:380–386.

53. Calabrese LH, Mallek JA. Primary angiitis of the central nervous system. Report of 8 new cases, review of the literature, and proposal for diagnostic criteria. *Medicine*. 1987;**67**:20–38.

54. Lanthier S, Lortie A, Michaud J, Laxer R, Jay V, deVeber G. Isolated angitis of the CNS in children. *Neurology*. 2001;**56**:837–842.

55. LaMancusa J, Steiman G. Suspected isolated angiitis causing stroke in a child. *Stroke*. 1990;**21**:1380.

56. Cupps TR, Moore PM, Fauci AS. Isolated angiitis of the central nervous system – prospective diagnostic and therapeutic experience. *Am J Med*. 1983;**74**:97–105.

57. Craven RS, French JK. Isolated angiitis of the central nervous system. *Ann Neurol*. 1985;**18**:263–265.

58. Barron TF, Ostrov BE, Zimmerman RA, Packer RJ. Isolated angiitis of CNS: treatment with pulse cyclophosphamide. *Pediatr Neurol*. 1993;**9**:73–75.

59. Abu-Shakra M, Khraishi M, Grosman H, Lewtas J, Cividino A, Keystone EC. Primary angiitis of the CNS diagnosed by angiography. *Q J Med*. 1994;**87**:351–358.

60. Birnbaum J, Hellmann DB. Primary angiitis of the central nervous system. *Arch Neurol*. 2009;**66**:704–709.

61. Nadeau SE. Neurologic manifestations of systemic vasculitis. *Neurol Clin*. 2002;**20**:123–150.

62. Bares M, Muchova M, Dufek M, Litzman J, Krupa P, Rektor I. Wegener's granulomatosis: ischemic stroke as the first clinical manifestation (case study). *J Neurol*. 2002;**249**:1593–1594.

63. Drachman DA. Neurological complications of Wegener's granulomatosis. *Arch Neurol*. 1963;**8**:145.

64. Nishino H, Rubino FA, Deremee RA, Swanson JW, Parissi JE. Neurological involvement in Wegener's granulomatosis: an analysis of 324 consecutive patients at the Mayo Clinic. *Ann Neurol*. 1993;**33**:4–9.

65. Satoh J, Miyasaka N, Yamada T, et al. Extensive cerebral infarction due to involvement of both anterior cerebral arteries by Wegener's granulomatosis. *Ann Rheum Dis*. 1988;**47**:606–611.

66. Savitz JM, Young MA, Ratan RR. Basilar artery occlusion in a young patient with Wegener's granulomatosis. *Stroke*. 1994;**25**:214–216.

67. Scully RE, Mark EJ, McNeely WF, Ebeling SH. Case records of the Massachusetts General Hospital. Weekly clinicopathological exercises. Case 9–1999. *N Engl J Med*. 1999;**340**:945–953.

68. Jennette JC, Falk RJ. Small-vessel vasculitis. *N Engl J Med*. 1997;**337**:1512–1523.

69. Fienberg R, Mark EJ, Goodman M, McCluskey RT, Niles JL. Correlation of antineutrophil cytoplasmic antibodies with the extrarenal histopathology of Wegener's (pathergic) granulomatosis and related forms of vasculitis. *Human Pathol*. 1993;**24**:160–168.

70. Granziera C, Michel P, Rossetti AO, Lurati F, Reymond S, Bogousslavsky J. Wegener granulomatosis presenting with haemorrhagic stroke in a young adult. *J Neurol*. 2005;**252**:615–616.

71. Murphy JM, Gomez-Anson B, Gillard JH, et al. Wegener granulomatosis: MR imaging findings in brain and meninges. *Radiology*. 1999;**213**:794–799.

72. Jayne DR, Esnault VL, Lockwood CM. ANCA anti-idiotype antibodies and the treatment of systemic vasculitis with intravenous immunoglobulin. *J Autoimmunity*. 1993;**6**:207–219.

73. Fieschi C, Rasura M, Anzini A, Beccia M. Central nervous system vasculitis. *J Neurol Sci*. 1998;**153**:159–171.

74. Rauta V, Tornroth T, Gronhagen-Riska C. Henoch-Schoenlein nephritis in adults-clinical features and outcomes in Finnish patients. *Clin Nephrol*. 2002;**58**:1–8.

75. Aita JA. Neurologic manifestations of Henoch-Schonlein purpura. *Nebraska Med J*. 1973;**58**:37.

76. Belman AL, Leicher CR, Moshe SL, Mezey AP. Neurologic manifestations of Schonlein-Henoch purpura: report of three cases and review of the literature. *Pediatrics*. 1985;**75**:687–692.

77. Clark JH, Fitzgerald JF. Hemorrhagic complications of Henoch-Schonlein syndrome. *J Pediatr Gastroent Nutr*. 1985;**4**:311–315.

78. Lewis IC, Philpott MG. Neurological complications in the Schonlein-Henoch syndrome. *Arch Dis Child*. 1956;**31**:369–371.

79. Chiaretti A, Caresta E, Piastra M, Pulitano S, Di RC. Cerebral hemorrhage in Henoch-Schoenlein syndrome. *Childs Nerv Syst*. 2002;**18**:365–367.

80. Giangiacomo J, Tsai CC. Dermal and glomerular deposition of IgA in anaphylactoid purpura. *Am J Dis Child*. 1977;**131**:981–983.

81. Younger DS. Vasculitis of the nervous system. *Curr Opin Neurol*. 2004;**17**:317–336.

82. Solling J. Circulating immune complexes in glomerulonephritis: a longitudinal study. *Clin Nephrol*. 1983;**20**:177–189.

83. Chen TC, Chung FR, Lee CH, Huang SC, Chen JB, Hsu KT. Successful treatment of crescentic glomerulonephritis associated with adult-onset Henoch-Schoenlein purpura by double-filtration plasmapheresis. *Clin Nephrol*. 2004;**61**:213–216.

84. Davenport J, Hart RG. Prosthetic valve endocarditis 1976–1987. Antibiotics, anticoagulation, and stroke. *Stroke*. 1990;**21**:993–999.

85. Ahuja GH, Jain N, Vijayaraghavan M, Roy S. Cerebral mycotic aneurysm of fungal origin. *J Neurosurg*. 1978;**49**:107–110.

86. Barrow DL, Prats AR. Infectious intracranial aneurysms: comparison of groups with and without endocarditis. *Neurosurgery*. 1990;**27**:562–573.

87. Hart RG, Foster JW, Luther MF, Kanter MC. Stroke in infective endocarditis. *Stroke*. 1990;**21**:695–700.

88. Griesemer DA, Barton LL, Reese CM, et al. Amebic meningoencephalitis caused by Balamuthia mandrillaris. *Pediatr Neurol*. 1994;**10**:249–254.

89. Riela AR, Roach ES. Choreoathetosis in an infant with tuberculous meningitis. *Arch Neurol*. 1982;**39**:596.

90. Pfister HW, Borasio GD, Dirnagl U, Bauer M, Einhaupl KM. Cerebrovascular complications of bacterial meningitis in adults. *Neurology*. 1992;**42**:1497–1505.

91. Snyder RD, Stovring J, Cushing AH, Davis LE, Hardy TL. Cerebral infarction in childhood bacterial meningitis. *J Neurol Neurosurg Psychiatry*. 1981;**44**:581–585.

92. Poltera AA. Vascular lesions in intracranial tuberculosis. *Path Microbiol*. 1975;**43**:192–194.

93. Kingsley DPE, Hendrickse WA, Kendall BE, Swash M, Singh V. Tuberculous meningitis: role of CT in management and prognosis. *J Neurol Neurosurg Psychiatry*. 1987;**50**:30–36.

94. Leiguarda R, Berthier M, Starkstein S, Nogues M, Lylyk P. Ischemic infarction in 25 children with tuberculous meningitis. *Stroke*. 1988;**19**:200–204.

95. Schoeman JF, Van Zyl LE, Laubscher JA, Donald PR. Serial CT scanning in childhood tuberculous meningitis: prognostic features in 198 cases. *J Child Neurol*. 1995;**10**:320–329.

96. Hsieh F-Y, Chia L-G, Shen W-C. Locations of cerebral infarctions in tuberculous meningitis. *Neurorad*. 1992;**34**:197–199.

97. Hilt DC, Buchholz D, Krumholz A, Weiss H, Wolinsky JS. Herpes zoster ophthalmicus and delayed contralateral hemiparesis caused by cerebral angiitis: diagnosis and management approaches. *Ann Neurol*. 1983;**14**:543–553.

98. Elble RJ. Intracerebral hemorrhage with herpes zoster ophthalmicus. *Ann Neurol*. 1983;**14**:591–592.

99. Hall S, Carlin L, Roach ES, McLean WT. Herpes zoster and central retinal artery occlusion. *Ann Neurol*. 1983;**13**:217.

100. Russman AN, Lederman RJ, Calabrese LH, Embi PJ, Forghani B, Gilden DH. Multifocal varicella-zoster virus vasculopathy without rash. *Arch Neurol*. 2003;**60**:1607–1609.

101. Doyle PW, Gibson G, Dolman CL. Herpes zoster ophthalmicus with contralateral hemiplegia: identification of cause. *Ann Neurol*. 1983;**14**:84–85.

102. Bodensteiner JB, Hille MR, Riggs JE. Clinical features of vascular thrombosis following varicella. *Am J Dis Child*. 1992;**146**:100–102.

103. Kamholz J, Tremblay G. Chickenpox with delayed contralateral hemiparesis caused by cerebral angiitis. *Ann Neurol*. 1985;**18**:358–360.

104. Sebire G, Meyer L, Chabrier S. Varicella as a risk factor for cerebral infarction in childhood: a case-control study. *Ann Neurol*. 1999;**45**:679–680.

105. Askalan R, Laughlin S, Mayank S, et al. Chickenpox and stroke in childhood. A study of frequency and causation. *Stroke*. 2001;**32**:1257–1262.

106. Caruso JM, Tung GA, Brown WD. Central nervous system and renal vasculitis associated with primary varicella infection in a child. *Pediatrics*. 2001;**107**:E9.

107. Kovacs SO, Kuban K, Strand R. Lateral medullary syndrome following varicella infection. *Am J Dis Child*. 1993;**147**:823–825.

108. Qureshi AI, Janssen RS, Karon JM, et al. Human immunodeficiency virus infection and stroke in young patients. *Arch Neurol*. 1997;**54**:1150–1153.

109. Evers S, Nabavi D, Rahmann A, Heese C, Reichelt D, Husstedt IW. Ischaemic cerebrovascular events in HIV infection: a cohort study. *Cerebrovasc Dis*. 2003;**15**:199–205.

110. Park YD, Belman AL, Kim TS, et al. Stroke in pediatric acquired immunodeficiency syndrome. *Ann Neurol*. 1990;**28**:303–311.

111. Nogueras C, Sala M, Sasal M, et al. Recurrent stroke as a manifestation of primary angiitis of the central nervous system in a patient infected with human immunodeficiency virus. *Arch Neurol*. 2002;**59**:468–473.

112. Husson RN, Saini R, Lewis LL, Butler KM, Patronas N, Pizzo PA. Cerebral artery aneurysms in children infected with human immunodeficiency virus. *J Pediatr*. 1992;**121**:927–930.

113. Crevits L, Van Dyke A, Vanhee F, Crevits JH. Carotid artery aneurysm in human immunodeficiency virus infection. *Clin Neurol Neurosurg*. 2005;**107**:404–407.

114. Brightbill TC, Ihmeidan IH, Post MJ, Berger JR, Katz DA. Neurosyphilis in HIV-positive and HIV-negative patients: neuroimaging findings. *AJNR Am J Neuroradiol*. 1995;**16**:703–711.

115. Burns DK. The neuropathology of pediatric acquired immunodeficiency syndrome. *J Child Neurol*. 1992;**7**:332–346.

116. Tyler KL, Sandberg E, Baum KF. Medial medullary syndrome and meningovascular syphilis: a case report in an HIV-infected man and a review of the literature. *Neurology*. 1994;**44**:2231–2235.

117. Timmermans M, Carr J. Neurosyphilis in the modern era. *J Neurol Neurosurg Psychiatry*. 2004;**75**:1727–1730.

118. Nakane H, Okada Y, Ibayashi S, Sadoshima S, Fujishima M. Brain infarction caused by syphilitic aortic aneurysm. A case report. *Angiology*. 1996;**47**:911–917.

119. Flint AC, Liberato BB, Anziska Y, Schantz-Dunn J, Wright CB. Meningovascular syphilis as a cause of basilar artery stenosis. *Neurology*. 2005;**64**:391–392.

120. Solis ST, Ebright JR. Stroke in a young woman with a history of gonorrhea. *Hosp Pract (Off Ed)*. 1996;**31**:140–142.

121. Umashankar G, Gupta V, Harik SI. Acute bilateral inferior cerebellar infarction in a patient with neurosyphilis. *Arch Neurol.* 2004;**61**:953–956.

122. Simon RP. Neurosyphilis. *Arch Neurol.* 1985;**42**:606–613.

123. Landi G, Villani F, Anzalone N. Variable angiographic findings in patients with stroke and neurosyphilis. *Stroke.* 1990;**21**:333–338.

124. Beal MF, O'Carroll CP, Kleinman GM, Grossman RI. Aspergillosis of the nervous system. *Neurology.* 1982;**32**:473–479.

125. Walsh TJ, Hier DB, Caplan LR. Aspergillosis of the central nervous system: clinicopathological analysis of 17 patients. *Ann Neurol.* 1985;**18**:574–582.

126. Iihara K, Makita Y, Nabeshima S, Tei T, Keyaki A, Nioka H. Aspergillosis of the central nervous system causing subarachnoid hemorrhage from mycotic aneurysm of the basilar artery – case report. *Neurol Med Chir (Tokyo).* 1990;**30**:618–623.

127. Chou SM, Chong YY, Kinkel R. A proposed pathogenetic process in the formation of Aspergillus mycotic aneurysm in the central nervous system. *Ann Acad Med Singapore.* 1993;**22**:518–525.

128. Carrazana EJ, Rossitch E Jr, Morris J. Isolated central nervous system aspergillosis in the acquired immunodeficiency syndrome. *Clin Neurol Neurosurg.* 1991;**93**:227–230.

129. Eucker J, Sezer O, Lehmann R, et al. Disseminated mucormycosis caused by Absidia corymbifera leading to cerebral vasculitis. *Infection.* 2000;**28**:246–250.

130. Seijo MM, Grandes IJ, Sanchez HJ, Garcia-Monco JC. Spontaneous brain hemorrhage associated with Lyme neuroborreliosis. *Neurologia.* 2001;**16**:43–45.

131. Defer G, Levy R, Brugieres P, Postic D, Degos JD. Lyme disease presenting as a stroke in the vertebrobasilar territory: MRI. *Neurorad.* 1993;**35**:529–531.

132. Brogan GX, Homan CS, Viccellio P. The enlarging clinical spectrum of Lyme disease: Lyme cerebral vasculitis, a new disease entity. *Ann Emerg Med.* 1990;**19**:572–576.

133. Hammers-Berggren S, Grondahl A, Karlsson M, von AM, Carlsson A, Stiernstedt G. Screening for neuroborreliosis in patients with stroke. *Stroke.* 1993;**24**:1393–1396.

134. Esdaile JM, Abrahamowicz M, Grodzicky T, et al. Traditional Framingham risk factors fail to fully account for accelerated atherosclerosis in systemic lupus erythematosus. *Arthritis Rheum.* 2001;**44**:2331–2337.

135. Appenzeller S, Cendes F, Costallat LTL. Epileptic seizures in systemic lupus erythematosis. *Neurology.* 2004;**63**:1808–1812.

136. Krishnan E. Stroke subtypes among young patients with systemic lupus erythematosus. *Am J Med.* 2005;**118**:1415.

137. Cervera R, Piette JC, Font J, et al. Antiphospholipid syndrome: clinical and immunologic manifestations and patterns of disease expression in a cohort of 1,000 patients. *Arthritis Rheum.* 2002;**46**:1019–1027.

138. Toloza SM, Uribe AG, McGwin G Jr, et al. Systemic lupus erythematosus in a multiethnic US cohort (LUMINA). XXIII. Baseline predictors of vascular events. *Arthritis Rheum.* 2004;**50**:3947–3957.

139. Jennings JE, Sundgren PC, Attwood J, McCune J, Maly P. Value of MRI of the brain in patients with systemic lupus erythematosis and neurologic disturbance. *Neurorad.* 2004;**46**:15–21.

140. Lampropoulos CE, Koutroumanidis M, Reynolds PPM, Manidakis I, Hughes GRV, D'Cruz DP. Electroencephalography in the assessment of neuropsychiatric manifestations in antiphospholipid syndrome and systemic lupus erythematosis. *Arthrit Rheumat.* 2005;**52**:841–846.

141. Lewis MA, Priestley BL. Transient neonatal Behçet's disease. *Arch Dis Child.* 1986;**61**:805–806.

142. Kone I, Berbis P, Palix C, Bernard JL. Familial Behçet's disease in children. A report of 3 cases (letter). *Clin Exp Rheumatol.* 1992;**10**:627–628.

143. Serdaroglu P. Behçet's disease and the nervous system. *J Neurol.* 1998;**245**:197–205.

144. Yazici H, Tuzun Y, Pazarli H, et al. Influence of age of onset and patient's sex on the prevalence and severity of manifestations of Behçet's syndrome. *Ann Rheum Dis.* 1984;**43**:783–789.

145. Haghighi AB, Pourmand R, Nikseresht AR. Neuro-Behçet disease. A review. *Neurologist.* 2005;**11**:80–89.

146. Silva A, Altintas A, Sap S. Behçet's syndrome and the nervous system. *Curr Opin Neurol.* 2004;**17**:347–357.

147. Krespi Y, Akman-Demir G, Poyraz M, et al. Cerebral vasculitis and ischaemic stroke in Behçet's disease: report of one case and review of the literature. *Eur J Neurol.* 2001;**8**:719–722.

148. Akman-Demir G, Serdaroglu A. Clinical patterns of neurological involvement in Behçet's disease: a study of 200 cases. *Brain.* 1999;**122**:2171–2181.

149. Kerr JS, Roach ES, Sinal SH, McWhorter JM. Intracranial arterial aneurysms complicating Behçet's disease. *J Child Neurol.* 1989;**4**:147–149.

150. Bahar S, Coban O, Gurvit H, Akman-Demir G, Gokyigit A. Spontaneous dissection of the extracranial vertebral artery with spinal subarachnoid hemorrhage in a patient with Behçet's disease. *Neuroradiology.* 1993;**35**:352–354.

151. Stern JM, Kesler SM. Raised intracranial pressure in a 16-year-old boy. Report of a case of Behçet's disease. *S African Med J.* 1989;**75**:243–244.

152. Wechsler B, Vidailhet M, Piette JC, et al. Cerebral venous thrombosis in Behçet's disease: clinical study and long-term follow-up of 25 cases. *Neurology.* 1992;**42**:614–618.

153. Sakane T, Takeno M, Suzuke N, Inaba G. Behçet's disease. *N Engl J Med.* 1999;**341**:1284–1291.

154. Espinosa G, Font J, Tassies D, et al. Vascular involvement in Behçet's disease: relation with thrombophilic factors, coagulation activation, and thrombomodulin. *Am J Med.* 2002;**112**:37–43.

155. Banna M, el-Ramahl K. Neurologic involvement in Behçet disease: imaging findings in 16 patients. *AJNR Am J Neuroradiol.* 1991;**12**:791–796.

156. Morrissey SP, Miller DH, Hermaszewski R, et al. Magnetic resonance imaging of the central nervous system in Behçet's disease. *Eur Neurol.* 1993;**33**:287–293.

157. Ramos M, Mandybur TI. Cerebral vasculitis in rheumatoid arthritis. *Arch Neurol.* 1975;**32**:271–275.

158. Chowdhry V, Kumar N, Lachance DH, Salomao DR, Luthra HS. An unusual presentation of rheumatoid meningitis. *J Neuroimaging.* 2005;**15**:286–288.

159. Graf WD, Milstein JM, Sherry DD. Stroke and mixed connective tissue disease. *J Child Neurol.* 1993;**8**:256–259.

160. Koh MS, Goh KY, Chen C, Howe HS. Cerebral infarct mimicking glioma in Sjögren's syndrome. *Hong Kong Med J.* 2002;**8**:292–294.

161. Nagahiro S, Mantani A, Yamada K, Ushio Y. Multiple cerebral arterial occlusions in a young patient with Sjögren's syndrome: case report. *Neurosurgery.* 1996;**38**:592–595.

162. Jimenez C, Rowe PC, Keene D. Cardiac and central nervous system vasculitis in a child with dermatomyositis. *J Child Neurol.* 1994;**9**:297–300.

163. Lucivero V, Mezzapesa DM, Petruzzellis M, Carella A, Lamberti P, Federico F. Ischemic stroke in progressive systemic sclerosis. *Neurol Sci.* 2004;**25**:230–233.

164. Kanzato N, Matsuzaki T, Komine Y, Saito M, Yoshio T, Suehara M. Localized scleroderma associated with progressing ischemic stroke. *J Neurol Sci.* 1999;**163**:86–89.

165. Alarcon F, Vanormelingen K, Moncayo J, Vinan I. Cerebral cysticercosis as a risk factor for stroke in young and middle-aged people. *Stroke.* 1992;**23**:1563–1565.

166. Barinagarrementeria F, Del Brutto OH. Lacunar syndrome due to neurocysticercosis. *Arch Neurol.* 1989;**46**:415–417.

167. Alarcon F, Hidalgo F, Moncayo J, Vinan I, Duenas G. Cerebral cysticercosis and stroke. *Stroke.* 1992;**23**:224–228.

168. Azad R, Gupta RK, Kumar S, et al. Is neurocysticercosis a risk factor in coexistent intracranial disease? An MRI based study. *J Neurol Neurosurg Psychiatry.* 2003;**74**:359–361.

169. Kobayashi M, Nishikimi N, Komori K. Current pathological and clinical aspects of Buerger's disease in Japan. *Ann Vasc Surg.* 2006;**20**:148–156.

170. Biller J, Asconape J, Challa VR, Toole JF, McLean WT. A case for cerebral thromboangiitis obliterans. *Stroke.* 1981;**12**:686–689.

171. Lie JT. Visceral intestinal Buerger's disease. *Int J Cardiol.* 1998;**66**(Suppl 1):S249–S256.

172. Inzelberg R, Bornstein NM, Korczyn AD. Cerebrovascular symptoms in thromboangiitis obliterans. *Acta Neurol Scand.* 1989;**80**:347–350.

173. No YJ, Lee EM, Lee DH, Kim JS. Cerebral angiographic findings in thromboangiitis obliterans. *Neurorad.* 2005;**47**:912–915.

174. Drake ME Jr. Winiwarter-Buerger disease ('thromboangiitis obliterans') with cerebral involvement. *JAMA.* 1982;**248**:1870–1872.

175. Shionoya S. Diagnostic criteria of Buerger's disease. *Int J Cardiol.* 1998;**66**(Suppl 1):S243–S245.

176. Matchev S, Petrov V, Batchvarova V, Maljakova A, Doneva S. Transcranial Doppler velocities in patients with thromboangiitis obliterans. *Angiology.* 1997;**48**:535–544.

177. Mills JL Sr. Buerger's disease in the 21st century: diagnosis, clinical features, and therapy. *Semin Vasc Surg.* 2003;**16**:179–189.

178. Kurata A, Franke FE, Machinami R, Schulz A. Thromboangiitis obliterans: classic and new morphological features. *Virchows Arch.* 2000;**436**:59–67.

179. Eichhorn J, Sima D, Lindschau C, et al. Antiendothelial cell antibodies in thromboangiitis obliterans. *Am J Med Sci.* 1998;**315**:17–23.

180. Sasaki S, Sakuma M, Yasuda K. Current status of thromboangiitis obliterans (Buerger's disease) in Japan. *Int J Cardiol.* 2000;**75**(Suppl 1):S175–S181.

181. Lau H, Cheng SW. Buerger's disease in Hong Kong: a review of 89 cases. *Aust NZ J Surg.* 1997;**67**:264–269.

182. Bozkurt AK, Koksal C, Demirbas MY, et al. A randomized trial of intravenous iloprost (a stable prostacyclin analogue) versus lumbar sympathectomy in the management of Buerger's disease. *Int Angiol.* 2006;**25**:162–168.

183. Nakajima N. The change in concept and surgical treatment on Buerger's disease – personal experience and review. *Int J Cardiol.* 1998;**66**(Suppl 1):S273–S280.

11

Hematological Disorders and Hypercoagulable States

Careful investigation of the blood proves that, in addition to the usual elements, there exist pale granular masses, which on closer inspection present a corpuscular appearance. In size they vary greatly from half or a quarter that of a white blood-corpuscle, to enormous masses. They have a compact look . . . while in specimens examined without any reagents the filaments of fibrin adhere to them.

William Osler
Description of platelets

Blood is a mobile organ that has evolved over the eons for efficient transportation of oxygen and nutrients to all the cells in the body. Its many properties and its contents can have such far-reaching effects on neuronal function that the brain microcirculation has developed a barrier for selective interchange between blood and brain. The blood serves to distribute nutrients to the brain while removing by-products of metabolism. In this regard, the brain is unique because of an interposed blood-brain barrier to free metabolic exchange that preserves homeostasis by keeping the microenvironment surrounding the neurons very carefully controlled. Not surprisingly, disruption of this finely balanced system in either direction can lead to cerebrovascular compromise.

Aberrations of hematologic function generate cerebrovascular complications of different types and via various mechanisms. Hemoglobinopathies, for example, cause both large vessel vasculopathy and small vessel occlusion and can promote either infarction or hemorrhage. Similarly, severe thrombocytopenia is a risk factor for intracerebral hemorrhage, and thrombocytosis (thrombocythemia) may lead to microvascular occlusion. Depending on which aspect of the process is disturbed, coagulation abnormalities can promote either thrombosis or hemorrhage. To complicate things further, many hematological abnormalities remain quiescent unless they occur in tandem with other risk factors. In this chapter we will review some of the major hematological abnormalities that play a role in cerebrovascular disease.

HEMOGLOBIN DISORDERS

Sickle cell disease (SCD) is an autosomal recessive condition first described by James B. Herrick in 1910.[1] Sickle cell disease results from a single amino acid substitution of valine for glutamic acid in the beta hemoglobin chain. About 8% to 10% of African Americans carry the gene for SCD, and roughly one in 500 have the disease. SCD occurs in other populations whose ancestors originated in sub-Saharan Africa, including persons in Cuba, Saudi Arabia, India, Turkey, Greece, and Italy, among others. SCD is more common than other hemoglobinopathies but also more likely to cause an ischemic or hemorrhagic stroke than the other hemoglobinopathies.[2]

Pathophysiology of Stroke Due to SCD

SCD promotes multiple forms of cerebrovascular disease. The large arteries, in particular the distal internal carotids, develop progressive endothelial proliferation and fibrosis, eventually producing significant distal hemodynamic effects (Figure 11-1).[3] How SCD leads to large vessel stenosis is debated, but some practitioners suspect that it may result from occlusion of the vasa vasorum by abnormal red blood cells. Large infarctions result from progressive occlusion of the large arteries. Some individuals develop progressive stenosis of the distal intracranial internal carotid arteries with distal collateral vessels, or moyamoya syndrome (see Chapter 13). Watershed infarctions are less common than large vessel occlusions, but both types of stroke trace their origins to large artery disease.[4] Additionally, small cerebral vessels may be obstructed by abnormal red blood cells. Whether a large or small vessel is involved, the individual with SCD has decreased perfusion reserve because of the often severe anemia and abnormal hemoglobin.

Occasional people have a mild phenotype, living into late adulthood with relatively few clinical manifestations of SCD. Many of these individuals persist in making an unusual amount of fetal hemoglobin, which is unaffected by the SCD mutation. Individuals with SCD in some families are more likely to have a stroke than affected individuals in other families, which suggests that there might be additional genetic risk factors that influence the risk of stroke due to SCD.[5] In all probability, this shift in the stroke risk results from an interplay between several different genes that influence cell adhesion, coagulation, and vascular response to injury.[6]

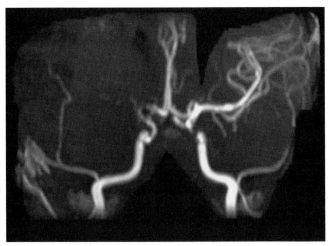

Figure 11-1. Magnetic resonance angiogram from an individual with sickle cell disease reveals right internal carotid artery occlusion with nonvisualization of the right middle cerebral artery. The left internal carotid artery is stenotic but less severely affected. Photograph courtesy of Dr. Geoffrey Heyer.

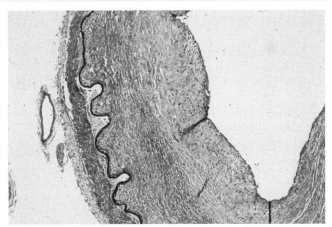

Figure 11-2. Section from the proximal middle cerebral artery of an individual with sickle cell disease. Note the asymmetrical endothelial and subendothelial hyperplasia. Reprinted with permission from Riela and Roach.[217]

Clinical Features of SCD

Aside from the potential occurrence of systemic SCD complications (e.g., severe pain, priapism, or chest syndrome) at the time of the stroke, there is nothing unique about the clinical manifestations of stroke due to SCD. The internal carotid arteries and its branches bear the brunt of the disease (Figure 11-2), and stroke more often occurs in the anterior circulation. The middle cerebral artery territory is more often affected than the anterior cerebral or posterior cerebral artery territories. Small infarctions, many of them clinically silent, may occur anywhere in the brain or spinal cord.[7]

Although most strokes due to SCD are ischemic, some individuals develop intraparenchymal or subarachnoid hemorrhage. A substantial number of these patients are found to have underlying structural vascular lesions, so it is appropriate to do a thorough evaluation for causes of hemorrhage in addition to the SCD.[8,9]

Occasionally, individuals with SCD may develop intracranial sinovenous thrombosis or a spinal cord infarction.[10] Subarachnoid and intracerebral hemorrhages also occur in the context of intracranial sinovenous thrombosis as well as after rupture of an intracranial aneurysm. Some intraparenchymal hemorrhages represent hemorrhagic conversion of an infarction.

Patients with a time-averaged mean blood flow velocity of 200 cm/second or more on transcranial Doppler (TCD) have an estimated 10% annual stroke risk.[11–13] Other predictors of stroke due to SCD include low hemoglobin levels, high white blood cell count, systemic hypertension, earlier silent brain infarction, and history of chest crisis.[2]

Management of SCD

Recently published recommendations for the management of the cerebrovascular complications of SCD are summarized in Table 11-1. Individuals with an acute ischemic stroke should be optimally hydrated, and hypoxemia and arterial hypotension should be corrected.[8] Periodic transfusions limit the production of sickle hemoglobin and dramatically reduce the likelihood of ischemic stroke, but transfusions also subject the patient to the danger of hepatic and cardiac damage from iron overload if effective chelation is not maintained. Because of the high rate of additional strokes, regular transfusions to reduce the level of sickle hemoglobin below 30% have been used for many years following the first stroke due to SCD.[14] More recently, similar transfusion regimens have been recommended as primary prevention for individuals whose TCD findings indicate a similarly high stroke risk due to SCD.[11,15] Unfortunately, cessation of the transfusions results in a return to the higher risk level.[12,16,17] There is some evidence that shifting to less frequent transfusions might lower the risk of iron overload while still offering some stroke protection.[18] It is unclear whether transfusions reduce the risk of hemorrhage due to SCD.

Chronic administration of hydroxyurea lowers average-mean blood flow velocity in individuals with SCD, increases the fetal hemoglobin level, improves the anemia, and may reduce the risk of stroke and other complications.[19,20] It is not yet clear to what extent hydroxyurea prevents primary or secondary stroke, but it circumvents the problem of iron overload from transfusions, and its long-term use is well tolerated.[19,21] Hydroxyurea is a reasonable option in patients who cannot tolerate long-term transfusion therapy and possibly for selected other individuals.[8]

Revascularization procedures (see Chapter 13) have been done in individuals with moyamoya syndrome due to SCD who have not responded to more conservative measures.[22,23] For individuals with suitable donors, bone marrow transplantation provides long-term reduction of stroke risk and other SCD complications.[24]

Sickle Cell Trait

Flying at high altitudes in a depressurized airplane is a well-known hazard for individuals who are heterozygous for the sickle hemoglobin gene (sickle cell trait). These individuals may also develop splenic infarction and heat stroke in situations that promote oxygen desaturation, such as high altitude or prolonged strenuous activity.[25–27] However, whether sickle cell trait is a stroke risk factor in day-to-day life is debated.[28–30]

Table 11-1: Recommendations for Sickle Cell Disease Management

Class I recommendations

1. Acute management of ischemic stroke due to SCD should include optimal hydration, correction of hypoxemia, and correction of systemic hypotension.

2. Periodic transfusions to reduce the percentage of sickle hemoglobin are effective for reducing the risk of stroke in children 2 to 16 years of age with abnormal TCD results due to SCD and are recommended.

3. Children with SCD and a confirmed cerebral infarction should be placed on a regular program of red cell transfusion in conjunction with measures to prevent iron overload.

4. Reducing the percentage of sickle hemoglobin with transfusions before performing catheter angiography is indicated in an individual with SCD.

Class II recommendations

1. For acute cerebral infarction, exchange transfusion designed to reduce Hb S to < 30% total hemoglobin is reasonable.

2. In children with SCD and an intracranial hemorrhage, it is reasonable to evaluate for a structural vascular lesion.

3. In children with SCD, it is reasonable to repeat a normal TCD annually and to repeat an abnormal study in 1 month. Borderline and mildly abnormal TCD studies may be repeated in 3 to 6 months.

4. Hydroxyurea may be considered in children and young adults with SCD and stroke who cannot continue on long-term transfusion.

5. Bone marrow transplantation may be considered for children with SCD.

6. Surgical revascularization procedures may be considered as a last resort in children with SCD who continue to have cerebrovascular dysfunction despite optimal medical management.

Adapted from Roach et al. with permission.[8]
Class I: Should be pursued because the benefits clearly exceed the risks. Class II: Reasonable to consider because benefits probably exceed the risks, but additional studies with focused or age-specific objectives are needed.

Although periodic case reports document young adults with a stroke and no obvious risk factors other than sickle cell trait, heterozygosity for sickle hemoglobin is so common that the odds of a coincidental stroke are not trivial. Considering the large number of people who carry the abnormal gene and the paucity of well-documented patients with both sickle cell trait and a stroke, it seems unlikely that the heterozygosity for the sickle hemoglobin gene alone is a noteworthy stroke risk factor.[30]

Other Hemoglobinopathies

Hemoglobin C is relatively common, and it causes dysfunction when it occurs in conjunction with hemoglobin S (hemoglobin SC). However, individuals with hemoglobin SC disease tend to have a milder phenotype and a lower incidence of stroke than those with homozygous SCD.[31] Hemoglobin SC disease also has a higher incidence of retinopathy than SCD.

Dozens of allelic variants of the beta globulin A gene have been reported, but these are generally not associated with stroke.

Thalassemia

A variety of neurologic signs and symptoms occur in individuals with thalassemia major, but stroke is relatively uncommon. Focal ischemic brain lesions were found in only two of 138 patients in one series.[32] However, individuals with sickle cell–thalassemia mimic the clinical pattern of SCD patients.

RED BLOOD CELL DISORDERS

Red blood cells contain hemoglobin within a moldable membrane. As they flow through progressively smaller tubes, the stream characteristics change. In the large arteries the cells are about evenly distributed throughout the lumen, but, at bifurcations and with diminishing lumen area, the majority of cells travel more centrally in the stream surrounded concentrically by a boundary layer of plasma. At this point branching of the arterial tree causes plasma skimming, resulting in differences in the proportion of cells to plasma in different branches. Red cells traverse capillaries one at a time in extremely rapid succession, their contour being molded by the vessel walls as the cells progress.

Red blood cell concentration and hemoglobin content may be increased or decreased as in polycythemia or anemia. At high shear rates, red cell membrane malleability is the main determinant for viscosity, whereas at low rates it is red cell aggregability. These may cause neurologic complications, in some cases related solely to the absence of sufficient oxygen-carrying capacity, and, in others, to increased viscosity with reduction in the rate of flow.

Anemia

An anemia that develops gradually over a prolonged interval is less likely to cause symptoms than one of more rapid onset. Severe anemia tends to produce diffuse neurological symptoms similar to those of hypoxemia. Occasional individuals with anemia develop intermittent focal neurological deficits that resolve following transfusion.[33] Marked anemia can contribute to focal brain dysfunction distal to a coexisting arterial stenosis.

Polycythemia

Erythrocytosis occurs either as a primary disorder or as a reaction to chronic hypoxemia, as occurs in pulmonary disorders or cyanotic heart lesions. Primary polycythemia, or *polycythemia rubra vera,* is a myeloproliferative disorder that often features excessive production of all cellular blood constituents. Familial polycythemia is a rare autosomal dominant condition that most often results from a mutation of the erythropoietin receptor gene.[34–36] A few families without an erythropoietin receptor gene mutation have an autosomal recessive form of polycythemia.[37] Patients with unexplained polycythemia should also be screened for a Janus kinase 2 (JAK2) mutation, a dominant gain of function mutation that can be detected in the majority of individuals with polycythemia vera as well as in about a fourth of the people with essential thrombocythemia.[38]

Polycythemia increases the blood viscosity in a logarithmic fashion and eventually decreases the cerebral blood flow.[39] Patients with polycythemia vera have an added risk due to the co-occurrence of thrombocytosis.[40] In one retrospective analysis of 1,213 polycythemia vera patients who were followed for at least 20 years, 485 patients (41%) had one or more venous or arterial thromboses. The incidence of thrombosis in this cohort was 3.4% per year.[41]

Untreated patients are at increased risk for arterial, microcirculatory, and venous occlusion. Thus, the neurological manifestations include focal infarctions and diffuse microvascular signs as well as increased intracranial pressure from sinovenous occlusion. Chorea is well documented.[42–44]

Acutely, phlebotomy can be used to lower the blood viscosity. When feasible, the underlying cause of the polycythemia should be corrected. Low-dose aspirin can reduce the risk of thrombotic complications from polycythemia vera.[45] Cytoreduction therapy reduces the likelihood of thrombotic events but carries a risk of drug-induced neoplasm.[41]

Paroxysmal Nocturnal Hemoglobinuria

Paroxysmal nocturnal hemoglobinuria is a rare condition that results from an acquired stem cell mutation of the *PIGA* gene (on chromosome Xp22.1), leading to impaired synthesis of a transmembrane glycolipid called the glycosyl-phosphatidylinositol anchor. The anchor molecule covalently binds to an assortment of cell surface proteins, including various proteins that protect the cell from complement lysis.[46,47] The membrane abnormality affects all of the progeny of the abnormal stem cells, including the platelets and leucocytes in addition to the red blood cells. The proportion of abnormal circulating cells largely determines the severity of the disease, so the symptoms may gradually worsen or even resolve in response to the fate of the mutated stem cell line.[48,49]

Paroxysmal nocturnal hemoglobinuria most often manifests in young adults but can occur at any age. The typical morning hemoglobinuria may result from increased hemolysis because of sleep-related respiratory acidosis, and the hematuria is made more obvious by overnight concentration of the urine. Other exacerbations of the hemoglobinuria result from increased hemolysis during periods of increased complement activity, as might occur during an infection. Some people with paroxysmal nocturnal hemoglobinuria do not develop major complications. Although arterial occlusion or hemorrhage can occur, venous thrombosis is the more likely cerebrovascular complication.[50–54] A few women have developed dural sinus thrombosis associated with pregnancy or while taking oral contraceptives.[55,56] Some individuals develop aplastic anemia or leukemia.[49,54,57]

Blood transfusions, iron therapy, and antibiotics may be needed. Anticoagulants or thrombolytic agents may be useful in patients with thrombosis. Corticosteroids may be of use especially during acute exacerbations of the disease. Eculizumab reduces intravascular hemolysis and improves symptoms in individuals with paroxysmal nocturnal hemoglobinuria. This agent is a human monoclonal antibody that targets the C5 component of complement and inhibits complement activation.[58] Bone marrow transplantation may be curative.

HYPERVISCOSITY SYNDROME

The effects of increased viscosity on the circulation was discussed even before Stephen Hales's 1753 observation: "But the resistance which the blood meets in those capillary passages, may be greatly varied, either by different degrees of viscidity or fluidity of the blood, or by the several degrees of constriction or relaxation of these fine vessels."[59] Two and a half centuries later, viscosity's contribution to stroke is still not fully understood.

Viscosity and vessel diameter are the main determinants of flow of nonparticulate liquids through straight tubes, a relationship that is expressed by the Hagen-Poiseuille equation. However, this formula does not apply seamlessly to a particle-laden fluid like blood. In normal blood the red blood cells are the main determinant of viscosity. With this model, flow depends on the propelling pressure (cardiac output) and flow resistance (in blood this is determined by the vascular resistance and the blood's viscosity).[60]

Although this formula applies well to plasma, the determinants of whole blood flow are much more complex because of the presence of myriad blood cells that cause friction against the vessel wall. This resistance, the shear rate, is inversely proportional to the vessel radius. Force per unit area of a fluid layer is shear stress and is defined as the ratio of shear stress to shear rate. Increasing viscosity requires greater shear stress to achieve the same shear rate and flow velocity.[60]

Clinically significant hyperviscosity results from very large numbers of circulating blood cells or in the face of large amounts of asymmetrical high molecular weight molecules in the serum that alter the conformational properties of the blood. Modest fluctuations in the hematocrit around normal physiologic values have a limited effect on the blood's viscosity, but increasing numbers of circulating red blood cells generate a logarithmic increase in viscosity.[60] However, even modest increases in viscosity can be clinically important in individuals with other stroke risk factors.[61]

White cells and platelets normally have a near-negligible effect on blood viscosity, but viscosity can increase dramatically during a leukemia blast crisis or with severe thrombocythemia. Hyperviscosity syndrome also occurs with Waldenstrom's macroglobulinemia, multiple myeloma, and other malignancies.[62,63] Stroke following intravenous infusion of immunoglobulin (IVIG) has been described.[64,65]

The neurological manifestations of hyperviscosity syndrome tend to feature signs of diffuse neurological dysfunction, such as headache, vertigo, altered mental status, and seizures. Retinopathy and focal ischemic strokes also occur.[62]

PLATELET DISORDERS

Hemostasis is the combined process that halts bleeding after an injury to small blood vessels, such as capillaries, venules, and small arterioles. Normal hemostasis involves the vessel wall, platelets, and the blood coagulation factors. After disruption of the vascular endothelium, platelets rapidly adhere to the exposed subendothelial collagen at the site of injury. Adherence is mediated by von Willebrand factor and platelet surface glycoprotein Ib. Activated platelets secrete their granule contents (Ca^{++}, adenosine diphosphate, and serotonin) and form thromboxane A_2. These messengers recruit additional platelets, enhance vasoconstriction, and make available the fibrinogen receptors on platelets. Fibrinogen then binds to these surface receptors, the glycoprotein IIb/IIIa, and acts as an intercellular bridge in the formation of platelet aggregates, temporarily arresting the flow of blood.

Simultaneously the exposure of the plasma coagulation proteins to the newly exposed subendothelial tissue initiates blood coagulation. The coagulation system is composed of linked proenzymes that are activated sequentially. Nonenzymatic cofactors, phospholipids, divalent cations, and receptors on the surface membrane of activated platelets or endothelial cells play important roles in blood coagulation.

Platelets contain several constituents that promote clotting: calcium, adenosine diphosphate (ADP), heparin-neutralizing factors, and prostaglandins. When the platelets come into contact with collagen, as occurs in ulcerated atheromatous plaques, they swell, fuse, and adhere to the denuded area while liberating ADP, generating further platelet aggregation. This interaction is fostered by glycoproteins in the platelet membrane, which act as receptor sites for fibrinogen and von Willebrand factor. This process continues until equilibrium between adhesion aggregation and counterbalancing thrombolysis occurs. Platelets are the source of most of the prostaglandins and its derivative thromboxane A_2, a potent vasoconstrictor that is the stimulus for platelet aggregation.

Depending on the specific nature of the platelet abnormality, neurologic complications can be either occlusive (with thrombocytosis and excessive platelet aggregability) or hemorrhagic (with thrombocytopenia and functional platelet abnormalities). Whether or not symptoms occur in a given individual depends largely on the severity of the platelet disorder. Some individuals also have coexisting conditions that increase the likelihood of complications related to platelet dysfunction, such as atherosclerosis and elevated plasma lipids. Additionally, hyperaggregability may develop following bleeding, thrombosis, or injury in another location, such as after myocardial infarction or cerebral infarction.

Thrombocytopenia

Modestly low platelet counts are often clinically insignificant, but individuals whose platelet count dips below 50,000/mm³ sometimes develop intracranial hemorrhage or other significant hemorrhagic complications. Spontaneous intracranial hemorrhage is unusual unless the platelet count falls below 20,000/mm³, although individuals with less severe thrombocytopenia may have significant bleeding after relatively minor trauma. The risk of hemorrhagic complications is largely independent of the cause of the thrombocytopenia.

The most common cause of acquired thrombocytopenia is the use of various cancer chemotherapy agents. These individuals usually have anemia and leucopenia as well as thrombocytopenia, but intracranial hemorrhage due solely to chemotherapy is relatively rare. Leukemia patients who present with a strikingly

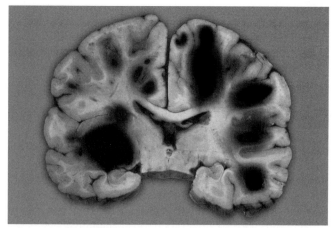

Figure 11-3. Multiple white matter hemorrhages in a patient with acute leukemia.

elevated white cell count coupled with severe thrombocytopenia are also at risk for intracerebral hemorrhage (Figure 11-3). In contrast, some individuals develop a hypercoagulable state with their malignancy, so there is also a risk of cerebral infarction.

Thrombocytopenia is a well-recognized complication of heparin administration. Early-onset heparin-induced thrombocytopenia is common but typically mild and asymptomatic.[66] Immune-mediated thrombocytopenia is more severe, and typically occurs after several days of heparin therapy.[66] It occurs in about 1% to 5% of patients receiving heparin.[67] Heparin induces endothelial injury and increased platelet aggregation and consumption.[68] Most patients remain asymptomatic, but when symptoms occur, they are usually thrombotic rather than hemorrhagic and more likely to involve the venous system than the arterial circulation. Platelet transfusions may worsen the problem and should be avoided.

Thrombocytopenia is common in individuals with persistently high serum valproic acid levels. The severity of the valproate-induced thrombocytopenia typically increases with increasing serum valproate levels and with higher doses, although occasional individuals have an idiosyncratic thrombocytopenia due to valproate. Most individuals have mild thrombocytopenia with limited clinical significance, but those with very high valproate levels for a prolonged interval sometimes develop severe thrombocytopenia.[69] The platelet count promptly improves, the valproate level drops, and individuals with a normal platelet count can tolerate neurosurgery without difficulty.[70]

Severe isoimmune thrombocytopenic purpura (ITP) can result in intracerebral hemorrhage.[71] Brain hemorrhage due to ITP does not usually occur with platelet counts above 20,000/mm³. Brain hemorrhage later in the course of ITP frequently coincides with a systemic infection, probably because the infection stimulates the production of antiplatelet antibodies and causes an additional drop in the platelet count.[72,73] Antiplatelet antibodies can cross the placenta and induce thrombocytopenia in neonates, sometimes leading to intracerebral hemorrhage.[74,75]

Therapy of Thrombocytopenia

In cases of immune-mediated heparin-induced thrombocytopenia, management requires discontinuation of the offending drug and administration of either argatroban or recombinant hirudin (lepirudin). Patients with thrombocytopenia due to medication use should ideally stop taking the drug. In instances where the drug's use is vital to the patient's well-being and the platelet count is seriously reduced, the dose can be lowered or the treatment temporarily halted. These individuals should also try to avoid nonsteroidal agents as well as situations with a major risk of trauma. Platelet transfusions may be considered in individuals with severe thrombocytopenia or in people with less severe thrombocytopenia who are facing surgery.

Asymptomatic individuals with ITP whose platelet count is only modestly decreased can be followed clinically. Those who are more severely affected may benefit from corticosteroids, although the thrombocytopenia often recurs when treatment is halted. Infusions of intravenous immune globulin may be effective when prednisone is not.[76] For individuals with chronic ITP, splenectomy results in an immediate remission in 77% of the patients and a long-term remission in 66%.[77]

Thrombocythemia

Thrombocythemia is defined by a platelet count of over 600,000/mm³, and platelet counts may exceed 1,000,000/mm³ in some individuals. Reactive thrombocytosis is a nonspecific abnormality and occurs in individuals with various conditions, including iron deficiency anemia, malignancies, inflammatory bowel disease, collagen vascular disorders, and hemolysis. Extremely elevated platelet counts can occur with myeloproliferative disorders such as polycythemia vera and chronic myelogenous leukemia. Elevated platelet counts can also occur as a rebound phenomenon after splenectomy or following suppression of thrombopoiesis.

Essential thrombocythemia is a clonal myeloproliferative disorder resulting from chronic overproduction of platelets. Most people with essential thrombocythemia are over 50 years of age, but it occasionally occurs in younger individuals.[78–80] The natural history of essential thrombocythemia is not well defined. Many patients with essential thrombocythemia have a normal life span, but some individuals eventually develop either polycythemia vera or idiopathic myelofibrosis.

Most people with thrombocytosis remain asymptomatic, especially when their platelet count is only modestly elevated. However, neurological dysfunction sometimes develops even with a modestly elevated platelet count.[81] Ischemic arterial stroke and intracranial sinovenous thrombosis have been documented in individuals with thrombocythemia, but transient and poorly localizing neurological symptoms are far more common.[82,83] Sudden-onset paresthesias, dysarthria, scintillating scotomas, monocular visual loss, and transient unsteadiness are commonly reported, but the individual attacks last only seconds or minutes.[78,83] These symptoms characteristically occur in conjunction with a headache, giving each episode a striking resemblance to complicated migraine.[84]

Therapy of Thrombocytosis

Asymptomatic individuals with modestly elevated platelet counts require no therapy. Symptomatic individuals usually respond to reduction of the platelet count, and low-dose aspirin minimizes the neurologic symptoms. Warfarin, in contrast, is not effective.[83,84]

Consumption Coagulopathy – Disseminated Intravascular Coagulation

With disseminated intravascular coagulation (DIC), excessive intravascular coagulation consumes the circulating coagulation factors, causing a hemorrhagic diathesis. The inciting stimulus is the release of thromboplastin or a thromboplastin-like substance into the bloodstream, converting prothrombin to thrombin, which then activates platelets, fibrinogen, and factors V and VIII. Fibrinogen is then converted into fibrin, consuming the available prothrombin, factor V, and antihemophilia globulin. This process leads to a low fibrinogen level and a prolonged prothrombin time along with the presence of fibrinogen split products in the blood.

Among the reported causes of DIC are missed abortion, endotoxic shock, septicemia, acute pancreatitis, incompatible blood transfusions, carcinomatosis, trauma, and insect or snake bites.[85–88] Patients with acute DIC are critically ill, but some individuals have a more indolent and chronic form of DIC. Characteristic initial signs of DIC are cutaneous ecchymoses, oozing from venipuncture sites, hematuria, and epistaxis. In fulminant cases there is multiple organ failure.[89] DIC can cause tissue infarction due to microvascular thrombi, hemorrhage secondary to platelet destruction and consumption of coagulation factors, or a combination of hemorrhage and infarction.[86]

Intravenous heparin in gradually escalating doses may benefit some categories of DIC patients. However, heparin therapy may aggravate bleeding due to DIC, a particular problem in individuals with trauma, hepatic failure, or those with severe hemostatic compromise. Heparin is contraindicated in patients with a brain hemorrhage and in individuals whose platelet count cannot be maintained above 20,000/dl. Naturally, the cause of the DIC should be corrected whenever possible.

Thrombotic Thrombocytopenic Purpura

Neurological signs and symptoms occur in about half of the individuals with thrombotic thrombocytopenic purpura (TTP); these typically include altered mental status, seizures, and various focal neurological deficits.[90] Small multifocal brain lesions (Figure 11-4) from microcirculatory disruption are the most common pattern, but larger focal lesions are relatively common as well. TTP occurs in response to various infections and is more common during and just after pregnancy. Several drugs

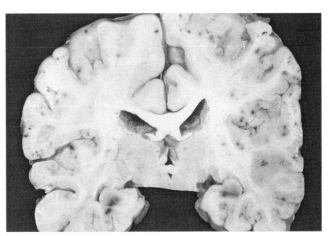

Figure 11-4. Multiple petechial lesions due to TTP.

evidently increase the risk of developing TTP, including cyclosporine, quinine, ticlopidine, and clopidogrel.[91–93]

An autosomal recessive form of TTP results from a mutation of the ADAMT13 gene that codes for von Willebrand factor-cleaving protease.[94] This protease activity is also severely reduced in some cases of acquired TTP, evidently because of auto-antibodies targeting the protease.[95]

Plasma exchange, with or without the addition of corticosteroids, is effective for most individuals with TTP.[96] Potential TTP-inducing drugs should be stopped. Platelet transfusions should be avoided in people with TTP.[97]

Qualitative Platelet Disorders

Drug-Induced Platelet Dysfunction

Qualitative platelet disorders are characterized by a significant bleeding history in an individual with a normal platelet count, normal coagulation tests, and a prolonged bleeding time. Several inherited disorders of platelet function have been described, but acquired platelet dysfunction due to various medications is more common.[98] The number of drugs with the potential to alter platelet function is far too long to review in detail; the reader is referred to the comprehensive review by George and Shattil.[98] In addition to numerous medications, certain foods (e.g., onions and garlic) and spices (e.g., cumin, cloves, ginger, and turmeric) sometimes affect platelet function. Fortunately most patients do not develop clinically significant bleeding.[98]

Clinical manifestations of impaired platelet function often occur in individuals taking a drug for therapeutic platelet inhibition, such as aspirin, clopidogrel, and ticlopidine (see Chapter 25). The drugs most commonly responsible for impaired platelet function are aspirin and other nonsteroidal anti-inflammatory drugs. Aspirin irreversibly acetylates the platelet enzyme cyclo-oxygenase and blocks thromboxane A_2 production. Because the platelet cannot synthesize proteins de novo, it remains inhibited for its life span. Nonaspirin, nonsteroidal anti-inflammatory drugs, in contrast, reversibly alter platelet function by inhibiting cyclo-oxygenase. Unlike aspirin, the platelet effect from these agents lasts only while the drug remains in the circulation.

Antibiotics that contain a β-lactam ring often induce a dose-dependent prolongation of the bleeding time and alter both platelet aggregation and activation.[99] Half to three-fourths of the individuals taking large doses of these agents develop abnormal platelet aggregation.[99–101] In most individuals the platelet antagonist effect of antibiotics is not clinically significant, but the antiplatelet effect tends to be more pronounced in debilitated individuals or those with coexisting impairment of hemostasis.[102]

Von Willebrand Disease

Von Willebrand disease results from a defective or absent glycoprotein (von Willebrand factor) whose function is to bind and stabilize inactive factor VIII and to bind to activated platelet receptors and help them adhere to damaged endothelium. About 1% of the population has some form of von Willebrand disease, but fortunately most individuals have few clinical manifestations. The disorder occurs with equal frequency in men and women, but it is diagnosed somewhat more often in women, probably because abnormal bleeding during menstruation triggers a diagnostic evaluation in an otherwise oligosymptomatic individual.

Four types and several subtypes of von Willebrand disease have been defined, and several different mutations have been identified.[103] About 75% of the people with von Willebrand disease have type 1, which features low levels of von Willebrand factor and mild clinical features. Type 2 is characterized by abnormally functioning von Willebrand factor, whereas individuals with the rare autosomal recessive type 3 have severe manifestations due to absent von Willebrand factor and very low factor VIII levels.[104] Additionally, the platelet-type von Willebrand disease (also called pseudo–von Willebrand disease) results from a platelet-binding defect instead of deficient von Willebrand factor. Sadler has reviewed the von Willebrand classification scheme in detail.[103] There are also acquired forms of von Willebrand disease.[105]

Despite the diffuse bleeding tendency that accompanies the severe forms of von Willebrand disease, reports of intracranial hemorrhage are relatively unusual, and some of the reported patients with intracranial hemorrhage had prior trauma or a second coagulation defect.[106] However, recent reports suggest that somewhat reduced levels of von Willebrand factor occur in individuals with an intracerebral hemorrhage, even in the absence of von Willebrand disease, and that increased factor levels may correlate with the risk of ischemic stroke.[106,107]

Sticky Platelet Syndrome

Hyperaggregable platelets occur with various acquired disorders, but the *sticky platelet syndrome* is an autosomal dominant disorder that is characterized by platelet hyperaggregability on exposure to ADP and/or epinephrine.[108,109] Blockage of a vessel by platelet aggregates generates transient ischemic attacks, stroke, myocardial infarction, retinal artery thrombosis, and peripheral vessel occlusion. Symptoms often arise during or after a period of emotional stress. Low-dose aspirin improves both the clinical symptoms and the platelet hyperaggregability of sticky platelet syndrome.[108,109]

Hyperhomocysteinemia

Homocysteine is toxic to the vascular endothelium and promotes early atherosclerosis and thromboembolism, but there is also evidence that hyperhomocysteinemia induces platelet aggregation.[110–112] The most common hereditary cause of homocystinuria is deficient cystathionine β-synthase, but a few cases are due to homozygous mutations of methylene tetrahydrofolate reductase (MTHFR) or methionine synthase. Individuals who are heterozygous are usually asymptomatic; the *MTHFR* gene has several common (i.e., 10% of the U.S. population) polymorphisms that cause a mild increase in the serum homocysteine.[113] Whether these *MTHFR* alleles increase the risk of thrombosis is debatable. The homocysteine level also tends to creep up with increasing age, possibly facilitating the development of atherosclerosis. The clinical manifestations, pathogenesis, and treatment of homocysteine-related conditions are presented in Chapter 21.

HYPEREOSINOPHILIC SYNDROME

Although hypereosinophilia occurs in individuals with parasitic infections, malignancy, drug reactions, and many other disorders, the modest increase in the eosinophil count that typically occurs with these conditions does not cause neurological dysfunction. Individuals with essential hypereosinophilia, in contrast, can have extremely elevated eosinophil counts and develop cardiac or neurological dysfunction.[114,115] By convention, a threefold eosinophil increase exceeding 1500/mm³ for at least 6 months in an individual with no apparent reason for eosinophilia is diagnostic of essential eosinophilia. The eosinophil proliferation can be either polyclonal or monoclonal.[116] Familial hypereosinophilia is occasionally documented.[117]

Neurological complications of eosinophilia arise via more than one mechanism and involve either the central or the peripheral nervous system. Focal brain infarction is less common than diffuse brain dysfunction manifested by psychosis, cognitive impairment, and seizures.[118] In Moore's series of 52 patients with hypereosinophilia, seven developed encephalopathy and 23 had peripheral neuropathy.[115] Imaging studies reveal a watershed infarction pattern. Brain biopsy findings include infarction with reactive gliosis and abundant intravascular eosinophils.[119]

The eosinophils probably secrete cytotoxins that induce microcirculatory dysfunction. Additionally, some individuals generate emboli from the endocardium and cardiac valves whereas others develop a hypercoagulable state.[119] Hypereosinophilia may facilitate coagulation in individuals with hereditary thrombophilias.[120]

HYPERCOAGULABLE STATES

Hypercoagulability is a state in which the clotting mechanisms shift the hemostatic balance toward inappropriate or excessive platelet/fibrin deposition and lead to arterial or venous thrombosis in response to a vascular injury that would not usually trigger thrombus formation.

The coagulation system is a finely tuned balance of surface-associated interacting enzymes and cofactors that generate thrombin at sites of vascular injury. Thrombin converts soluble fibrinogen to insoluble fibrin, activates factor XIII that causes the clot formation, and activates both platelets and endothelial cells by proteolytic digestion. Thrombin potentiates clot formation through activation of factors VIII and V and inhibits it through activation of the protein C system. The major deterrents to pathologic thrombin generation are the protein C system, antithrombin, and the tissue factor pathway inhibitor. In addition, the fibrinolysis generates serine protease plasmin by the action of tPA on plasminogen, promoting dissolution of the fibrin clot.

Hypercoagulable states can be hereditary or occur in a variety of clinical settings, including pregnancy, use of oral contraceptives, the nephrotic syndrome, diabetes mellitus, trauma, surgery, immobilization, and infections. There is no single mechanism that explains how each of these conditions increases coagulation. It is clear, however, that the occurrence of more than one congenital or acquired risk factor in the same individual greatly increases the likelihood of thrombosis.

The process of normal and abnormal hemostasis is too complex to allow a comprehensive discussion in this book, but some of the more important disorders are discussed in more detail below. Table 11-2 lists some of the acquired conditions that contribute to increased thrombosis, and a more complete survey of the coagulation pathway and its dysfunction is provided by Lichman and colleagues.[121]

Antithrombin Deficiency

Antithrombin is a plasma serine protease inhibitor that is synthesized by the liver and strongly catalyzed by the presence of

Table 11-2: Acquired Causes of Increased Thrombosis

Cancer

Pregnancy

Oral contraceptives

Ovarian hyperstimulation syndrome

Polycythemia vera

Thrombocythemia

Nephrotic syndrome

Myeloproliferative disorders

Hyperlipidemia

Hyperhomocysteinemia

Heparin-induced thrombocytopenia

Diabetes mellitus

Inflammatory bowel disease

Paroxysmal nocturnal hemoglobinuria

Postoperative state

Thrombotic thrombocytopenic purpura

Trauma

Vasculitis

Antiphospholipid antibody syndrome

Medications (e.g., L-asparaginase)

heparin on the endothelial cells. It inhibits thrombin as well as factors IXa, Xa, XIa, and XIIa. It also inactivates kallikrein and plasmin.[122] A deficiency state can be inherited as an autosomal dominant trait or acquired due to nephrotic syndrome, protein-losing enteropathy, hepatic disease, estrogen use, L-asparaginase treatment, or extensive surgery or burns.[123] Antithrombin has been divided into types I and II. In type I deficiency there is reduced synthesis of the antithrombin molecule. Type II deficiency is due to the presence of a dysfunctional antithrombin molecule, typically from a point mutation. The prevalence of antithrombin deficiency has been estimated to be 1 in 2,000 to 1 in 5,000 individuals, but its frequency among individuals with recurrent or extensive thrombosis is 2% to 3%.[124]

Venous thrombosis occurs far more often than arterial occlusion in individuals with antithrombin deficiency. Not all individuals develop symptoms, and those who do typically manifest in early to middle adulthood.[125,126] Thrombosis is more likely to occur around the time of surgery or during pregnancy or the postpartum period.[126,127] Homozygous antithrombin deficiency is rare, typically presenting in neonates as widespread venous and arterial thromboses. Antithrombin deficiency carries a higher risk of thrombosis than factor V Leiden, protein C deficiency, or protein S deficiency.[127,128] As with other disorders that increase the likelihood of thrombosis, the risk of clotting increases substantially when antithrombin deficiency occurs in an individual with other coagulation risk factors.[129,130]

Asymptomatic individuals are not usually treated. Those with a thrombosis are typically given heparin followed by long-term anticoagulation with warfarin.[122,131] However, both unfractionated heparin and low-molecular-weight heparin may be less reliable because they require antithrombin for proper function. After heparin therapy, there may be a 10% to 15% decrease in antithrombin levels and rebound hypercoagulability after discontinuation. Homozygous patients may require fresh frozen plasma or antithrombin concentrates.

Protein C Deficiency

Protein C is a vitamin K–dependent serine protease that circulates in an inactive form. Activation is accomplished by a specific enzymatic complex consisting of thrombin and the endothelial cell surface protein thrombomodulin. Activated protein C, together with its cofactor protein S, is then able to cleave and inactivate factors V and VIII.[132] Protein C deficiency can be either inherited or acquired. Acquired protein C deficiency results from the same causes as acquired antithrombin deficiency, except that protein C levels are not usually decreased in nephrotic syndrome.

Some individuals with protein C deficiency have few problems. Esmon suggests that patients with protein C levels below 40% of normal are more likely to have thrombotic complications.[132] In the acute phase of thrombosis, plasma levels of both protein C and protein S tend to be low. If the protein levels remain low several months after the acute thrombosis and there is no reason to suspect an acquired deficiency, hereditary protein C or protein S deficiency is likely.[133]

Similar to other hypercoagulable states, heterozygous protein C deficiency is more likely to cause venous thrombosis than arterial occlusion.[134] In general, protein C deficiency is not a common cause for arterial stroke, but it is more likely in younger stroke patients or in those with other coagulation defects. In one consecutive series of 50 patients less than 45 years of age with unexplained arterial ischemic stroke, three individuals (6%) had hereditary protein C deficiency.[135] Homozygous protein C deficiency presents as widespread venous and arterial thromboses and death in the newborn period.[136,137]

Treatment with heparin followed by warfarin or subcutaneous low-molecular-weight heparin is probably justified for individuals with thrombosis due to protein C or protein S deficiency.[138,139] Warfarin can induce skin necrosis in patients with deficits of natural anticoagulants, so it is prudent to initiate treatment with small doses.[140,141]

Protein S Deficiency

Protein S is a vitamin K–dependent plasma protein that acts as a cofactor for protein C.[132] Both protein C and S are plasma glycoproteins synthesized in the liver. Protein S functions as a cofactor for activated protein C because it activates factor Va and factor VIIIa. About half of plasma protein S is in the active form, and the other half is bound to the C4B-binding protein.

Like protein C, protein S deficiency can be either inherited as an autosomal dominant trait or acquired. Both total and free protein S decrease steadily throughout a normal pregnancy, reaching their lowest levels at term. This may partly explain the increased frequency of postpartum thrombosis. Protein S levels are also lower among smokers, in people with hepatic disease, and following therapy with L-asparaginase.[142,143] The risk of pathologic thrombosis due to hereditary protein S deficiency is increased fivefold.[144]

Individuals with deficient protein S are more likely to have a cerebral venous thrombosis than an arterial occlusion; the authors have seen one patient with a cerebral hemorrhage secondary to a sagittal sinus thrombosis in a patient with protein S deficiency. One study of 36 consecutive young adults with unexplained cerebral infarction found five (13.9%) patients with protein S deficiency.[145]

Prothrombin Gene Mutation

The most common genetic variation affecting prothrombin (factor II) is a guanine to adenine transition at the 20210 nucleotide position in an untranslated region of the prothrombin gene.[146] The resulting prothrombin is normal in structure but increased in amount. This prothrombin mutation is inherited as an autosomal dominant trait. Heterozygosity for the prothrombin G20210A allele occurs in an estimated 1.2% of the Caucasian population and in 0.5% of African Americans. Homozygosity for the prothrombin G20210A mutation is estimated to occur once in every 10,000 individuals. Although the prothrombin G20210A allele increases circulating normal prothrombin and thus increases the likelihood of thrombosis, less common mutations that reduce either the amount or the function of circulating prothrombin instead promote bleeding complications.[147,148]

Heterozygotes for the prothrombin G20210A allele have a 2–6-fold increased risk of venous thrombosis but little increased risk of arterial thrombosis, myocardial infarction, or pregnancy-related complications.[146,149–151] However, individuals who carry both the common prothrombin mutation and another coagulation-promoting gene (e.g., a factor V Leiden mutation) have a 10-fold increase in the odds ratio for venous thrombosis and a 16-fold increase when taking oral contraceptives.[151]

Factor V Leiden Mutation

Factor V has a dominantly inherited variant that increases the likelihood of thrombosis. Known as factor V Leiden after the city of its discovery, it is the most common genetic abnormality of coagulation. Heterozygosity for factor V Leiden varies by ethnicity. In the United States, factor V Leiden occurs in 5.27% of Caucasians, 2.21% of Hispanic Americans, 1.23% of African Americans, 0.45% of Asian Americans, and 1.25% of Native Americans.[152] This genetically altered form of factor V is not readily degraded by activated protein C, enhancing the downstream production of thrombin and fibrin.

The risk of abnormal thrombosis due to a heterozygous factor V Leiden mutation varies in different reports, but it appears to be lower than the risk from deficiencies of antithrombin, protein C, or protein S.[128] One study analyzed over a thousand relatives of people with mutations of factor V Leiden or prothrombin; it noted an annual incidence of venous thrombosis of 0.19% for heterozygotes of the factor V Leiden mutation and 0.13% for carriers of the prothrombin gene 20210A mutation.[153] However, the risk of thrombosis increases dramatically in individuals who are homozygous for factor V Leiden. The clotting risk also increases when factor V Leiden is coupled with other hereditary or acquired prothrombotic states. The risk of thrombosis due to factor V Leiden increases during pregnancy or while taking estrogen-containing oral contraceptives.[127,151] Recent surgery and cigarette smoking increase its risk as well. Similarly, the clotting risk from a factor V Leiden mutation increases sharply when coupled with other hereditary coagulation abnormalities such as a prothrombin mutation or deficient protein C or protein S.

Most factor V Leiden mutation carriers remain asymptomatic, and many of the individuals who develop thrombotic complications have one or more thrombotic risk factors in addition to the factor V mutation. Most of the thromboses in individuals with a factor V Leiden mutation are venous rather than arterial. Deep vein thrombosis, pulmonary embolism, and dural sinus thrombosis all occur.

Disorders of Plasminogen and Fibrinolysis

Dysplasminogenemia, hypoplasminogenemia, decreased synthesis or release of tissue plasminogen activator, and increased concentrations of plasminogen activator inhibitor have all been reported as rare causes of recurrent familial thromboembolic disease associated with impaired fibrinolysis. Congenital plasminogen deficiency is inherited as an autosomal dominant trait. The plasminogen is more likely to be dysfunctional than absent. Congenital deficiency of tPA appears to be an extremely uncommon problem, as is defective release of tPA.

These individuals typically begin to experience thrombotic events in their late teenage years although some people remain asymptomatic. Both intracranial arterial and venous occlusions occur, but venous thromboses are more common.[154,155]

Therapy has included the use of heparin, warfarin, antiplatelet agents, and thrombolysis. However, if plasminogen levels are decreased significantly, thrombolytic therapy may be ineffective.

Antiphospholipid Antibodies

Antiphospholipid antibodies (APLAs) are a group of polyclonal immunoglobulins directed against phospholipid moieties of platelets, endothelial cells, and components of the coagulation pathway. Most people with APLAs remain asymptomatic, and these individuals should be distinguished from those with *antiphospholipid antibody syndrome*.[156] The clinical manifestations of APLA syndrome include thrombocytopenia, fetal loss, and a hypercoagulable state. Lupus anticoagulant and anticardiolipin antibodies are the APLAs with the most clinical relevance, but the presence of other autoantibodies could explain some of the uncommon clinical findings in these individuals.

Lupus anticoagulant was first identified in individuals with systemic lupus erythematosus (SLE), but it has now been linked to other autoimmune diseases, neoplasms, infections, and the use of certain drugs (e.g., phenothiazines, procainamide, quinidine, phenytoin, and hydralazine). It is sometimes difficult to know whether APLAs have clinical significance because they occur in 2% to 5% of the general population, usually not in conjunction with an underlying disorder. The prevalence of APLAs increases with age, exceeding 10% in individuals older than 70 years. Additionally, although thrombotic complications occur in about 10% of the patients with SLE, some of them have strokes or other vascular complications that are clearly unrelated to APLAs.[157,158]

Lupus anticoagulants inhibit the prothrombin activator complex and prolong the partial thromboplastin time (PTT) and so might be predicted to promote hemorrhage.[159] Paradoxically, APLAs are generally linked to arterial or venous cerebral thrombosis rather than hemorrhage.[160] However, the neurologic manifestations of APLAs are not very specific: they have been identified in individuals with transient ischemic attacks (TIAs), retinal and cerebral arterial and venous thrombosis, optic neuritis, migraine, chorea, seizures, dementia, Sneddon syndrome, and neuropsychiatric disorders.[161]

Sneddon syndrome is characterized by livedo reticularis, frequent migraine-like headaches, transient ischemic attacks, vertigo, and the frequent occurrence of APLAs.[162] The frequency of cerebral infarction and TIAs due to Sneddon syndrome has not been established.[163] Large artery occlusion is relatively uncommon with Sneddon syndrome, but small infarctions in the cerebral cortex and white matter are evident pathologically and radiographically.[164,165]

Therapy of Antiphospholipid Antibody Syndrome

Anticoagulants are often indicated in patients who have APAS and recurrent venous thromboembolism.[166] There is no evidence to support the use of high-intensity (e.g., international normalized ratio > 3.0) warfarin. The best therapeutic strategy for preventing stroke in patients who have APAS remains unclear. In patients who have stroke and APAS, aspirin is as effective as moderate-intensity warfarin for preventing recurrent cerebral ischemia. The usefulness of clopidogrel or the combination of extended-release dipyridamole and aspirin has not been proven in patients that have APAS and ischemic stroke.

Pregnancy and Oral Contraceptives

Both arterial and venous occlusions occur in individuals taking oral contraceptives, although preparations with lower hormone concentrations carry less risk. Hypercoagulability induced by estrogen is multifactorial, including diminished vascular tone, which promotes stasis, decreased antithrombin, and increased levels of fibrinogen and factors II, VII, IX, and X. The relative contribution of each of these changes is debated.

The risk of stroke is also increased during pregnancy and the postpartum period. Pregnancy increases the risk of stroke by 13-fold compared to nonpregnant young women.[167,168] Increased thrombin-antithrombin levels and decreased protein S levels occur during normal pregnancy.[169] Thrombotic complications of pregnancy are presented in more detail in Chapter 23.

Cryoglobulins

Circulating agglutinins may result in hypercoagulability and thrombosis. Cryoglobulinemia usually results from a mixture of IgG and IgM immunoglobulins. These develop particularly with multiple myeloma, collagen vascular disease, and Waldenstrom's macroglobulinemia. Typical presenting manifestations include encephalopathy, cutaneous purpura, Raynaud syndrome, arthralgia or arthritis, and dysfunction of the liver and kidneys. Some patients develop peripheral neuropathy and recurrent ischemic strokes.

In most instances the clinical manifestations of cryoglobulinemia stem from obstruction of the microcirculation by precipitated cryoglobulins. At times, hyperviscosity syndrome develops with cold agglutination, defective clotting, and a reaction to precipitated protein with vasoconstriction and secondary vascular and tissue damage.

Cryofibrinogenemia is exacerbated by exposure to cold. Its typical manifestations include headache, vertigo, Raynaud's phenomena, acrocyanosis, and livedo reticularis. The diagnosis is made by applying an ice cube to the skin, with the result being the production of a typical urticarial response.

Inflammatory Bowel Disease

Thrombosis occurs in some individuals with inflammatory bowel disease, but the frequency has not been established.[170–172] Sinovenous occlusion occurs more often than arterial thrombosis. A few patients have evidence of vasculitis.[173] Thrombocytosis and elevated fibrinogen or factor VIII have been demonstrated inconsistently.[174]

HEMORRHAGIC COAGULOPATHY

Intracranial hemorrhage can result from either hereditary or acquired coagulopathy. Factor VIII deficiency (hemophilia A) and factor IX deficiency (hemophilia B) are the most common hereditary coagulopathies to cause intracranial hemorrhage. However, brain hemorrhage (see Chapter 16) has been documented with various other coagulation disorders, including factor V deficiency,[175] factor XIII deficiency,[176] factor XI deficiency,[177] and congenital afibrinogenemia.[178] The severity of the bleeding disorder determines the likelihood of brain hemorrhage, not the specific deficiency.[179]

Similarly, there are numerous acquired coagulopathies that could lead to brain hemorrhage. A complete discussion of the causes of hemorrhagic coagulopathy is beyond the scope of this text, and we present some of the more clinically important disorders.

Hemophilia

Intracranial hemorrhage is the most feared complication in hemophiliac patients and the most common cause of death.[180,181] Before the availability of factor concentrates, intracranial hemorrhage occurred in up to 14% of hemophiliac patients.[182,183] Eyster and colleagues documented 71 individuals with a central nervous system hemorrhage among 2,500 hemophilia patients in their cooperative study,[184] and another report identified 156 episodes of central nervous system hemorrhage in a cohort of 1,410 individuals with hemophilia.[180]

Trauma precedes intracranial hemorrhage at least half of the time. However, the onset of symptoms can begin several days after an injury, and the trauma can be minor, making it difficult to be certain that a particular episode of trauma caused the hemorrhage.[180,184–186] Clearly the risk of brain hemorrhage is greater with more severe factor deficiencies. In one report 67 of 71 patients with an intracranial hemorrhage had severe or moderately severe (5% or less of normal activity) disease, but only four patients had mild or moderate disease severity (6% to 20% of normal factor activity).[184]

Treatment of Hemophilia

Hemophilia patients should eschew activities that are likely to cause head trauma and avoid antiplatelet drugs. Rapid factor replacement at the first suspicion of intracranial hemorrhage or immediately after head trauma reduces the likelihood of severe intracranial hemorrhage.[184,185] Early therapy is particularly important for patients with a severe factor deficiency.

Patients with possible intracranial hemorrhage should have treatment initiated pending completion of confirmatory tests. Eyster and colleagues recommend a single dose of factor replacement calculated to produce 40% to 50% of normal activity for severe hemophiliacs even after a minor injury. Treatment is started for mild hemophiliacs only if symptomatic or for more significant injuries. Surgical evacuation of subdural or epidural hemorrhages, after proper factor replacement, may be lifesaving.

Stem cell and gene replacement therapy have shown great promise for hemophilia but have yet to become clinically feasible.[187–189]

Dysfibrinogenemia

Fibrinogen is a large protein with two identical segments, each of which contains three polypeptide sections encoded by three different genes. Dysfibrinogenemia can be either hereditary or acquired. Inherited dysfibrinogenemia is genetically and phenotypically heterogeneous. Numerous autosomal dominant mutations have been identified, each resulting in the synthesis of a structurally and functionally abnormal fibrinogen molecule. Acquired dysfibrinogenemia has been described in individuals with hepatic dysfunction or multiple myeloma.[190,191]

An estimated 55% of the individuals with dysfibrinogenemia remain asymptomatic, whereas 25% have a bleeding tendency and 20% develop one or more thromboses. Those who develop a thrombus are more likely to have a venous thrombosis than an arterial occlusion.[192]

Vitamin K Deficiency

Vitamin K is a fat-soluble vitamin that is a cofactor for the biosynthesis of factors II, VII, IX, and X along with proteins C and S.[193,194] Symptomatic vitamin K deficiency is more likely to result from vitamin malabsorption or from prolonged use of antibiotics than an inadequate diet. Malabsorption of vitamin K and other fat-soluble vitamins can occur in individuals with celiac disease, cystic fibrosis, small bowel resection, and chronic cholestyramine use.[195,196]

Because vitamin K is utilized in the formation of both anticoagulant factors and proteins C and S, vitamin K deficiency could theoretically either enhance or inhibit coagulation.[194] However, vitamin K seems to be more important in the formation of the coagulation factors, so a deficiency state promotes hemorrhage.

Warfarin Toxicity

Warfarin and related compounds inhibit vitamin K epoxide reductase, an enzyme that normally recycles vitamin K to its reduced form following its oxidation during the biosynthesis of coagulation proteins. An inadequate supply of reduced vitamin K has much the same physiologic effect as vitamin K deficiency.

Individuals taking oral anticoagulants have an intracerebral hemorrhage rate of 0.3% to 0.6% per year.[197] The risk increases in people who are hypertensive, those with supratherapeutic INR values, and individuals taking a concomitant antiplatelet agent.[197] The risk of an intracranial hemorrhage also increases after an injury. Inadvertent or purposeful warfarin overdose can generate very high INR values, but more often warfarin's anticoagulation effect is bolstered by interaction with other drugs or herbal remedies.[198,199] Fortunately, the effects of warfarin can be reversed by the administration of vitamin K.[200–202]

Dozens of medications and herbal remedies increase or decrease the effectiveness of warfarin, interactions with obvious clinical implications. Some of the drugs that can increase the anticoagulant effect of warfarin include acetaminophen, amiodarone, cimetidine, ciprofloxacin, clofibrate, erythromycin, thyroid hormone, lovastatin, phenytoin, propranolol, tamoxifen, and the tricyclic antidepressants.[203,204] Among the drugs reported to reduce the anticoagulant effect of warfarin include antithyroid drugs, carbamazepine, cholestyramine, cyclophosphamide, oral contraceptives, barbiturates, furosemide, and spironolactone.[196]

Some herbal remedies enhance the effects of warfarin, and an estimated 30% of the patients being treated with warfarin admit to taking one or more such compounds.[198,205,206] Excessive consumption of vitamin K, of course, reduces the warfarin's effect, and wide fluctuations in the dietary consumption of foods rich in vitamin K can make it difficult to maintain stable anticoagulation.[207,208]

Ingestion of brodifacoum, a long-acting warfarin-like compound that is used in many rat poisons, can induce a severe and sometimes fatal coagulopathy.[209,210]

Hepatic Dysfunction

Individuals with hepatic disease carry an increased risk of both thrombotic and hemorrhagic complications due to aberrant synthesis of clotting factors, coagulation inhibitors, and fibrinolytic proteins.[211] The risk of a clinically significant coagulopathy increases in parallel with the severity of the hepatic dysfunction. Thrombocytopenia and DIC are also common in people with liver failure. Acute or chronic hepatic dysfunction impairs hepatic protein synthesis, leading to decreased production of most vitamin K–dependent factor levels but particularly of factor VII and protein C.[212] Some individuals have deficient vitamin K stores, and it may be hard to distinguish the contribution of inadequate vitamin K from that of impaired biosynthesis of coagulation factors by the diseased hepatocytes.[211]

Brain hemorrhage has been documented in people with liver failure. Administration of parenteral vitamin K may help those with inadequate vitamin stores. Antifibrinolytic agents may be helpful in some patients.[212] Recombinant factor VIIa infusion or fresh frozen plasma may be helpful.[211,213] Blonski and colleagues have reviewed the management of coagulopathy associated with hepatic dysfunction.[211]

Maternal Medications

Infants whose mothers take warfarin during the first trimester can have congenital defects, and exposure during the third trimester can produce severe coagulopathy.[214] Prenatal exposure to anticonvulsants such as phenytoin or phenobarbital can cause a severe vitamin K–dependent coagulopathy that requires a higher than usual vitamin supplementation to correct.[215,216] Animal studies suggest that the reduction of vitamin K–dependent coagulation factors is dose dependent and can be prevented by vitamin K supplementation during pregnancy.[215]

REFERENCES

1. Herrick JB. Peculiar elongated and sickle-shaped red blood corpuscles in a case of severe anemia. *Arch Intern Med.* 1910; **6**:517–521.

2. Ohene-Frempong K, Weiner SJ, Sleeper LA, et al. Cerebrovascular accidents in sickle cell disease: rates and risk factors. *Blood.* 1998;**91**:288–294.

3. Adams RJ, Nichols FT, McKie V, McVie K, Milner P, Gammal TE. Cerebral infarction in sickle cell anemia. Mechanism based on CT and MRI. *Neurology.* 1988;**38**:1012–1017.

4. Prengler M, Pavlakis SG, Prohovnik I, Adams RJ. Sickle cell disease: the neurological complications. *Ann Neurol.* 2002;**51**:543–552.

5. Driscoll MC, Hurlet A, Styles L, et al. Stroke risk in siblings with sickle cell anemia. *Blood.* 2003;**101**:2401–2404.

6. Hillery CA, Panepinto JA. Pathophysiology of stroke in sickle cell disease. *Microcirculation.* 2004;**11**:195–208.

7. Moser FG, Miller ST, Bello JA, et al. The spectrum of brain MR abnormalities in sickle-cell disease: a report from the Cooperative Study of Sickle Cell Disease. *AJNR Am J Neuroradiol.* 1996; **17**:965–972.

8. Roach ES, Golomb MR, Adams RJ, et al. Management of stroke in infants and children. A scientific statement for healthcare professionals from a special writing group of the Stroke Council, American Heart Association. *Stroke.* 2008;**39**:2644–2691.

9. Preul MC, Cendes F, Just N, Mohr G. Intracranial aneurysms and sickle cell anemia: multiplicity and propensity for the vertebrobasilar territory. *Neurosurgery.* 1998;**42**:971–977.

10. Rothman SM, Nelson JS. Spinal cord infarction in a patient with sickle cell anemia. *Neurology.* 1980;**30**:1072–1076.

11. Adams RJ, Pavlakis S, Roach ES. Sickle cell disease and stroke: primary prevention and transcranial Doppler. *Ann Neurol.* 2003;**54**:559–563.

12. Adams RJ, Brambilla DJ, Granger S, et al. Stroke and conversion to high risk in children screened with transcranial Doppler ultrasound during the STOP study. *Blood.* 2004;**103**:3689–3694.

13. Adams R, McKie V, Nichols F, et al. The use of transcranial ultrasonography to predict stroke in sickle cell disease. *N Engl J Med.* 1992;**326**:605–610.

14. Pegelow CH, Adams RJ, McKie V, et al. Risk of recurrent stroke in patients with sickle cell disease treated with erythrocyte transfusions. *J Pediatr.* 1995;**126**:896–899.

15. Adams RJ, McKie VC, Hsu L, et al. Stroke prevention trial in sickle cell anemia ("STOP"): study results. *N Engl J Med.* 1998; **339**:5–11.

16. Adams RJ, Brambilla D. Discontinuing prophylactic transfusions used to prevent stroke in sickle cell disease. *N Engl J Med.* 2005;**353**:2769–2778.

17. Wang WC, Kovnar EH, Tonkin IL, et al. High risk of recurrent stroke after discontinuance of five to twelve years of transfusion therapy in patients with sickle cell disease. *J Pediatr.* 1991;**118**: 377–382.

18. Miller ST, Jensen D, Rao SP. Less intensive long-term transfusion therapy for sickle cell anemia and cerebrovascular accident. *J Pediatr.* 1992;**120**:54–57.

19. Ware RE, Zimmerman SA, Sylvestre PB, et al. Prevention of secondary stroke and resolution of transfusional iron overload in children with sickle cell anemia using hydroxyurea and phlebotomy. *J Pediatr.* 2004;**145**:346–352.

20. Zimmerman SA, Schultz WH, Davis JS, et al. Sustained long-term hematologic efficacy of hydroxyurea at maximum tolerated dose in children with sickle cell disease. *Blood.* 2004;**103**: 2039–2045.

21. Gulbis B, Haberman D, Dufour D, et al. Hydroxyurea for sickle cell disease in children and for prevention of cerebrovascular events: the Belgian experience. *Blood.* 2005;**105**:2685–2690.

22. Scott RM, Smith JL, Robertson RL, Madsen JR, Soriano SG, Rockoff MA. Long-term outcome in children with moyamoya syndrome after cranial revascularization by pial synangiosis. *J Neurosurg.* 2004;**100**:142–149.

23. Hankinson TC, Bohman LE, Heyer G, et al. Surgical treatment of moyamoya syndrome in patients with sickle cell anemia: outcome following encephaloduroarteriosynangiosis. *J Neurosurg Pediatr.* 2008;**1**:211–216.

24. Walters MC, Storb R, Patience M, et al. Impact of bone marrow transplantation for symptomatic sickle cell disease: an interim report. Multicenter investigation of bone marrow transplantation for sickle cell disease. *Blood.* 2000;**95**:1918–1924.

25. Lane PA, Githens JH. Splenic syndrome at mountain altitudes in sickle cell trait. Its occurrence in nonblack persons. *JAMA.* 1985;**253**:2251–2254.

26. Kark JA, Posey DM, Schumacher HR, Ruehle CJ. Sickle-cell trait as a risk factor for sudden death in physical training. *N Engl J Med.* 1987;**317**:781–787.

27. Martin TW, Weisman IM, Zeballos RJ, Stephenson SR. Exercise and hypoxia increase sickling in venous blood from an exercising limb in individuals with sickle cell trait. *Am J Med.* 1989;**87**:48–56.

28. Dowling MM. Sickle cell trait is not a risk factor for stroke. *Arch Neurol.* 2005;**62**:1780–1781.

29. Golomb MR. Sickle cell trait is a risk factor for early stroke. *Arch Neurol.* 2005;**62**:1778–1779.

30. Roach ES. Sickle cell trait: innocent until proven guilty. *Arch Neurol.* 2005;**62**:1781–1782.

31. Portnoy BA, Herion JC. Neurological manifestations in sickle-cell disease – with a review of the literature and emphasis on the prevalence of hemiplegia. *Ann Intern Med.* 1972;**76**:643–652.

32. Logothetis J, Constantoulakis M, Economidou J, et al. Thalassemia major (homozygous beta-thalassemia) – a survey of 138 cases with emphasis on neurologic and muscular aspects. *Neurology.* 1972;**22**:294–304.

33. Siekert RG, Whisnant JP, Millikan CH. Anemia and intermittent focal cerebral arterial insufficiency. *Arch Neurol.* 1960;**3**:386–390.

34. Kralovics R, Indrak K, Stopka T, Berman BW, Prchal JF, Prchal JT. Two new EPO receptor mutations: truncated EPO receptors are most frequently associated with primary familial and congenital polycythemias. *Blood.* 1997;**90**:2057–2061.

35. Furukawa T, Narita M, Sakaue M, et al. Primary familial polycythaemia associated with a novel point mutation in the erythropoietin receptor. *Br J Haematol.* 1997;**99**:222–227.

36. Arcasoy MO, Degar BA, Harris KW, Forget BG. Familial erythrocytosis associated with a short deletion in the erythropoietin receptor gene. *Blood.* 1997;**89**:4628–4635.

37. Sergeyeva A, Gordeuk VR, Tokarev YN, Sokol L, Prchal JF, Prchal JT. Congenital polycythemia in Chuvashia. *Blood.* 1997;**89**:2148–2154.

38. Kralovics R, Passamonti F, Buser AS, et al. A gain-of-function mutation of JAK2 in myeloproliferative disorders. *N Engl J Med.* 2005;**352**:1779–1790.

39. Thomas DJ, du Boulay GH, Marshall J, et al. Cerebral blood-flow in polycythaemia. *Lancet.* 1977;**2**:161–163.

40. De S, V, Za T, Rossi E, et al. Recurrent thrombosis in patients with polycythemia vera and essential thrombocythemia: incidence, risk factors, and effect of treatments. *Haematologica.* 2008;**93**:372–380.

41. Polycythemia vera: the natural history of 1213 patients followed for 20 years. Gruppo Italiano Studio Policitemia. *Ann Intern Med.* 1995;**123**:656–664.

42. Midi I, Dib H, Koseoglu M, Afsar N, Gunal DI. Hemichorea associated with polycythaemia vera. *Neurol Sci.* 2006;**27**:439–441.

43. Mas JL, Gueguen B, Bouche P, Derouesne C, Varet B, Castaigne P. Chorea and polycythaemia. *J Neurol.* 1985;**232**:169–171.

44. Bruyn GW, Padberg G. Chorea and polycythaemia. *Eur Neurol.* 1984;**23**:26–33.

45. Landolfi R, Marchioli R, Kutti J, et al. Efficacy and safety of low-dose aspirin in polycythemia vera. *N Engl J Med.* 2004;**350**:114–124.

46. Mahoney JF, Urakaze M, Hall S, et al. Defective glycosylphosphatidylinositol anchor synthesis in paroxysmal nocturnal hemoglobinuria granulocytes. *Blood.* 1992;**79**:1400–1403.

47. Nafa K, Mason PJ, Hillmen P, Luzzatto L, Bessler M. Mutations in the PIG-A gene causing paroxysmal nocturnal hemoglobinuria are mainly of the frameshift type. *Blood.* 1995;**86**:4650–4655.

48. Luzzatto L, Gianfaldoni G. Recent advances in biological and clinical aspects of paroxysmal nocturnal hemoglobinuria. *Int J Hematol.* 2006;**84**:104–112.

49. Hillmen P, Lewis SM, Bessler M, Luzzatto L, Dacie JV. Natural history of paroxysmal nocturnal hemoglobinuria. *N Engl J Med.* 1995;**333**:1253–1258.

50. Donhowe SP, Lazaro RP. Dural sinus thrombosis in paroxysmal nocturnal hemoglobinuria. *Clin Neurol Neurosurg.* 1984;**86**:149–152.

51. Johnson RV, Kaplan SR, Blailock ZR. Cerebral venous thrombosis in paroxysmal nocturnal hemoglobinuria. *Neurology.* 1970;**20**:681–686.

52. Audebert HJ, Planck J, Eisenburg M, Schrezenmeier H, Haberl RL. Cerebral ischemic infarction in paroxysmal nocturnal hemoglobinuria report of 2 cases and updated review of 7 previously published patients. *J Neurol.* 2005;**252**:1379–1386.

53. al-Hakim M, Katirji B, Osorio I, Weisman R. Cerebral venous thrombosis in paroxysmal nocturnal hemoglobinuria: report of two cases. *Neurology.* 1993;**43**:742–746.

54. Devine DV, Gluck WL, Rosse WF, Weinberg JB. Acute myeloblastic leukemia in paroxysmal nocturnal hemoglobinuria. Evidence of evolution from the abnormal paroxysmal nocturnal hemoglobinuria clone. *J Clin Invest.* 1987;**79**:314–317.

55. Sterling ML, Lenton RJ, Sumerling MD. Cerebral vein thrombosis and the contraceptive pill in paroxysmal nocturnal haemoglobinuria. *Scot Med J.* 1980;**25**:243–244.

56. Spencer JAD. Paroxysmal nocturnal haemoglobinuria in pregnancy. *Brit J Obstet Gynecol.* 1980;**87**:246–248.

57. Teyssier JR, Pigeon F, Behar C, Pignon B, Blaise AM. Chromosomal subclonal evolution in paroxysmal nocturnal hemoglobinuria evolving into acute megakaryoblastic leukemia. *Cancer Genet Cytogenet.* 1987;**25**:259–264.

58. Hillmen P, Young NS, Schubert J, et al. The complement inhibitor eculizumab in paroxysmal nocturnal hemoglobinuria. *N Engl J Med.* 2006;**355**:1233–1243.

59. Clark-Kennedy AE. *Stephen Hales, D.D., F.RS. An Eigthteenth Century Biography.* Cambridge, England: Cambridge University Press; 1929.

60. Wood MH, Kee DB. Hemorheology of the cerebral circulation in stroke. *Stroke.* 1985;**16**:765–772.

61. Coull BM, Beamer N, de Garmo P, et al. Chronic blood hyperviscosity in subjects with acute stroke, transient ischemic attack, and risk factors for stroke. *Stroke.* 1991;**22**:162–168.

62. Park MS, Kim BC, Kim IK, et al. Cerebral infarction in IgG multiple myeloma with hyperviscosity. *J Korean Med Sci.* 2005;**20**:699–701.

63. Jovin TG, Boosupalli V, Zivkovic SA, Wechsler LR, Gebel JM. High titers of CA-125 may be associated with recurrent ischemic strokes in patients with cancer. *Neurology.* 2005;**64**:1944–1945.

64. Byrne NP, Henry JC, Herrmann DN, et al. Neuropathologic findings in a Guillain-Barre patient with strokes after IVIg therapy. *Neurology.* 2002;**59**:458–461.

65. Caress JB, Cartwright MS, Donofrio PD, Peacock JE Jr. The clinical features of 16 cases of stroke associated with administration of IVIg. *Neurology.* 2003;**60**:1822–1824.

66. Walther EU, Tiecks FP, Haberl RL. Cranial sinus thrombosis associated with essential thrombocytopenia followed by heparin associated thrombocytopenia. *Neurology.* 1996;**47**:300–301.

67. Atkinson JLD, Sundt TM, Kazmier FJ, Bowie EJW, Whisnant JP. Heparin-induced thrombocytopenia and thrombosis in ischemic stroke. *Mayo Clin Proc.* 1988;**63**:353–361.

68. Cines DB, Tomaski A, Tannenbaum S. Immune endothelial cell injury in heparin-associated thrombocytopenia. *N Engl J Med.* 1987;**316**:581–589.

69. Delgado MR, Riela AR, Mills J, Browne R, Roach ES. Thrombocytopenia secondary to high valproate levels in children with epilepsy. *J Child Neurol.* 1994;**9**:311–314.

70. Anderson GD, Lin Y-X, Berge C, Ojemann GA. Absence of bleeding complications in patients undergoing cortical surgery while receiving valproate treatment. *J Neurosurg.* 1997;**87**:252–256.

71. Humphries RP, Hockley AD, Freedman MH, Saunders EF. Management of intracerebral hemorrhage in idiopathic thrombocytopenic purpura. *J Neurosurg.* 1976;**45**:700–704.

72. Krivit W, Tate D, White JG, Robison LL. Idiopathic thrombocytopenic purpura and intracranial hemorrhage. *Pediatrics.* 1981;**67**:570–571.

73. Woerner SJ, Abildgaard CF, French BN. Intracranial hemorrhage in children with idiopathic thrombocytopenic purpura. *Pediatrics.* 1981;**67**:453–460.

74. Morales WJ, Stroup M. Intracranial hemorrhage in utero due to isoimmune neonatal thrombocytopenia. *Obstet Gynecol.* 1985;**65**:20–21S.

75. Sia CG, Amigo NC, Harper RG, Farahani G, Kochen J. Failure of cesarian section to prevent intracranial hemorrhage in siblings with isoimmune neonatal thrombocytopenia. *Am J Obstet Gynecol.* 1985;**153**:79–81.

76. Bussel JB, Pham LC, Aledort L, Nachman R. Maintenance treatment of adults with chronic refractory immune thrombocytopenic purpura using repeated intravenous infusions of gammaglobulin. *Blood.* 1988;**72**:121–127.

77. Schwartz J, Leber MD, Gillis S, Giunta A, Eldor A, Bussel JB. Long term follow-up after splenectomy performed for immune thrombocytopenic purpura (ITP). *Am J Hematol.* 2003;**72**:94–98.

78. Jabaily J, Iland HJ, Laszlo J, et al. Neurologic manifestations of essential thrombocythemia. *Ann Intern Med.* 1983;**99**:513–518.

79. McIntyre KJ, Hoagland HC, Silverstein MN, Petitt RM. Essential thrombocythemia in young adults. *Mayo Clin Proc.* 1991;**66**:149–154.

80. Hoagland HC, Silverstein MN. Primary thrombocythemia in the young patient. *Mayo Clin Proc.* 1978;**53**:578–580.

81. Regev A, Stark P, Blickstein D, Lahav M. Thrombotic complications in essential thrombocythemia with relatively low platelet counts. *Am J Hematol.* 1997;**56**:168–172.

82. Iob I, Scanarini M, Andrioli GC, Pardatscher K. Thrombosis of the superior sagittal sinus associated with idiopathic thrombocytosis. *Surg Neurol.* 1979;**11**:439–441.

83. Michiels JJ, Koudstaal PJ, Mulder AH, van Vliet HHDM. Transient neurologic and ocular manifestations in primary thrombocythemia. *Neurology.* 1993;**43**:1107–1110.

84. Koudstaal PJ, Koudstaal A. Neurologic and visual symptoms in essential thrombocythemia: efficacy of low-dose aspirin. *Semin Thromb Hemost.* 1997;**23**:365–370.

85. Kawanami T, Kurita K, Yamakawa M, Omoto E, Kato T. Cerebrovascular disease in acute leukemia: a clinicopathological study of 14 patients. *Intern Med.* 2002;**41**:1130–1134.

86. Rogers LR. Cerebrovascular complications in cancer patients. *Neurol Clin.* 2003;**21**:167–192.

87. Kitchens C, Eskin T. Fatality in a case of envenomation by Crotalus adamanteus initially successfully treated with polyvalent ovine antivenom followed by recurrence of defibrinogenation syndrome. *J Med Toxicol.* 2008;**4**:180–183.

88. Stein SC, Smith DH. Coagulopathy in traumatic brain injury. *Neurocrit Care.* 2004;**1**:479–488.

89. Hardaway RM. Organ damage in shock, disseminated intravascular coagulation, and stroke. *Compr Ther.* 1992;**18**:17–21.

90. Ridolfi RL, Bell WR. Thrombotic thrombocytopenic purpura. Report of 25 cases and review of the literature. *Medicine.* 1981;**60**:413–428.

91. Zakarija A, Bandarenko N, Pandey DK, et al. Clopidogrel-associated TTP: an update of pharmacovigilance efforts conducted by independent researchers, pharmaceutical suppliers, and the Food and Drug Administration. *Stroke.* 2004;**35**:533–537.

92. Medina PJ, Sipols JM, George JN. Drug-associated thrombotic thrombocytopenic purpura-hemolytic uremic syndrome. *Curr Opin Hematol.* 2001;**8**:286–293.

93. Zakarija A, Bennett C. Drug-induced thrombotic microangiopathy. *Semin Thromb Hemost.* 2005;**31**:681–690.

94. Furlan M, Robles R, Galbusera M, et al. von Willebrand factor-cleaving protease in thrombotic thrombocytopenic purpura and the hemolytic-uremic syndrome. *N Engl J Med.* 1998;**339**:1578–1584.

95. Lian EC. Pathogenesis of thrombotic thrombocytopenic purpura: ADAMTS13 deficiency and beyond. *Semin Thromb Hemost.* 2005;**31**:625–632.

96. Lammle B, Kremer Hovinga JA, Alberio L. Thrombotic thrombocytopenic purpura. *J Thromb Haemost.* 2005;**3**:1663–1675.

97. Harkness DR, Byrnes JJ, Lian EC, Williams WD, Hensley GT. Hazard of platelet transfusion in thrombotic thrombocytopenic purpura. *JAMA.* 1981;**246**:1931–1933.

98. George JN, Shattil SJ. The clinical importance of acquired abnormalities of platelet function. *N Engl J Med.* 1991;**324**:27–39.

99. Sattler FR, Weitekamp MR, Ballard JO. Potential for bleeding with the new beta-lactam antibiotics. *Ann Intern Med.* 1986;**105**:924–931.

100. Pillgram-Larsen J, Wisloff F, Jorgensen JJ, Godal HC, Semb G. Effect of high-dose ampicillin and cloxacillin on bleeding time and bleeding in open-heart surgery. *Scand J Thorac Cardiovasc Surg.* 1985;**19**:45–48.

101. Fass RJ, Copelan EA, Brandt JT, Moeschberger ML, Ashton JJ. Platelet-mediated bleeding caused by broad-spectrum penicillins. *J Infect Dis.* 1987;**155**:1242–1248.

102. Sattler FR, Weitekamp MR, Sayegh A, Ballard JO. Impaired hemostasis caused by beta-lactam antibiotics. *Am J Surg.* 1988;**155**:30–39.

103. Sadler JE. A revised classification of von Willebrand disease. For the Subcommittee on von Willebrand Factor of the Scientific and Standardization Committee of the International Society on Thrombosis and Haemostasis. *Thromb Haemost.* 1994;**71**:520–525.

104. Mannucci PM. How I treat patients with von Willebrand disease. *Blood.* 2001;**97**:1915–1919.

105. Franchini M, Lippi G. Acquired von Willebrand syndrome: an update. *Am J Hematol.* 2007;**82**:368–375.

106. Johansson L, Jansson JH, Stegmayr B, Nilsson TK, Hallmans G, Boman K. Hemostatic factors as risk markers for intracerebral hemorrhage: a prospective incident case-referent study. *Stroke.* 2004;**35**:826–830.

107. Bongers TN, de Maat MP, van Goor ML, et al. High von Willebrand factor levels increase the risk of first ischemic stroke:

influence of ADAMTS13, inflammation, and genetic variability. *Stroke*. 2006;**37**:2672–2677.

108. Mammen EF. Sticky platelet syndrome. *Semin Thromb Hemost*. 1999;**25**:361–365.

109. Frenkel EP, Mammen EF. Sticky platelet syndrome and thrombocythemia. *Hematol Oncol Clin N Am*. 2003;**17**:63–83.

110. Olas B, Kedzierska M, Wachowicz B. Comparative studies on homocysteine and its metabolite-homocysteine thiolactone action in blood platelets in vitro. *Platelets*. 2008;**19**:520–527.

111. Mohan IV, Jagroop IA, Mikhailidis DP, Stansby GP. Homocysteine activates platelets in vitro. *Clin Appl Thromb Hemost*. 2008;**14**:8–18.

112. Undas A, Stepien E, Plicner D, Zielinski L, Tracz W. Elevated total homocysteine is associated with increased platelet activation at the site of microvascular injury: effects of folic acid administration. *J Thromb Haemost*. 2007;**5**:1070–1072.

113. Schneider JA, Rees DC, Liu YT, Clegg JB. Worldwide distribution of a common methylenetetrahydrofolate reductase mutation. *Am J Hum Genet*. 1998;**62**:1258–1260.

114. Weller PF, Bubley GJ. The idiopathic hypereosinophilic syndrome. *Blood*. 1994;**83**:2759–2779.

115. Moore PM, Harley JB, Fauci AS. Neurologic dysfunction in the idiopathic hypereosinophilic syndrome. *Ann Intern Med*. 1985;**102**:109–114.

116. Chang HW, Leong KH, Koh DR, Lee SH. Clonality of isolated eosinophils in the hypereosinophilic syndrome. *Blood*. 1999;**93**:1651–1657.

117. Rioux JD, Stone VA, Daly MJ, et al. Familial eosinophilia maps to the cytokine gene cluster on human chromosomal region 5q31-q33. *Am J Hum Genet*. 1998;**63**:1086–1094.

118. Prick JJ, Gabreels-Festen AA, Korten JJ, van der Wiel TW. Neurological manifestations of the hypereosinophilic syndrome (HES). *Clin Neurol Neurosurg*. 1988;**90**:269–273.

119. Kwon SU, Kim JC, Kim JS. Sequential magnetic resonance imaging findings in hypereosinophilia-induced encephalopathy. *J Neurol*. 2001;**248**:279–284.

120. Mates M, Nesher G, Roth B, Rosenberg R, Heyd J, Hershko C. Transient severe eosinophilia precipitating massive venous thrombosis in a patient with hereditary thrombophilia. *Acta Haematol*. 2004;**112**:209–211.

121. Lichman MA, Beutler E, Kaushansky K, et al., eds. *Williams Hematology*. 6th ed. New York: McGraw-Hill; 2005.

122. Whitlock JA, Janco RL, Phillips JA. Inherited hypercoagulable states in children. *Am J Pediatr Hematol Oncol*. 1989;**11**:170–173.

123. Kucuk O, Kwaan HC, Gunnar W, Vazquez RM. Thromboembolic complications associated with L-asparaginase therapy. Etiologic role of low antithrombin III and plasminogen levels and therapeutic correction by fresh frozen plasma. *Cancer*. 1985;**55**:702–706.

124. Rosenberg RD. Actions and interactions of antithrombin and heparin. *N Engl J Med*. 1975;**292**:146–151.

125. Ueyama H, Hashimoto Y, Uchino M, et al. Progressing ischemic stroke in a homozygote with variant antithrombin III. *Stroke*. 1989;**20**:815–818.

126. Tuite P, Ahmad F, Grant I, Stewart JD, Carpenter S, Ethier R. Cerebral vein thrombosis due to hereditary antithrombin III deficiency. *Can J Neurol Sci*. 1993;**20**:158–161.

127. Martinelli I, de Stefano V, Taioli E, et al. Inherited thrombophilia and first venous thromboembolism during pregnancy and puerperium. *Thromb Haemost*. 2002;**87**:791–795.

128. Finazzi G, Barbui T. Different incidence of venous thrombosis in patients with inherited deficiencies of antithrombin III, protein C and protein S. *Thromb Haemost*. 1994;**71**:15–18.

129. Demers C, Ginsberg JS, Hirsh J, Henderson P, Blajchman MA. Thrombosis in antithrombin III deficient persons. *Ann Intern Med*. 1992;**116**:754–761.

130. Rosendaal FR. Venous thrombosis: a multicausal disease. *Lancet*. 1999;**353**:1167–1173.

131. Ambruso DR, Jacobson LJ, Hathaway WE. Inherited antithrombin III deficiency and cerebral thrombosis in a child. *Pediatrics*. 1980;**65**:125–131.

132. Esmon CT. Protein-C: biochemistry, physiology, and clinical implications. *Blood*. 1983;**62**:1155–1158.

133. Uysal S, Anlar B, Altay C, Kirazli S. Role of protein C in childhood cerebrovascular occlusive accidents. *Eur J Pediatr*. 1989;**149**:216–218.

134. Caballero FM, Buchanan GR. Abetalipoproteinemia presenting as severe vitamin K deficiency. *Pediatrics*. 1980;**65**:161–163.

135. Camerlingo M, Finazzi G, Casto L, Laffranchi C, Barbui T, Mamoli A. Inherited protein C deficiency and nonhemorrhagic arterial stroke in young adults. *Neurology*. 1991;**41**:1371–1373.

136. Pegelow CH, Curless R, Bradford B. Severe protein C deficiency in a newborn. *Am J Pediatr Hematol Oncol*. 1988;**10**:326–329.

137. Tarras S, Gadia C, Meister L, Roldan E, Gregorios JB. Homozygous protein C deficiency in a newborn: clinicopathologic correlation. *Arch Neurol*. 1988;**45**:214–216.

138. Broekman AW, Veltkamp JJ, Bertina RM. Congenital protein C deficiency and venous thromboembolism: a study of three Dutch families. *N Engl J Med*. 1983;**309**:340–344.

139. Green D, Otoya J, Oriba H, Rovner R. Protein S deficiency in middle-aged women with stroke. *Neurology*. 1992;**42**:1029–1033.

140. Moreb J, Kitchens CS. Acquired functional protein S deficiency, cerebral venous thrombosis, and coumarin skin necrosis in association with antiphospholipid syndrome: report of two cases. *Am J Med*. 1989;**87**:207–210.

141. Chan YC, Valenti D, Mansfield AO, Stansby G. Warfarin induced skin necrosis. *Br J Surg*. 2000;**87**:266–272.

142. Scott BD, Esmon CT, Comp PC. The natural anticoagulant protein S is decreased in male smokers. *Am Heart J*. 1991;**122**:76–80.

143. Lee JH, Kim SW, Sung KJ. Sagittal sinus thrombosis associated with transient free protein S deficiency after L-asparaginase treatment: case report and review of the literature. *Clin Neurol Neurosurg*. 2000;**102**:33–36.

144. Makris M, Leach M, Beauchamp NJ, et al. Genetic analysis, phenotypic diagnosis, and risk of venous thrombosis in families with inherited deficiencies of protein S. *Blood*. 2000;**95**:1935–1941.

145. Barinagarrementeria F, Cantu-Brito C, de la Pena A, Izaguirre R. Prothrombotic states in young people with idiopathic stroke. A prospective study. *Stroke*. 1994;**25**:287–290.

146. Poort SR, Rosendaal FR, Reitsma PH, Bertina RM. A common genetic variation in the 3′-untranslated region of the prothrombin gene is associated with elevated plasma prothrombin levels and an increase in venous thrombosis. *Blood*. 1996;**88**:3698–3703.

147. Poort SR, Michiels JJ, Reitsma PH, Bertina RM. Homozygosity for a novel missense mutation in the prothrombin gene causing a severe bleeding disorder. *Thromb Haemost*. 1994;**72**:819–824.

148. Poort SR, Landolfi R, Bertina RM. Compound heterozygosity for two novel missense mutations in the prothrombin gene in a patient with a severe bleeding tendency. *Thromb Haemost*. 1997;**77**:610–615.

149. Bank I, Libourel EJ, Middeldorp S, et al. Prothrombin 20210A mutation: a mild risk factor for venous thromboembolism but not for arterial thrombotic disease and pregnancy-related

complications in a family study. *Arch Intern Med.* 2004;**164**:1932–1937.

150. Miles JS, Miletich JP, Goldhaber SZ, Hennekens CH, Ridker PM. G20210A mutation in the prothrombin gene and the risk of recurrent venous thromboembolism. *J Am Coll Cardiol.* 2001;**37**:215–218.

151. Martinelli I, Taioli E, Bucciarelli P, Akhavan S, Mannucci PM. Interaction between the G20210A mutation of the prothrombin gene and oral contraceptive use in deep vein thrombosis. *Arterioscler Thromb Vasc Biol.* 1999;**19**:700–703.

152. Ridker PM, Miletich JP, Hennekens CH, Buring JE. Ethnic distribution of factor V Leiden in 4047 men and women. Implications for venous thromboembolism screening. *JAMA.* 1997;**277**:1305–1307.

153. Martinelli I, Bucciarelli P, Margaglione M, de Stefano V, Castaman G, Mannucci PM. The risk of venous thromboembolism in family members with mutations in the genes of factor V or prothrombin or both. *Br J Haematol.* 2000;**111**:1223–1229.

154. Munts AG, van Genderen PJ, Dippel DW, van Kooten F, Koudstaal PJ. Coagulation disorders in young adults with acute cerebral ischaemia. *J Neurol.* 1998;**245**:21–25.

155. Dolan G, Greaves M, Cooper P, Preston FE. Thrombovascular disease and familial plasminogen deficiency: a report of three kindreds. *Br J Haematol.* 1988;**70**:417–421.

156. Pierangeli SS, Chen PP, Gonzalez EB. Antiphospholipid antibodies and the antiphospholipid syndrome: an update on treatment and pathogenic mechanisms. *Curr Opin Hematol.* 2006;**13**:366–375.

157. Mitsias P, Levine SR. Large cerebral vessel occlusive disease in systemic lupus erythematosus. *Neurology.* 1994;**44**:385–393.

158. Levine SR, Diaczok IM, Deegan MJ, et al. Recurrent stroke associated with thymoma and anticardiolipin antibodies. *Arch Neurol.* 1987;**44**:678–679.

159. Hart RG, Miller VT, Coull BM. Cerebral infarction associated with lupus anticoagulants – preliminary report. *Stroke.* 1984;**15**:114–118.

160. Mueh JR, Herbst KD, Rapaport SI. Thrombosis in patients with the lupus anticoagulant. *Ann Intern Med.* 1980;**92**:156–159.

161. Levine SR, Welch KMA. The spectrum of neurologic disease associated with antiphospholipid antibodies. Lupus anticoagulants and anticardiolipin antibodies. *Arch Neurol.* 1987;**44**:876–883.

162. Rumpl E, Neuhofer J, Pallua A, et al. Cerebrovascular lesions and livedo reticularis (Sneddon's syndrome) – a progressive cerebrovascular disorder? *J Neurol.* 1985;**231**:324–330.

163. Stockhammer G, Felber SR, Zelger B, et al. Sneddon's syndrome: diagnosis by skin biopsy and MRI in 17 patients. *Stroke.* 1993;**24**:685–690.

164. Hilton DA, Footitt D. Neuropathological findings in Sneddon's syndrome. *Neurology.* 2003;**60**:1181–1182.

165. Boesch SM, Plorer AL, Auer AJ, et al. The natural course of Sneddon syndrome: clinical and magnetic resonance imaging findings in a prospective six year observation study. *J Neurol Neurosurg Psychiatry.* 2003;**74**:542–544.

166. Dafer RM, Biller J. Antiphospholipid syndrome: role of antiphospholipid antibodies in neurology. *Hematol Oncol Clin N Am.* 2008;**22**:95–105.

167. Fox MW, Harms RW, Davis DH. Selected neurologic complications of pregnancy. *Mayo Clin Proc.* 1990;**65**:1595–1618.

168. Weibers DO. Ischemic cerebrovascular complications of pregnancy. *Arch Neurol.* 1985;**42**:1106–1113.

169. de Boer K, ten Cate JW, Sturk A, Borm JJJ, Treffers PE. Enhanced thrombin generation in normal and hypertensive pregnancy. *Am J Obstet Gynecol.* 1989;**160**:95–100.

170. Mayeux R, Fahn S. Strokes and ulcerative colitis. *Neurology.* 1978;**28**:571–574.

171. Standridge S, de los Reyes E. Inflammatory bowel disease and cerebrovascular arterial and venous thromboembolic events in 4 pediatric patients: a case series and review of the literature. *J Child Neurol.* 2008;**23**:59–66.

172. Younes-Mhenni S, Derex L, Berruyer M, et al. Large-artery stroke in a young patient with Crohn's disease. Role of vitamin B6 deficiency-induced hyperhomocysteinemia. *J Neurol Sci.* 2004;**221**:113–115.

173. Nomoto T, Nagao T, Hirabayashi K, et al. Cerebral arteriopathy with extracranial artery involvement in a patient with ulcerative colitis. *J Neurol Sci.* 2006;**243**:87–89.

174. Schneiderman JH, Sharpe JA, Sutton DMC. Cerebral and retinal vascular complications of inflammatory bowel disease. *Ann Neurol.* 1979;**5**:331–337.

175. Findler G, Aldor A, Hadani M, Sahar A, Feinsod M. Traumatic intracranial hemorrhage in children with rare coagulation disorders. *J Neurosurg.* 1982;**57**:775–778.

176. Hanna M. Congenital deficiency of factor XIII: report of a family from Newfoundland with associated mild deficiency of factor XII. *Pediatrics.* 1970;**46**:611–619.

177. Siao D, Seetapah A, Ryman A, Guerin V, Mesli A, Maurette P. Optimal management of an aneurysmal subarachnoid hemorrhage in a patient with known factor XI deficiency: a case report. *Clin Appl Thromb Hemost.* 2008;**14**:108–111.

178. Montgomery R, Natelson SE. Afibrinogenemia with intracerebral hematoma. *Am J Dis Child.* 1977;**131**:555–556.

179. Hoyer LW. Hemophilia A. *N Engl J Med.* 1994;**330**:38–47.

180. de Tezanos Pinto M, Fernandez J, Perez Bianco PR. Update on 156 episodes of central nervous system bleeding in hemophiliacs. *Haemostasis.* 1992;**22**:259–267.

181. Larsson SA, Wiechel B. Deaths in Swedish hemophiliacs, 1957–1980. *Acta Med Scand.* 1983;**214**:199–206.

182. Silverstein A. Intracranial bleeding in hemophilia. *Arch Neurol.* 1960;**3**:141–157.

183. Kerr CB. Intracranial haemorrhage in hemophilia. *J Neurol Neurosurg Psychiatry.* 1964;**27**:166–173.

184. Eyster ME, Gill FM, Blatt PM, Hilgartner MW, Ballard JO, Kinney TR. Central nervous system bleeding in hemophiliacs. *Blood.* 1978;**51**:1179–1188.

185. Andes WA, Wulff K, Smith WB. Head trauma in hemophilia: a prospective study. *Arch Intern Med.* 1984;**144**:1981–1983.

186. Seeler RA, Imana RB. Intracranial hemorrhage in patients with hemophilia. *J Neurosurg.* 1973;**39**:181–185.

187. Murphy SL, High KA. Gene therapy for haemophilia. *Br J Haematol.* 2008;**140**:479–487.

188. Fewell JG. Factor IX gene therapy for hemophilia. *Methods Mol Biol.* 2008;**423**:375–382.

189. Doering CB. Retroviral modification of mesenchymal stem cells for gene therapy of hemophilia. *Methods Mol Biol.* 2008;**433**:203–212.

190. Kotlin R, Sobotkova A, Riedel T, et al. Acquired dysfibrinogenemia secondary to multiple myeloma. *Acta Haematol.* 2008;**120**:75–81.

191. Francis JL, Armstrong DJ. Acquired dysfibrinogenaemia in liver disease. *J Clin Pathol.* 1982;**35**:667–672.

192. Hayes T. Dysfibrinogenemia and thrombosis. *Arch Pathol Lab Med.* 2002;**126**:1387–1390.

193. Ferland G, Sadowski JA, O'Brien ME. Dietary induced subclinical vitamin K deficiency in normal human subjects. *J Clin Invest.* 1993;**91**:1761–1768.

194. Shirakawa Y, Shirahata A, Fukuda M. Differences in reactivity to vitamin K administration of the vitamin K-dependent procoagulant factors, protein C and S, and osteocalcin. *Semin Thromb Hemost.* 2000;**26**:119–126.

195. Al-Terkait F, Charalambous H. Severe coagulopathy secondary to vitamin K deficiency in patient with small-bowel resection and rectal cancer. *Lancet Oncol.* 2006;**7**:188.

196. Vroonhof K, van Rijn HJ, van Hattum J. Vitamin K deficiency and bleeding after long-term use of cholestyramine. *Neth J Med.* 2003;**61**:19–21.

197. Hart RG, Tonarelli SB, Pearce LA. Avoiding central nervous system bleeding during antithrombotic therapy: recent data and ideas. *Stroke.* 2005;**36**:1588–1593.

198. Samuels N. Herbal remedies and anticoagulant therapy. *Thromb Haemost.* 2005;**93**:3–7.

199. Brandin H, Myrberg O, Rundlof T, Arvidsson AK, Brenning G. Adverse effects by artificial grapefruit seed extract products in patients on warfarin therapy. *Eur J Clin Pharmacol.* 2007;**63**:565–570.

200. Crowther MA, Douketis JD, Schnurr T, et al. Oral vitamin K lowers the international normalized ratio more rapidly than subcutaneous vitamin K in the treatment of warfarin-associated coagulopathy. A randomized, controlled trial. *Ann Intern Med.* 2002;**137**:251–254.

201. Gunther KE, Conway G, Leibach L, Crowther MA. Low-dose oral vitamin K is safe and effective for outpatient management of patients with an INR > 10. *Thromb Res.* 2004;**113**:205–209.

202. Dentali F, Ageno W. Management of coumarin-associated coagulopathy in the non-bleeding patient: a systematic review. *Haematologica.* 2004;**89**:857–862.

203. Ellis RJ, Mayo MS, Bodensteiner DM. Ciprofloxacin-warfarin coagulopathy: a case series. *Am J Hematol.* 2000;**63**:28–31.

204. Chute JP, Ryan CP, Sladek G, Shakir KM. Exacerbation of warfarin-induced anticoagulation by hyperthyroidism. *Endocr Pract.* 1997;**3**:77–79.

205. Wittkowsky AK. Dietary supplements, herbs and oral anticoagulants: the nature of the evidence. *J Thromb Thrombolysis.* 2008;**25**:72–77.

206. Elmer GW, Lafferty WE, Tyree PT, Lind BK. Potential interactions between complementary/alternative products and conventional medicines in a Medicare population. *Ann Pharmacother.* 2007;**41**:1617–1624.

207. Schulman S. Clinical practice. Care of patients receiving long-term anticoagulant therapy. *N Engl J Med.* 2003;**349**:675–683.

208. Marcason W. Vitamin K: what are the current dietary recommendations for patients taking coumadin? *J Am Diet Assoc.* 2007;**107**:2022.

209. Olmos V, Lopez CM. Brodifacoum poisoning with toxicokinetic data. *Clin Toxicol (Phila).* 2007;**45**:487–489.

210. Kruse JA, Carlson RW. Fatal rodenticide poisoning with brodifacoum. *Ann Emerg Med.* 1992;**21**:331–336.

211. Blonski W, Siropaides T, Reddy KR. Coagulopathy in liver disease. *Curr Treat Options Gastroenterol.* 2007;**10**:464–473.

212. Mammen EF. Coagulation defects in liver disease. *Med Clin N Am.* 1994;**78**:545–554.

213. Kaul V, Munoz SJ. Coagulopathy of liver disease. *Curr Treat Options Gastroenterol.* 2000;**3**:433–438.

214. Stevenson RE, Burton OM, Ferlauto GJ, Taylor HA. Hazards of oral anticoagulants during pregnancy. *JAMA.* 1980;**243**:1549–1551.

215. Solomon GE, Hilgartner MW, Kutt H. Coagulation defects caused by diphenylhydantoin. *Neurology.* 1972;**22**:1165–1171.

216. Blyer WA, Skinner AL. Fatal neonatal hemorrhage after maternal anticonvulsant therapy. *JAMA.* 1976;**235**:626–627.

217. Riela AR, Roach ES. Etiology of stroke in children. *J Child Neurol.* 1993;**8**:201–220.

12

Arterial Dissection

Disease often tells its secrets in a casual parenthesis.

Wilfred Trotter

When the force of the blood column flowing through an artery separates the intima from the media, a dissecting hematoma is formed. Most dissections do not result in arterial dilatation, but, if they do, it is a dissecting aneurysm.

ETIOLOGY AND PATHOGENESIS

Even a small tear in the intima can enlarge as the bloodstream burrows circumferentially, proximally, and distally beneath the flap. As dissection continues, blood beneath the intima progressively reduces the size of the arterial lumen and may eventually occlude it. Some dissections reenter the main channel to create a so-called double-barreled artery; others perforate through the media into the surrounding adventitia, forming a false aneurysm (pseudoaneurysm) or causing death from massive bleeding.

Arterial dissection causes ischemic infarction via multiple mechanisms.[1–6] If the lumen size is significantly compromised, reduced brain perfusion distal to the dissection site rapidly leads to ischemic infarction unless there is sufficient collateral circulation to maintain adequate perfusion. Thrombosis of the artery at the dissection site can also occur well after the dissection occurs. Alternatively, an infarction can develop days or weeks later because of an artery-to-artery embolism of a clot that forms at the dissection site.

Cervicocephalic arterial dissections (CCADs) may be spontaneous or traumatic.[7] Either penetrating injuries or blunt injuries associated with sudden stretching or torsion of the vessel due to trauma or during strenuous exertion may tear the intima and lead to dissection. Trauma to the neck from a non-penetrating blow or a hyperextension injury, as in a vehicular accident, is common. Following a hyperextension injury, the vertebral arteries can be traumatized by the movement of the atlas on the odontoid, resulting in distal dissection. The lateral process of C1 can injure the internal carotid from behind. Blunt force injuries may cause a linear transverse tear of the intima, followed by a retraction of its margins and separation from the media. The rent causes a thrombus that may extend or embolize. Most often the lesion lies at or within 3 cm of the bifurcation of the common carotid artery, but a few lesions begin more distally in the internal carotid artery.

Dissection has been documented following chiropractic manipulation and after periods of repetitive neck movements. Most of these reports describe one or two patients, however, and it has been estimated that only one vertebral artery (VA) dissection occurs during every 6 million cervical spine manipulations.[8–10]

Occasional individuals develop an arterial dissection after trauma to the aortic arch or its branches by angiography catheters or surgery on adjacent tissues. Because of the retropharyngeal course of the internal carotid artery, a dissection of this artery sometimes follows an intra-oral injury. Stroke following intra-oral trauma has been observed following tonsillar surgery or in individuals who fall face forward with a popsicle, toothbrush, or similar object in their mouth.[11,12]

Dissections of cervical and cerebral arteries may account for 5% or more of ischemic strokes in young adults, and the estimated recurrence rate for CCAD is 1% per year.[13] The overall incidence is about 3.6–4.4 per 100,000. Carotid artery dissections have been reported in 2.6–2.9 individuals per 100,000 per year, whereas spontaneous vertebral artery dissections have been reported in 1–1.5 per 100,000.[14]

CCADs are more often extracranial than intracranial. Extracranial dissections most commonly involve the media or subadventitia, whereas intracranial dissections usually involve the intima and media. Most extracranial internal carotid artery (ICA) dissections occur in the pharyngeal and distal segments and often extend up to the level of the skull base (foramen lacerum); the most frequently involved segment in individuals with vertebral artery dissection is either the V_1 segment or the V_3 segment. Regarding intracranial dissections, ICA dissections are most common supraclinoid, but intracranial dissections of the posterior circulation involve the distal VA (V4 segment) or the basilar artery. CCADs may involve a single or multiple vessels; multivessel dissections have been noted in 16% to 28% of cases.

A number of underlying conditions (Table 12-1) increase the likelihood of spontaneous arterial dissection, but a specific

Table 12-1: Reported Associations of Dissection of the Cervicocephalic Arteries

Fibromuscular dysplasia (FMD)

Extreme vessel tortuosity and/or redundancy (kinks, loops, coils)

Marfan syndrome

Ehlers-Danlos syndrome (vascular type)

Pseudoxanthoma elasticum

Type I collagen point mutation

Mutations of type III procollagen gene

Cystic medial necrosis (Marfan syndrome, lentiginosis)

Alpha-1 antitrypsin deficiency

Familial lentiginosis

Osteogenesis imperfecta type I

Hyperhomocysteinemia

Recent infections (usually upper respiratory)

Migraines

Oral contraceptives

Moyamoya

Meningovascular lues

Torsion or acceleration injuries

Excessive neck movements[a]

Cerebral angiography

Carotid endarterectomy

Blunt pharyngeal injuries

Post-partum

Cervical spine procedures

Chiropractic manipulation[b]

Miscellaneous

---

[a] Including sudden stretching, or prolonged rotation, extension, or flexion of the neck.

[b] More important with VA dissections.

risk factor and/or association is not identified in many individuals with a spontaneous CCAD.[15–18] CCADs have been reported with a variety of vascular and connective tissue disorders, including fibromuscular dysplasia (FMD), Marfan disease, vascular Ehlers-Danlos syndrome (vascular type), pseudoxanthoma elasticum, type I collagen mutation, osteogenesis imperfecta type I, lentiginosis, moyamoya disease (see Chapter 13), and aberrant vessel configuration (i.e., tortuosity, kinks, loops, and coils). The likelihood of dissection may be increased with meningovascular lues, certain arteritides, hyperhomocysteinemia, and recent infections. Alpha-1-antitrypsin deficiency has been associated with intracranial aneurysms and FMD, but whether this deficiency also increases the likelihood of CCAD is uncertain.

INTRATHORACIC DISSECTION

Spontaneous intrathoracic dissections occur most frequently in the ascending aorta of hypertensive men over the age of 50, although pregnant women are also at increased risk. Patients with a bicuspid aortic valve also have an increased risk of aortic dissection compared to the general population. Aortic dissection can be classified using the Stanford or DeBakey classification scheme. In the Standford classification, type A dissections include the ascending aorta, and type B are dissections excluding the ascending aorta. The DeBakey classification subdivides aortic dissections, with type I involving the entire aorta, type II involving only the ascending aorta, and type III excluding the ascending aorta and arch.

Most often the intimal tear is spontaneous and unrelated to exertion. The symptoms mimic those of myocardial infarction with excruciating substernal pain which may radiate into the arms, shoulders, back, neck, or jaw. About half the patients with acute dissection of the aortic arch are extremely ill and in shock. Others have no symptoms at the onset and come to the physician with signs secondary to obstruction of the aortic branches.[19–24]

As a rule, neurologic deficits appear shortly after the onset, in contrast to the delayed onset of embolic phenomena after myocardial infarction. Coma occurs in about one-third of the cases, and focal neurologic signs may occur as a result of dissection of the carotid arteries, or the arteries supplying the spinal cord. Extension upward along the brachiocephalic or a carotid artery may cause contralateral hemiplegia, absence of the carotid pulse, homolateral blindness, and pallor of the retina. Other complications include possible ischemic peripheral neuropathy with a flaccid anesthetic extremity. Paraplegia due to spinal cord infarction caused by obstruction of the intercostal or lumbar arteries may develop. The cord levels involved vary from T2 to L5.

The dissection can cause stenosis or occlusion of the coronary, brachiocephalic, left carotid, and the left subclavian arteries. Diagnosis must first be suspected, so that ultrasonography, computed tomography (CT), or magnetic resonance (MR) of the mediastinum with intravenous contrast enhancement of the great vessels can be done.[25,26]

CAROTID OR VERTEBRAL ARTERY DISSECTION

The cervical portions of the carotid arteries, the brachiocephalic artery, vertebral arteries, or, at times, the left subclavian artery proximal to the origin of the vertebral artery may also undergo spontaneous or traumatic dissection. A tear in the subclavian artery may be initiated by hyperextending and wrenching the arm, and there are reports of dissection of the carotid artery following sudden blows to the neck that do not damage the skin.

Tenderness or pain over the carotid (carotidynia) and homolateral fronto-temporal or hemicranial cephalgia followed by Horner syndrome is the classic clinical presentation of carotid artery dissection. Some individuals develop hemispheric transient ischemic attacks (TIAs) or homolateral amaurosis fugax after carotid dissection. Ipsilateral cephalgia and neck pain may precede ischemic stroke for days or even weeks.[27,28] Cranial nerve involvement of the hypoglossal nerve (CN XII) is frequently observed, followed by compromise of cranial nerves IX–X, XI, V, VII, VI, and III in that order.[29] Brainstem symptoms and signs (often a lateral medullary syndrome), cerebellar symptoms, and ipsilateral occipital headache and neck pain are

Table 12.2: Clinical Picture of Extracranial CCADs

Ipsilateral headache

Ocular/orbital pain

Jaw pain

Carotidynia

Lightheadedness and syncope

Pulsatile tinnitus

Eyelid ptosis, miosis, and anhydrosis (Horner syndrome)

Dysgeusia

Scintillations

Amaurosis fugax

Branch retinal artery occlusion (BRAO)

Central retinal artery occlusion (CRAO)

Anterior and posterior ischemic optic neuropathy (AION, PION)

Cranial nerve palsies

Cerebral infarction

Brainstem/cerebellar infarction

Spinal cord infarction

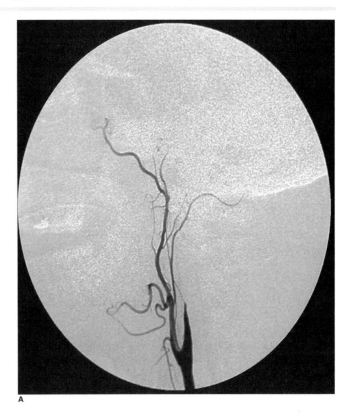

the most common clinical findings in spontaneous dissections of the vertebral arteries. Horner syndrome may occur in one-third of patients with VA dissections. Uncommon findings may include manifestations of spinal cord ischemia or locked-in syndrome. Table 12-2 summarizes the most commonly observed clinical features of extracranial CCADs.

INTRACRANIAL DISSECTION

Head trauma can stretch the intracranial arteries at the base of the brain sufficiently to rupture the intima and create an arterial dissection. The basilar and the internal carotid arteries above the clinoid processes are particularly susceptible to this type of injury. Occlusion of a cerebral artery hours or even weeks after trauma to the head may be secondary to dissecting hematoma or may result from subintimal hemorrhage into an atheromatous plaque. As to clinical characteristics, intracranial carotid artery dissections differ from extracranial cervical artery dissections. In general, patients with intracranial dissections are younger and have more severe strokes. Subarachnoid or intracerebral hemorrhage can accompany intracranial dissection, causing a dilemma regarding anticoagulation.[30–32]

DIAGNOSIS OF ARTERIAL DISSECTION

The radiographic hallmark of a CCAD is gradual tapering of the lumen, and this can be confirmed via several different studies.[33–37] MR angiography reveals a long irregular stenosis beginning distal to the carotid sinus and often extending to the base of the skull. This has been termed the crescent sign. It is often accompanied by a pseudoaneurysm in the upper carotid near the skull base. Intracranial dissection through the petrous and cavernous portions of the internal carotid occurs only rarely. Ultrasound and MR angiography are sensitive methods to detect

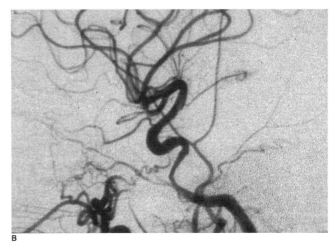

Figure 12-1. A: Catheter cerebral angiogram demonstrating a "pencil" tapering occlusion of the left internal carotid artery secondary to a dissection. B: Another patient has gradual narrowing of the internal carotid artery following cervical trauma, the angiographic "string sign" of a CCAD.

carotid dissection.[38–41] Catheter angiography accurately depicts the tapering or occlusion of an arterial dissection.[42–45] However, CT angiography is an attractive alternative because it is noninvasive and it is almost as reliable as catheter angiography in patients with an arterial dissection.[46–48] In some instances the characteristic aneurysmal dilatation of the cervical carotid near the base of the skull can be identified.

The characteristic appearance of CCAD on catheter angiography is gradual tapering of the artery (Figure 12-1), either to complete occlusion (the "pencil sign") or to a long narrowed segment (the "string sign"). Aneurysmal dilatation of the artery

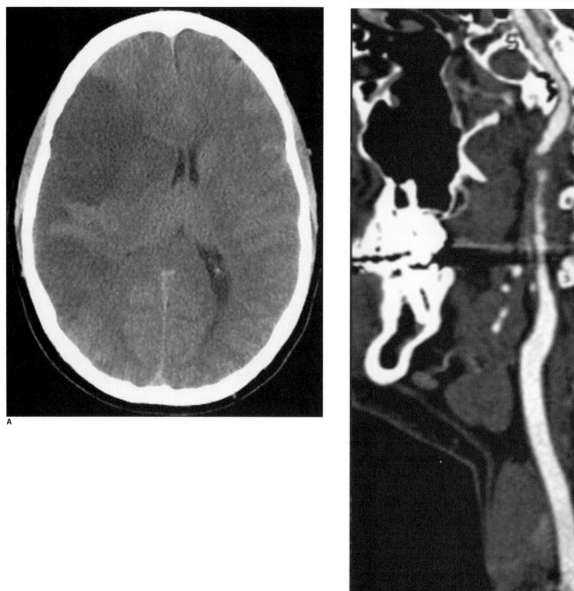

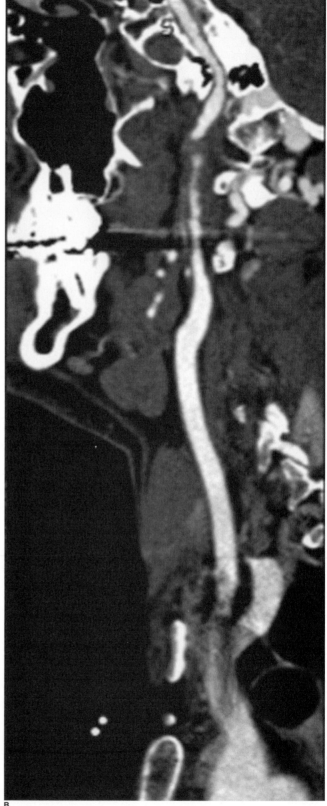

Figure 12-2. A: Cranial CT from a 46-year-old man shows a large, irregular hypodensity within the right middle cerebral artery territory with adjacent ventricular compression and midline shift. B: CT angiography confirms an arterial dissection of his right internal carotid artery beginning about 2 cm above the carotid bifurcation where the artery begins to taper and extending to within 1.5 cm of the skull base.

distal to the stenotic lumen is diagnostic of CCAD. These pseudoaneurysms are extremely ominous looking, but, surprisingly, their natural history is one of healing and subsequent disappearance of the aneurysm. The danger with these lesions is that during the course of the dissection the stagnated blood can form a clot and embolize. Increasingly, CCAD is confirmed by CT angiography, which shows many of the same findings less invasively (Figure 12-2). Reconstructed images from CT angiograms offer exquisite anatomical detail (Figure 5-4).

COURSE AND PROGNOSIS

The rate of recurrent ischemic events and/or recurrent dissections among patients with CCADs is low (about 1% per year in an initially uninvolved artery).[48] In carotid dissection the lumen usually remains patent although stenosed, and, after an interval, the clot may resorb, the false passage closes, and normal flow may be reestablished. In some cases, however, the thrombus intrudes into the lumen and casts emboli to the brain, or the artery dissects through the carotid canal and into the carotid siphon, where it can cause disastrous cerebral infarction.

MANAGEMENT ISSUES

Intravenous tPA should be considered in patients with extracranial CCADs associated with acute ischemic strokes within 4.5 hours of onset of symptoms (see Chapter 25). Randomized clinical trials comparing anticoagulation and aspirin in patients with extracranial CCAD have not been completed. Anticoagulation with heparin (UFH or LMWH) followed by warfarin (target INR = 2.0–3.0 is often recommended for the first 3 to 6 months in an effort to decrease the risk of recurrent stroke. Alternatively, an antiplatelet agent may be substituted for heparin or warfarin.[49–51] We generally avoid anticoagulation in patients with intracranial CCADs because these patients may have associated subarachnoid hemorrhage.

Interventional endovascular angioplasty using stents is emerging as the treatment of choice to close the false passage. If the artery occludes, bypass procedures may be needed. In all cases risk factor reduction, including control of blood pressure, is indicated.[52–53]

REFERENCES

1. Hart RG, Easton JD. Dissections of cervical and cerebral arteries. *Neurol Clin.* 1983;**1**:155–182.
2. Saver JL, Easton JDH, Hart RG. Dissection and trauma of cervicocerebral arteries. In: Barnett HJM, Mohr JP, Stein BM, Yatsu FM, eds. *Stroke, Pathophysiology, Diagnosis and Management.* 2nd ed. New York: Churchill Livingstone; 1992;**24**:671–688.
3. Mokri B, Piepgras DG, Houser OW. Traumatic dissections of the extracranial internal carotid artery. *J Neurosurg.* 1988;**68**: 189–197.
4. Mokri B. Traumatic and spontaneous extracranial internal carotid artery dissections. *J Neurol.* 1990;**237**:356–361.
5. Biller J, Hingtgen WL, Adams HP Jr, Smoker WR, Godersky JC, Toffol GJ. Cervicocephalic arterial dissections. A ten-year experience. *Arch Neurol.* 1986;**43**(12):1234–1238.
6. Schievink WI, Mokri B, O'Fallon WM. Recurrent spontaneous cervical-artery dissection. *N Engl J Med.* 1994;**330**:393–397.
7. Didier L, Debetle S, Lucas C, Leclerc X. Cervical artery dissection. In: Aminoff MJ, Boller F, Swaab DR, eds. *Handbook of Clinical Neurology.* 93 (3rd Series). *Stroke,* Part II. *Clinical Manifestations and Pathogenesis* (Fisher M, ed.). Edinburgh: Elsevier; 2009: 751–766.
8. Haldeman S, Carey P, Townsend M, Papadopoulos C. Clinical perceptions of the risk of vertebral artery dissection after cervical manipulation: the effect of referral bias. *Spine J.* 2002;**2**:334–342.
9. Rothwell DM, Bondy SJ, Williams JI. Chiropractic manipulation and stroke: a population-based case-control study. *Stroke.* 2001;**32**:1054–1060.
10. Nadgir RN, Loevner LA, Ahmed T, et al. Simultaneous bilateral internal carotid and vertebral artery dissection following chiropractic manipulation: case report and review of the literature. *Neurorad.* 2003;**45**:311–314.
11. Woodhurst WB, Robertson WD, Thompson GB. Carotid injury due to intraoral trauma: case report and review of the literature. *Neurosurgery.* 1980;**6**:559–563.
12. Pearl PL. Childhood stroke following intraoral trauma. *J Pediatr.* 1987;**110**:574–575.
13. Schievink WI, Roiter V. Epidemiology of cervical artery dissection. *Front Neurol Neurosci.* 2005;**20**:12–15.
14. Lee VH, Brown RD Jr, Mandrekar JN, Mokri B. Incidence and outcome of cervical artery dissection: a population-based study. *Neurology.* 2006;**67**:1809–1812.
15. Brandt T, Grond-Ginsbach C. Spontaneous cervical artery dissection. From risk factors toward pathogenesis. *Stroke.* 2002;**33**: 657–658.
16. Brandt T, Hausser I, Orberk E, Grau A, Hartschuh W, Anton-Lamprecht I, Hacke W. Ultrastructural connective tissue abnormalities in patients with spontaneous cervicocerebral artery dissections. *Ann Neurol.* 1998;**44**:281–285.
17. Brandt T, Orberk E, Weber R, et al. Pathogenesis of cervical artery dissections: association with connective tissue abnormalities. *Neurology.* 2001;**57**:24–30.
18. Caso V, Paciaroni M, Bogousslavsky J. Environmental factors and cervical artery dissection. *Front Neurol Neurosci.* 2005;**20**:44–53.
19. DeSanctis RW, Doroghazi RM, Austen WG, et al. Aortic dissection. *N Engl J Med.* 1990;**317**:1060–1100.
20. Hagan PG, Nienaber CA, Isselbacher EM, et al. The International Registry of Acute Aortic dissection (IRAD): new insights into an old disease. *JAMA.* 2000;**283**:897–903.
21. Spittell PC, Spittell JA Jr, Joyce JW, et al. Clinical features and differential diagnosis of aortic dissection: experience with 236 cases (1980 through 1990). *Mayo Clin Proc.* 1993;**68**:642–651.
22. Meszaros I, Morocz J, Szlavi J, et al. Epidemiology and clinicopathology of aortic dissection: a population-based longitudinal study over 27 years. *Chest.* 2000;**117**:1271.
23. DeBakey ME, McCollum CH, Crawford ES, et al. Dissection and dissecting aneurysms of the aorta. Twenty-year follow-up of five hundred twenty-seven patients treated surgically. *Surgery.* 1982;**92**: 1118–1134.
24. Mikich B. Dissection of the aorta. A new approach. *Heart.* 2003; **89**(1):6–8.
25. Wilbers CRH, Carrol CL, Hnilica MA. Optimal diagnostic imaging of aortic dissection. *Tex Heart Inst J.* 1990;**17**:271–278.
26. Erbel R, Alfonso F, Boileau C, et al. Diagnosis and management of aortic dissection. *Eur Heart J.* 2001;**22**(18):1642–1681.
27. Biousse V, D'Anglejan-Chatillon J, Massiou H, Bousser MG. Head pain in non-traumatic carotid artery dissection: a series of 65 patients. *Cephalalgia.* 1994;**14**:33–36.
28. Dziewas R, Konrad C, Drager B, et al. Cervical artery dissection – clinical features, risk factors, therapy and outcome in 126 patients. *J Neurol.* 2003;**250**:1179–1184.
29. Mokri B, Schievink WI, Olsen KD, Piepgras DG. Spontaneous dissection of the cervical internal carotid artery. Presentation with lower cranial nerve palsies. *Arch Otolaryngol Head Neck Surg.* 1992;**118**(4):431–435.

30. Farrell MA, Gilbert JJ, Kaufmann JC. Fatal intracranial arterial dissection: clinical pathological correlation. *J Neurol Neurosurg Psychiatry*. 1985;**48**:111–121.

31. Murakami K, Takahashi N, Matsumura N, Umezawa K, Midorikawa H, Nishijima M. Vertebrobasilar artery dissection presenting with simultaneous subarachnoid hemorrhage and brain stem infarction: case report. *Surg Neurol*. 2003;**59**:18–22.

32. Ramgren B, Cronqvist M, Romner B, Brandt L, Holtas S, Larsson EM. Vertebrobasilar dissection with subarachnoid hemorrhage: a retrospective study of 29 patients. *Neurorad*. 2005;**47**:97–104.

33. Auer A, Felber S, Schmidauer C, Waldenberger P, Aichner F. Magnetic resonance angiographic and clinical features of extracranial vertebral artery dissection. *J Neurol Neurosurg Psychiatry*. 1998;**64**:474–481.

34. Phan T, Huston J III, Bernstein MA, Riederer SJ, Brown RD Jr. Contrast-enhanced magnetic resonance angiography of the cervical vessels: experience with 422 patients. *Stroke*. 2001;**32**:2282–2286.

35. Oelerich M, Stogbauer F, Kurlemann G, Schul C, Schuierer G. Craniocervical artery dissection: MR imaging and MR angiographic findings. *Eur Radiol*. 1999;**9**:1385–1391.

36. Bryan RN, Levy LM, Whitlow WD, Killian JM, Preziosi TJ, Rosario JA. Diagnosis of acute cerebral infarction: comparison of CT and MR imaging. *AJNR Am J Neuroradiol*. 1991;**12**:611–620.

37. Kasner SE, Hankins LL, Bratina P, Morgenstern LB. Magnetic resonance angiography demonstrates vascular healing of carotid and vertebral artery dissection. *Stroke*. 1997;**28**:1993–1997.

38. Bakke SJ, Smith H-J, Kerty E, Dahl A. Cervicocranial artery dissection. Detection by Doppler ultrasound and MR angiography. *Acta Radiol*. 1996;**37**:529–534.

39. Bartels E, Flugel KA. Evaluation of extracranial vertebral artery dissection with duplex color-flow imaging. *Stroke*. 1996;**27**:290–295.

40. deBray JM, Lhoste P, Dubas F, Emile J, Saumet J-L. Ultrasonic features of extracranial carotid dissections: 47 cases studied by angiography. *J Ultrasound Med*. 1994;**13**:659–664.

41. Dittrich R, Dziewas R, Ritter MA, et al. Negative ultrasound findings in patients with cervical artery dissection. Negative ultrasound in CAD. *J Neurol*. 2006;**253**:424–433.

42. Nakagawa K, Touho H, Morisako T, et al. Long-term follow-up study of unruptured bertebral artery dissection: clinical outcomes and serial angiographic findings. *J Neurosurg*. 2000;**93**:19–25.

43. Katzen BT. Current status of digital angiography in vascular imaging. *Radiol Clin N Am*. 1995;**33**:1–14.

44. Hosoya T, Adachi M, Yamaguchi K, Haku T, Kayama T, Kato T. Clinical and neuroradiological features of intracranial vertebrobasilar artery dissection. *Stroke*. 1997;**28**:1993–1997.

45. Houser OW, Mokri B, Sundt TM Jr, Baker HL Jr, Reese DF. Spontaneous cervical cephalic arterial dissection and its residuum: angiographic spectrum. *AJNR Am J Neuroradiol*.1984;**5**:27–34.

46. Vertinsky AT, Schwartz NE, Fischbein NJ, Rosenberg J, Albers GW, Zaharchuk G. Comparison of multidetector CT angiography and MR imaging of cervical artery dissection. *AJNR Am J Neuroradiol*. 2008;**29**:1753–1760.

47. Elijovich L, Kazmi K, Gauvrit JY, Law M. The emerging role of multidetector row CT angiography in the diagnosis of cervical arterial dissection: preliminary study. *Neurorad*. 2006;**48**:606–612.

48. Nunez DB Jr, Torres-Leon M, Munera F. Vascular injuries of the neck and thoracic inlet: helical CT-angiographic correlation. *Radiographics*. 2004;**24**:1087–1098.

49. Schievink WI. The treatment of spontaneous carotid and vertebral artery dissections. *Curr Opin Cardiol*. 2000;**15**:316–321.

50. Arnold M, Nedeltchev K, Sturzenegger M, et al. Thrombolysis in patients with acute stroke caused by cervical artery dissection. Analysis of 9 patients and review of the literature. *Arch Neurol*. 2002;**59**:549–553.

51. Derex L, Nighoghossian N, Turjman F, et al. Intravenous tPA in acute ischemic stroke related to internal carotid artery dissection. *Neurology*. 2000;**54**:2159–2161.

52. Halbach VV, Higashida RT, Dowd CF, et al. Endovascular treatment of cerebral artery dissections and pseudoaneurysms. *J Neurosurg*. 1993;**79**:183–191.

53. Saito R, Ezura M, Takahashi A, Yoshimoto T. Combined neuroendovascular stenting and coil embolization for cervical carotid artery dissection causing symptomatic mass effect. *Surg Neurol*. 2000;**53**:318–322.

13

Moyamoya and Other Vasculopathies

In 1956 the author encountered an unusual angiogram showing a diffuse intracranial vascular network without the usual cerebral vascular pattern. Although a precise interpretation of this angiogram was impossible, it was postulated that it must represent very unusual cerebral hemodynamics. Further clinical investigation suggested to us that these interesting vascular patterns represented collateral channels resulting from impaired blood flow through the circle of Willis.

Tatsuyuki Kudo

Moyamoya disease is a chronic, typically progressive vasculopathy that is characterized by progressive stenosis and occlusion of the internal carotid arteries with secondary development of distal collateral branches. In addition to moyamoya disease, this chapter summarizes several other vasculopathies that sometimes lead to stroke, including radiation vasculopathy, fibromuscular dysplasia, and malignant atrophic papulosis. The conditions presented here are noninflammatory and nonatheromatous, although moyamoya disease overlaps some of the hereditary conditions presented in Chapter 21.

MOYAMOYA

The term *moyamoya* is a Japanese expression meaning "hazy, like a cloud of smoke drifting through the air," referring to the often hazy appearance of the distal collateral network on angiography.[1] By custom, individuals with an accepted moyamoya risk factor (Table 13-1) are said to have *moyamoya syndrome,* and people with idiopathic disease are characterized as having *moyamoya disease.*[2]

Clinical Features of Moyamoya

The Japanese Research Committee on moyamoya proposed criteria for the diagnosis of moyamoya disease. These require (1) stenosis involving the region of the internal cerebral artery bifurcation and proximal portions of the anterior and middle cerebral arteries, (2) the development of dilated basal collateral arteries, and (3) bilateral vascular abnormalities.[2] Early in the course, however, unilateral stenosis is relatively common,

although many of these individuals later develop bilateral stenosis.[3] There may be few distal collateral vessels at the time of diagnosis. In addition, comparable changes in the posterior circulation are relatively common.[4]

Moyamoya affects both adults and children, but its clinical features are to some extent age dependent. Children with moyamoya typically have ischemic complications. Adults also have ischemic strokes but are more likely to develop hemorrhagic complications.[5–7] In one report of 505 individuals, almost two-thirds of the adults with moyamoya had an intracranial hemorrhage, and a similar percentage of the children had an ischemic infarction.[8] Many of the adults with hemorrhage have had an earlier infarction as well.

In addition to focal neurological deficits from infarction or hemorrhage, individuals with moyamoya can develop transient ischemic attacks, alternating hemiparesis, headaches, seizures, dystonia, chorea, speech deterioration, and progressive cognitive deterioration.[9,10] Recurrent stroke and transient ischemic attacks are most likely to occur during the first few years after the onset of symptoms, but some individuals have long asymptomatic intervals between bouts of clinical dysfunction. Recurrent attacks may be precipitated by crying, hyperventilation, cough, or fever.[11,12]

Intraparenchymal, subarachnoid, and intraventricular hemorrhage are more common in adults than children.[7,13–15] Several individuals with moyamoya disease have developed an intracranial aneurysm, but most individuals with an intracranial hemorrhage due to moyamoya do not have an aneurysm.[16,17] The occurrence of an intracranial hemorrhage does not bode well for a person with moyamoya. In one report of 28 patients with hemorrhage due to moyamoya disease, for example, five (17.9%) patients died from the initial hemorrhage, two died from other causes, and six (28.6% of the remaining 21) went on to have a second hemorrhage.[15] Although several reports have suggested an increased risk of hemorrhage during pregnancy, Komiyama and colleagues reviewed 53 pregnant patients and concluded that the risk of hemorrhage is not increased.[18]

Moyamoya has been described in individuals with various other conditions (Table 13-1), although its occurrence with another condition could be coincidental when only one or two

Table 13-1: Disorders Reported with Moyamoya Syndrome

	Number of Patients
No associated conditions (idiopathic)	66
Neurofibromatosis type 1 (NF 1)	16
Asian heritage	16
Cranial therapeutic radiation	15
Down syndrome	10
Congenital cardiac anomaly, previously operated	7
Renal artery stenosis	4
Hemoglobinopathy (2 sickle cell, 1 "Bryn Mawr")	3
(Other hematologic: 1 spherocytosis, 1 ITP)	2
Giant cervico-facial hemangiomas	3
Shunted hydrocephalus	3
Arterial hypertension on medication	3
Hyperthyroidism (one with Grave disease)	2

Table modified from Roach et al.[61] with permission.
Other syndromes with one patient each: Reye's (remote), Williams, Alagille, cloacal extrophy, renal artery fibromuscular dysplasia, and congenital cytomegalic inclusion virus infection (remote). Two patients had unclassified syndromic presentations. There were four African Americans, two of whom had sickle cell disease.

patients have been reported. The evidence is more robust for other conditions, such as Down syndrome, sickle cell disease, neurofibromatosis, cranial radiotherapy, and Fanconi's anemia.[19–22] Most individuals with moyamoya, however, do not have a recognized cause.

Incidence and Distribution

Moyamoya disease is far more common among Asians than in other individuals, but it occurs in all ethnic groups.[23,24] The age at presentation is bimodal, with a childhood peak between 6 and 14 years of age and an adult peak between 30 and 40 years.[8] About half of the patients are diagnosed by age 10. Moyamoya disease is the most common cause of pediatric stroke in Japan, and there it affects females almost twice as often as males.[25] The estimated prevalence of moyamoya disease in Japan is just over 3 per 100,000 population and an incidence rate of 0.35 per year per 100,000 individuals.[25] In contrast, the estimated incidence of moyamoya disease in the United States is only 0.086 individuals per 100,000 individuals per year, although the rate among Asian Americans is much higher.[26] The incidence ratios compared to American whites were 4.6 for Asian Americans, 2.2 for African Americans, and 0.5 for Hispanics.[26]

Diagnosis of Moyamoya

Confirmation of moyamoya requires the demonstration of stenosis or occlusion of the distal internal carotid arteries and the distal arterial collateral network (Table 13-2). The arterial abnormalities are typically bilateral, even in individuals with

Table 13-2: Angiographic Stages of Moyamoya Disease[164]

Stage I	Stenosis of both intracranial carotid arteries
Stage II	Moyamoya vessels develop at the base of the brain as the carotids narrow
Stage III	Moyamoya vessels become prominent as the anterior circulation becomes progressively stenotic and occluded
Stage IV	Moyamoya vessels begin to involve the posterior circulation
Stage V	Moyamoya vessels begin to diminish
Stage VI	Moyamoya vessels disappear, and the brain receives blood through abnormal extracranial-intracranial anastomoses

unilateral signs or symptoms,[27] but some individuals with moyamoya have unilateral carotid artery stenosis or even normal findings at the time of presentation.[28,29]

Moyamoya can be confirmed by catheter angiography (Figure 13-1) or noninvasively by either magnetic resonance angiography (MRA) (Figure 13-2) or computed tomography (CT) angiography.[30–32] Magnetic resonance studies have largely replaced catheter angiography in the diagnosis of moyamoya. With magnetic resonance imaging (MRI), the absence of flow voids in both distal internal carotid arteries together with prominent dilated collateral vessels within the thalamus and basal ganglia are diagnostic of moyamoya. Coupling MRI and MRA offers a reliable noninvasive means of diagnosis.[31,33,34]

The external carotid branches and the posterior circulation are sometimes involved, but the internal carotid artery and its

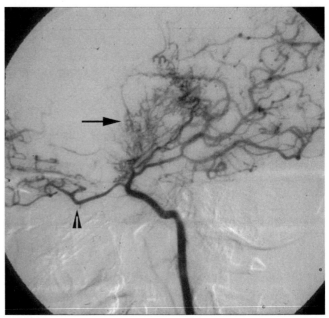

Figure 13-1. A catheter angiogram reveals occlusion of the distal internal carotid artery, dilated collateral vessels (*arrow*) distal to the carotid occlusion, and an enlarged ophthalmic artery (*arrowhead*). These are classic findings of moyamoya syndrome, in this instance caused by irradiation. Reprinted with permission from Roach and Riela.[165]

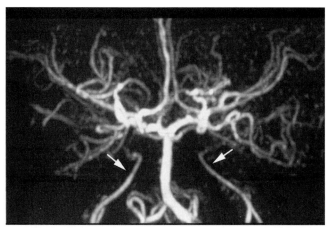

Figure 13-2. MRA from an individual with moyamoya disease reveals bilateral internal carotid artery occlusion (*arrows*). The middle and anterior cerebral arteries are presumably filled via collateral vessels.

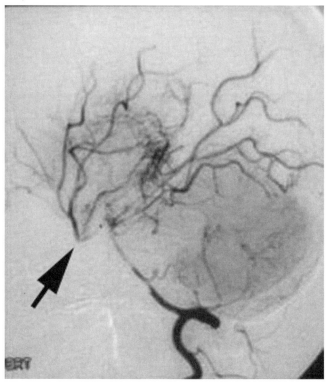

Figure 13-3. Catheter angiogram of the vertebral artery from a patient with bilateral internal carotid artery occlusions due to moyamoya disease. Note the filling of the middle cerebral artery (*arrow*) via the basilar artery as a result of carotid occlusion.

branches are consistently affected.[35,36] The vertebral artery often enlarges to provide additional flow. The main branches of the occluded internal carotid artery may receive enough collateral circulation to be visible on imaging studies (Figure 13-3). The basal telangiectatic network is visualized angiographically as the "puff of smoke" for which moyamoya syndrome is named (Figure 13-1). Serial angiograms demonstrate progression of the vascular lesion in some individuals, but the angiographic manifestations do not change in others.[37] Transcranial Doppler is a practical way to follow moyamoya patients and to assess their course following surgery.[38,39]

Infarctions are often multiple and bilateral. Although larger infarctions and hemorrhages are evident with CT, MRI more reliably demonstrated smaller infarctions.[40] Acute infarcts are best seen using diffusion-weighted MRI. With MRI the proximal anterior and middle cerebral arteries may not be visible following contrast infusion, and tortuous distal collateral vessels may be apparent.

Techniques to assess cerebral perfusion have been increasingly utilized in individuals with moyamoya disease. Single-photon emission computed tomography (SPECT) with acetazolamide challenge, MR perfusion imaging, xenon-enhanced CT, and positron emission tomography (PET) provide a measure of resting cerebral perfusion and blood flow reserve in people with moyamoya disease.[38,41–45] Asymptomatic individuals who have good cerebral blood flow reserve demonstrated by SPECT or PET may not need to undergo immediate revascularization surgery, especially in the absence of progressive arterial stenosis.[46,47] These studies also offer a means of demonstrating improved perfusion following surgery.[48–50]

Electroencephalography characteristically reveals slowing of the background rhythm after cessation of hyperventilation (the "rebuild-up" phenomenon). It may also capture spike discharges in individuals who are prone to have epileptic seizures.[51]

Pathology of Moyamoya

The internal carotid arteries bear the brunt of moyamoya syndrome, but the proximal anterior and middle cerebral arteries are often stenotic as well.[52] Less commonly, the posterior cerebral artery or the external carotid branches are affected.[53,54]

Microscopic findings include eccentric intimal thickening and deterioration and duplication of the internal elastic lamina (Figure 13-4).[55] The dilated capillary network can be seen microscopically.[27,56] Small mural thrombi are sometimes identified adjacent to areas of abnormal intimal thickening and edema, most often located in the larger intracranial arteries. Fibrin and platelet microthrombi have been identified in distal vessels.[57]

Pathophysiology

The pathophysiology of moyamoya is neither well defined nor particularly uniform, but genetic factors clearly play a key role. There is substantial evidence that moyamoya susceptibility is genetically mediated, although not necessarily as a single genetic trait. Aside from the high incidence of moyamoya disease in Japan and Korea, an estimated 7% to 12% of moyamoya disease cases are familial, and it sometimes occurs in identical twins.[25,58–60] Moyamoya has been associated with certain human leukocyte antigen (HLA) haplotypes including the B40 HLA antigen in patients younger than 10 years old and the B52 HLA antigen in older patients. It has also been associated with the AW24, BW46, B51-DR4, and BW54 antigens.[61]

Ikeda and associates[62] did a total genome search and mapped a gene for familial moyamoya disease to chromosome 3p24-p26. Others have suggested additional links to chromosome 6,[63] to 17q25,[64] and to 8q23.[65] Yamamoto and colleagues[66] found increased elastin gene expression in arterial smooth muscle cells taken from individuals with moyamoya disease. Together these findings suggest that several genes may increase the susceptibility to moyamoya disease and that more than one molecular mechanism may be involved.

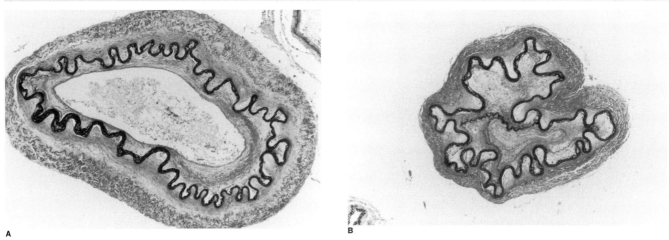

A

B

Figure 13-4. Intimal hyperplasia (A) and occlusion (B) of the internal carotid artery from two individuals with moyamoya disease.

Ischemic stroke sometimes occurs in "watershed" areas, suggesting poor perfusion from arterial stenosis.[40] The tendency for hyperventilation and dehydration to promote stroke could result in further deterioration of brain perfusion during these periods. Other individuals deteriorate via a series of discrete episodes, and there is evidence that some infarctions result from artery-to-artery embolism.[57,67] This observation has enormous implications: the surgical methods now used to increase cerebral blood flow, even if effective, may not prevent embolism.

Treatment of Moyamoya

The natural history of untreated moyamoya disease is not well delineated, so its prognosis and response to therapy are difficult to predict. Some individuals with moyamoya do well for prolonged periods without treatment, and others do poorly even after surgery. Despite an extensive literature on moyamoya, there are no randomized clinical trials to guide therapy.[68] Moreover, many individuals with moyamoya do relatively well even without treatment, making it harder to gauge the effects of treatment in the absence of well-designed trials. In one report, for example, three-fourths of the moyamoya patients reported normal daily activities or working ability even before being treated.[25] Few studies have directly compared medical and surgical therapy for moyamoya. One Japanese report found no significant outcome difference between medically and surgically treated moyamoya patients.[69] By some estimates, however, over a third of the moyamoya patients who were initially managed conservatively eventually underwent surgery as a result of progressive symptoms. One approach in clinically stable individuals is to defer surgery if the SPECT scan indicates adequate blood flow reserve.[46]

A recent consensus paper on childhood stroke made several specific recommendations (Table 13-3) regarding the diagnosis and treatment of moyamoya.[61] An assortment of surgical procedures designed to increase perfusion has been described. Although none of these procedures have been thoroughly studied in a controlled clinical trial, surgical revascularization is now commonly recommended.[61,68]

Adults and older children typically undergo direct anastomosis of the superficial temporal artery to the middle cerebral artery (STA-MCA). Direct bypass techniques are technically more difficult in small children, who instead undergo an indirect bypass procedure such as encephaloduroarteriosynangiosis (EDAS), in which the temporal artery and an attached galeal strip are positioned near the cerebral cortex.[70,71] Increased cerebral blood flow can sometimes be demonstrated after these procedures, and many of the patients seem to stabilize. Potential surgical complications include postoperative ischemic stroke, intracerebral hemorrhage, and spontaneous or traumatic subdural hematoma.

It is not clear whether revascularization after hemorrhage reduces the likelihood of additional hemorrhages due to moyamoya.[69,72–74] Because hemorrhage due to moyamoya occurs more often in adults, it is perhaps not surprising that surgery done late in the course to prevent bleeding would be ineffective. Whether earlier surgery done in younger individuals reduces the risk of hemorrhage later is uncertain.

Various medical treatments have been utilized, including corticosteroids, vasodilators, and antiplatelet agents. One Japanese report found no significant outcome difference between medically and surgically treated moyamoya patients.[69] Dehydration and pain-induced hyperventilation should be avoided.[75,76] Calcium channel blockers have been used in individuals with intractable headaches or recurrent transient ischemic attacks. Antiplatelet agents are sometimes prescribed for moyamoya patients with relatively mild disease or for those who are considered a poor surgical risk, but there are few data demonstrating either short- or long-term efficacy. Antiplatelet agents have been used in individuals with ischemic symptoms due to suspected micro-emboli from the site of arterial stenosis and for patients undergoing revascularization procedures.[22,61] Anticoagulants such as warfarin are not generally used because of the risk of hemorrhage due to moyamoya.

RADIATION VASCULOPATHY

Clinical Features

Stenosis and occlusion of the cervicocephalic arteries are common following radiotherapy of head and neck tumors.[77,78] Radiation vasculopathy often presents years after treatment.[79,80] Many patients remain asymptomatic, so the incidence of postradiotherapy vasculopathy is unknown.[81,82] The symptoms of radiation vasculopathy depend on the affected artery and

Table 13-3: Recommendations for Treatment of Moyamoya Disease

Class I recommendations

1. Different revascularization techniques are useful to effectively reduce the risk of stroke due to moyamoya disease. However, despite a vast literature on moyamoya, there are no controlled clinical trials to guide the selection of therapy.

2. Indirect revascularization techniques are generally preferable and should be used in younger children whose small caliber vessels make direct anastomosis difficult, whereas direct bypass techniques are preferable in older individuals.

3. Revascularization surgery is useful for moyamoya. Indications for revascularization surgery include progressive ischemic symptoms or evidence of inadequate blood flow or cerebral perfusion reserve in an individual without a contraindication to surgery.

Class II recommendations

1. Transcranial Doppler may be useful in the evaluation and follow-up of individuals with moyamoya.

2. Techniques to minimize anxiety and pain during hospitalizations may reduce the likelihood of stroke caused by hyperventilation-induced vasoconstriction in individuals with moyamoya.

3. Management of systemic hypotension, hypovolemia, hyperthermia, and hypocarbia during the intraoperative and perioperative periods may reduce the risk of perioperative stroke in individuals with moyamoya disease.

4. Aspirin may be considered in individuals with moyamoya following revascularization surgery or in asymptomatic individuals for whom surgery is not anticipated.

5. Techniques to measure cerebral perfusion and blood flow reserve may assist in the evaluation and follow-up of individuals with moyamoya disease.

Class III recommendations

1. Except in selected individuals with frequent TIAs or multiple infarctions despite antiplatelet therapy and surgery, anticoagulants are not recommended for most individuals with moyamoya because of the risk of hemorrhage as well as the difficulty of maintaining therapeutic levels in children.

2. In the absence of a strong family history of moyamoya disease or medical conditions that predispose to moyamoya syndrome, there is insufficient evidence to justify screening studies for moyamoya disease in asymptomatic individuals or in relatives of patients with moyamoya syndrome.

Adapted from Roach et al. with permission.[61]

Class I: Should be pursued because the benefits clearly exceed the risks. Class II: Reasonable to consider because benefits probably exceed the risks, but additional studies with focused or age-specific objectives are needed. Class III: Should not be pursued because the risks exceed the benefits.

whether the lesion is ischemic or hemorrhagic, and the presentation can be confusing because the vascular symptoms must be distinguished from those of recurrent tumor as well as from the effects of radiation on the brain parenchyma. There can be a long interval (up to two or three decades) between the radiotherapy and the onset of vascular symptoms.[79,83,84]

Stenosis and occlusion of the cervicocephalic arteries after radiotherapy of cervical tumors can induce atherosclerosis-like changes that predispose the individual to stroke.[85] In one report 10% of the individuals undergoing cervical or cranial radiotherapy developed greater than 70% stenosis in one or both internal carotid arteries within 6 years of therapy.[86] Similarly, individuals less than 60 years of age have a 12% cumulative stroke risk after cervical radiotherapy, and both hypertension and diabetes mellitus increase the risk of stroke in these individuals.[87] The clinical pattern of radiotherapy-induced vasculopathy of the internal carotid arteries can resemble either atherosclerosis or moyamoya syndrome.[88,89]

As might be predicted, radiation-induced moyamoya syndrome occurs most often following radiotherapy of tumors near the internal carotid arteries.[83,90] The irradiated lesion was located near the basal portion of the cerebral hemispheres in all 14 of the radiation-induced moyamoya patients in one report.[91] Vasculopathy has also been described in individuals treated with more precise radiosurgery.[92]

Vasculopathy after radiotherapy is more likely to be recognized in young patients, in part because of their greater incidence of tumors near the intracranial carotid arteries. In one report of 41 patients with post-radiotherapy cranial vasculopathy, 77% of the patients were less than 18 years old at the time they developed vascular symptoms, and 49% were less than 4 years old.[89]

Occasional patients develop intracerebral hemorrhage following radiotherapy,[77,80,84,93] and subarachnoid hemorrhage due to a ruptured aneurysm or pseudoaneurysm has also been reported.[84,94–96] Some individuals have vascular stenosis as well as an aneurysm.[84] Aneurysms are sometimes multiple and are more common in adults.[84,97]

Hemorrhage can also result from a cavernous malformation, which appears to develop with some regularity after cranial radiotherapy.[98–102] In one study 10 of 297 (3%) patients developed a new cavernous malformation following radiotherapy.[103] Cavernous malformation of the spinal cord following radiotherapy has also been described.[104,105]

Pathology

Endothelial cells are especially susceptible to the effects of radiotherapy.[106] Small arteries and capillaries are the vessels most likely to be injured, but large arteries are also affected and tend to be more clinically significant.[106] Histopathology demonstrates subendothelial fibrosis, interruption of the internal elastic lamina, and stenosis or occlusion of the lumen.[81] With large artery stenosis, irregular telangiectatic dilatations of the distal vessels occur, similar to those in idiopathic moyamoya.

Treatment

As with moyamoya disease, it is probably prudent to avoid hyperventilation and dehydration in individuals with radiation vasculopathy. Both endarterectomy and endovascular procedures have been used to repair radiotherapy-induced aneurysms and carotid vasculopathy.[85,106–109] A few patients have undergone revascularization procedures (see the discussion of moyamoya above).[110,111] One report suggested that anticoagulation with heparin and warfarin might be able to reverse radiation-induced cerebral radionecrosis and myelopathy in patients.[112] Hyperbaric oxygen therapy has been suggested, but its value remains unproven.[113]

FIBROMUSCULAR DYSPLASIA

Fibromuscular dysplasia (FMD) is a segmental, nonatheromatous, noninflammatory angiopathy affecting medium to large arteries. It was first described in 1938 by Ledbetter and Burkland, who described a hypertensive patient with renal artery stenosis caused by overgrowth of smooth muscle.[114] FMD affects the internal carotid artery about half as frequently as it does the renal artery, and both carotid arteries are affected in some individuals. Although FMD has been increasingly recognized in recent years because of improved neuroimaging methods, the factors culminating in FMD are poorly understood and probably heterogeneous. There is no evidence of an underlying systemic illness, although the striking predominance of women with FMD suggests a hormonal effect.

Because FMD is a relatively common incidental finding on imaging studies, its contribution to cerebrovascular dysfunction is not precisely known. Among people undergoing cerebral angiography for a variety of reasons, FMD is identified in 0.25% to 1%.[115] Two-thirds of these individuals have no symptoms that are attributable to the FMD, which suggests that most patients are probably never identified and remain asymptomatic.[116,117]

Some data suggest a familial predisposition to FMD.[118] In some families FMD may be inherited as an autosomal dominant trait with reduced penetrance in males, but complete ascertainment is impossible, and most cases are probably sporadic.[119,120] FMD seems to occur with increased frequency in individuals with alpha-1-antitrypsin deficiency, a defect that also promotes aneurysm formation.[121]

Clinical Features

Women are much more likely to have FMD than men. In three series with a combined 113 individuals with FMD, there were only nine men (8%).[117,120,122] FMD is most often identified in young adults.

Cerebral ischemia can result from arterial stenosis, thromboembolism, or arterial dissection.[123] Even when FMD is present, it is sometimes hard to be certain of its significance, especially in individuals with other stroke risk factors. About half of the symptomatic individuals with FMD have a transient ischemic attack (TIA) or an ischemic infarction.[122] However, actual occlusion of the involved artery is unusual, suggesting thromboembolism may be the cause of TIA or infarction. The risk of arterial dissection is also higher in individuals with FMD, providing yet another mechanism for cerebrovascular dysfunction.

In some series intracranial aneurysms have been documented in up to a quarter of the individuals with cervicocephalic FMD.[116,117,122,124,125] However, a meta-analysis of 498 patients culled from 17 published reports estimated the aneurysm risk due to FMD at 7.3%, a number that is not nearly as high as earlier reports have suggested.[126] Patients with concomitant hypertension due to renal artery FMD may have an increased risk of aneurysmal rupture.[127] At least one patient developed a carotid-cavernous fistula.[115]

Diagnosis of FMD

The diagnosis of FMD can be confirmed by ultrasound, CT angiography, MRA, or catheter angiography.[128,129] Osborn and Anderson suggested the following angiographic classification for cervicocephalic FMD: type 1 FMD (the most common subtype) is characterized by the classic "string of beads" angiographic pattern that is formed by alternating segments of arterial constriction and dilatation (Figure 13-5), type 2 FMD (7% of patients) is characterized by stenosis of long segments of the artery, and type 3 FMD (4% of patients) is defined by focal or multifocal arterial stenosis.[116] Because of its distinctive radiographic pattern, the diagnosis of type 1 FMD is generally more obvious than that of type 2 or type 3.

At least in some individuals, FMD is not a static lesion.[130] In one cohort of 32 FMD patients, progression of the FMD occurred in two of the six individuals who underwent repeat cerebral angiography.[122] Conversion from type 1 FMD to type 2 FMD has also been documented.[128]

Pathology

FMD can involve predominantly the media, the intima, or the adventitia. The most common form of FMD results from medial hyperplasia and fibrosis and accounts for over 90% of the FMD cases.[129,131] The common beadlike angiographic pattern is created by concentric rings of smooth muscle hyperplasia and fibrous proliferation. The carotid sinus and proximal 3 cm of the internal carotid are seldom involved. Intimal proliferation causes weblike bands of concentric narrowing of the lumen. This rare form of FMD is characterized by intimal thickening and degeneration of the internal elastic membrane. Adventitial FMD results from adventitial and periarterial fibrosis.[115,129]

Management

The natural history of FMD is unknown, and thus it is difficult to make precise treatment recommendations. Asymptomatic patients with FMD should be observed, but avoidance of other risk factors for cerebrovascular disease seems prudent. How frequently asymptomatic patients with FMD should be reassessed and the effectiveness of antiplatelet agents in preventing ischemic stroke are unknown.[132]

Surgical intervention is usually unnecessary, but symptomatic patients may benefit from angioplasty or stenting.[123,124,130] Aneurysms should be repaired if accessible (Chapter 17), and repair of stenotic renal arteries may prevent complications from hypertension.[133]

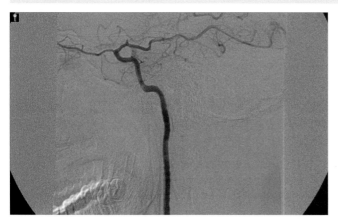

Figure 13-5. Catheter angiogram showing an irregular "string of beads" appearance of the common carotid artery due to fibromuscular dysplasia.

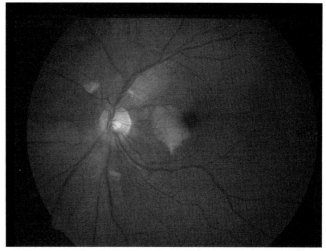

Figure 13-6. Retinal infarction due to branch retinal artery occlusions in an individual with Susac syndrome. Reprinted with permission from Roach and Riela.[165]

SUSAC SYNDROME

Microangiopathy of the brain, retina, and cochlea is variously known as Susac syndrome, RED-M (retinopathy, encephalopathy, and deafness-associated microangiopathy) syndrome, the SICRET (small infarction of cochlear, retinal, and encephalitic tissue) syndrome, or retinochocleocerebral vasculopathy. Although the pathogenesis of Susac syndrome is not fully understood, it is included here because of its characterization as an autoimmune microvascular endotheliopathy.[134,135]

Symptoms of Susac syndrome include migraine-like headaches, visual loss, vertigo, tinnitus, and symmetrical sensorineural hearing loss of the low and medium frequencies. Branch retinal artery occlusion (Figure 13-6) is a classic finding of Susac syndrome. Encephalopathy, confusion, memory loss, and psychiatric disturbance are also common. Ataxia, dysarthria, or signs of corticospinal tract dysfunction may also occur. There is a three to one female predominance, and it most often occurs between 20 and 40 years of age. Susac syndrome is unrelated to arterial hypertension or diabetes and is often misdiagnosed as multiple sclerosis, acute disseminated encephalomyelitis (ADEM), or SLE.[136,137]

Small multifocal hyperintense white matter lesions are evident on T_2-weighted MRI sequences. These lesions occur most often in the white matter and have a predilection for the central fibers of the corpus callosum.[135,138] The lesions typically enhance during the acute period and may also involve the thalamus and basal ganglia. The MRI lesions probably represent small infarcts because brain biopsy specimens contain multifocal brain microinfarcts in both gray and white matter. The cerebrospinal fluid may be normal or show mild protein elevation, and a mild lymphocytic pleocytosis may occur. Fluorescein angiography confirms the branch retinal artery occlusions.

Successful treatment of Susac syndrome requires immunosuppression. High-dose corticosteroid therapy is the first line of therapy, but intravenous immunoglobulin, mycophenolate mofetil, and cyclophosphamide may also be useful.[134] Plasmapheresis, calcium channel blockers, and platelet antiaggregants have been suggested, although the evidence in their favor is scant. Oral contraceptives should probably be avoided. There is no role for anticoagulant therapy.

MALIGNANT ATROPHIC PAPULOSIS

Malignant atrophic papulosis (MAP, also known as Kohlmeier-Degos disease or Degos disease) is an often progressive vasculopathy characterized by occlusion of small arteries and arterioles that in turn lead to infarctions in various organs.[139] It was once thought to have a uniformly poor prognosis (hence the term *malignant*),[140,141] but it has become apparent that there is a benign cutaneous variant of MAP as well as the more malignant systemic variant with multiple organ infarctions in addition to the skin lesions.[142,143] Individuals of all ages develop MAP, but it occurs most often in young adults.[144,145] Despite scattered familial clusters, most cases are sporadic.[146–148]

Clinical Features

The first symptoms of MAP are usually nonspecific (e.g., malaise, fever, or weight loss).[149] Skin lesions begin as an erythematous papule, then within a few days its center becomes white, flattened, and scaly.[142] These lesions occur more often on the neck, trunk, or proximal extremities, and lesions in various stages of development are present at the same time. The onset of gastrointestinal or neurological signs often heralds a deteriorating phase of the illness.[150]

An estimated 20% to 60% of MAP patients develop neurological impairment due to arterial occlusion within the central or peripheral nervous system,[139,151] although given the recent recognition of chronic and milder forms of the disease, this estimate is probably high. Symptoms include headache, seizures, and cognitive deterioration. Various focal neurological deficits have been recorded.[151–155]

Cranial MRI demonstrates meningeal thickening and ischemic brain lesions in individuals with neurological involvement.[151,156] Angiography is typically normal, but occasional reports document stenosis, ectasia, or aneurysms of the peripheral artery branches.[156] The diagnosis is confirmed by skin biopsy.

Pathology of MAP

The skin lesions have a characteristic inverted wedge-shaped dermal infarction.[157] Multiple infarctions of the brain and other organs are typical in individuals with systemic disease.[144] MAP typically affects small arteries and arterioles,[152] but both veins and capillaries can be involved.[158] Typical histological findings include endothelial swelling, vacuolization, fibrous intimal proliferation, and fibrinoid necrosis.[149,159]

Several pathogenic mechanisms have been suggested, but none of them fully explain the disorder. Mild inflammatory perivascular changes have been described in a few patients,[144,149] but the paucity of perivascular inflammation suggests that MAP should be characterized as a vasculopathy rather than a vasculitis. High and colleagues[157] theorized that the vascular abnormalities of MAP might be a nonspecific end point of several different processes and not a distinct pathologic entity. This concept might help to explain the co-occurrence of MAP with an array of other conditions, such as systemic lupus erythematosus, rheumatoid arthritis, anticardiolipin antibodies, and dermatomyositis. Immune complex deposition has been documented in affected humans and in a mouse model of MAP, and some authors characterize MAP as an immune-mediated, noninflammatory disorder.[160]

Treatment

Anticoagulation does not prevent the recurrence of neurological or gastrointestinal complications and might be disastrous should a gastrointestinal hemorrhage occur. One patient with increased platelet aggregation seemed to improve after starting aspirin and dipyridamole,[161] but another patient failed to respond to these agents.[162] Corticosteroids and other immunosuppressant agents are ineffective, and one patient, in fact, worsened after starting immunosuppression after renal transplantation.[163] Thus, the treatment for patients with the systemic form of MAP is unsatisfactory.

REFERENCES

1. Suzuki J, Takaku A. Cerebrovascular "moyamoya" disease. *Arch Neurol.* 1969;**20**:288–299.
2. Ikeda E, Hosoda Y. Spontaneous occlusion of the circle of Willis (cerebrovascular moyamoya disease): with special reference to its clinicopathological identity. *Brain Dev.* 1992;**14**:251–254.
3. Kawano T, Fukui M, Hashimoto N, Yonekawa Y. Follow-up study of patients with "unilateral" moyamoya disease. *Neurol Med Chir (Tokyo).* 1994;**34**:744–747.
4. Yamada I, Himeno Y, Suzuki S, Matsushima Y. Posterior circulation in moyamoya disease: angiographic study. *Radiology.* 1995;**197**:239–246.
5. Levin S. Moyamoya disease. *Develop Med Child Neurol.* 1982;**24**:850–859.
6. Yilmaz EY, Pritz MB, Bruno A, Lopez-Yunez A, Biller J. Moyamoya: Indiana University Medical Center experience. *Arch Neurol.* 2001;**58**:1274–1278.
7. Chiu D, Shedden P, Bratina P, Grotta JC. Clinical features of moyamoya disease in the United States. *Stroke.* 1998;**29**:1347–1351.
8. Han DH, Kwon OK, Byun BJ, et al. A co-operative study: clinical characteristics of 334 Korean patients with moyamoya disease treated at neurosurgical institutes (1976–1994). The Korean Society for Cerebrovascular Disease. *Acta Neurochir (Wien).* 2000;**142**:1263–1273.
9. Lyoo CH, Oh SH, Joo JY, Chung TS, Lee MS. Hemidystonia and hemichoreoathetosis as an initial manifestation of moyamoya disease. *Arch Neurol.* 2000;**57**:1510–1512.
10. Seol HJ, Wang KC, Kim SK, Hwang YS, Kim KJ, Cho BK. Headache in pediatric moyamoya disease: review of 204 consecutive cases. *J Neurosurg.* 2005;**103**:439–442.
11. Kurokawa T, Tomita S, Ueda K, et al. Prognosis of occlusive disease of the circle of Willis (moyamoya disease) in children. *Pediatr Neurol.* 1985;**1**:274–277.
12. Kim HY, Chung CS, Lee J, Han DH, Lee KH. Hyperventilation-induced limb shaking TIA in moyamoya disease. *Neurology.* 2003;**60**:137–139.
13. Aylett SE, Britton JA, De Sousa CMCP. Down syndrome and moyamoya disease: presentation with subarachnoid hemorrhage. *Pediatr Neurol.* 1996;**14**:259–261.
14. Takahashi M, Saito Y, Konno K. Intraventricular hemorrhage in childhood moyamoya disease. *J Comput Assist Tomogr.* 1980;**4**:117–120.
15. Yoshida Y, Yoshimoto T, Shirane R, Sakurai Y. Clinical course, surgical management, and long-term outcome of moyamoya patients with rebleeding after an episode of intracerebral hemorrhage: an extensive follow-up study. *Stroke.* 1999;**30**:2272–2276.
16. Nagamine Y, Takahashi S, Sonobe M. Multiple intracranial aneurysms associated with moyamoya disease. *J Neurosurg.* 1981;**54**:673–676.
17. Adams HP, Kassell NF, Wisoff HS, Drake CG. Intracranial saccular aneurysm and moyamoya disease. *Stroke.* 1979;**10**:174–179.
18. Komiyama M, Yasui T, Kitano S, Sakamoto H, Fujitani K, Matsuo S. Moyamoya disease and pregnancy: case report and review of the literature. *Neurosurgery.* 1998;**43**:360–368.
19. Pavlakis SG, Verlander PC, Gould RJ, Strimling BC, Auerbach AD. Fanconi anemia and moyamoya: evidence for an association. *Neurology.* 1995;**45**:998–1000.
20. Cramer SC, Robertson RL, Dooling EC, Scott RM. Moyamoya and Down syndrome. Clinical and radiological features. *Stroke.* 1996;**27**:2131–2135.
21. Jea A, Smith ER, Robertson R, Scott RM. Moyamoya syndrome associated with Down syndrome: outcome after surgical revascularization. *Pediatrics.* 2005;**116**:e694–e701.
22. Scott RM, Smith JL, Robertson RL, Madsen JR, Soriano SG, Rockoff MA. Long-term outcome in children with moyamoya syndrome after cranial revascularization by pial synangiosis. *J Neurosurg.* 2004;**100**:142–149.
23. Makayo PZ, Rapoport AM, Fleming RJ. Moya-moya disease in black adults. *Arch Neurol.* 1977;**34**:130.
24. Schoenberg BS, Mellinger JF, Schoenberg DG, Barringer FS. Moyamoya disease presenting as a seizure disorder. *Arch Neurol.* 1977;**34**:511–512.
25. Wakai K, Tamakoshi A, Ikezaki K, et al. Epidemiological features of moyamoya disease in Japan: findings from a nationwide survey. *Clin Neurol Neurosurg.* 1997;**99**(Suppl 2):S1–S5.
26. Uchino K, Johnston SC, Becker KJ, Tirschwell DL. Moyamoya disease in Washington State and California. *Neurology.* 2005;**65**:956–958.
27. Halonen H, Halonen V, Donner M, Iivanainen M, Vuolio M, Makinen J. Occlusive disease of intracranial main arteries with collateral networks in children. *Neuropadiatrie.* 1973;**4**:187–206.
28. Houkin K, Abe H, Yoshimoto T, Takahashi A. Is "unilateral" moyamoya disease different from moyamoya disease? *J Neurosurg.* 1996;**85**:772–776.
29. Matsushima T, Inoue T, Natori Y, et al. Children with unilateral occlusion or stenosis of the ICA associated with surrounding

moyamoya vessels – "unilateral" moyamoya disease. *Acta Neurochir (Wien)*. 1994;**131**:196–202.

30. Yamada I, Matsushima Y, Suzuki S. Moyamoya disease: diagnosis with three-dimensional time-of-flight angiography. *Radiology*. 1992;**184**:773–778.

31. Yoon HK, Shin HJ, Lee M, Byun HS, Na DG, Han BK. MR angiography of moyamoya disease before and after encephaloduroarteriosynangiosis. *Am J Roentgenol*. 2000;**174**:195–200.

32. Saeki N, Silva MN, Kubota M, Takanashi JI, Nakazaki S, Yamaura A. Comparative performance of magnetic resonance angiography and conventional angiography in moyamoya disease. *J Clin Neurosci*. 2000;**7**:112–115.

33. Yamada I, Suzuki S, Matsushima Y. Moyamoya disease: comparison of assessment with MR angiography and MR imaging versus conventional angiography. *Radiology*. 1995;**196**:211–218.

34. Houkin K, Aoki T, Takahashi A, Abe H. Diagnosis of moyamoya disease with magnetic resonance angiography. *Stroke*. 1994;**25**:2159–2164.

35. Hoshimaru M, Kikuchi H. Involvement of the external carotid arteries in moyamoya disease: neuroradiological evaluation of 66 patients. *Neurosurgery*. 1992;**31**:398–400.

36. Ikezaki K, Loftus CM, eds. *Moyamoya Disease*. Rolling Meadows, IL: American Association of Neurological Surgeons; 2001.

37. Handa J, Handa H. Progressive cerebral arterial occlusive disease: analysis of 27 cases. *Neuroradiology*. 1972;**3**:119–133.

38. Takase K, Kashihara M, Hashimoto T. Transcranial Doppler ultrasonography in patients with moyamoya disease. *Clin Neurol Neurosurg*. 1997;**99**(Suppl 2):S101–S105.

39. Morgenstern C, Griewing B, Muller-Esch G, Zeller JA, Kessler C. Transcranial power-mode duplex ultrasound in two patients with moyamoya syndrome. *J Neuroimaging*. 1997;**7**:190–192.

40. Bruno A, Yuh WTC, Biller J, Adams HP, Cornell SH. Magnetic resonance imaging in young adults with cerebral infarction due to moyamoya. *Arch Neurol*. 1988;**45**:303–306.

41. Ikezaki K, Matsushima T, Kuwabara Y, Suzuki SO, Nomura T, Fukui M. Cerebral circulation and oxygen metabolism in childhood moyamoya disease: a perioperative positron emission tomography study. *J Neurosurg*. 1994;**81**:843–850.

42. Nambu K, Suzuki R, Hirakawa K. Cerebral blood flow: measurement with xenon-enhanced dynamic helical CT. *Radiology*. 1995;**195**:53–57.

43. Kuwabara Y, Ichiya Y, Sasaki M, et al. Response to hypercapnia in moyamoya disease. Cerebrovascular response to hypercapnia in pediatric and adult patients with moyamoya disease. *Stroke*. 1997;**28**:701–707.

44. Hoshi H, Ohnishi T, Jinnouchi S, et al. Cerebral blood flow study in patients with moyamoya disease evaluated by IMP SPECT. *J Nucl Med*. 1994;**35**:44–50.

45. Nakagawara J, Takeda R, Suematsu K, Nakamura J. Quantification of regional cerebral blood flow and vascular reserve in childhood moyamoya disease using [123I]IMP-ARG method. *Clin Neurol Neurosurg*. 1997;**99**(Suppl 2):S96–S99.

46. Ikezaki K. A rational approach to treatment of moyamoya disease in childhood. *J Child Neurol*. 2000;**15**:350–356.

47. Katano H, Sugiyama N, Yamada K. Simple delineation of misery perfusion areas by superimposition of PET on PET images. *Br J Neurosurg*. 1998;**12**:353–357.

48. Kuwabara Y, Ichiya Y, Sasaki M, et al. Cerebral hemodynamics and metabolism in moyamoya disease – a positron emission tomography study. *Clin Neurol Neurosurg*. 1997;**99**(Suppl 2):S74–S78.

49. Han DH, Nam DH, Oh CW. Moyamoya disease in adults: characteristics of clinical presentation and outcome after encephaloduro-arterio-synangiosis. *Clin Neurol Neurosurg*. 1997;**99**(Suppl 2):S151–S155.

50. Honda M, Ezaki Y, Kitagawa N, Tsutsumi K, Ogawa Y, Nagata I. Quantification of the regional cerebral blood flow and vascular reserve in moyamoya disease using split-dose iodoamphetamine I 123 single-photon emission computed tomography. *Surg Neurol*. 2006;**66**:155–159.

51. Kurlmann G, Fahrendorf G, Krings W, Sciuk J, Palm D. Characteristic EEG findings in childhood moyamoya syndrome. *Neurosurg Rev*. 1992;**15**:57–60.

52. Maki Y, Enomoto T. Moyamoya disease. *Child's Nerv Syst*. 1988;**4**:204–212.

53. Tashima-Kurita S, Matsushima T, Kato M, et al. Moyamoya disease: posterior cerebral artery occlusion and pattern-reversal visual evoked potential. *Arch Neurol*. 1989;**46**:550–553.

54. Satoh S, Shibuya H, Suzuki S. Analysis of the angiographic findings in childhood cases of moyamoya disease. *Neuroradiology*. 1988;**30**:111–119.

55. Fukui M, Kono S, Sueishi K, Ikezaki K. Moyamoya disease. *Neuropathology*. 2000;**20**(Suppl):S61–S64.

56. Carlson CB, Harvey FH, Loop J. Progressive alternating hemiplegia in early childhood with basal arterial stenosis and telangiectasia (moyamoya syndrome). *Neurology*. 1973;**23**:734–744.

57. Yamashita M, Oka K, Tanaka K. Cervico-cephalic arterial thrombi and thromboemboli in moyamoya disease – possible correlation with progressive intimal thickening in the intracranial major arteries. *Stroke*. 1984;**15**:264–270.

58. Andreone V, Ciarmiello A, Fusco C, Ambrosanio G, Florio C, Linfante I. Moyamoya disease in Italian monozygotic twins. *Neurology*. 1999;**53**:1332–1335.

59. Kitahara T, Ariga N, Yamaura A, Makino H, Maki Y. Familial occurrence of moya-moya disease: report of three Japanese families. *J Neurol Neurosurg Psychiatry*. 1979;**42**:208–214.

60. Hamada JI, Yoshioka S, Nakahara T, Marubayashi T, Ushio Y. Clinical features of moyamoya disease in sibling relations under 15 years of age. *Acta Neurochir (Wien)*. 1998;**140**:455–458.

61. Roach ES, Golomb MR, Adams RJ, et al. Management of stroke in infants and children. A scientific statement for healthcare professionals from a special writing group of the Stroke Council, American Heart Association. *Stroke*. 2008;**39**:2644–2691.

62. Ikeda H, Sasaki T, Yoshimoto T, Fukui M, Arinami T. Mapping of a familial moyamoya disease gene to chromosome 3p24.2-p26. *Am J Hum Genet*. 1999;**64**:533–537.

63. Inoue TK, Ikezaki K, Sasazuki T, Matsushima T, Fukui M. Linkage analysis of moyamoya disease on chromosome 6. *J Child Neurol*. 2000;**15**:179–182.

64. Yamauchi T, Tada M, Houkin K, et al. Linkage of familial moyamoya disease (spontaneous occlusion of the circle of Willis) to chromosome 17q25. *Stroke*. 2000;**31**:930–935.

65. Sakurai K, Horiuchi Y, Ikeda H, et al. A novel susceptibility locus for moyamoya disease on chromosome 8q23. *J Hum Genet*. 2004;**49**:278–281.

66. Yamamoto M, Aoyagi M, Tajima S, et al. Increase in elastin gene expression and protein synthesis in arterial smooth muscle cells derived from patients with Moyamoya disease. *Stroke*. 1997;**28**:1733–1738.

67. Horn P, Bueltmann E, Buch CV, Schmiedek P. Arterio-embolic ischemic stroke in children with moyamoya disease. *Childs Nerv Syst*. 2005;**21**:104–107.

68. Fung LW, Thompson D, Ganesan V. Revascularisation surgery for paediatric moyamoya: a review of the literature. *Childs Nerv Syst*. 2005;**21**:358–364.

69. Fujii K, Ikezaki K, Irikura K, Miyasaka Y, Fukui M. The efficacy of bypass surgery for the patients with hemorrhagic moyamoya disease. *Clin Neurol Neurosurg*. 1997;**99**(Suppl 2):S194–S195.

70. Houkin K, Kuroda S, Ishikawa T, Abe H. Neovascularization (angiogenesis) after revascularization in moyamoya disease.

Which technique is most useful for moyamoya disease? *Acta Neurochir (Wien)*. 2000;**142**:269–276.

71. Golby AJ, Marks MP, Thompson RC, Steinberg GK. Direct and combined revascularization in pediatric moyamoya disease. *Neurosurgery*. 1999;**45**:50–58.

72. Aoki N. Cerebrovascular bypass surgery for the treatment of moyamoya disease: unsatisfactory outcome in the patients presenting with hemorrhage. *Surg Neurol*. 1993;**40**:372–377.

73. Kawaguchi S, Okuno S, Sakaki T. Effect of direct arterial bypass on the prevention of future stroke in patients with the hemorrhagic variety of moyamoya disease. *J Neurosurg*. 2000;**93**:397–401.

74. Saeki N, Nakazaki S, Kubota M, et al. Hemorrhagic type moyamoya disease. *Clin Neurol Neurosurg*. 1997;**99**(Suppl 2): S196–S201.

75. Sakamoto T, Kawaguchi M, Kurehara K, Kitaguchi K, Furuya H, Karasawa J. Postoperative neurological deterioration following the revascularization surgery in children with moyamoya disease. *J Neurosurg Anesthesiol*. 1998;**10**:37–41.

76. Nomura S, Kashiwagi S, Uetsuka S, Uchida T, Kubota H, Ito H. Perioperative management protocols for children with moyamoya disease. *Childs Nerv Syst*. 2001;**17**:270–274.

77. Allen JC, Miller DC, Budzilovich GN, Epstein FJ. Brain and spinal cord hemorrhage in long-term survivors of malignant pediatric brain tumors: a possible late effect of therapy. *Neurology*. 1991;**41**:148–150.

78. Kreisl TN, Toothaker T, Karimi S, DeAngelis LM. Ischemic stroke in patients with primary brain tumors. *Neurology*. 2008;**70**:2314–2320.

79. Grenier Y, Tomita T, Marymont MH, Byrd S, Burrowes DM. Late postirradiation occlusive vasculopathy in childhood medulloblastoma. Report of two cases. *J Neurosurg*. 1998;**89**:460–464.

80. Lee JK, Chelvarajah R, King A, David KM. Rare presentations of delayed radiation injury: a lobar hematoma and a cystic space-occupying lesion appearing more than 15 years after cranial radiotherapy: report of two cases. *Neurosurgery*. 2004;**54**:1010–1013.

81. Mitchell WG, Fishman LS, Miller JH, et al. Stroke as a late sequela of cranial irradiation for childhood brain tumors. *J Child Neurol*. 1991;**6**:128–133.

82. Marcel M, Leys D, Mounier-Vehier F, et al. Clinical outcome in patients with high-grade internal carotid artery stenosis after irradiation. *Neurology*. 2005;**65**:959–961.

83. Servo A, Puranen M. Moyamoya syndrome as a complication of radiation therapy. *J Neurosurg*. 1978;**48**:1026–1029.

84. Maruyama K, Mishima K, Saito N, Fujimaki T, Sasaki T, Kirino T. Radiation-induced aneurysm and moyamoya vessels presenting with subarachnoid haemorrhage. *Acta Neurochir (Wien)*. 2000;**142**:139–143.

85. Rockman CB, Riles TS, Fisher FS, Adelman MA, Lamparello PJ. The surgical management of carotid artery stenosis in patients with previous neck irradiation. *Am J Surg*. 1996;**172**:191–195.

86. Cheng SW, Wu LL, Ting AC, Lau H, Lam LK, Wei WI. Irradiation-induced extracranial carotid stenosis in patients with head and neck malignancies. *Am J Surg*. 1999;**178**:323–328.

87. Dorresteijn LD, Kappelle AC, Boogerd W, et al. Increased risk of ischemic stroke after radiotherapy on the neck in patients younger than 60 years. *J Clin Oncol*. 2002;**20**:282–288.

88. Kestle JRW, Hoffman HJ, Mock AR. Moyamoya phenomenon after radiation for optic glioma. *J Neurosurg*. 1993;**79**:32–35.

89. Bitzer M, Topka H. Progressive cerebral occlusive disease after radiation therapy. *Stroke*. 1995;**26**:131–136.

90. Mori K, Takeuchi J, Ishikawa M, Handa H, Toyama M, Yamaki T. Occlusive arteriopathy and brain tumor. *J Neurosurg*. 1978;**49**: 22–35.

91. Okuno T, Prensky AL, Gado M. The moyamoya syndrome associated with irradiation of an optic glioma in children: report of

two cases and review of the literature. *Pediatr Neurol*. 1985;**1**:311–316.

92. Kaido T, Hoshida T, Uranishi R, et al. Radiosurgery-induced brain tumor. Case report. *J Neurosurg*. 2001;**95**:710–713.

93. Chung E, Bodensteiner JB, Hogg JP. Spontaneous intracerebral hemorrhage: a very late delayed effect of radiation therapy. *J Child Neurol*. 1992;**7**:259–263.

94. Azzarelli B, Moore J, Gilmor R, Muller J, Edwards M, Mealey J. Multiple fusiform aneurysms following curative radiation therapy foe suprasellar germinoma. *J Neurosurg*. 1984;**61**:1141–1145.

95. Benson PJ, Sung JH. Cerebral aneurysms following radiotherapy for medulloblastoma. *J Neurosurg*. 1989;**70**:545–550.

96. Auyeung KM, Lui WM, Chow LC, Chan FL. Massive epistaxis related to petrous carotid artery pseudoaneurysm after radiation therapy: emergency treatment with covered stent in two cases. *Am J Neuroradiol*. 2003;**24**:1449–1452.

97. Nishi T, Maksukado Y, Kodama T, Hiraki T. Multiple intracranial aneurysms following radiation therapy for pituitary adenoma. *Neural Med Chir (Tokyo)*. 1987;**27**:336–341.

98. Detwiler PW, Porter RW, Zabramski JM, Spetzler RF. De novo formation of a central nervous system cavernous malformation: implications for predicting risk of hemorrhage. Case report and review of the literature. *J Neurosurg*. 1997;**87**:629–632.

99. Furuse M, Miyatake SI, Kuroiwa T. Cavernous malformation after radiation therapy for astrocytoma in adult patients: report of 2 cases. *Acta Neurochir (Wien)*. 2005;**147**:1097–1101.

100. Pozzati E, Giangaspero F, Marliani F, Acciarri N. Occult cerebrovascular malformations after irradiation. *Neurosurgery*. 1996; **39**:677–684.

101. Casey ATH, Marsh HT, Utley M, Utley D. Intracranial aneurysm formation following radiotherapy. *Br J Neurosurg*. 1993;**7**:575–579.

102. Maeder P, Gudinchet F, Meuli R, de Tribolet N. Development of a cavernous malformation of the brain. *AJNR Am J Neuroradiol*. 1998;**19**:1141–1143.

103. Burn S, Gunny R, Phipps K, Gaze M, Hayward R. Incidence of cavernoma development in children after radiotherapy for brain tumors. *J Neurosurg*. 2007;**106**:379–383.

104. Yoshino M, Morita A, Shibahara J, Kirino T. Radiation-induced spinal cord cavernous malformation. Case report. *J Neurosurg*. 2005;**102**:101–104.

105. Maraire JN, Abdulrauf SI, Berger S, Knisely J, Awad IA. De novo development of a cavernous malformation of the spinal cord following spinal axis radiation. Case report. *J Neurosurg*. 1999; **90**:234–238.

106. Fajardo LF, Berthrong M. Vascular lesions following radiation. *Pathol Annu*. 1988;**23**:297–330.

107. Murakami N, Tsukahara T, Toda H, Kawakami O, Hatano T. Radiation-induced cerebral aneurysm successfully treated with endovascular coil embolization. *Acta Neurochir*. 2002;**82**(Suppl): 55–58.

108. Koenigsberg RA, Grandinetti LM, Freeman LP, McCormick D, Tsai F. Endovascular repair of radiation-induced bilateral common carotid artery stenosis and pseudoaneurysms: a case report. *Surg Neurol*. 2001;**55**:347–352.

109. Harrod-Kim P, Kadkhodayan Y, Derdeyn CP, Cross DT III, Moran CJ. Outcomes of carotid angioplasty and stenting for radiation-associated stenosis. *AJNR Am J Neuroradiol*. 2005; **26**:1781–1788.

110. Ishikawa T, Houkin K, Yoshimoto T, Abe H. Vasoreconstructive surgery for radiation-induced vasculopathy in childhood. *Surg Neurol*. 1997;**48**:620–626.

111. Leseche G, Castier Y, Chataigner O, et al. Carotid artery revascularization through a radiated field. *J Vasc Surg*. 2003;**38**:244–250.

112. Glantz MJ, Burger PC, Friedman AH, Radtke RA, Massey EW, Schold SC. Treatment of radiation-induced nervous system injury with heparin and warfarin. *Neurology*. 1994;**44**:2020–2027.

113. Chuba PJ, Aronin P, Bhambhani K, et al. Hyperbaric oxygen therapy for radiation-induced brain injury in children. *Cancer*. 1997;**80**:2005–2012.

114. Ledbetter WF, Burkland CF. Hypertension in unilateral renal disease. *J Urol*. 1938;**39**:611–626.

115. Bellot J, Gherardi R, Poirier J, Lacour P, Debrun G, Barbizet J. Fibromuscular dysplasia of cervico-cephalic arteries with multiple dissections and a carotid-cavernous fistula. A pathological study. *Stroke*. 1985;**16**:255–261.

116. Osborn AG, Anderson RE. Angiographic spectrum of cervical and intracranial fibromuscular dysplasia. *Stroke*. 1977;**8**:617–626.

117. Sandok BA, Houser OW, Baker HL, Holley KE. Fibromuscular dysplasia. *Arch Neurol*. 1971;**24**:462–466.

118. Perdu J, Boutouyrie P, Bourgain C, et al. Inheritance of arterial lesions in renal fibromuscular dysplasia. *J Hum Hypertens*. 2007;**21**:393–400.

119. Mettinger KL. Fibromuscular dysplasia and the brain 2. Current concept of the disease. *Stroke*. 1982;**13**:53–58.

120. Mettinger KL, Ericson K. Fibromuscular dysplasia and the brain. Observations on angiographic, clinical, and genetic characteristics. *Stroke*. 1982;**13**:46–52.

121. Schievink WI, Meyer FB, Parisi JE, Wijdicks EF. Fibromuscular dysplasia of the internal carotid artery associated with alpha1-antitrypsin deficiency. *Neurosurgery*. 1998;**43**:229–233.

122. So EL, Toole JF, Dalal P, Moody DM. Cephalic fibromuscular dysplasia in 32 patients: clinical findings and radiologic features. *Arch Neurol*. 1981;**38**:619–622.

123. Van Damme H, Sakalihasan N, Limet R. Fibromuscular dysplasia of the internal carotid artery. Personal experience with 13 cases and literature review. *Acta Chir Belg*. 1999;**99**:163–168.

124. Chiche L, Bahnini A, Koskas F, Kieffer E. Occlusive fibromuscular disease of arteries supplying the brain: results of surgical treatment. *Ann Vasc Surg*. 1997;**11**:496–504.

125. Wesen CA, Elliott BM. Fibromuscular dysplasia of the carotid arteries. *Am J Surg*. 1986;**151**:448–451.

126. Cloft HJ, Kallmes DF, Kallmes MH, Goldstein JH, Jensen ME, Dion JE. Prevalence of cerebral aneurysms in patients with fibromuscular dysplasia: a reassessment. *J Neurosurg*. 1998;**88**:436–440.

127. Belber CJ, Hoffman RB. The syndrome of intracranial aneurysm associated with fibromuscular hyperplasia of the renal arteries. *J Neurosurg*. 1969;**28**:556–559.

128. Sell JJ, Seigel RS, Orrison WW, Roberts WS. Angiographic pattern change in fibromuscular dysplasia. *Angiology*. 1995;**46**:165–168.

129. Furie DM, Tien RD. Fibromuscular dysplasia of arteries of the head and neck: imaging findings. *AJR Am J Roentgenol*. 1994;**162**:1205–1209.

130. So EL, Toole JF, Moody DM, Challa VR. Cerebral embolism from septal fibromuscular dysplasia of the common carotid artery. *Ann Neurol*. 1979;**6**:75–78.

131. Harrison EG Jr, McCormack LJ. Pathologic classification of renal arterial disease in renovascular hypertension. *Mayo Clin Proc*. 1971;**46**:161–167.

132. Leary MC, Finley A, Caplan LR. Cerebrovascular complications of fibromuscular dysplasia. *Curr Treat Options Cardiovasc Med*. 2004;**6**:237–248.

133. Manninen HI, Koivisto T, Saari T, et al. Dissecting aneurysms of all four cervicocranial arteries in fibromuscular dysplasia: treatment with self-expanding endovascular stents, coil emboliza-

tion, and surgical ligation. *AJNR Am J Neuroradiol*. 1997;**18**:1216–1220.

134. Rennebohm RM, Egan RA, Susac JO. Treatment of Susac's syndrome. *Curr Treat Options Neurol*. 2008;**10**:67–74.

135. Susac JO, Egan RA, Rennebohm RM, Lubow M. Susac's syndrome: 1975–2005 microangiopathy/autoimmune endotheliopathy. *J Neurol Sci*. 2007;**257**:270–272.

136. Petty GW, Engel AG, Younge BR, et al. Retinocochleocerebral vasculopathy. *Medicine (Baltimore)*. 1998;**77**:12–40.

137. Hahn JS, Lannin WC, Sarwal MM. Microangiopathy of brain, retina, and inner ear (Susac's syndrome) in an adolescent female presenting as acute disseminated encephalomyelitis. *Pediatrics*. 2004;**114**:276–281.

138. Susac JO. Susac's syndrome. *AJNR Am J Neuroradiol*. 2004;**25**:351–352.

139. Roach ES. Malignant atrophic papulosis. In: Vinken PJ, Bruyn GW, Klawans HL, eds. *Handbook of Clinical Neurology. Volume 11: Vascular Diseases*, Part III. Amsterdam: Elsevier; 1989:275–283.

140. Degos R. Malignant atrophic papulosis: a fatal cutaneo-intestinal syndrome. *Br J Dermatol*. 1954;**66**:304–307.

141. Sidi E, Reinberg A, Spinasse B, Hincky M. Lethal cutaneous and gastrointestinal arteriolar thrombosis (malignant atrophying papulosis of Degos). *JAMA*. 1960;**174**:1170–1173.

142. Scheinfeld N. Malignant atrophic papulosis. *Clin Exp Dermatol*. 2007;**32**:483–487.

143. Zamiri M, Jarrett P, Snow J. Benign cutaneous Degos disease. *Int J Dermatol*. 2005;**44**:654–656.

144. Rosemberg S, Lopes MBS, Sotto MN, Graudenz MS. Childhood Degos disease with prominent neurological symptoms: report of a clinicopathological case. *J Child Neurol*. 1987;**3**:42–46.

145. Torrelo A, Sevilla J, Mediero IG, Candelas D, Zambrano A. Malignant atrophic papulosis in an infant. *Br J Dermatol*. 2002;**146**:916–918.

146. Kisch LS, Bruynzeel DP. Six cases of malignant atrophic papulosis (Degos' disease) occurring in one family. *Br J Dermatol*. 1984;**111**:469–471.

147. Katz SK, Mudd LJ, Roenigk HH Jr. Malignant atrophic papulosis (Degos' disease) involving three generations of a family. *J Am Acad Dermatol*. 1997;**37**:480–484.

148. Habbema L, Kisch LS, Starink TM. Familial malignant atrophic papulosis (Degos' disease) – additional evidence for heredity and a benign course. *Br J Dermatol*. 1986;**114**:134–135.

149. Horner FA, Myers GJ, Stumpf DA, Oseroff BJ, Choi BH. Malignant atrophic papulosis (Kohlmeier-Degos disease) in childhood. *Neurology*. 1976;**26**:317–321.

150. Leslie TA, Goldsmith PC, Thompson AJ, Dowd PM. Degos disease and spastic paraplegia. *Clin Exp Dermatol*. 1993;**18**:344–346.

151. Amato C, Ferri R, Elia M, et al. Nervous system involvement in Degos disease. *AJNR Am J Neuroradiol*. 2005;**26**:646–649.

152. McFarland HR, Wood WG, Drowns BV, Meneses ACO. Papulosis atrophicans maligna (Kohlmeier-Degos disease): a disseminated occlusive vasculopathy. *Ann Neurol*. 1978;**3**:388–392.

153. Petit WA, Soso MJ, Higman H. Degos disease: neurologic complications and cerebral angiography. *Neurology*. 1982;**32**:1305–1309.

154. Culicchia CF, Gol A, Erickson EE. Diffuse central nervous system involvement in papulosis atrophicans maligna. *Neurology*. 1962;**12**:503–509.

155. Dastur DK, Singhal BS, Shroff HJ. CNS involvement in malignant atrophic papulosis (Kohlmeier-Degos disease): vasculopathy and coagulopathy. *J Neurol Neurosurg Psychiatry*. 1981;**44**:156–160.

156. Yoshikowa H, Maruta T, Yokoji H, Takamori M, Yachie A, Torii Y. Degos' disease: radiological and immunological aspects. *Acta Neurol Scand*. 1996;**94**:353–356.

157. High WA, Arada J, Patel SB, Cockerell CJ, Costner MI. Is Degos' disease a clinical and histological end point rather

than a specific disease? *J Amer Acad Dermatol*. 2004;**50**:895–899.

158. Warot P, Caron JC, Lehembre P, Houcke M. Maladie de Degos a forme cerebrale. *Rev Neurol (Paris)*. 1977;**133**:353–358.

159. Vanderhaeghen JJ, Joffroy A, Achten G, Warszawski M, Reyknaers H. Lesions vasculaires dans la papulose atrophiante maligne de Degos atteinte disseminee du systeme nerveux avec infiltration lipidique de l'intima des arteres sous-arachnoidiennes. *Pathol Europ*. 1968;**3**:1–26.

160. Molenaar WM, Rosman JB, Donker AJ, Houthoff HJ. The pathology and pathogenesis of malignant atrophic papulosis (Degos' disease). A case study with reference to other vascular disorders. *Pathol Res Pract*. 1987;**182**:98–106.

161. Stahl D, Thomsen K, Hou-Jensen K. Malignant atrophic papulosis. Treatment with aspirin and dipyridamole. *Arch Dermatol*. 1978;**114**:1687–1689.

162. Pallesen RM, Rasmussen NR. Malignant atrophic papulosis-Degos' syndrome. *Acta Chir Scand*. 1979;**145**:279–283.

163. Powell J, Bordea C, Wojnarowska F, Farrell AM, Morris PJ. Benign familial Degos disease worsening during immunosupression. *Br J Dermatol*. 1999;**141**:524–527.

164. Suzuki J, Takaku A. Cerebrovascular "moyamoya" disease. Disease showing abnormal net-like vessels in base of brain. *Arch Neurol*. 1969;**20**:288–299.

165. Roach ES, Riela AR. *Pediatric Cerebrovascular Disorders*. 2nd ed. New York: Futura; 1995.

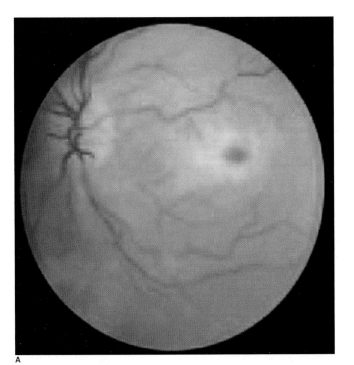

A

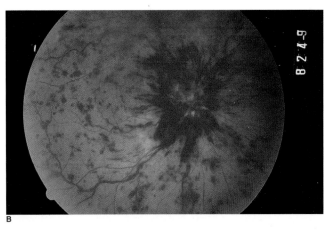

B

Figure 2-3. A: Retinal appearance after a central retinal artery occlusion. Note the cloudy appearance of the retina, the indistinctness of the retinal arteries, and the cherry-red macular lesion. B: Retinal findings following thrombosis of the central retinal vein include retinal edema and perivenous hemorrhage.

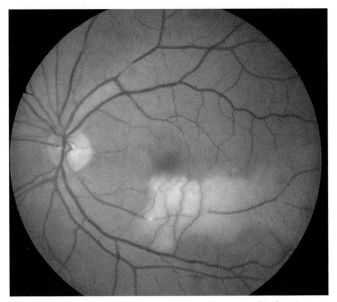

Figure 2-4. Retinal embolus with secondary retinal infarction.

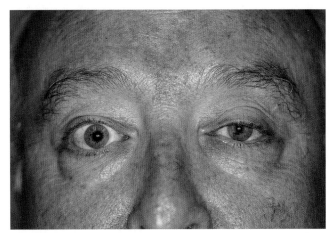

Figure 2-5. Left miosis and ptosis due to an oculosympathetic paresis, or partial Horner syndrome. Photograph courtesy of Dr. Carol Zimmerman.

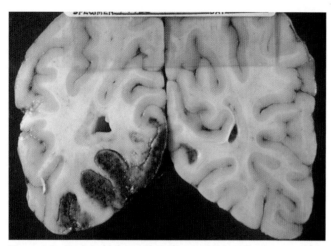

Figure 4-2. Occipital lobe gyriform hemorrhagic infarction secondary to uncal herniation causing compression of the posterior cerebral artery.

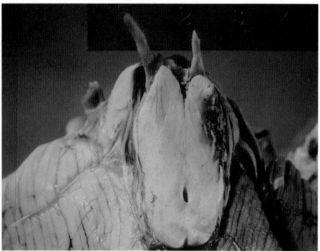

Figure 4-3. Coronal specimen shows necrosis of the contralateral cerebral peduncle due to uncal herniation (Kernohan's notch syndrome) caused by a large hemorrhagic infarction with uncal herniation.

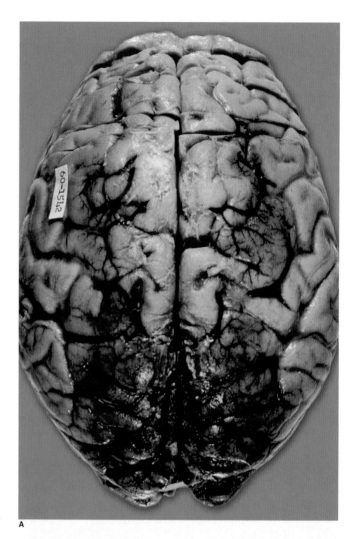

A

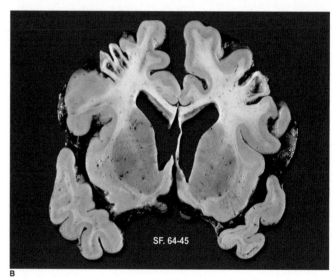

B

Figure 4-4. A: Pathological specimen demonstrates a watershed infarct of both cerebral hemispheres. B: Coronal brain section demonstrates selective parasagittal necrosis.

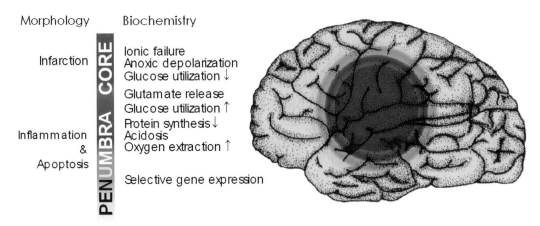

Morphology   Biochemistry

Infarction   Ionic failure
              Anoxic depolarization
              Glucose utilization ↓

              Glutamate release
              Glucose utilization ↑
              Protein synthesis ↓
Inflammation Acidosis
    &   Oxygen extraction ↑
Apoptosis

              Selective gene expression

Figure 4-5. The ischemic penumbra can enlarge over time. Early intervention aims at restoring function of this area of viable tissue. Reprinted with permission from Dirnagl et al. 1999.

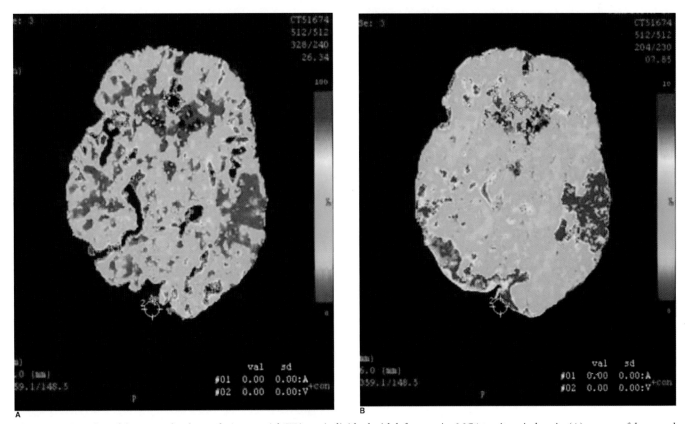

Figure 4-6. Imaging of the penumbra by perfusion cranial CT in an individual with left posterior MCA territory ischemia: (A) an area of decreased CBF (*dark blue*), (B) increased MTT of the contrast agent (*red*). The noncontrast cranial CT was within normal limits before and following the administration of tPA.

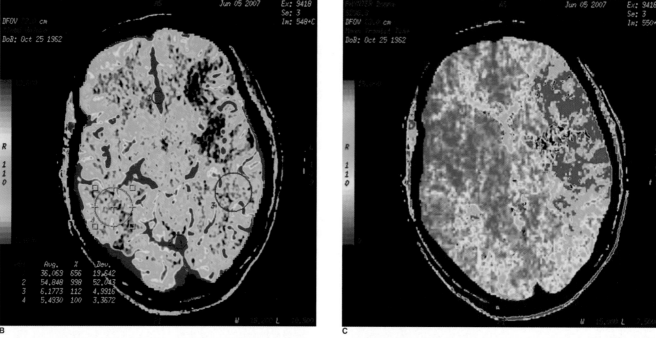

Figure 5-3. Perfusion CT studies from a patient who presented at the end of the three-hour time limit for thrombolysis and instead underwent mechanical thrombectomy and intra-arterial thrombolysis. Her studies show matching areas of cerebral blood volume (B), and decreased mean transit time (C) within the left middle cerebral artery territory, findings that collectively suggest a completed infarct without evidence of an ischemic penumbra.

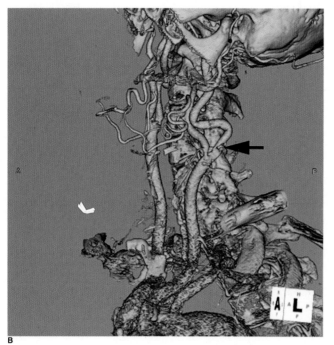

Figure 5-4. B: A three-dimensional reconstruction of the cervical arteries shows this same lesion more clearly (*arrow*) and better demonstrates an out-pouching of contrast along the posterior aspect of the proximal left internal carotid artery consistent with a small dissection.

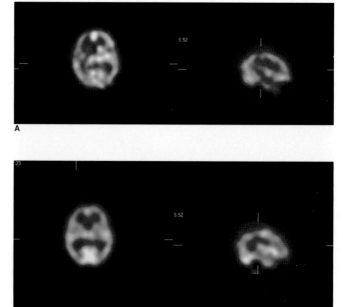

Figure 5-8. Single photon emission tomography (SPECT) scan images in the transaxial and sagittal planes done both with (A) and without (B) intravenous acetazolamide infusion. After intravenous acetazolamide, there is decreased perfusion in the right hemisphere primarily in a watershed region. A repeat study a few days later without acetazolamide (B) shows an improved, although not yet normal, perfusion pattern.

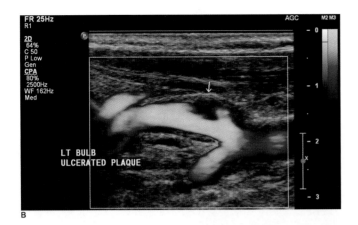

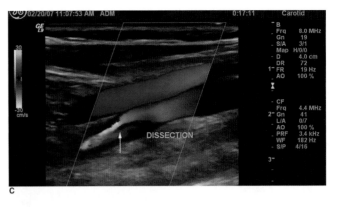

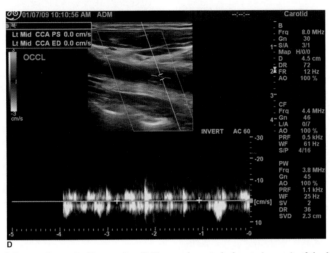

Figure 5-10. Ultrasound depiction of the cervicocephalic arteries. B: Large ulcerated plaque (*arrow*) of the left carotid artery bifurcation. C: Dissection of the right internal carotid artery (*red*). A flap (*arrow*) divides the true and false lumen. D: With occlusion of the left common carotid artery there is no detectable color flow within the vascular lumen, and the spectral analysis shows absent arterial flow. Ultrasound images are courtesy of the Vascular Laboratory at Penn State College of Medicine, Hershey, Pennsylvania.

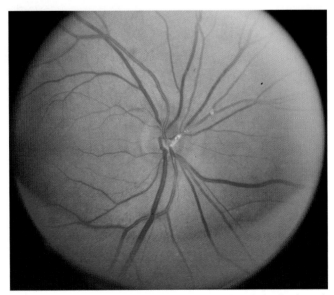

Figure 6-1. Retinal photograph shows an embolism lodged at branch point of a retinal artery. Photograph courtesy of Dr. Nick Hogan.

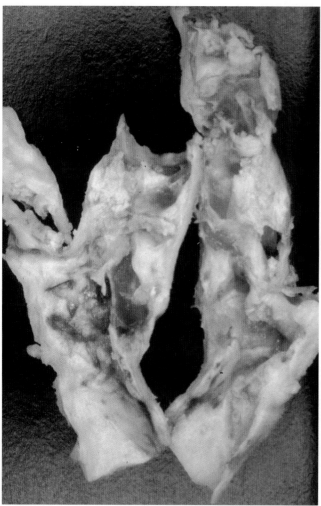

Figure 7-2. A carotid artery plaque removed at endarterectomy reveals an irregular, fibrin-coated luminal surface. Photograph courtesy of Dr. David Lefkowitz.

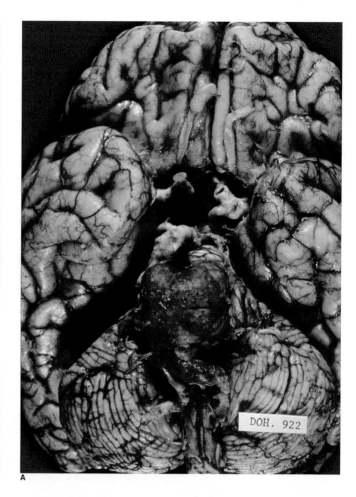

A

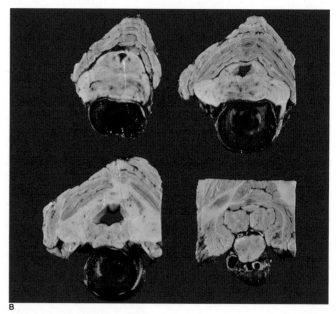

B

Figure 7-3. A: A large, fusiform, dolichoectatic basilar artery aneurysm resulting from atherosclerosis. B: In cross section, there is thrombus within the lesion with preservation of the lumen within the center of the clot. Note the indentation of the brainstem.

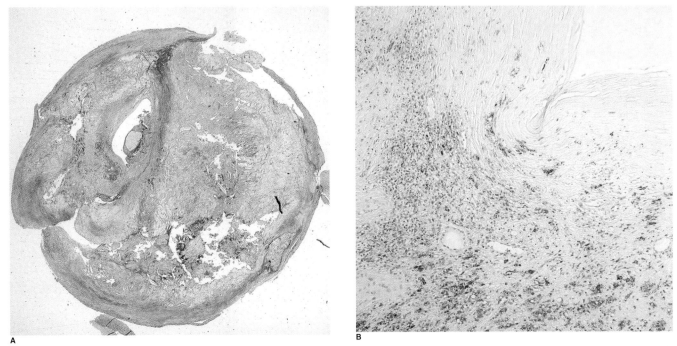

A

B

Figure 7-5. A: The carotid artery lumen is almost occluded by extensive lipid-laden plaque-containing cholesterol crystals (Picro-Serius red collagen stain with × 20 magnification). B: CD-68 stained carotid plaque demonstrates heavy macrophage infiltration (× 100). These findings predict a lower likelihood of carotid artery restenosis after endarterectomy. Reprinted with permission from Hellings et al. 2008.

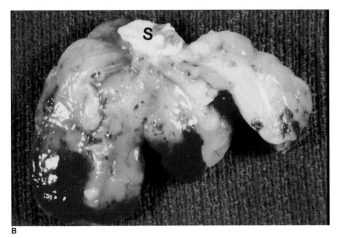

B

Figure 8-4. B: Surgically removed atrial myxoma specimen. Note the pedunculated nature of the tumor and the associated thrombus. Reprinted with permission from Bayir et al. 1999.

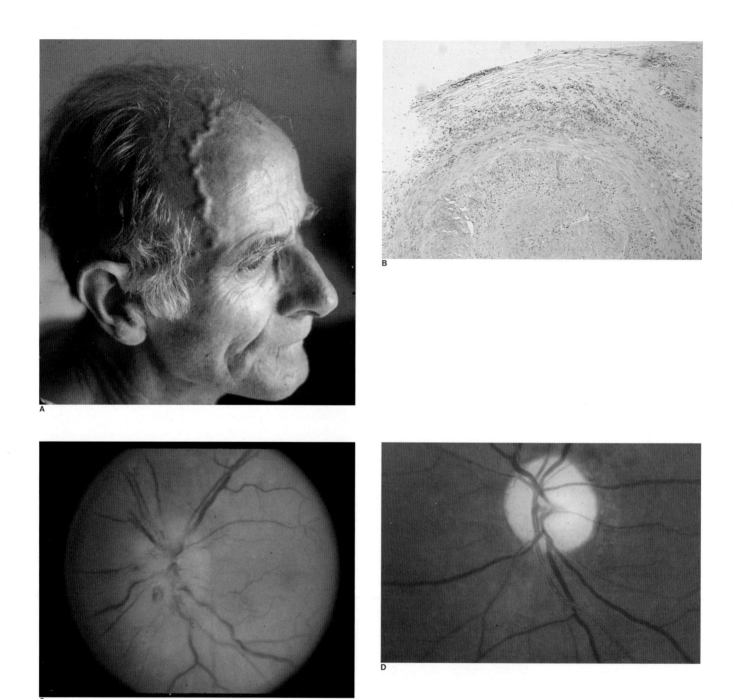

Figure 10-1. A: Striking enlargement of the right temporal artery due to giant cell arteritis in a 70-year-old man with a 6-month history of frontal headache and weight loss. B: Temporal artery biopsy from a patient with giant cell arteritis showing lymphocytic infiltration and lumen occlusion. C: Optic nerve edema and infarction due to giant cell arteritis. D: Chronic optic atrophy following acute visual loss due to giant cell arteritis . Parts C and D courtesy of Dr. Carol F. Zimmerman.

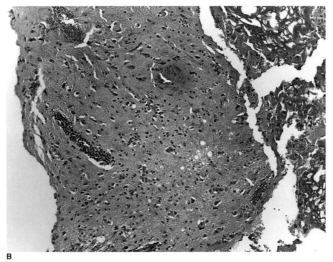

B

Figure 10-3. B: Biopsy of this patient's right temporal lobe showed perivascular mononuclear lymphocytic and plasma cell infiltrates suggestive of primary cerebral arteritis. Although not well shown in this picture, the brain tissue around some of these vessels contained reactive astrocytes and degenerating neurons (hematoxylin-eosin, original magnification × 400).

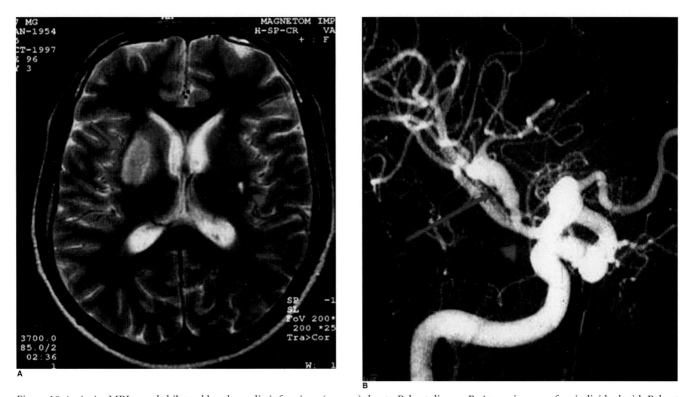

Figure 10-4. A: An MRI reveals bilateral basal ganglia infarctions (arrows) due to Behçet disease. B: An angiogram of an individual with Behçet disease shows subtle stenosis (arrowhead) of the proximal right middle cerebral artery and aneurysmal dilatation of a middle cerebral branch (arrow). Reprinted with permission from Krepsi et al. 2001. Photographs courtesy of Professor Gulsen Akman-Demir.

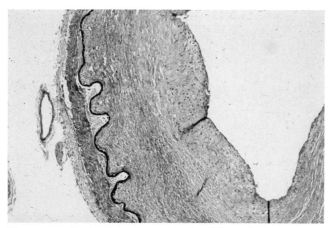

Figure 11-2. Section from the proximal middle cerebral artery of an individual with sickle cell disease. Note the asymmetrical endothelial and subendothelial hyperplasia. Reprinted with permission from Riela and Roach 1993.

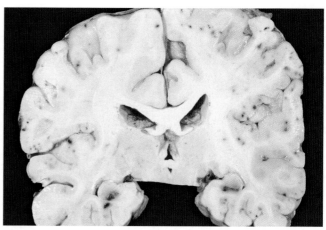

Figure 11-4. Multiple petechial lesions due to TTP.

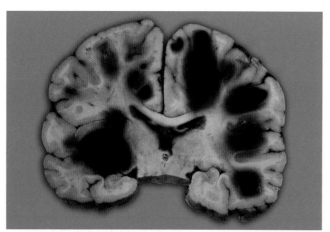

Figure 11-3. Multiple white matter hemorrhages in a patient with acute leukemia.

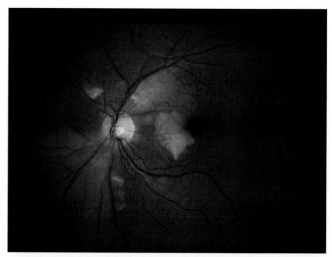

Figure 13-6. Retinal infarction due to branch retinal artery occlusions in an individual with Susac syndrome. Reprinted with permission from Roach and Riela 1995.

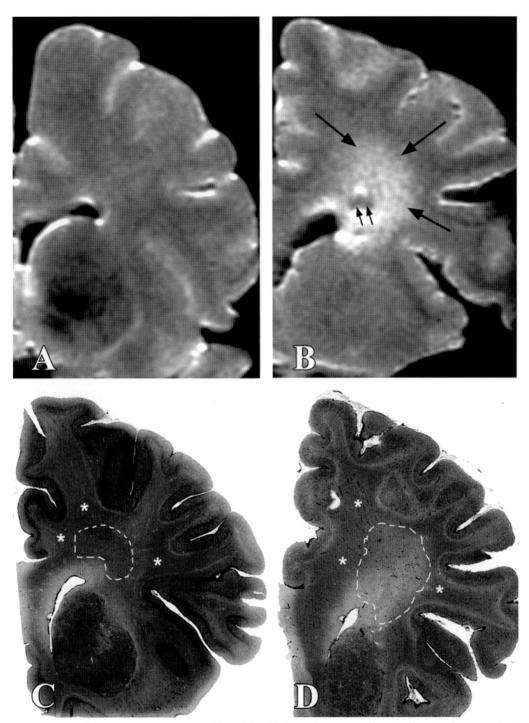

Figure 15-1. White matter appearance on T_2-weighted MRI and corresponding alkaline phophatase-stained section in a patient with leukoaraiosis (B and D) and a healthy individual (A and C). Dotted lines represent areas of sampling for vascular density analysis. Areas with asterisk (*) indicate unaffected white matter. Reprinted with permission from Moody et al. 2004.

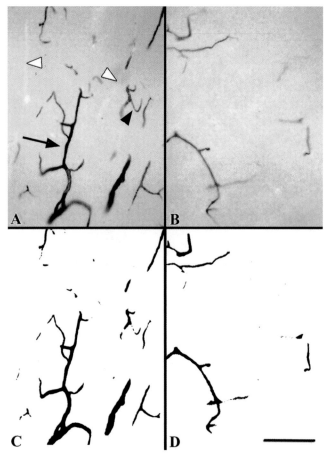

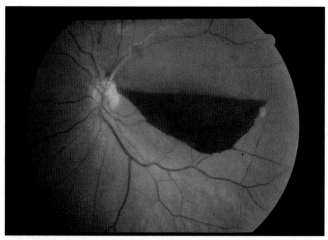

Figure 17-2. Preretinal hemorrhages are common in individuals with SAH. Because of their frequent keel-shaped appearance they are sometimes called "boat hemorrhages."

Figure 15-2. Density of afferent cerebral vessels in white matter of a healthy individual (A, alkaline phosphatase-stain and C, binary image) and in a leukoaraiotic lesion of a patient with ischemic small vessel disease (B, alkaline phophatase-stain and D, binary image). Arteriolar and capillary density is significantly decreased in areas of leukoaraiosis. Reprinted with permission from Moody et al. 2004.

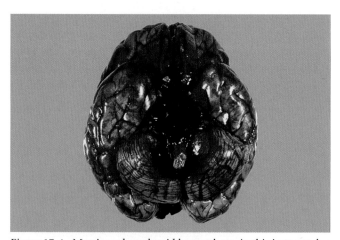

Figure 17-4. Massive subarachnoid hemorrhage, in this instance due to a ruptured aneurysm. The base of the brain is encased in blood, and the convexities are blood tinged.

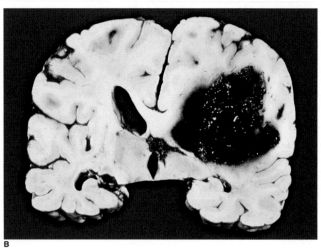

Figure 16-1. B: Coronal brain section (from a patient with hypertension) reveals a large putaminal hemorrhage with ventricular penetration and mass effect.

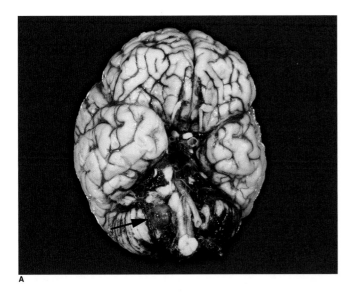

A

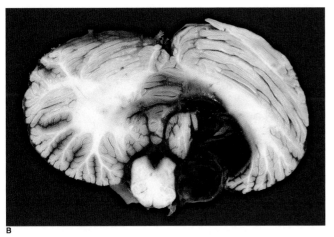

B

Figure 17-6. A: Aneurysm of the posterior inferior cerebellar artery (*arrow*). B: In addition to subarachnoid and intraparenchymal hemorrhage, the aneurysm also caused brainstem and cerebellar compression.

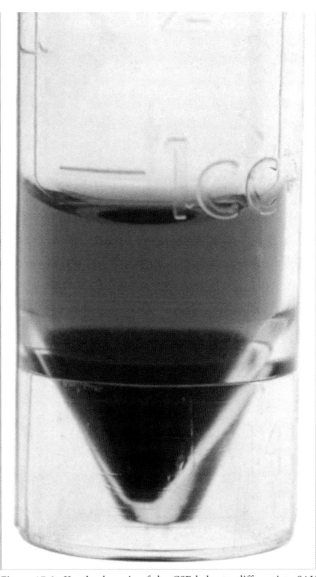

Figure 17-9. Xanthochromia of the CSF helps to differentiate SAH from a traumatic lumbar puncture.

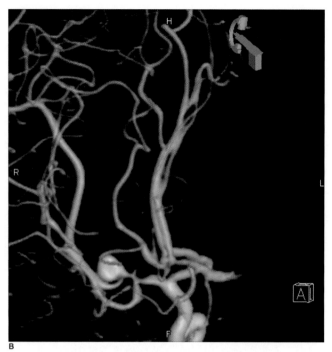

B

Figure 17-10. B: An angiogram depicts a three-dimensional reconstruction of an aneurysm and its relationship to nearby arteries. Photograph courtesy of Dr. Louis Carragine.

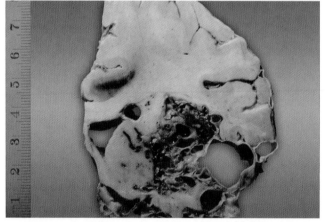

Figure 18-1. Coronal brain specimen showing a large AVM. Note the disorganized array of vessels of varying sizes.

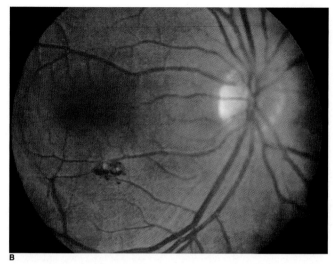

B

Figure 18-6. B: A cavernous lesion of the retina. Multiple brain and retinal cavernous malformations are often inherited as an autosomal dominant trait.

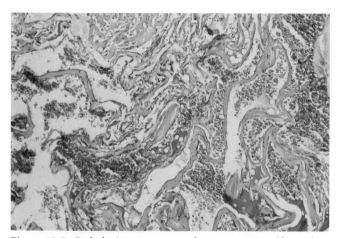

Figure 18-7. Pathologic appearance of a cavernous malformation. Note the large, thin-walled vessels in this cavernous malformation.

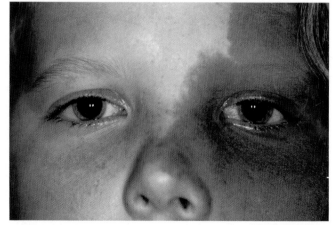

Figure 18-8. Typical facial cutaneous nevus of an individual with Sturge-Weber syndrome. Reprinted with permission from Riela and Roach 2004.

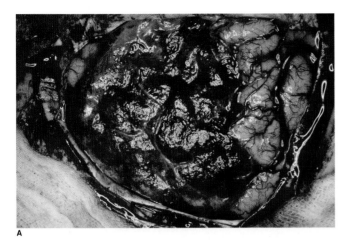

A

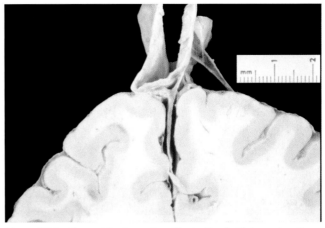

Figure 19-1. Coronal brain section illustrating bridging veins. Rupture of these vessels, as a result of a sudden change in the velocity of the head, may lead to subdural hemorrhage.

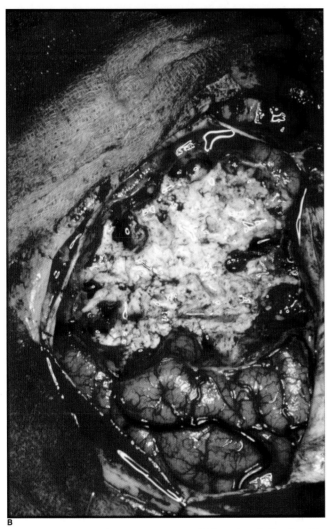

B

Figure 18-9. A: The leptomeninges are thickened and discolored by increased vascularity in this operative photograph of an individual with Sturge-Weber syndrome. B: This same patient is shown after surgical resection of the lesion.

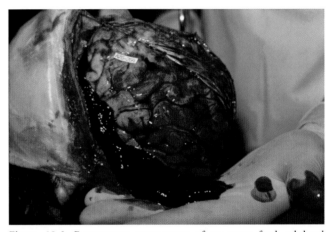

Figure 19-2. Postmortem appearance of an acute fatal subdural hematoma.

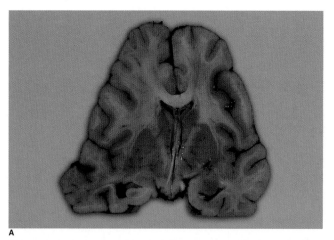

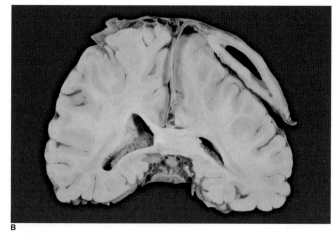

Figure 19-3. A: Compression and displacement of both cerebral hemispheres due to bilateral chronic subdural hematomas. B: Coronal section illustrates an ossified chronic subdural hematoma that has displaced the adjacent cerebral hemisphere.

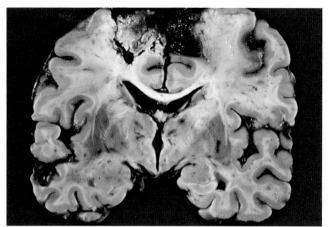

Figure 20-2. Coronal brain specimen shows bilateral hemispheric hemorrhagic infarctions due to a thrombosed sagittal sinus.

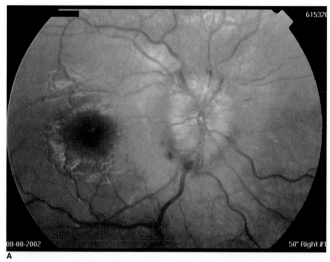

Figure 20-3. A: Papilledema. Reprinted with permission from Bari et al. 2005.

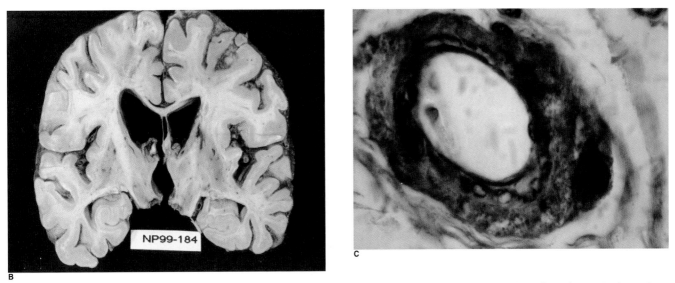

Figure 21-1. B: The brain of an individual with CADASIL has numerous small lesions in the white matter and confluent lesions in the periventricular region. C: Microscopic sections reveal the characteristic perivascular osmophilic changes of CADASIL.

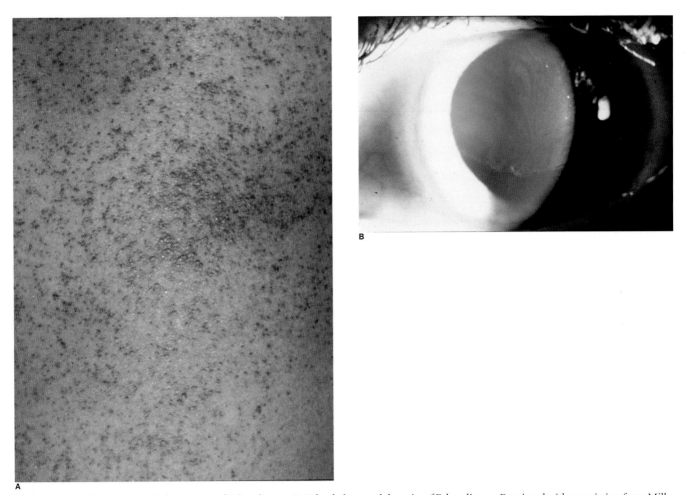

Figure 21-2. A: Cutaneous angiokeratomas of Fabry disease. B: Whorled corneal deposits of Fabry disease. Reprinted with permission from Miller and Roach 2000.

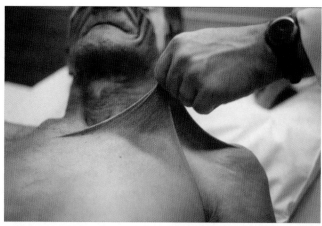

Figure 21-3. Hyperelastic skin is not characteristic of the vascular subtype (type IV) of Ehlers-Danlos syndrome, the only subtype that frequently causes vascular complications. Reprinted with permission from Roach and Riela 1995.

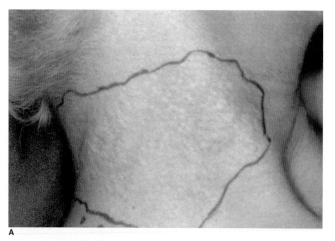

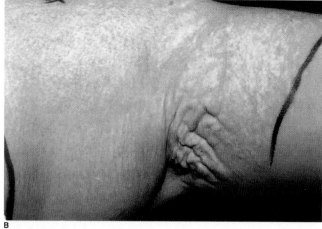

Figure 21-4. A: Characteristic cutaneous appearance of PXE on the neck of an individual with PXE (outlined in red). B: Redundant skin folds in the axilla due to PXE. Reprinted with permission from Neldner and Roach 2004.

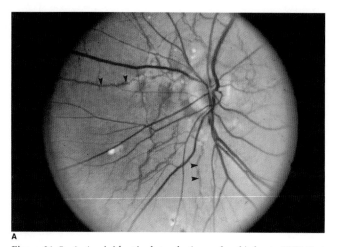

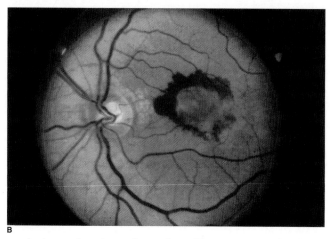

Figure 21-5. A: Angioid retinal streaks (*arrowheads*) due to PXE. B: Acute macular hemorrhage in another patient with PXE. Reprinted with permission from Neldner and Roach 2004.

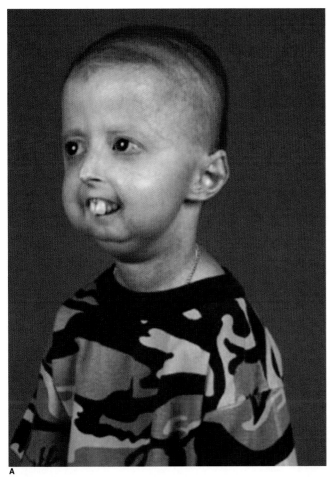

A

Figure 21-7. A: Physical characteristics of an individual with progeria at about 9 years of age. Note the aged appearance due to stooped shoulders, skin laxity, and alopecia.

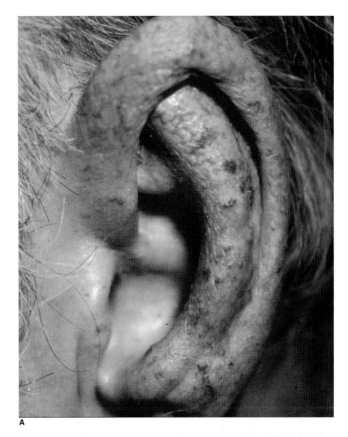

A

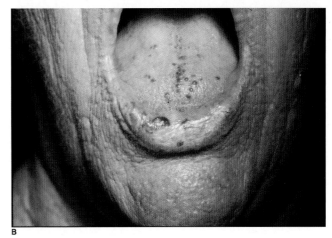

B

Figure 21-8. Cutaneous telangiectasias of the ear (A) and lips and tongue (B) due to hereditary hemorrhagic telangiectasia. Reprinted with permission from Dowling 2004.

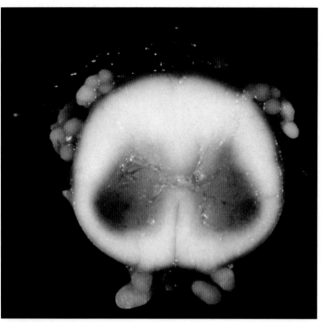

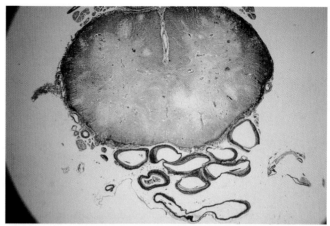

Figure 24-5. Subacute necrotic myelopathy due to an AVM (Foix-Alajouanine syndrome). Note the dilated AVM vessels anterior to the spinal cord and the widespread necrosis within the spinal cord.

Figure 24-4. Cross section of the spinal cord shows hypoxic–ischemic myelopathy of the central portion of the cord.

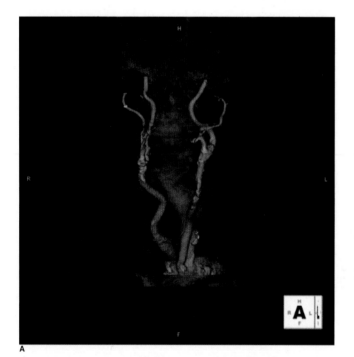

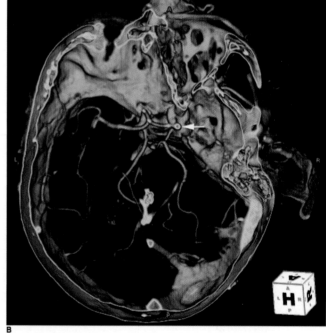

Figure 25-4. CTA is a useful diagnostic tool to rapidly assess the cerebrovascular circulation in stroke patients. A: CTA of the neck showing areas of atherosclerotic plaques in both carotid systems. There is no flow-limiting stenosis. B: CTA of the intracranial circulation showing proximal occlusion of the left M1 segment of the MCA (*arrow*).

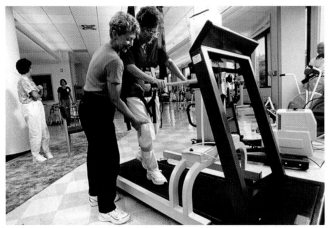

Figure 26-3. Patient with a stroke in the left anterior cerebral artery distribution with weakness in right leg undergoing gait training using treadmill with partial body weight support.

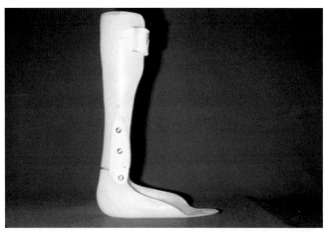

Figure 26-4. A custom-fabricated, lightweight ankle-foot orthosis with a hinged ankle joint. The joint allows free active dorsiflexion but prevents excessive plantar flexion.

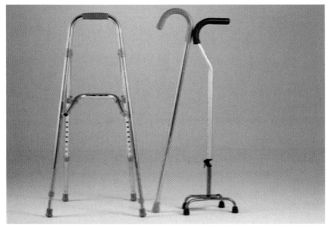

Figure 26-5. Several commonly used assistive devices for ambulation after hemiparesis, including (from right to left) a hemiwalker (walker cane), standard J-neck cane, and four-pronged quad cane.

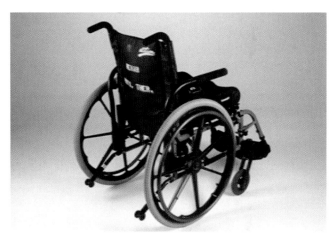

Figure 26-6. A wheelchair with standard foam cushion and commonly prescribed features, including swing-away leg rests, wheel grips to facilitate propulsion, pneumatic tires, and anti-tip bars.

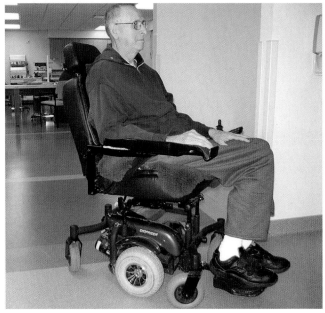

Figure 26-7. Nonambulatory patient with right hemiparesis who uses a power wheelchair. Note arm trough for support of paretic arm.

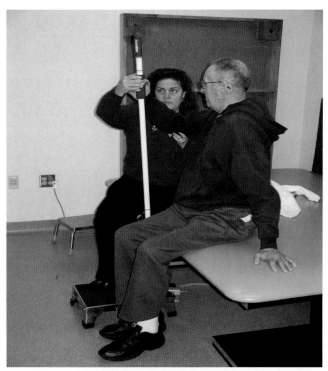

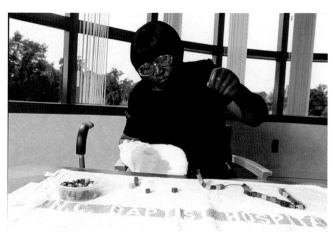

Figure 26-9. Patient with left hemiparesis receiving constraint-induced movement therapy (CIMT). She is repetitively placing beads on a string, a very difficult task for her. Note "mitt" on her right hand to prevent its involvement in this task.

Figure 26-8. Therapist working with patient with paretic arm, spasticity, and shoulder pain. Goals are strengthening, improved active range of motion, decreased hypertonicity, and decreased shoulder pain.

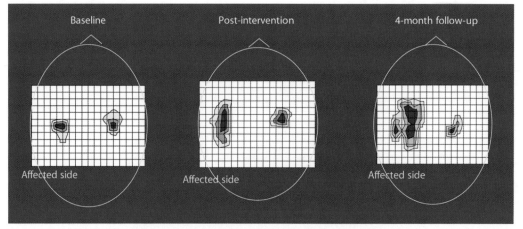

Figure 26-10. Longitudinal changes in a two-dimensional motor map obtained by using transcranial magnetic stimulation (TMS) over the motor cortex of each hemisphere in a patient receiving CIMT after stroke. The grid size is 1 cm, and motor responses at each scalp position are coded by intensity (relative to the maximal response). Note expansion of the motor map over the affected hemisphere associated with CIMT, which persists at 4 months.

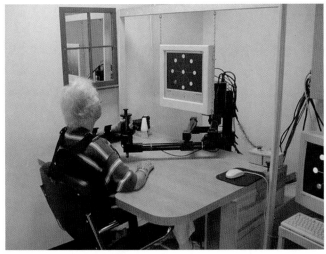

Figure 26-11. Patient undergoing robot-assisted training following stroke. The patient is presented with a visual stimulus on the computer screen and asked to move the cursor to the stimulus. Used with permission of Dr. Igo Krebs.

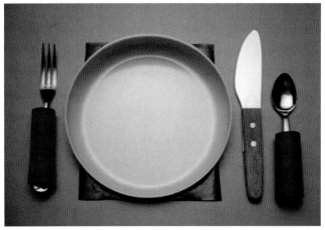

Figure 26-13. Adapted eating utensils, including built-up handles on spoon and fork, a rocker knife for one-handed cutting, a plate with raised edge, and a special surface to prevent the plate from sliding on the table.

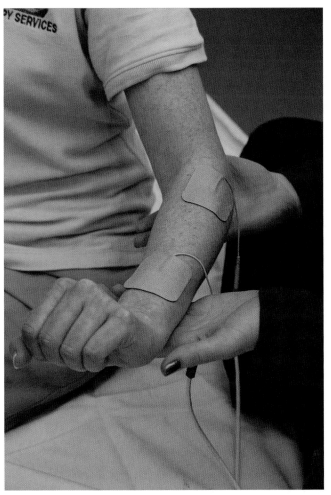

Figure 26-12. Functional electrical stimulation applied over the wrist extensors to facilitate motor movement.

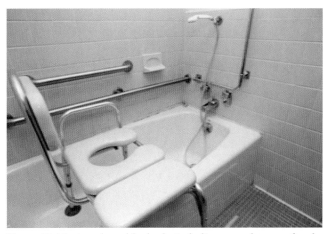

Figure 26-14. An adapted bathtub, including several types of grab-bars, a hand-held shower nozzle, and bathtub transfer bench on which the patient may safely sit.

14

Migraine and Related Disorders

Disease is from of old and nothing about it has changed. It is we who change as we learn to recognize what was formerly imperceptible.

Jean-Martin Charcot

Migraine is perhaps the most common neurologic complaint, and it ranks among the 10 most common disabling disorders worldwide. Migraine affects approximately 13% of the adult population in Western countries. Prevalence is highest between the ages of 25 and 55. The number of migraine sufferers in the United States is estimated to be 25 to 28 million.[1] Migraine is symptomatic in women (15–18%) far more often than in men (5–6%) and often begins during childhood or adolescence. The occurrence of migraine attacks strongly correlates to hormonal fluctuations, as with menses. The likelihood of a migraine attack is also elevated with ovulation. Often migraine abates during pregnancy. After menopause the prevalence of migraine lessens as well.

CLINICAL FEATURES OF MIGRAINE

The migraine process has four phases: prodrome, aura, headache (pain), and postdrome. Migraine may occur with or without aura; many patients have both patterns with different headaches. Formerly known as classic migraine, migraine with aura (Table 14-1) accounts for only 15% to 20% of migraine, whereas migraine without aura (Table 14-2) or common migraine accounts for 80% to 85% of the attacks. Migraine without aura may be episodic or chronic. The most common type of aura is visual. Most visual auras are positive (scintillating scotomata) and last less than 60 minutes. Auras may also be sensory, motor, aphasic, or auditory. Auras may also be somatosensory and characterized by spreading numbness or tingling involving the ipsilateral side of the face and the ipsilateral upper limb (cheiro-oral migraine) and may occur in succession. Photophobia or phonophobia are often present, and allodynia may occur.

MIGRAINE VARIANTS

An important migraine variant is basilar-type migraine, formerly known as Bickerstaff migraine or basilar artery migraine. This disorder affects mainly adolescent girls or young women. A basilar-type aura is often manifested by vertigo, dysarthria, tinnitus, diplopia, bilateral visual symptoms or bilateral paresthesias, transient loss of consciousness, hypoacusia, and rarely ataxia.

Migraine sufferers may also experience episodic vertigo (migraine-associated vertigo), a condition that is often misdiagnosed. A few of these patients with migraine-related vertigo may experience tinnitus and low-frequency hearing loss. It must be emphasized that isolated vertigo lasting a few minutes may also precede posterior circulation infarcts. Benign paroxysmal vertigo of childhood is thought to be related to migraines.

Another migraine variant is retinal migraine, also known as ophthalmic or ocular migraine. This is characterized by recurrent attacks of transient monocular blindness in young adults and often is attributable to vasospasm of the choroidal or retinal arteries.

Ophthalmoplegic migraine, currently classified as cranial neuralgia, is a rare disorder, associated with migraine-like attacks, periorbital pain, and ophthalmoplegia, most often due to an oculomotor (CN III) paresis. Occasionally the sixth cranial nerve may be involved. Involvement of the trochlear nerve (CN IV) is extremely rare.

MIGRAINE AND STROKE

Several studies have suggested that migraine is associated with an increased incidence of stroke.[2–6] Epidemiological studies suggest a nonrandom association of migraine with stroke, particularly among young women with migraine with aura. The risk is further increased among women with arterial hypertension, tobacco use, and use of oral contraceptives. Evaluation of these patients may be quite challenging, and the evaluation should be thorough. The overlap of migraine and stroke raises a complex bidirectional relation and relevant and potentially serious clinical connotations. Is it ischemia-induced migraine with aura, or rather migraine-associated ischemic migrainous infarction? Migraine has a unique pathophysiology, including both central and peripheral elements, which are likely to be linked. Activation of the trigeminovascular system releases inflammatory peptides into the dura, causing "neurogenic inflammation" in the course of migraine.

Table 14-1: IHS Criteria for Migraine with Aura

At least two attacks fulfilling the criteria below

Aura consists of one of following, no motor weakness:

- Fully reversible visual symptoms including positive and or negative features
- Fully reversible sensory symptoms including positive and or negative features
- Fully reversible dysphasic speech disturbance

At least two of the following:

- Homonymous visual symptoms and/or unilateral sensory symptoms
- At least one aura symptom develops gradually over 5 minutes, and/or different symptoms occur in succession over > 5 minutes

Headache fulfills criteria for migraine without aura

Not attributable to another disease

Table 14-2: IHS Criteria for Migraine without Aura

At last five attacks

Headache attacks lasting 4–72 hours

Headache with at least two of the following:

- Unilateral location
- Pulsating quality
- Moderate to severe pain
- Aggravation by physical activity or by its avoidance

During headache at least one of the following:

- Nausea and/or vomiting
- Photophobia and phonophobia

Not attributed to another disorder

The possible association between migraine headache and stroke was evaluated by the Physician's Health Study; physicians reporting migraine had an increased risk of subsequent stroke compared with those not reporting migraines.[7] In a large prospective study from the Women's Health Study, there was no overall association of stroke with migraine or migraine with aura.[8] However, this study and several retrospective and case-control studies have described an association of migraine with aura and stroke in women. In the Women's Health Study, the hazard ratio for ischemic stroke was 2.25 (95% CI 1.30–3.91) for women under age 55 who reported a history of migraine with aura, but the absolute risk increase was low, with 3.8 additional cases per year per 10,000 women.

To establish a diagnosis of migrainous infarction, the International Headache Society Classification and Diagnostic Criteria (ICHD-2) requires that the index attack in a patient with migraine with aura be typical of a previous attack, except that one or more aura symptoms persist longer than 60 minutes. In addition, there must be neuroimaging confirmation of an

Table 14-3: Diagnostic Criteria for Migrainous Infarction[16]

Previously established diagnosis of migraine with aura

Infarction must occur during the course of a typical migraine attack

Symptoms and signs must be present and fully reversed within 7 days from onset and/or associated with neuroimaging confirmation of ischemic infarction

Other causes of infarction need to be excluded by appropriate investigations

ischemic infarction.[9] This definition implies that a firm diagnosis of migraine with aura has been made in the past. Also, the clinical manifestations judged to be the result of a migrainous infarction must be those typical of previous attacks for that individual. Finally, other causes of infarction (cervicocephalic arterial dissections, thrombophilic states, patent foramen ovale, etc.), including those related to migraine therapy, have to be excluded by appropriate investigations (Table 14-3).

Migrainous infarction is a rare event considering the high prevalence of migraine in the general population. The overall incidence has been estimated at 3.36 per 100,000 population per year. In the Barcelona Stroke Registry (Sagrat Cor Hospital) migrainous infarction accounted for only 0.6% of all first-ever acute strokes, 0.8% of ischemic stroke, 12.8% of ischemic strokes of unusual etiology, and 13.7% of ischemic strokes in young adults 45 years of age or younger.[10]

SYMPTOMATIC HEADACHE

Headache occurs commonly as a consequence of cerebrovascular dysfunction, and it may be difficult to distinguish symptomatic headache in these individuals from a migraine attack. Headache is reported in approximately 17% to 34% of cases of ischemic stroke. Pain is common with posterior circulation strokes but rare with lacunar infarcts. Headache may accompany embolic or thrombotic causes of stroke, but it is strongly associated with cervicocephalic arterial dissections (Chapter 12).

In the Lausanne Stroke Registry, headache at stroke onset was reported by 18% of the patients overall, including 14% of those with anterior circulation strokes and 29% of those with posterior circulation strokes. Headache was reported by one-third of patients with intracranial hemorrhage (37% with infratentorial hemorrhage and 36% with supratentorial bleeds) and by only 16% with infarcts. Only 9% of patients with first-ever stroke attributed to lacunar infarct reported headaches, whereas headaches were reported in 15% of patients with middle cerebral artery (MCA) territory infarcts.[11] The Barcelona investigators observed that a mesencephalic location, nausea and vomiting, female gender, diabetes mellitus, and age were independent variables associated with lacunar infarcts and headaches.[12]

Migraines also can be a prominent symptom in the antiphospholipid antibody syndrome (Chapter 11); other clinical manifestations include venous or arterial thromboses, recurrent miscarriages, and thrombocytopenia. Because symptomatic migraine attacks are more frequent than migraine-induced ischemic insults, the presence of headache with a stroke is therefore not sufficient to make the diagnosis of migraine as the cause of the patient's symptoms.[13] Furthermore, patchy subcortical abnormalities on MRI in patients with migraine with aura should be interpreted with caution. MRI studies in patients with migraines with aura often show nonspecific T_2W and FLAIR white matter hyperintensities involving supratentorial and infratentorial compartments, more commonly involving the pons.

PATHOGENESIS OF MIGRAINOUS STROKE

The pathogenesis of migrainous infarction remains controversial. Cerebral infarcts complicating migraine are mostly cortical and involve the distribution of the posterior cerebral artery (PCA). The usual scenario of migrainous infarction is one of recurrent episodes of gradual buildup of unilateral throbbing headaches, associated with stereotyped visual phenomena occurring in both visual fields simultaneously, in one of which a hemianopic field loss becomes permanent. Anterior circulation infarctions may also occur. Likewise migrainous infarctions may involve two different vascular territories concomitantly or sequentially.[4,14] Others have reported an increased risk of cerebellar infarcts among people with migraine with aura. Most lesions were multiple, and were more prevalent in border zone regions.[15]

Migrainous infarctions have been subdivided as definite when all the International Headache Society criteria are fulfilled and possible when some, but not all, criteria are fulfilled. Patients with migrainous infarction are at increased risk for recurrent stroke.[16] Although the risk of stroke due to migraine appears to be low, it is hard to quantitate the risk of migraine as a comorbidity, contributing to the risk of stroke in individuals who have other disorders.

GENETICS OF MIGRAINE

Major advances on the exact role of genetics and stroke risk and the genetics of migraine have occurred in the last decade. Most migraine patients have one or more first-degree relatives with migraine. Furthermore, identical twins are twice as likely to have migraine as fraternal twins.[17] In addition to the familial nature of migraine itself, specific genes that are responsible for familial hemiplegic migraine have been identified, and several other genetic conditions that promote cerebrovascular lesions have migraine-like headache as a prominent early symptom.

Cerebral autosomal dominant arteriopathy with subcortical infarcts and leukoencephalopathy (CADASIL) is a familial non-arteriosclerotic, nonamyloid cerebral microangiopathy that is often accompanied by migraine-like headaches with or without aura, recurrent subcortical ischemic infarctions starting in mid-adulthood, cognitive decline, executive dysfunction, subcortical dementia, and early white matter hyperintensities on MRI (Chapter 21). A characteristic neuroimaging marker is the presence of bilateral temporal polar hyperintensities. The external capsule and corpus callosum are also frequently affected. A reversible acute encephalopathy presenting with acute confusion, fever, coma, and seizures (CADASIL coma) may be a rare occurrence.[18] CADASIL is caused by simple missense mutations or small deletions in the *Notch3* gene on chromosome 19q12 encoding a transmembrane receptor Notch 3. Pathologically, there is a characteristic granular osmophilic material in arterial walls, including dermal arteries (Figure 21–1C).[19]

A subtype of migraine with aura, known as familial hemiplegic migraine (FHM), features a familial pattern of transient weakness or frank paralysis in the setting of a migrainous aura. The neurological deficit typically resolves after most attacks, but they may be permanent. One of the three genes for FHM is adjacent to the CADASIL gene.[20] Familial hemiplegic migraine typically begins during the first three decades, and headache duration is typically considerable longer in FHM than migraine with aura.[21] Three genes have been associated with FHM: *CACNA1A* (*FHM1*, chromosome locus 19p13), *ATP1A2* (*FHM2*, chromosome locus 1q21-q23), and *SCN1A* (*FHM3*, chromosome locus 2q24). Altered ion channel gating has been proposed as a common pathophysiological mechanism in FHM.[22]

The newer acronym CADASILM, cerebral autosomal dominant arteriopathy with subcortical infarcts, leukoencephalopathy, and migraine, refers to a subvariety of CADASIL characterized by the high frequency of migraines, frequency of psychotic disorders, and early neurologic manifestations.[23] Conversely, in cerebral autosomal recessive arteriopathy with subcortical infarcts and leukoencephalopathy (CARASIL), also known as Maeda syndrome and not linked to the *Notch3* gene, there is early-onset alopecia, lumbago, spondylosis deformans, lack of migraines, and no granular eosinophilic material in the vessel walls.

Mitochondrial encephalomyopathy, lactic acidosis, and stroke-like episodes (MELAS) is a progressive multisystemic disorder associated with several different mitochondrial mutations, most commonly an A to G point mutation at position 3243 of their transfer RNA-leu gene.[24] The ischemic lesions of MELAS do not usually correspond to a single large cerebral vessel territory, but they do tend to occur in the parietal and occipital lobes. Some patients develop tonic-clonic or myoclonic seizures, ataxia, recurrent migraines, short stature, sensorineural hearing loss, diabetes mellitus, ragged-red fiber myopathy, and lactic acidemia. The clinical manifestations and pathophysiology of MELAS are presented in more detail in Chapter 21.

MANAGEMENT OF THE MIGRAINEUR WITH STROKE

For individuals with typical migraine triggers, it is prudent to avoid foods containing vasoactive substances (e.g., chocolate, cheese, foods with nitrite preservatives), alcohol, tobacco, and estrogens. Arterial hypertension, if present, should be controlled. In theory, elimination of either migraine or stroke risk factors might lessen the likelihood of a given migraine attack resulting in a stroke.

Intravenous (IV) diphenhydramine, IV chlorpromazine or prochlorperazine, or IV valproate sodium (diluted in normal saline) may help to resolve an acute migraine attack. Intramuscular or IV ketorolac is sometimes useful. We avoid the use of opioids, butalbital containing preparations, and isometheptene mucate containing compounds in the routine management of these patients.

Daily aspirin is sometimes effective in preventing migraine. Nonsteroidal anti-inflammatory drugs may be useful for migraine attacks, but their frequent use should be discouraged because rebound headaches occur in some individuals. Metoclopramide may be helpful in treating migraine-associated nausea; the combination of aspirin and metoclopramide may be valuable. A wide range of other drugs are often used for prophylaxis, including beta blockers, calcium channel blockers, amitriptyline, nortriptyline, divalproex sodium, sodium valproate, topiramate, flunarizine, and pizotifen (the last two are not available in the

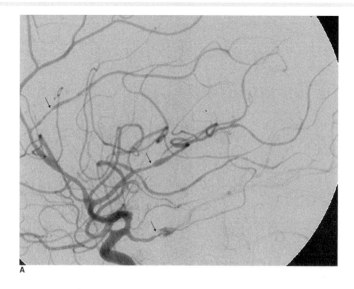

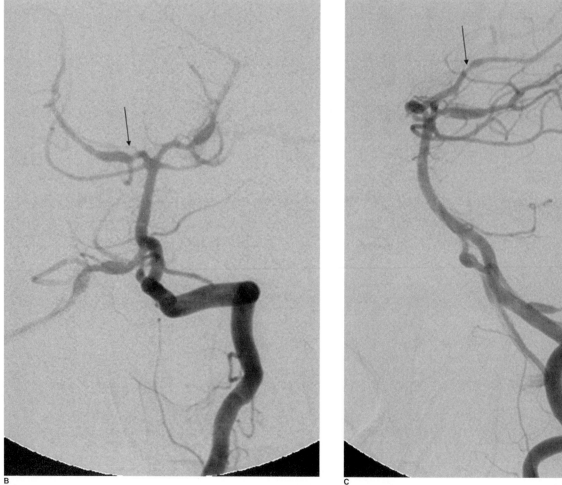

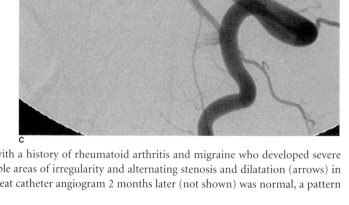

Figure 14-1. A–C: Catheter angiogram (from a 35-year-old woman with a history of rheumatoid arthritis and migraine who developed severe headaches, right sided numbness, and speech hesitation) shows multiple areas of irregularity and alternating stenosis and dilatation (arrows) in arteries of the anterior (A) and posterior (B and C) circulations. A repeat catheter angiogram 2 months later (not shown) was normal, a pattern that is typical of Call-Fleming syndrome.

United States). Other touted agents include gabapentin, butterbur, riboflavin, and magnesium.

Triptan agents (5-hydroxytryptophan [5-HT]1B/1D agonists) should probably be avoided in individuals with cardiac or cerebrovascular disease or in people with hemiplegic or basilar-type migraine.[25–27] Likewise, the use of nonselective 5-HT1 agonists such as ergotamine or dihydroergotamine is not recommended in these individuals.

CALL-FLEMING SYNDROME

Call or Call-Fleming syndrome is a rare, reversible multifocal segmental vasoconstriction of the cerebral arteries (Figure 14-1).[28] It most commonly occurs among women (female to male ratio 2–3 to 1) who are aged 20 to 50 years. Typical symptoms include "thunderclap" headaches, nausea, and photophobia, followed in some individuals by focal neurologic deficits or seizures. The signs and symptoms typically resolve spontaneously within two to six weeks and the angiographic abnormalities clear within twelve weeks.

Evaluation of Call-Fleming Syndrome

Blood and cerebrospinal fluid studies are typically normal but may help to eliminate other conditions. Magnetic resonance imaging can identify an ischemic stroke or intracranial hemorrhage. Serial transcranial Doppler studies can be used to monitor blood flow velocities and to assess the severity of vasospasm and the potential risk of cerebral infarction.

Angiographic narrowing of the intracranial arteries is a nonspecific finding that has been described with a wide array of conditions.[28] The rapid reversibility of the vasospasm of Call-Fleming syndrome differentiates it from intracranial atherosclerosis, inflammatory vasculitides (Chapter 10), and cervicocephalic fibromuscular dysplasia (Chapter 13) and neoplastic angioendotheliosis.[29,30] Transient vasospasm (early or delayed) occurs after aneurysmal subarachnoid hemorrhage (Chapter 17) and following surgical manipulation of the intracranial arteries, but the clinical diagnosis is seldom a mystery in these situations.

Pathophysiology of Call-Fleming Syndrome

The pathophysiology of Call-Fleming syndrome is not well understood. Most patients have a history of migraine, and it is not certain whether the syndrome is a distinct entity or a particularly severe variant of migraine. Pregnancy or the postpartum state may precipitate the syndrome, and Call-Fleming syndrome is probably synonymous with postpartum angiopathy (see Chapter 23). Exposure to certain diet pills, antidepressants, or other vasoactive drugs may initiate the attacks.[31,32]

Some authors use Call-Fleming syndrome to describe vasospasm following subarachnoid hemorrhage or other conditions, but the term will remain more useful if it is narrowly applied to isolated reversible vasospasm of the cerebral vessels.

Therapy of Call-Fleming Syndrome

No specific treatment has been established, but intravenous magnesium, calcium channel blockers (nimodipine or verapamil), and a short course of corticosteroids are often used.[33] Another report advocated the use of nimodipine and dantrolene.[34]

REFERENCES

1. Lipton RB, Diamond S, Reed M, et al. American migraine study II. Prevalence, burden, and health care utilization for migraine in the United States. *Headache*. 2000;**40**:416.
2. Connor RCR. Complicated migraine. *Lancet*. 1962;**2**:1072–1075.
3. Spaccavento LJ, Solomon GD. Migraine as an etiology of stroke in young adults. *Headache*. 1984;**24**:19–22.
4. Broderick JP, Swanson JW. Migraine-related strokes. *Arch Neurol*. 1987;**44**:858–871.
5. Welch KMA, Levine SR. Migraine-related stroke in the context of the international Headache Society classification of head pain. *Arch Neurol*. 1990;**47**:458–462.
6. Linetsky E, Leker R, Ben Hur T. Headache characteristics in patients after migrainous stroke. *Neurology*. 2001;**57**:130–132.
7. Buring JE, Hebert P, Romero J, et al. Migraine and subsequent risk of stroke in the Physician's Health Study. *Arch Neurol*. 1995;**52**:129–134.
8. Kurth T, Shouke MA, Kase CS, et al. Migraine headache and the risk of stroke in women: a prospective study. *Neurology*. 2005;**64**:1020–1026.
9. The international classification of headache disorders: second edition. *Cephalalgia*. 2004;**24**:1–160.
10. Arboix A, Massons J, Garcia-Eroles L, et al. Migrainous cerebral infarction in the Sagrat Cor Hospital of Barcelona Stroke Registry. *Cephalalgia*. 2003;**23**:389–394.
11. Kumral E, Bogousslavsky J, Van Melle G, et al. Headaches at stroke onset: the Lausanne Stroke Registry. *J Neurol Neurosurg Psychiatry*. 1995;**58**:490–492.
12. Arboix A, Garcia-Tralliro O, Garcia-Eroles L, et al. Stroke-related headache: a clinical study in lacunar infarction. *Headache*. 2005;**45**:1345–1392.
13. Olesen J, Friberg L, Olsen TJ, et al. Ischemic-induced symptomatic migraine attacks may be more frequent than migraine-induced ischemic insults. *Brain*. 1993;**116**:187–202.
14. Tang S-C, Jeng J-S, Liu H-M, Yip P-K. Migrainous infarction involving two different arterial territories: report of two cases. *Acta Neurol Taiwan*. 2004;**13**:20–23.
15. Kruit MC, Launer L, Ferrari MD, van Buchen MA. Infarcts in the posterior circulation territory in migraine: the population-based MRI CAMERA study. *Brain*. 2005;**128**:2068–2077.
16. Rothrock J, North J, Madden K, et al. Migraine and migrainous stroke: risk factors and prognosis. *Neurology*. 1993;**42**:2473–2476.
17. Silberstein SD, Lipton RB, Goadsby PJ. *Headache in Clinical Practice*. 2nd ed. London: Martin Dunitz; 2002.
18. Schon F, Martin RJ, Prevett M, et al. "CADASIL coma" an underdiagnosed acute encephalopathy. *J Neurol Neurosurg Psychiatry*. 2003;**74**:249–252.
19. Kalimo H, Ruchoux MM, Vitanen M, et al. CADASIL: a common form of hereditary arteriopathy causing brain infarct and dementia. *Brain Pathol*. 2002;**12**:371–384.
20. Hutchinson M, O'Riordan J, Javed M, et al. Familial hemiplegic migraine and autosomal dominant arteriopathy with leukoencephalopathy (CADASIL). *Ann Neurol*. 1995;**38**:816–824.
21. Thomsen LL, Eriksen MK, Roemmer SF, et al. A population-based study of familial hemiplegic migraine suggests revised diagnostic criteria. *Brain*. 2002;**125**:1379–1391.
22. Kraus RL, Sinnegger MJ, Koschak A, et al. Three new familial hemiplegic migraine mutants affect P/Q-type Ca2+ channel kinetics. *J Biol Chem*. 2000;**275**:9239–9293.
23. Verin M, Rolland Y, Landgraf F, et al. New phenotype of the cerebral autosomal dominant arteriopathy mapped to chromosome 19: migraine as the prominent clinical feature. *J Neurol Neurosurg Psychiatry*. 1995;**59**:579–585.

24. Enter C, Muller-Hocker J, Kurlemann G, et al. A specific point mutation in the mitochondrial genome of Caucasians with MELAS. *Hum. Genet.* 1988;**88**:233–236.

25. Snow V, Weiss K, Wall EM, et al. Pharmacologic management of acute attacks of migraine and prevention of migraine headache. *Ann Int Med.* 2002;**137**:840–849.

26. Evers S. Treatment of migraine with prophylactic drugs. *Expert Opin Pharmacother.* 2008;**9**:2565–2573.

27. Goadsby PJ. Current concepts on the pathophysiology of migraine. *Neurol Clin.* 1997;**15**:24–42.

28. Calabrese LH, Dodick DW, Schwedt TJ, Singhal AB. Narrative review: reversible cerebral vasoconstriction syndromes. *Ann Intern Med.* 2007;**146**:34–44.

29. Knight RS, Anslow P, Theaker JM. Neoplastic angioendotheliosis: a case of subacute dementia with unusual cerebral CT appearances and a review of the literature. *J Neurol Neurosurg Psychiatry.* 1987;**50**:1022–1028.

30. Williams DB, Lyons MK, Yanagihara T, Colgan JP, Banks PM. Cerebral angiotropic large cell lymphoma (neoplastic angioendotheliosis): therapeutic considerations. *J Neurol Sci.* 1991;**103**: 16–21.

31. Noskin O, Jafarimojarrad E, Libman RB, Nelson JL. Diffuse cerebral vasoconstriction (Call-Fleming syndrome) and stroke associated with antidepressants. *Neurology.* 2006;**67**:159–160.

32. Singhal AB, Caviness VS, Begleiter AF, Mark EJ, Rordorf G, Koroshetz WJ. Cerebral vasoconstriction and stroke after use of serotonergic drugs. *Neurology.* 2002;**58**:130–133.

33. Nowak DA, Rodiek SO, Henneken S, et al. Reversible segmental cerebral vasoconstriction (Call-Fleming syndrome): are calcium channel inhibitors a potential treatment option? *Cephalalgia.* 2003;**23**:218–222.

34. Salomone S, Soydan G, Moskowitz MA, Sims JR. Inhibition of cerebral vasoconstriction by dantrolene and nimodipine. *Neurocrit Care.* 2009;**10**:93–102.

15

Vascular Dementia

To me old age is always fifteen years older than I am.

Bernard Baruch

If the brain was so simple that we could understand it, we would be so simple that we couldn't.

Watson Lyall

With the global aging of the population, the incidence and prevalence of vascular dementia will continue to increase.[1] This is not surprising because atherosclerosis, which is one of the key mechanisms for its development, remains a primary cause of death and disability worldwide.[2] Following Alzheimer disease, vascular dementia is the second most common form of dementia affecting people 65 years and older.[3–7] However, inconsistencies in its diagnostic and pathological criteria complicate reliable epidemiologic estimates of incidence and prevalence rates.[8] At least a third of individuals with dementia have pure vascular disease, and an estimated 15% have a combination of Alzheimer disease and vascular dementia, now termed mixed dementia. Furthermore, the concept that vascular disease is an important contributor to the pathogenesis of Alzheimer disease has recently reemerged.[9,10]

Before the seminal description in 1906 by Alzheimer and Kraepelin,[11] dementia was thought to stem from cerebrovascular atherosclerosis. Subsequently the recognition of a neurodegenerative disorder causing dementia, however, overshadowed previous observations that brain vascular disease was often demonstrated in Alzheimer patients at autopsy. Multi-infarct dementia, as it was dubbed, was thereafter considered rare, and the vascular etiology of dementia remained underrecognized for more than half a century. Modern pathological studies and brain-imaging techniques have sparked renewed interest in the vascular contribution to dementia, and the distinction between Alzheimer disease and vascular dementia is becoming increasingly more complex. For example, 50% to 80% of patients with Alzheimer disease have structural vascular changes or cerebral infarctions.[12] Furthermore, Alzheimer disease and vascular dementia seem to share many of the same vascular risk factors.

Thus, the diagnosis of vascular dementia often remains challenging and its therapy limited to modification of traditional vascular risk factors, or rarely, the treatment of a specific underlying medical, cardiac, or vascular disorder. Much like stroke in general, vascular dementia has multiple risk factors. It can be caused by different mechanisms of cerebral ischemia affecting different cerebral vessels and cerebral vascular territories or by hemorrhagic strokes (Table 15-1). Vascular dementia can be suspected in multiple clinical and radiological situations (Table 15-2). Diagnosis might be complicated by the presence of depression, underlying medical co-morbidities causing cognitive compromise, superimposed toxic-metabolic derangements, or use of medications, such as antihypertensives, cardiac agents, sedatives, or psychotropic compounds. With increasing age, dementia is often multifactorial, and the differential diagnosis is therefore broad.

Table 15-1: Anatomic Distribution of Vascular Dementia

Dementia Type	Vessels Affected	Lesion Location
Cortical	Superficial arterioles/ leptomeningeal vessels	Superficial cortical infarction and hemorrhage
	Large extracranial arteries	Watershed infarction
	Medium-sized intracranial arteries	Infarction in vascular territory of MCA/ACA/ PCA and their branches
Subcortical	Arterioles/capillaries	Leukoaraiosis of periventricular white matter and corona radiata
	Long penetrating arteries	Lacunar state with infarctions in basal ganglia, internal capsule, thalamus
Mixed	Small and large vessel disease	

Table 15-2: Selected Causes of Vascular Dementia

Atherosclerosis

- Atherothrombosis or atheroembolism of large extracranial vessels
- Intracranial atherosclerosis of large and medium sized arteries

Intracranial microangiopathy (small vessel disease)

- Lypohyalinosis
- Microatheroma
- Embolism

Cardioembolic stroke

- Arrhythmias, especially atrial fibrillation
- Valvular heart disease
- Cardiomyopathies with left ventricular thrombus
- Congestive heart failure
- Infective endocarditis
- Atrial myxoma
- Other cardiac sources

Systemic disorders

- Arterial hypertension
- Diabetes mellitus

Hypoxia or hemodynamic compromise

- Cardiopulmonary arrest
- Recurrent hypotension with syncope
- Severe pulmonary disease
- Obstructive sleep apnea
- AVM with regional steal phenomena

Hematological and coagulation disorders

- Sickle cell disease
- Polycythemia
- Thrombocytosis
- Antiphospholipid antibody syndrome (including Sneddon syndrome)
- Inherited and acquired hypercoagulable states

Vascular inflammation

- SLE and other connective tissue diseases
- Sjogren syndrome
- Polyarteritis nodoasa
- Churg Strauss syndrome
- Neuro-Behcet's
- Isolated CNS angiitis

Infectious disease

- Neurosyphilis
- Chagas disease
- Infective endocarditis with emboli

Non-atherosclerotic cerebrovascular disorders

- Cervicocephalic arterial dissection
- Moyamoya syndrome/disease
- Radiation induced cerebral vasculopathy
- Neoplastic angioendotheliomatosis

Miscellaneous hereditary disorders

- MELAS
- MERFF
- CADASIL
- Cerebral amyloid angiopathy
- Other inherited microangiopathies
- Progeria

AVM = arteriovenous malformation; CNS = central nervous system; SLE = Systemic lupus erythematosus; MELAS = mitochondrial encephalomyopathy, lactic acidosis, and stroke-like episodes; MERFF = myoclonic epilepsy with ragged red fibers; CADASIL = cerebral autosomal dominant arteriopathy with subcortical infarcts and leukoencephalopathy.

Criteria and testing instruments commonly used for the diagnosis of vascular dementia are listed in Table 15-3, but none of the current criteria are evidence based, often leaving the diagnosis of vascular dementia in question. Diagnostic criteria and tools with improved sensitivity and specificity need to be developed and validated. Currently the inter-rater variability is high, and the diagnostic criteria cannot be used interchangeably.[13] Another important shortcoming is the fact that diagnostic instruments now used in clinical practice tend to identify patients with more advanced stages of dementia, making it

Table 15-3: Diagnostic Criteria for Vascular Dementia

Diagnostic Instruments	Clinical Criteria
HIS	Ischemia score: Abrupt onset, stepwise decline, fluctuating course, nocturnal confusion, relative preservation of personality, depression, somatic complaints, emotional incontinence, history of hypertension, history of strokes, associated atherosclerosis, focal neurological signs and symptoms
ADDTC	Evidence of ≥ 2 ischemic strokes by history or neurological signs and/or neuroimaging studies (CT or T_1-weighted MRI) or occurrence of a single stroke with clearly documented temporal relationship to onset of dementia and evidence of ≥ 1 infarct outside the cerebellum by neuroimaging
NINDS-AIREN	Focal neurological signs and evidence of relevant infarct by brain MRI including multiple large-vessel infarcts or single strategically placed infarct or multiple basal ganglia and white matter lacunes or extensive periventricular white matter lesions or combination thereof and a relationship of the above manifested by one or more of the following: dementia onset within 3 months after a recognized stroke, abrupt deterioration or fluctuation or stepwise progression of cognitive deficits
DSM-IV	Cognitive deficits, including memory impairment, aphasia, apraxia, agnosia, executive dysfunction causing a significant impairment in social or occupational functioning representing a significant decline from a previous level of function and focal neurological signs and symptoms or laboratory evidence of cerebrovascular disease affecting cortex or subcortical structures that are etiologically related to the disturbance
ICD-10	Deficits in higher cognitive function are unequally distributed, and focal neurological signs and evidence from history, examination, or tests of significant cerebrovascular disease etiologically related to the dementia (e.g., history of stroke, evidence of infarct)

ADDTC = Alzheimer Disease Diagnostic and Treatment Centers; DSM-IV = *Diagnostic and Statistical Manual of Mental Disorders*, 4th ed.; HIS = Hachinski Ischemic Score; ICD-10 = *International Classification of Diseases*, 10th ed.; NINDS-AIREN = National Institute of Neurological Disorders and Stroke – Association Internationale pour la Recherche et l'Enseignement en Neurosciences.

difficult to modify early risk factors for individuals with mild vascular cognitive impairment. Nevertheless, early diagnosis and intervention is essential because morbidity and mortality in patients with vascular dementia are high; the median survival is only 3.3 years after diagnosis.[14] Vascular dementia has significant implications, with a five-year survival rate of only 39% compared to 75% for age-matched controls without cognitive impairment.

RISK FACTORS FOR VASCULAR DEMENTIA

Age is the main risk factor for the development of dementia. About 0.3% to 1% of the population aged 60 to 64 years have dementia; the risk then doubles every 5 years to affect about half of the individuals 95 years of age and older.[6] Men are more commonly affected than women. A higher frequency of vascular dementia has been reported in individuals with lower education, those living in rural areas, and those in certain geographic regions, such as Russia and parts of Asia.[1,15] Vascular dementia causes an estimated 50% of dementia in Japan, 20% to 40% in Europe, and about 15% in Latin America. However, it is unclear if these differences are due to genetic and/or environmental factors or to the use of different diagnostic criteria.

There is a higher risk of vascular dementia among individuals with family members who also have vascular dementia. The role of genetic polymorphisms as independent risk factors for vascular dementia is now being explored, and multiple candidate genes are under active investigation (see Table 15-4). The hereditary component of vascular dementia is likely to be polygenetic, so the search for candidate genes will require large sample sizes and screening for a multitude of candidate genes. Known hereditary disorders that feature vascular dementia

include cerebral autosomal dominant arteriopathy with subcortical infarcts and leukoencephalopathy (CADASIL), familial forms of cerebral amyloid angiopathy, and the autosomal recessive inherited form of arteriopathy with subcortical infarcts and leukoencephalopathy (CARASIL).

Traditional vascular risk factors are associated with vascular dementia as well as with Alzheimer disease. Among these arterial hypertension, diabetes mellitus, and hyperlipidemia are major risks of cerebrovascular atherosclerosis with cerebral infarctions and leukoaraiosis. The presence of vascular risk factors in the fourth decade is associated with a 20% to 40% increased risk of dementia later in life. Individuals with arterial hypertension in their 40s have a 24% greater risk to develop dementia, and those with diabetes have a 46% higher risk, while those with hypercholesterolemia and smokers are 42% and 26%, respectively, more likely to develop dementia. The higher the number of vascular risk factors present during midlife, the greater the risk for vascular dementia during the following decades.[16]

Ischemic stroke and vascular dementia share risk factors, and a previous stroke is a risk factor for vascular dementia. Following a stroke, about 25% of patients develop dementia within a year, and the incidence of dementia is about nine times higher in stroke patients than in age-matched controls. If cerebral infarctions are found in a patient with dementia, a complete stroke evaluation should be performed (see Chapter 5). Treatment of traditional vascular risk factors is the cornerstone of therapy, so vascular dementia patients should be screened for diabetes, hypertension, hyperlipidemia, tobacco use, and cardiac disease, among other factors. The association of vascular dementia with nontraditional risk factors such as intercellular adhesion molecules (ICAM), high-sensitivity C-reactive protein (hsCRP), angiotensin-converting enzyme (ACE), plasminogen

Table 15-4: Vascular Dementia Risk Factors

Demographic

- Older age

- Race/ethnic group (Asian)

- Male gender

- Geography (rural, geographic regions)

Traditional modifiable vascular risks

- Hypertension

- Tobacco use

- Heart disease

- Diabetes

- Hyperlipidemia

Genetic factors

- Apolipoprotein E

- Mutations in *Notch3* gene (CADASIL)

- CARASIL

- Cerebral amyloid angiopathy (amyloid precursor protein)

Genes regulating:

- Atherogenesis

- Hemostasis and rheology (fibrin)

Endothelial function and angiogenesis (VEGF)

Lipid metabolism (glutathione S-transferase omega-1, sterol regulatory element binding protein-2)

Rennin-angiotensinsystem (ACE D/D)

Inflammation (polymorphism for intercellular adhesion molecule-1 E/K gene, IL-6)

Possible other risk factors

- Previous stroke (hemorrhagic or ischemic)

- Menopause, on hormone replacement therapy

- Hyperhomocysteinemia

- Consumption of high amounts of alcohol (?)

- Platelet antiaggregant use (?)

- Stress

- Depression

- Exposure to pesticides/herbicides, liquid plastic/rubber (?)

? = Relationship not clearly established or conflicting study data available.

activator inhibitor-1, or other markers of inflammation is less well established. Clearly, new sensitive and specific biomarkers for vascular dementia need to be identified.

PATHOPHYSIOLOGY

Memory and cognitive performance in an elderly individual require structural integrity of the brain but are also influenced by genetic and environmental factors as well as key life experiences. To some extent, decline in cognition correlates with the usual age-related loss of brain volume. The cognitive capacity at any time is determined by the initial endowment of the individual minus declines due to neuronal apoptosis, previous brain trauma by injury, exposure to drugs and toxins, vascular disease, and impairment of neuroplasticity. Cognitive consequences of multiple vascular lesions are cumulative and lead to a stepwise deterioration with intermittent phases of relatively stable cognitive performance. According to this "cognitive reserve theory" cerebral vascular disease not only leads to primary brain injury but also aggravates the clinical manifestations of concomitant neurodegenerative diseases, resulting in earlier symptom onset, faster disease progression, and more severe course.

Until recently the term muli-infarct dementia was used to describe the dementia syndromes caused by cerebrovascular disorders, especially those due to small vessel disease and large vessel atherothrombotic brain infarcts. This has been replaced by the term vascular dementia, because not only multiple infarcts but also other vascular abnormalities, including single strategically located infarcts (thalamus, caudate nucleus, lenticular nucleus, angular gyrus, and genu of the internal capsule) and hemorrhages (subdural, subarachnoid, parenchymatous), play a role in pathogenesis. For example, white matter hypoperfusion causing cumulative ischemic lesions with subsequent functional denervation may result in vascular dementia. But single infarcts or hemorrhages, located in a critical brain region, may also cause or exacerbate dementia.

Elderly individuals who have enjoyed exceptional good mental and physical health may have cerebral blood flow (CBF) and metabolism values similar to those of 25-year-old people, but on average CBF as well as glucose and oxygen consumption decrease with age. Positron emission tomography (PET) provides semiquantitative measures of both regional cerebral blood flow (rCBF) and cerebral metabolic rate for oxygen ($CMRO_2$). Lenzi and coworkers reported an age-related decrease in rCBF approximating 3.2 ml/100 mg/min per decade, whereas there was a lesser correlation between $CMRO_2$ and age.[17,18] In the aged individual, rCBF and $CMRO_2$ are both decreased, especially in the fronto-temporo-sylvian and parieto-occipital regions. Thus, the decrease in $CMRO_2$ with age appears to be real but not linear, and a likely explanation may be cell death and/or diminished metabolism. The degree of flow reduction observed in vascular dementia roughly parallels the severity of cognitive impairment. Brain areas previously affected by stroke have decreased regional cerebral perfusion, oxygenation, and metabolism. Xenon[133]-based perfusion studies in patients with leukoaraiosis suggest diminished white matter perfusion,[19] and areas of ischemic leukoaraiosis show lower perfusion compared to nonaffected white matter.[20]

The pathophysiology of leukoaraiosis is not completely understood. However, there is growing evidence that the vast majority of cases of leukoaraiosis are caused by ischemia due to damage of small cerebral blood vessels including the arterioles and capillaries,[21–23] although alternative mechanisms have been entertained.[24–27] The microvascular distribution causes region-specific vulnerability of the brain, which can be amplified by anatomical changes of penetrating arterioles due to atherosclerosis, hyalinosis, or vascular tortuosity, changes that are at least partly due to aging and hypertension.[28] White matter derives its blood supply from relatively long arterioles that travel several

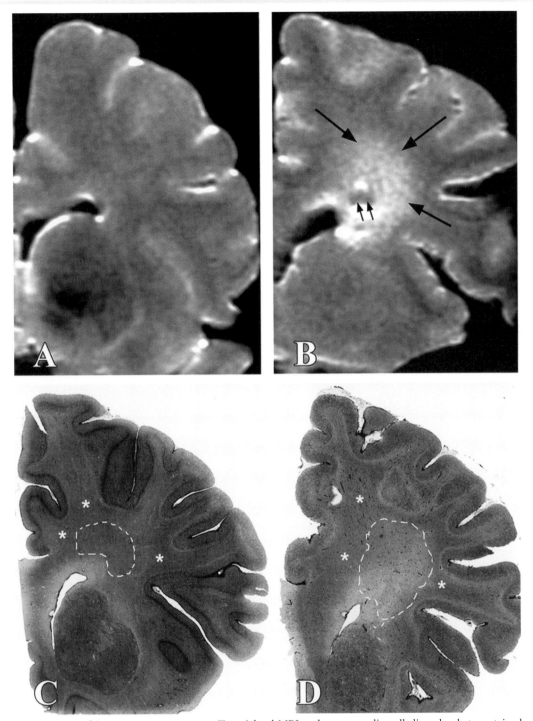

Figure 15-1. White matter appearance on T_2-weighted MRI and corresponding alkaline phophatase-stained section in a patient with leukoaraiosis (B and D) and a healthy individual (A and C). Dotted lines represent areas of sampling for vascular density analysis. Areas with asterisk (*) indicate unaffected white matter. Reprinted with permission from Moody et al.[29]

centimeters before reaching their final destination. Relatively high perfusion pressures are required to supply blood to these dependent vascular territories, and excessive blood pressure reduction in elderly individuals may promote ischemic/hypoxic brain injury. The paucity of collaterals between the vascular systems creates watershed zones that are prone to ischemic injury. In aging individuals there is a reduction of the intracranial blood flow velocity as well as the number of afferent small arteries,

arterioles, and capillaries in the white matter. Moody and coworkers estimated an approximately 26% reduction of vascular density per decade in healthy individuals between the ages of 57 and 90 years.[29] Individuals with leukoaraiosis have a significantly lower vascular density in affected white matter compared to age-matched controls, providing a possible anatomical explanation for the occurrence of ischemic white matter disease in the elderly (Figures 15-1 and 15-2).

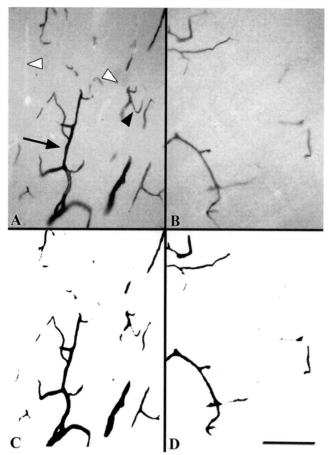

Figure 15-2. Density of afferent cerebral vessels in white matter of a healthy individual (A, alkaline phosphatase-stain and C, binary image) and in a leukoaraiotic lesion of a patient with ischemic small vessel disease (B, alkaline phophatase-stain and D, binary image). Arteriolar and capillary density is significantly decreased in areas of leukoaraiosis. Reprinted with permission from Moody et al.[29]

Table 15-5: Differential Diagnosis of Vascular Dementia

Clinical diagnoses
- Alzheimer disease
- Dementia with Lewy bodies
- Fronto-temporal dementia
- Parkinson disease
- Normal pressure hydrocephalus
- Depression
- CNS malignancy

White matter lesions on brain MRI
- Normal aging
- Unidentified bright objects (UBOs)
- Multiple sclerosis
- Acute disseminated encephalomyelitis (ADEM)
- AIDS dementia complex
- Progressive multifocal leukoencephalopathy (PML)
- Creutzfeldt-Jakob disease
- Subacute sclerosing panencephalitis (SSPE)
- Cerebral vasculitis
- Sarcoidosis
- Migraine-associated changes
- CADASIL
- Hypertensive encephalopathy
- Encephalopathy associated with renal or hepatic failure
- Leukoencephalopathy with drug use, toxins, or chemotherapeutic agents
- Radiation leukoencephalopathy
- Diffuse axonal injury
- Leukodystrophies
- Lipid storage diseases
- Mucopolysaccharidoses
- Carbon monoxide poisoning

Gradient echo signal abnormalities on MRI suggesting cerebral amyloid angiopathy
- Multiple cavernous malformations
- CADASIL and other cerebral microangiopathies
- Vasculitis
- Leptomeningeal hemosiderosis
- Calcium and iron deposits
- Primary or metastatic brain tumors
- Normal vascular flow voids

Postmortem studies of leukoaraiosis have shown a decreased number of axons, rarefaction of myelin, increased perivascular spaces, and gliosis.[30,31] These results, together with the observation that some individuals with leukoaraiosis have little or no cognitive impairment,[32–34] suggest that the neurological and histological abnormalities associated with leukoaraiosis are relatively nonspecific.[35] On the other hand, the most consistent pathological observation in leukoaraiosis is most likely due to ischemic demyelination.[24] Narrowing and damage of the small arterioles has almost always been detected in areas of leukoaraiosis,[23,30,31,36] which is strongly associated with traditional risk factors for vascular disease.[37–39] Alterations of the small cerebral vessels due to arterial hypertension, hyperlipidemia, diabetes mellitus, or amyloid depositions increase the capillary wall thickness of the microvasculature. Deep penetrating arteries become tortuous and elongated, causing a decrease in distal perfusion pressure and increase in the diffusion length for oxygen and other metabolites.[28,40] Decreased capillary density additionally results in reduced brain oxygenation, which depends on the number, distribution, and exchange surface of capillaries.

Episodes of diminished perfusion pressure in individuals with impaired cerebral autoregulation during transient nocturnal hypotension or in association with low cardiac output may result in recurrent ischemic/hypoxic injury. These episodes may be sufficient to cause alteration of the white matter visible on brain MRIs but may not necessarily cause frank tissue necrosis.

DIAGNOSIS

Early diagnosis of vascular dementia is important because risk factor modifications may halt or slow disease progression. At times it is difficult to be certain about the presence of cognitive impairment because the initial symptoms are often subtle and nonspecific. The diagnosis depends on the type and quality of reported cognitive difficulties by the affected individual and his or her family.

Cognition and functional status are more precisely assessed by neuropsychological testing. Although there is currently no infallible standard for vascular dementia screening, neuropsychological testing allows the cognitive skills of an individual to be compared to normative data from age-matched groups. Cognitive decline is then assessed by comparing function relative to previous test performance.

The pattern and severity of cognitive impairment are influenced by lesion location, lesion burden (i.e., the combined number and size of the lesions), and severity of accompanying cerebral atrophy. Large artery disease results in loss of function within the affected portion of the brain. Small artery disease often results in mental slowing, loss of executive function, and Parkinson-like symptoms such as rigidity or disturbance of gait, and emotional or psychiatric abnormalities.

Although vascular dementia may present acutely, the course typically fluctuates, with relatively long intervals of stable cognitive function punctuated by sudden declines. Signs and symptoms depend on stroke location and often include hemiparesis, hemisensory deficits, visual abnormalities, pseudobulbar signs, hyperreflexia, and presence of pathological reflexes (e.g., grasp, palmomental, or snout reflex). Because of the anatomical location of ischemic lesions in the anterior and median fiber tracts of the deep white matter, many individuals with leukoaraiosis develop a fronto-subcortical disconnection syndrome resulting in abnormal information-processing speed and impaired executive frontal functions.[41–43]

Clinical manifestations of vascular dementia are diverse. Vascular dementia eventually impairs memory, with a decreased ability to acquire new information or to recall learned material. Aphasia, apraxia, agnosia, abulia, executive dysfunction, and apathy occur as well. Focal neurological findings, hemineglect, visuospatial and constructional impairments, confusion, agitation, depression, or emotional lability are frequently present. Neuroimaging studies typically demonstrate one or more infarctions or leukoaraiosis.

DIFFERENTIAL DIAGNOSIS

In early stages of vascular dementia, the pattern of cognitive impairment is often dominated by frontal and subcortical dysfunction. The cognitive decline can be saltatory, whereas individuals with Alzheimer disease typically decline more gradually and have more pronounced dysfunction of memory, language disturbance, apraxia, and visuospatial disorientation. Ultimately the two conditions cannot be reliably distinguished at the bedside, particularly in the early stages.

Leukoaraiosis may produce a clinical picture that resembles Parkinson disease or normal pressure hydrocephalus. Other important differential diagnoses include toxic-metabolic encephalopathy due to the use of drugs, vitamin B_{12} (cobalamin) deficiency, thyroid disease, fronto-temporal dementias, dementia with Lewy bodies, brain tumors, central nervous system infections, depression, or head injury (Table 15-5). Evaluation for causes of dementia is important especially at the time of presentation or when there is a sudden functional deterioration that could signal the presence of a treatable condition.

DIAGNOSTIC EVALUATION

Patients often present at an advanced stage of dementia after family members become aware of the cognitive dysfunction and after the individual's social or occupational function declines. The diagnostic evaluation should focus on a detailed history provided by the patient and a reliable third party who knows the individual well enough to comment on the presence, type, and severity of cognitive difficulties. During the interview, information about activities of daily living (ADLs) and social, community, and intellectual activities should be obtained. Memory, language, orientation, judgment, and problem-solving abilities and changes in behavior and/or personality should be assessed.

Although it is not disease specific and often reflects rather advanced cognitive impairment, the Mini-Mental Status Examination (MMSE) may provide a preliminary assessment of the severity and pattern of cognitive dysfunction and supply a baseline score of cognitive function. However, the MMSE is not sensitive for frontal and executive deficits and is unreliable when assessing subcortical vascular cognitive impairment. Although no one test is sensitive or disease specific for mild stages of vascular dementia, the diagnostic criteria in Table 15-3 allow one to create a working hypothesis and differential diagnosis.

LABORATORY STUDIES

Laboratory evaluation should include tests for vascular risk factors as well as studies to eliminate other causes of dementia. Evaluation should concentrate on the identification of potentially treatable conditions. Useful studies include a complete blood count as well as a comprehensive metabolic panel to assess kidney and liver function, electrolytes, glucose level, and lipid profile. Additional studies include determination of serum TSH, B_{12} and folate levels, syphilis serology, erythrocyte sedimentation rate, plasma ammonia level, and homocysteine level.

With an atypical presentation or if an infectious, inflammatory, or neoplastic etiology is suspected, analysis of the cerebrospinal fluid (CSF) is indicated. Measurement of CSF opening pressure and removal of at least 20 ml of CSF with evaluation of gait and cognitive function pre- and postlumbar puncture are essential for the evaluation of possible normal pressure hydrocephalus. An EEG might demonstrate epileptiform discharges in an individual with intermittent episodes of confusion or worsening of mental status. If vascular dementia is suspected based on clinical evaluation and imaging studies, detailed neuropsychological testing can provide a baseline assessment of cognitive function with which to compare follow-up evaluations and to identify individuals who may benefit from cognitive rehabilitation or treatment of possible coexisting Alzheimer disease.

NEUROIMAGING STUDIES

Patients with suspected vascular dementia should have a brain MRI with contrast infusion (if there is no contraindication) to

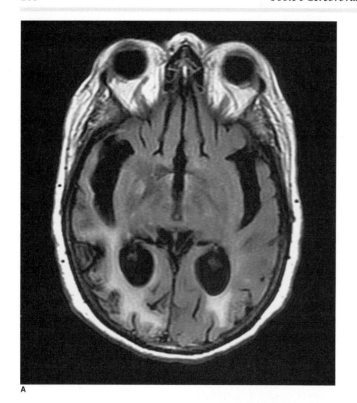

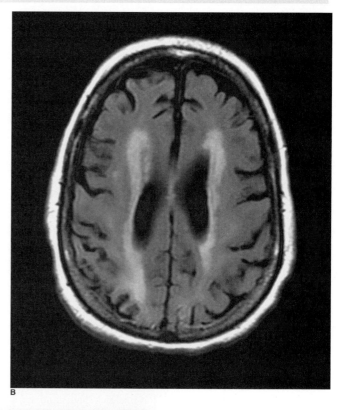

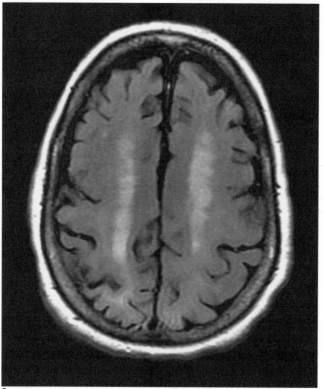

Figure 15-3. A, B, and C: MRI of the brain shows cortical atrophy and chronic ischemic changes of the white matter in a patient with vascular dementia. The patient was a 63-year-old woman with history of hypertension and cognitive impairment.

assess the extent, acuity, and location of cerebrovascular lesions and to exclude other causes of dementia, such as a tumor, hydrocephalus, or infection. Neuroimaging techniques used in the evaluation of cerebrovascular disease are discussed in Chapter 5.

Individuals with Alzheimer disease, at least in the early stages of decline, have regional temporo-parietal hypoperfusion and diminished metabolic rates. In contrast, vascular dementia appears to be characterized by early impairment of the cerebral autoregulation and a more diffuse and often asymmetric reduction in cortical and subcortical CBF and metabolism on functional imaging studies.[44,45] Measurement of acetazolamide-induced vasoreactivity with PET may be useful in the differentiation of vascular dementia from other forms of dementia.[46] However, no imaging study is able to reliably confirm vascular dementia, and, in advanced disease stages, functional and structural imaging studies often fail to differentiate Alzheimer disease and vascular dementia. In the future functional neuroimaging modalities may be able to identify individuals at risk to develop dementia long before the clinical onset of the disease.[47]

Standard brain MRI sequences in vascular dementia show infarctions of different sizes and in different vascular territories along with increasingly severe cerebral atrophy (Figure 15-3). Fluid-attenuation inversion recovery (FLAIR) and T_2-weighted MRI sequences are highly sensitive to leukoaraiosis, and gradient-echo MRI is now commonly used to identify patients with microbleeds and intracranial hemorrhages. More advanced imaging sequences will help to identify early white and gray matter perfusion and structural changes associated with the development of vascular dementia.

NEUROPATHOLOGY

The pathological substrate of vascular dementia is diffuse and, extensive research is still needed to better characterize valid morphological criteria.[48] Neurofibrillary plaques and tangles as well as amyloid depositions can be found in the brain of patients with Alzheimer disease but also in those with vascular dementia or in healthy elderly individuals. None of the pathological findings is disease specific, and there is a significant overlap between vascular and neurodegenerative disease mechanisms.[49] Vascular dementia is a heterogeneous group of disorders, so the resulting brain imaging and neuropathological correlates are heterogeneous as well.

Often there is a disparity between the clinical manifestations and the pathology findings. The clinical effect of vascular brain injury depends on location, number, and size of vascular lesions, presence of additional brain pathology, and, to some degree, the volume of damaged brain tissue (i.e., the "lesion burden").

Endothelial dysfunction and vessel wall alteration can be caused by many pathological processes, including atherosclerosis, deposition of amyloid, fibromuscular dysplasia, mural dissection, angiitis, or other acquired or inherited forms of arteriopathies affecting vessels of different caliber.[50] Thromboembolism, progressive vessel occlusion, hemodynamic impairment, and global hypoxia are the main underlying pathophysiological mechanisms.

Autopsy studies demonstrate infarctions in the territory of large and small-to-medium-sized vessels leading to coagulation necrosis, surrounding apoptotic cell death, and eventually brain cavitation. At times hemorrhages are found within these lesions, suggesting reperfusion injury, hemorrhagic transformation, or venous occlusion. Damage of penetrating arteries and arterioles, mostly associated with traditional vascular risk factors, causes lacunar cavitations. These lesions typically measure less than 1.5 cm in diameter and occur in the basal ganglia, brainstem, and white matter. Watershed lesions are of similar appearance and are observed between vascular territories of large brain-supplying arteries or between the cortex and the white matter.

Cortical laminar necrosis indicates global hypoperfusion due to episodes of sustained systemic hypotension or cardiac arrest and selectively involves layers of the cerebral and cerebellar cortex that are most susceptible to decreased perfusion and oxygenation. Reactive gliosis and incomplete ischemic necrosis due to global ischemia and poor brain perfusion occur in selected areas of the hippocampus. White matter ischemic disease is accompanied by rarefaction of myelin, loss of axons, cavitations and enlarged Virchow-Robin spaces, reactive gliosis, and structural alteration of small cerebral blood vessels.

SUBTYPES OF VASCULAR DEMENTIA

Vascular dementia is usually acquired during later life and can result from disease of medium-sized to large arteries or from arterioles, capillaries and venules, or veins. The topographic approach allows us to classify vascular dementia into multi-infarct dementia, strategically placed infarcts, multiple subcortical lacunar infarcts, leukoaraiosis, Binswanger disease, a combination of the above, single or multiple hemorrhages, and mixed dementia with coexistence of vascular dementia and Alzheimer disease. Patients with mixed dementia or multiple lesions often have a variety of vascular risk factors and medical co-morbidities.

POST-STROKE DEMENTIA

Multiple ischemic infarctions, often of different acuity, are scattered throughout cortical and subcortical structures following the distribution of the major cerebral arteries. They are often caused by cardiac or arterial embolism with arterial branch occlusion. High-grade stenosis of the internal carotid or vertebral arteries in the setting of transient hemodynamic compromise results in watershed infarctions. Infarction of the anterior, middle, or posterior cerebral arteries can cause dementia associated with classic cortical findings, such as neglect, aphasia, focal motor and sensory deficits, or apraxia (see Chapter 2).

Strategically located infarcts resulting in cognitive impairment are commonly found in the thalamus and/or frontal white matter or in the basal ganglia. With involvement of the angular gyrus, one observes impaired memory and judgment, language dysfunction affecting reading and writing, impairment of mathematical and constructional skills, as well as disorientation in space. Vascular dementia can also result from lesions in the dominant anterior cerebral and posterior cerebral artery territories, the dominant caudate nucleus, the anterior internal capsule, the hippocampus and parahippocampal formation, the amygdala, the fronto-cingulate gyrus, and the basal forebrain.

Multiple subcortical lacunar infarctions, attributable to occlusion of the deep penetrating arterioles of the white matter and the lenticulostriate arteries, often cause psychomotor impairment, urinary incontinence, depression, and impaired memory and attention.

WHITE MATTER ISCHEMIC DISEASE (LEUKOARAIOSIS)

In 1894 Binswanger described a severe and progressive form of subcortical dementia, later termed Binswanger disease by Alzheimer.[51] Binswanger's initial report referred to eight patients but provided details of the clinical course and macroscopic pathology of only one patient. It was Alzheimer who first described the histopathology. Leukoaraiosis is characterized by lacunar infarcts of the basal ganglia, internal capsule, and white matter

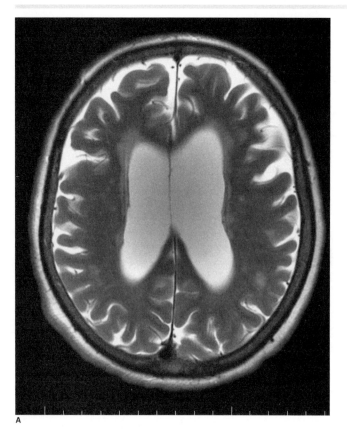
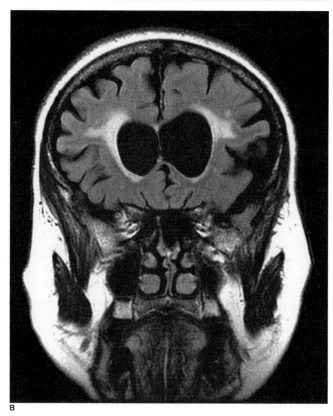

Figure 15-4. A: Axial T$_2$-weighted MRI from a 78-year-old woman with hypertension, hyperlipidemia, diabetes, and progressive dementia shows extensive leukoaraiosis. B: Coronal FLAIR image shows extensive white matter hyperintensity in the periventricular white matter, cerebral atrophy, and compensatory ventricular enlargement.

due to severe arteriosclerosis of small cerebral vessels. Affected individuals typically experience a gradual loss of memory, deterioration of intellectual abilities, strokes, seizures at times, behavioral disturbances, incontinence, and abnormal gait.

This disorder was originally thought to be rare, and only about 150 cases had been reported in the literature between the original description by Binswanger and 1988.[52] However, with the wide availability of neuroimaging modalities it became apparent that ischemic white matter disease is common and has an increasing frequency and severity with age (Figure 15-4). In 1987 the term *leukoaraiosis* was introduced by Hachinski and coworkers to describe these lesions.[53,54] The concept of leukoaraiosis now encompasses Binswanger disease, a condition that is characterized by rather extensive ischemic white matter lesions and lacunar infarctions.

Leukoaraiosis, initially coined to describe areas of hypoattenuation on cranial CT, refers to corresponding hyperintense signals on T$_2$-weighted or FLAIR sequences in the deep periventricular white matter and the centrum semiovale. Previously considered unimportant, especially with few lesions present, it is now known that these lesions are predictive of stroke and dementia. Because those signal abnormalities on MRI are nonspecific and can be observed in various clinical conditions, the presence of white matter abnormalities in the elderly does not precisely parallel the extent of cognitive impairment. Table 15-5 summarizes the differential diagnosis of common white matter abnormalities found in brain MRI.

Risk factors for leukoaraiosis include arterial hypertension and other traditional stroke risk factors, normal pressure hydrocephalus, history of brain injury, and previous cerebral infarctions, especially lacunar infarctions. The reported frequency of leukoaraiosis varies widely,[55,56] but it is common in MRI-based studies. MRI is a highly sensitive technique for the detection of even subtle and potentially reversible changes in white matter. Some individuals with few leukoaraiotic lesions have no cognitive or neurological manifestation on examination; others have gait abnormalities, cognitive impairment, pathological reflexes, and frontal lobe dysfunction due to functional disconnection syndromes of fronto-subcortical structures.[57,58]

Because ischemic lesions are distributed in the border zones of the deep white matter with typical sparing of subcortical U-fibers and the corpus callosum, it has been suggested that they are due to watershed infarctions caused by a combination of atherosclerosis of small penetrators and episodic decrease in cerebral perfusion pressure.[59] Postmortem examination reveals focal edema and loss of white matter, particularly in the temporal, parietal, and occipital lobes. Patients with leukoaraiosis also show structural damage of white matter veins, which can be stenotic or occluded by collagen.[60] The ventricular system is dilated, and the brain shows generalized atrophy. There is usually evidence of diffuse atherosclerosis, with thickened and hyalinized arteries and arterioles.

INHERITED ISCHEMIC WHITE MATTER DISORDERS WITH VASCULAR DEMENTIA

CADASIL and CARASIL (Maeda syndrome) are familial diseases of white matter. They lead to cognitive impairment and dementia. Both have their onset early in life, usually in the third decade, and affect arteries and arterioles of the white matter and leptomeninges.[61] CADASIL usually presents initially with migraines, which are frequently associated with aura. These are followed by cerebral infarctions and stroke-like episodes about a decade later. In advanced cases dementia, psychiatric manifestations, gait disturbance, urinary incontinence, pseudobulbar palsy, and rarely seizures develop.[62] Multiple confluent infarctions of the white matter can be seen on MRI, and less commonly hemorrhages can occur.

In 1993 Tournier-Lasserve and coworkers linked CADASIL to chromosome 19, and in 1996 a *Notch3* gene mutation was identified. The mutated gene is expressed in smooth muscle cell of the vasculature of multiple organs, including the brain, muscle, and skin.[63–65] However, the central nervous system (CNS) bears the brunt of the clinical manifestations. Since the 1990s several CADASIL families worldwide have been described. The disorder is evidently rare, occurring with an estimated frequency of 1:100,000.

Diagnosis is confirmed with screening for the *Notch3* gene mutation. Less reliably, the diagnosis is supported by typical electron microscopic findings in skin or, preferably, muscle tissue. Skin biopsies can be false negative in up to 50% of individuals, probably because skin contains fewer vascular smooth muscle cells than does muscle.[66] Expression of the aberrant *Notch3* gene causes accumulation of granular osmophilic deposits in the vessel walls, damaging typically arteries of less than 400 μm in diameter, arterioles, and capillaries (Figure 21-1).

Neurological symptoms and signs are probably due to progressive occlusion and leakage of these vessels. The course is progressive with poor prognosis, often leading to death in the sixth decade. Treatment is symptomatic because no curative therapy is presently available.

CARASIL, first described in Japan by Maeda and coworkers in 1976, causes damage to small cerebral vessels with subsequent white matter ischemic disease and vascular dementia.[61] Granular osmophilic deposits or amyloid is not found, but rather there is severe arteriosclerotic disease with media degeneration, intimal thickening, splitting of the internal elastic lamina, and luminal narrowing and obstruction. The underlying genetic defect is unknown. Like CADASIL, the disease has a relatively early onset and is not associated with traditional atherosclerotic risk factors. Clinically, patients present with subcortical vascular dementia, psychiatric disturbances, and pseudobulbar, pyramidal, and extrapyramidal signs as well as symptoms indicative of extensive white matter disease. Characteristically these patients also have alopecia, severe intervertebral disc disease, and spinal deformities. No effective treatment is available, and death often occurs in the fifth or sixth decade of life. Additional information on CARASIL and CADASIL is provided in Chapter 21.

HEMORRHAGIC STROKES

Analogous to ischemic strokes, single or multiple intracranial hemorrhages (subdural, subarachnoid, intraparenchymatous) can cause cognitive impairment. In the elderly cerebral hemorrhages commonly occur as consequence of arterial hypertension with bleeds into the basal ganglia, thalamus, or the brain parenchyma, also termed lobar hemorrhages. Other causes include CNS bleeding from intracranial aneurysms, arteriovenous malformations, or hemorrhagic diathesis (Chapter 16).

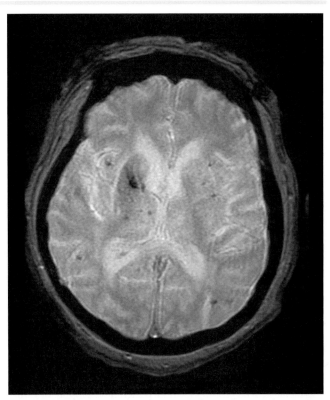

Figure 15-5. Patient with intracranial hemorrhage. Echo-gradient MRI shows multiple hypointensities caused by microbleeds from cerebral amyloid angiopathy.

CEREBRAL AMYLOID ANGIOPATHY

Vascular cognitive impairment, intracranial hemorrhages, and leukoaraiosis may occur with cerebral amyloid angiopathy (CAA). Up to a third of intracranial hemorrhages in the elderly are caused by CAA.[67,68] Those hemorrhages are often recurrent and can consist of microbleeds, primarily located in the cortex or at the cortical/subcortical junction or manifest as extensive lobar parenchymal bleedings (Figure 15-5). Microbleeds associated with CAA often cause only mild transient neurological symptoms, whereas macrobleeds often result in persistent focal neurological deficits.

Increasingly frequent with age, CAA is found in the brain of 10% to 40% of elderly individuals and in approximately 80% of patients with Alzheimer disease in autopsy series. Deposits of β-amyloid in CAA are predominantly detected in cortical and leptomeningeal capillaries, small arterioles, and arteries, whereas in Alzheimer disease β-amyloid accumulates in the brain parenchyma. Although both conditions can coexist, only a subgroup of Alzheimer disease patients have intracranial hemorrhages from advanced CAA. Conversely, most elderly patients with intracranial hemorrhages due to CAA do not have Alzheimer disease. Interestingly, cognitive impairment and cerebral hemorrhages can also be observed with parenchymal and vascular β-amyloid depositions associated with Down syndrome.[69]

Advanced white matter disease is commonly seen in patients with CAA, and patients with CAA and Alzheimer disease are more severely demented than those without CAA.[70] It remains to be answered whether cognitive impairment in CAA is due to ischemic white matter and/or hemorrhagic lesions or due to vascular and parenchymal β-amyloid depositions mediating a neurotoxic effect.

Clinically CAA is characterized by recurrent lobar cerebral hemorrhages and cognitive impairment, often in elderly normotensive individuals. In advanced stages there is evidence of recurrent intracranial hemorrhages of different acuity and rather extensive leukoaraiosis on neuroimaging studies. Acquired CAA can rarely cause a rapidly progressive course, characterized by rapid cognitive deterioration, seizures, and extensive leukoaraiosis occurring in combination with CAA-related vasculitis that at times responds to immunosuppressive therapy.

Hereditary forms of CAA are due to a mutation in the β-amyloid precursor protein. Affected individuals typically present between 30 and 60 years of age, have a more severe clinical course with rapid onset of dementia and recurrent hemorrhages, and, in contrast to some forms of acquired CAA, are not associated with ApoE 2 and 4 polymorphisms. The diagnostic yield of leptomeningeal and cortical biopsy has limited sensitivity and specificity and does not result in effective treatment.

MICROBLEEDS

There is growing interest in the clinical significance of microbleeds that are frequently observed on gradient-echo MRI. Previously considered clinically silent, it has recently become apparent that microbleeds from different etiologies can result in cognitive impairment, and more specifically executive frontal dysfunction.[71,72] Most microbleeds in the elderly are associated with CAA or with hypertensive vasculopathy and result from vessel damage due to amyloid depositions or fibrohyalinosis with rupture of small vessels less than 200 μm in diameter. The underlying pathophysiology of microbleeds seems similar to that of ischemic small vessel disease of the white matter. Individuals with microbleeds are more likely to smoke, be hypertensive, and have a history of ischemic strokes. MRI often demonstrates extensive associated leukoaraiosis and a high frequency of lacunar infarctions. These lesions are associated with advanced age and male gender.[73–76] The appearance of microhemorrhages on brain MRI needs to be differentiated from normal vascular flow voids, cavernous malformations, or accumulation of calcium or iron, such as in subpial siderosis. Microbleeds occur in CADASIL and other small vessel cerebral vasculopathies.

Cerebral microhemorrhages may be a marker for small vessel disease burden and parallel the presence of modifiable risk factors. Whereas treatment of hypertension may have no clear effect on the course of hemorrhages due to CAA, microbleeding associated with traditional vascular risk factors allow the opportunity for treatment and prevention of disease progression. Patients with microbleeds may be at high risk for intracranial hemorrhages. The use of antiplatelet agents, anticoagulants, or thrombolytics requires caution in this population.[77] However, prospective studies are needed to assess whether the presence of cerebral microbleeds potentiates the risk for intracranial hemorrhage among patients treated with these agents.

MIXED DEMENTIA

Mixed dementia (vascular and degenerative), first described by Delay and colleagues in 1962,[78] is responsible for at least 15% of individuals with dementia. Others have suggested that a mixed vascular and degenerative dementia may actually be the most frequent form of dementia. Although the definition of mixed dementia is open to discussion,[79–82] it is best characterized pathologically. Autopsy studies demonstrate extracellular amyloid plaques and intracellular neurofibrillary tangles occurring in conjunction with cerebral infarctions, lacunes, and leukoaraiosis. Mixed dementia can be difficult to diagnose and should be suspected in individuals with signs and symptoms typical for Alzheimer disease who have accompanying focal neurological deficits and evidence of stroke on neuroimaging studies. Strokes can be ischemic or hemorrhagic because patients with Alzheimer disease at times have CAA.

Patients with mixed dementia frequently have vascular risk factors such as arterial hypertension, tobacco use, diabetes, or history of heart disease. The apolipoprotein E (APOE) ε4 genotype is associated with increased risk for Alzheimer disease as well as atherosclerosis and may suggest a potential link between neurodegenerative and cerebrovascular disease.[83,84] Not surprisingly, patients with mixed dementia have more severe cognitive function and worse clinical outcome than individuals with pure Alzheimer disease.[85–87]

An estimated 50% to 80% of Alzheimer disease patients have ischemic white matter lesions on brain MRI.[88] The incidence of leukoariosis detected by MRI is considerably higher in patients with Alzheimer disease than in age-matched unaffected controls.[89] Coffman reported that asymptomatic descendants of patients with Alzheimer disease also have significant higher rates of leukoaraiosis compared to age-matched controls without family history of Alzheimer disease.[90] Neuropathological studies indicate that microvascular amyloid depositions may cause leukoaraiosis in this population.[91] Additionally, patients with Alzheimer disease frequently show strong tortuosities and multiplications and aneurysms of small arterioles and capillaries,[92] which suggests that a variety of synergistic factors may lead to ischemic white matter disease in these patients. A primary neurodegenerative disorder may cause apoptosis leading to Wallerian degeneration with rarefaction of myelin, axonal death, and pallor of the white matter. Damage to the ultrastructure of small blood vessels due to amyloid depositions or lipohyalinosis induced by hypertension, diabetes, and other vascular injury could result in incomplete infarctions and impaired autoregulatory capacity of the cerebral circulation, especially with recurrent episodes of systemic hypotension. Therapy should thus focus on both pharmacological treatment of Alzheimer disease and modification of vascular risk factors.

THERAPY AND PREVENTION

Treatment of vascular risk factors such as arterial hypertension or diabetes may prevent or at least delay the development of vascular dementia, mixed dementia, and possibly even Alzheimer disease.[93] Early recognition of cognitive impairment and identification of modifiable vascular risk factors is therefore essential. Therapeutic goals should focus on slowing or arresting cognitive decline and on improvement of cognitive status, behavior, and overall function. Overlying anxiety or depression may also require appropriate intervention. Contributing medical conditions need to be identified and treated. The use of psychotropic agents and medications with adverse effects on the central nervous or cardiovascular system needs to be critically reviewed.

The cholinesterase inhibitors donepezil, rivastigmine, and galantamine have been used in the treatment of vascular dementia, but the reslts are, at best, modest. Daily doses of 5 mg and 10 mg of donepezil showed a statistically significant but clinically meager improvement of cognition, global functioning (in the 5 mg group only), and ADLs in a 24-week multicenter randomized, placebo-controlled trial.[94,95] Galantamine, a cholinesterase inhibitor and central modulator of nicotinergic receptors, used in daily doses of 24 mg over 6 months modestly improved cognition, global functioning, and behavioral symptoms in patients with vascular dementia.[96] In small trials rivastigmine also improved cognition and behavioral symptoms in vascular dementia and mixed dementia.[97,98] Results of a multicenter trial examining the efficacy and safety of rivastigmine in patients with probable vascular dementia are pending.

Cholinesterase inhibitors and the N-methyl-D-aspartate (NMDA) receptor antagonist memantine may provide a modest benefit in a few individuals with vascular dementia. However, the observation period during these trials was relatively brief, and the clinical assessment tools were largely based on scales developed for Alzheimer disease. Moreover, the great heterogeneity in the subtypes of vascular dementia makes it difficult to choose appropriate functional scales to assess changes in cognition and daily function related to pharmacological treatment. In two randomized, multicenter trials, 20 mg of daily memantine for 6 months led to improved cognition, especially in patients with advanced vascular dementia and in the subgroup with small vessel ischemic disease on neuroimaging studies.[99,100] Memantine also showed a possible benefit in the treatment of mixed dementia.[101] Cholinesterase inhibitors as well as memantine are relatively well tolerated and may transiently benefit cognition, function, and behavioral symptoms in some individuals. Nevertheless, the agents appear to have no long-term benefit, and additional studies are needed.

Small studies using antiplatelet agents, ergot derivatives, nootropics, vasoactive agents, antioxidants, serotonin, xanthine derivatives, and calcium antagonists showed mostly negative results but are limited by methodological shortcomings. A large multicenter trial showed no benefit for the highly touted ginko biloba in patients with Alzheimer disease. Individuals taking propentofylline, used experimentally in Canada and Europe for patients with mild to moderate vascular dementia, had symptomatic improvement and possibly slower disease progression.[102,103] The evidence for a beneficial effect for the calcium channel blocker nimodipine is weak.[104]

Several studies have examined the link between blood pressure control and cognition, but these studies are limited by lack of appropriate diagnostic tools for vascular dementia and by early vascular cognitive impairment and unknown subclassifications of vascular dementia subtypes. The SHEP trial showed that the diuretic chlorthalidone lowered the risk of ischemic stroke, but it had no influence on dementia onset.[105] In contrast, the rate of dementia over a five-year follow-up period was lowered by 50% by use of the calcium channel blocker nitrendipine in the Syst-Eur study.[106] The number needed to treat was 1,000 patients over 5 years to prevent 20 cases of dementia by lowering the systolic blood pressure by 7 mm Hg and the diastolic blood pressure by 3.2 mm Hg. The PROGRESS trial compared perindopril (ACE-inhibitor), or perindopril plus indapamide (thiazide diuretic), with placebo for the prevention of stroke and vascular dementia. It demonstrated no reduction of dementia over 3.9 years, but there was a significant but clinically small decrease in cognitive decline.[107] The SCOPE trial showed a trend for dementia reduction on the ACE inhibitor canderartan cilexetil,[108] and the FOCUS study showed that felodipine or enalapril significantly improved cognitive function at 1–2 and 24 weeks,

which suggests that blood pressure control ≤ 140/90 in the elderly reduces cognitive decline.[109] However, vigorous control of blood pressure in the elderly needs to be critically evaluated because excessive reduction of the systemic blood pressure in an elderly individual with decreased cerebral perfusion and impaired cerebral autoregulation may promote vascular dementia due to leukoariosis or infarction.

Although the presence of traditional vascular risk factors increases the event rate of stroke and hence the risk of vascular dementia, relatively little is known about how the treatment of diabetes, hyperhomocysteinemia, or dyslipidemia affects cognition and, more specifically, vascular dementia. Although it is accepted that individuals with diabetes mellitus have a greater risk of cognitive decline, the relation between diabetes, treatment of elevated glucose levels, and the development of vascular dementia are not well understood. Optimal control of diabetes mellitus is prudent for multiple reasons, perhaps including delayed development of vascular dementia.[110,111] Hyperhomocysteinemia may be associated with cognitive decline, but its role in the development of vascular dementia has not been established.[112,113]

Elevated levels of serum total cholesterol, LDL, and lipoprotein(a) are risk factors for both stroke and Alzheimer disease. However, their relative contribution to cognitive decline may depend on the presence of additional genetic cofactors such as apolipoprotein E, and it is uncertain whether the statins slow the development or the progression of vascular dementia.[114]

Prevention and early treatment of vascular cognitive impairment should also address a healthy diet, stress reduction, and physical exercise. Increased fish consumption, regular physical activity, and reduction of stress have all shown to contribute to the prevention of dementia.[115–120] The use of hormonal therapy in elderly women needs to be critically assessed because there is evidence that women on hormone replacement show increased risk of dementia. In the WHIMS study women received either 0.625 mg of estrogen daily or a combination of 0.625 mg estrogen/progestin at 2.5 mg daily. Women on hormonal replacement had a significant higher risk to develop dementia than those who did not take the hormones. The WHIMS study included 8.5% women with vascular dementia and 19% with mixed dementia; it concluded that hormonal replacement therapy is not indicated for dementia in women 65 years or older. There also is a significantly increased risk of stroke and myocardial infarction for women on hormonal replacement therapy. Future research should focus on the development of new compounds for prevention and therapy for vascular dementia.

REFERENCES

1. Fratliglioni L, De Ronchi D, Agüero-Torres H. Worldwide prevalence and incidence of dementia. *Drugs Aging.* 1999;**15**:365–375.
2. World Health Organization. *The ICD-10 Classification of Mental and Behavioral Disorders: Clinical Descriptions and Disorders for Diagnostic Guidelines.* Geneva, Switzerland: World Health Organization; 1992.
3. Winker MA Aging: a global issue. *JAMA.* 1997;**278**:1377.
4. Rocca WA, Hofman A, Brayne C, et al. The prevalence of vascular dementia in Europe: facts and fragments from 1980–1990 studies: EURODEM-Prevalence Research Group. *Ann Neurol.* 1991;**30**:817–824.

5. Jorm AF. Cross-national comparisons of the occurrence of Alzheimer's and vascular dementias. *Eur Arch Psychiatry Clin Neurosci.* 1991;**240**:218–222.

6. Ott A, Breteler MM, van Harskamp F, et al. Incidence and risk of dementia: the Rotterdam Study. *Am J Epidemiol.* 1998;**147**: 574–580.

7. Herbert R, Brayne C. Epidemiology of vascular dementia. *Neuroepidemiology.* 1995;**14**:240–257.

8. Chu HC, Victoroff JI, Margolin D, et al. Criteria for the diagnosis of ischemic vascular dementia proposed by the State of California Alzheimer's Disease Diagnostic and Treatment Centers. *Neurology.* 1992;**42**:473–489.

9. Jellinger KA, Attems J. Prevalence and pathogenic role of cerebrovascular lesions in Alzheimer disease. *J Neurol Sci.* 2005;**229–230**:37–41.

10. de la Torre JC. Alzheimer disease as a vascular disorder: nosological evidence. *Stroke.* 2002;**33**:1152–1162.

11. Alzheimer A. (1907). About a peculiar disease of the cerebral cortex. (translated by Jarvik L., Greenson H). *Alzheimer Dis Assoc Disord.* 1987;**1**:7–8.

12. Jellinger KA. Pathology and pathophysiology of vascular cognitive impairment: a critical update. *Panminerva Med.* 2004;**46**: 217–226.

13. Pohjasvaara T, Mäntylä R, Ylikoski R, et al. Comparison of different clinical criteria (DS-111, ADDTC, ICD-10, NINDS-AIREN, DSM-IV) for the diagnosis of vascular dementia. *Stroke.* 2000;**31**:2952–2957.

14. Wolfson C, Wolfson DB, Asgharian M, et al. A reevaluation of the duration of survival after the onset of dementia. *N Engl J Med.* 2001;**344**:1111–1116.

15. Neyenhuis DL, Gorelick PB. Vascular dementia: a contemporary review of epidemiology, diagnosis, prevention, and treatment. *J Am Geriatr Soc.* 1998;**46**:1437–1438.

16. Whitmer RA, Sidney S, Selby J, et al. Midlife cardiovascular risk factors and risk of dementia in late life. *Neurology.* 2005;**64**: 277–281.

17. Lenzi GL, Jones T, Moss S. The relationship between regional oxygen utilization and cerebral blood flow in multi-infarct dementia. *Acta Neurol Scand.* 1997;**64**(Suppl):248–249.

18. Shaw TG, Mortel KF, Meyer JS, et al. Cerebral blood flow changes in benign aging and cerebrovascular disease. *Neurology.* 1984; **34**:855–862.

19. Fazekas F, Niederkorn K, Schmidt R, et al. White matter signal abnormalities in normal individuals: correlation with carotid ultrasonography, cerebral blood flow measurements, and cerebrovascular risk factors. *Stroke.* 1988;**19**:1285–1288.

20. Markus HS, Lythgoe DJ, Ostegaard L, et al. Reduced cerebral blood flow in white matter in ischaemic leukoaraiosis demonstrated using quantitative exogenous contrast based perfusion MRI. *J Neurol Neurosurg Psychiatry.* 2000;**69**:48–53.

21. Furuta A, Ishii N, Nishihara Y, Horie A. Medullary arteries in aging and dementia. *Stroke.* 1991;**22**:442–446.

22. Ostrow PT, Miller LL. Pathology of small artery disease. *Adv Neurol.* 1993;**62**:93–123.

23. Fazekas F, Kleinert R, Offenbacher H, et al. Pathologic correlates of incidental MRI white matter signal hypertensities. *Neurology.* 1993;**43**:1683–1689.

24. Pantoni L, Garcia JH. Pathogenesis of leukoaraiosis: a review. *Stroke.* 1997;**28**:652–659.

25. Román GC. White matter lesions and normal-pressure hydrocephalus: Binswanger's disease or Hakim syndrome? *AJNR Am J Neuroradiol.* 1991;**12**:40–41.

26. Graff-Radford NR, Godersky JC. Idiopathic normal pressure hydrocephalus and systemic hypertension. *Neurology.* 1987; **37**:868–871.

27. Feigin I, Popoff N. Neuropathological changes late in cerebral edema: the relationship to trauma, hypertensive disease and Binswanger's encephalopathy. *J Neuropathol Exp Neurol.* 1963; **22**:500–511.

28. Spangler KM, Challa VR, Moody DM, Bell MA. Arteriolar tortuosity of the white matter in aging and hypertension: a microradiographic study. *J Neuropathol Exp Neurol.* 1994;**53**:22–26.

29. Moody DM, Thore CR, Anstrom JA, et al. Quantification of afferent vessels shows reduced brain vascular density in subjects with leukoaraiosis. *Radiology.* 2004;**233**:883–890.

30. Leifer D, Buonanno FS, Richardson EP Jr. Clinicopathologic correlations of cranial magnetic resonance imaging of periventricular white matter. *Neurology.* 1990;**40**:911–918.

31. van Swieten JC, van den Hout JHW, van Ketel BA, et al. Periventricular lesions in the white matter on magnetic resonance imaging in the elderly: a morphometric correlation with arteriolosclerosis and dilated perivascular spaces. *Brain.* 1991;**114**:761–774.

32. Erkinjuntti T, Gao F, Lee DH, et al. Lack of difference in brain hypertensities between patients with early Alzheimer's disease and control subjects. *Arch Neurol.* 1994;**51**:260–268.

33. Hendrie HC, Farlow MR, Austom GM, Edwards MK, Williams MA. Foci of increased T2 signal intensity on brain MR scans of healthy elderly subjects. *AJNR Am J Neuroradiol.* 1989;**10**:703–707.

34. Hunt AL, Orrison WW, Yeo RA, et al. Clinical significance of MRI white matter lesions in the elderly. *Neurology.* 1989;**39**:1470–1474.

35. Pantoni L, Garcia JH. The significance of cerebral white matter abnormalities 100 years after Binswanger's report: a review. *Stroke.* 1995;**26**:1293–1301.

36. Breteler MB, van Swieten JC, Bots ML, et al. Cerebral white matter lesions, vascular risk factors and cognitive function in a population-based study: the Rotterdam Study. *Neurology.* 1994;**44**:1246–1252.

37. Inzitari D, Diaz F, Fox A, et al. Vascular risk factors and leukoaraiosis. *Arch Neurol.* 1987;**44**:42–47.

38. Cadelo M, Inzitari D, Pracucci G, Masalchi M. Predictors of leukoaraiosis in elderly neurological patients. *Cerebrovasc Dis.* 1991;**1**:345–351.

39. Ljindgren A, Roijer A, Rudling O, et al. Cerebral lesions on magnetic resonance imaging, heart, disease, and vascular risk factors in subjects without stroke. *Stroke.* 1994;**25**:929–934.

40. Moody DM, Santamore WP, Bell MA. Does the tortuosity in cerebral arterioles impair down-autoregulation in hypertensive and elderly normotensive: a hypothesis and computer model. *Clin Neurosurg.* 1990;**37**:372–387.

41. Prins ND, van Dijk EJ, Den Heijer T, et al. Cerebral small-vessel disease and decline in information processing speed, executive function and memory. *Brain.* 2005;**128**:2034–2041.

42. DeGroot JC, de Leeuw FF, Oudkerk M, et al. Cerebral white matter lesions and cognitive function: the Rotterdam Scan Study. *Ann Neurol.* 2000;**47**:145–151.

43. Wolfe N, Linn R, Babikian VL, et al. Frontal systems impairment following multiple lacunar infarcts. *Arch Neurol.* 1990;**47**: 129–132.

44. Tohgi H, Yonezawa H, Takahashi S, et al. Cerebral blood flow and oxygen metabolism in senile dementia of Alzeheimer's type and vascular dementia with deep white matter changes. *Neuroradiology.* 1998;**40**:131–137.

45. Pavics L, Grunwald F, Reichmann K, et al. Regional cerebral blood flow single-photon emission tomography with 99mTc-HMPAO and the acetazolamide test in the evaluation of vascular and Alzheimer's dementia. *Eur J Nucl Med.* 1999;**26**: 239–245.

46. De Rueck J, Decoo D, Haenbroekx MC, et al. Acetazolamide vasoreactivity in vascular dementia: a positron emission tomography study. *Eur Neurol.* 1999;**41**:31–36.

47. Drzezga A, Grimmer T, Riemenschneider M, et al. Prediction of individual clinical outcome in MCI by means of genetic assessment and (18)F-FDG PET. *J Nucl Med.* 2005;**46**:1625–1632.

48. Jellinger KA. Alpha-synuclein lesions in normal aging, Parkinson disease, and Alzheimer disease: evidence from the Baltimore Longitudinal Study of Aging (BLSA). *J Neuropathol Sci.* 2005; **65**:554.

49. Pantoni L. Subtypes of vascular dementia and their pathogenesis: a critical overview. In: Bowler J, Hachninski V, eds. *Vascular Cognitive Impairment-Preventable Dementia.* New York: Oxford University Press; 2003:217–219.

50. Garcia JH, Brown GG. Vascular dementia: neuropathologic alterations and metabolic brain changes. *J Neurol Sci.* 1992; **109**:121–131.

51. Blass J, Hoyer S, Nitsch R. A translation of Otto Binswanger's article, "The delineation of the generalized progressive paralyses." 1894. *Arch Neurol.* 1991;**48**:961–972.

52. Schorer CE, Rodin E. Binswanger's disease: a complete translation. *J Geriatr Psychiatr Neurol.* 1990;**3**:61–66.

53. Hachinski VC, Potter P, Merskey H. *Leuko-ariosis. Arch Neurol.* 1987;**44**:21–23.

54. Román GC. Senile dementia of the Binswanger type: a vascular form of dementia in the elderly. *JAMA.* 1987;**258**:1782–1788.

55. Longstreth WT Jr, Arnold AM, Beauchamp NJ Jr, et al. Incidence, manifestations, and predictors of worsening white matter on serial cranial magnetic resonance imaging in the elderly: the Cardiovascular Health Study. *Stroke.* 2005;**36**: 56–61.

56. Fazekas FC. Magnetic resonance signal abnormalities in asymptomatic individuals: prevalence and functional correlates. *Eur Neurol.* 1989;**29**:164–166.

57. McPherson SE. Neuropsychological aspects of vascular dementia. *Brain Cogn.* 1996;**31**:269–282.

58. Graham NL, Emery T, Hodges JR. Distinctive cognitive profiles in Alzheimer's disease and subcortical vascular dementia. *J Neurol Neursurg Psychiatry.* 2004;**75**:61–71.

59. Brown WR, Moody DM, Thore CR, Challa VR. Cerebrovascular pathology in Alzheimer's disease and leukoaraiosis. *Ann NY Acad Sci.* 2000;**903**:39–45.

60. Moody DM, Brown WR, Challa VR, Ghazi-Birry HS, Reboussin DM. Cerebral microvascular alterations in aging, leukoaraiosis, and Alzheimer's disease. *Ann NY Acad Sci.* 1997;**26**: 103–116.

61. Arima K, Yanagawa S, Ito N, Ikeda S. Cerebral arterial pathology of CADASIL and CARRASIL (Maeda syndrome). *Neuropathology.* 2003;**23**:327–334.

62. Davous P. Cadasil: a review with proposed diagnostic criteria. *Eur J Neurol.* 1998;**5**:219–233.

63. Bousser MG, Tournier-Lasserve E. Summary of the proceedings of the First International Workshop on CADASIL. Paris, May 19–21, 1993. *Stroke.* 1994;**25**:704–707.

64. Tournier-Lasserve E, Joutel A, Melki J, et al. Cerebral autosomal dominant arteriopathy with subcortical infarcts and leukoencephalopathy maps to chromosome 19q12. *Nat Genet.* 1993; **3**:256–259.

65. Joutel A, Corpechot C, Docros A, et al. Notch3 mutations in CADASIL, a hereditary adult-onset condition causing stroke and dementia. *Nature.* 1996;**383**:707–710.

66. Markus HS, Martin RJ, Simpson MA, et al. Diagnostic strategies in CADASIL. *Neurology.* 2002;**59**:1134–1138.

67. Greenberg SM. Cerebral amyloid angiopathy: prospects for clinical diagnosis and treatment. *Neurology.* 1998;**51**:690–694.

68. Kase CS. Cerebral amyloid angiopathy. In: Kase CS, Caplan LR, eds. *Intracerebral Hemorrhage.* Boston: Butterworth-Heinemann; 1994:179–200.

69. McCarron MO, Nicoll JA, Graham DI. A quartet of Down's syndrome, Alzheimer's disease, cerebral amyloid angiopathy, and cerebral hemorrhage: interacting genetic risk factors. *J Neurol Neurosurg Psychiatry.* 1998;**65**:405–406.

70. Pfeiffer LA, White LR, Ross GW, et al. Cerebral amyloid angiopathy and cognitive function: the HAAS autopsy study. *Neurology.* 2002;**58**:1629–1634.

71. Werring DJ, Frazer DN, Coward LJ, et al. Cognitive dysfunction in patients with cerebral microbleeds on T_2*-weighted gradient-echo MRI. *Brain.* 2004;**127**:2265–2275.

72. Cordonnier C, van der Flier WM, Sluimer JD, et al. Prevalence and severity of microbleeds in a memory clinic setting. *Neurology.* 2006;**66**:1356–1360.

73. Lesnik Oberstein SA, van den Boom R, van Buchem MA, et al. Cerebral microbleeds in CADASIL. *Neurology.* 2001;**57**:1066–1070.

74. Dichgans M, Holtmannspotter M, Herzog J, Peters N, et al. Cerebral microbleeds in CADASIL: a gradient-echo magnetic resonance imaging and autopsy study. *Stroke.* 2002;**33**:67–71.

75. Roob G, Schmidt R, Kapeller P, et al. MRI evidence of past cerebral microbleeds in a healthy elderly population. *Neurology.* 1999;**52**:991–994.

76. Jeerakathil T, Wolf PA, Beiser A, et al. Stroke risk profile predicts white matter hyperintensity volume: the Framingham Study. *Stroke.* 2004;**35**:1857–1861.

77. Eckman MH, Rosand J, Knudsen KA, et al. Can patients be anticoagulated after intracerebral hemorrhage? A decision analysis. *Stroke.* 2003;**34**:1710–1716.

78. Delay J, Brion S. Les Démence senile mixte. In: Delay J, Brion S, eds. *Démences Tardives.* Paris: Masson; 1962:195–201.

79. Tomlinson BE, Blessed G, Roth M. Observations on the brains of demented old people. *J Neurol Sci.* 1970;**11**:205–242.

80. Mölsa PK, Paljarvi L, Rinne JO, Rinne UK, Sako E. Validity of clinical diagnosis in dementia: a prospective clinicopathological study. *Neurol Neurosurg Psychiatry.* 1985;**48**:1085–1090.

81. Chui H, Victoroff JI, Margolin D, et al. Criteria for the diagnosis of ischemic vascular dementia proposed by the State of California Alzeheimer's Disease Diagnostic and Treatment Centers. *Neurology.* 1992;**42**:473–480.

82. Román GC, Tatemichi TK, Erkinjuntti T, et al. Vascular dementia: diagnostic criteria for research studies: report of the NINDS-AIREN International Workshop. *Neurology.* 1993;**43**: 250–260.

83. Casserly I, Topol E. Convergence of atherosclerosis and Alzehimer's disease: inflammation, cholesterol, and misfolded proteins. *Lancet.* 2004;**363**:1139–1146.

84. Haan MN, Shemanski L, Jagust WJ, et al. The role of APOE epsilon4 in modulating effects of other risk factors for cognitive decline in elderly persons. *JAMA.* 1999;**282**:40–46.

85. Snowdon DA, Greiner LH, Mortimer JA, et al. Brain infarction and the clinical expression of Alzheimer disease: the Nun Study. *JAMA.* 1997;**277**:813–817.

86. Zekry D, Duyckaerts C, Moulias R, et al. Degenerative and vascular lesions of the brain have synergistic effects in dementia of the elderly. *Acta Neuropath.* 2002;**103**:481–487.

87. Esiri MM, Nagy Z, Smith MZ, et al. Cerebrovascular disease and threshold for dementia in the early stages of Alzheimer's disease. *Lancet.* 1999;**354**:919–920.

88. Janota I, Mirsen TR, Hachinski VC, et al. Neuropathologic correlates of leukoaraiosis. *Arch Neurol.* 1989;**46**:1124–1128.

89. Kawamura J, Meyer JS, Terayama Y, Weathers S. Leukoaraiosis correlates with cerebral hypoperfusion in vascular dementia. *Stroke.* 1991;**22**:609–614.

90. Coffman JA, Torello MW, Bornstein RA, et al. Leukoaraiosis in asymptomatic adult offspring of individuals with Alzheimer's disease. *Biol Psychiatry*. 1990;**27**:1244–1248.

91. Thal DR, Ghebremedhin E, Orantes M, Wiestler OD. Vascular pathology in Alzheimer disease: correlation of cerebral amyloid angiopathy and arteriosclerosis/lipohyalinosis with cognitive decline. *J Neuropathol Exp Neurol*. 2003;**63**: 1287–1301.

92. Brown WR, Moody DM, Tytell M, et al. Microembolic brain injuries from cardiac surgery: are they seeds of future Alzheimer's disease? *Ann NY Acad Sci*. 1997;**26**:386–389.

93. Erkinjuntti T, Román, GC, Gauthier S, et al. Emerging therapies for vascular dementia and vascular cognitive impairment. *Stroke*. 2004;**35**:1010–1017.

94. Black S, Román GC, Geldmacher DS, et al. Efficacy and tolerability of donepezil in vascular dementia: positive results of a 24-week, multicenter, international, randomized, placebo-controlled clinical trial. *Stroke*. 2003;**34**:2323–2330.

95. Wilkinson D, Doody R, Helme R, et al. Donepezil in vascular dementia: a randomized, placebo-controlled study. *Neurology*. 2003;**61**:479–486.

96. Erkinjuntti T, Kurz A, Gauthier S, et al. Efficacy of galantamine in probably vascular dementia and Alzheimer's disease combined with cerebrovascular disease: a randomized trial. *Lancet*. 2002;**359**:1283–1290.

97. Moretti R, Torre P, Antonello RM, et al. Rivastigmine in subcortical vascular dementia: an open 22-month study. *J Neurol Sci*. 2002;**203–204**:141–146.

98. Kumar V, Anad R, Messina J, et al. An efficacy and safety analysis of Exelon in Alzheimer's disease patients with concurrent vascular risk factors. *Eur J Neurol*. 2000;**7**:159–169.

99. Orgogozo JM, Rigaud AS, Stoffler A, et al. Efficacy and safety of memantine in patients with mild to moderate vascular dementia: a randomized, placebo-controlled trial (MMM 300). *Stroke*. 2002;**33**:1834–1839.

100. Wilcock G, Mobius HJ, Stoffler A. MMM 500 group; a double-blind, placebo-controlled multicentre study of memantine in mild to moderate vascular dementia (MMM500). *Internat Clin Psychopharmacol*. 2002;**17**:297–305.

101. Görtelmeyer R, Erbler H. Memantine in the treatment of mild to moderate dementia syndrome: a double-blind placebo-controlled study. *Arzneimittelforschung*. 1992;**42**:904–913.

102. Kittner B. Clinical trials of propentofylline in vascular dementia: European/Canadian Propentofylline Study Group. *Alzheimer Dis Associat Disord*. 1999;**13**(Suppl 3):S166–S171.

103. Mielke R, Möller H-J, Erkinjuntti T, et al. Propentofylline in the treatment of vascular dementia and Alzheimer-type dementia: overview of phase I and phase II clinical trials. *Alzheimer Dis Associat Disord*. 1998;**12**(Suppl 2):29–35.

104. Pantoni L, del Ser T, Soglian AG, et al. Efficacy and safety of nimodipine in subcortical vascular dementia: a randomized placebo-controlled trial. *Stroke*. 2005;**36**:619–624.

105. SHEP Cooperative Research Group. Prevention of stroke by antihypertensive drug treatment in older persons with isolated systolic hypertension: final results of the Systolic Hypertension in the Elderly Program (SHEP). SHEP Cooperative Research Group. *JAMA*. 1991;**265**:3255–3264.

106. Forette F, Seux ML, Stassen JA, et al. The prevention of dementia with antihypertensive treatment: new evidence from the Systolic Hypertension in Europe (Syst-Eur) study. *Arch Intern Med*. 2002;**162**:2046–2052.

107. Tzourio C, Anderson C, PROGRESS Management Committee. Blood pressure reduction and risk of dementia in patients with stroke: rationale of the dementia assessment in PROGRESS (Perindopril Protection Against Recurrent Stroke Study). PROGRESS Management Committee. *J Hypertens*. 2000; **18**(Suppl):S21–S24.

108. Lithel H, Hansson L, Skoog I, et al. The Study on Cognition and Prognosis in the Elderly (SCOPE): outcomes in patients not receiving add-on therapy after randomization. *J Hypertens*. 2004;**22**:1605–1612.

109. Jacobson EJ, Salehmoghaddam S, Dorman JA, et al. The effect of blood pressure control on cognitive function (the FOCUS Study). *Am J Hypertens*. 2001;**14**(Suppl):55A–56A.

110. Biessels GJ, Staekenborg S, Brunner E, Brayne C, Scheltens P. Risk of dementia in diabetes mellitus: a systematic review. *Lancet Neurol*. 2006;**5**:64–74.

111. Cuckierman T, Gerstein HC, Williamson JD. Cognitive decline and dementia in diabetes: systematic overview of prospective observational studies. *Diabetologia*. 2005;**48**:2460–2469.

112. Hassan A, Hunt BJ, O'Sullivan M, Bell R, et al. Homocysteine is a risk factor for cerebral small vessel disease, acting via endothelial dysfunction. *Brain*. 2004;**127**:212–219.

113. McMahon JA, Green TJ, Skeaff CM, et al. A controlled trial of homocysteine lowering and cognitive performance. *N Engl J Med*. 2006;**354**:2764–2772.

114. Del Parigi A, Panza F, Capurso C, Solfrizzi V. Nutritional factors, cognitive decline, and dementia. *Brain Res Bull*. 2006;**69**: 1–19.

115. Seeman TE, Singer BH, Rowe JW, Horwitz RI, McEwen BS. Price of adaptation: allostatic load and its health consequences. MacArthur studies of successful aging. *Arch Intern Med*. 1997; **157**:2259–2268.

116. Laurin D, Verreait R, Lindsay J, MacPherson K, Rockwood K. Physical activity and risk of cognitive impairment and dementia in elderly persons. *Arch Neurol*. 2001;**58**:498–504.

117. Colcombe SJ, Erickson KI, Raz N, et al. Aerobic fitness reduces brain tissue loss in aging humans. *J Gerontol A Biol Sci Med Sci*. 2003;**58**:176–180.

118. Yaffe K, Barnes D, Nevitt M, et al. A prospective study of physical activity and cognitive decline in elderly women: women who walk. *Arch Intern Med*. 2001;**161**:1703–1708.

119. Kalmijn S, Launer LJ, Ott A, et al. Dietary fat intake and the risk of incident dementia in the Rotterdam Study. *Ann Neurol*. 1997;**42**:776–792.

120. Kalmijn S, Feskens EJ, Launer LJ, Kromhout D. Polyunsaturated fatty acids, antioxidants, and cognitive function in very old men. *Am J Epidemiol*. 1997;**145**:33–41.

16

Intracerebral Hemorrhage

To kill an error is as good a service as, and sometimes even
better than, the establishing of a new truth or fact.

Charles Darwin

Nontraumatic intracerebral hemorrhage (ICH) accounts for
approximately 10% to 15% of all strokes in Western countries
but occurs relatively more often in other parts of the world.[1–3]
Because hemorrhagic stroke often causes such devastating
neurological dysfunction, it contributes disproportionately to
stroke's cost to family and society.

Intracerebral hemorrhage remains easier to prevent than to
treat, because many of its risk factors, such as arterial hypertension,
smoking and excessive alcohol consumption, are controllable.[4]
The decline in hemorrhagic stroke mortality in recent years is
largely attributable to better identification and treatment of individuals
with systemic hypertension rather than advances in stroke
treatment.[5,6] But with an aging population, we are likely to see a
substantial increase in the absolute number of people with ICH.[7]

The causes of nontraumatic ICH are legion. Some of the
more frequent disorders are discussed in this chapter, and Table
16-1 provides a more complete listing of the known or suspected
risk factors for ICH. Intracranial aneurysms, subarachnoid
hemorrhage, and arteriovenous malformations (AVMs) are
presented in the following two chapters.

CLINICAL FEATURES OF INTRACEREBRAL
HEMORRHAGE

The clinical spectrum of ICH is much broader than the classic
constellation of acute-onset severe headache progressing rapidly
to decreased consciousness. As might be expected, the volume
of an ICH, its location, direction of spread, and the rapidity
with which it develops play a prominent role in determining the
clinical presentation and outcome. Depending on the location
and size of the hemorrhage, approximately half of the patients
have headache, nausea, and vomiting. Patients may exhibit a
variable level of alertness. Seizures are common with lobar hemorrhages.
Individuals with a large ICH that accumulates rapidly
are likely to present with catastrophic neurological dysfunction,
whereas those with a smaller ICH in the same location are less

likely to be comatose but more likely to have focal neurological
deficits.[8] The location of the lesion largely determines the specific
array of focal neurological deficits that occur with a given
hemorrhage. The anatomical structures most likely to be
involved in spontaneous ICH are putamen, thalamus, lobar
subcortical white matter, cerebellum, pons, and caudate nucleus.
Occasional people have multiple hemorrhages at the same time
but in different anatomic locations.[9] Not surprisingly, their
prognosis is worse than for individuals with a single lesion.

The neurologic signs generated by an ICH overlap those of
a similarly placed ischemic infarction (see Chapter 3). Without
modern imaging techniques, it is nearly impossible to distinguish
with absolute confidence ICH from ischemic stroke.
Patients with either condition can experience acute headache,
and those with a brainstem infarction, in particular, often have
altered consciousness. Likewise, a small ICH may cause a focal
neurological deficit without headache or stupor. The occurrence
of both hemorrhage and infarction in the same individual adds
another layer of complexity. An individual with a minimally
symptomatic ischemic infarction, for example, sometimes deteriorates
dramatically because hemorrhagic transformation of
the infarction occurs. Similarly, an ischemic infarction can
develop adjacent to a hemorrhage after the arterial blood supply
to the area is compromised by the hemorrhage. Systemic disorders
that promote hemorrhage can play an independent role in
the clinical presentation, influence the location of the lesion,
and determine the risk of recurrent hemorrhage.

In this section we describe some of the subtypes of ICH, and
in the following chapter we present the clinical manifestations
of subarachnoid hemorrhage (SAH).

Putaminal Hemorrhage

About 33% of ICHs due to hypertension occur in the putamen
(Figure 16-1). The initial manifestation of a putaminal hemorrhage
is typically an abrupt onset of hemiplegia contralateral to
the hematoma, often accompanied by headache, vomiting, and
a decreasing level of alertness. Gaze preference and contralateral
homonymous hemianopia are the rule. In dominant putaminal
lesions, aphasia is common, but its characteristics vary with the

Table 16-1: Risk Factors for Spontaneous Intracerebral Hemorrhage

Arterial hypertension

- Essential
- Secondary

Aneurysms

- Saccular
- Infective
- Traumatic
- Neoplastic

Vascular malformations

- Arteriovenous malformations
- Capillary telangiectasias
- Cavernous malformations
- Developmental venous anomalies

Bleeding diatheses

- Leukemia
- Thrombocytopenia
- Disseminated intravascular coagulation
- Polycythemia
- Hyperviscosity syndromes
- Hemophilia
- Hypoprothrombinemia
- Afibrinogenemia
- Selective factor deficiencies
- Von Willebrand disease
- Sickle cell anemia
- Antiplatelet therapy
- Anticoagulant therapy (heparin, warfarin)
- Thrombolytic therapy

Cerebral amyloid angiopathy

Arteritis/arteriopathies

- Infectious vasculitis
- Multisystem vasculitis
- Isolated CNS angiitis
- Moyamoya disease

Drug-related

- Amphetamines
- Cocaine
- Phenylpropanolamine
- Talwin-pyribenzamine
- Phencyclidine
- Heroin
- MAOI
- Alcohol

Intracranial tumors

- Primary malignant or benign
- Metastatic

Cerebral venous occlusive disease

Miscellaneous risk factors

- After carotid endarterectomy
- After extracranial/intracranial stenting procedures
- After neurosurgery (e.g. DBE implantation)
- After spinal anesthesia
- Postmyelography
- Lightning stroke
- Heat stroke
- Fat embolism
- After painful dental procedures
- Protracted migraine
- Methanol intoxication

Hemorrhagic transformation of infarction

Adapted with permission from Biller and Shah.[119]
CNS = central nervous system; DBE = deep brain electrode; MAOI = monoamine oxidase inhibitors.

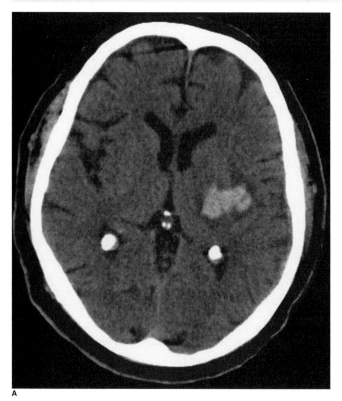

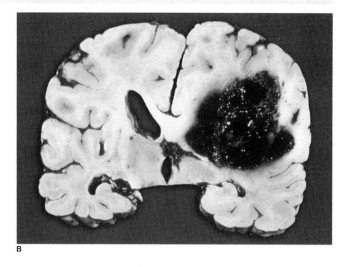

Figure 16-1. A: Cranial CT from a 68-year-old man with chronic arterial hypertension shows a hemorrhage in the left putamen. B: Coronal brain section (from a different patient with hypertension) reveals a large putaminal hemorrhage with ventricular penetration and mass effect.

size and placement of the lesion. Right putaminal hemorrhages cause apractagnosia, left visual neglect, and constructional apraxia.

Lobar Hemorrhage

About a quarter of all ICHs occur in the subcortical white matter and affect mainly one cerebral lobe. Most lobar hematomas involve the posterior brain regions, primarily the parietal, temporal, and occipital lobes. Individuals with lobar hematomas (Figure 16-2) usually present with sudden-onset headache and a focal neurological deficit, not unlike patients with hemorrhages in other locations. However, lobar hematomas differ in several important ways. Because lobar hemorrhages involve the cerebral cortex, affected individuals are more likely to develop epileptic seizures and to have deficits of higher cortical function than patients with more deeply seated hematomas.

Patients with lobar hematomas generally have a better prognosis than those with a brainstem or putaminal hemorrhage even though the lobar hemorrhage is often larger. The risk of recurrent hemorrhage is higher in individuals with a lobar hemorrhage than it is in patients with a brainstem or basal ganglia hemorrhage, probably because of the array of underlying conditions that cause lobar hematomas but perhaps also because more people with a lobar hemorrhage survive the initial hemorrhage.

Chronic hypertension may be responsible for many lobar hemorrhages, but it is not nearly so dominant a risk factor as in other locations. The etiology of lobar hemorrhage in one series of 26 patients included hypertension (eight patients), metastatic tumor (one patient), and two patients each with coagulopathy due to warfarin and with an AVM.[10] Cerebral amyloid angiopathy

(CAA) was documented in six of 29 patients with lobar hemorrhage in another series.[11]

Frontal lobe hemorrhages are typically accompanied by headache, contralateral hemiparesis, and conjugate eye deviation toward the diseased hemisphere.[10] Severity of motor findings varies with the size of the hematoma and proximity to the motor cortex. Focal motor seizures may also occur.

Parietal lobe hemorrhages (Figure 16-2) can be accompanied by pain in the homolateral temple or above the ear, moderate contralateral sensory loss, neglect of the contralateral visual field, and mild to moderate hemiparesis. A lesion in the dominant parietal lobe may be accompanied by Gerstmann syndrome, whereas hemineglect, constructional, and dressing apraxias are more common with a lobar hemorrhage of the nondominant parietal lobe.

Occipital lobe hemorrhages classically cause ipsilateral orbital region pain. Contralateral homonymous hemianopia is usually present.[10]

Temporal lobe hemorrhages may generate a contralateral homonymous hemianopia or superior quadrantanopia if the hematoma enlarges enough to encroach on the optic radiations. Pain near the homolateral ear may occur. If the dominant temporal lobe is involved, Wernicke's aphasia may develop.

Thalamic Hemorrhages

About 20% of ICHs occur in the thalamus, and bilateral thalamic hemorrhages may occur, especially in individuals with hypertension (Figure 16-3). Thalamic hemorrhages often begin with contralateral hemisensory loss, variable weakness, and altered consciousness.[8,12] If the adjacent internal capsule is

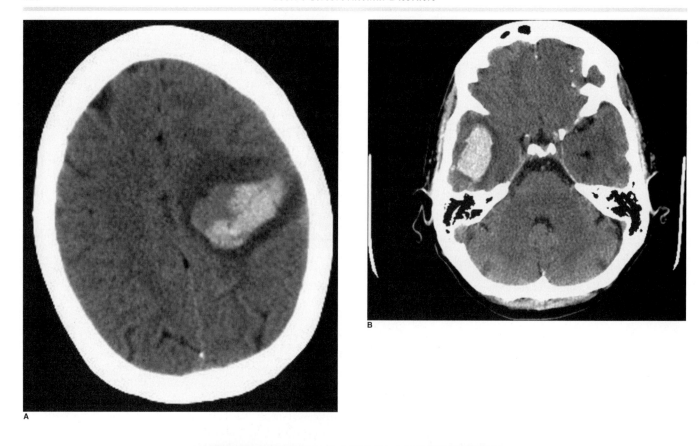

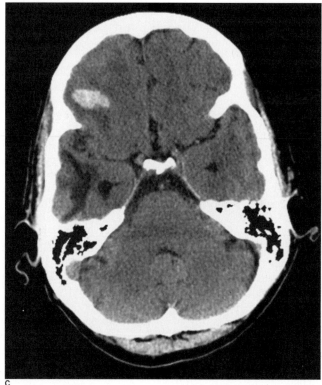

Figure 16-2. Cranial CT demonstrates lobar hemorrhage in the parietal lobe (A), temporal lobe (B), and frontal lobe (C). The parietal lobe hemorrhage was due to a cavernous malformation, while the temporal and frontal lesions resulted from amyloid angiopathy.

involved, there is contralateral hemiparesis or hemiplegia. Upward extension may cause contralateral hemianopia. Medial extension causes hemorrhage into the third ventricle. Inferior extension causes the pupils to be small and sluggishly reactive to light. If the subthalamic-diencephalic regions are involved, there may be downward and inward deviation of the eyes with paralysis of upward gaze. The eyes may be tonically deviated away from the thalamic hemorrhage. Pathologic lid retraction occurs with damage to the posterior commissure. Other neuro-ophthalmological abnormalities may include nystagmus retractorius, skew deviation, and ocular tilt.

Patients with dominant thalamic hemorrhages may develop a subcortical type of aphasia with severe anomia and relative preservation of comprehension and repetition after an initial period of mutism or near-mutism. When the nondominant thalamus is involved, anosognosia is often present. If blood leaks into the third ventricle, the resulting clot can block the aqueduct of Sylvius and cause obstructive hydrocephalus.

Prognosis of thalamic hemorrhage is directly related to the size of the lesion: a thalamic hemorrhage greater than 3 cm in diameter is often fatal.

Caudate Hemorrhages

Spontaneous hematomas of the head of the caudate nucleus account for about 5% of all primary ICHs. Rupture into the ventricles may cause symptoms mimicking SAH. Sometimes the hemorrhage extends to neighboring structures, causing hemiparesis, hemisensory symptoms, gaze palsy, cognitive symptoms, and/or oculosympathetic disturbances. Outcome of a caudate hemorrhage is usually favorable provided that intraventricular extension of the hemorrhage does not occur.

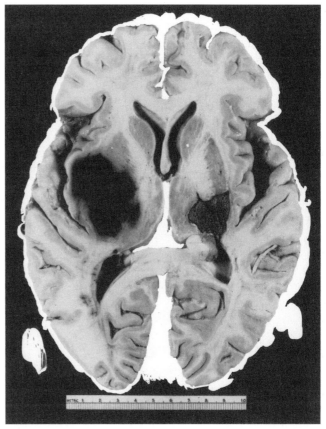

Figure 16-3. Horizontal brain section showing bilateral hemorrhages: an older lesion of the thalamus on the right and a new hemorrhage into the corpus striatum on the left.

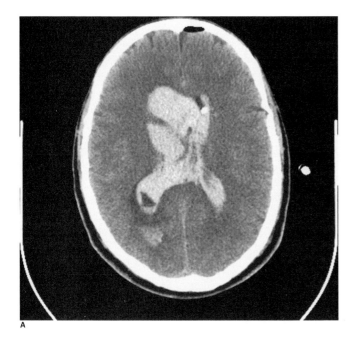

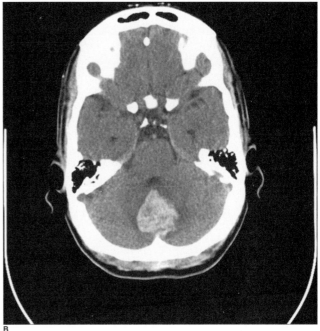

Figure 16-4. A: Cranial CT depicts a right thalamic hemorrhage dissecting into the ventricles to cause massive intraventricular hemorrhage and hydrocephalus. A left ventricular drain has partially decompressed the left ventricle and a fluid-fluid level is evident in the lateral horns of the right lateral ventricle. B: Cranial CT demonstrates a 3-cm acute parenchymal hemorrhage centered in the superior cerebellar vermis, extending into the medial aspect of the left cerebellar hemisphere.

Intraventricular Hemorrhage

Intraventricular hemorrhage (IVH; Figure 16-4 A) may be primary or secondary. Primary IVH accounts for some 3% of ICHs. SAH and IVH often occur together, which is not surprising given the communication between these two spaces.[13] The clinical presentation of primary IVH resembles that of SAH (Chapter 17) with sudden onset of a severe headache and impaired consciousness.[14] In alert patients survival is common, but functional recovery is often incomplete.[13]

Hematomas that remain confined to the subependymal region may be asymptomatic or present as a mass lesion or with contralateral weakness. These lesions often resolve spontaneously and leave no residual dysfunction.

Causes of primary IVH often overlap with those of ICH. Arterial hypertension causes IVH infrequently, but AVMs, cavernous malformations, tumors, and coagulopathies are regularly reported. As anterior communicating artery aneurysms are separated from the third ventricle by only the thin-walled lamina terminalis, rupture of an aneurysm in this location commonly leads to prominent IVH.

Cerebellar Hemorrhages

Cerebellar hemorrhage (Figure 16-4 B) accounts for 8% to 10% of all spontaneous ICHs. The most common cause of spontaneous cerebellar hemorrhage is arterial hypertension.[15] Cerebellar hemorrhages related to hypertension tend to occur in the area of the dentate nucleus and may spread to involve the ipsilateral cerebellar hemisphere and peduncles or rupture into the IV ventricle. The hemorrhage rarely extends into the brainstem. Other causes of cerebellar hemorrhage include blood dyscrasias, coagulopathies, AVMs, or tumors.

Cerebellar hemorrhage is typically heralded by headaches, dizziness, vertigo, and repeated vomiting. Inability to stand or walk, truncal or appendicular ataxia, an ipsilateral gaze palsy, and ipsilateral CN VII palsy may be present.[15] The hematoma may dissect into the brainstem or extrude into the subarachnoid space or the fourth ventricle. Swelling from the hematoma and the surrounding edema can be dramatic enough to cause herniation of the cerebellar tonsils into the foramen magnum with brainstem compression or, less commonly, upward herniation through the tentorial incisura with midbrain compression. Nuchal rigidity can signify either brainstem herniation into the foramen magnum or presence of subarachnoid bleeding.

When there is pontine compression by a cerebellar hemorrhage, the clinical manifestations closely resemble those of a pontine hemorrhage, with coma, flaccid tetraplegia, small reactive pupils, ocular bobbing, and signs of an autonomic abnormality (including hyperpyrexia and respiratory abnormality).

Death sometimes ensues rapidly, but the clinical picture is more often that of an expanding posterior fossa tumor with bilateral corticospinal tract signs and increased intracranial pressure (ICP). The most consistent signs of impending clinical deterioration after a cerebellar hemorrhage are acute hydrocephalus and location of the hemorrhage in the vermis with compression of ventricular and subarachnoid flow.[16] Prompt recognition of a cerebellar hemorrhage is essential because emergency surgical decompression can be lifesaving.[17]

Pontine Hemorrhages

Approximately 7% of ICHs occur in the pons. Bleeding in the pons typically begins at the junction of the basis pontis with the tegmentum, usually at the midpontine level. Sudden onset of coma, without premonitory warning or headaches, is the rule, and death may occur within hours.[18] Bilateral long-tract signs and decerebrate rigidity are commonplace. In the earlier stages contralateral hemiplegia may be accompanied by homolateral facial paralysis or other cranial nerve palsies. In contrast to hemispheric lesions, pontine hemorrhage is usually characterized by permanent deviation of the eyes and head away from the side of the lesion and impairment of eye movement reflexes during caloric or oculocephalic stimulation. Bilateral, horizontal gaze paralysis with ocular bobbing, characterized by rapid conjugate downward movements of the eyes followed by a slow upward drive to primary position, may occur.

In the later stages a pentad of poor prognostic "P" factors develops: paralysis, pulsus parvus, pinpoint pupils, pyrexia, and periodic respiration. These late signs are so characteristic of a pontine lesion that the only conditions that remain to be considered are drug overdosage and intraventricular hemorrhage.

Damage to the lateral basis pontis may cause a pure motor hemiparesis. Hemorrhages in the lateral pontine tegmentum may account for an ipsilateral conjugate gaze paresis, ipsilateral internuclear ophthalmoplegia, the "one-and-a-half" syndrome, and ocular bobbing. Lateral tegmental hemorrhages may cause ipsilateral hemiataxia with contralateral hemiparesis and hemisensory deficits.

Midbrain Hemorrhage

Primary hemorrhage into the midbrain (Figure 16-5) is extraordinarily rare. When it does occur, it results in ipsilateral oculomotor paralysis and contralateral long-tract signs (Weber syndrome).[19] If the hemorrhage enlarges, these signs become bilateral; involvement of the ascending reticular activating system causes coma, and blockage of the aqueduct of Sylvius causes hydrocephalus and acute elevation of ICP.

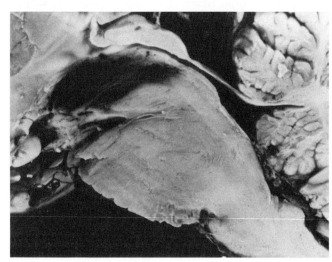

Figure 16-5. Sagittal section of the brain showing a midbrain hemorrhage.

Medulla Oblongata Hemorrhage

Medulla oblongata hemorrhage is rare. Its main symptoms include vertigo, headache, long tract signs, dysphagia, and dysarthria.

ETIOLOGY OF ICH

There are numerous conditions that increase the risk of ICH, and these risk factors are summarized in Table 16-1. Several of the more common reasons for ICH are discussed individually in this section. In general, the causes of nontraumatic ICH fall into four categories:

1. Abnormal arteries unable to withstand normal systemic arterial pressure. Included in this group are congenital vascular defects such as arteriovenous malformations and intracranial aneurysms along with acquired conditions such as arteritis.
2. Clotting abnormalities that fail to contain what would otherwise be minor bleeding, such as inherited or acquired coagulopathies or severe thrombocytopenia.
3. Sustained elevation of arterial blood pressure. A brief increase in blood pressure does not typically cause a hemorrhage, although transiently elevated blood pressure may be problematic in individuals with coexisting blood vessel lesions.
4. Increased venous pressure due to obstruction of venous outflow, typically due to back pressure from an intracranial venous thrombosis.

Naturally, some individuals do not fit neatly into any one of the above categories, as in the person with an intracranial AVM as well as systemic hypertension. Nevertheless, this is a useful way to conceptualize the causes of intraparenchymal brain hemorrhage.

Arterial Hypertension

Arterial hypertension increases the risk of both ICH and ischemic infarction, and, in each case normalization of the blood pressure lowers the stroke risk.[20,21] In most cases hemorrhage originates from penetrating arteries, some of which plunge into brain parenchyma perpendicular to the course of the superficial cortical vessels from which they arise. Hypertensive hemorrhages occur most often in the putamen, thalamus, cerebellum, or pons.

Stroke risk increases with severity of hypertension and with the length of time that the individual has been hypertensive. In one series of 68 children and adolescents with spontaneous ICH, for example, none of the patients had a history of systemic hypertension.[22] Transient increases in systemic blood pressure do not normally create difficulty for individuals with an AVM.[23] This is not necessarily true for individuals with an aneurysm or when the pressure elevation is higher or more prolonged. Furthermore, among adults with treated hypertension, hypokalemia (defined as a potassium equal to or less than 3.4 mmol/L) in the year before a stroke was associated with an increased risk of ischemic and hemorrhagic stroke.

Bleeding due to chronic arterial hypertension probably results from the rupture of an arteriole weakened by the effects of prolonged arterial hypertension. Hypertension induces proliferation of arteriolar smooth muscle followed by apoptotic smooth muscle cell death and then collagen deposition. The collagen-laden arteriole is less contractile and prone to develop ectatic areas.[24] Over time the arterioles lengthen and develop dilated, tortuous, looped, or corkscrew shapes. Traditionally these dilated areas have been characterized as Charcot-Bouchard aneurysms, but Challa and colleagues could not demonstrate true Charcot-Bouchard aneurysms in any of the 35 autopsied hypertensive patients, among whom four spontaneous ICHs had occurred. Instead, coils, twists, and knuckles in arterioles that mimicked aneurysm were demonstrated.[25]

Central Nervous System Vascular Malformations

Intracranial aneurysms (Chapter 17), cavernous malformations, and AVMs (Chapter 18) all cause ICH. Although bleeding from these lesions can occur at any age, individuals with ICH due to any of these lesions tend to be younger than the average patient with a hypertensive ICH. Not only do these lesions tend to bleed before old age, but other causes of hemorrhage, notably chronic arterial hypertension and CAA, tend to cause hemorrhage later in life.

Each of these vascular lesions can cause subarachnoid, intraparenchymal, or intraventricular bleeding, either alone or in combination. But despite their overlapping clinical manifestations, aneurysms, AVMs, and cavernous malformations each have distinct clinical tendencies. Saccular aneurysms usually lie within the subarachnoid space, so SAH almost always occurs when an aneurysm ruptures, even when there is also intraparenchymal hemorrhage. In contrast, aneurysms resulting from infective emboli or from a cardiac myxoma tend to occur in the distal arterial branches, so hemorrhage from these aneurysms tends to be intraparenchymal. Hemorrhage from an AVM usually accumulates within the brain parenchyma surrounding the AVM, and subarachnoid bleeding is variable. Cavernous malformations (Figure 16-6) also cause intraparenchymal hemorrhage, but the low pressure within these lesions tends to cause less severe clinical manifestations than occurs with an aneurysm or an AVM.

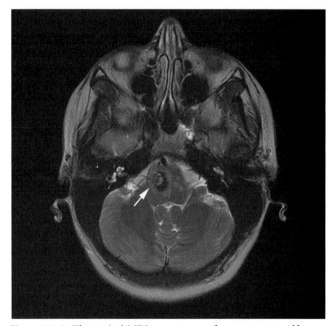

Figure 16-6. The typical MRI appearance of a cavernous malformation, in this case in the right pontine region. Note the lesion's characteristic high signal core that is surrounded by a dark ring of residual methemoglobin from one or more earlier hemorrhages.

Although brain hemorrhage has also been attributed to developmental venous anomalies (DVAs), these structures are functional anatomical variants that almost never bleed. However, they often occur in proximity to a small cavernous malformation, so a brain hemorrhage adjacent to a DVA should prompt a meticulous search for one of these lesions.

About 20% of individuals with an intracranial aneurysm have more than one aneurysm, and multiple AVMs are occasionally documented. Familial intracranial aneurysms are well described, and multiple cavernous malformations are inherited as an autosomal dominant trait in some families.[26–29]

Identification and treatment of an intracranial aneurysm or AVM in a patient with an ICH is vital because of the potentially devastating effects of a second hemorrhage. Small aneurysms or AVMs can be missed even with catheter angiography, especially when they occur near a hemorrhage. When there is no apparent explanation for an acute ICH, it is reasonable to repeat a catheter angiogram once the hemorrhage has begun to resolve.

Hemorrhagic Infarction

Any ischemic stroke can become hemorrhagic and confluent, broadening the list of potential causes of an intraparenchymal hemorrhage dramatically to include many of the causes of ischemic stroke. Hemorrhage within an existing infarction probably results when blood flow is restored to infarcted tissue whose damaged blood vessels can no longer withstand the force of the systemic blood pressure. Dissolution of a proximal clot by natural thrombolysis may be responsible for most hemorrhagic transformations, although existing collateral channels may play a role as well.[30] Initially there are multiple petechial hemorrhages that gradually enlarge and coalesce (Figure 16-7). Hemorrhagic infarction occurs more often after an embolic infarction than after thrombotic infarction and occurs more frequently with larger infarctions.[31,32] Hemorrhage can be identified in up to two-thirds of patients with ischemic strokes by magnetic

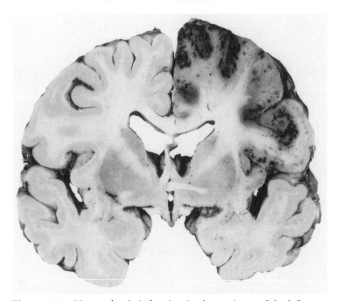

Figure 16-7. Hemorrhagic infarction in the territory of the left anterior and middle cerebral arteries caused by a thrombosis of the intracranial internal carotid artery. Note the gyral swelling and the confluent petechial hemorrhages.

resonance imaging (MRI) but the vast majority of these lesions do not cause additional symptoms.[31] The likelihood of a hemorrhagic conversion increases when blood flow is restored long after the infarction takes place, as evidenced by the increased risk of hemorrhage when tissue plasminogen activator (tPA) administration is delayed.

Hemorrhage after Cerebral Sinovenous Thrombosis

Intraparenchymal hemorrhage is common after cerebral sinovenous thrombosis (CVST; see Chapter 20). The hemorrhage typically develops in the region being drained by the thrombosed venous channel, presumably because of a combination of tissue damage and increased venous pressure in the region affected by the thrombosis. The initial presentation is determined by which venous sinus or venous channel is occluded. Frequent manifestations include headache, seizures, and visual disturbances. Although hemorrhage secondary to CSVT can have serious consequences, patients who survive often recover fully.

Coagulation Disorders

Numerous congenital and acquired coagulation disorders have been documented in individuals with hemorrhagic stroke. Hemorrhagic stroke occurs in some individuals treated with therapeutic agents such as warfarin and tissue plasminogen activator. In addition, acquired coagulopathies (e.g., due to hepatic dysfunction) and congenital coagulation defects (e.g., hemophilia or von Willebrand disease) can cause an ICH (see Chapter 11). As a general rule, the risk of hemorrhagic stroke increases in direct proportion to the severity of the coagulopathy, and the specific nature of the bleeding tendency is less important.

Symptomatic ICH has been reported among 0.4% to 1.3% of patients with myocardial infarction treated with alteplase.[33–35] In the 1995 NINDS study of tPA for ischemic stroke, symptomatic ICH within 36 hours of the index stroke occurred in 6.4% of the subjects who received tPA, but only in 0.6% of the individuals in the placebo arm.[36] Nevertheless, the individuals receiving tPA were at least 30% more likely to have little or no disability 3 months after their stroke, and the overall outcome at 3 months was enough to offset the risk of hemorrhage when the drug is given within 3 hours of symptom onset.[36,37] Subsequent trials suggest that tPA is beneficial when given up to 4.5 hours after the onset of symptoms.[38] The ability to identify individuals at high risk for hemorrhage might allow the use of tPA to be safely broadened by not treating the high-risk patients (see Chapter 25). Predictors of a higher risk of hemorrhage include, in addition to delayed drug administration, a large lesion, greater severity on the stroke-rating scale (NIHSS), higher baseline blood glucose levels, advanced age, and a hyperdense artery sign.[39,40]

With the widespread use of long-term oral anticoagulation for the prevention of cardioembolic stroke, the number of individuals with hemorrhagic stroke due to anticoagulation has increased. One study estimated that the number of people taking an anticoagulant who developed a hemorrhagic stroke increased from 0.8 per 100,000 in 1988 to 4.4 per 100,000 in 1999.[41] The increased risk of hemorrhage while taking warfarin appears to be justified by studies showing a significant reduction in the ischemic stroke risk in patients with atrial fibrillation who take warfarin. Nevertheless, the dose should be monitored closely because hemorrhage risk seems to increase in proportion to the degree of anticoagulation.

The actual risk of intracranial bleeding due to anticoagulants or antiplatelet drugs may not be as high as once suspected, and their use may be justified in some situations even when there is existing ICH. In one small series, for example, none of the 12 patients who developed a hemorrhagic infarction while taking warfarin or heparin for embolism prevention deteriorated despite continued anticoagulation.[42] Similarly, antiplatelet agents did not promote recurrent hemorrhage in a cohort of 46 individuals with a previous brain hemorrhage who later began taking antiplatelet agents for cardiac disease.[43] Neither of these series is large enough to be conclusive, but they do suggest that a recent or remote history of ICH is not an absolute contraindication when the risk from recurrent embolism or thrombosis is high.

Newborns are at risk for hemorrhage from vitamin K deficiency, but hemorrhagic disease of the newborn has become rare in countries where supplemental vitamin K is routinely given right after birth.[44,45] Babies whose mothers took phenobarbital, phenytoin, or other selected medications during pregnancy often require a higher dose of supplemental vitamin K to prevent neonatal hemorrhage.[46–49] It is reasonable in this situation to provide supplemental vitamin K during pregnancy.

Platelet Disorders

Thrombocytopenia (Chapter 11) is unlikely to cause a spontaneous hemorrhagic stroke unless the platelet count is extremely low, usually less than 20,000/mm³. Thrombocytopenia results from either inadequate production of platelets by the bone marrow or too rapid destruction of the platelets once they are circulating. Examples of inadequate production would include aplastic anemia or destruction of the megakaryocytes by chemotherapeutic agents, whereas excessive turnover results from isoimmune thrombocytopenia (ITP), thrombotic thrombocytopenic purpura (TTP), and hemolytic-uremic syndrome. Brain hemorrhage has been documented with all of these conditions, but not usually until the platelet count has become very low.

As with the coagulation disorders, a platelet count that would not be low enough to cause a spontaneous life-threatening condition can be problematic when coupled with trauma. Similarly, moderate thrombocytopenia may delay needed surgery or a lumbar puncture until a platelet transfusion can be given.

Abnormal platelet function can increase the risk of hemorrhagic stroke even when the platelet count is normal or only slightly reduced, as occurs with the administration of antiplatelet agents for stroke and heart attack prevention. The risk of hemorrhagic stroke from the use of prophylactic aspirin or other antiplatelet agent is relatively low and no doubt more than compensated by the reduction in the risk of ischemic stroke and myocardial infarction. Nevertheless, most large trials of antiplatelet agents report a small increase in the risk of hemorrhagic complications.

Hyperperfusion Syndrome

Brain hemorrhage or hemorrhagic infarction occasionally occurs in the setting of cerebral hyperperfusion syndrome following revascularization of the carotid or vertebral arteries with endarterectomy or stenting.[50–52] In a review of 2,452 consecutive endarterectomies, Wilson and Ammar identified five hemorrhagic strokes, a rate of only 0.20% (however, these cases represented 13.5% of all postoperative neurological complications).[53] Hemorrhage probably occurs more often when surgery is done on an acutely occluded artery than a stenotic one.[54]

The symptoms of the hyperperfusion syndrome depend on the vascular territory affected, but often include headache, seizures, new focal neurological deficits, and confusion.[55] Radiographic studies may remain normal or reveal edema, infarction, or hemorrhage.[55]

The pathophysiology of hemorrhage following perfusion restoration is probably multifactorial. Blood flow studies suggest that the distal brain perfusion may double in some individuals following an endarterectomy, and loss of normal autoregulatory function during the period preceding surgery may impair the brain's ability to adjust to this sudden augmentation of perfusion.[50] The situation is further complicated by the occurrence of systemic hypertension in some individuals following carotid endarterectomy.[56] When perioperative ischemia was present at the time of the procedure, a subsequent hemorrhage may result in much the same fashion as a hemorrhagic infarction. The use of perioperative anticoagulants may play a role in some individuals.[57] Single photon emission tomography (SPECT) sometimes documents a striking increase in perfusion in individuals who remain asymptomatic.[52,58]

Implanted Electrodes

Seijo and associates reported an ICH in 3.3% of 130 Parkinson disease patients with 272 deep-brain–stimulating electrodes.[59] In another study of 259 patients with 567 implanted electrodes, Sansur and colleagues documented symptomatic hemorrhage in 1.2% but noted that the risk of sustaining a permanent neurologic deficit was only 0.7%.[60] Because of the disabling nature of Parkinson disease and the fact that such stimulators tend to be inserted after appropriate medication has failed, this is probably an acceptable risk.

Cerebral Amyloid Angiopathy

Cerebral amyloid angiopathy results from the deposition of ß-amyloid into arteries of the cerebral cortex and the leptomeninges. Neumann was the first to suggest a link between cerebral amyloid angiopathy and ICH in a 1960 description of a 45-year-old woman with severe amyloid angiopathy who had two lobar hemorrhages plus numerous additional petechial hemorrhages.[61] Cerebral amyloid angiopathy is now recognized as a common cause of lobar brain hemorrhage, but it is almost certainly underrecognized. Although the majority of patients with hemorrhage due to cerebral amyloid angiopathy are seen sporadically, several familial forms of cerebral amyloid angiopathy and brain hemorrhage have been identified.[62–65] A mutation of the amyloid precursor protein gene on chromosome 21q21 can result in either familial cerebral amyloid angiopathy or an autosomal dominant form of Alzheimer disease. The epsilon 2 and epsilon 4 alleles of the apolipoprotein E (APOE) gene similarly predisposes to hemorrhage from cerebral amyloid angiopathy.[66,67]

Cerebral amyloid angiopathy should be suspected in elderly individuals who present with a lobar brain hemorrhage in the absence of other risk factors for hemorrhage. Many of these individuals already have cognitive impairment by the time the hemorrhage occurs.[68] Knudsen and colleagues diagnosed cerebral amyloid angiopathy with the Boston diagnostic criteria in 13 of 39 individuals with primary lobar cerebral hemorrhage, and the diagnosis was pathologically confirmed in all 13 of these patients.[69] These authors conclude that an antemortem diagnosis of cerebral amyloid angiopathy is feasible using the established clinical diagnostic criteria. Individuals with the familial form of amyloid angiopathy tend to develop symptoms two or three decades earlier than those with the sporadic form.[70]

Okazaki and colleagues summarized 23 patients aged 60 to 97 years old at the time of autopsy who had significant cerebrovascular amyloid deposits.[68] All 23 of the individuals in this series had multiple small cortical infarctions and hemorrhages, and nine patients, only two of whom had a history of systemic hypertension, had died because of a large cerebral hemorrhage.[68]

Pathological findings of cerebral amyloid angiopathy include amyloid deposition in the media and intima of cortical and leptomeningeal arteries.[68] Amyloid deposition can be seen in large and medium-sized arteries as well as the smaller vessels, but the resulting luminal stenosis may result in the smaller vessels becoming symptomatic earlier and more often than the larger ones.[68] There are typically multiple small cortical infarctions and small hemorrhagic lesions. Over time, the severity of the vascular changes and the number of cortical lesions increase.[71]

The presence of the APOE epsilon 2 allele may increase the likelihood of brain hemorrhage due to hypertension, trauma, or antithrombotic agents.[67,72] Effective therapy for cerebral amyloid angiopathy is not currently available.

Hemorrhage within Brain Tumors

Acute intraparenchymal brain hemorrhage is relatively common among individuals with brain tumors.[73–75] Licata and Turazzi identified 110 patients with an intracranial tumor who developed symptomatic intraparenchymal brain hematomas.[76] This subgroup represented 4.4% of their 2,514 patients with hemorrhagic stroke who underwent surgery and 1.5% of the individuals with brain tumors. In large case series of children with ICH, the frequency of hemorrhagic transformation of tumors is between 13% and 15%.[22,77]

Tumors that are associated with hemorrhage often tend to be high-grade malignancies, so, not surprisingly, the prognosis for these individuals is poor.[76,78] Highly malignant tumors are more likely to develop necrotic areas as the rapid tumor growth outstrips the available blood supply, probably explaining the occurrence of hemorrhage within the tumor.

The presence of an underlying tumor has significant implications for the patient's treatment and prognosis. Tumor-associated hemorrhage should be considered particularly when the patient has no apparent risk factors for brain hemorrhage. It can be difficult to recognize the tumor mingled with hemorrhage and edema, but MRI with contrast infusion seems to be more reliable at this task than computed tomography (CT).

Drug-Induced Hemorrhage

Intracranial hemorrhage has been described after the use of amphetamines or cocaine, either intravenously or by mouth.[79–82] One patient's brain biopsy showed lymphocytic infiltration, endothelial thickening, and deposition of an amorphous material in and around the vessel walls.[83] Additional evidence is provided by angiographic studies that show an irregular beaded appearance of some of the intracranial arteries as well as with segmental changes in the caliber of the vessels, suggesting diffuse spasm.

Phenylpropanolamine (PPA) was used for decades as a nasal decongestant and, at a higher dose, a diet aid. The initial publications tying PPA to hemorrhagic stroke were largely case reports, and one analysis of thousands of individuals from a single health maintenance organization failed to show an increased stroke risk.[84] The drug was removed from the U.S. market several years ago after a case-controlled study found a slightly increased risk of hemorrhage in women taking PPA as a diet aid (but not in men or in individuals taking it for respiratory infections).[85] Although the methodology of this study left several issues unanswered, the drug's removal from the market renders these questions largely moot. There have been similar anecdotal reports suggesting that ephedra might cause stroke, but a case-controlled analysis failed to demonstrate an increased stroke risk.[86] The excessive consumption of alcohol also increases the risk of hemorrhagic stroke.[4,87]

Moyamoya Disease

Adults with moyamoya tend to develop intraparenchymal or subarachnoid hemorrhage, although, like children, adults are also at risk for ischemic stroke due to moyamoya.[88,89] Moyamoya disease typically begins as a progressive occlusive vasculopathy of both terminal internal carotid arteries, followed later by the development of a network of dilated collateral vessels in the basal ganglia region distal to the stenotic internal carotid arteries. Hemorrhage in adults with moyamoya tends to occur in this region or into the subarachnoid space. Hemorrhage in some of these individuals arises from an aneurysm.[90–93] In other patients the hemorrhage evidently arises directly from the dilated collateral vessels in the absence of an aneurysm, presumably as a result of years of dilatation and distention of these collateral channels.[94] There is some evidence that the risk of hemorrhage may increase during pregnancy.[95,96] Moyamoya is presented in more detail in Chapter 13.

PATHOPHYSIOLOGY

Most brain hemorrhages begin as a liquid hematoma that expands within the brain parenchyma and then dissects along fiber tracts. As the lesion expands, the surrounding tissue is compressed, and nearby traversing venules and capillaries are torn. The vessels ruptured by the accumulating clot add their complement of blood, and the process accelerates. As the process continues, compression of the adjacent brain and vasculature results in secondary infarction, edema, and transtentorial herniation.

Clotting and spasm of the bleeding arteries may slow the accumulation of blood. The pressure within the area may increase sufficiently to tamponade further extravasation of blood. Most of the bleeding occurs in the first 3 hours, but later rebleeding may occur as natural thrombolysis occurs and the vasospasm relaxes. The average blood volume is about 35 ml (i.e., ping-pong-ball sized), and if the accumulating blood exceeds 60 ml, many of the patients die. The outlook is more favorable for lobar hemorrhages.

Lobar hemorrhages tend to be larger than those originating in the basal ganglia. Most large ICHs are fatal, death being caused by rupture into the ventricular system or by swelling of such degree that it causes herniation of the mesial portions of the temporal lobes through the incisura of the tentorium cerebelli. The resulting displacement and compression of the midbrain ruptures veins and small arterioles in its upper portion, leading to arteriolar and venous hemorrhage into the midbrain and pons and, eventually, death. In patients who survive, the blood is eventually reabsorbed, leaving a cavity or fibrous tissue.

In some instances, especially when the lesion is small, the hemorrhage is reabsorbed, leaving a lake of dark chocolate-colored fluid surrounded by a fibroglial wall. Laminated clots, some with calcification, are indicative of repeated hemorrhages.

DIAGNOSTIC EVALUATION

Differential Diagnosis

In the typical patient, the diagnosis of an ICH is straightforward. However, several entities can mimic the signs and symptoms of an ICH, including SAH, CSVT, ischemic infarction, meningitis, encephalitis, and hypertensive encephalopathy. Each of these conditions can present with sudden headache, decreased sensorium, and increased ICP. In addition, sudden deterioration in a previously asymptomatic individual with a brain tumor or abscess can be confused with an ICH. Acute deterioration due to an undiagnosed mass lesion is relatively common and is most often due to hemorrhage within the lesion, compression of a nearby vessel, or herniation of brain tissue.

In a comatose patient, the absence of localizing signs favors a diagnosis of ICH over infarction. Transient unconsciousness initially followed by progressive deterioration of the sensorium is more often due to an intracranial hematoma than a cerebral infarction. Although the differentiation of hemorrhage from infarction by history and examination is often impossible, imaging studies usually make it obvious.

Signs of meningeal irritation suggest SAH, but these signs also occur because of impending tonsillar cerebellar herniation or meningitis. Obvious papilledema immediately after the onset of symptoms suggests that elevated ICP was already present when the clinical deterioration occurred, which in turn would favor a tumor, hypertensive encephalopathy, CSVT, or a brain abscess. Although patients with SAH sometimes develop fever, a high fever at time of presentation is more suggestive of meningitis, encephalitis, or abscess.

Hypertensive encephalopathy typically causes headache, focal neurologic signs, papilledema, and retinal hemorrhages (see Chapter 9). Although occasional patients with hypertensive encephalopathy were not previously known to be hypertensive, most of these individuals will have had headache or other symptoms before their deterioration.

Paraclinical Evaluation of ICH

Ancillary evaluation in patients with ICH is shown in Table 16-2. A prothrombin time and activated partial thromboplastin time should identify individuals with bleeding tendencies due to a coagulopathy, and a complete blood count should identify individuals with thrombocytopenia or leukocytosis (typically in the range of 15,000/mm³). Individuals with long-standing arterial hypertension may have uremia and proteinuria.

Computed Tomography

CT and MRI are presented in greater detail in Chapter 5, but their role in the evaluation of ICH will be briefly reviewed here.

Table 16-2: Para-clinical Evaluation in Intracerebral Hemorrhage

All patients

1. Complete blood count with platelet count
2. Prothrombin time (INR)
3. Activated partial thromboplastin time (aPTT)
4. Erythrocyte sedimentation rate
5. Comprehensive metabolic profile (CMP)
6. Chest roentgenogram
7. Electrocardiogram
8. Unenhanced computed tomography (CT)

Selected patients

1. Blood cultures
2. Drug screen
3. Antinuclear antibody assay
4. Sickle cell screen
5. Hemoglobin electrophoresis
6. Serum fibrinogen
7. Fibrinogen split products
8. Type and screen
9. HIV titer
10. Magnetic resonance imaging of the brain (MRI)
11. Magnetic resonance angiography (MRA)
12. Magnetic resonance venography (MRV)
13. Computed tomographic angiography (CTA)
14. Catheter cerebral angiography

Adapted from Biller and Shah with permission.[119]
HIV = human immunodeficiency virus; INR = international normalized ratio.

Because of its rapid image acquisition time, widespread availability, and the acute nature of the patient's presentation, CT (Figure 16-4) is almost always the first imaging study to be done when a hemorrhagic stroke is suspected.[97] The high density of a recent intraparenchymal or extra-axial hemorrhage is obvious unless the lesion is very small. In addition, a CT will depict midline shift, brain herniation, enlarged or trapped cerebral ventricles, and, most of the time, SAH. CT sometimes provides clues about the reason for the hemorrhage, especially with the addition of intravenous contrast media, which can help to identify an aneurysm or an AVM.

As the blood breaks down, its density diminishes. The acute hemorrhage clears within about a month, leaving a cavitary lesion with decreased density at the site of the original clot. During this transition from high density to low density, however, there may be a transient period in which the lesion's density is virtually identical to that of the surrounding brain. If the scan is done several days after the stroke, this is density can be confusing.

As the density of the clot decreases, there may be an increase in the surrounding edema and mass effect, presumably because of the osmotic effects of the proteinaceous liquefying clot. At times a transient ring of contrast enhancement develops.

Magnetic Resonance Imaging

Gradient-echo MRI sequences can almost always demonstrate acute ICH. For the first three to five days, T_1-weighted images show a hematoma core that is occasionally hyperintense. Within 2 to 3 days of onset, a parenchymal reaction to intracerebral hematoma often becomes apparent. This reaction consists of a prolongation of both T_1 and T_2, primarily in adjacent white matter, and probably represents associated cerebral edema.

Within about a week, the hematoma cavity begins to develop a short T_1 signal, giving the lesion a hyperintense signal on T_1-weighted images. This change in the T_1 signal of the hematoma core may represent a proton relaxation enhancement effect attributable to the appearance of methemoglobin within the hematoma.

Soon after the above changes occur, the brain parenchyma immediately adjacent to the hematoma begins to form a thin rim of markedly hypointense T_2-weighted signal and isotense or slightly hypointense T_1 signal, attributable to a proton relaxation enhancement effect of intracellular hemosiderin.

Lumbar Puncture

Lumbar puncture is usually ill-advised in individuals with an ICH, so examination of the cerebrospinal fluid (CSF) is not often attempted when this diagnosis is suspected. The examination of the CSF in individuals with suspected subarachnoid hemorrhage is discussed in Chapter 17.

Catheter Cerebral Angiography

Many patients with ICH or SAH are too unstable initially to be taken to the angiography suite. For those who are stable enough to tolerate the procedure and have no obvious cause for their hemorrhage, catheter cerebral angiography is indicated.[97] Cloft and colleagues estimated that the risk of neurological complications from catheter angiography was only 0.07% when done to assess SAH, intracranial aneurysms, or AVMs, a risk that is lower than the complication rate for patients with ischemic stroke.[98]

The yield of catheter angiography diminishes when there is an obvious explanation for the hemorrhage, and in such patients it is acceptable to omit angiography. For example, an individual with long-standing, uncontrolled hypertension before developing a typical hypertensive thalamic or putaminal hemorrhage probably does not benefit from catheter angiography; in this setting arteriography would add a small risk but with little likelihood of finding information that alters therapy.

In contrast, an unexplained ICH should be fully investigated, because the discovery of an aneurysm or AVM would have major therapeutic and prognostic implications.[97] Assuming the individual regains good function following the initial hemorrhage, that person's long-term outlook depends greatly on whether another hemorrhage occurs, and the obliteration of an aneurysm or AVM before another hemorrhage occurs is a major accomplishment.

When they adequately answer the questions at hand, investigation with CT or MR angiographic techniques may suffice. But these studies do not depict smaller aneurysms or AVMs as reliably as catheter angiography nor do they demonstrate lesions of the smaller arteries such as arteritis. Magnetic resonance venography, in contrast, is a very effective means for demonstrating sinovenous occlusion.

INCIDENCE AND DISTRIBUTION

The incidence of ICH in the African American population is almost twice as high as it is among the Caucasian population, and most of this difference is due to hemorrhage among young and middle-aged individuals with hemorrhage in the deep cerebral and brainstem regions where hypertensive stroke typically occurs.[99,100]

The proportion of hemorrhagic stroke may be considerably higher in some non-Western countries. In Nigeria, for example, almost half of the individuals admitted for stroke to a university teaching hospital had a hemorrhagic lesion.[101] If the individuals with SAH in this cohort are added to those with ICH, together they constitute a small majority of the stroke patients. The proportion of stroke patients with hemorrhage was not this high in a smaller study from Iran, but at 33% the frequency of hemorrhagic stroke in this region was still substantially higher than in Western countries.[102] In China the frequency of stroke as well as the incidence of hemorrhagic stroke is higher than in Western countries, although the number of individuals with hemorrhagic stroke has declined in recent years.[103] It is unclear to what extent these geographic variations stem from ascertainment bias in the studies reporting them, differences in the medial care in various countries, or unique risks for hemorrhage within the different populations.

Since the introduction of CT, small hematomas are routinely identified that once would have been miscategorized as an ischemic stroke. Similarly, the introduction of gradient echo MRI, a very sensitive test for small hemorrhagic lesions, has resulted in many individuals with smaller hemorrhagic lesions being identified. The combined effect of CT and MRI has been to add many individuals with smaller hemorrhages to the assessment pool whose hemorrhage would probably not have been identified in the past. This addition of smaller hemorrhages with, one assumes, better outcome may be partly responsible for the apparent decline in mortality from hemorrhagic stroke. Before CT the mortality after a brain hemorrhage was estimated to be 50% to 70%. Since the routine use of CT, the 30-day mortality for hemorrhagic stroke has declined to 30% to 40%. No doubt some of this is due to improvements in patient care, but it is hard to be certain that the outcome of patients with more severe hemorrhages has improved dramatically.[5]

The incidence of ICH has diminished in recent decades mainly because of more effective identification and treatment of individuals with systemic hypertension. The fatality rate for ICH has diminished because of a combination of improved treatment methods and the addition of a large number of milder cases into the mix.

PROGNOSIS OF INTRACEREBRAL HEMORRHAGE

The prognosis after an ICH depends above all on the size and location of the hematoma.[104] Individuals with smaller hemorrhages fare better than those with large lesions, and hematomas in the cerebrum tend to cause less permanent dysfunction than a similar-sized lesion in the brainstem. In some individuals the reason for the hemorrhage plays a substantial role in the prognosis.

A major determining factor in the prognosis following ICH is the risk of additional hemorrhages, because even if the patient recovers fully after the initial hemorrhage, a second or third hemorrhage is likely to be devastating. Naturally, the risk of subsequent bleeding episodes is greatly dependent on why the hemorrhage occurred and on how effectively the risk factors can be treated. In one study the mortality rate following a second hemorrhage was 32%, not too different from the rate after a first hemorrhage.[105] Nevertheless, with each hemorrhage, more and more people will be left incapacitated.

Some individuals with an ICH seem stable at the time of presentation only to undergo clinical deterioration a few hours later. There are clearly multiple factors that contribute to this delayed clinical deterioration. Predictors of clinical deterioration include enlargement of the hematoma, intraventricular extension of the hemorrhage, and high systolic blood pressure 48 hours after presentation.[3]

Franke and colleagues conducted a prospective study of 157 patients with a supratentorial ICH and found that 24% of the patients died within 2 days, 43% within 30 days, and 53% within 1 year.[106] Generally, the mortality tends to increase with hematoma volume, midline shift, high blood pressure combined with impaired consciousness on hospital admission, and age. Sex makes no difference in outcome. At the end of a year, there was no difference between the 120 surviving hemorrhagic stroke patients in this series and a group of ischemic stroke patients with a similar level of initial neurological dysfunction.[106]

The prognosis after a primary intraventricular hemorrhage is not necessarily poor because the blood may have an egress from the brain without permanently damaging the parenchyma and resulting in neurologic deficit. However, the prognosis is worse in the individuals who have a concomitant intraparenchymal hemorrhage. For patients with a primary hemorrhage of the caudate, as well as those who have small, circumscribed thalamic hemorrhages, the prognosis is relatively good.

The outlook for individuals with large pontine hemorrhages is generally poor. The immediate mortality is often due to the hemorrhage itself, which causes brainstem compression. Patients who survive the initial period often develop pneumonia, gastric hemorrhage, and electrolyte disturbance from inappropriate secretion of antidiuretic hormone (SIADH) or central salt wasting syndrome. Other complications include pulmonary embolism, sometimes life-threatening cardiac dysrhythmias, and myocardial infarction. Between the damage to the pons and the subsequent complications, the prognosis is poor for both survival and return of neurological function. However, despite the often dismal prognosis of individuals with a brainstem hemorrhage, some patients make a near complete recovery.[107]

TREATMENT OF INTRACEREBRAL HEMORRHAGE

Medical Therapy

A suspected ICH is a medical emergency, and the patient must be promptly evaluated by experienced physicians with access to appropriate diagnostic and treatment modalities. Medical treatment of patients consists primarily of maintaining adequate oxygenation and appropriate blood pressures and preventing

Table 16-3: Medical Management of Intracranial Pressure in Intracerebral Hemorrhage

Correction of factors exacerbating increased ICP

- Hypercarbia
- Hypoxia
- Hyperthermia
- Acidosis
- Hypotension
- Hypovolemia
- Hyponatremia
- Pain control

Positional factors

- Avoid head and neck positions compressing jugular veins
- Avoid flat supine position; elevate head of bed 30 degrees (if no contraindications)

Medical therapy

- Endotracheal intubation and mechanical ventilation, if Glasgow Coma Scale < 8
- Hyperventilate to $PaCO_2$ of 35 ± 3 mm Hg (if herniation seems likely)
- Hyperosmolar therapy with mannitol (20% solution), 1 g/kg over 30 min
- Maintenance dose: 0.25–0.5 g/kg over 30–60 minutes every 4–6 hour, depending on clinical course, serum osmolality, and ICP measurements, maintain serum osmolality between 300 and 320 mosm/L
- Consider hypertonic saline if needed (3% or 23.4%)
- Maintain CPP = 60–70 mm Hg

Fluid restriction

- Avoid glucose solutions, use normal saline, maintain euvolemia
- Replace urinary losses with normal saline in patients receiving mannitol

CPP = cerebral perfusion pressure; ICP = intracranial pressure.

further compromise due to increased ICP or brain herniation. If there are signs of respiratory depression (Glasgow coma score of < 8) or raised ICP and impending herniation, intubation, hyperventilation, and intravenous osmotherapy with mannitol or hypertonic saline are indicated (Table 16-3). Endotracheal intubation facilitates adequate oxygenation and makes it possible to reduce the $PaCO_2$ in an individual with increased intracranial pressure.

It is reasonable to administer a stool softener and to sedate an agitated patient, especially when the hemorrhage resulted from an AVM or an intracranial aneurysm that might rebleed in response to agitation or a Valsalva maneuver. Effective control of arterial hypertension in individuals with an ICH may limit the eventual hematoma size.[108] Seizures should also be treated because of their potential to increase the ICP, but there is debate about whether to start antiepileptic agents prophylactically.[97]

Fever is common among stroke patients and can arise either from infection or as a febrile response to the brain injury. In a third of febrile stroke patients no infection can be identified even after a thorough evaluation.[109] Individuals with SAH have a higher rate of noninfectious fever than other stroke patients, and individuals in the same unit with traumatic brain injury who develop fever have a higher rate of documented infection.[109] Obviously infections must be treated, but it is also important to address noninfectious fevers given the possible negative effect of temperature elevation on neurological outcome in this setting.[97]

Control of Risk Factors

For patients who survive the initial ICH, one important determinant of the individual's long-term prognosis is the likelihood of additional hemorrhages. The occurrence of additional hemorrhages, in turn, depends in large measure on the presence of hemorrhage risk factors and whether the effect of these factors can be reduced or eliminated. Thus, adequate control of arterial hypertension is essential. The mean arterial blood pressure (MABP) must be maintained above 90 mm Hg in an effort to maintain a cerebral perfusion pressure (CPP) greater than 70 mm Hg. Nicardipine, labetalol, or esmolol are acceptable choices. Sodium nitroprusside is best avoided because it can cause ICP elevation. Arteriovenous malformations and aneurysms should be repaired or at least stabilized. Effective treatment of the thrombocytopenia, arteritis, or coagulopathy that caused the initial hemorrhage should in theory lower the individual's risk of having another hemorrhage.

Warfarin-related ICH is often treated with fresh frozen plasma and vitamin K. Prothrombin complex concentrate or recombinant factor VII (rFVIIa) concentrate have also been proposed as a faster approach to reverse warfarin-related anticoagulation under these circumstances. Heparin-related ICH is reversed with protamine sulfate. For patients with thrombolytic-related ICH, some experts recommend platelets (6–8 units), cryoprecipitate containing factor VIII (10 units), as well as fresh frozen plasma.[110]

Surgical Options

Surgical decompression of a cerebellar hemorrhage in an effort to prevent brainstem compression is a well-accepted approach, and surgery is the best approach for all but the smallest subdural or epidural hemorrhages. Surgical decompression is often attempted to relieve other herniation syndromes or to assist with the control of increased ICP. Nevertheless, there is no proven value for surgery for most individuals with an intraparenchymal brain hemorrhage.[97] Batjer and colleagues, for example, conducted an early prospective randomized trial of evacuation of hypertensive putaminal hemorrhage in 21 individuals but were unable to demonstrate any advantage of surgery compared to optimal medical management.[111] Similarly, Tan and associates found no benefit from hematoma evacuation in 34 individuals with basal ganglia hemorrhage.[112]

Rabinstein and colleagues analyzed 26 consecutive patients who underwent clot evacuation after acutely deteriorating because of a nontraumatic ICH.[113] All of the comatose patients with loss of upper brainstem reflexes and extensor posturing died despite surgery, and no one without corneal or oculocephalic reflexes before surgery regained independent function. Altogether, 56% of these 26 patients died despite surgery, 22% remained severely incapacitated, and 22% regained functional independence. However, given that the favorable outcome group had less severe neurological dysfunction before surgery, they may have recovered even without surgery. Bilbao and colleagues summarized a prospective but nonrandomized trial of 356 individuals with nontraumatic intraparenchymal hemorrhage and concluded that surgery offered no benefit.[114]

Mendelow and colleagues summarized a randomized trial of hematoma evacuation in 1,033 individuals with nontraumatic intraparenchymal hemorrhage (the International Surgical Trial in Intracerebral Hemorrhage, or STICH).[1] The patients were segregated into good and poor prognosis groups based on their clinical findings at time of study entry, then randomized to undergo clot evacuation within 24 hours (n = 503) or to receive conservative medical therapy (n = 530). Twenty-six percent of the individuals whose clot was evacuated had a favorable outcome at 6 months, whereas 24% of the individuals in the medical therapy arm did as well.[1] The authors concluded that there was no overall benefit from surgery.[115,116]

So although there may be a limited role for surgery in a few situations, there is little evidence that surgical evacuation of an ICH is beneficial in unselected patients. Surgery might be useful for lobar hemorrhage patients, and additional clinical trials are ongoing.[117] The STICH trial indicated that surgery is beneficial for individuals with intraventricular hemorrhage and hydrocephalus.[118]

Treatment of aneurysms, AVMs, and cavernous malformations reduces the likelihood of a potentially devastating recurrent hemorrhage. A variety of techniques are used to occlude AVMs and aneurysms, including clipping of aneurysms, resection and occlusion of AVMs, and endovascular occlusion techniques for either. These techniques are considered in Chapters 17 and 18.

REFERENCES

1. Mendelow AD, Gregson BA, Fernandes HM, et al. Early surgery versus initial conservative treatment in patients with spontaneous supratentorial intracerebral haematomas in the International Surgical Trial in Intracerebral Haemorrhage (STICH): a randomised trial. *Lancet.* 2005;**365**:387–397.

2. Dennis MS. Outcome after brain haemorrhage. *Cerebrovasc Dis.* 2003;**16**(Suppl)1:9–13.

3. Leira R, Davalos A, Silva Y, et al. Early neurologic deterioration in intracerebral hemorrhage: predictors and associated factors. *Neurology.* 2004;**63**:461–467.

4. Feldmann E, Broderick JP, Kernan WN, et al. Major risk factors for intracerebral hemorrhage in the young are modifiable. *Stroke.* 2005;**36**:1881–1885.

5. Hsieh PC, Awad IA, Getch CC, Bendok BR, Rosenblatt SS, Batjer HH. Current updates in perioperative management of intracerebral hemorrhage. *Neurol Clin.* 2006;**24**:745–764.

6. Sturgeon JD, Folsom AR. Trends in hospitalization rate, hospital case fatality, and mortality rate of stroke by subtype in Minneapolis–St. Paul, 1980–2002. *Neuroepidemiology.* 2007;**28**:39–45.

7. Carolei A, Sacco S, De SF, Marini C. Epidemiology of stroke. *Clin Exp Hypertens.* 2002;**24**:479–483.

8. Shintani S, Tsuruoka S, Shiigai T. Pure sensory stroke caused by a cerebral hemorrhage: clinical-radiologic correlations in seven patients. *AJNR Am J Neuroradiol.* 2000;**21**:515–520.

9. Yen CP, Lin CL, Kwan AL, et al. Simultaneous multiple hypertensive intracerebral haemorrhages. *Acta Neurochir (Wien).* 2005;**147**:393–399.

10. Ropper AH, Davis KR. Lobar cerebral hemorrhages: acute clinical syndromes in 26 cases. *Ann Neurol.* 1980;**8**:141–147.

11. Wakai S, Kumakura N, Nagai M. Lobar intracerebral hemorrhage. A clinical, radiographic, and pathological study of 29 consecutive operated cases with negative angiography. *J Neurosurg.* 1992;**76**:231–238.

12. Saez de Ocariz MM, Nader JA, Santos JA, Bautista M. Thalamic vascular lesions. Risk factors and clinical course for infarcts and hemorrhages. *Stroke.* 1996;**27**:1530–1536.

13. Gates PC, Barnett HJ, Vinters HV, Simonsen RL, Siu K. Primary intraventricular hemorrhage in adults. *Stroke.* 1986;**17**:872–877.

14. Marti-Fabregas J, Piles S, Guardia E, Marti-Vilalta JL. Spontaneous primary intraventricular hemorrhage: clinical data, etiology and outcome. *J Neurol.* 1999;**246**:287–291.

15. Weisberg LA. Acute cerebellar hemorrhage and CT evidence of tight posterior fossa. *Neurology.* 1986;**36**:858–860.

16. St Louis EK, Wijdicks EF, Li H. Predicting neurologic deterioration in patients with cerebellar hematomas. *Neurology.* 1998;**51**: 1364–1369.

17. Mathew P, Teasdale G, Bannan A, Oluoch-Olunya D. Neurosurgical management of cerebellar haematoma and infarct. *J Neurol Neurosurg Psychiatry.* 1995;**59**:287–292.

18. Lapchak PA, Araujo DM. Advances in hemorrhagic stroke therapy: conventional and novel approaches. *Expert Opin Emerg Drugs.* 2007;**12**:389–406.

19. Mizuguchi M, Kano H, Narita M, Chen R-F, Bessho F. Weber syndrome caused by intracerebral hemorrhage in a hemophiliac boy. *Brain Dev.* 1993;**15**:446–447.

20. SHEP Cooperative Research Group. Prevention of stroke by antihypertensive drug treatment in older persons with isolated systolic hypertension. Final results of the Systolic Hypertension in the Elderly Program (SHEP). *JAMA.* 1991;**265**:3255–3264.

21. Zia E, Hedblad B, Pessah-Rasmussen H, Berglund G, Janzon L, Engstrom G. Blood pressure in relation to the incidence of cerebral infarction and intracerebral hemorrhage. Hypertensive hemorrhage: debated nomenclature is still relevant. *Stroke.* 2007;**38**:2681–2685.

22. Al-Jarallah M, Al-Rifai T, Riela AR, Roach ES. Spontaneous intraparenchymal hemorrhage in children: a study of 68 patients. *J Child Neurol.* 2000;**15**:284–289.

23. Szabo MD, Crosby G, Sundaram P, Dodson BA, Kjellberg RN. Hypertension does not cause spontaneous hemorrhage of intracranial arteriovenous malformations. *Anesthesiology.* 1989; **70**:761–763.

24. Auer RN, Sutherland GR. Primary intracerebral hemorrhage: pathophysiology. *Can J Neurol Sci.* 2005;**32**(Suppl 2):S3–12.

25. Challa VR, Moody DM, Bell MA. The Charcot-Bouchard aneurysm controversy: impact of a new histologic technique. *J Neuropathol Exp Neurol.* 1992;**51**:264–271.

26. Acosta-Rua GJ. Familial incidence of ruptured intracranial aneurysms. *Arch Neurol.* 1978;**35**:675–677.

27. Lozano AM, Leblanc R. Familial intracranial aneurysms. *J Neurosurg.* 1987;**66**:522–528.

28. Morooka Y, Waga S. Familial intracranial aneurysms: report of four families. *Surg Neurol.* 1983;**19**:260–262.

29. ter Berg HWM, Dippel DWJ, Limburg M, Schievink WI, van Gijn J. Familial intracranial aneurysms – a review. *Stroke.* 1992;**23**:1024–1030.

30. Moulin T, Crepin-Leblond T, Chopard JL, Bogousslavsky J. Hemorrhagic infarcts. *Eur Neurol.* 1994;**34**:64–77.

31. Hornig CR, Bauer T, Simon C, Trittmacher S, Dorndorf W. Hemorrhagic transformation in cardioembolic cerebral infarction. *Stroke.* 1993;**24**:465–468.

32. Ott BR, Zamani A, Kleefield J, Funkenstein HH. The clinical spectrum of hemorrhagic infarction. *Stroke.* 1986;**17**:630–637.

33. Sloan MA. Neurologic complications of thrombolytic therapy. In: Biller J, ed. *Iatrogenic Neurology.* Boston: Butterworth-Heinemann; 1998:335–378.

34. Gurwitz JH, Gore JM, Goldberg RJ, et al. Risk for intracranial hemorrhage after tissue plasminogen activator treatment for acute myocardial infarction. Participants in the National Registry of Myocardial Infarction 2. *Ann Intern Med.* 1998;**129**:597–604.

35. Brass LM, Lichtman JH, Wang Y, Gurwitz JH, Radford MJ, Krumholz HM. Intracranial hemorrhage associated with thrombolytic therapy for elderly patients with acute myocardial infarction: results from the Cooperative Cardiovascular Project. *Stroke.* 2000;**31**:1802–1811.

36. National Institute of Neurological Disorders and Stroke rt-PA Stroke Study Group. Tissue plasminogen activator for acute ischemic stroke. *N Engl J Med.* 1995;**333**:1581–1587.

37. Koennecke HC, Nohr R, Leistner S, Marx P. Intravenous tPA for ischemic stroke team performance over time, safety, and efficacy in a single-center, 2-year experience. *Stroke.* 2001;**32**:1074–1078.

38. Del Zoppo GJ, Saver JL, Jauch EC, Adams HPJr. Expansion of the time window for treatment of acute ischemic stroke with intravenous tissue plasminogen activator: a science advisory from the American Heart Association/American Stroke Association. *Stroke.* 2009;**40**:2945–2948.

39. Lansberg MG, Thijs VN, Bammer R, et al. Risk factors of symptomatic intracerebral hemorrhage after tPA therapy for acute stroke. *Stroke.* 2007;**38**:2275–2278.

40. Derex L, Hermier M, Adeleine P, et al. Clinical and imaging predictors of intracerebral haemorrhage in stroke patients treated with intravenous tissue plasminogen activator. *J Neurol Neurosurg Psychiatry.* 2005;**76**:70–75.

41. Flaherty ML, Kissela B, Woo D, et al. The increasing incidence of anticoagulant-associated intracerebral hemorrhage. *Neurology.* 2007;**68**:116–121.

42. Pessin MS, Estol CJ, Lafranchise F, Caplan LR. Safety of anticoagulation after hemorrhagic infarction. *Neurology.* 1993;**43**: 1298–1303.

43. Viswanathan A, Rakich SM, Engel C, et al. Antiplatelet use after intracerebral hemorrhage. *Neurology.* 2006;**66**:206–209.

44. Chaou WT, Chou ML, Eitzman DV. Intracranial hemorrhage and vitamin K deficiency in early infancy. *J Pediatr.* 1984;**105**: 880–884.

45. Takeshita M, Kagawa M, Izawa M, Kitamura K. Hemorrhagic stroke in infancy, childhood, and adolescence. *Surg Neurol.* 1986;**26**:496–500.

46. Solomon GE, Hilgartner MW, Kutt H. Coagulation defects caused by diphenylhydantoin. *Neurology.* 1972;**22**:1165–1171.

47. Kuban KCK, Leviton A, Krishnamoorthy KS, et al. Neonatal intracranial hemorrhage and phenobarbital. *Pediatrics.* 1986;**77**: 443–450.

48. Kohler HG. Haemorrhage in the newborn of epileptic mothers. *Lancet.* 1966;**1**:267.

49. Mountain KR, Hirsh J, Gallus AS. Neonatal coagulation defect due to anticonvulsant drug treatment in pregnancy. *Lancet.* 1970; **1**:265–268.

50. Scozzafava J, Hussain MS, Yeo T, Jeerakathil T, Brindley PG. Case report: aggressive blood pressure management for carotid endarterectomy hyperperfusion syndrome. *Can J Anaesth.* 2006;**53**: 764–768.

51. Rezende MT, Spelle L, Mounayer C, Piotin M, Abud DG, Moret J. Hyperperfusion syndrome after stenting for intracranial vertebral stenosis. *Stroke.* 2006;**37**:e12–e14.

52. Ogasawara K, Inoue T, Kobayashi M, Endo H, Fukuda T, Ogawa A. Intracerebral hemorrhage after carotid endarterectomy associated with asymptomatic perioperative cerebral ischemia detected

by cerebral perfusion imaging: case report. *Surg Neurol.* 2004;**62**: 319–322.

53. Wilson PV, Ammar AD. The incidence of ischemic stroke versus intracerebral hemorrhage after carotid endarterectomy: a review of 2452 cases. *Ann Vasc Surg.* 2005;**19**:1–4.

54. Weis-Muller BT, Huber R, Spivak-Dats A, Turowski B, Siebler M, Sandmann W. Symptomatic acute occlusion of the internal carotid artery: reappraisal of urgent vascular reconstruction based on current stroke imaging. *J Vasc Surg.* 2008;**47**:752–759.

55. Naylor AR, Evans J, Thompson MM, et al. Seizures after carotid endarterectomy: hyperperfusion, dysautoregulation or hypertensive encephalopathy? *Eur J Vasc Endovasc Surg.* 2003;**26**:39–44.

56. Chobanian AV, Bakris GL, Black HR, et al. Seventh report of the Joint National Committee on Prevention, Detection, Evaluation, and Treatment of High Blood Pressure. *Hypertension.* 2003; **42**:1206–1252.

57. Henderson RD, Phan TG, Piepgras DG, Wijdicks EF. Mechanisms of intracerebral hemorrhage after carotid endarterectomy. *J Neurosurg.* 2001;**95**:964–969.

58. Ogasawara K, Inoue T, Kobayashi M, et al. Cerebral hyperperfusion following carotid endarterectomy: diagnostic utility of intraoperative transcranial Doppler ultrasonography compared with single-photon emission computed tomography study. *AJNR Am J Neuroradiol.* 2005;**26**:252–257.

59. Seijo FJ, Varez-Vega MA, Gutierrez JC, Fdez-Glez F, Lozano B. Complications in subthalamic nucleus stimulation surgery for treatment of Parkinson's disease. Review of 272 procedures. *Acta Neurochir (Wien).* 2007;**149**:867–875.

60. Sansur CA, Frysinger RC, Pouratian N, et al. Incidence of symptomatic hemorrhage after stereotactic electrode placement. *J Neurosurg.* 2007;**107**:998–1003.

61. Neumann MA. Combined amyloid vascular changes and argyrophilic plaques in the central nervous system. *J Neuropathol Exp Neurol.* 1960;**19**:370–382.

62. Maat-Schieman M, Roos R, van Duinen S. Hereditary cerebral hemorrhage with amyloidosis-Dutch type. *Neuropathology.* 2005;**25**:288–297.

63. Nishitsuji K, Tomiyama T, Ishibashi K, et al. Cerebral vascular accumulation of Dutch-type Abeta42, but not wild-type Abeta42, in hereditary cerebral hemorrhage with amyloidosis, Dutch type. *J Neurosci Res.* 2007;**85**:2917–2923.

64. Kumar-Singh S. Cerebral amyloid angiopathy: pathogenetic mechanisms and link to dense amyloid plaques. *Genes Brain Behav.* 2008;**7**(Suppl 1):67–82.

65. Greenberg SM, Shin Y, Grabowski TJ, et al. Hemorrhagic stroke associated with the Iowa amyloid precursor protein mutation. *Neurology.* 2003;**60**:1020–1022.

66. O'Donnell HC, Rosand J, Knudsen KA, et al. Apolipoprotein E genotype and the risk of recurrent lobar intracerebral hemorrhage. *N Engl J Med.* 2000;**342**:240–245.

67. Rosand J, Hylek EM, O'Donnell HC, Greenberg SM. Warfarin-associated hemorrhage and cerebral amyloid angiopathy: a genetic and pathologic study. *Neurology.* 2000;**55**:947–951.

68. Okazaki H, Reagan TJ, Campbell RJ. Clinicopathologic studies of primary cerebral amyloid angiopathy. *Mayo Clin Proc.* 1979; **54**:22–31.

69. Knudsen KA, Rosand J, Karluk D, Greenberg SM. Clinical diagnosis of cerebral amyloid angiopathy: validation of the Boston criteria. *Neurology.* 2001;**56**:537–539.

70. Zhang-Nunes SX, Maat-Schieman ML, van Duinen SG, Roos RA, Frosch MP, Greenberg SM. The cerebral beta-amyloid angiopathies: hereditary and sporadic. *Brain Pathol.* 2006;**16**:30–39.

71. Chen YW, Gurol ME, Rosand J, et al. Progression of white matter lesions and hemorrhages in cerebral amyloid angiopathy. *Neurology.* 2006;**67**:83–87.

72. McCarron MO, Nicoll JA, Ironside JW, Love S, Alberts MJ, Bone I. Cerebral amyloid angiopathy-related hemorrhage. Interaction of APOE epsilon2 with putative clinical risk factors. *Stroke.* 1999;**30**:1643–1646.

73. Takekawa Y, Umezawa T, Ueno Y, Sawada T, Kobayashi M. A case of undifferentiated glioma in a 70-year-old woman. *Brain Tumor Pathol.* 2001;**18**:55–60.

74. Nishimuta Y, Niiro M, Kamezawa T, Ishimaru K, Yokoyama S, Kuratsu J. Pontine malignant astrocytoma with hemorrhagic onset – case report. *Neurol Med Chir (Tokyo).* 2003;**43**:404–408.

75. Yoshida D, Kogiku M, Noha M, Takahashi H, Teramoto A. A case of pleomorphic xanthoastrocytoma presenting with massive tumoral hemorrhage. *J Neurooncol.* 2005;**71**:169–171.

76. Licata B, Turazzi S. Bleeding cerebral neoplasms with symptomatic hematoma. *J Neurosurg Sci.* 2003;**47**:201–210.

77. Lo WD, Lee J, Rusin J, Perkins E, Roach ES. Intracranial hemorrhage in children: an evolving spectrum. *Arch Neurol.* 2008;**65**: 1629–1633.

78. Nguyen TT, Wray AC, Laidlaw JD. Midbrain and thalamic haemorrhage as first presentation of intracerebral glioma. *J Clin Neurosci.* 2005;**12**:946–949.

79. Golbe LI, Merkin MD. Cerebral infarction in a user of free-base cocaine ("crack"). *Neurology.* 1986;**36**:1602–1604.

80. Levine SR, Brust JCM, Futrell N, et al. Cerebrovascular complications of the use of the "crack" form of alkaloidal cocaine. *N Engl J Med.* 1990;**323**:699–704.

81. Kaye BR, Fainstat M. Cerebral vasculitis associated with cocaine abuse. *JAMA.* 1987;**258**:2104–2106.

82. Westover AN, McBride S, Haley RW. Stroke in young adults who abuse amphetamines or cocaine: a population-based study of hospitalized patients. *Arch Gen Psychiatry.* 2007;**64**:495–502.

83. Fredericks RK, Lefkowitz DS, Challa VR, Troost BT. Cerebral vasculitis associated with cocaine abuse. *Stroke.* 1991;**22**:1437–1439.

84. Jick H, Aselton P, Hunter JR. Phenylpropanolamine and cerebral haemorrhage. *Lancet.* 1984;**1**:1017.

85. Kernan WN, Viscoli CM, Brass LM, et al. Phenylpropanolamine and the risk of hemorrhagic stroke. *N Engl J Med.* 2000;**343**:1826–1832.

86. Morgenstern LB, Viscoli CM, Kernan WN, et al. Use of ephedra-containing products and risk for hemorrhagic stroke. *Neurology.* 2003;**60**:132–135.

87. Sacco RL. Alcohol and stroke risk: an elusive dose-response relationship. *Ann Neurol.* 2007;**62**:551–552.

88. Fukui M, Kono S, Sueishi K, Ikezaki K. Moyamoya disease. *Neuropathology.* 2000;**20**(Suppl):S61–S64.

89. Houkin K, Kamiyama H, Abe H, Takahashi A, Kuroda S. Surgical therapy for adult moyamoya disease. Can surgical revascularization prevent the recurrence of intracerebral hemorrhage? *Stroke.* 1996;**27**:1342–1346.

90. Adams HP Jr, Kassell NF, Wisoff HS, Drake CG. Intracranial saccular aneurysm and moyamoya disease. *Stroke.* 1979;**10**:174–179.

91. Ali MJ, Bendok BR, Getch CC, Gottardi-Littell NR, Mindea S, Batjer HH. Surgical management of a ruptured posterior choroidal intraventricular aneurysm associated with moyamoya disease using frameless stereotaxy: case report and review of the literature. *Neurosurgery.* 2004;**54**:1019–1024.

92. Borota L, Marinkovic S, Bajic R, Kovacevic M. Intracranial aneurysms associated with moyamoya disease. *Neurol Med Chir (Tokyo).* 1996;**36**:860–864.

93. Hamada J, Hashimoto N, Tsukahara T. Moyamoya disease with repeated intraventricular hemorrhage due to aneurysm rupture. Report of two cases. *J Neurosurg.* 1994;**80**:328–331.

94. Aoki N. Caudate head hemorrhage caused by asymptomatic occlusion of the middle cerebral artery. *Surg Neurol.* 1987;**27**:173–176.

95. Hashimoto K, Fujii K, Nishimura K, Kibe M, Kishikawa T. Occlusive cerebrovascular disease with moyamoya vessels and intracranial hemorrhage during pregnancy – case report and review of the literature. *Neurol Med Chir (Tokyo).* 1988;**28**:588–593.

96. Enomoto H, Goto H. Moyamoya disease presenting as intracerebral hemorrhage during pregnancy: case report and review of the literature. *Neurosurgery.* 1987;**20**:33–35.

97. Broderick JP, Adams HP Jr, Barsan W, et al. Guidelines for the management of spontaneous intracerebral hemorrhage: a statement for healthcare professionals from a special writing group of the Stroke Council, American Heart Association. *Stroke.* 1999;**30**:905–915.

98. Cloft HJ, Joseph GJ, Dion JE. Risk of cerebral angiography in patients with subarachnoid hemorrhage, cerebral aneurysm, and arteriovenous malformation: a meta-analysis. *Stroke.* 1999;**30**:317–320.

99. Flaherty ML, Woo D, Haverbusch M, et al. Racial variations in location and risk of intracerebral hemorrhage. *Stroke.* 2005;**36**:934–937.

100. Smeeton NC, Heuschmann PU, Rudd AG, et al. Incidence of hemorrhagic stroke in black Caribbean, black African, and white populations: the South London stroke register, 1995–2004. *Stroke.* 2007;**38**:3133–3138.

101. Ogun SA, Ojini FI, Ogungbo B, Kolapo KO, Danesi MA. Stroke in south west Nigeria: a 10-year review. *Stroke.* 2005;**36**:1120–1122.

102. Ahangar AA, Ashraf Vaghefi SB, Ramaezani M. Epidemiological evaluation of stroke in Babol, northern Iran (2001–2003). *Eur Neurol.* **2005**;54:93–97.

103. Jiang B, Wang WZ, Chen H, et al. Incidence and trends of stroke and its subtypes in China: results from three large cities. *Stroke.* 2006;**37**:63–68.

104. Inagawa T, Ohbayashi N, Takechi A, Shibukawa M, Yahara K. Primary intracerebral hemorrhage in Izumo City, Japan: incidence rates and outcome in relation to the site of hemorrhage. *Neurosurgery.* 2003;**53**:1283–1297.

105. Gonzalez-Duarte A, Cantu C, Ruiz-Sandoval JL, Barinagarrementeria F. Recurrent primary cerebral hemorrhage: frequency, mechanisms, and prognosis. *Stroke.* 1998;**29**:1802–1805.

106. Franke CL, van Swieten JC, Algra A, van Gijn J. Prognostic factors in patients with intracerebral haematoma. *J Neurol Neurosurg Psychiatry.* 1992;**55**:653–657.

107. Bryan R, Weisberg L. Prolonged survival with good functional recovery in 3 patients with computed tomographic evidence of brain stem hemorrhage. *Comput Radiol.* 1982;**6**:43–48.

108. Anderson CS, Huang Y, Wang JG, et al. Intensive blood pressure reduction in acute cerebral haemorrhage trial (INTERACT): a randomised pilot trial. *Lancet Neurol.* 2008;**7**:391–399.

109. Rabinstein AA, Sandhu K. Non-infectious fever in the neurological intensive care unit: incidence, causes and predictors. *J Neurol Neurosurg Psychiatry.* 2007;**78**:1278–1280.

110. Manno EM, Atkinson JL, Fulgham JR, Wijdicks EF. Emerging medical and surgical management strategies in the evaluation and treatment of intracerebral hemorrhage. *Mayo Clin Proc.* 2005;**80**:420–433.

111. Batjer HH, Reisch JS, Allen BC, Plaizier LJ, Su CJ. Failure of surgery to improve outcome in hypertensive putaminal hemorrhage: a prospective randomized trial. *Arch Neurol.* 1990;**47**:1103–1106.

112. Tan ST, Ng PY, Yeo TT, Wong SH, Ong PL, Venketasubramanian N. Hypertensive basal ganglia hemorrhage: a prospective study comparing surgical and nonsurgical management. *Surg Neurol.* 2001;**56**:287–293.

113. Rabinstein AA, Atkinson JL, Wijdicks EF. Emergency craniotomy in patients worsening due to expanded cerebral hematoma: to what purpose? *Neurology.* 2002;**58**:1367–1372.

114. Bilbao G, Garibi J, Pomposo I, et al. A prospective study of a series of 356 patients with supratentorial spontaneous intracranial haematomas treated in a neurosurgical department. *Acta Neurochir (Wien).* 2005;**147**:823–829.

115. Wartenberg KE, Mayer SA. The STICH trial: the end of surgical intervention for supratentorial intracerebral hemorrhage? *Curr Neurol Neurosci Rep.* 2005;**5**:473–475.

116. Broderick JP. The STICH trial: what does it tell us and where do we go from here? *Stroke.* 2005;**36**:1619–1620.

117. Mendelow AD, Unterberg A. Surgical treatment of intracerebral haemorrhage. *Curr Opin Crit Care.* 2007;**13**:169–174.

118. Bhattathiri PS, Gregson B, Prasad KS, Mendelow AD. Intraventricular hemorrhage and hydrocephalus after spontaneous intracerebral hemorrhage: results from the STICH trial. *Acta Neurochir* 2006;**96**(Suppl):65–68.

119. Biller J, Shah MV. Intracerebral hemorrhage. In: Rakel RE, ed. *Conn's Current Therapy.* Philadelphia: W. B. Saunders Company; 1997:877–880.

17

Subarachnoid Hemorrhage and Aneurysms

The difficulty lies, not in the new ideas, but in escaping the old ones, which ramify, for those brought up as most of us have been, into every corner of our minds.

John Maynard Keynes

Subarachnoid hemorrhage (SAH) can be primary or secondary. Primary SAH results when an artery or vein ruptures directly into the subarachnoid space. Secondary SAH occurs when an intracerebral hemorrhage dissects through the brain parenchyma into the subarachnoid or intraventricular spaces.

Aneurysms are abnormal localized dilatations of the wall and lumen of an artery or vein. They are "false" if all tunica layers are ectatic and "true" if the intima herniates through the muscularis of the arterial wall, forming a balloon-shaped structure. The most common cause of SAH is trauma. By far the single-most-common cause of nontraumatic SAH (Table 17-1) is rupture of a cerebral saccular aneurysm. For this reason we will present SAH and intracerebral aneurysm together. Venous aneurysms and carotid-cavernous fistulas are considered in Chapter 18.

SUBARACHNOID HEMORRHAGE

Symptoms of Subarachnoid Hemorrhage

The classic presentation of an SAH is with sudden-onset, excruciating headache, often described as the worst headache ever experienced. The pain is aggravated by neck flexion, head movement, and the Valsalva maneuver, as well as by sound and light. The patient seeks relief by lying quietly. Consciousness may remain, especially with smaller hemorrhages. Increasing hemorrhage volume leads to greater symptom severity, including irritability, confusion, disorientation, or coma. Diplopia or blurred vision is common.

Patients with SAH sometimes report an atypical or particularly severe headache during the interval preceding the SAH.[1,2] This "sentinel" headache probably results from minor leakage of blood into the subarachnoid space or hemorrhage into the wall of the aneurysm. Sentinel headaches typically occur within a month preceding the diagnosed SAH.[3,4] Warning symptoms

occur in 15% to 40% of the patients with SAH, but their significance is often overlooked.[5–8]

A sentinel headache offers a window of opportunity to correct an intracranial aneurysm before a devastating SAH. Linn and colleagues, for example, analyzed 148 individuals with sudden-onset, severe headaches.[9] Thirty-seven (25%) had an SAH, but 18 others had another etiology for the headache, and the remaining 93 individuals had benign "thunderclap" headache.[9] When assessing individuals with sudden-onset headaches, it is wise to avoid overreliance on cranial computed tomography (CT) and to develop a low threshold for doing a lumbar puncture (LP).

Sometimes the headache is mild, and the patient seeks medical attention for symptoms secondary to meningeal irritation or increased intracranial pressure such as vomiting, fever, diplopia, or altered consciousness. Such a clinical picture may suggest meningitis or encephalitis, but the SAH is usually revealed by CT (Figure 17-1), magnetic resonance imaging (MRI), or LP.

With spinal subarachnoid hemorrhages, the patient typically develops sudden, sharp back pain (*coup-de-poignard*), which may radiate down one or both legs and may be accompanied by motor and sensory abnormality of the lower limbs with acute retention of urine. Opisthotonic posturing occasionally occurs. When these signs and symptoms dominate, they suggest that the SAH has arisen within the spinal canal. Among the causes of primary spinal SAH are intraspinal AVMs or cavernous malformations (see Chapter 18).

Focal or generalized seizures may develop at the time of the SAH or soon thereafter. Seizures at the onset of SAH do not invariably herald permanent cerebral dysfunction or a long-term risk of epilepsy. A long-standing history of convulsions suggests the possibility of other underlying brain diseases, for instance, AVM or tumor.

Physical Findings

These depend mostly on the severity of the SAH, but the site and the rapidity of blood accumulation also play a role in the clinical presentation. Arterial blood spurting under high pressure from a ruptured aneurysm may cause a very different

Table 17-1: Causes of Nontraumatic Subarachnoid Hemorrhage

Aneurysm
- Saccular
- Fusiform
- Infective
- Neoplastic

Other CNS vascular lesions
- Arteriovenous malformation
- Dural arteriovenous fistula
- Cavernous malformations
- Developmental venous anomaly
- Capillary telangiectasia

Perimesencephalic SAH

Intracranial arterial dissection (especially vertebral artery)

Intracerebral hemorrhage

Cerebral venous thrombosis

Pituitary apoplexy

Intracranial neoplasm

Hematological and coagulation disorders
- Thrombocytopenia
- Coagulation defects
- Anticoagulant therapy
- Thrombolytic therapy
- Disseminated intravascular coagulation
- Sickle cell disease

Infections

Sepsis

Meningo-encephalitis

Infective endocarditis

Vasculopathy/vasculitis

Cerebral amyloid angiopathy

Moyamoya disease

Collagen vascular disorders

Henoch-Schönlein purpura

Drug abuse

No identifiable etiology

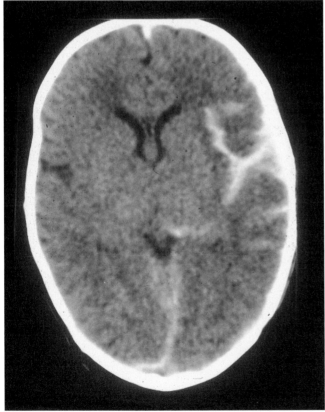

Figure 17-1. Computed tomography scan shows subarachnoid hemorrhage. Concentration of the hemorrhage within the Sylvian fissure is typical of a ruptured middle cerebral artery bifurcation aneurysm.

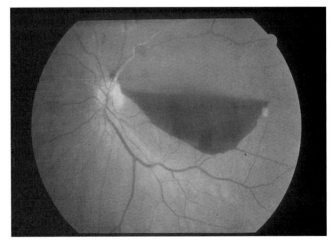

Figure 17-2. Preretinal hemorrhages are common in individuals with SAH. Because of their frequent keel-shaped appearance they are sometimes called "boat hemorrhages."

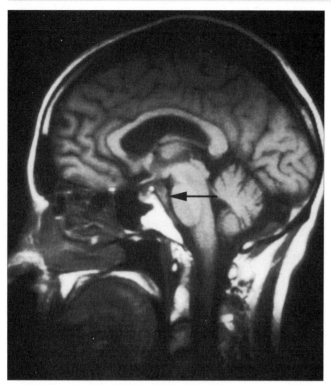

Figure 17-3. Nonaneurysmal perimesencephalic SAH (*arrow*) has a lower risk or rebleeding and a better prognosis.

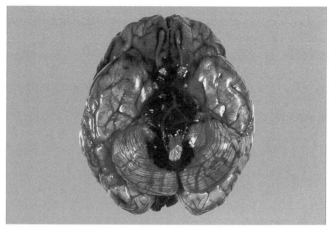

Figure 17-4. Massive subarachnoid hemorrhage, in this instance due to a ruptured aneurysm. The base of the brain is encased in blood, and the convexities are blood tinged.

clinical pattern than venous blood oozing from a ruptured vein. Another factor that may contribute to the clinical picture is vasospasm of the arteries surrounded by subarachnoid blood.

During the hours after hemorrhage onset, the level of consciousness may vary from normal to deeply comatose. If coma occurs, it usually develops soon after aneurysmal rupture or later in the course of the illness because of cerebral vasospasm or rebleeding. Disorientation, amnesia, delirium, and confabulation are common in the acute stages but usually disappear within a week. Confusion persisting longer than several weeks is an ominous sign, suggestive of permanent deficit.

Nuchal rigidity and other signs of meningeal irritation usually develop within 24 hours. Low-grade fever is common. At times arterial hypertension occurs as a result of acutely increased intracranial pressure (ICP), impaction of the cerebellum against the medulla, or stimulation of brainstem vasopressor reflexes.

Almost any cranial nerve may be affected. The oculomotor nerve (CN III) and the abducens nerve (CN VI) are affected most often. Abnormalities of the abducens nerve are of little localizing value, but involvement of the oculomotor nerve suggests an aneurysm located at the junction of the posterior communicating and internal carotid arteries. Of the many signs of oculomotor dysfunction, the first to appear is usually pupillary dilatation, so the size, shape, and reactivity of the pupils must be examined repeatedly.

Funduscopy may show preretinal hemorrhages (Figure 17-2). Although these are characteristic of SAH, they are not pathognomonic because they can be caused by any acute rise in ICP. Papilledema may develop. In one study of 100 consecutive SAH patients, 17 individuals had intraocular hemorrhage and 8 also had vitreous hemorrhage (Terson syndrome).[10] Terson syndrome is more likely to occur in patients with more severe SAH, and most of the patients with Terson syndrome have preretinal hemorrhages as well.[11]

Focal neurological deficits may result from (a) cerebral vasospasm in the neighboring or distant arteries with consequent cerebral ischemia, (b) intracerebral hemorrhage, (c) local pressure on the brain due to a localized subarachnoid hematoma, or (d) cerebral edema.

A cranial bruit suggests high flow from an underlying arteriovenous malformation (AVM) or arteriovenous fistula rather than a saccular aneurysm.

Risk Factors and Differential Diagnosis of SAH

Once a diagnosis of SAH has been established, its etiology must be promptly determined. Saccular aneurysms are the most likely cause of nontraumatic SAH. In the cooperative study of intracranial aneurysms and SAH, 54% of the SAHs were due to ruptured aneurysm.[12]

Individuals with a perimesencephalic SAH (also known as pre-truncal hemorrhage) represent an important SAH subgroup.[13] In these patients the SAH is centered in the interpeduncular fossa and ambient cisterns (Figure 17-3). The likelihood of an aneurysm is much lower in these individuals, and, consequently, their risk of rebleeding is lower than in individuals with aneurysmal SAH. As a result, their long-term prognosis is also much better.[14] Perimesencephalic nonaneurysmal SAH may arise from compromised veins or capillaries.[13]

Although SAH is seldom the sole manifestation of blood dyscrasias, all patients should be examined for petechiae or purpura and for evidence of mucocutaneous or internal bleeding. Severe platelet or coagulation dysfunction may predispose to

Table 17-2: Hunt and Hess Classification of SAH[21,22]

Grade	Description
1	Asymptomatic or mild headache, slight nuchal rigidity
2	Moderate to severe headache, nuchal rigidity, no neurological deficit other than cranial nerve palsy
3	Drowsiness, confusion, or mild focal neurological deficit
4	Stupor, moderate to severe hemiparesis, possible early decerebrate rigidity, and vegetative disturbances
5	Deep coma, decerebrate rigidity, and moribund appearance

Add a grade for serious medical disease (arterial hypertension, diabetes mellitus, severe atherosclerosis, COPD, or severe vasospasm on angiography)
Modified criteria adds the following:
0 = Unruptured aneurysm
1A = No acute meningeal or brain reaction in a patient with a fixed deficit

Table 17-3: World Federation of Neurological Surgeons SAH Grading System[20]

WFNS Grade	GCS	Motor Deficit
0	15	Unruptured aneurysm
1	15	Absent
2	13–14	Absent
3	13–14	Present
4	7–12	Present or absent
5	3–6	Present or absent

Table 17-4: The Glasgow Coma Scale[19]

Category	Parameter	Score[a]
Eyes	Open spontaneously	4
	Open to verbal command	3
	Open to pain	2
	No eye opening	1
Best Motor Response	Obeys to verbal command	6
	Localizes to painful stimulus	5
	Flexion withdrawal to pain	4
	Abnormal flexion (decorticate rigidity) to pain	3
	Abnormal extension (decerebrate rigidity) to pain	2
	No response	1
Best verbal response	Oriented and converses	5
	Disoriented and converses	4
	Inappropriate words	3
	Incomprehensible sounds	2
	No response	1

[a] Total the score from each axis to obtain a final comprehensive grade.

Table 17-5: Fisher CT Classification of Subarachnoid Hemorrhage[23]

Group	Description
1	No blood detected
2	Diffuse deposition or thin layer of blood with all vertical layers of blood (interhemispheric fissure, insular cistern, and ambient cistern) being less than 1 mm thick
3	Localized clots or vertical layers of blood more than 1 mm in thickness (or both)
4	Diffuse or no subarachnoid blood but with intracerebral or ventricular clots

both SAH and intracerebral hemorrhage, either spontaneously or in response to minor trauma. Sickle cell disease can lead to SAH, either with or without aneurysmal rupture.[15] Brain tumors occasionally lead to SAH. Neoplasms most likely to cause SAH are ependymoma, meningioma, glioblastoma multiforme, melanoma, or choriocarcinoma.

Intracranial arterial dissection sometimes leads to SAH. Cerebral amyloid angiopathy is a potential cause of SAH among elderly individuals.[16–18] Moyamoya disease can lead to SAH but more typically causes intracerebral hemorrhage. Cortical thrombophlebitis due to bacterial meningitis or vasculitis is a rare cause of SAH. Causes of SAH are outlined in Table 17-1.

Obviously other conditions that result in sudden onset of severe headache or acute mental status change must be considered in the differential diagnosis of SAH. The presenting manifestations of SAH are not always typical, and the initial symptoms are sometimes difficult to elicit from a patient with altered mental status, so the differential diagnosis is broad. Acute bacterial or viral meningitis often feature severe headache, photophobia, and meningismus, although the headache usually does not begin as explosively as with SAH. Similarly, viral encephalitis can cause severe headache and mental status change. When papilledema and retinal hemorrhages occur in a patient with clouded consciousness, the clinical picture may suggest hypertensive encephalopathy. If the patient is pregnant, eclampsia or pituitary apoplexy might be considered (see Chapter 23).

Pathophysiology of Subarachnoid Hemorrhage

Subarachnoid bleeding (Figure 17-4) is followed quickly by increased ICP, decreased cerebral blood flow (CBF), increased cerebral blood volume or oxygen extraction, which suggests arteriolar constriction and dilatation of the microcirculation. At times ICP can approach the range of diastolic arterial blood pressure. Thereafter, other mechanisms, particularly brain edema, blockage of CSF drainage, and impaired venous drainage perpetuate the pathophysiologic cycle of events. Vasoparalysis of distal cerebral arterioles may allow transmission of arterial pressure directly to the brain with disruption of the blood-brain barrier and consequent cerebral edema and sudden rise of ICP. Elevation of the ICP may compress the site of bleeding, providing time for clotting to occur, but once the ICP begins to exceed the blood's perfusion pressure blood flow fails.

Grading of Aneurysmal SAH

Numerous clinical grading scales for aneurysmal SAH patients have been devised in an effort to improve prognostication and stratify treatment risks.[19] Collectively, SAH patients with increased severity scores tend to do poorly. Clinical severity grades, however, are often used to stratify the level of clinical severity of the individuals enrolled in research studies.[19] The two most often cited SAH grading systems are those of Hunt and Hess and a scale developed under the auspices of the World Federation of Neurological Surgeons.[20,21] Both scales have subjective aspects but are widely recognized and simple to apply over a broad range of clinical severity.

The 1968 Hunt and Hess score (Table 17-2) was conceived as a way to estimate the surgical risk and select the optimal time for surgery.[21,22] Subsequently, Hunt and Kosnik modified the scale, adding Grade 0 for individuals with an unruptured aneurysm and Grade 1a for individuals with a fixed neurological deficit without acute meningeal or other clinical signs.[22] The 1988 WFNS scale (Table 17-3) was derived from the Glasgow Coma Scale (Table 17-4), but its approach was underpinned by relevant data from the International Cooperative Aneurysm Study. In addition, Fisher and colleagues developed a CT-based SAH classification scale (Table 17-5) that provides a standardized approach to categorizing the severity of SAH.[23]

The Hunt-Hess grade at presentation correlates with mortality: 30% for Grade 1, 40% for Grade 2, 50% for Grade 3, 80% for Grade 4, and 90% for Grade 5. Predictors of rebleeding in a multiple logistic regression model of factors present on admission included only Hunt-Hess grade and larger aneurysmal size.[24]

INCIDENCE OF SAH AND ANEURYSM

Incidence of SAH

The annual incidence of nontraumatic SAH in one study was 6 per 100,000 individuals per year.[25] However, the reported incidence varies considerably, in part because of case selection and methodology as well as differences in the population under study. For example, an increased incidence has been reported in the Japanese and Finnish populations.[26,27] In Sweden the overall incidence of SAH was 12.4 per 100,000 person-years, and the rate increased with age, ranging from 6.4/100,000 person-years among individuals between 30 and 39 years of age to 25.8/100,000 person-years among individuals older than 80 years.[28]

Incidence of Aneurysm

Unruptured, asymptomatic intracranial saccular aneurysms are incidental findings in about 5% of autopsies.[29] Similarly, among 400 volunteers who had a systematic evaluation with digital subtraction angiography, CT, MRI, and magnetic resonance angiography (MRA), there were 26 individuals (6.5%) with 27

asymptomatic, unruptured aneurysms.[30] In this study individuals with a family history of SAH had an even higher incidence of unruptured aneurysms (17.9%).

Individuals with an intracranial aneurysm often have one or more additional intracranial aneurysms. In one cohort of 1,314 patients with aneurysm, for example, 302 (23%) had at least one additional intracranial aneurysm.[31] In addition, AVMs or other vascular lesions sometimes occur in individuals with intracranial aneurysms.[32]

SACCULAR ANEURYSMS

Pathogenesis of Saccular Aneurysms

Saccular aneurysms are usually acquired lesions. Traditionally intracranial aneurysms have been classified as small (equal to or less than 12 mm), large (13–24 mm), and giant (equal to or greater than 25 mm). Saccular aneurysms are relatively uncommon in infants and children. Half or more of the individuals with a symptomatic aneurysm are past the age of 40 when symptoms first occur, and many people with an aneurysm remain asymptomatic.

The course of an intracranial aneurysm in a given individual is unpredictable. Smoking cigarettes increases the likelihood of an aneurysm rupturing.[33] A history of arterial hypertension also increases the odds of aneurysm rupture, but not as dramatically as a long smoking history (more than 10 pack years).[33] Hypertension also increases the odds of having giant and multiple aneurysms.[34,35]

In a few individuals an intracranial aneurysm is associated with vascular Ehlers-Danlos syndrome (type IV) or pseudoxanthoma elasticum.[36,37] However, most patients with an intracranial aneurysm do not have an associated connective tissue disorder.

Before age 40 the anatomical site of aneurysm formation is about the same for men and women. Thereafter, the most likely site of aneurysm formation in women is at the junction between the internal carotid and posterior communicating artery, whereas 40% of SAHs in men are due to anterior communicating artery aneurysms. Women are also more likely to develop intracavernous carotid artery aneurysms. For further delineation of the sites of aneurysms, see Table 17-6.

Clinical Features of Aneurysms

By far the most common presentation of an intracranial aneurysm is SAH. In rare instances the hemorrhage from a ruptured aneurysm is purely intraparenchymal or subdural.[38] About 10% of aneurysms rupture during sleep, over half during periods of exertion, and a third during other normal daily activities. Contrary to common belief, intermittent or chronic headache rarely results from an unruptured intracranial aneurysm. Occasionally an aneurysm of the infraclinoid internal carotid artery can cause pain in the first or second divisions of the trigeminal nerve.

Aneurysms most often burst after they have reached 5 to 10 mm in diameter, but there is a wide variation in the size of the aneurysm at the time of rupture. Many people harboring an intracranial aneurysm remain asymptomatic throughout life. Some aneurysms enlarge very slowly, reaching a large size before rupturing. These lesions typically cause no symptoms at first, but because of their large size and strategic location, some produce symptoms and signs by compressing adjacent brain or cranial nerves or by obstruction of the CSF pathways. In the aggregate

Table 17-6: Distribution of Single Aneurysms Associated with SAH

Aneurysm Site	Number	Percentage of Total
Internal carotid artery		
Intracavernous	2	N
Below posterior communicating junction	101	4.3
Region of posterior communicating junction	576	25
Posterior communicating to bifurcation	101	4.3
Bifurcation of internal carotid	106	4.5
Subtotal	**886**	**38**
Anterior cerebral artery		
Proximal to anterior communicating artery	35	1.5
Anterior communicating artery region	711	30.3
Distal to anterior communicating artery	66	2.8
Segment not specified	36	1.5
Subtotal	**848**	**36**
Middle cerebral artery		
Proximal to main branches	91	3.9
Region of main branches	307	13.1
Distal to main branches	32	1.4
Segment not specified	58	2.5
Subtotal	**488**	**21**
Posterior cerebral artery		
Main trunk	7	N
At basilar junction	4	N
Segment not specified	10	N
Subtotal	**21**	**0.9**
Basilar artery		
Apical bifurcation	48	2
Main trunk	19	0.8
Subtotal	**67**	**2.8**
Vertebral artery		
Proximal to basilar	8	N
At basilar junction	3	N
Segment not specified	9	N
Subtotal	**20**	**0.9**
Cerebellar arteries		
Posterior inferior	11	N
Superior	6	N
Anterior inferior	2	N
Subtotal	**19**	**0.8**
Total	2,349	100

Adapted with permission from Locksley et al.[224]
SAH = subarachnoid hemorrhage; N = negligible.

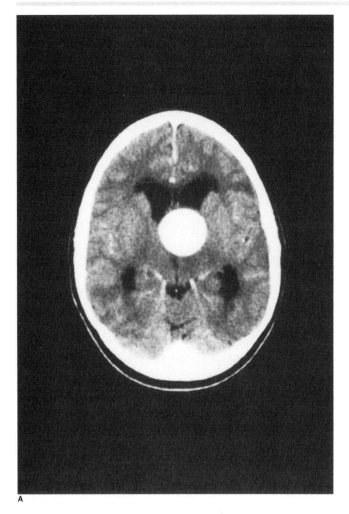

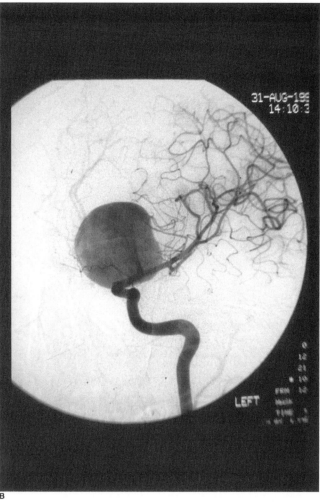

Figure 17-5. A: Cranial CT with contrast depicts a giant aneurysm filling the third ventricle and displacing the lateral ventricles. B: Catheter angiogram shows the aneurysm arising near the junction of the internal carotid artery and the middle cerebral artery.

about 10% of saccular aneurysms present with symptoms and signs of pressure on an adjacent structure (Figure 17-5).

Transient ischemic attacks or ischemic infarction may occur in the distribution of the aneurysmal artery, perhaps resulting from artery-to-artery embolism of a clot originating within the aneurysm.[39,40] In addition, vasospasm of the involved or adjacent arteries following an SAH can produce an ischemic infarction of the tissue distal to the aneurysm.

Pregnancy per se does not seem to be associated with increased risk of aneurysmal rupture, but labor may be. The risk of aneurysmal rupture may be exacerbated by the coexistence of arterial hypertension due to eclampsia. Aneurysms were responsible for 77% of the intracranial hemorrhages during pregnancy in one summary of 154 individuals. Surgical treatment of the aneurysm was associated with lower maternal and fetal mortality.[41] Women with an intracranial aneurysm who deliver by Cesarean section fare no better than those who opt for vaginal delivery (see Chapter 23).

ANEURYSM SYNDROMES

Most aneurysms of the cerebral circulation present with SAH and thus have very similar initial signs and symptoms. The general

signs and symptoms of SAH have already been presented. Some aneurysms, however, develop location-specific clinical findings. The salient features of aneurysms of individual vessels are described briefly in the following pages. It should be emphasized, however, that these descriptions are intended to serve only as guides to the anatomic location of intracranial aneurysms because the clinical features of these lesions show a great deal of variation and overlap depending on their size, shape, and type and the directions in which they enlarge.

Cervical Internal Carotid Artery

Aneurysms of the cervical portion of the internal carotid artery typically arise near the common carotid bifurcation but may occur anywhere along the vessel, including the carotid canal. Larger aneurysms that arise above the ramus of the mandible typically bulge medially to form a mass in the lateral pharynx, whereas those below it present as a neck mass.[42] Cervical aneurysms must be distinguished from arterial kinks, coils, or pseudo-aneurysms.

Extracranial internal carotid artery aneurysms typically cause headache, carotidynia, and oculosympathetic paresis (Horner syndrome). These lesions may be pulsatile and tender.[43] Ischemic symptoms occur more often with extracranial carotid aneurysms than with intracranial aneurysms.[42,43] Bleeding into the pharynx may occur, especially during surgical procedures in the region.

Carotid Canal

Aneurysms of the carotid canal are rare.[44] If the lesion extends into the middle ear, the patient experiences ear pain, recurrent otitis media, and deafness. Intrapetrous aneurysms can compress the trigeminal nerve or ganglion and cause facial pain resembling tic douloureux. The location of these aneurysms adjacent to the middle ear makes them especially important for individuals undergoing middle ear surgery.[44]

Infraclinoid Intracavernous Carotid Artery

Retro-orbital pain and diplopia are the most common presenting symptoms.[45] The extent of trigeminal nerve involvement depends on the exact position of the aneurysm within the sinus. Anterior lesions cause pain and hypalgesia restricted to the ophthalmic division (V1); those located in the midportion of the sinus involve both the ophthalmic (V1) and the maxillary division (V2); posteriorly placed or very large aneurysms may involve all three divisions of the trigeminal nerve. Very large aneurysms may simulate a pituitary neoplasm and produce hypopituitarism. Infraclinoid aneurysms are more likely to rupture into the cavernous sinus than into the subarachnoid space, resulting in a carotid-cavernous fistula (Figure 18-5) that may spare the patient's life but cause pain and loss of vision.[46,47]

Supraclinoid Internal Carotid Artery

Aneurysms arising from the internal carotid artery after it emerges from the cavernous sinus may project in any direction and, therefore, produce a variety of clinical signs. They often rupture. Because the internal carotid travels between the optic nerve and the optic chiasm medially and the oculomotor nerve laterally, supraclinoid aneurysms may produce a CN III palsy or variable defects in vision.[48] Long-standing pressure on the optic nerve produces unilateral optic atrophy and compression of the optic chiasm, leading to visual field defects that may mimic pituitary adenoma. Very large aneurysms occasionally produce unilateral anosmia. Aneurysms of the terminal portion of the internal carotid are more common in individuals with genetic disorders such as pseudoxanthoma elasticum and vascular Ehlers-Danlos syndrome.[49,50]

Middle Cerebral Artery

Almost 14% of aneurysms arise from the first or second division of the middle cerebral artery within the depth of the Sylvian fissure. Bifurcation middle cerebral artery aneurysms do not produce extraocular palsies. Their cardinal features are hemiplegia, dysphasia, visual field defects, and/or focal seizures. One or more of these signs may develop suddenly as a result of hemorrhage or vasospasm of the arterial tree or insidiously because of pressures on the adjacent cortex produced by slow expansion of the sac.

Anterior Cerebral Artery

Large aneurysms of the proximal anterior cerebral artery can produce amaurosis or anosmia, but most are asymptomatic until they rupture. Suprachiasmatic pressure may rarely lead to altitudinal visual field defects. Rupture into the frontal lobe can cause behavioral change and paralysis of the contralateral lower limb. An aneurysm at the bifurcation of the callosal marginal and pericallosal arteries is the only distal location for a saccular aneurysm found with any frequency and occurs in about 5% of ruptured aneurysms. In other locations aneurysms situated peripherally are usually infective (septic).

Anterior Communicating Artery

About 30% of aneurysms arise from the anterior communicating artery. These lesions are usually silent until they rupture, but suprachiasmatic pressure from large lesions can cause lower visual field defects. The anterior communicating artery lies just anterior to the lamina terminalis, the thin anterior wall of the third ventricle. Consequently, upward rupture of an aneurysm in this location often leads to intraventricular hemorrhage with profound mental change, akinetic mutism, or immediate coma. Akinetic mutism, which may be permanent, is a sequel to rupture or it can become apparent following intracranial surgery. This complication presumably results from infarction of the region of the septum, medial forebrain bundle, or fornix. Blood in the supraoptic area may promote inappropriate antidiuretic hormone secretion.

Posterior Communicating Artery

Aneurysms of the posterior communicating artery constitute 29% of all aneurysms and most commonly occur at the junction of this vessel with the internal carotid (Table 17-6). The posterior communicating artery lies adjacent to CN III, so an aneurysm of this vessel often results in oculomotor nerve paralysis with pupillary involvement.[51,52]

Posterior Cerebral Artery

Aneurysms of the posterior cerebral artery may be saccular or fusiform.[53] They account for less than 1% of all intracranial aneurysms.[54] Depending on their size and location along the course of the posterior cerebral artery, these aneurysms may produce midbrain cranial nerve palsies, sensory disturbance, or visual field quadrantanopia.[55–57] Giant aneurysms of the proximal posterior cerebral artery may compress the brainstem and produce signs of bulbar dysfunction.

Basilar Artery

Basilar artery aneurysms make up 10% of intracranial aneurysms but only 3% of the aneurysmal SAH. They may involve the basilar bifurcation (tip), the basilar/superior cerebellar artery junction, or the basilar artery trunk, in that order. They also occur at the vertebral/posterior inferior cerebellar artery (PICA) junction or at the junction of the vertebral arteries. Aneurysms of the basilar artery may be fusiform or saccular. Fusiform aneurysms occasionally rupture, and they sometimes lead to ischemic stroke because of artery-to-artery embolism.[58] The tortuosity of fusiform aneurysms can cause compression palsies of adjacent cranial nerves, dysfunction of the nearby ascending or descending tracts, or obstructive hydrocephalus. Tic douloureux and hemifacial spasm may be the initial manifestation. Saccular aneurysms of the basilar artery may rupture, causing severe suboccipital pain, decerebrate rigidity, and bulbar paralysis, which is often fatal.

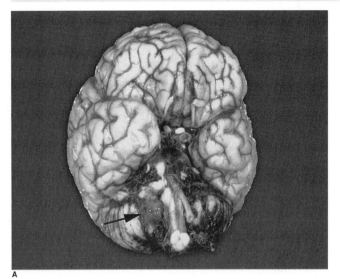

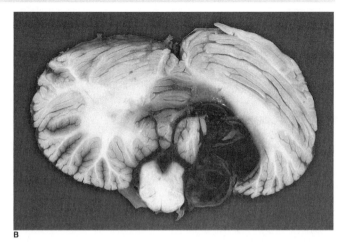

Figure 17-6. A: Aneurysm of the posterior inferior cerebellar artery (*arrow*). B: In addition to subarachnoid and intraparenchymal hemorrhage, the aneurysm also caused brainstem and cerebellar compression.

Vertebral Artery

Aneurysms of the vertebral artery are unusual, accounting for less than 1–2% of all intracranial aneurysms. The symptoms they produce resemble those of basilar artery aneurysm. In addition, they may lead to attacks of a Ménière-like syndrome, ataxia, or signs of bulbar involvement. Some aneurysms of the vertebral artery protrude into the cervical canal, producing bulbar and spinal cord involvement (foramen magnum syndrome).

Cerebellar Arteries

Aneurysms of the cerebellar arteries are rare.[59] In addition to SAH, these aneurysms can compress the brainstem or cranial nerves. Palsy of the oculomotor and, at times, abducens nerve may be caused by aneurysms of the proximal portion of the superior cerebellar artery. Aneurysms of the anterior inferior cerebellar artery sometimes compress the lower cranial nerves.[60] Large aneurysms of the posterior inferior cerebellar artery (Figure 17-6) may simulate tumor of the foramen magnum.[61,62] Some aneurysms of the cerebellar arteries produce no localizing signs other than those of an expanding, bleeding lesion in the posterior cranial fossa.

DISORDERS ASSOCIATED WITH INTRACRANIAL ANEURYSM

Intracranial aneurysms have been identified among individuals with various congenital or acquired disorders. Although the aneurysm risk for some of these conditions is well accepted, in other instances the link is at best tenuous. The signs and symptoms of an aneurysm in these individuals are not unique, although some of the conditions may be associated with an earlier occurrence of intracranial bleeding or a predisposition to arterial dissection or other complications. Some of the disorders with an acknowledged aneurysm risk are presented individually below, and others are summarized in Table 17-7.

Coarctation of the Aorta

The association of cerebral aneurysms and coarctation of the aorta was first mentioned by Eppinger in an 1871 autopsy report. However, one early survey identified only three individuals with definite and two with probable aneurysms among 200 patients with aortic coarctation (2.5%), a number that is roughly the same as in the general population.[63] Conversely, Connolly and colleagues screened 100 coarctation patients with MRA and identified cerebral aneurysms in 10 individuals.[64] Despite the congenital nature of aortic coarctation, individuals with an associated intracranial aneurysm seldom become symptomatic until after adolescence.

Fibromuscular Dysplasia

Individuals with fibromuscular dysplasia (FMD; see Chapter 13) have an increased risk of harboring an intracranial aneurysm. Sandok and colleagues identified 13 individuals with an intracranial aneurysm among 44 people with fibromuscular dysplasia (30%), although only six of these lesions had ruptured.[65] In another report 19 of 37 (51%) fibromuscular dysplasia patients had one or more cerebral aneurysms, although in most other cohorts the frequency is considerably lower.[66] Recent reports suggest that the prevalence of asymptomatic cerebral aneurysms among individuals with fibromuscular dysplasia is about 7%, which is greater than that of the general population but much less than many of the early reports suggested.[67]

Autosomal Dominant Polycystic Kidney Disease

Autosomal dominant polycystic kidney disease is caused by mutations of *PKD1* (chromosome 16) or *PKD2* (chromosome 4). A mutation of either of these genes can lead to an intracranial aneurysm. The risk of developing an intracranial aneurysm is increased substantially above that of unaffected individuals.[68] Although the exact pathophysiology of aneurysm formation due to polycystic kidney disease is not well understood, PKD1 knockout mice exhibit vascular instability and blood vessel

Table 17-7: Conditions Associated with Intracranial Aneurysm

Takayasu Arteritis[225]

Atrial myxoma[135]

Infective endocarditis[119]

Behçet disease[226]

Coarctation of the aorta[64]

Ehlers-Danlos syndrome (especially type IV)

Familial aneurysms[98]

Fibromuscular dysplasia[67]

Human immunodeficiency virus[131]

Marfan syndrome[226]

Moyamoya disease[89]

Neurofibromatosis type 1[229,230]

PHACES syndrome[83]

Autosomal dominant polycystic kidney disease[68]

Pompe disease[230]

Pseudoxanthoma elasticum[90,91]

Sickle cell disease[231]

rupture.[69] Occasional individuals with tuberous sclerosis complex develop intracerebral aneurysms.[70–72] One of the two genes that cause tuberous sclerosis (*TSC2*) is located adjacent to the polycystic kidney disease gene *PKD1* on chromosome 16, creating a possible explanation for the aneurysms that sometimes accompany tuberous sclerosis complex.

Most patients with autosomal dominant polycystic kidney disease and intracerebral aneurysms do not develop symptoms from the aneurysm until after the second decade.[73,74] The majority of the aneurysms in people with polycystic kidney disease occur in the anterior circulation, especially in the branches of the middle cerebral artery.[75,76] Multiple aneurysms in the same individual are common: about a quarter of the patients have more than one aneurysm.[76] There is evidence that individuals with polycystic kidney disease who have a relative with both polycystic kidney disease and a ruptured aneurysm may be at still greater risk of developing a symptomatic aneurysm.[68]

Ehlers-Danlos Syndrome

Ehlers-Danlos syndrome is subdivided into several subtypes based on the inheritance pattern, clinical features, and various defects in collagen synthesis.[77,78] Most individuals with an intracranial aneurysm related to Ehlers-Danlos syndrome, however, have vascular Ehlers-Danlos syndrome (type IV), an autosomal dominant defect of type III collagen, the major form of collagen found in blood vessels. The collagen defect of vascular Ehlers-Danlos results from a mutation of the *COL3A1* gene.[79] Although type III collagen is the major collagen found in blood vessels, aneurysm patients who do not have features of Ehlers-Danlos syndrome do not have *COL3A1* mutations.[80] Occasional individuals with Ehlers-Danlos type I or type VI develop an intracranial aneurysm.

Hyperelastic skin (Figure 21–3) and hyperextensible joints are not striking features of vascular Ehlers-Danlos syndrome, so the diagnosis is often made only after a major vascular complication. The intracranial segment of the internal carotid artery (Figure 17-7) is the site most likely to develop an aneurysm.[37] Additional information about Ehlers-Danlos syndrome is presented in Chapter 21.

Marfan Syndrome

The extent to which Marfan syndrome increases the risk of an intracranial aneurysm is debatable (see Chapter 21). Although individuals with Marfan syndrome have an increased risk of aortic aneurysms, in larger case series, very few individuals with Marfan syndrome develop an intracranial aneurysm.[81,82]

Other Possible Aneurysm Associations

Anomalies in the circle of Willis or persistent fetal patterns are about twice as frequent in patients with saccular aneurysms as in the rest of the population. Both anomalous intracranial arteries and aneurysms occur in individuals with the PHACE syndrome (PHACE is an acronym for posterior fossa brain malformations, hemangiomas of the face, anomalous arteries, cardiac defects, and eye lesions). In one report 13% of the individuals with the PHACE syndrome had an intracranial aneurysm.[83]

Perhaps not surprisingly given the frequency of intracranial aneurysms, an estimated 1.1% of individuals with cerebral aneurysms have concurrent AVMs.[84,85] There are occasional reports of aneurysms arising several years after cranial irradiation.[86,87] Aneurysms sometimes occur in patients with moyamoya disease (see Chapter 13) or those with sickle cell disease (see Chapter 11).[88,89] Intracranial aneurysms sometimes occur in individuals with neurofibromatosis type 1 and those with pseudoxanthoma elasticum (see Chapter 21).[90,91]

Familial Intracranial Aneurysms

Familial clusters of individuals with one or more intracranial aneurysms are more common than once suspected.[92] Familial occurrence of SAH has also been described, but many of these individuals prove to have an aneurysm when careful catheter angiography is done.[93] A few families with five or six affected individuals have been described, but, more commonly, two or three siblings are affected.[94,95] Individuals with familial intracranial aneurysms tend to become symptomatic at an earlier age than other people with sporadic aneurysms. Familial aneurysms often involve the anterior circulation and are often smaller at the time of rupture. Multiple aneurysms and "mirror image" lesions (involving the same artery in the opposite hemisphere) occur in 26% and 13%, respectively.[94,96]

The likelihood of an aneurysm patient having a similarly affected family member varies in different series, perhaps reflecting differences in ascertainment methods.[92] In a study from Scotland, only 2% of the individuals with an SAH or an intracerebral aneurysm had a similarly affected family member.[97] Kojima and colleagues studied 8,680 individuals with MRA, including a subgroup of 380 individuals who had a family member with an intracranial aneurysm.[98] In this series the likelihood of an aneurysm was 10% among the relatives of the aneurysm patients and 6.8% among the remaining cohort. Kim and colleagues found an aneurysm in at least one family member of 20% of their patients regardless of ethnicity.[99] The risk seems

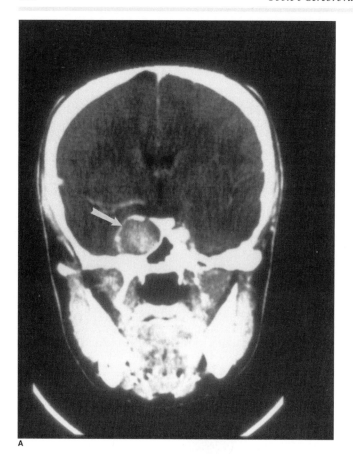

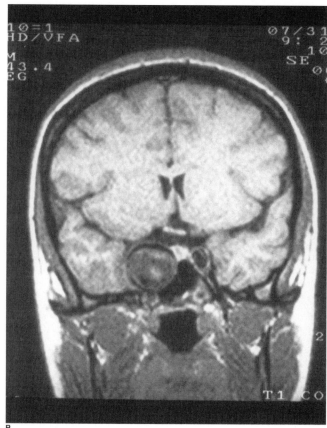

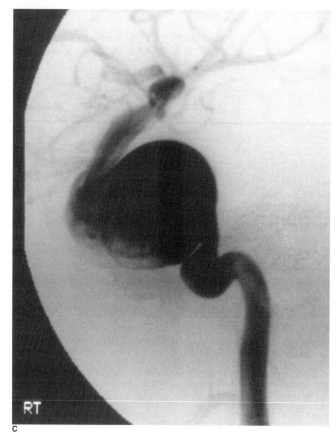

Figure 17-7. A: Coronal CT with contrast (from an 18-year-old with vascular Ehlers-Danlos syndrome) shows a giant aneurysm (*arrow*) of the right intracavernous carotid artery. B: Coronal T_1-weighted magnetic resonance scan demonstrates the same lesion as well as a smaller intracavernous aneurysm on the other side. C: Catheter angiography of the right internal carotid artery shows the intracavernous carotid artery aneurysm. Reprinted with permission from Roach and Zimmerman.[223]

higher in first-degree relatives and in families with multiple affected members.

Rational evaluation of family members is problematic.[100–102] Noninvasive imaging methods make it feasible to screen asymptomatic individuals who are at increased risk for intracerebral aneurysms, and repeated examinations are justifiable when the risk is particularly high.[103] The aneurysm risk is greater among first-degree relatives, especially first-degree relatives who smoke or have hypertension. Screening with MRA is justified, especially in first-degree relatives who smoke and those with hypertension.[95,104,105] Unfortunately, small aneurysms can still be missed, and new aneurysms may appear later, so screening does not benefit everyone.

There is genetic heterogeneity among individuals with familial aneurysms, and the pathophysiology of these lesions is not fully understood.[106,107] One autopsy study noted degeneration of the arterial elastic fibers in individuals with familial aneurysms,[93] and in some families specific haplotypes of the elastin gene seem to correlate with aneurysm susceptibility.[108] In a Japanese cohort, alterations of the COL1A2 gene encoding type I collagen were identified.[109] Another study identified a polymorphism of the LOXL2 gene, one of a group of genes that promote cross-linkage of elastin and collagen.[110] Nongenetic factors, such as cigarette smoking and arterial hypertension, evidently help to determine which individuals with a susceptibility gene become symptomatic.[111]

OTHER ANEURYSM TYPES

Fusiform Aneurysms

Like saccular aneurysms, fusiform aneurysms often remain asymptomatic. When symptoms do result from a fusiform aneurysm, they are more likely to stem from compression of the adjacent brain structures than from aneurysm rupture and subarachnoid hemorrhage. In one series of 120 patients, the aneurysm created a mass effect in 50% of the patients, whereas only 20% presented with hemorrhage.[112]

Individuals with fusiform aneurysms are prone to develop ischemic symptoms compared to people with a saccular aneurysm. Eight of 120 patients described by Drake and Peerless, for example, developed ischemic infarction or transient ischemic attacks.[112] Strokes can result from embolism from the aneurysm to a distal branch of the artery or from occlusion of local penetrating branches originating near the aneurysm.[58] Stroke following thrombosis of the aneurysm itself has been described.[113]

Fusiform aneurysms typically affect large vessels – the basilar, vertebral, and internal carotid arteries. Unlike saccular aneurysms, which have a strong predilection for the carotid circulation, fusiform aneurysms are more likely to occur in the posterior circulation. In one review of 120 patients with fusiform aneurysms, for example, 95 lesions were present in the posterior circulation versus only 25 in the anterior circulation.[112]

Although fusiform aneurysms are often assumed to arise because of atherosclerosis, the available evidence for this notion is sparse. Atherosclerosis is striking in some individuals. However, in the Drake and Peerless series of 120 patients, only six individuals had prominent atherosclerosis, and three others had another known arteriopathy. Moreover, patients in this cohort were, on average, younger than would have been predicted for atherosclerosis, and fusiform aneurysms have been described even in children. More likely, fusiform aneurysms develop because of nonatheromatous degenerative changes within the artery.

Infective Aneurysms

The term mycotic aneurysm is a misnomer inasmuch as these lesions most often result from bacterial rather than fungal infections. Fungal aneurysms sometimes occur in immuno-compromised patients or with sinusitis or trauma. Antibiotic treatment of infective endocarditis has greatly reduced the frequency of infective aneurysms. In one center infectious aneurysms accounted for 4% of all aneurysms,[114] but they should be suspected in individuals with a subarachnoid or intracerebral hemorrhage who have a structural heart lesion, history of intravenous drug abuse, or chronic pulmonary infection. A few patients have infectious aneurysms in conjunction with lung infections, trauma, or meningitis.[115,116]

Pathophysiology of Infective Aneurysms

Aneurysms resulting from infective endocarditis are typically due to various strains of Streptococcus or Staphylococcus, whereas the organisms from other sources tend to be more diverse.[117] The most common site for an infectious aneurysm is the middle cerebral artery branches either in the Sylvian fissure or distal to it.[118,119] Multiple infected emboli can produce multiple aneurysms, and the lesions are classically located in the more distal arterial branches where the embolism comes to rest.[120,121]

Infective aneurysms occur when the wall of an intracranial artery is weakened by inflammation and infection due to an infective embolus.[118,122] Less virulent organisms produce the localized inflammation and arterial wall damage that leads to aneurysm formation, whereas more virulent organisms result in meningitis or brain abscess. Microscopic examination reveals inflammation and necrosis of the expanding arterial wall.

Clinical Findings

Because of the conditions that foster infective aneurysms, the patient is often ill-appearing and febrile. Cardiac murmurs, pulmonary dysfunction, skin lesions, and other signs of the underlying disease state may be apparent.

An infective aneurysm can produce isolated SAH, but the tendency of infectious aneurysms to involve the more distal artery branches also increases their likelihood of causing an intracerebral hemorrhage when the aneurysm ruptures. The clinical picture is sometimes complicated by focal cerebritis, an abscess, or the occurrence of an adjacent ischemic infarction before the aneurysm formation.[123–125] If the weakened arterial wall ruptures, hemorrhagic bacterial meningitis may result.

Human Immunodeficiency Virus

Human immunodeficiency virus (HIV) can cause intracranial vascular changes that promote ischemic stroke.[126–128] A number of case reports, mostly describing children, have documented the occurrence of intracranial aneurysms in HIV-infected individuals.[129,130] One report documented two HIV-infected children with an intracranial aneurysm among a cohort of 250 individuals who were HIV-infected.[131]

In addition to the aneurysm, postmortem studies demonstrate ectasia of the arteries of the circle of Willis, medial fibrosis, loss of the muscularis, intimal hyperplasia, and destruction of the internal elastic lamina without prominent inflammation.[129,132] It seems plausible that the progressive structural damage to the vessel wall over an extended period of time could allow the aneurysm to form.

Neoplastic Aneurysms

Atrial myxomas are uncommon, but the occurrence of intracerebral aneurysms in affected individuals is well documented.[133–135] Aneurysms develop in arteries that have been infiltrated and weakened by embolized myxoma cells.[136] Intracranial aneurysms due to myxomas occur predominantly in the middle cerebral artery territory, but many individuals have multiple aneurysms involving either the intracranial or systemic arteries.[137] Both saccular and fusiform aneurysms have been identified.[138,139] Like infectious emboli, tumor emboli tend to lodge in the distal arterial branches, increasing the chances of an intraparenchymal brain hemorrhage when the lesion ruptures.[140]

Individuals with an atrial myxoma are also at risk for ischemic stroke from blood clot or tumor embolism (Figure 8-4), so one or more ischemic infarctions may be identified in an individual with a myxomatous aneurysm.[135,141] Seeded tumor cells may continue to damage the arterial wall over time, and new intracranial aneurysms can arise years after the successful removal of the cardiac tumor.[139,140,142] However, some neoplastic aneurysms remain stable over time, whereas others enlarge steadily until rupture occurs.[143]

Neoplastic aneurysms also occasionally occur because of metastatic choriocarcinoma,[144,145] bronchogenic carcinoma,[146,147] or other tumors. Primary intracranial tumors occasionally lead to aneurysm formation in an adjacent artery,[148] and aneurysms rarely develop following radiation therapy of an intracranial mass.[149]

NATURAL HISTORY OF ANEURYSMS

Knowledge of the natural history of unruptured intracranial aneurysms allows clinicians to make sound therapeutic and prognostic judgments based on the likelihood of the aneurysm's rupture over the course of the individual's remaining lifetime. Obviously, risk of treatment should not exceed the risk of hemorrhage, but the likelihood of the eventual aneurysmal rupture varies among different "natural history" studies. The risk of hemorrhage also increases as the size of an aneurysm increases. Jane and colleagues estimated that 1% of the individuals with an asymptomatic aneurysm or an unruptured secondary aneurysm will develop an SAH each year.[150] Juvela and associates identified 33 instances of first-time SAH among 142 patients who were tracked for 2,575 patient years, for an estimated annual rupture rate of 1.3%. These authors found a cumulative bleeding rate of 10.5% at 10 years, 23% at 20 years, and 30.3% at 30 years after diagnosis.[151]

Other reports, however, suggest a lower rate of rupture. In one cohort of 1,449 patients with 1,937 unruptured aneurysms, the annual aneurysm rupture rate was less than 0.05% per year among individuals who had lesions that were less than 10 mm in diameter and who had not had a prior SAH from another aneurysm.[29] In this same cohort, the frequency of aneurysm rupture among individuals with a lesion diameter greater than 10 mm but less than 25 mm was 0.5% per year, but the frequency surged to 6% in people with aneurysms greater than 25 mm in diameter.[29]

Cigarette smoking and arterial hypertension, along with larger aneurysm size, increase the likelihood of an aneurysm rupture.[151,152] Patients who have used cocaine tend to have an SAH at a younger age and have a worse outcome than other aneurysm patients.[153] Older individuals and those with larger aneurysms are less likely to survive a ruptured aneurysm.[154] People with a fatal SAH also tend to have had higher systolic blood pressure values and a higher prevalence of arterial hypertension.[154]

Once the initial SAH occurs, the risk of additional bleeding from an unrepaired aneurysm is very high. The risk of rebleeding is highest within the first 24 hours of the initial bleed. Untreated, about half of patients who survive an aneurysm-related SAH will have a second hemorrhage within 6 months. Thereafter, the risk of rebleeding diminishes to about 3% per year.[150]

PATHOLOGY OF SACCULAR ANEURYSMS

Aneurysm Location

Most saccular aneurysms arise near the bifurcations of arteries. About 85% are located on the internal carotid or its branches and the anterior communicating artery, and 15% arise from the vertebral-basilar system. Of those in the carotid distribution, over 30% are in the anterior cerebral communicating complex, 13% on the middle cerebral, 8% on the ophthalmic artery or cavernous carotid, and another 20% at the origin of the posterior communicating artery. Of the 15% from the vertebral basilar system, 3% arise directly from vertebral arteries or PICA, 2% from the superior cerebellar artery, and 7% from the top of the basilar. Aneurysms in children are more likely to affect the intracranial carotid artery and the posterior circulation.

About 20% of the time, multiple aneurysms occur in the same individual, and up to 40% of these are bilateral in symmetrical locations. Because saccular aneurysms originate near arterial bifurcation sites, it is often difficult to specify which of the two arteries gave rise to the aneurysm. The distributions given above depend, to some extent, on whether the data were collected at autopsy, by catheter arteriography, or at surgery.

Macroscopic Appearance

Most saccular aneurysms lie within the subarachnoid space (Figure 17-6), but as they enlarge, a portion of the aneurysm may extend into the brain parenchyma. Except in rare instances, aneurysmal rupture leads to SAH. Intraparenchymal hemorrhage may result from either dissection of blood from the subarachnoid space or from rupture of the aneurysm directly into the substance of the brain. In general, the larger the aneurysm, the more likely it is to rupture, although large-diameter aneurysms may create a mass effect without rupture.[155]

Saccular aneurysms classically arise from their parent vessel by a narrow stalk or neck, but in many cases the junction is broad-based and even wider than its dome. Most saccular aneurysms are pea-sized, but they may be as small as a pinhead or bigger than a walnut. Occasional aneurysms reach gigantic proportions, sometimes compressing cranial nerves, distorting the nearby brain substance, or even eroding adjacent bone. Some sacs enlarge over time, whereas others seem to remain static.

The sac of a large aneurysm is often partially filled with laminated, organized, or organizing blood clot, a factor that may slow progressive enlargement and subsequent rupture of the aneurysm. The rupture usually occurs at the apex of the aneurysm, often at the site of a small diverticulum.[156] Some enlarging saccular aneurysms become complex biloculated or multiloculated lesions with multiple fragile blebs. However, small aneurysms can rupture and not be apparent on visual inspection because they are obscured by subarachnoid blood. At autopsy or surgery, brownish pigmentation, fibrous thickening, and adhesions of surrounding tissues are evidence of a previous hemorrhage.[157]

Microscopic Appearance

If bleeding has occurred previously, the aneurysm may be surrounded by phagocytes containing hemosiderin, lymphocytic infiltration, and fibrous thickening. The muscular coat of the artery stops at the neck of the aneurysm, whereas the degenerated internal elastic membrane continues for a short distance into the aneurysmal sac.[157–159] Calcification may develop within the aneurysm wall. The wall of the aneurysm is made up of fibrous tissue continuous with the intima and adventitia of the parent artery. Thus, the aneurysm wall consists of an endothelial lining, fibrous tissue, and adventitia. Electron microscopic studies confirm fragmentation of the internal elastic lamina at its junction with the aneurysmal sac and diminished elastic tissue. The basement membrane underneath the endothelium is frequently thickened and reticulated, and degenerative changes and necrosis of the muscle are evident.[160]

Defects in the media are often present at multiple cerebral arterial bifurcation sites, even in individuals who do not have an aneurysm.[161] Why an aneurysm develops in some individuals with these congenital defects but not in others is uncertain, but, in all probability, the defective area is further compromised over time by hemodynamic wear and tear. Systemic hypertension may contribute to the formation of aneurysms in older patients and increase the rate of rebleeding of a ruptured aneurysm.[162] As yet unknown genetic or metabolic factors may play a role in determining which individuals with vascular defects actually develop an aneurysm.

Infectious aneurysms are distinguished from other aneurysms microscopically by the intense local inflammatory reaction.[163,164] An abscess may form about the aneurysm site, and the offending organism can sometimes be seen or cultured. The arterial media and elastica are damaged, but the acute nature of this process is usually apparent.

DIAGNOSTIC STUDIES

The clinical features of SAH are dramatic, but not all patients with a sudden-onset, severe headache have an SAH. Even after the diagnosis of SAH has been confirmed, one must still identify the cause of the hemorrhage and the anatomic origin of the bleeding to develop an appropriate treatment plan. These goals can usually be achieved with the aid of CT, catheter angiography, and other diagnostic procedures. More information about specific diagnostic procedures is provided in Chapter 5.

Computed Tomography

When done within 24 hours of the ictus, CT depicts the SAH (Figure 17-1) in most patients.[165,166] However, the sensitivity of CT quickly diminishes as the subarachnoid blood is cleared and the cerebrospinal fluid (CSF) hemoglobin concentration drops. Only 76% of the hemorrhages are detectable by 2 days after the ictus, and just over half of the hemorrhages are detectable after 5 days.[165] Additionally, CT provides a useful means of estimating the amount of bleeding, and it is often the severity of the hem-

orrhage that determines the patient's eventual outcome. Individuals with more severe SAH on the initial CT have a greater likelihood of developing delayed cerebral ischemia due to vasospasm.[167] Computed tomography can depict hydrocephalus, impending cerebral herniation, and other complications of SAH. Larger aneurysms or AVMs are often apparent on CT, but it does not reliably exclude smaller lesions.

The densest area of subarachnoid blood on the initial CT is to some extent predictive of the site of a bleeding aneurysm.[168] This is an important determination in individuals with multiple intracranial aneurysms whose site of bleeding may not be otherwise apparent. Prominent intraventricular hemorrhage with less prominent bleeding in the subarachnoid space suggests the rupture of an anterior communicating artery aneurysm, but, in the absence of intraventricular bleeding, the hemorrhage from these aneurysms tends to be basilar or interhemispheric. Dense hemorrhage within the Sylvian fissure suggests an aneurysm of the middle cerebral artery trifurcation. Intraparenchymal brain hemorrhage due to a ruptured aneurysm, not surprisingly, usually occurs near the aneurysm. The pattern and quantity of bleeding on the initial CT is a better predictor of aneurysms of the middle cerebral and anterior communicating arteries than those at other sites.[168] An SAH that is located predominantly in the perimesencephalic area (Figure 17-3) is also important to recognize, because these individuals have a much lower aneurysm risk and a much better prognosis.

A high-quality CT scan with contrast infusion will sometimes depict an aneurysm (Figure 17-8 A), particularly one greater than 4 mm in diameter. A dense clot within the aneurysmal sac or a curvilinear calcification within the aneurysm wall may be apparent. Routine CT, however, is not a sensitive means of detecting smaller aneurysms, and even larger lesions may not be readily apparent in the setting of a severe SAH.

Diffuse cerebral edema can be present at the time of presentation or develop later in the course. The presence of global edema is a predictor of both mortality and poor outcome.[169] Cerebral edema is more likely to occur in an individual with coma or higher-grade SAH as well as in patients who require the use of vasopressors.[169]

CT Angiography

In experienced hands CT angiography has good sensitivity and specificity in the detection of aneurysms. In most reports, however, the reliability of CT angiography lags slightly behind that of catheter angiography, especially for the detection of smaller aneurysms and in defining the relationship of the aneurysm to adjacent vessels.[170–172] CT angiography is noninvasive and provides information about the aneurysm's anatomic relationship to bony structures that is not possible with either catheter angiography or MRA. The level of confidence in the use of CT angiography is likely to depend greatly on a physician's accumulated experience with the technique and with the clinical situation.

In one report of 136 individuals with 244 intracranial aneurysms, the sensitivity and specificity of CT angiography for aneurysms were 98.0% and 99.1%, respectively. The authors concluded that CT angiography is a reasonable substitute for catheter angiography, even for smaller aneurysms.[173] In other series, however, the reliability of CT angiography is not quite as good and also somewhat interpreter dependent.[170] Chappell and colleagues concluded from their meta-analysis of CT angiography comparison studies that digital subtraction angiography

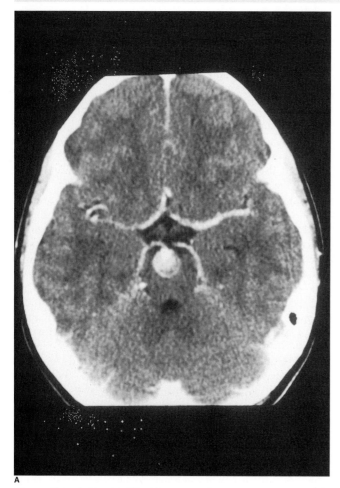

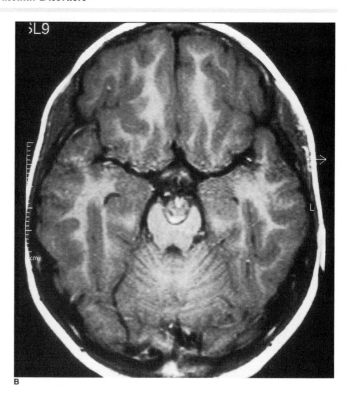

Figure 17-8. A: Cranial CT with contrast showing an aneurysm of the rostral basilar artery. B: The same aneurysm is evident on MRI.

remains more reliable, but that CT angiography may be sufficient in some situations and is safer.[174]

Magnetic Resonance Imaging

The wall of an intracranial aneurysm is sometimes apparent on
brain MRI (Figure 17-8 B), but this imaging modality is not a
reliable way to test for an intracranial aneurysm.[175] In occasional
individuals an aneurysm that is not apparent with catheter
angiography is seen on MRI, probably because thrombus within
the aneurysmal sac precludes contrast filling of the aneurysm
during angiography.

   With the appropriate imaging sequences, SAH is often visible on cranial MRI.[176] However, MRI is not as reliable as CT for
demonstrating SAH. Furthermore, CT is often more readily
available in emergency situations, and images are readily available within a few minutes. For these reasons, unenhanced CT
remains the preferred initial test for SAH. Nevertheless, MRI is
more sensitive than CT in depicting ischemic lesions that sometimes result from SAH-related vasospasm or after endovascular
or surgical procedures.[177–179]

Magnetic Resonance Angiography

Although larger intracranial aneurysms can be identified with
MRA, this test is not as reliable as either catheter angiography or

CT angiography when the aneurysm is smaller or more peripherally located. However, noninvasiveness and lack of radiation
of MRA make it ideal for the repeated testing of individuals at
high risk of aneurysm formation or those already known to
have an aneurysm. Once the vascular tree has been fully characterized by catheter angiography, MRA can be an effective means
of tracking the lesion's status. Infective aneurysms can be followed by repeated MRA to assess for possible resolution during
antimicrobial therapy.[180]

Lumbar Puncture

An SAH is occasionally confirmed with an LP that is not apparent on CT.[181] Whether a patient with a normal CT should
undergo an LP depends on the level of clinical suspicion for
SAH, but it is usually unnecessary to examine the CSF once an
SAH has been convincingly demonstrated on a neuroimaging
procedure. Given the high frequency of ruptured intracranial
aneurysms among individuals with SAH, it is often better to
avoid potentially stressful or uncomfortable procedures that
could perhaps trigger additional bleeding.

   The opening pressure is usually elevated, and the CSF is
almost always bloody (usually > 100,000 RBCs/ml). Although
hemorrhage may not be visible to the naked eye when there are
fewer than 200 red blood cells/mm³ of CSF, clear fluid ordinarily
means that there is no SAH. The presence of xanthochromic

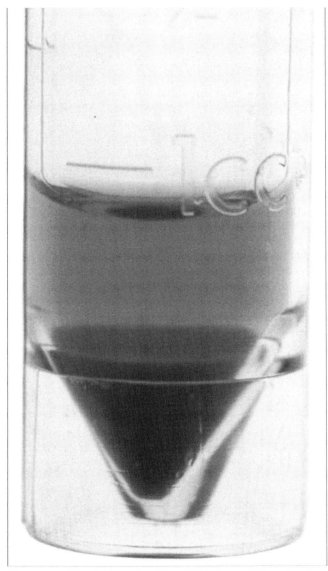

Figure 17-9. Xanthochromia of the CSF helps to differentiate SAH from a traumatic lumbar puncture.

fluid (Figure 17-9) helps to distinguish an SAH from a traumatic LP.[166] The protein content is typically elevated and the CSF glucose normal. Mild pleocytosis sometimes occurs, but high numbers of leukocytes in the setting of an SAH suggest an infective aneurysm or herpetic encephalitis. In very rare instances the fluid may remain clear when an intracranial aneurysm ruptures directly into the subdural space, when the hemorrhage remains loculated in the subarachnoid space because of previous adhesions, or when an LP has been performed too soon for blood to equilibrate with the CSF in the subarachnoid space.

Catheter Arteriography

Despite the appeal of less invasive tests, catheter angiography (see Chapter 5) remains the most reliable way to confirm an intracranial aneurysm. Catheter cerebral angiography is particularly valuable for detecting smaller aneurysms or lesions of the smaller peripheral arteries, neither of which are reliably visualized by noninvasive vascular imaging. In one analysis of 2,899 patients undergoing cerebral catheter angiography, the overall complication rate was 1.3%, but the frequency of permanent morbidity was only 0.5%.[182]

The artery that is most likely to harbor the ruptured intracranial aneurysm should be studied first in the event that the procedure has to be terminated before completion. However, because so many sites can be involved and because of the frequent occurrence of multiple intracranial aneurysms in the same individual, it is prudent to carefully image both the carotid and the vertebrobasilar circulations to ensure that all sources of bleeding have been identified.[183] When more than one aneurysm is present, the lesion that is larger and has an irregular contour is often the one that was responsible for the hemorrhage.[184]

Given the small size and distal location of many infective aneurysms, catheter angiography probably remains the most accurate way to assess individuals at high risk (e.g., those with infective endocarditis) or those whose clinical features suggest an infective aneurysm. It is reasonable to undertake a catheter angiogram in such individuals even in the absence of a hemorrhage. Once the aneurysms have been identified, however, CT or MR techniques may be adequate to monitor the lesions in patients who are undergoing treatment and evidently doing well.[185]

Catheter angiography may fail to reveal an aneurysm in some individuals with an initial SAH due to an aneurysm, and a second or even a third angiogram may be necessary to properly identify the source of the bleeding.[186,187] Even at autopsy no cause can be established in some individuals with SAH.[59] Unless the subarachnoid blood is more concentrated in a particular area, the search for the responsible vessel can be daunting, especially in the absence of an aneurysm. A small vascular lesion can be obliterated by the very hemorrhage it created, disappearing without a trace in the mass of blood that now surrounds it. Moreover, most autopsies do not include examination of the venous system or spinal subarachnoid space, and, yet, hemorrhage may originate in either.

In some individuals there is a small ectatic out-pouching at the junction of the internal carotid and the posterior communicating artery.[188–190] These infundibula are usually less than 2 mm in diameter and have a rounded or pyramidal-shaped configuration with no neck. A few of these ectatic areas enlarge progressively and ultimately develop into saccular aneurysms, but, for the most part, they have little clinical significance.

Screening for Aneurysms

Should asymptomatic individuals with an increased aneurysm risk undergo diagnostic surveillance studies? The answer depends on an individual's perceived aneurysm risk and the invasiveness of the tests to be employed. To justify diagnostic screening, the benefit from early diagnosis and treatment of an aneurysm must exceed the combined risks of the diagnostic study and therapy, although this concern is more relevant to catheter angiography than other studies. It is also hard to justify surveillance angiography in an individual who is either unwilling or unable to undergo treatment in the event that an aneurysm is discovered.

The decision to do surveillance studies is likely to hinge in part on the invasiveness of the study being contemplated. Although CT and MR angiography procedures offer the allure of noninvasiveness, neither test is as accurate as a good-quality catheter angiogram, especially when the lesion is small or located in the peripheral vasculature. On the other hand, CT or MR angiography may be an adequate way to track the size of an aneurysm that is already known to be present.

Given the high frequency of multiple aneurysms and the observation that some of these lesions become apparent well after the patient's initial SAH, it might seem reasonable to look for additional aneurysms in individuals with a prior ruptured aneurysm. Additionally, periodic imaging might identify an aneurysm that has recurred after treatment. In practice, the yield for surveillance screening is relatively low except in selected situations.

Although most of the individuals with autosomal dominant polycystic renal disease who develop intracranial aneurysms remain asymptomatic until adulthood, we recommend screening with MRA or CTA when the diagnosis of polycystic kidney disease is established.[191,192] Unfortunately, smaller aneurysms can be missed or develop later.[193,194] Catheter angiography should be considered in patients with an abnormal or questionable MRA or suggestive neurologic symptoms. The mutation site on *PKD1* may predict an individual's aneurysm risk.[195] If confirmed, this finding could alter the approach to aneurysm screening in these individuals.

MANAGEMENT PRINCIPLES

Subarachnoid Hemorrhage and Neurological Complications

Every effort should be made to prevent recurrent aneurysmal SAH. Careful attention should be paid to pain control and to blood pressure management. Anxious patients may benefit from a sedative. A stool softener is appropriate. A seizure in an individual with an unsecured ruptured aneurysm could have devastating consequences. Patients who experience seizures are treated with appropriate antiepileptic drugs, but the routine prophylactic administration of these agents remains controversial. There is little evidence that prophylactic corticosteroids are beneficial.[196]

The occurrence of rebleeding peaks within 24 hours from the index SAH. Antifibrinolytic therapy reduces the risk of rebleeding, but it does so at the expense of an increased risk of cerebral vasospasm and hydrocephalus.

Acute hydrocephalus is a common complication of SAH, and hydrocephalus is especially common in the setting of intraventricular hemorrhage.[197] Hydrocephalus is also more common among individuals whose blood is concentrated in the basilar and lateral regions and those with a large amount of subarachnoid blood regardless of its location.[198] Ventricular drainage may be needed to relieve the pressure of hydrocephalus.

Cerebral vasospasm has a peak incidence between 6–8 days after aneurysmal SAH. Management involves administration of calcium channel blockers, hypertensive/hypervolemic therapy, and endovascular therapy. In a meta-analysis of seven trials of nimodipine in patients with subarachnoid hemorrhage, the drug reduced the risk of ischemic deficits due to SAH and increased the likelihood of a good outcome.[199] The mortality was slightly reduced, although this trend did not reach statistical significance.

Saccular Aneurysms

A multimodal, multidisciplinary approach is recommended for the optimal treatment of aneurysm patients. Both operative and endovascular aneurysm techniques yield good results, but a multimodal group endeavor with decision making by a team of neuro-endovascular interventionalists, neurologists, and neurosurgeons offers the best opportunity for optimal patient management.[200,201] This multidisciplinary approach allows the team to select the best therapeutic option for each patient or to combine operative and endovascular techniques in the same individual. In practice, the choice of therapy often depends as much on the expertise and experience of the practitioners as on the nature of the aneurysm, and the proportion of aneurysm patients who undergo endovascular treatment is increasing.[202]

In general, aneurysm therapy is designed to isolate the aneurysm or reduce the arterial pressure within it, to strengthen its walls by encasing material around it, or to promote thrombosis in it. The transcranial approach has been greatly aided by improved anesthetic techniques, the use of dehydrating agents to better control the intracranial pressure, and the induction of controlled hypotension and hypothermia. Endovascular therapy continues to rapidly evolve, spurred both by technical improvements and by the increasing experience and expertise of the physicians who perform it.[202]

The optimal neurosurgical aneurysm treatment is to place a clip across the isthmus between the aneurysm and its parent vessel. Other surgical techniques include isolating the aneurysm between two clips placed on the parent vessel and reinforcing the wall of the aneurysm by wrapping or encasing it. Aneurysm clipping or other operative techniques are best suited for aneurysms of the distal branches of the anterior, middle, or posterior cerebral artery as well as for aneurysms with wide necks that open directly into a high-pressure, high-flow artery, such as the carotid or top of the basilar artery.[203]

Endovascular placement of detachable platinum coils or other material inside the aneurysm with secondary lesion thrombosis greatly reduces the likelihood of aneurysm rupture (Figure 17-10). Endovascular treatment is attractive because it avoids craniotomy and is tolerated by some patients who would be unable to withstand a neurosurgical procedure. Aneurysms that are secured in this fashion can recanalize, but the treatment failure rate is generally comparable to that of neurosurgery, at least for the first few years.[204] Endovascular techniques are ideal for patients who are too ill or debilitated to tolerate surgery or for lesions that are not easily clipped, such as an intracavernous carotid artery aneurysm. A combined approach is ideal for complex lesions that are not easily managed entirely by either endovascular or operative therapy. Even more distal aneurysms can sometimes be secured with endovascular techniques.[205] The success rate for endovascular coil treatment of a ruptured aneurysm is comparable to that of neurosurgical therapy, although the patient is more likely to be free of disability a year after treatment with platinum coils than with neurosurgery.[206,207]

Because recurrent hemorrhage is most likely to occur within 1 day of the initial rupture, an aneurysm should usually be repaired as soon as the source of the bleeding has been identified and the patient is stable enough to tolerate treatment.[208] For alert patients, early treatment has always been recommended. Early surgery or endovascular treatment is also being performed on individuals with higher-grade hemorrhages.[208,209] The reduction in rebleeding episodes with early aneurysm surgery in these patients is evidently sufficient to offset any increased operative morbidity.[210] In addition, the availability of less invasive endovascular techniques makes treatment of sicker patients more feasible.

Fusiform Aneurysms

Because fusiform aneurysms are elongated and have no defined neck, they are often more difficult to manage with the surgical

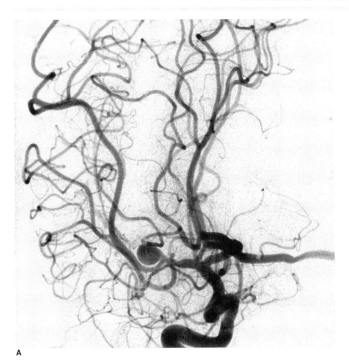
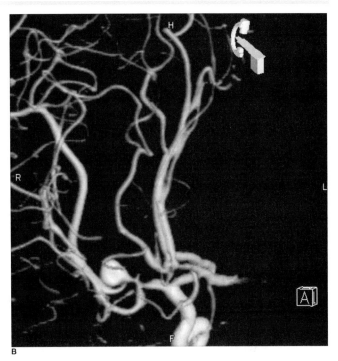

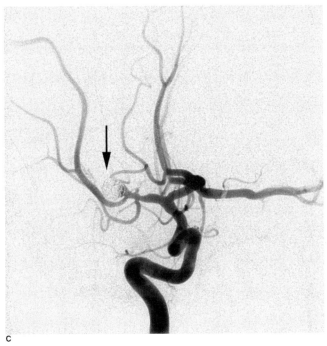

Figure 17-10. A: A catheter angiogram depicts a right middle cerebral artery aneurysm. B: Three-dimensional CT reconstruction of the same aneurysm demonstrates its relationship to nearby arteries. C: The lesion is no longer filled after placement of platinum coils. Photographs courtesy of Dr. Louis Carragine.

and endovascular techniques that are used for saccular aneurysms. Nevertheless, the majority of patients do reasonably well, one suspects, because of the indolent nature of these lesions as much as the effectiveness of the available therapy. If the collateral circulation is adequate, a fusiform aneurysm can be "trapped" – isolating the aneurysm from its blood supply by occluding the affected artery both proximal and distal to the lesion.[112,201] This approach requires that there be adequate collateral blood flow to the brain distal to the occluded artery as well as an alternate source of blood to replace penetrating branches from the isolated segment of the artery. When successful, this technique reduces the likelihood of aneurysm rupture as well as the potential for artery-to-artery embolism and stroke. Trapping the aneurysm may also keep the mass effect from worsening. Techniques to encase and stabilize the aneurysm reduce the likelihood of hemorrhage and the progression of the mass effect but do nothing to prevent embolism. In recent years the combination of endovascular and operative techniques has been successfully adapted for use with fusiform aneurysms.[211]

Infective Aneurysms

Treatment of individuals with an infective aneurysm provides unique challenges. The distal location of many infectious aneurysms can make both surgery and endovascular procedures more difficult. The often debilitated condition of patients with infective endocarditis, impaired immunity, or a history of intravenous drug use add to the difficulty.[119] The underlying infection must be aggressively treated regardless of what is done for the aneurysm, and, to this end, it is imperative to identify the responsible organism to optimize antimicrobial therapy.

Some infective aneurysms involute with long-term antimicrobial treatment and do not rupture or rebleed.[119] This conservative approach is particularly attractive when there are multiple unruptured infective aneurysms, when the patient is too ill to undergo a major procedure, and when the aneurysm is in a location that is difficult to reach. As with other aneurysms, however, the deferral of definitive therapy for infective aneurysms can be disastrous, and in general lesions that have bled should be occluded if feasible.[125,212] Persistence of an aneurysm after 2 months of antibiotics or the development of symptoms are indications for surgery.[185]

The distal location of some infectious aneurysms can make both surgical management and endovascular procedures more difficult. Endovascular techniques have been increasingly utilized, especially in individuals with intracranial infectious aneurysms associated with infective endocarditis, who may also require cardiac surgery with cardiopulmonary bypass.[119,125,213]

Unruptured Aneurysms

An individual with an incidentally discovered aneurysm is typically asymptomatic and may be destined to remain so, but if the aneurysm ruptures, the result is often disastrous. The appropriate approach depends on the size and location of the aneurysm, age and family history of the patient, ability of the patient to tolerate treatment, and experience of the treating physicians.[214,215]

Mizoi and colleagues analyzed their experience with 139 patients who had one or more incidentally discovered intracranial aneurysms.[216] Eight (16%) of their 49 patients who were managed conservatively later had an SAH during the 4.3 year average follow-up interval, and seven of these eight patients died from the aneurysm rupture. In contrast, 99 other individuals with a total of 119 intracranial aneurysms underwent surgery with no significant operative complications and no subsequent SAH.[216] King and colleagues performed a meta-analysis on 733 individuals who had undergone elective surgery for an asymptomatic unruptured intracranial aneurysm.[217] Thirty patients (4.1%) had a postoperative neurological deficit and 7 (1%) died, leading the authors to conclude that elective surgery caries an acceptable risk given the devastating results of many SAHs.[217]

Clearly the decision to undertake an elective aneurysm repair hinges on the perceived risk of leaving the lesion alone versus the treatment risk specific to a particular medical center. The bleeding risk from small aneurysms is low, but a lesion larger than 10 mm or one that has grown should probably be repaired.[214] Similarly, a previous symptomatic aneurysm or one or more first-degree relatives with an aneurysm argue for treatment. Given the cumulative risk of aneurysmal rupture over several years and the often devastating results of such a catastrophe, more aggressive therapy is probably justified in younger individuals.[30]

Thus, the optimal management approach for individuals with an incidentally discovered aneurysm depends on the size and number of the lesions (larger aneurysms may be more likely to rupture, generating greater urgency to repair them), the anatomic location of the aneurysm (which will influence the difficulty of both surgery and endovascular procedures), and the age and well-being of the patient.[216] Whether or not an incidental aneurysm is secured, every effort should be made to control modifiable risk factors, such as smoking and systemic hypertension.

Treatment Outcome

Intact survival following an SAH depends largely on the severity of the initial hemorrhage and whether additional hemorrhages occur. Patients who undergo surgery when asymptomatic have few complications.[216] Most of the time, however, it is the initial SAH that leads to the diagnosis of an aneurysm, and in many instances the initial hemorrhage is severe. Occasional patients undergoing aneurysm surgery develop orbital infarction syndrome, thought to result from hypoperfusion of the ophthalmic artery and its branches.[218] However, the likelihood of a good outcome has improved in recent years, probably because of improved techniques to manage cerebral vasospasm as well as the increasing availability of endovascular therapies.[219]

The volume of the hemorrhage is the single biggest predictor of death. In one report 21 of 36 (58%) aneurysm-related deaths were attributed to the initial SAH, and about half of the remaining deaths were due to rebleeding.[220] Although delayed vasospasm contributes to the short-term and long-term morbidity of SAH, vasospasm accounted for only two of the 36 (5.5.%) deaths due to SAH in this series.[220]

As might be predicted, individuals with multiple intracranial aneurysms tend to do worse than those with a single aneurysm, and, treatment results become increasingly worse in proportion to the number of additional aneurysms.[31] A second SAH resulting from rupture of another aneurysm no doubt adds to the morbidity and mortality of these individuals, but much of the poorer outcome is due to manipulation of the cerebral arteries during multiple aneurysm surgery.[31]

Epilepsy may occur after aneurysm surgery. In one series 14 (8%) of 183 individuals developed epilepsy within 2 years of aneurysm surgery.[198] Factors increasing the likelihood of post-treatment epilepsy included a middle cerebral artery aneurysm, postoperative cerebral vasospasm, and cortical infarctions.

Unfortunately, varying degrees of long-term cognitive impairment occur following an aneurysm repair.[221] In one series of 37 people who had undergone a single intracranial aneurysm repair at least 6 months earlier, 65% were left with impaired executive function or memory.[222] The long-term cognitive function was worse in individuals with postoperative neurologic events and in those with preoperative rebleeding.

REFERENCES

1. Verweij RD, Wijdicks EFM, van Gijn J. Warning headache in aneurysmal subarachnoid hemorrhage. A case-control study. *Arch Neurol.* 1994;**45**:1019–1020.

2. Ostergaard JR. Warning leak in subarachnoid haemorrhage. *BMJ.* 1990;**301**:190–191.

3. de Falco FA. Sentinel headache. *Neurol Sci* 2004;**25**(Suppl 3):S215–S217.

4. Leblanc R. The minor leak preceding subarachnoid hemorrhage. *J Neurosurg.* 1987;**66**:35–39.

5. Bassi P, Bandera R, Loiero M, Tognoni G, Mangoni A. Warning signs in subarachnoid hemorrhage: a cooperative study. *Acta Neurol Scand.* 1991;**84**:277–281.

6. Juvela S. Minor leak before rupture of an intracranial aneurysm and subarachnoid hemorrhage of unknown etiology. *Neurosurgery.* 1992;**30**:7–11.

7. Hauerberg J, Andersen BB, Eskesen V, Rosenorn J, Schmidt K. Importance of the recognition of a warning leak as a sign of a ruptured intracranial aneurysm. *Acta Neurol Scand.* 1991;**83**:61–64.

8. Polmear A. Sentinal headache in aneurysmal subarachnoid hemorrhage: what is the true incidence? *Cephalalgia.* 2003;**23**:935–941.

9. Linn FH, Wijdicks EF, van der Graff Y, et al. Prospective study of sentinel headache in aneurysmal subarachnoid haemorrhage. *Lancet.* 1994;**344**:590–593.

10. Kuhn F, Morris R, Witherspoon CD, Mester V. Terson syndrome. Results of vitrectomy and the significance of vitreous hemorrhage in patients with subarachnoid hemorrhage. *Ophthalmology.* 1998;**105**:472–477.

11. Ness T, Janknecht P, Berghorn C. Frequency of ocular hemorrhages in patients with subarachnoidal hemorrhage. *Graefes Arch Clin Exp Ophthalmol.* 2005;**243**:859–862.

12. *Intracranial Aneurysms and Subarachnoid Hemorrhage: A Cooperative Study.* Philadelphia: J. B. Lippincott Company; 1969.

13. Vermeulen M, Lindsay KW, van Gijn J. *Subarachnoid Hemorrhage.* London: W. B. Saunders Company; 1992.

14. Rinkel GJ, Wijdicks EF, Vermeulen M, et al. The clinical course of perimesencephalic nonaneurysmal subarachnoid hemorrhage. *Ann Neurol.* 1991;**29**:463–468.

15. Batjer HH, Adamson TE, Bowman GW. Sickle cell disease and aneurysmal subarachnoid hemorrhage. *Surg Neurol.* 1991;**36**:145–149.

16. Yamada M, Itoh Y, Otomo E, Hayakawa M, Miyatake T. Subarachnoid haemorrhage in the elderly: a necropsy study of the association with cerebral amyloid angiopathy. *J Neurol Neurosurg Psychiatry.* 1993;**56**:543–547.

17. Takeda S, Yamazaki K, Miyakawa T, et al. Subcortical hematoma caused by cerebral amyloid angiopathy: does the first evidence of hemorrhage occur in the subarachnoid space? *Neuropathology.* 2003;**23**:254–261.

18. Linn J, Herms J, Dichgans M, et al. Subarachnoid hemosiderosis and superficial cortical hemosiderosis in cerebral amyloid angiopathy. *AJNR Am J Neuroradiol.* 2008;**29**:184–186.

19. Rosen DS, Macdonald RL. Subarachnoid hemorrhage grading scales: a systematic review. *Neurocrit Care.* 2005;**2**:110–118.

20. Report of World Federation of Neurological Surgeons Committee on a Universal Subarachnoid Hemorrhage Grading Scale. *J Neurosurg.* 1988;**68**:985–986.

21. Hunt WE, Hess RM. Surgical risk as related to time of intervention in the repair of intracranial aneurysms. *J Neurosurg.* 1968;**28**:14–20.

22. Hunt WE, Kosnik EJ. Timing and perioperative care in intracranial aneurysm surgery. *Clin Neurosurg.* 1974;**21**:79–89.

23. Fisher CM, Kistler JP, Davis JM. Relation of cerebral vasospasm to subarachnoid hemorrhage visualized by computerized tomographic scanning. *Neurosurgery.* 1980;**6**:1–9.

24. Naidech AM, Janjua N, Kreiter KT, et al. Predictors and impact of aneurysm rebleeding after subarachnoid hemorrhage. *Arch Neurol.* 2005; **62**:410–416.

25. Broderick JP, Brott T, Tomsick T, Miller R, Huster G. Intracerebral hemorrhage more than twice as common as subarachnoid hemorrhage. *J Neurosurg.* 1993;**78**:188–191.

26. Pakarinen S. Incidence, aetiology, and prognosis of primary subarachnoid haemorrhage. A study based on 589 cases diagnosed in a defined urban population during a defined period. *Acta Neurol Scand.* 1967;**43**(Suppl):1–28.

27. Inagawa T, Ishikawa S, Aoki H, Takahashi M, Yoshimoto H. Aneurysmal subarachnoid hemorrhage in Izumo City and Shimane Prefecture of Japan. Incidence. *Stroke.* 1988;**19**:170–175.

28. Koffijberg H, Buskens E, Granath F, et al. Subarachnoid haemorrhage in Sweden 1987–2002: regional incidence and case fatality rates. *J Neurol Neurosurg Psychiatry.* 2008;**79**:294–299.

29. International Study of Unruptured Intracranial Aneurysms Investigators. Unruptured intracranial aneurysms – risk of rupture and risks of surgical intervention. *N Engl J Med.* 1998;**339**:1725–1733.

30. Nakagawa T, Hashi K. The incidence and treatment of asymptomatic, unruptured cerebral aneurysms. *J Neurosurg.* 1994;**80**:217–223.

31. Rinne J, Hernesniemi J, Niskanen M, Vapalahti M. Management outcome for multiple intracranial aneurysms. *Neurosurgery.* 1995;**36**:31–37.

32. Batjer H, Suss RA, Samson D. Intracranial arteriovenous malformations associated with aneurysms. *Neurosurgery.* 1986;**18**:29–35.

33. Adamson J, Humphries SE, Ostergaard JR, Voldby B, Richards P, Powell JT. Are cerebral aneurysms atherosclerotic? *Stroke.* 1994;**25**:963–966.

34. Sloan MA, Price TR, Foulkes MA, et al. Circadian rhythmicity of stroke onset. Intracerebral and subarachnoid hemorrhage. *Stroke.* 1992;**23**:1420–1426.

35. Kleinpeter G, Schatzer R, Bock F. Is blood pressure really a trigger for the circadian rhythm of subarachnoid hemorrhage? *Stroke.* 1995;**26**:1805–1810.

36. Pretorius ME, Butler IJ. Neurologic manifestations of Ehlers-Danlos syndrome. *Neurology.* 1983;**33**:1087–1089.

37. Rubinstein MK, Cohen NH. Ehlers-Danlos syndrome associated with multiple intracranial aneurysms. *Neurology.* 1964;**14**:125–132.

38. Thai QA, Raza SM, Pradilla G, Tamargo RJ. Aneurysmal rupture without subarachnoid hemorrhage: case series and literature review. *Neurosurgery.* 2005;**57**:225–229.

39. Przelomski MM, Fisher M, Davidson RI, Jones HR, Marcus EM. Unruptured intracranial aneurysm and transient focal cerebral ischemia: a follow-up study. *Neurology.* 1986;**36**:584–587.

40. Fisher M, Davidson RI, Marcus EM. Transient focal cerebral ischemia as a presenting manifestation of unruptured cerebral aneurysms. *Ann Neurol.* 1980;**8**:367–372.

41. Dias MS, Sekhar LN. Intracranial hemorrhage from aneurysms and arteriovenous malformations during pregnancy and the puerperium. *Neurosurgery.* 1990;**27**:855–865.

42. Larson JJ, Tew JM Jr, Tomsick TA, van Loveren HR. Treatment of aneurysms of the internal carotid artery by intravascular balloon occlusion: long-term follow-up of 58 patients. *Neurosurgery.* 1995;**36**:26–30.

43. Mokri B, Piepgras DG, Sundt TM Jr, Pearson BW. Extracranial internal carotid artery aneurysms. *Mayo Clin Proc.* 1982;**57**:310–321.

44. Frank E, Brown BM, Wilson DF. Asymptomatic fusiform aneurysm of the petrous carotid artery in a patient with von Recklinghausen's neurofibromatosis. *Surg Neurol.* 1989;**32**:75–78.

45. Hahn CD, Nicolle DA, Lownie SP, Drake CG. Giant cavernous carotid aneurysms: clinical presentation in fifty-seven cases. *J Neuroophthalmol.* 2000;**20**:253–258.

46. Goldenberg-Cohen N, Curry C, Miller NR, Tamargo RJ, Murphy KP. Long term visual and neurological prognosis in patients with treated and untreated cavernous sinus aneurysms. *J Neurol Neurosurg Psychiatry.* 2004;**75**:863–867.

47. Kupersmith MJ, Hurst R, Berenstein A, Choi IS, Jafar J, Ransohoff J. The benign course of cavernous carotid artery aneurysms. *J Neurosurg.* 1992;**77**:690–693.

48. Birchall D, Khangure MS, McAuliffe W. Resolution of third nerve paresis after endovascular management of aneurysms of the posterior communicating artery. *AJNR Am J Neuroradiol.* 1999;**20**:411–413.

49. Desal HA, Toulgoat F, Raoul S, et al. Ehlers-Danlos syndrome type IV and recurrent carotid-cavernous fistula: review of the literature, endovascular approach, technique and difficulties. *Neuroradiology.* 2005;**47**:300–304.

50. Dixon JM. Angioid streaks and pseudoxanthoma elasticum with aneurysm of the internal carotid artery. *Am J Ophthalmol.* 1951;**34**:1322–1323.

51. Fujiwara S, Fujii K, Nishio S, Matsushima T, Fukui M. Oculomotor nerve palsy in patients with cerebral aneurysms. *Neurosurg Rev.* 1989;**12**:123–132.

52. White JB, Layton KF, Cloft HJ. Isolated third nerve palsy associated with a ruptured anterior communicating artery aneurysm. *Neurocrit Care.* 2007;**7**:260–262.

53. Selviaridis P, Spiliotopoulos A, Antoniadis C, Kontopoulos V, Foroglou G. Fusiform aneurysm of the posterior cerebral artery: report of two cases. *Acta Neurochir (Wien).* 2002;**144**:295–299.

54. van Rooij WJ, Sluzewski M, Beute GN. Endovascular treatment of posterior cerebral artery aneurysms. *AJNR Am J Neuroradiol.* 2006;**27**:300–305.

55. Hall JK, Jacobs DA, Movsas T, Galetta SL. Fourth nerve palsy, homonymous hemianopia, and hemisensory deficit caused by a proximal posterior cerebral artery aneurysm. *J Neuroophthalmol.* 2002;**22**:95–98.

56. Hamada J, Morioka M, Yano S, Todaka T, Kai Y, Kuratsu J. Clinical features of aneurysms of the posterior cerebral artery: a 15-year experience with 21 cases. *Neurosurgery.* 2005;**56**:662–670.

57. Taylor CL, Kopitnik TA Jr, Samson DS, Purdy PD. Treatment and outcome in 30 patients with posterior cerebral artery aneurysms. *J Neurosurg.* 2003;**99**:15–22.

58. Pessin MS, Chimowitz MI, Levine SR, et al. Stroke in patients with fusiform vertebrobasilar aneurysms. *Neurology.* 1989;**39**:16–21.

59. Matsushita Y, Kawabata S, Kamo M, et al. Ruptured aneurysm at the cortical segment of the posterior inferior cerebellar artery. *J Clin Neurosci.* 2006;**13**:777–781.

60. Kamii H, Ogawa A, Sakurai Y, Kayama T. [Anterior inferior cerebellar artery aneurysm with a sudden onset of caudal cranial nerve symptoms]. *No Shinkei Geka.* 1989;**17**:387–391.

61. Dernbach PD, Sila CA, Little JR. Giant and multiple aneurysms of the distal posterior inferior cerebellar artery. *Neurosurgery.* 1988;**22**:309–312.

62. Yamamoto I, Tsugane R, Ohya M, Sato O, Ogura K, Hara M. Peripheral aneurysms of the posterior inferior cerebellar artery. *Neurosurgery.* 1984;**15**:839–845.

63. Tyler HR, Clark DB. Neurologic complications in patients with coarctation of aorta. *Neurology.* 1958;**8**:712–718.

64. Connolly HM, Huston J III, Brown RD Jr, Warnes CA, Ammash NM, Tajik AJ. Intracranial aneurysms in patients with coarctation of the aorta: a prospective magnetic resonance angiographic study of 100 patients. *Mayo Clin Proc.* 2003;**78**:1491–1499.

65. Sandok BA, Houser OW, Baker HL, Holley KE. Fibromuscular dysplasia. *Arch Neurol.* 1971;**24**:462–466.

66. Mettinger KL, Ericson K. Fibromuscular dysplasia and the brain. Observations on angiographic, clinical, and genetic characteristics. *Stroke.* 1982;**13**:46–52.

67. Cloft HJ, Kallmes DF, Kallmes MH, Goldstein JH, Jensen ME, Dion JE. Prevalence of cerebral aneurysms in patients with fibromuscular dysplasia: a reassessment. *J Neurosurg.* 1998;**88**:436–440.

68. Belz MM, Hughes RL, Kaehny WD, et al. Familial clustering of ruptured intracranial aneurysms in autosomal dominant polycystic kidney disease. *Am J Kidney Dis.* 2001;**38**:770–776.

69. Kim K, Drummond I, Ibraghimov-Beskrovnaya O, Klinger K, Arnaout MA. Polycystin 1 is required for the structural integrity of blood vessels. *Proc Natl Acad Sci USA.* 2000;**97**:1731–1736.

70. Brill CB, Peyster RG, Hoover ED, Keller MS. Giant intracranial aneurysm in a child with tuberous sclerosis: CT demonstration. *J Comput Assist Tomogr.* 1985;**9**:377–380.

71. Blumenkopf B, Huggins MJ. Tuberous sclerosis and multiple intracranial aneurysms. *Neurosurgery.* 1985;**17**:797–800.

72. Beltramello A, Puppini G, Bricolo A, et al. Does the tuberous sclerosis complex include intracranial aneurysms? A case report with a review of the literature. *Pediatr Radiol.* 1999;**29**:206–211.

73. Chapman AB, Rubinstein D, Hughes R, et al. Intracranial aneurysms in autosomal dominant polycystic kidney disease. *N Engl J Med.* 1992;**327**:916–920.

74. Lozano AM, Leblanc R. Cerebral aneurysms and polycystic kidney disease: a critical review. *Can J Neurol Sci.* 1992;**19**:222–227.

75. Chauveau D, Pirson Y, Verellen-Dumoulin C, Macnicol A, Gonzalo A, Grunfeld JP. Intracranial aneurysms in autosomal dominant polycystic kidney disease. *Kidney Int.* 1994;**45**:1140–1146.

76. Schievink WI, Torres VE, Piepgras DG, Wiebers DO. Saccular intracranial aneurysms in autosomal dominant polycystic kidney disease. *J Am Soc Nephrol.* 1992;**3**:88–95.

77. Krog M, Almgren B, Eriksson I, Nordstrom S. Vascular complications in the Ehlers-Danlos syndrome. *Acta Chir Scand.* 1983;**149**:279–282.

78. Hunter GC, Malone JM, Moore WS, Misiorowski DL, Chvapil M. Vascular manifestations in patients with Ehlers-Danlos syndrome. *Arch Surg.* 1982;**117**:495–498.

79. Germain DP, Herrera-Guzman Y. Vascular Ehlers-Danlos syndrome. *Ann Genet.* 2004;**47**:1–9.

80. Kuivaniemi H, Prokop DJ, Wu Y, et al. Exclusion of mutations in the gene for type III collagen (COL3A1) as a common cause of intracranial aneurysms or cervical artery dissections: results from sequence analysis of the coding sequences of type III collagen from 55 unrelated patients. *Neurology.* 1993;**43**:2652–2658.

81. Conway JE, Hutchins GM, Tamargo RJ. Marfan syndrome is not associated with intracranial aneurysms. *Stroke.* 1999;**30**:1632–1636.

82. Wityk RJ, Zanferrari C, Oppenheimer S. Neurovascular complications of Marfan syndrome: a retrospective, hospital-based study. *Stroke.* 2002;**33**:680–684.

83. Heyer GL, Dowling MM, Licht DJ, et al. The cerebral vasculopathy of PHACES syndrome. *Stroke.* 2008;**39**:308–316.

84. Perret G, Nishioka H. Report on the cooperative study of intracranial aneurysms and subarachnoid hemorrhage. *J Neurosurg.* 1966;**25**:467–490.

85. Halim AX, Singh V, Johnston SC, et al. Characteristics of brain arteriovenous malformations with coexisting aneurysms: a comparison of two referral centers. *Stroke.* 2002;**33**:675–679.

86. Azzarelli B, Moore J, Gilmor R, Muller J, Edwards M, Mealey J. Multiple fusiform aneurysms following curative radiation therapy foe suprasellar germinoma. *J Neurosurg.* 1984;**61**:1141–1145.

87. Benson PJ, Sung JH. Cerebral aneurysms following radiotherapy for medulloblastoma. *J Neurosurg.* 1989;**70**:545–550.

88. Adams HP Jr, Kassell NF, Wisoff HS, Drake CG. Intracranial saccular aneurysm and moyamoya disease. *Stroke.* 1979;**10**:174–179.

89. Chen ST, Liu YH, Hsu CY, Hogan EL, Ryu SJ. Moyamoya disease in Taiwan. *Stroke.* 1988;**19**:53–59.

90. Rios-Montenegro EN, Behrens MM, Hoyt WF. Pseudoxanthoma elasticum. *Arch Neurol.* 1972;**26**:151–155.

91. Munyer TP, Margulis AR. Pseudoxanthoma elasticum with internal carotid artery aneurysm. *Am J Roentgenol.* 1981;**136**:1023–1029.

92. Schievink WI. Genetics of intracranial aneurysms. *Neurosurgery.* 1997;**40**:651–663.

93. Schievink WI, Parisi JE, Pipegras DG. Familial intracranial aneurysms: an autopsy study. *Neurosurgery.* 1997;**41**:1247–1252.

94. Kasuya H, Onda H, Takeshita M, Hori T, Takakura K. Clinical features of intracranial aneurysms in siblings. *Neurosurgery.* 2000;**46**:1301–1305.

95. Raaymakers TW, Rinkel GJ, Ramos LM. Initial and follow-up screening for aneurysms in families with familial subarachnoid hemorrhage. *Neurology.* 1998;**51**:1125–1130.

96. Ruigrok YM, Rinkel GJ, Algra A, Raaymakers TW, van Gijn J. Characteristics of intracranial aneurysms in patients with familial subarachnoid hemorrhage. *Neurology.* 2004;**62**:891–894.

97. Teasdale GM, Wardlaw JM, White PM, Murray G, Teasdale EM, Easton V. The familial risk of subarachnoid haemorrhage. *Brain.* 2005;**128**:1677–1685.

98. Kojima M, Nagasawa S, Lee YE, Takeichi Y, Tsuda E, Mabuchi N. Asymptomatic familial cerebral aneurysms. *Neurosurgery.* 1998;**43**:776–781.

99. Kim DH, Van GG, Milewicz DM. Incidence of familial intracranial aneurysms in 200 patients: comparison among Caucasian, African-American, and Hispanic populations. *Neurosurgery.* 2003;**53**:302–308.

100. Crawley F, Clifton A, Brown MM. Should we screen for familial intracranial aneurysm? *Stroke.* 1999;**30**:312–316.

101. White PM, Lindsay KW, Teasdale E, Teasdale GM, Wardlaw JM. Should we screen for familial intracranial aneurysm? *Stroke.* 1999;**30**:2241–2242.

102. Roberts G, Nanra J, Phillips J. Screening for familial intracranial aneurysm: resource implications. *Br J Neurosurg.* 1999;**13**:395–398.

103. Brown BM, Soldevilla F. MR angiography and surgery for unruptured familial intracranial aneurysms in persons with a family history of cerebral aneurysms. *Am J Roentgenol.* 1999;**173**:133–138.

104. Ronkainen A, Miettinen H, Karkola K, et al. Risk of harboring an unruptured intracranial aneurysm. *Stroke.* 1998;**29**:359–362.

105. Brown RD, Huston J, Hornung R, et al. Screening for brain aneurysm in the Familial Intracranial Aneurysm study: frequency and predictors of lesion detection. *J Neurosurg.* 2008;**108**:1132–1138.

106. Hofer A, Hermans M, Kubassek N, et al. Elastin polymorphism haplotype and intracranial aneurysms are not associated in Central Europe. *Stroke.* 2003;**34**:1207–1211.

107. Foroud T, Sauerbeck L, Brown R, et al. Genome screen to detect linkage to intracranial aneurysm susceptibility genes. The Familial Intracranial Aneurysm (FIA) Study. *Stroke.* 2008;**39**:1434–1440.

108. Ruigrok YM, Seitz U, Wolterink S, Rinkel GJ, Wijmenga C, Urban Z. Association of polymorphisms and haplotypes in the elastin gene in Dutch patients with sporadic aneurysmal subarachnoid hemorrhage. *Stroke.* 2004;**35**:2064–2068.

109. Yoneyama T, Kasuya H, Onda H, et al. Collagen type I alpha2 (COL1A2) is the susceptible gene for intracranial aneurysms. *Stroke.* 2004;**35**:443–448.

110. Akagawa H, Narita A, Yamada H, et al. Systematic screening of lysyl oxidase-like (LOXL) family genes demonstrates that LOXL2 is a susceptibility gene to intracranial aneurysms. *Hum Genet.* 2007;**121**:377–387.

111. Connolly ES Jr, Choudhri TF, Mack WJ, et al. Influence of smoking, hypertension, and sex on the phenotypic expression of familial intracranial aneurysms in siblings. *Neurosurgery.* 2001;**48**:64–68.

112. Drake CG, Peerless SJ. Giant fusiform intracranial aneurysms: review of 120 patients treated surgically from 1965 to 1992. *J Neurosurg.* 1997;**87**:141–162.

113. Watanabe T, Sato K, Yoshimoto T. Basilar artery occlusion caused by thrombosis of atherosclerotic fusiform aneurysm of the basilar artery. *Stroke.* 1994;**25**:1068–1070.

114. Frazee JG, Cahan LD, Winter J. Bacterial intracranial aneurysms. *J Neurosurg.* 1980;**53**:633–641.

115. Heidelberger KP, Layton WM, Fisher RG. Middle cerebral mycotic aneurysms complicating posttraumatic pseudomonas meningitis. *J Neurosurg.* 1968;**29**:631–635.

116. Ho CL, Deruytter MJ. CNS aspergillosis with mycotic aneurysm, cerebral granuloma and infarction. *Acta Neurochir (Wien).* 2004;**146**:851–856.

117. Barrow DL, Prats AR. Infectious intracranial aneurysms: comparison of groups with and without endocarditis. *Neurosurgery.* 1990;**27**:562–573.

118. Roach MR, Drake CG. Ruptured cerebral aneurysms caused by micro-organisms. *N Engl J Med.* 1965;**273**:240–244.

119. Nakahara I, Taha MM, Higashi T et al. Different modalities of treatment of intracranial mycotic aneurysms: report of 4 cases. *Surg Neurol.* 2006;**66**:405–409.

120. Takeshita M, Kagawa M, Kubo O, et al. Clinicopathological study of bacterial intracranial aneurysms. *Neurol Med Chir (Tokyo).* 1991;**31**:508–513.

121. Bohmfalk GL, Story JL, Wissenger JP, Brown WE. Bacterial intracranial aneurysm. *J Neurosurg.* 1978;**48**:369–382.

122. Molinari GF, Smith BS, Goldstein MN, Satran R. Pathogenesis of cerebral mycotic aneurysms. *Neurology.* 1973;**23**:325–332.

123. Cole DG, Buchbinder BR, Richardson EP. Case 10-1993: a 67 year-old man with mitral regurgitation and an abrupt onset of ataxia and fever. *N Eng J Med.* 1993;**328**:717–725.

124. Bakshi R, Wright PD, Kinkel PR, et al. Cranial magnetic resonance imaging findings in bacterial endocarditis: the neuroimaging spectrum of septic brain embolization demonstrated in twelve patients. *J Neuroimag.* 1999;**9**:78–84.

125. Peters PJ, Harrison T, Lennox JL. A dangerous dilemma: management of infectious intracranial aneurysms complicating endocarditis. *Lancet Infect Dis.* 2006;**6**:742–748.

126. Tipping B, de Villiers L, Wainwright H, Candy S, Bryer A. Stroke in patients with human immunodeficiency virus infection. *J Neurol Neurosurg Psychiatry.* 2007;**78**:1320–1324.

127. Connor MD, Lammie GA, Bell JE, Warlow CP, Simmonds P, Brettle RD. Cerebral infarction in adult AIDS patients: observations from the Edinburgh HIV Autopsy Cohort. *Stroke.* 2000;**31**:2117–2126.

128. Evers S, Nabavi D, Rahmann A, Heese C, Reichelt D, Husstedt IW. Ischaemic cerebrovascular events in HIV infection: a cohort study. *Cerebrovasc Dis.* 2003;**15**:199–205.

129. Lang C, Jacobi G, Kreuz W, et al. Rapid development of giant aneurysm at the base of the brain in an 8-year-old boy with perinatal HIV infection. *Acta Histochem* 1992;**42**(Suppl):83–90.

130. Bonkowsky JL, Christenson JC, Nixon GW, Pavia AT. Cerebral aneurysms in a child with acquired immune deficiency syndrome during rapid immune reconstitution. *J Child Neurol.* 2002;**17**:457–460.

131. Husson RN, Saini R, Lewis LL, Butler KM, Patronas N, Pizzo PA. Cerebral artery aneurysms in children infected with human immunodeficiency virus. *J Pediatr.* 1992;**121**:927–930.

132. Dubrovsky T, Curless R, Scott G, et al. Cerebral aneurysmal arteriopathy in childhood AIDS. *Neurology.* 1998;**51**:560–565.

133. Burton C, Johnston J. Multiple cerebral aneurysms and cardiac myxoma. *N Engl J Med.* 1970;**282**:35–36.

134. Bobo H, Evans OB. Intracranial aneurysms in a child with recurrent atrial myxoma. *J Child Neurol.* 1987;**3**:230–232.

135. Sabolek M, Bachus-Banaschak K, Bachus R, Arnold G, Storch A. Multiple cerebral aneurysms as delayed complication of left cardiac myxoma: a case report and review. *Acta Neurol Scand.* 2005;**111**:345–350.

136. Furuya K, Sasaki T, Yoshimoto Y, Okada Y, Fujimaki T, Kirino T. Histologically verified cerebral aneurysm formation secondary to embolism from cardiac myxoma. Case report. *J Neurosurg.* 1995;**83**:170–173.

137. Knepper LE, Biller J, Adams HP, Bruno A. Neurologic manifestations of atrial myxoma. A 12-year experience and review. *Stroke.* 1988;**19**:1435–1440.

138. Fujita K, Yanaka K, Kamezaki T, Noguchi M, Nose T. Ruptured middle cerebral artery aneurysm with intramural myxoid degeneration in a child. *Pediatr Neurosurg.* 2003;**39**:108–111.

139. Oguz KK, Firat MM, Cila A. Fusiform aneurysms detected 5 years after removal of an atrial myxoma. *Neurorad.* 2001;**43**:990–992.

140. Jean WC, Walski-Easton SM, Nussbaum ES. Multiple intracranial aneurysms as delayed complications of an atrial myxoma: case report. *Neurosurgery.* 2001;**49**:200–202.

141. Lee VH, Connolly HM, Brown RD Jr. Central nervous system manifestations of cardiac myxoma. *Arch Neurol.* 2007;**64**:1115–1120.

142. Gonsalves CG, Nidecker AC. Cerebral aneurysms and cardiac myxoma. *J Can Assoc Radiol.* 1979;**30**:127–128.

143. Josephson SA, Johnston SC. Multiple stable fusiform intracranial aneurysms following atrial myxoma. *Neurology.* 2005;**64**:526.

144. Hove B, Andersen BB, Christiansen TM. Intracranial oncotic aneurysms from choriocarcinoma. Case report and review of the literature. *Neurorad.* 1990;**32**:526–528.

145. Weir B, MacDonald N, Mielke B. Intracranial vascular complications of choriocarcinoma. *Neurosurgery.* 1978;**2**:138–142.

146. Murata J, Sawamura Y, Takahashi A, Abe H, Saitoh H. Intracerebral hemorrhage caused by a neoplastic aneurysm from small-cell lung carcinoma: case report. *Neurosurgery.* 1993;**32**:124–126.

147. Ho KL. Neoplastic aneurysm and intracranial hemorrhage. *Cancer.* 1982;**50**:2935–2940.

148. Raskind R. An intracranial arterial aneurysm associated with a recurrent meningioma. Report of a case. *J Neurosurg.* 1965;**23**:622–625.

149. Scodary DJ, Tew JM Jr, Thomas GM, Tomsick T, Liwnicz BH. Radiation-induced cerebral aneurysms. *Acta Neurochir (Wien).* 1990;**102**:141–144.

150. Jane JA, Kassell NF, Torner JC, Winn HR. The natural history of aneurysms and arteriovenous malformations. *J Neurosurg.* 1985;**62**:321–323.

151. Juvela S, Porras M, Poussa K. Natural history of unruptured intracranial aneurysms: probability of and risk factors for aneurysm rupture. *J Neurosurg.* 2008;**108**:1052–1060.

152. Juvela S. Natural history of unruptured intracranial aneurysms: risks for aneurysm formation, growth, and rupture. *Acta Neurochir.* 2002;**82**(Suppl):27–30.

153. Vannemreddy P, Caldito G, Willis B, Nanda A. Influence of cocaine on ruptured intracranial aneurysms: a case control study of poor prognostic indicators. *J Neurosurg.* 2008;**108**:470–476.

154. Juvela S. Prehemorrhage risk factors for fatal intracranial aneurysm rupture. *Stroke.* 2003;**34**:1852–1857.

155. Amacher AL, Drake CG. Cerebral artery aneurysms in infancy, childhood and adolescence. *Childs Brain.* 1975;**1**:72–80.

156. Chason JL, Hindman WM. Berry aneurysms of the circle of Willis. *Neurology.* 1958;**8**:41–44.

157. Crawford T. Some observations on the pathogenesis and natural history of intracranial aneurysms. *J Neurol Neurosurg Psychiatry.* 1959;**22**:259–266.

158. Grode ML, Saunders M, Carton CA. Subarachnoid hemorrhage secondary to ruptured aneurysms in infants. *J Neurosurg.* 1978;**49**:898–902.

159. Kamm RC. Aneurysm of the posterior inferior cerebellar artery of a 5-year-old girl. *Am J Dis Child.* 1975;**129**:1437–1439.

160. Stehbens WE. Ultrastructure of aneurysms. *Arch Neurol.* 1975;**32**:798–807.

161. Sahs AL. Observations on the pathology of saccular aneurysms. *J Neurosurg.* 1966;**24**:792–806.

162. McCormick WF, Schmalstieg EJ. The relationship of arterial hypertension to intracranial aneurysms. *Arch Neurol.* 1977;**34**:285–287.

163. Bell WE, Butler C. Cerebral mycotic aneurysms in children. *Neurology.* 1968;**18**:81–86.

164. Ahuja GH, Jain N, Vijayaraghavan M, Roy S. Cerebral mycotic aneurysm of fungal origin. *J Neurosurg.* 1978;**49**:107–110.

165. Kassell NF, Torner JC, Haley EC Jr, Jane JA, Adams HP, Kongable GL. The International Cooperative Study on the Timing of Aneurysm Surgery. Part 1: overall management results. *J Neurosurg.* 1990;**73**:18–36.

166. Edlow JA, Caplan LR. Avoiding pitfalls in the diagnosis of subarachnoid hemorrhage. *N Engl J Med.* 2000;**342**:29–36.

167. Brouwers PJ, Dippel DW, Vermeulen M, Lindsay KW, Hasan D, van Gijn J. Amount of blood on computed tomography as an independent predictor after aneurysm rupture. *Stroke.* 1993;**24**:809–814.

168. Karttunen AI, Jartti PH, Ukkola VA, Sajanti J, Haapea M. Value of the quantity and distribution of subarachnoid haemorrhage on CT in the localization of a ruptured cerebral aneurysm. *Acta Neurochir (Wien).* 2003;**145**:655–661.

169. Claassen J, Carhuapoma JR, Kreiter KT, Du EY, Connolly ES, Mayer SA. Global cerebral edema after subarachnoid hemorrhage: frequency, predictors, and impact on outcome. *Stroke.* 2002;**33**:1225–1232.

170. Jayaraman MV, Mayo-Smith WW, Tung GA, et al. Detection of intracranial aneurysms: multi-detector row CT angiography compared with DSA. *Radiology.* 2004;**230**:510–518.

171. Taschner CA, Thines L, Lernout M, Lejeune JP, Leclerc X. Treatment decision in ruptured intracranial aneurysms: comparison between multi-detector row CT angiography and digital subtraction angiography. *J Neuroradiol.* 2007;**34**:243–249.

172. Baxter AB, Cohen WA, Maravilla KR. Imaging of intracranial aneurysms and subarachnoid hemorrhage. *Neurosurg Clin N Am.* 1998;**9**:445–462.

173. Chen W, Yang Y, Xing W, Qiu J, Peng Y. Sixteen-row multislice computed tomography angiography in the diagnosis and characterization of intracranial aneurysms: comparison with conventional angiography and intraoperative findings. *J Neurosurg.* 2008;**108**:1184–1191.

174. Chappell ET, Moure FC, Good MC. Comparison of computed tomographic angiography with digital subtraction angiography in the diagnosis of cerebral aneurysms: a meta-analysis. *Neurosurgery*. 2003;**52**:624–631.

175. Vernooij MW, Ikram MA, Tanghe HL, et al. Incidental findings on brain MRI in the general population. *N Engl J Med*. 2007;**357**:1821–1828.

176. Fiebach JB, Schellinger PD, Geletneky K, et al. MRI in acute subarachnoid haemorrhage; findings with a standardised stroke protocol. *Neuroradiology*. 2004;**46**:44–48.

177. Shimoda M, Takeuchi M, Tominaga J, Oda S, Kumasaka A, Tsugane R. Asymptomatic versus symptomatic infarcts from vasospasm in patients with subarachnoid hemorrhage: serial magnetic resonance imaging. *Neurosurgery*. 2001;**49**:1341–1348.

178. Weidauer S, Lanfermann H, Raabe A, Zanella F, Seifert V, Beck J. Impairment of cerebral perfusion and infarct patterns attributable to vasospasm after aneurysmal subarachnoid hemorrhage: a prospective MRI and DSA study. *Stroke*. 2007;**38**:1831–1836.

179. Kivisaari RP, Salonen O, Servo A, Autti T, Hernesniemi J, Ohman J. MR imaging after aneurysmal subarachnoid hemorrhage and surgery: a long-term follow-up study. *AJNR Am J Neuroradiol*. 2001;**22**:1143–1148.

180. Lubicz B, Levivier M, Sadeghi N, Emonts P, Baleriaux D. Immediate intracranial aneurysm occlusion after embolization with detachable coils: a comparison between MR angiography and intra-arterial digital subtraction angiography. *J Neuroradiol*. 2007;**34**:190–197.

181. van der Wee N, Rinkel GJ, Hasan D, van GJ. Detection of subarachnoid haemorrhage on early CT: is lumbar puncture still needed after a negative scan? *J Neurol Neurosurg Psychiatry*. 1995;**58**:357–359.

182. Willinsky RA, Taylor SM, Terbrugge K, Farb RI, Tomlinson G, Montanera W. Neurologic complications of cerebral angiography: prospective analysis of 2,899 procedures and review of the literature. *Radiology*. 2003;**227**:522–528.

183. Rosenorn J, Eskesen V, Madsen F, Schmidt K. Importance of cerebral pan-angiography for detection of multiple aneurysms in patients with aneurysmal subarachnoid haemorrhage. *Acta Neurol Scand*. 1993;**87**:215–218.

184. Nehls DG, Flom RA, Carter LP, Spetzler RF. Multiple intracranial aneurysms: Determining the site of rupture. *J Neurosurg*. 1985;**63**:342–348.

185. Ahmadi J, Tung H, Giannotta SL, Destian S. Monitoring of infectious intracranial aneurysms by sequential computed tomographic/magnetic resonance imaging studies. *Neurosurgery*. 1993;**32**:45–50.

186. Rinkel GJE, van Gijn J, Wijdicks EFM. Subarachnoid hemorrhage without detectable aneurysm. *Stroke*. 1993;**24**:1403–1409.

187. Duong H, Melancon D, Tampieri D, Ethier R. The negative angiogram in subarachnoid haemorrhage. *Neuroradiology*. 1996;**38**:15–19.

188. Fox JL, Baiz TC, Jakoby RK. Differentiation of aneurism from infundibulum of the posterior communicating artery. *J Neurosurg*. 1964;**21**:135–138.

189. Kaufmann TJ, Razack N, Cloft HJ, Kallmes DF. Dimpled appearance of a posterior communicating artery saccule: an angiographic indicator of arterial infundibula. *Am J Roentgenol*. 2005;**185**:1358–1360.

190. Hohlrieder M, Spiegel M, Hinterhoelzl J, et al. Cerebral vasospasm and ischaemic infarction in clipped and coiled intracranial aneurysm patients. *Eur J Neurol*. 2002;**9**:389–399.

191. Huston J III, Torres VE, Wiebers DO, Schievink WI. Follow-up of intracranial aneurysms in autosomal dominant polycystic kidney disease by magnetic resonance angiography. *J Am Soc Nephrol*. 1996;**7**:2135–2141.

192. Butler WE, Barker FG, Crowell RM. Patients with polycystic kidney disease would benefit from routine magnetic resonance angiographic screening for intracerebral aneurysms: a decision analysis. *Neurosurgery*. 1996;**38**:506–515.

193. Nakajima F, Shibahara N, Arai M, Ueda H, Katsuoka Y. Ruptured cerebral aneurysm not detected by magnetic resonance angiography in juvenile autosomal dominant polycystic kidney. *Int J Urol*. 2000;**7**:153–156.

194. Schievink WI, Prendergast V, Zabramski JM. Rupture of a previously documented small asymptomatic intracranial aneurysm in a patient with autosomal dominant polycystic kidney disease. Case report. *J Neurosurg*. 1998;**89**:479–482.

195. Rossetti S, Chauveau D, Kubly V, et al. Association of mutation position in polycystic kidney disease 1 (PKD1) gene and development of a vascular phenotype. *Lancet*. 2003;**361**:2196–2201.

196. Feigin VL, Anderson N, Rinkel GJ, Algra A, van Gijn J, Bennett DA. Corticosteroids for aneurysmal subarachnoid haemorrhage and primary intracerebral haemorrhage. *Cochrane Database Syst Rev*. 2005; CD004583.

197. Jartti P, Karttunen A, Jartti A, Ukkola V, Sajanti J, Pyhtinen J. Factors related to acute hydrocephalus after subarachnoid hemorrhage. *Acta Radiol*. 2004;**45**:333–339.

198. Ukkola V, Heikkinen ER. Epilepsy after operative treatment of ruptured cerebral aneurysms. *Acta Neurochir (Wien)*. 1990;**106**:115–118.

199. Barker FG, Ogilvy CS. Efficacy of prophylactic nimodipine for delayed ischemic deficit after subarachnoid hemorrhage: a metaanalysis. *J Neurosurg*. 1996;**84**:405–414.

200. Hamada J, Kai Y, Morioka M, Yano S, Todaka T, Ushio Y. Multimodal treatment of ruptured dissecting aneurysms of the vertebral artery during the acute stage. *J Neurosurg*. 2003;**99**:960–966.

201. Johnston SC, Higashida RT, Barrow DL, et al. Recommendations for the endovascular treatment of intracranial aneurysms: a statement for healthcare professionals from the Committee on Cerebrovascular Imaging of the American Heart Association Council on Cardiovascular Radiology. *Stroke*. 2002;**33**:2536–2544.

202. Gnanalingham KK, Apostolopoulos V, Barazi S, O'Neill K. The impact of the international subarachnoid aneurysm trial (ISAT) on the management of aneurysmal subarachnoid haemorrhage in a neurosurgical unit in the UK. *Clin Neurol Neurosurg*. 2006;**108**:117–123.

203. Raftopoulos C, Goffette P, Vaz G, et al. Surgical clipping may lead to better results than coil embolization: results from a series of 101 consecutive unruptured intracranial aneurysms. *Neurosurgery*. 2003;**52**:1280–1287.

204. Kawabe T, Tenjin H, Hayashi Y, Kakita K, Kubo S. Midterm prevention of rebleeding by Guglielmi detachable coils in ruptured intracranial aneurysms less than 10 mm. *Clin Neurol Neurosurg*. 2006;**108**:163–167.

205. Andreou A, Ioannidis I, Mitsos A. Endovascular treatment of peripheral intracranial aneurysms. *AJNR Am J Neuroradiol*. 2007;**28**:355–361.

206. Molyneux A, Kerr R, Stratton I, et al. International Subarachnoid Aneurysm Trial (ISAT) of neurosurgical clipping versus endovascular coiling in 2143 patients with ruptured intracranial aneurysms: a randomised trial. *Lancet*. 2002;**360**:1267–1274.

207. Lubicz B, Baleriaux D, Lefranc F, Brotchi J, Bruneau M, Levivier M. Endovascular treatment of intracranial aneurysms as the first therapeutic option. *J Neuroradiol*. 2007;**34**:250–259.

208. Sorteberg W, Slettebo H, Eide PK, Stubhaug A, Sorteberg A. Surgical treatment of aneurysmal subarachnoid haemorrhage in the presence of 24-h endovascular availability: management and results. *Br J Neurosurg*. 2008;**22**:53–62.

209. Fogelholm R, Hernesniemi J, Vapalahti M. Impact of early surgery on outcome after aneurysmal subarachnoid hemorrhage: a population-based study. *Stroke.* 1993;**24**:1649–1654.

210. Kassell NF, Torner JC, Jane JA, Haley EC Jr, Adams HP. The International Cooperative Study on the Timing of Aneurysm Surgery. Part 2: surgical results. *J Neurosurg.* 1990;**73**:37–47.

211. Coert BA, Chang SD, Do HM, Marks MP, Steinberg GK. Surgical and endovascular management of symptomatic posterior circulation fusiform aneurysms. *J Neurosurg.* 2007;**106**:855–865.

212. Bingham WF. Treatment of mycotic intracranial aneurysms. *J Neurosurg.* 1977;**46**:428–437.

213. Hara Y, Hosoda K, Wada T, Kimura H, Kohmura E. Endovascular treatment for a unusually large mycotic aneurysm manifesting as intracerebral hemorrhage – case report. *Neurol Med Chir (Tokyo).* 2006;**46**:544–547.

214. Bederson JB, Awad IA, Wiebers DO, et al. Recommendations for the management of patients with unruptured intracranial aneurysms: a statement for healthcare professionals from the Stroke Council of the American Heart Association. *Stroke.* 2000;**31**:2742–2750.

215. Johnston SC, Wilson CB, Halbach VV, et al. Endovascular and surgical treatment of unruptured cerebral aneurysms: comparison of risks. *Ann Neurol.* 2000;**48**:11–19.

216. Mizoi K, Yoshimoto T, Nagamine Y, Kayama T, Koshu K. How to treat incidental cerebral aneurysms: a review of 139 consecutive cases. *Surg Neurol.* 1995;**44**:114–120.

217. King JT, Berlin JA, Flamm ES. Morbidity and mortality from elective surgery for asymptomatic, unruptured, intracranial aneurysms: a meta-analysis. *J Neurosurg.* 1994;**81**:837–842.

218. Zimmerman CF, Van Patten PD, Golnik KC, Kopitnik TA Jr, Anand R. Orbital infarction syndrome after surgery for intracranial aneurysms. *Ophthalmology.* 1995;**102**:594–598.

219. Le Roux PD, Elliott JP, Downey L, et al. Improved outcome after rupture of anterior circulation aneurysms: a retrospective 10-year review of 224 good-grade patients. *J Neurosurg.* 1995;**83**:394–402.

220. Broderick JP, Brott TG, Duldner JE, Tomsick T, Leach A. Initial and recurrent bleeding are the major causes of death following subarachnoid hemorrhage. *Stroke.* 1994;**25**:1342–1347.

221. Stenhouse LM, Knight RG, Longmore BE, Bishara SN. Long-term cognitive deficits in patients after surgery on aneurysms of the anterior communicating artery. *J Neurol Neurosurg Psychiatry.* 1991;**54**:909–914.

222. Tidswell P, Dias PS, Sagar HJ, Mayes AR, Battersby RD. Cognitive outcome after aneurysm rupture: relationship to aneurysm site and perioperative complications. *Neurology.* 1995;**45**:875–882.

223. Roach ES, Zimmerman CF. Ehlers-Danlos syndrome. In: Bogousslavsky J, Caplan LR, eds. *Cerebrovascular Syndromes.* London: Oxford University Press; 1995:491–496.

224. Locksley HB. Natural history of subarachnoid hemorrhage, intracranial aneurysms and arteriovenous malformations. Based on 6368 cases in the Cooperative Study. *J Neurosurg.* 1966; **25**:219–239.

225. Takayama K, Nakagawa H, Iwasaki S, et al. Multiple cerebral aneurysms associated with Takayasu arteritis successfully treated with coil embolization. *Radiat Med.* 2008;**26**:33–38.

226. Aktas EG, Kaplan M, Ozveren MF. Basilar artery aneurysm associated with Behçet's Disease: a case report. *Turk Neurosurg.* 2008;**18**:35–38.

227. Schievink WI, Parisi JE, Piepgras DG, Michels VV. Intracranial aneurysms in Marfan's syndrome: an autopsy study. *Neurosurgery.* 1997;**41**:866–870.

228. Rosser TL, Vezina G, Packer RJ. Cerebrovascular abnormalities in a population of children with neurofibromatosis type 1. *Neurology.* 2005;**64**:553–555.

229. Rizzo JF, Lessell S. Cerebrovascular abnormalities in neurofibromatosis type 1. *Neurology.* 1994;**44**:1000–1002.

230. Laforet P, Petiot P, Nicolino M, et al. Dilative arteriopathy and basilar artery dolichoectasia complicating late-onset Pompe disease. *Neurology.* 2008;**70**:2063–2066.

231. Vicari P, Choairy AC, Siufi GC, Arantes AM, Fonseca JR, Figueiredo MS. Embolization of intracranial aneurysms and sickle cell disease. *Am J Hematol.* 2004;**76**:83–84.

18

Intracranial Vascular Malformations

In the last analysis, we see only what we are ready to see, what we have been taught to see. We eliminate and ignore everything that is not part of our prejudices.

Jean-Martin Charcot

Vascular malformations of the central nervous system include arteriovenous malformations (AVMs), cavernous malformations, developmental venous anomalies, and capillary telangiectasias.[1,2] AVMs differ from other vascular lesions by their direct anastomosis of arterial and venous channels without an intervening capillary bed.[3] Cavernous malformations are thin-walled sinusoidal lesions without prominent arterial or venous connections. Developmental venous anomalies are structurally anomalous venous channels that have little risk of hemorrhage unless they occur together with other vascular lesions. Capillary telangiectasias, characterized by dilated capillaries with intervening normal brain parenchyma, are low-risk lesions and are not considered in detail.

In this chapter we review the clinical manifestations, diagnosis, and management of AVMs, cavernous-carotid fistulas, cavernous malformations, and the Sturge-Weber syndrome.

ARTERIOVENOUS MALFORMATIONS

Arteriovenous malformations are abnormal complexes of arteries and veins (with no capillary phase) and their connecting channels that typically cause shunting of arterial blood directly into the venous circulation.[4] The frequency of AVMs in the general population is estimated to be 0.1%.[5,6] However, AVMs can remain asymptomatic and are sometimes found incidentally at autopsy, so the exact incidence has not been pinpointed. There is a slight male predominance among symptomatic patients.[7]

Clinical Features of AVMs

The two most common modes of presentation of an AVM are intracranial hemorrhage and epileptic seizures. A few patients with a history of epilepsy later develop a hemorrhage. Both intraparenchymal hemorrhage and subarachnoid hemorrhage (SAH) occur because of AVMs, but intracerebral hemorrhage is about twice as frequent as SAH.[8] Both intracerebral hemorrhage and SAH sometimes occur in the same individual. In addition, patients with a dural-based arteriovenous fistula sometimes develop a subdural hemorrhage. The general signs and symptoms of intracerebral and subarachnoid hemorrhage are presented in Chapters 16 and 17 and will not be restated here aside from a few unique features.

The clinical manifestations of AVMs vary in different reports, but intracranial hemorrhage and epileptic seizures are the two most frequent problems. In the series of 125 AVM patients described in 1957 by Olivecrona and Ladenheim, 50 patients (40%) presented with seizures, and 48 patients (39%) developed intracranial bleeding. The other 27 patients (20%) in this series presented with complaints such as headaches or dizziness.[9] Among the 131 AVM patients summarized by Fults and Kelly, 68 (51.9%) presented with hemorrhage, 36 (27.5%) were evaluated for seizures, and eight (6.1%) were seen for headaches.[10] A smattering of patients presented because of a bruit or various neurological symptoms.

Patients with an intracranial hemorrhage due to an AVM tend to do better than individuals whose hemorrhage resulted from an aneurysm. In one study of 115 AVM patients, 54 (47%) had no residual neurological deficit, and another 43 (37%) remained independent after the hemorrhage. Only 18 patients were listed as moderately to severely disabled.[11] This favorable prognosis following an AVM-related hemorrhage may be due to bleeding under lower pressure with an AVM than with an aneurysm.

Not surprisingly, seizures due to an AVM typically begin focally. Focal motor seizures and complex partial seizures are the most common seizure types, but secondary generalization of the seizures may happen so rapidly that it is impossible to distinguish focal from generalized seizures on purely clinical grounds. Vascular malformations involving the temporal lobe cause seizures twice as often as lesions at other sites.[12]

Episodic migraine-like headaches, without signs of intracranial hemorrhage, are the initial symptom in 15% to 20% of individuals with an AVM.[9,13] This is about the same headache frequency as occurs in the general population, so it is likely that some of the AVM patients have coincidental migraine. However, headaches seem to be particularly frequent and severe in some AVM patients, and the headache sometimes resolves after the AVM is obliterated.[14] Conceivably, AVM-induced blood flow alterations could exacerbate headaches in individuals who are susceptible. When vascular headache and seizures occur in the same patient, the possibility of an AVM should be considered. Other concerning signs include particularly severe headaches, consistent aggravation of the headaches by strenuous activity, and a fixed headache location.

Some individuals with a large AVM show signs of cognitive impairment.[15,16] Usually the changes are subtle – a change in personality or mild memory loss – but a few patients develop progressive dementia. This decline probably results from chronic diversion of blood from the cerebral tissues because it is often associated with some degree of cortical atrophy, either regional or generalized. In addition to altered cognition, this intracranial steal phenomenon may also be responsible for the seizures and frequent headaches that occur in some patients.

Wyburn-Mason syndrome (Bonnet-Dechaume-Blanc syndrome) is a rare condition characterized by often multiple AVMs of the brain, orbit, and retina.[17] An orbital AVM may extend posteriorly adjacent to the anterior visual pathway.[18] Occasionally the malformation extends to the skin near the orbit.[19]

An AVM in infants or neonates can present with high output cardiac failure or with hydrocephalus as well as with hemorrhage (see Chapter 22).

The hemorrhage risk from an AMV does not increase markedly during pregnancy.[20] The likelihood of a woman with an AVM having an intracranial hemorrhage during a given pregnancy is 3.5%.[20]

Physical Findings of an AVM

An unruptured AVM creates few physical signs. Depending on the location of the AVM, various focal neurological deficits occur after an intracerebral hemorrhage. These signs must be distinguished from an ischemic or postepileptic phenomenon (Todd's paralysis). In individuals with large malformations since childhood or those with a hemorrhage at an early age, the contralateral side of the body may fail to develop and be smaller than the normal side.

A cranial bruit occurs in up to a quarter of the patients, and the likelihood of hearing a bruit is directly proportional to the diligence of the examiner. The size of the lesion, rather than its location, determines the presence or absence of a bruit. Bruits are often absent during the acute phase of an intracranial hemorrhage, probably because of altered hemodynamics produced by vasospasm.

Occasionally an intracranial AVM communicates with the extracranial arteries, usually those of the external carotid system, resulting in dilated, tortuous face and scalp veins with cirsoid aneurysms. The dilated superficial vessels are pulsatile and have a palpable thrill.[9]

Pathologic Findings

Macroscopic Appearance

AVMs vary in size and can be found anywhere within the nervous system. Some are large enough to replace most of a lobe (Figure 18-1). Others are so small that they are difficult to see with the unaided eye and are discovered only on microscopic analysis after a hemorrhage has occurred.[21,22] During life,

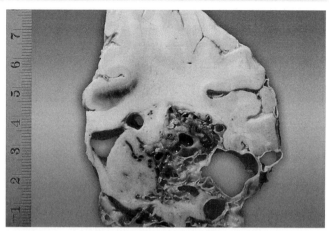

Figure 18-1. Coronal brain specimen showing a large AVM. Note the disorganized array of vessels of varying sizes.

the vessels of the larger lesions are markedly enlarged, tortuous, and distended with blood, resembling the writhing appearance of a can of worms. It is impossible to visually distinguish the arteries from the veins.[3] Because oxygenated blood is shunted directly to the veins without passing through a capillary bed, the veins often contain bright red blood under relatively high pressure.

The neighboring gyri and underlying parenchyma have hemosiderin deposits, indicating the occurrence of earlier, sometimes asymptomatic, hemorrhages. The lesion may be located predominantly or partially on the surface of the cerebral hemispheres or deep in the basal ganglia, thalamus, brainstem, cerebellum, or spinal cord. Infratentorial AVMs account for about 10% of the AVMs of the nervous system, with the remaining lesions divided evenly between the two hemispheres. Some individuals have multiple brain AVMs, sometimes in widely separated locations within the nervous system. Larger lesions can extend through the gray and white matter of a cerebral hemisphere in the shape of a cone with the base on the cortex and the apex pointing toward the ventricle. A few patients also have vascular anomalies in other viscera or in the skin.

Microscopic Appearance

Microscopic examination reveals dilated, thin-walled vessels. The internal elastic lamina is largely missing, the muscularis is poorly developed, and the collagen within the vessel wall is disorganized.[3,23,24] The abnormalities tend to be more pronounced in the veins and shunting vessels than in the feeding arteries, but, even microscopically, it may be difficult to clearly differentiate arteries from arterialized veins. The walls of the feeding and draining vessels are often thin in one place and thickened by intimal hypertrophy sufficient to block the lumen in others. Calcium deposits are often found adjacent to the abnormal vessels. Some individuals have venous thrombosis or evidence of prior hemorrhage or infarction with gliosis, cortical atrophy, or hemosiderin deposition.[3]

Pathophysiology of AVMs

During embryogenesis, the cerebral vasculature normally begins as a uniform capillary mesh that, through the atrophy of some channels and the enlargement of others, evolves into the adult pattern. Malformations represent the persistence of these primitive vascular channels, which gradually enlarge and carry blood directly from arteries to veins without an intervening capillary.[25]

Although AVMs have a congenital origin, they are not always static lesions. They often enlarge slowly over many years as blood shunted through the abnormal channels gains access to an adjacent meshwork of abnormal vessels. Sometimes the lesion expands quickly and dramatically.[26] AVMs are sometimes documented in individuals with a previously normal angiogram following surgery.[27] Complete spontaneous involution of the lesion occurs in about 1% of the individuals with an AVM.[28,29] Angiographic disappearance is more likely to occur in patients who present with a hemorrhage due to a small AVMs with few feeding arteries. Disappearance of an AVM in these individuals may result from the lesion's thrombosis, which, in turn, is due to venous outflow obstruction secondary to a hemorrhage.[28,30,31]

Small AVMs do not usually cause ischemic symptoms, but large shunts can divert enough blood from the arterial circulation to generate an intracerebral steal phenomenon and cause ischemia of the adjacent brain tissue. The reduced peripheral vascular resistance lowers the diastolic pressure within the cranial arteries. Cerebral blood flow may be increased as much as 50% to 100%, but despite this vastly increased overall blood flow, tissue perfusion may be markedly reduced. Consequently, chronic ischemia may result in progressive cognitive impairment, seizures, and cortical atrophy.

One or more aneurysms, either within the AVM complex (intranidal) or involving an artery proximal to the AVM, are often documented in individuals with an AVM.[32,33] Neither aneurysm location altered the odds of having presented with a hemorrhage from the AVM, but the presence of an intranidal aneurysm increased the risk of rebleeding sufficiently to make it a useful therapeutic target.[32,33] Stenosis of the feeding arteries lessens the likelihood of hemorrhage, while venous stenosis increases the hemorrhage rate.[33]

Patients who are older at the time of AVM diagnosis are more likely to have a hemorrhage soon after diagnosis than younger individuals.[12] Patients with a bleeding AVM are more likely to have systemic hypertension than other AVM patients. Angiographic predictors of bleeding due to an AVM include a deeply situated lesion, the presence of deep draining veins, location of the lesion in the posterior fossa, and a paucity of draining veins.[34–37] In most studies small lesions are more likely to bleed than larger ones.[12,35,37] Most of these factors have one thing in common that could explain their effect on the AVM – each tends to increase the intralesional pressure.[37] Although smoking cigarettes increases the hemorrhage risk in people

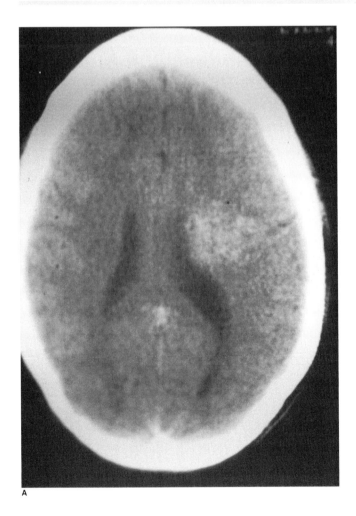

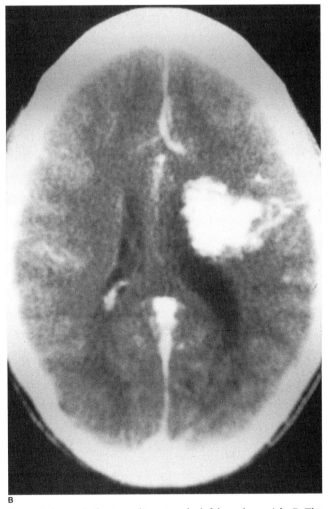

Figure 18-2. A: Cranial CT without contrast reveals a poorly demarcated AVM with faint calcification adjacent to the left lateral ventricle. B: The lesion is obvious after the addition of contrast. Catheter angiography subsequently confirmed the presence of an AVM.

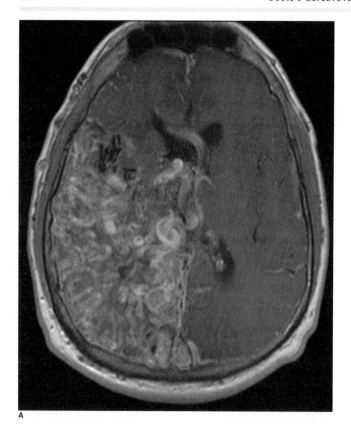
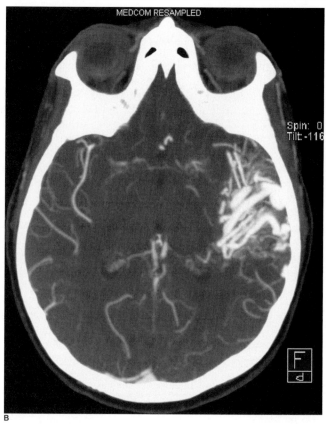

Figure 18-3. A: Cranial MRI shows the myriad serpiginous vessels of a large AVM of the right posterior hemisphere. B: CTA from another patient with an incidental, unruptured AVM within the left temporal lobe. The lesion was supplied predominately from the left middle cerebral artery and drained into the superficial venous system.

with intracranial aneurysms, it seems to have no effect on the bleeding risk due to an AVM.[35]

Occasional individuals with multiple, separate intracranial AVMs are documented.[38,39] Nevertheless, no genetic predisposition to the development of AVMs is known except in individuals with hereditary hemorrhagic telangiectasia (Osler-Weber-Rendu disease).[40,41] The risk of an AVM in individuals with hereditary hemorrhagic telangiectasia is not known precisely. In one report 7.9% of the individuals with HHT and some type of neurological involvement had an AVM, and another 16.7% had cerebral telangiectasia or angiomas.[42] Hereditary hemorrhagic telangiectasia should be considered in individuals with multiple arteriovenous malformations of the nervous system.[43–45] Hereditary hemorrhagic telangiectasia is considered in more detail in Chapter 21.

Diagnosis of AVMs

The differential diagnosis depends greatly on an individual's presenting signs and symptoms. Any patient with an unexplained intracerebral hemorrhage or SAH could have an AVM, so the differential list is long (see Chapters 16 and 17). As a rule the younger the patient with an intracerebral hemorrhage, the more likely he or she is to have an AVM. Similarly, an AVM is occasionally the cause of either epilepsy or headache. Individuals with an AVM can usually be identified with neuroimaging studies (see Chapter 5).

Computed Tomography

Computed tomography (CT) reliably demonstrates the intracranial hemorrhage that often brings an AVM to attention, and some AVMs are highlighted vividly with the addition of CT contrast (Figure 18-2). AVMs often contain calcium deposits that are evident on CT. Unless large tortuous vessels of the malformation are apparent, however, CT cannot reliably distinguish a small AVM from an associated hemorrhage or from tumors or other lesions.[46]

An intracranial AVM can be identified with computed tomographic angiography (CTA) (Figure 18-3), although catheter angiography still offers superior visualization of the lesion's sources of blood supply before therapy. Kokkinis and colleagues compared digital subtraction angiography to CTA in 198 individuals with SAH. Both tests detected the 15 patients with an AVM, and CTA detected 176 of 179 aneurysms (178 aneurysms were detected with digital subtraction angiography).[47]

Magnetic Resonance Imaging

Most sizable AVMs can be demonstrated with contrast-enhanced magnetic resonance imaging (MRI), although the nature of the lesion is not always apparent without other tests. The dilated, serpiginous vessels of larger AVMs are sometimes apparent even on noncontrast MRI as a signal void created by the rapidly moving blood within the lesion. Other AVMs have a characteristic honeycomb appearance created by the feeding arteries and draining veins.[48] The brain parenchyma near an

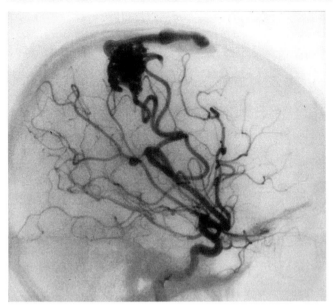

Figure 18-4. Catheter angiogram demonstrates an AVM. Note the simultaneous filling of arteries and veins.

AVM sometimes shows signs of prior hemorrhage or evidence of ischemic injury or gliosis. Small AVMs are not always apparent on MRI, and, as with CT, it can be difficult to differentiate a small AVM that is surrounded by acute hemorrhage. However, MRI and CT occasionally show evidence of an AVM that is not apparent with catheter angiography because of the effects of vasospasm or local pressure effects.[49]

Catheter Angiography

Although evidence of an AVM is often identified with CT or MRI and the lesion can be characterized by CTA, catheter arteriography remains the optimal procedure for the characterization of an AVM in preparation for treatment. The best angiographic evidence of an AVM is large feeding arteries and the premature filling of draining veins (Figure 18-4). Signs of an AVM are (a) a very short arterial phase in any or all of the arterial branches, (b) a tangle of opacified arteries and veins, and (c) unusually rapid filling of veins, which appear opacified during the "capillary" phase. Both carotid systems and the vertebral-basilar system should be studied to characterize the number and source of the feeding vessels and to ensure that there is only one AVM.

Small AVMs are not always apparent angiographically, especially in the presence of a subarachnoid or intracerebral hemorrhage. In some of these individuals, the angiographic contrast is unable to penetrate the AVM because of spasm or thrombosis of the afferent arteries or their tamponade by an adjacent hematoma, and the test may need to be repeated after the acute stage has passed.[50] In other people the AVM may be too small to identify angiographically, or it was destroyed by the very hemorrhage it created.[51,52]

Course and Prognosis

The natural history of AVMs is not precisely known because the symptomatic lesions that can be obliterated usually are. Occasional AVMs are identified as incidental findings on autopsy or on neurodiagnostic studies. Follow-up studies typically include

symptomatic patients whose AVMs were eliminated as well as those whose lesions were not amenable to therapy. A few older reports retrospectively analyzed groups of untreated patients, and it is clear even from these potentially biased cohorts that the long-term risk from untreated AVMs is substantial.

In one cohort of 217 unoperated AVM patients, there was a projected 20-year hemorrhage risk of 42%, a 27% risk of developing epilepsy, and a 29% risk of death.[12] Overall, the annual risk of hemorrhage in this cohort was about 2% per year except for a slightly higher risk during the first 2 years after initial presentation. Individuals who presented with an intracranial hemorrhage had a 51% risk of a second hemorrhage over the 20-year observation period versus a 31% risk of hemorrhage for the subgroup with another initial clinical presentation.[12] In another cohort of 83 AVM patients who did not undergo definitive therapy, a second hemorrhage occurred in 67.4% of the patients whose initial presentation included a hemorrhage. The rate of rebleeding was 17.9% for the first year after the initial hemorrhage, declining to 3% per year after 5 years, and to 2% per year after 10 years.[10] In a prospectively followed cohort of 166 unoperated AVM patients, Ondra and colleagues noted a 4% per year hemorrhage risk and a 1% per year death rate.[53]

Treatment of AVMs

The goal of treatment is obliteration of the AVM. Seizures per se are not an indication for surgery as long as they can be controlled with medication. There are three main techniques to definitively treat an intracranial AVM: surgical removal, endovascular embolism, and focused radiation. The most appropriate approach for a given patient will depend on the size and location of the AVM, the patient's condition, and the experience of the physicians caring for the patient. When all three techniques are available, they can be selectively applied, singly or in combination, to best suit the patient's situation.

AVM Surgery

The grading system developed by Spetzler and Martin helps to determine the likelihood of successful surgery for an AVM. In their system the feasibility of surgical removal of an AVM depends on the lesion's size (small < 3 cm; medium 3–6 cm; large > 6 cm), location (noneloquent versus eloquent areas), and configuration of venous drainage (deep versus superficial).[54] Surgical results are best in medically stable patients with smaller, uncomplicated lesions. In contrast, patients with large or deep-seated malformations tend to have a higher operative morbidity and an increased risk of long-term dysfunction. In one study of 112 AVM patients who underwent surgery, there were four deaths (3.6%) that were attributed to surgery (three due to intraoperative hemorrhage), and 24 patients (21%) had complications.[55] Of the 43 patients in this cohort who were neurologically normal before surgery, one died and eight people had at least a minor neurological deficit. Thus, postoperative neurological deficits are common but tend to improve with time.[56] Although there are occasional exceptions, the recurrence rate of an AVM in an individual with a normal postoperative angiogram is low.[27]

Endovascular Procedures

In skilled hands some AVMs can be completely or partially occluded by selective catheterization and flow-directed embolism of various particulate or liquid embolizing agents. Various materials have been used to occlude AVMs, including metal coils, detachable balloons, bucrylate (isobutyl-2-cyanoacrylate), and polyvinyl alcohol particles. In many patients a combined approach with embolization followed by surgery or radiotherapy is more successful than embolization alone.[57-59]

Arterial embolization via selective catheterization may help reduce the size of a large malformation in preparation for surgery and reduce the likelihood of hemorrhage during surgery. Embolization is also used in patients who are medically unstable or whose lesions are not appropriate for surgery. Even when an embolism procedure appears to be successful, the malformation sometimes returns, either because the occluded arteries recanalize or collateral channels form.

Endovascular procedures are not without risks. The most often reported complications of endovascular AVM treatment are intracerebral hemorrhage and ischemic infarction. Hemorrhage occurring during or soon after the embolism procedure probably stems from alteration of hemodynamic factors within the lesion. In one series over a third of the patients had radiographic evidence of pulmonary embolism of the material used to occlude the AVM.[60]

Radiosurgery

Radiosurgery can be an effective treatment for AVM patients for whom surgery or endovascular procedures are not feasible. Radiation is focused on the area of the AVM, avoiding the surrounding brain as much as possible using gamma knife, linear accelerators, or proton beam radiation.

Radiosurgery is often used for AVMs in the thalamus, basal ganglia, and brainstem that can not be treated with surgery or with endovascular techniques. Radiosurgery is also utilized after surgery or endovascular procedures in an effort to eliminate any remaining portions of the lesion. Deep-seated AVMs are particularly problematic, because they are more likely to hemorrhage, more likely to cause a significant deficit when the hemorrhage occurs, and more difficult to treat.[61] In one series of 56 patients with these lesions, obliteration of the AVM was achieved in 24 patients (43%).[62] Seven patients (12%) had a hemorrhage despite treatment, and permanent radiation-related complications occurred in six (12%) of the 51 surviving patients. These results seem disappointing until one considers the hemorrhage risk in these individuals and the lack of effective alternative therapies.[62]

Radiosurgery is often avoided with large AVMs because of concern about toxicity, but it can sometimes be applied to larger AVMs with a staged approach using multiple treatments.[63,64]

CAROTID-CAVERNOUS FISTULA

While coursing through the cavernous sinus, the internal carotid artery has the unique feature of being surrounded by venous blood, separated only by the arterial wall and a thin venous endothelium. Any breach in the continuity of these tissues results in a carotid-cavernous fistula. This exceptional anatomic configuration explains why carotid-cavernous fistulas account for most acquired intracranial arterio-venous shunts.

Carotid-cavernous fistulas are classified as direct or indirect types based on their angiographic findings.[65] Direct fistulas, which make up over 90% of the lesions, shunt blood from the internal carotid artery immediately into the cavernous sinus. Indirect fistulas describe a shunt between dural arteries and the cavernous sinus.

Etiology

Three-fourths of carotid-cavernous fistulas develop after head trauma, often after a fracture of the floor of the middle cranial fossa exerts tension on the carotid siphon and ruptures it.[66-68] The second most common cause is rupture of saccular aneurysms of the internal carotid artery within the cavernous sinus.[69,70] In one series of 100 consecutive carotid-cavernous fistulas, 76 resulted from trauma, 22 were due to a ruptured aneurysm, and two were iatrogenic.[71] Carotid-cavernous fistulas occasionally begin after blunt neck trauma.[72] Carotid dissection has been documented both with and without an accompanying skull fracture.[73] Bilateral carotid-cavernous fistulas have been documented after trauma[74] or in individuals with internal carotid artery aneurysms due to Ehlers-Danlos syndrome type IV.[75-77] Other rare causes include dural AVMs and collagen vascular diseases. Iatrogenic carotid-cavernous fistulas have developed in conjunction with therapeutic embolism procedures,[78-80] transsphenoidal pituitary surgery,[81] carotid endarterectomy,[82] and maxillectomy.[83] In a few individuals no definite cause can be pinpointed.

Clinical Features

Traumatic fistulas are more common in men, whereas spontaneous fistulas develop far more often in women. The female predominance of spontaneous carotid-cavernous fistulas probably stems from the higher frequency of intracavernous carotid artery aneurysms in women. In one series of 174 such aneurysm patients, for example, there were 161 women but only 13 men.[84] In posttraumatic cases, symptoms and signs usually appear within 24 hours after the injury but are occasionally delayed for several weeks or months when an initially small fistula slowly enlarges. Facial soft tissue injury and trauma-related impairment of consciousness can obscure the diagnosis initially.

The clinical manifestations of a carotid-cavernous fistula depend largely on the amount of blood flowing through the fistula. The onset of symptoms is usually abrupt, and the patient may report feeling or hearing an intracranial "pop." However, fistulas with low-flow shunts can generate more subtle findings. Some small fistulas gradually enlarge, and, with increasing flow, more severe signs and symptoms occur. Spontaneous closure of the fistula is more likely to occur with low-flow shunts.[85]

A carotid-cavernous fistula sometimes presents with isolated cranial nerve dysfunction, most commonly an abducens palsy.[86,87] It may be painless or accompanied by severe pain in the distribution of the first division of the trigeminal nerve and loss of vision.[88,89] Headache resembling migraine is sometimes the only initial symptom.[90,91] Eighty percent of the patients hear a bruit that is synchronous with the heartbeat.[71] The examiner similarly may hear a continuous murmur with systolic accentuation over the orbit and may detect a thrill.

Ipsilateral proptosis and chemosis develop quickly after a high-flow carotid-cavernous fistula develops, but individuals with a low-flow fistula do not always develop eye signs. Bilateral proptosis can occur because of the connection between the two cavernous sinuses via the circular sinus. Subconjunctival hemorrhage and papilledema are variable findings.[92] The retina is cyanotic with distended, hyperpulsatile veins. Retinal hemorrhage, retinal detachment, and central retinal artery occlusion have been described.[93,94] Visual loss results from these complications or from secondary glaucoma. Without adequate treatment, visual loss eventually occurs in most individuals with a carotid-cavernous fistula, although the risk is not as great among individuals whose fistula is promptly diagnosed and treated.[67,95] In some individuals the vision improves once the fistula is occluded.[96,97]

Occasional patients develop an intracerebral or a subarachnoid hemorrhage in conjunction with a carotid-cavernous fistula, presumably because the internal carotid lesion extends into the cranial cavity above the cavernous sinus or from leakage of blood under high pressure from the cavernous sinus.[98,99] If the fistula diverts huge quantities of blood from internal carotid artery, flow to its distal branches can be sufficiently compromised that signs of cerebral ischemia develop.

Diagnosis

The diagnosis of a carotid-cavernous fistula is obvious in an individual with pulsatile exophthalmos and a continuous orbital bruit.[100] Only the rare AVM in the orbit produces the same clinical picture. An unruptured aneurysm of the carotid siphon does not cause a bruit or conjunctival injection, although it may cause unilateral headache and cranial neuropathy. Thrombosis of the inferior petrosal vein can cause engorgement of the superior ophthalmic vein with proptosis and chemosis, but the eye is not pulsatile and there is no bruit. The Tolosa-Hunt syndrome causes periorbital pain and dysfunction of the cranial nerves that course through the wall of the cavernous sinus, but there is no bruit and proptosis does not occur.[101]

The diagnosis of carotid-cavernous fistula can usually be confirmed with neuroimaging studies, although the findings are more obvious with higher-flow lesions. With high-volume shunts, the cavernous sinus and its tributaries are enlarged on contrast-enhanced CT and MRI. Transcranial Doppler can document the increased flow velocity and can be used to determine which arteries at the base of the brain are affected. The fistula is apparent with magnetic resonance angiography or CTA.[102,103]

Catheter angiography (Figure 18-5 A) confirms the diagnosis of a carotid-cavernous fistula and allows one to better analyze the structure of the lesion before attempting to close it. When the fistula has already been confirmed with other studies, the angiogram can be done in conjunction with the endovascular treatment. With a large fistula, the anterior or the middle cerebral artery fails to fill because all the contrast material is being diverted into the cavernous sinus.

Treatment

About 10% of carotid-cavernous fistulas close without therapy, and spontaneous closure is more likely to occur with low-flow lesions. Neurologic and ophthalmologic dysfunction persist in some individuals even after the fistula is occluded, whereas in others fistula closure results in resolution of some or all clinical manifestations. There have been occasional reports of fistula closure during catheter angiography without embolization.[104]

The aim of therapy is to eliminate the fistula while maintaining perfusion of the internal carotid artery branches. The location of the carotid artery lesion within the cavernous sinus makes a direct surgical approach all but impossible. In 1935 Walter Dandy clipped the carotid artery in an effort to trap a carotid-cavernous fistula.[105] Although carotid occlusion is still necessary in rare instances, most fistulas are now treated with endovascular techniques. The first report of endovascular occlusion of a carotid-cavernous fistula was in 1930 by Brooks, who inserted a piece of muscle tissue into the carotid artery to occlude the fistula.[106] Variations of the muscle embolism technique were used until the development of detachable balloons almost four decades after Brooks's original report.

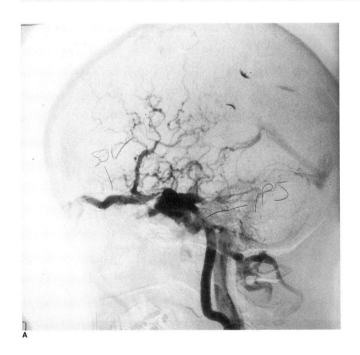
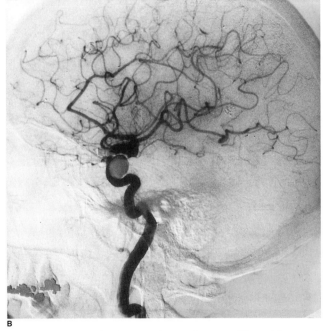

Figure 18-5. A: Catheter angiogram of the internal carotid artery confirms a carotid-cavernous fistula. Note the simultaneous filling of the carotid artery, dilated retinal vein, cavernous sinus, and straight sinus. B: After an intravascular balloon implant, the fistula is closed.

The treatment of choice for carotid-cavernous fistulas is now endovascular occlusion of the fistula (Figure 18-5 B), and the results are generally good. In one report of 98 consecutive patients with 100 carotid-cavernous fistulas that were treated with detachable balloons, 88 fistulas (in 86 patients) were successfully occluded, and blood flow in the carotid artery was successfully preserved in 66 of the 88 treated fistulas.[71] Platinum coils are sometimes used, especially in individuals whose fistula resulted from a ruptured intracavernous carotid artery aneurysm.[69,107,108] Recurrent fistulas can arise when a balloon deflates or when the arterial lesion recurs in an adjacent location.[109]

When the carotid artery is either inaccessible or excessively fragile (as with Ehlers-Danlos syndrome), transvenous access to the cavernous sinus via the superior orbital vein has been employed.[72,110] For complex fistulas that cannot be obliterated solely with a carotid artery approach, a combined arterial and venous approach is sometimes useful.[111,112] Embolism procedures are also used to occlude fistulas involving the lateral and sigmoid sinuses.[113]

CAVERNOUS MALFORMATIONS

A *cavernous malformation* is a complex of thin-walled, dilated vessels that are not separated by brain parenchyma and do not communicate directly with the arterial system. The synonymous terms *cavernous angioma, cavernous hemangioma,* and *cavernoma* suggest a neoplastic lesion, and, for this reason, the term *cavernous malformation* is preferable. These lesions occur in an estimated 0.5% of the population.[114]

Clinical Features of Cavernous Malformations

Cavernous malformations typically present with epileptic seizures, a clinical or radiographic mass lesion, or signs of intraparenchymal hemorrhage. Symptoms most often begin in mid-adulthood but can occur at any age. In the 138 individuals with histologically verified cavernous malformations summarized by Simard and colleagues, 49 people were initially evaluated for seizures, 49 were evaluated for a mass lesion, and 40 were seen for clinical signs of an intracranial hemorrhage.[115] In the 68 individuals with one or more cavernous malformations summarized by Moriarity and colleagues, 65% presented with headache, 49% presented with seizures, and 46% were evaluated because of a focal neurological deficit (some patients were listed in more than one category).[114] Cavernous malformations are increasingly identified because of the widespread use of neurodiagnostic studies.

Because cavernous malformations are low-pressure venous lesions, hemorrhagic lesions are generally less destructive than the intraparenchymal hemorrhages that occur with AVMs. Occasional patients develop SAH.[116] The location of the lesion plays a large role in determining the signs and symptoms that accompany a cavernous malformation. The most common site for these lesions is the cerebral white matter, but they also occur in the brainstem, cerebellum, and spinal cord. A few reports document cavernous malformations within the ventricular system.[117] About half of the patients have more than one cavernous malformation.

In a prospective study of 68 patients, Moriarity and colleagues estimated the risk of hemorrhage from a cavernous malformation to be 3.1% per person-year and the likelihood of new-onset seizures to be 2.4% per person-year.[114] Females in the study had a higher hemorrhage rate than males (4.2% per patient-year versus 0.9% per patient-year). The combined rate of new-onset seizures and hemorrhage in this study (5.5% per person-year) is similar to the 4.2% rate found in the study by Porter and colleagues.[118] Among these patients a hemorrhage at presentation did not increase the likelihood of a subsequent hemorrhage.[114]

Familial Cavernous Malformations

The familial occurrence of cavernous malformations was first suspected decades ago.[119–122] Among unselected individuals with one or more cavernous malformations of the nervous system, about a fifth have a positive family history of these lesions.[114] However, given the frequency of asymptomatic malformations and the subtlety of the findings in others, this estimate is likely to be low. Individuals with familial cavernous malformations are three times more likely to have multiple lesions (Figure 18-6 A) than patients without affected family members.[114] Some individuals with familial disease also have lesions of the retina (Figure 18-6 B) and other organs.[123] Familial cavernous malformations, like their sporadic counterparts, typically present with seizures or ICH.

Familial cerebral cavernous malformation is transmitted as an autosomal dominant trait and occurs more often among Mexican Americans.[124] There is genetic heterogeneity with at least three different disease-causing genes. The *CCM1* (or *KRIT1*) gene on chromosome 7q11.2-q21 is responsible for about 40% of the familial cavernous malformation families and almost all of those affect Mexican Americans.[124,125] Other families have mutations of the *CCM2* gene on chromosome 7p15-p13 and the *CCM3* (*PDCD10*) gene on chromosome 3q25.2–27.[126,127] These account for 20% and 40% of the families, respectively.[127,128]

Pathology of Cavernous Malformations

Cavernous malformations are irregular sinusoidal vascular channels without prominent feeding arteries or venous drainage (Figure 18-7). It is this absence of well-formed feeding arteries and draining veins that distinguishes a cavernous malformation from an AVM. The lesion size increases after each hemorrhage, but generally they range from 1 to 4 cm in diameter. The abnormal vessels contain endothelium and a fine adventitia of connective tissue but no muscular or elastic elements.[115,129] Calcium deposits commonly occur within the vessel walls. Acute hemorrhage or evidence of previous hemorrhage is sometimes noted at autopsy or in surgical specimens; in some patients the vascular lesion cannot be identified even at autopsy because it has been destroyed by hemorrhage.[121,130]

Diagnosis of Cavernous Malformations

Cavernous malformations typically have a central increased signal intensity surrounded by a dark ring of hemosiderin on T_2-weighted MRI (Figure 18-6).[131] Increased signal intensity on both T_1-weighted and T_2-weighted MRI sequences occur with a subacute hemorrhage. Lesion enlargement due to repeated small hemorrhages may generate progressive symptoms like those of a neoplasm. Even with MRI, a cavernous lesion may be difficult to recognize in the absence of the residual hemosiderin from a previous hemorrhage. Because of its specificity and low risk, MRI is ideal for initial diagnosis and for screening family members.[129] Abnormalities are more likely to be found in older individuals.[132]

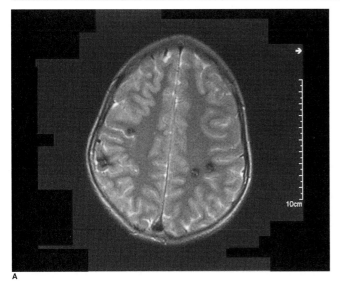
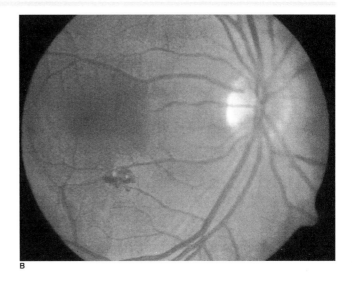

Figure 18-6. A: Cranial MRI showing multiple cavernous malformations of the cerebral hemispheres. The characteristic variegated appearance of the cavernous malformation on MRI results from hemosiderin left from earlier hemorrhages. B: This same patient has a cavernous lesion of the retina. Multiple brain and retinal cavernous malformations are often inherited as an autosomal dominant trait.

This classic appearance makes MRI more reliable in the diagnosis of these lesions than CT or catheter angiography.[131,133] In the absence of an acute hemorrhage, CT can be normal or nonspecific, showing only an irregular low-density lesion with faint contrast enhancement.[129] An acute hemorrhage is usually apparent with CT, and any calcium deposition within the lesion is also apparent, but CT is unlikely to allow a confident diagnosis.

Because of the paucity of arterial blood flow to a cavernous malformation, catheter angiography is often normal or its findings subtle and nonspecific.[21] In one collection of 115 patients who had arteriography, 31 studies were normal and another 55 had only an avascular mass.[115] Most of the remaining patients had subtle findings.

Treatment of Cavernous Malformations

Cavernous malformations that are accessible can be excised. The risk from surgery varies with the site of the lesion, and surgery is not always an option for lesions located in the brainstem or spinal cord.[134] Similarly, elective removal of numerous scattered cavernous malformations is not practical, although the one or two that are causing dysfunction can be removed even when multiple lesions are present. Removal of the lesion prevents further episodes of bleeding and usually stops seizures and other symptoms.[135]

Stereotactic radiosurgery can be used to reduce the bleeding risk of cavernous malformations that are not approachable by surgery.[136] However, the benefit from radiotherapy may be delayed, and treating numerous lesions may not be feasible.[137]

STURGE-WEBER SYNDROME

Also known as encephalofacial angiomatosis, Sturge-Weber syndrome is characterized by a leptomeningeal angioma with abnormal draining veins of one or both cerebral hemispheres and by an ipsilateral angioma (port wine stain or nevus flammeus) of the upper face. The cortex underlying the leptomeningeal hemangioma is often atrophic, and signs of neurological disturbance (e.g., seizures, hemiparesis, mental retardation, or visual field defects) may occur. Sturge-Weber syndrome is seldom difficult to diagnose, but it is often hard to predict or treat effectively. This difficulty is due to the highly variable phenotype of Sturge-Weber syndrome and the lack of effective treatment for some of its more serious features.

Clinical Features of Sturge-Weber Syndrome

Almost all patients with Sturge-Weber syndrome have a facial cutaneous hemangioma (port wine stain) on the forehead or around the eye ipsilateral to the intracranial abnormality (Figure 18-8). Although the facial nevus of Sturge-Weber syndrome is often described by its occurrence within the first division of the trigeminal nerve, in reality this pattern is related to the common embryologic origins of the facial and brain vasculature.

Individuals with a cutaneous hemangioma not affecting the upper face have little chance of developing the neurological complications of Sturge-Weber syndrome, and only about 15% of the individuals with a typical forehead nevus ever develop evidence of brain involvement.[138–140] However, occasional patients have typical intracranial findings of Sturge-Weber syndrome in the absence of a nevus. Bilateral upper facial involvement is relatively common, and the nevus can extend onto the trunk and extremities. Over a period of years, the skin lesion tends to thicken and darken in color.[141] By adulthood the surface of the nevus may become raised and irregular.

The classic neurological manifestations of Sturge-Weber syndrome include epilepsy, mental retardation, and various focal neurological deficits. Epilepsy occurs in most patients, but some patients respond well to medication. Typically seizures begin explosively in conjunction with an acute febrile illness at several months of age.[141] Seizures are often very difficult to control during the acute phase, only to resolve after a few days with or without the continued use of an antiepileptic medication. Many patients are eventually left with frequent seizures that are refractory to medication. Status epilepticus is common in these patients and can result in death.

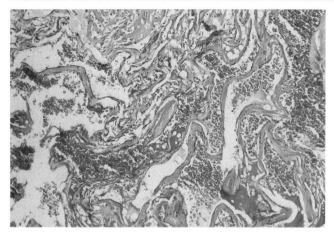

Figure 18-7. Pathologic appearance of a cavernous malformation. Note the large, thin-walled vessels in this cavernous malformation.

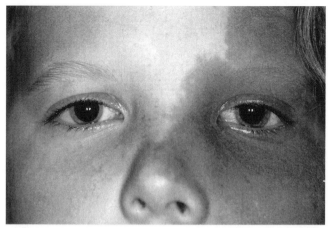

Figure 18-8. Typical facial cutaneous nevus of an individual with Sturge-Weber syndrome. Reprinted with permission from Riela and Roach.[157]

Mental retardation was once thought to be almost universal among patients with Sturge-Weber syndrome, but the phenotype is extremely variable, and about half of the patients remain cognitively intact. Some individuals have normal cognition but abnormal behavior, poor impulse control, or reduced attentiveness.[141]

Hemispheric involvement frequently results in contralateral spastic hemiparesis, sensory loss, and homonymous hemianopia. If the hemiparesis begins early in life, growth of the contralateral limbs is often stunted.

The most serious ocular findings are ipsilateral choroid hemangioma and glaucoma.[141] One of the most striking ocular signs is the presence of dilated, engorged tortuous episcleral vessels. In rare cases angiomatosis involves the iris on the side of the facial nevus, causing it to be darker than the other. Buphthalmos and amblyopia are present in some newborns, evidently because of prenatal onset glaucoma. Glaucoma occurs in 30% to 71% of the individuals with Sturge-Weber syndrome.[142] Most patients with glaucoma are identified during the first few years of life, but occasionally glaucoma due to Sturge-Weber syndrome develops in adulthood.[143] The intracranial angioma is frequently found in the occipital region, and, not surprisingly, visual field defects are common.

Pathologic Findings

The occipital and parietal lobes are affected more often than the frontal lobes. Cortical atrophy adjacent to the leptomeningeal angioma is typical, and the involved hemisphere is often smaller than the normal one. The leptomeninges are thickened and discolored by increased vascularity (Figure 18-9). Angiomatous vessels may obliterate the subarachnoid space, and the tortuous deep-draining veins that are evident radiographically can also be seen in pathologic specimens.[144] There is often calcification of the vessels in the angioma and in the cortex of the adjacent brain, causing a gritty sensation when the brain is cut with a knife.

Microscopic features include neuronal loss and gliosis that, like the abnormal vessels, often extend beyond the area of obvious abnormality.[144] Angiomatous vessels sometimes extend into the superficial brain parenchyma. The ipsilateral choroid plexus is often involved. Microscopically the abnormal vessels are variably sized thin-walled veins with a single layer of endothelial

cells.[144,145] Some of the vessels are narrowed or occluded by progressive hyalinization and subendothelial proliferation.[144,146] The typical gyriform calcification results from deposition of calcium within the outer cortical layers.[144,145]

Pathogenesis of Sturge-Weber Syndrome

Although Sturge-Weber syndrome was first described over a century ago, its pathogenesis remains poorly understood. The anatomic distribution of the angiomatous vessels is explained by their common embryologic origins. During embryologic development, the primordial vascular plexus splits into an inner layer supplying the brain and retina and an outer layer supplying the meninges, choroid, and face. Because this plexus does not form in similar fashion in the hindbrain, a hemangioma of the occipital skin is not associated with angiomatosis of the structures lying in the posterior fossa.

Clinical and pathological evidence suggests that the vascular lesions of Sturge-Weber syndrome are dynamic structures. The cutaneous and leptomeningeal angiomas gradually thicken and proliferate. The gradual occlusion of the intracranial vessels may result in chronic venous stasis with anoxic injury of the adjacent brain. In addition, occlusion of cortical and deep veins may be responsible for the episodes of acute neurological dysfunction that characterize Sturge-Weber syndrome.[141]

Sturge-Weber syndrome occurs sporadically, although somatic mosaicism could be responsible.[147] Immunohistochemical studies demonstrate up-regulation of the nuclear hypoxia-inducible factor (HIF) protein in the abnormal vessels from individuals with Sturge-Weber syndrome. HIF, in turn, induces vascular endothelial growth factor (VEGF), although the significance of this finding is not yet known.[148]

Diagnosis of Sturge-Weber Syndrome

Although the cutaneous manifestations of Sturge-Weber syndrome are straightforward, most individuals with an upper facial lesion do not have neurological involvement. Those who are destined to develop neurological dysfunction from Sturge-Weber syndrome usually remain asymptomatic for several months after birth. Neuroimaging studies will usually distinguish the individuals who have the complete syndrome from those with only the cutaneous features.

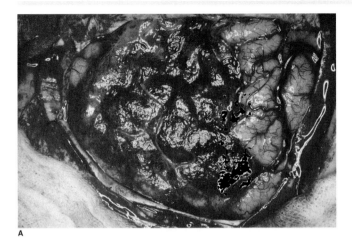

A

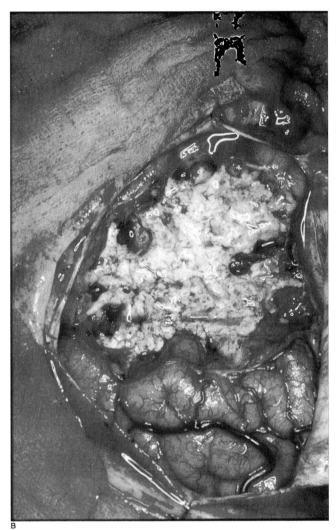

B

Figure 18-9. A: The leptomeninges are thickened and discolored by increased vascularity in this operative photograph of an individual with Sturge-Weber syndrome. B: This same patient is shown after surgical resection of the lesion.

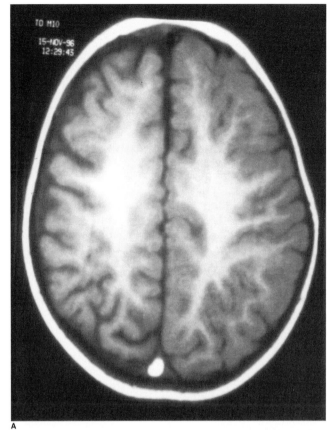

A

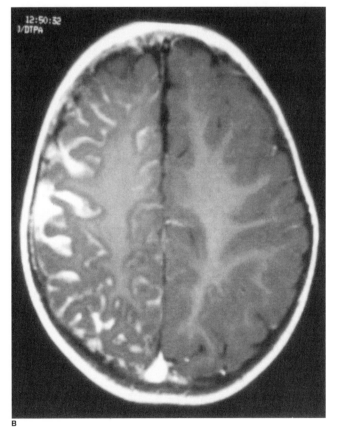

B

Figure 18-10. A: Normal T$_1$-weighted MRI without contrast of an individual with Sturge-Weber syndrome. B: The addition of gadolinium contrast reveals extensive parenchymal and leptomeningeal angiomatosis. Reprinted with permission from Roach and Bodensteiner.[158]

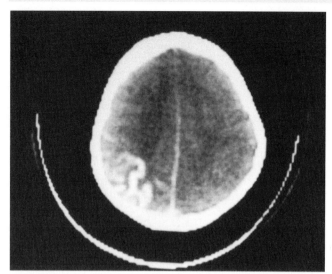

Figure 18-11. Cranial CT from a patient with Sturge-Weber syndrome shows a gyriform pattern of calcification in the parietal-occipital region. Reprinted with permission from Garcia et al.[151]

The PHACE syndrome is sometimes confused with Sturge-Weber syndrome. PHACE is an acronym for posterior fossa brain malformations, hemangiomas of the face, anomalous arteries, cardiac defects, and eye lesions. In one report 13% of the individuals with the PHACE syndrome had an intracranial aneurysm.[149,150] Neither aneurysms nor structural brain anomalies are characteristic of Sturge-Weber syndrome.

Magnetic resonance imaging with gadolinium contrast (Figure 18-10) is the most reliable way to detect the abnormal brain vasculature of Sturge-Weber syndrome. The abnormal vessels include both a leptomeningeal angioma as well as abnormal venous channels within the brain parenchyma. Noncontrasted MRI may also show cerebral atrophy, enlargement of the choroid plexus, or evidence of calcification, but MRI can be normal until the addition of contrast, especially in younger patients. The abnormal vessels are more likely to occur posteriorly, but any part of the cerebral hemispheres can be affected. Not surprisingly, individuals who have bilateral or extensive abnormalities of the brain vasculature tend to have more severe clinical manifestations than those with very focal lesions.

Although CT does not depict the abnormal blood vessels of Sturge-Weber syndrome as well as MRI, it does effectively show the brain calcifications that characterize Sturge-Weber syndrome (Figure 18-11). However, brain calcification may not be present during the early stages when the diagnosis might still be in question. The classic calcification appearance is a double-contoured pattern resulting from calcium deposition within the gyri adjacent to the vascular lesion. This pattern of calcification is sometimes evident even on plain X-rays as the classic *tram track* pattern, but, in many patients, the calcification is irregular and more diffuse.

Catheter angiography is now seldom performed on patients with Sturge-Weber syndrome. It does not reveal striking abnormalities of the arteries, but the superficial veins tend to be sparse, and abnormalities of the deep-draining veins are evident.[151]

Management of Sturge-Weber Syndrome

Most individuals with Sturge-Weber syndrome require medication for epilepsy, and, in many of these individuals, the seizures can be adequately controlled. Individuals with intractable seizures can be treated surgically (Figure 18-9). It is reasonable to first try antiepileptic medication and reserve surgery for patients who have significant dysfunction from seizures despite medication.[152] However, surgery should be done without delay once it is apparent that medicine is unlikely to work.

Some patients with Sturge-Weber syndrome have episodic focal neurological deficits without seizures, and it can be difficult to distinguish these episodes from post-ictal deficits. These episodes and the progressive neurologic dysfunction might result from venous occlusions or microcirculatory obstruction, although this is a hard concept to prove. Based on this model, some physicians prescribe antiplatelet therapy with daily aspirin.

Periodic measurement of the intraocular pressure and treatment of glaucoma may prevent blindness. The cosmetic impact of the facial nevus can be lessened with vascular-specific pulsed dye laser treatments.

DEVELOPMENTAL VENOUS ANOMALIES

A developmental venous anomaly (DVA) is a structurally anomalous but still functioning network of dilated venous channels.[153] As such, these lesions carry little risk unless they are associated with a cavernous malformation or an AVM. DVAs constitute two-thirds of all intracerebral vascular anomalies identified pathologically.[153] However, based on the frequency with which DVAs occur as incidental findings on neuroimaging studies, these lesions are exceedingly common, much more so than once suspected.

DVAs have been documented in individuals with epilepsy as well as those with cerebral hemorrhage.[130] However, the frequent occurrence of cerebral dysplasia adjacent to DVAs is a more likely explanation for the epilepsy, and most of the hemorrhagic lesions arise from a nearby cavernous malformation or AVM rather than the DVA per se. As a percentage of all DVAs, these mixed vascular lesions, with features of cavernous malformation, DVAs, and/or AVMs, are relatively uncommon.[154–156] Nevertheless, mixed vascular lesions probably account for most of the hemorrhages in people with a DVA.

Curling and Kelly calculated a 0.022% per person-year risk of intracranial hemorrhage from a DVA.[153] Even this low number may overstate the risk once the mixed vascular lesions are excluded.

REFERENCES

1. McCormick WF. The pathology of vascular ("arteriovenous") malformations. *J Neurosurg*. 1966;**24**:807–816.
2. *Intracranial Arteriovenous Malformations*. New York: Informa Health Care; 2006.
3. Stein BM, Wolpert SM. Arteriovenous malformations of the brain I: current concepts and treatment. *Arch Neurol*. 1980;**37**:1–5.
4. Friedlander RM. Clinical practice. Arteriovenous malformations of the brain. *N Engl J Med*. 2007;**356**:2704–2712.
5. Hofmeister C, Stapf C, Hartmann A, et al. Demographic, morphological, and clinical characteristics of 1289 patients with brain arteriovenous malformation. *Stroke*. 2000;**31**:1307–1310.
6. Arteriovenous malformations of the brain in adults. *N Engl J Med*. 1999;**340**:1812–1818.
7. Brown RD Jr, Wiebers DO, Forbes G, et al. The natural history of unruptured intracranial arteriovenous malformations. *J Neurosurg*. 1988;**68**:352–357.

8. Brown RD Jr, Wiebers DO, Torner JC, O'Fallon WM. Frequency of intracranial hemorrhage as a presenting symptom and subtype analysis: a population-based study of intracranial vascular malformations in Olmsted Country, Minnesota. *J Neurosurg.* 1996; **85**:29–32.

9. Olivecrona H, Ladenheim J. *Congenital Arteriovenous Aneurysms of the Carotid and Vertebral Arterial Systems.* Berlin: Springer; 1957.

10. Fults D, Kelly DL. Natural history of arteriovenous malformations of the brain: a clinical study. *Neurosurgery.* 1984;**15**: 658–662.

11. Hartmann A, Mast H, Mohr JP, et al. Morbidity of intracranial hemorrhage in patients with cerebral arteriovenous malformation. *Stroke.* 1998;**29**:931–934.

12. Crawford PM, West CR, Chadwick DW, Shaw MDM. Arteriovenous malformations of the brain: natural history in unoperated patients. *J Neurol Neurosurg Psychiatry.* 1986;**49**:1–10.

13. So SC. Cerebral arteriovenous malformations in children. *Childs Brain.* 1978;**4**:242–250.

14. Troost BT, Mark LE, Maroon JC. Resolution of classic migraine after removal of an occipital lobe AVM. *Ann Neurol.* 1979;**5**: 199–201.

15. Marks MP, Lane B, Steinberg G, Chang P. Vascular characteristics of intracerebral arteriovenous malformations in patients with clinical steal. *AJNR Am J Neuroradiol.* 1991;**12**:489–496.

16. Sheth RD, Bodensteiner JB. Progressive neurologic impairment from an arteriovenous malformation vascular steal. *Pediatr Neurol.* 1995;**13**:352–354.

17. Wyburn-Mason R. Arteriovenous aneurysm of mid-brain and retina, facial naevi and mental changes. *Brain.* 1943;**66**:12–203.

18. Hopen G, Smith JL, Hoff JT, Quencer R. The Wyburn-Mason syndrome- concomitant chiasmal and fundus vascular malformations. *J Clin Neuroophthalmol.* 1983;**3**:53–62.

19. Ponce FA, Han PP, Spetzler RF, Canady A, Feiz-Erfan I. Associated arteriovenous malformation of the orbit and brain: a case of Wyburn-Mason syndrome without retinal involvement. Case report. *J Neurosurg.* 2001;**95**:346–349.

20. Horton JC, Chambers WA, Lyons SL, Adams RD, Kjellberg RN. Pregnancy and the risk of hemorrhage from cerebral arteriovenous malformations. *Neurosurgery.* 1990;**27**:867–871.

21. Becker DH, Townsend JJ, Kramer RA, Newton TH. Occult cerebrovascular malformations. A series of 18 histologically verified cases with negative angiography. *Brain.* 1979;**102**:249–287.

22. Crawford JV, Russell DS. Cryptic arteriovenous and venous hamartomas of the brain. *J Neurol Neurosurg Psychiatry.* 1956; **19**:1–11.

23. Yamashita Y, Nakamura Y, Okudera T, et al. Neuroradiological and pathological studies on neonatal aneurysmal vein of Galen. *J Child Neurol.* 1990;**5**:45–48.

24. Wong JH, Awad IA, Kim JH. Ultrastructural pathological features of cerebrovascular malformations: a preliminary report. *Neurosurgery.* 2000;**46**:1454–1459.

25. Kaplan HA, Aronson SM, Browder EJ. Vascular malformations of the brain – an anatomic study. *J Neurosurg.* 1961;**18**:630–635.

26. Wakabayashi S, Ohno K, Shishido T, Tamaki M, Matsushima Y, Hirakawa K. Marked growth of a cerebral arteriovenous malformation: case report and review of the literature. *Neurosurgery.* 1991;**29**:920–923.

27. Kader A, Goodrich JT, Sonstein WJ, Stein BM, Carmel PW, Michelsen WJ. Recurrent cerebral arteriovenous malformations after negative postoperative angiograms. *J Neurosurg.* 1996;**85**: 14–18.

28. Wakai S, Chen CH, Wu KY, Chiu CW. Spontaneous regression of a cerebral arteriovenous malformation. Report of a case and review of the literature. *Arch Neurol.* 1983;**40**:377–380.

29. Patel MC, Hodgson TJ, Kemeny AA, Forster DM. Spontaneous obliteration of pial arteriovenous malformations: a review of 27 cases. *AJNR Am J Neuroradiol.* 2001;**22**:531–536.

30. Krapf H, Siekmann R, Freudenstein D, Kuker W, Skalej M. Spontaneous occlusion of a cerebral arteriovenous malformation: angiography and MR imaging follow-up and review of the literature. *AJNR Am J Neuroradiol.* 2001;**22**:1556–1560.

31. Abdulrauf SI, Malik GM, Awad IA. Spontaneous angiographic obliteration of cerebral arteriovenous malformations. *Neurosurgery.* 1999;**44**:280–287.

32. Meisel HJ, Mansmann U, Alvarez H, Rodesch G, Brock M, Lasjaunias P. Cerebral arteriovenous malformations and associated aneurysms: analysis of 305 cases from a series of 662 patients. *Neurosurgery.* 2000;**46**:793–800.

33. Mansmann U, Meisel J, Brock M, Rodesch G, Alvarez H, Lasjaunias P. Factors associated with intracranial hemorrhage in cases of cerebral arteriovenous malformation. *Neurosurgery.* 2000; **46**:272–279.

34. Stefani MA, Porter PJ, TerBrugge KG, Montanera W, Willinsky RA, Wallace MC. Angioarchitectural factors present in brain arteriovenous malformations associated with hemorrhagic presentation. *Stroke.* 2002;**33**:920–924.

35. Langer DJ, Lasner TM, Hurst RW, Flamm ES, Zager EL, King JT Jr. Hypertension, small size, and deep venous drainage are associated with risk of hemorrhagic presentation of cerebral arteriovenous malformations. *Neurosurgery.* 1998;**42**:481–486.

36. Stefani MA, Porter PJ, TerBrugge KG, Montanera W, Willinsky RA, Wallace MC. Large and deep brain arteriovenous malformations are associated with risk of future hemorrhage. *Stroke.* 2002;**33**:1220–1224.

37. Duong DH, Young WL, Vang MC, et al. Feeding artery pressure and venous drainage pattern are primary determinants of hemorrhage from cerebral arteriovenous malformations. *Stroke.* 1998;**29**:1167–1176.

38. Reddy K, West M, McClarty B. Multiple intracerebral arteriovenous malformations: a case report and literature review. *Surg Neurol.* 1987;**27**:495–499.

39. Mizutani T, Tanaka H, Aruga T. Multiple arteriovenous malformations located in the cerebellum, posterior fossa, spinal cord, dura, and scalp with associated port-wine stain and supratentorial venous anomaly. *Neurosurgery.* 1992;**31**:137–140.

40. Lesser BA, Wendt D, Miks VM, Norum RA. Identical twins with hereditary hemorrhagic telangiectasia concordant for cerebrovascular arteriovenous malformations. *Am J Med.* 1986;**81**: 931–934.

41. Letteboer TG, Mager JJ, Snijder RJ, et al. Genotype-phenotype relationship in hereditary haemorrhagic telangiectasia. *J Med Genet.* 2006;**43**:371–377.

42. Roman G, Fisher M, Perl DP, Poser CM. Neurological manifestations of hereditary hemorrhagic telangiectasia (Rendu-Osler-Weber disease): report of 2 cases and review of the literature. *Ann Neurol.* 1978;**4**:130–144.

43. Aesch B, Lioret E, De Toffol B, Jan M. Multiple cerebral angiomas and Rendu-Osler-Weber disease: case report. *Neurosurgery.* 1991;**29**:599–602.

44. Willinsky RA, Lasjaunias P, Terbrugge K, Burrows P. Multiple cerebral arteriovenous malformations (AVMs). Review of our experience from 203 patients with cerebral vascular lesions. *Neuroradiology.* 1990;**32**:207–210.

45. Iizuka Y, Rodesch G, Garcia-Monaco R, et al. Multiple cerebral arteriovenous shunts in children: report of 13 cases. *Child's Nerv Syst.* 1992;**8**:437–444.

46. Song WZ, Mao BY, Hu BF, Liu YH, Sun H, Mao Q. Intraventricular vascular malformations mimicking tumors: case reports and review of the literature. *J Neurol Sci.* 2008;**266**:63–69.

47. Kokkinis C, Vlychou M, Zavras GM, Hadjigeorgiou GM, Papadimitriou A, Fezoulidis IV. The role of 3D-computed tomography angiography (3D-CTA) in investigation of spontaneous subarachnoid haemorrhage: comparison with digital subtraction angiography (DSA) and surgical findings. *Br J Neurosurg.* 2008;**22**:71–78.

48. Nussel F, Wegmuller H, Huber P. Comparison of magnetic resonance angiography, magnetic resonance imaging and conventional angiography in cerebral arteriovenous malformation. *Neurorad.* 1991;**33**:56–61.

49. Lemme-Plaghos L, Kucharczyk W, Brant-Zawadzki M, et al. MRI of angiographically occult vascular malformations. *Am J Roentgenol.* 1986;**146**:1223–1228.

50. Lobato RD, Perez C, Rivas JJ, Cordobes F. Clinical, radiological, and pathological spectrum of angiographically occult intracranial vascular malformations. *J Neurosurg.* 1988;**68**:518–531.

51. Cohen HC, Tucker WS, Humphreys RP, Perrin RJ. Angiographically cryptic histologically verified cerebrovascular malformations. *Neurosurgery.* 1982;**10**:704–714.

52. Ogilvy CS, Heros RC, Ojemann RG, New PF. Angiographically occult arteriovenous malformations. *J Neurosurg.* 1988;**69**:350–355.

53. Ondra SL, Troupp H, George ED, Schwab K. The natural history of symptomatic arteriovenous malformations of the brain: a 24-year follow-up assessment. *J Neurosurg.* 1990;**73**:387–391.

54. Spetzler RF, Martin NA. A proposed grading system for arteriovenous malformations. *J Neurosurg.* 1986;**65**:476–483.

55. Morgan MK, Johnston IH, Hallinan JM, Weber NC. Complications of surgery for arteriovenous malformations of the brain. *J Neurosurg.* 1993;**78**:176–182.

56. Heros RC, Korosue K, Diebold PM. Surgical excision of cerebral arteriovenous malformations: late results. *Neurosurgery.* 1990;**26**:570–578.

57. Vinuela F, Dion JE, Duckwiler G, et al. Combined endovascular embolization and surgery in the management of cerebral arteriovenous malformations: experience with 101 cases. *J Neurosurg.* 1991;**75**:856–864.

58. Paulsen RD, Steinberg GK, Norbash AM, Marcellus ML, Marks MP. Embolization of basal ganglia and thalamic arteriovenous malformations. *Neurosurgery.* 1999;**44**:991–996.

59. Fox AJ, Pelz DM, Lee DH. Arteriovenous malformations of the brain: recent results of endovascular therapy. *Radiology.* 1990;**177**:51–57.

60. Kjellin IB, Boechat MI, Vinuela F, Westra SJ, Duckwiler GR. Pulmonary emboli following therapeutic embolization of cerebral arteriovenous malformations in children. *Pediatr Radiol.* 2000;**30**:279–283.

61. Fleetwood IG, Marcellus ML, Levy RP, Marks MP, Steinberg GK. Deep arteriovenous malformations of the basal ganglia and thalamus: natural history. *J Neurosurg.* 2003;**98**:747–750.

62. Pollock BE, Gorman DA, Brown PD. Radiosurgery for arteriovenous malformations of the basal ganglia, thalamus, and brainstem. *J Neurosurg.* 2004;**100**:210–214.

63. Pendl G, Unger F, Papaefthymiou G, Eustacchio S. Staged radiosurgical treatment for large benign cerebral lesions. *J Neurosurg.* 2000;**93**(Suppl 3):107–112.

64. Pan DH, Guo WY, Chung WY, Shiau CY, Chang YC, Wang LW. Gamma knife radiosurgery as a single treatment modality for large cerebral arteriovenous malformations. *J Neurosurg.* 2000;**93** (Suppl 3):113–119.

65. Barrow DL, Spector RH, Braun IF, Landman JA, Tindall SC, Tindall GT. Classification and treatment of spontaneous carotid-cavernous sinus fistulas. *J Neurosurg.* 1985;**62**:248–256.

66. Bavinzski G, Killer M, Knosp E, Ferraz-Leite H, Gruber A, Richling B. False aneurysms of the intracavernous carotid artery – report of 7 cases. *Acta Neurochir (Wien).* 1997;**139**:37–43.

67. Fabian TS, Woody JD, Ciraulo DL, et al. Posttraumatic carotid cavernous fistula: frequency analysis of signs, symptoms, and disability outcomes after angiographic embolization. *J Trauma.* 1999;**47**:275–281.

68. Liang W, Xiaofeng Y, Weiguo L, Wusi Q, Gang S, Xuesheng Z. Traumatic carotid cavernous fistula accompanying basilar skull fracture: a study on the incidence of traumatic carotid cavernous fistula in the patients with basilar skull fracture and the prognostic analysis about traumatic carotid cavernous fistula. *J Trauma.* 2007;**63**:1014–1020.

69. Wanke I, Doerfler A, Stolke D, Forsting M. Carotid cavernous fistula due to a ruptured intracavernous aneurysm of the internal carotid artery: treatment with selective endovascular occlusion of the aneurysm. *J Neurol Neurosurg Psychiatry.* 2001;**71**:784–787.

70. van Rooij WJ, Sluzewski M, Beute GN. Ruptured cavernous sinus aneurysms causing carotid cavernous fistula: incidence, clinical presentation, treatment, and outcome. *AJNR Am J Neuroradiol.* 2006;**27**:185–189.

71. Lewis AI, Tomsick TA, Tew JM Jr. Management of 100 consecutive direct carotid-cavernous fistulas: results of treatment with detachable balloons. *Neurosurgery.* 1995;**36**:239–244.

72. Berlis A, Klisch J, Spetzger U, Faist M, Schumacher M. Carotid cavernous fistula: embolization via a bilateral superior ophthalmic vein approach. *AJNR Am J Neuroradiol.* 2002;**23**:1736–1738.

73. Yong RL, Heran NS. Traumatic carotid cavernous fistula with bilateral carotid artery and vertebral artery dissections. *Acta Neurochir (Wien).* 2005;**147**:1109–1113.

74. Luo CB, Teng MM, Chang FC, Sheu MH, Guo WY, Chang CY. Bilateral traumatic carotid-cavernous fistulae: strategies for endovascular treatment. *Acta Neurochir (Wien).* 2007;**149**:675–680.

75. Koh JH, Kim JS, Hong SC, et al. Skin manifestations, multiple aneurysms, and carotid-cavernous fistula in Ehlers-Danlos syndrome type IV. *Circulation.* 1999;**100**:e57–e58.

76. Kanner AA, Maimon S, Rappaport ZH. Treatment of spontaneous carotid-cavernous fistula in Ehlers-Danlos syndrome by transvenous occlusion with Guglielmi detachable coils. Case report and review of the literature. *J Neurosurg.* 2000;**93**:689–692.

77. Chuman H, Trobe JD, Petty EM, et al. Spontaneous direct carotid-cavernous fistula in Ehlers-Danlos syndrome type IV: two case reports and a review of the literature. *J Neuroophthalmol.* 2002;**22**:75–81.

78. Barr JD, Mathis JM, Horton JA. Iatrogenic carotid-cavernous fistula occurring after embolization of a cavernous sinus meningioma. *AJNR Am J Neuroradiol.* 1995;**16**:483–485.

79. Phatouros CC, Halbach VV, Malek AM, Dowd CF, Higashida RT. Simultaneous subarachnoid hemorrhage and carotid cavernous fistula after rupture of a paraclinoid aneurysm during balloon-assisted coil embolization. *AJNR Am J Neuroradiol.* 1999;**20**:1100–1102.

80. Liang W, Xiaofeng Y, Weiguo L, et al. Bilateral traumatic carotid cavernous fistula: the manifestations, transvascular embolization and prevention of the vascular complications after therapeutic embolization. *J Craniofac Surg.* 2007;**18**:74–77.

81. Dolenc VV, Lipovsek M, Slokan S. Traumatic aneurysm and carotid-cavernous fistula following transsphenoidal approach to a pituitary adenoma: treatment by transcranial operation. *Br J Neurosurg.* 1999;**13**:185–188.

82. Ou RJ, Lee AG. Direct carotid-cavernous fistula following carotid endarterectomy. *Can J Ophthalmol.* 1999;**34**:401–406.

83. Holmes JD, Dierks EJ. Carotid-cavernous fistula after partial maxillectomy: case report. *J Oral Maxillofac Surg.* 2001;**59**:102–105.

84. Kupersmith MJ, Stiebel-Kalish H, Huna-Baron R, et al. Cavernous carotid aneurysms rarely cause subarachnoid hemorrhage or major neurologic morbidity. *J Stroke Cerebrovasc Dis.* 2002; **11**:9–14.

85. Alkhani A, Willinsky R, Terbrugge K. Spontaneous resolution of bilateral traumatic carotid cavernous fistulas and development of trans-sellar intercarotid vascular communication: case report. *Surg Neurol.* 1999;**52**:627–629.

86. Kurata A, Takano M, Tokiwa K, Miyasaka Y, Yada K, Kan S. Spontaneous carotid cavernous fistula presenting only with cranial nerve palsies. *AJNR Am J Neuroradiol.* 1993;**14**:1097–1101.

87. Jensen RW, Chuman H, Trobe JD, Deveikis JP. Facial and trigeminal neuropathies in cavernous sinus fistulas. *J Neuroophthalmol.* 2004;**24**:34–38.

88. Goldenberg-Cohen N, Curry C, Miller NR, Tamargo RJ, Murphy KP. Long term visual and neurological prognosis in patients with treated and untreated cavernous sinus aneurysms. *J Neurol Neurosurg Psychiatry.* 2004;**75**:863–867.

89. Kupersmith MJ, Hurst R, Berenstein A, Choi IS, Jafar J, Ransohoff J. The benign course of cavernous carotid artery aneurysms. *J Neurosurg.* 1992;**77**:690–693.

90. Evans RW, Schiffman JS. Headache as the only symptom of a spontaneous dural carotid-cavernous fistula. *Headache.* 2005; **45**:1256–1259.

91. Yamada SM, Masahira N, Shimizu K. A migraine-like headache induced by carotid-cavernous fistula. *Headache.* 2007;**47**: 289–293.

92. Pong JC, Lam DK, Lai JS. Spontaneous subconjunctival haemorrhage secondary to carotid-cavernous fistula. *Clin Experiment Ophthalmol.* 2008;**36**:90–91.

93. Choi HY, Newman NJ, Biousse V, Hill DC, Costarides AP. Serous retinal detachment following carotid-cavernous fistula. *Br J Ophthalmol.* 2006;**90**:1440.

94. Pillai GS, Ghose S, Singh N, Garodia VK, Puthassery R, Manjunatha NP. Central retinal artery occlusion in dural carotid cavernous fistula. *Retina.* 2002;**22**:493–494.

95. Sanders MD, Hoyt WF. Hypoxic ocular sequelae of carotid-cavernous fistulae. *Br J Ophthalmol.* 1969;**53**:82–97.

96. Das S, Bendok BR, Novakovic RL, et al. Return of vision after transarterial coiling of a carotid cavernous sinus fistula: case report. *Surg Neurol.* 2006;**66**:82–85.

97. Albuquerque FC, Heinz GW, McDougall CG. Reversal of blindness after transvenous embolization of a carotid-cavernous fistula: case report. *Neurosurgery.* 2003;**52**:233–236.

98. Hiramatsu K, Utsumi S, Kyoi K, et al. Intracerebral hemorrhage in carotid-cavernous fistula. *Neurorad.* 1991;**33**:67–69.

99. Lee AG, Mawad ME, Baskin DS. Fatal subarachnoid hemorrhage from the rupture of a totally intracavernous carotid artery aneurysm: case report. *Neurosurgery.* 1996;**38**:596–598.

100. Zimmerman CF, Batjer HH, Purdy P, Samson D, Kopitnik T, Carstens GJ. Ehlers-Danlos syndrome type IV: neuro-ophthalmic manifestations and management. *Ophthalmology.* 1994;**101S**: 133.

101. Miwa H, Koshimura I, Mizuno Y. Recurrent cranial neuropathy as a clinical presentation of idiopathic inflammation of the dura mater: a possible relationship to Tolosa-Hunt syndrome and cranial pachymeningitis. *J Neurol Sci.* 1998;**154**:101–105.

102. Vattoth S, Cherian J, Pandey T. Magnetic resonance angiographic demonstration of carotid-cavernous fistula using elliptical centric time resolved imaging of contrast kinetics (EC-TRICKS). *Magn Reson Imaging.* 2007;**25**:1227–1231.

103. Coskun O, Hamon M, Catroux G, Gosme L, Courtheoux P, Theron J. Carotid-cavernous fistulas: diagnosis with spiral CT angiography. *AJNR Am J Neuroradiol.* 2000;**21**:712–716.

104. Luo CB, Teng MM, Chang FC, Chang CY. Spontaneous thrombosis and complete disappearance of traumatic carotid-cavernous fistulas after angiography. *J Chin Med Assoc.* 2005; **68**:487–490.

105. Dandy W. The treatment of carotid-cavernous arterio-venous aneurysms. *Ann Surg.* 1935;**102**:916–920.

106. Brooks B. The treatment of traumatic arterio-venous fistula. *South Med J.* 1930;**23**:100–106.

107. Eddleman CS, Surdell D, Miller J, Shaibani A, Bendok BR. Endovascular management of a ruptured cavernous carotid artery aneurysm associated with a carotid cavernous fistula with an intracranial self-expanding microstent and hydrogel-coated coil embolization: case report and review of the literature. *Surg Neurol.* 2007;**68**:562–567.

108. Moron FE, Klucznik RP, Mawad ME, Strother CM. Endovascular treatment of high-flow carotid cavernous fistulas by stent-assisted coil placement. *AJNR Am J Neuroradiol.* 2005;**26**:1399–1404.

109. Lee ST, Hsu HH, Ng SH, Wong HF. Recurrent traumatic carotid-cavernous fistula caused by rupture of the detachable balloon. *J Trauma.* 1998;**45**:969–971.

110. Hollands JK, Santarius T, Kirkpatrick PJ, Higgins JN. Treatment of a direct carotid-cavernous fistula in a patient with type IV Ehlers-Danlos syndrome: a novel approach. *Neurorad.* 2006; **48**:491–494.

111. Russell EJ, Reddy V, Rovin R. Combined arterial and venous approaches for cure of carotid-cavernous sinus fistula in a patient with fibromuscular dysplasia. *Skull Base Surg.* 1994;**4**: 103–109.

112. Men S, Ozturk H, Hekimoglu B, Sekerci Z. Traumatic carotid-cavernous fistula treated by combined transarterial and transvenous coil embolization and associated cavernous internal carotid artery dissection treated with stent placement. Case report. *J Neurosurg.* 2003;**99**:584–586.

113. Dawson RC III, Joseph GJ, Owens DS, Barrow DL. Transvenous embolization as the primary therapy for arteriovenous fistulas of the lateral and sigmoid sinuses. *AJNR Am J Neuroradiol.* 1998;**19**:571–576.

114. Moriarity JL, Wetzel M, Clatterbuck RE, et al. The natural history of cavernous malformations: a prospective study of 68 patients. *Neurosurgery.* 1999;**44**:1166–1171.

115. Simard JM, Garcia-Bengochea F, Ballenger WE, Mickle JP, Quisling RG. Cavernous angioma: a review of 126 collected and 12 new clinical cases. *Neurosurgery.* 1986;**18**:162–172.

116. Acciarri N, Padovani R, Pozzati E, Gaist G, Manetto V. Spinal cavernous angioma: a rare cause of subarachnoid hemorrhage. *Surg Neurol.* 1992;**37**:453–456.

117. Iwasa H, Indel I, Sato F. Intraventricular cavernous hemangioma. *J Neurosurg.* 1983;**59**:153–157.

118. Porter PJ, Wilinsky RA, Harper W, Wallace MC. Cerebral cavernous malformations: natural history and prognosis after clinical deterioration with or without hemorrhage. *J Neurosurg.* 1997;**87**:190–197.

119. Michael JC, Levin PM. Multiple telangiectasias of brain: a discussion of hereditary factors in their development. *Arch Neurol Psychiatry.* 1936;**36**:514–536.

120. Kidd HA, Cumings JN. Cerebral angiomata in an Icelandic family. *Lancet.* 1947;**1**:747–748.

121. Bicknell JM, Carlow TJ, Kornfeld M, Stovring J, Turner P. Familial cavernous angiomas. *Arch Neurol.* 1978;**35**:746–749.

122. Clark JV. Familial occurrence of cavernous angiomata of the brain. *J Neurol Neurosurg Psychiatry.* 1970;**33**:871–876.

123. Dobyns WB, Michels VV, Groover RV, et al. Familial cavernous malformations of the central nervous system and retina. *Ann Neurol.* 1987;**21**:578–583.

124. Gunel M, Awad IA, Finberg K, et al. A founder mutation as a cause of cerebral cavernous malformation in Hispanic Americans. *N Engl J Med.* 1996;**334**:946–951.

125. Laberge-le CS, Jung HH, Labauge P, et al. Truncating mutations in CCM1, encoding KRIT1, cause hereditary cavernous angiomas. *Nat Genet.* 1999;**23**:189–193.

126. Bergametti F, Denier C, Labauge P, et al. Mutations within the programmed cell death 10 gene cause cerebral cavernous malformations. *Am J Hum Genet.* 2005;**76**:42–51.

127. Craig HD, Gunel M, Cepeda O, et al. Multilocus linkage identifies two new loci for a mendelian form of stroke, cerebral cavernous malformation, at 7p15–13 and 3q25.2–27. *Hum Mol Genet.* 1998;**7**:1851–1858.

128. Laurans MS, DiLuna ML, Shin D, et al. Mutational analysis of 206 families with cavernous malformations. *J Neurosurg.* 2003;**99**:38–43.

129. Rigamonti D, Hadley MN, Drayer BP, et al. Cerebral cavernous malformations: incidence and familial occurrence. *N Engl J Med.* 1988;**319**:343–347.

130. Zeller RS, Chutorian AM. Vascular malformations of the pons in children. *Neurology.* 1975;**28**:776–780.

131. Rigamonti D, Drayer BP, Johnson PC, Hadley MN, Zabramski J, Spetzler RF. The MRI appearance of cavernous malformations (angiomas). *J Neurosurg.* 1987;**67**:518–524.

132. Labauge P, Laberge S, Brunereau L, Levy C, Tournier-Lasserve E. Hereditary cerebral cavernous angiomas: clinical and genetic features in 57 French families. Société Française de Neurochirurgie. *Lancet.* 1998;**352**:1892–1897.

133. Requena I, Arias M, Lopez-Ibor L, et al. Cavernomas of the central nervous system: clinical and neuroimaging manifestations in 47 patients. *J Neurol Neurosurg Psychiatry.* 1991;**54**:590–594.

134. Amin-Hanjani S, Ogilvy CS, Ojemann RG, Crowell RM. Risks of surgical management for cavernous malformations of the nervous system. *Neurosurgery.* 1998;**42**:1220–1227.

135. Churchyard A, Khangure M, Grainger K. Cerebral cavernous angioma: a potentially benign condition? Successful treatment in 16 cases. *J Neurol Neurosurg Psychiatry.* 1992;**55**:1040–1045.

136. Pollock BE, Garces YI, Stafford SL, Foote RL, Schomberg PJ, Link MJ. Stereotactic radiosurgery for cavernous malformations. *J Neurosurg.* 2000;**93**:987–991.

137. Karlsson B, Kihlstrom L, Lindquist C, Ericson K, Steiner L. Radiosurgery for cavernous malformations. *J Neurosurg.* 1998;**88**:293–297.

138. Enjolras O, Riche MC, Merland JJ. Facial port-wine stains and Sturge-Weber syndrome. *Pediatrics.* 1985;**76**:48–51.

139. Tallman B, Tan OT, Morelli JG, et al. Location of port-wine stains and the likelihood of ophthalmic and/or central nervous system complications. *Pediatrics.* 1991;**87**:323–327.

140. Uram M, Zubillaga C. The cutaneous manifestations of Sturge-Weber syndrome. *J Clin Neuroophthalmol.* 1982;**2**:245–248.

141. Bodensteiner JB, Roach ES (eds). *Sturge-Weber Syndrome.* Mt Freedom, NJ: Sturge-Weber Foundation; 1999.

142. Sullivan TJ, Clarke MP, Morin JD. The ocular manifestations of the Sturge-Weber syndrome. *J Pediatr Ophthal Strabismus.* 1992;**29**:349–356.

143. Sujansky E, Conradi S. Sturge-Weber syndrome: age of onset of seizures and glaucoma and the prognosis for affected children. *J Child Neurol.* 1995;**10**:49–58.

144. Wohlwill FJ, Yakovlev PI. Histopathology of meningo-facial angiomatosis (Sturge-Weber's disease). *J Neuropathol Exp Neurol.* 1957;**16**:341–364.

145. Di Trapani G, Di Rocco C, Abbamondi AL, Caldarelli M, Pocchiari M. Light microscopy and ultrastructural studies of Sturge-Weber disease. *Brain.* 1982;**9**:23–36.

146. Norman MG, Schoene WC. The ultrastructure of Sturge-Weber disease. *Acta Neuropathol.* 1977;**37**:199–205.

147. Huq AH, Chugani DC, Hukku B, Serajee FJ. Evidence of somatic mosaicism in Sturge-Weber syndrome. *Neurology.* 2002;**59**:780–782.

148. Comati A, Beck H, Halliday W, Snipes GJ, Plate KH, Acker T. Upregulation of hypoxia-inducible factor (HIF)-1alpha and HIF-2alpha in leptomeningeal vascular malformations of Sturge-Weber syndrome. *J Neuropathol Exp Neurol.* 2007;**66**:86–97.

149. Heyer GL, Dowling MM, Licht DJ, et al. The cerebral vasculopathy of PHACES syndrome. *Stroke.* 2008;**39**:308–316.

150. Heyer GL, Millar WS, Ghatan S, Garzon MC. The neurologic aspects of PHACE: case report and review of the literature. *Pediatr Neurol.* 2006;**35**:419–424.

151. Garcia JC, Roach ES, McLean WT. Recurrent thrombotic deterioration in the Sturge-Weber syndrome. *Childs Brain.* 1981;**8**:427–433.

152. Roach ES, Riela AR, Chugani HT, Shinnar S, Bodensteiner JB, Freeman J. Sturge-Weber syndrome: recommendations for surgery. *J Child Neurol.* 1994;**9**:190–193.

153. Curling OD, Kelly DL. The natural history of intracranial cavernous and venous malformations. *Prospect Neurol Surg.* 1990;**1**:19–43.

154. Sasaki O, Tanaka R, Koike T, Koide A, Koizumi T, Ogawa H. Excision of cavernous angioma with preservation of coexisting venous angioma. *J Neurosurg.* 1991;**75**:461–464.

155. Rigamonti D, Spetzler RF. The association of venous and cavernous malformations. Report of four cases and discussion of the pathophysiological, diagnostic, and therapeutic implications. *Acta Neurochir.* 1988;**92**:100–105.

156. Awad IA, Robinson JR, Mohanty S, Estes ML. Mixed vascular malformations of the brain: clinical and pathogenetic considerations. *Neurosurgery.* 1993;**33**:179–188.

157. Riela AR, Roach ES. Sturge-Weber syndrome. In: Roach ES, Miller VS, eds. *Neurocutaneous Disorders.* Cambridge, England: Cambridge University Press; 2004:179–185.

158. Roach ES, Bodensteiner JB. Neurologic manifestations of Sturge-Weber syndrome. In: Bodensteiner JB, Roach ES, eds. *Sturge-Weber Syndrome.* Mt Freedom, NJ: Sturge-Weber Foundation; 1999:27–38.

19

Subdural and Epidural Hematomas

Sometimes a great wound or concussion of the head, especially which happens by falling headlong from an high place, brings a prejudice and weakness to the animal faculty, dulling the understanding.

Thomas Willis

Intracranial bleeding can occur in the subdural or epidural spaces, the subarachnoid space, the brain, the ventricular system, or the pituitary gland. Subdural hematomas arise between the dura and the arachnoid membranes, whereas epidural hematomas form in the potential space between the dura and the skull.[1] Intracerebral, subarachnoid, and intraventricular hemorrhages are presented in Chapters 16 and 17.

SUBDURAL HEMATOMA

The finding of trephine holes in the skulls of Neanderthals and of ancient Egyptians suggests that subdural hematomas could have been treated since prehistoric times, although one suspects that any relief of a subdural hematoma in this setting was likely a matter of luck. However, the earliest recognition of acute subdural hematoma as a clinical entity is attributed to the French surgeon Ambroise Paré. Thomas Willis and Johann Jacob Wepfer also recognized chronic subdural hematomas.[2]

Subdural hematomas may be acute, subacute, or chronic.[3,4] Acute subdural hematomas have been arbitrarily defined as those presenting within 48 hours of onset. Subacute subdural hematomas present 3 to 14 days after onset, whereas chronic subdural hematomas present 15 days or more after onset.[1] Large symptomatic acute subdural hematomas require immediate surgical intervention to prevent rapid clinical deterioration and death. Subacute and chronic subdural hematomas are less urgent but provide unique diagnostic and therapeutic challenges.

ETIOLOGY AND PATHOGENESIS

Situated between the dura mater and the arachnoid membranes is a potential space (the subdural space), across which cortical (bridging) veins drain blood from the brain into the dural sinuses (Figure 19-1). If these veins rupture, blood dissecting between these membranes enlarges the space in all directions, and eventually a mass large enough to compress adjacent portions of the brain may be created. If rupture of the arachnoid membrane occurs as well, cerebrospinal fluid (CSF) can seep into the hematoma from the subarachnoid space and add to its bulk. In occasional patients trauma tears the arachnoid without rupturing the veins, so that a collection of CSF forms in the subdural space (subdural hygroma). In other instances the blood in a subdural hematoma is resorbed, leaving a yellow-tinged, clear effusion with a protein content much higher than that of normal CSF.

Closed head injury, with or without fracture, is responsible for the vast majority of subdural hematomas, although "spontaneous" hematoma, unrelated to known trauma, does occur. When the moving head suddenly strikes an object, or when the stationary head is displaced by a blow, the brain moves within the skull. One result may be rupture of the cortical veins that drain blood from the hemispheres into the intra-dural venous sinuses. The effect of displacement of the brain within the cranium is usually greatest in the parasagittal region, where these cortical draining veins are longest and have the least support.

The severity of injury necessary to produce a subdural hematoma varies considerably. Severe injuries with skull fracture may not be associated with subdural hematoma, and chronic subdural hematoma may follow mild trauma to the head. The initial injury often does not cause loss of consciousness and is sometimes so trivial that the patient forgets the episode, which occurred long before symptoms appear. At times, subdural hematomas are produced by trivial injuries that merely jar the head. Small subdural hematomas may also be produced by intracranial surgery, but these rarely grow large enough to cause symptoms. Some subdural hematomas might result from an acute rise in venous pressure, such as that caused by vigorous coughing or straining.

Subdural hematoma is more common among the elderly because the cerebral atrophy that often accompanies aging increases the gap across which the bridging veins (Figure 19-1) must traverse. Subdural hematoma is also more common in

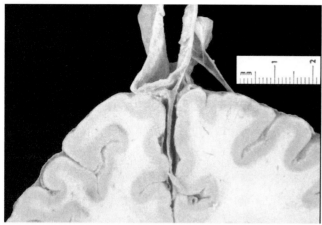

Figure 19-1. Coronal brain section illustrating bridging veins. Rupture of these vessels, as a result of a sudden change in the velocity of the head, may lead to subdural hemorrhage.

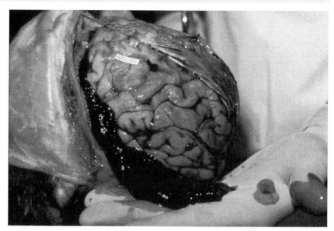

Figure 19-2. Postmortem appearance of an acute fatal subdural hematoma.

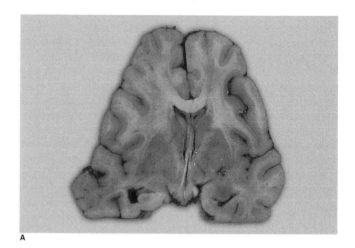

A

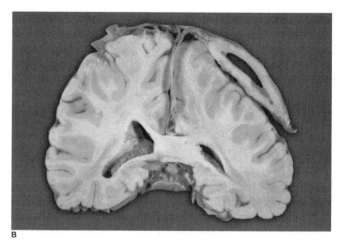

B

Figure 19-3. A: Compression and displacement of both cerebral hemispheres due to bilateral chronic subdural hematomas. B: Coronal section illustrates an ossified chronic subdural hematoma that has displaced the adjacent cerebral hemisphere.

men, perhaps because men sustain more head injuries than women. Individuals taking anticoagulant medications may develop subdural hematoma following minor head injury because of their abnormal clotting mechanisms.[5,6] Patients on long-term hemodialysis for chronic renal failure or individuals with chronic alcohol dependence, epilepsy (which increases the risk of falls), and low CSF pressure (intracranial hypotension) are also predisposed to subdural hematoma formation. Subdural hematomas rarely complicate ruptured intracranial aneurysms or arteriovenous malformations, intracranial meningiomas, dural metastases, neurosurgical intervention, coagulopathies, bone marrow transplantation, and systemic thrombolysis for myocardial infarction.[7-13]

Why does a subdural hematoma increase in size? The answer to this question is not definitely known. Some pathologists postulate that the high protein content of the serum, augmented by protein released from degenerating cellular elements of the blood, draws CSF into the subdural space through the semipermeable arachnoid membrane. A more likely explanation is that oozing from the vascular membrane causes the progressive enlargement. Because of its relative avascularity and lack of lymphatic drainage, the arachnoid membrane has little resorptive capacity, and the process of resorption takes place through the moderately vascularized dura mater. When the rate of uptake is so slow that fluid accumulates faster than it can be removed, progressive enlargement occurs.[14]

Pathologic Findings

Site

Subdural hematomas are most likely to develop where the veins crossing the subdural space are longest. Thus many subdural hematomas occur in the frontoparietal region after injury to the superior cerebral veins draining into the superior sagittal sinus. About 10% to 20% of these patients have bilateral subdural hematomas. Another common location for a subdural hematoma is the tip of the temporal lobe (arising from the inferior cerebral veins draining into the sphenoparietal sinus). Less commonly subdural hemorrhage occurs beneath the frontal or temporal lobes, and rarely do they accumulate between the hemispheres or in the posterior fossa.

Gross Appearance

The appearance of a subdural hematoma evolves over time. When seen at surgery or autopsy, the dura overlying a hematoma has a bluish-green hue. Beneath the dura lies a glistening brown outer membrane.[15,16] When this is stripped and the mass is removed, a shiny inner membrane stippled with petechial hemorrhages can be seen. The mass composing a hematoma usually contains fluid (from a film to as much as 500 ml) surrounded by fibrin clot (Figure 19-2). The pia-arachnoid membrane usually lies free of the inner membrane, although in long-standing cases some adhesions may occur.

The portion of brain underlying the hematoma is usually compressed and is discolored by bilirubin. Large subdural hematomas compress and displace the underlying brain and sometimes result in herniation through the tentorial notch. Chronic subdural hematomas may calcify (Figure 19-3). Eventually the tissue adjacent to the hematoma becomes atrophic.[17–18]

Microscopic Appearance

The outer membrane, 1 to 5 mm thick and adherent to the dura, is composed of granulation tissue containing fibroblasts, new blood vessels, histiocytes, pigment, and occasional red and white blood cells. A characteristic feature of this layer is the presence of thin-walled, sinus-like vessels; some pathologists believe that these contribute to the progressive enlargement of the hematoma by oozing fresh blood into the cavity. The inner membrane, which is almost completely avascular, consists of a layer of mesothelial cells lying on a sheet of connective tissue. The fluid portion of the hematoma, supported in a fibrin network, contains red blood cells in various stages of disintegration.

Although hematomas are usually well organized after four to six weeks, the time required for the formation of the encapsulating membranes varies from about two to seven weeks.

CLINICAL FEATURES OF SUBDURAL HEMATOMA

The classic signs and symptoms of subdural hematoma result from increased intracranial pressure (ICP) and from compression of the adjacent brain. However, the specific clinical features of subdural hematomas are somewhat age specific.

In Infants

Subdural hematomas are bilateral in about 80% of infants, compared to only 10% to 20% in adults. In many instances no history of trauma is obtainable. Traumatic delivery is often blamed in neonates, but there is no consistent pattern of prematurity, difficult delivery, or birth presentation to support a birth-related injury in most patients. A few infants prove to have a coagulation defect, arteriovenous fistula, or other explanation for the subdural. Unless there is an obvious cause, an infant with a subdural hematoma should be evaluated for child abuse ("nonaccidental trauma," "inflicted trauma," or "shaken-baby syndrome"). These subdural hemorrhages often occur in the parieto-occipital convexity or in the posterior interhemispheric fissure.[19–22] Many of the infants also have subarachnoid and retinal hemorrhages. These injuries result more often from shaking the child than from a direct blow to the head.

Symptoms and signs depend on the size of the hematoma, whether it is unilateral or bilateral, and on its chronicity. One must also consider the possibility of cumulative neurological injuries as well as injuries to other organ systems. When the subdural hematoma results from nonaccidental injury, the history is almost always clouded by inaccurate and misleading information from the caregivers, and it is often the disparity between the history and the child's findings that raises suspicion. Infants with chronic subdural hematomas often have nonspecific symptoms such as feeding problems, vomiting, or failure to thrive. Others lose developmental milestones or develop generalized or focal seizures. An infant with a larger acute subdural hematoma usually presents more dramatically, with circulatory collapse, apnea, stupor, or coma.

The majority of these infants do not have obvious bruising or other external injuries, although it is important to document these lesions when they occur. Shaking an infant sufficiently to cause a subdural or subarachnoid hemorrhage typically causes retinal hemorrhages as well. These are typically bilateral and can assume any shape. Lethargy and irritability are common, often alternating in the same child. Infants with extensive retinal hemorrhages may not see. Common neurological findings include hypotonia or hypertonia, hemiparesis, brisk reflexes, altered consciousness, and sluggish pupillary light reflexes. The anterior fontanel is often tense and bulging unless the infant is dehydrated. Macrocephaly occurs in about a quarter of the infants with a chronic subdural hematoma.[19–22]

The subdural hematoma is confirmed with cranial computed tomography (CT), which sometimes shows evidence of a skull fracture as well. A skeletal survey may reveal multiple rib fractures and metaphyseal fractures, and the presence of fractures of differing ages is pathognomonic of child abuse. Acute intracranial blood loss may be sufficient to cause anemia in infants. A lumbar puncture is not usually undertaken in individuals with a sizable subdural hematoma. When CSF is examined, however, it is often bloody or xanthochromic because of the frequent coexistence of subarachnoid hemorrhage in these infants (Figure 17-9).

An infant with unexplained retinal and intracranial hemorrhages must be admitted to the hospital to ensure his safety and to facilitate a systematic evaluation for injuries as well as potential nontraumatic causes for the hemorrhage. The proper authorities should be notified when there is suspicion of child abuse.

Children

Clinical features in children are similar to those seen in adults. The cause of the subdural hematoma is more likely to be attributable to a specific traumatic event or underlying risk factor in children than is the case in infants or in the elderly. Chronic subdural hematomas in children typically present with headaches, deterioration of school performance, or behavior change.

Neuroimaging rarely shows expansion of one side of the middle cranial fossa and thinning of the inner table (a finding not seen in adults). The expansion of the middle cranial fossa as well as the proptosis and bulging of the temporal region is caused by a forward and upward displacement of the still malleable sphenoid bone.

Adults

Subdural hematomas produce local effects related to their site and general effects secondary to their mass. Headache is the most prominent symptom in more than 80% of patients. It is usually incapacitating but may fluctuate in intensity. Pain may be diffuse or localized over the site of the hematoma and is often exacerbated by coughing, stooping, or straining. At the height of the headache, nausea and vomiting are common.

In the early stages it is notoriously difficult to locate or even lateralize a subdural hematoma solely on the basis of physical findings. As the hematoma enlarges, the headaches become more severe, and signs of neurologic dysfunction develop. The latter usually consist of mild paresis of the contralateral arm and leg together with speech difficulty if the hematoma lies over the dominant hemisphere. Focal or generalized seizures may occur. In more than 90% of all cases, lateralizing signs have developed before the diagnosis is made.

Later findings of a subdural hematoma include drowsiness, inability to concentrate, deterioration of memory, confusion, and disorientation. These changes are often more noticeable to friends and relatives than to the patient. Further enlargement of the hematoma may trigger stupor or coma. Signs of increased ICP include papilledema, slowing of the pulse and respirations, and elevation of the blood pressure.[23–24]

The Elderly

The cerebral atrophy that usually accompanies old age causes widening of the subdural space and makes the bridging veins more susceptible to rupture. Loss of pliability of the veins that occurs with advancing age further increases the hazard of rupture. In the elderly the cognitive deterioration that often dominates the clinical picture with a subdural hematoma may be incorrectly attributed to senility. Neurologic abnormalities, if present, are often incorrectly attributed to a "stroke" or a "neurodegenerative" dementing process.

When a patient develops signs of cerebral damage concomitant with head injury, it is sometimes difficult to be sure whether the neurological deficit is due to the injury or whether the head injury resulted from a fall following a spontaneous (nontraumatic) cerebrovascular episode. With the increased susceptibility of elderly individuals to develop subdural hematomas, a high index of suspicion leading to prompt CT or magnetic resonance imaging (MRI) is appropriate.[24,25]

ACUTE "SPONTANEOUS" SUBDURAL HEMATOMA

Recently attention has been drawn to a newly recognized cause of subdural hemorrhage – the rupture of a small artery on the convexity of the cerebrum. The pathogenesis is as yet unclear, but it has been postulated that at the time of head injury a small asymptomatic venous subdural hematoma is formed. Following absorption of this subdural blood, adhesions develop between the dura mater and the cortical surface, entrapping a small cortical artery. Later these adhesions bind the artery, and in a later, often minor, blow to the head, the brain is displaced and the artery torn, resulting in an acute subdural hemorrhage.

In such instances patients present with an abrupt onset of headache, vomiting, progressive deterioration in consciousness, and signs of meningeal irritation. On examination, the patient usually has a dilated pupil and ipsilateral hemiparesis due to displacement of the brain with compression of the peduncle against the incisura. At times, ipsilateral hemisensory loss and ipsilateral homonymous hemianopia caused by compression of the posterior cerebral artery against the incisura of the opposite side are seen. In some cases papilledema is evident.

The diagnosis of acute subdural hematoma caused by arterial bleeding is confirmed by carotid angiography, and the lesion is treated by evacuating the subdural blood and clipping the spurting artery.

DIFFERENTIAL DIAGNOSIS

Errors in the diagnosis of subdural hematoma are common. Symptoms of subdural hematoma that are often mistakenly attributed to other conditions include changes in cognition in the elderly patients, repeated seizures in patients with epilepsy, behavior changes in young people, and symptoms suggestive of inebriation in patients with alcohol dependence. Other conditions frequently confused with subdural hematoma are intracranial neoplasms and strokes.[1]

Because subdural hematoma is one of the few reversible causes of dementia, correct diagnosis is of paramount importance. Aside from the history of earlier head injury, three clinical signs should strongly suggest a diagnosis of subdural hematoma: (1) daily or even hourly fluctuations in the symptoms, especially those of drowsiness, confusion, and headache; (2) focal signs of hemispheric involvement, such as motor weakness, sensory changes, and aphasia; and (3) the prominence of mental aberration in comparison to signs related to the corticospinal tract. Unfortunately, these differentiating features are not very reliable, and a high index of suspicion is prudent.

DIAGNOSTIC EVALUATION

Both CT and MRI reliably demonstrate acute and chronic subdural hematomas (Figures 19-4 and 19-5) along with accompanying complications such as intracerebral hemorrhage or brain herniation. Gradient-echo MRI may demonstrate the presence of blood products.[25–26] A lumbar puncture is generally contraindicated because of the risk of herniation.

COURSE AND PROGNOSIS

In spite of their frequency, the natural history of chronic subdural hematomas is not fully known. Many are diagnosed and removed surgically; others are not suspected until they are found as incidental abnormalities at autopsy; still others are resorbed completely without ever causing symptoms. Some chronic subdurals become quiescent and calcify (Figure 19-3).[27] Most chronic subdural hematomas ultimately produce signs of an expanding intracranial lesion, with or without collapse of the underlying brain.

Left untreated, a large subdural hematoma may cause a combination of intellectual deterioration, hemiparesis, and seizures followed by coma and death from compression of the midbrain (from herniation of the hippocampus through the incisura of the tentorium cerebelli). A fluctuating downhill course is typical and is probably related to alterations in the volume of fluid within the membranes. In some patients sudden, unexplained death occurs. Even if the hematoma stabilizes, mental deterioration, headache, and recurrent convulsions may persist.

TREATMENT

The fact that a few patients may live for years with a chronic subdural hematoma does not diminish the importance of prompt diagnosis and therapy. Small asymptomatic lesions can be followed pending evidence of enlargement. For larger lesions, treatment consists of draining the fluid portion through bur holes or removing the solid portions of the clot and the membranes via craniotomy. The rare case of a subdural hematoma in the posterior fossa requires occipital bur holes on each side or a suboccipital craniotomy.

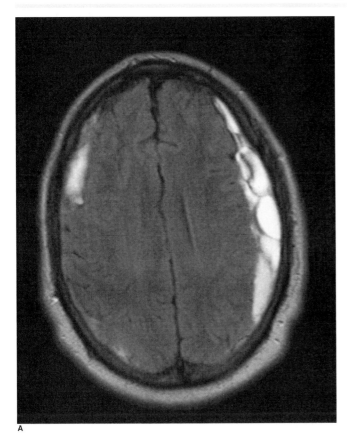

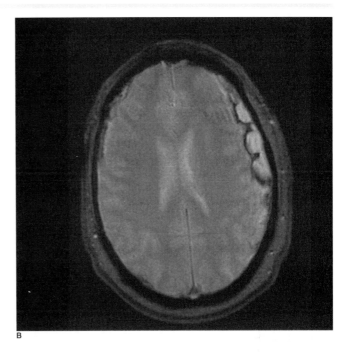

Figure 19-4. A and B: Cranial MRI (from a 47-year-old man with alcohol dependence, thrombocytopenia, and focal seizures) shows bilateral subacute convexity subdural hematomas, larger on the left than the right. There is sulcal effacement but no midline shift.

In most instances prompt removal of a subdural hematoma is a therapeutic triumph because the patient promptly returns to baseline function following surgery. When the underlying brain fails to reexpand after surgery, however, the results are not so gratifying, although the patient's function often stabilizes. Lingering cognitive deficits, seizures, and hemiparesis may result from residual brain atrophy or unexpanded brain.[28–32]

Asymptomatic infants with a small subdural hematoma can be watched closely. Larger acute or subacute hematomas need to be removed. For patients in stable condition who have large chronic bilateral subdural hematomas, daily removal of 10 to 14 ml of fluid from first one and then the other side on alternate days is recommended if the condition of the patient permits the elective approach. In an emergency greater volumes may be removed simultaneously from the two sides. If the lesion fails to resolve with this conservative approach, shunt procedures may be needed. As much of the membrane as possible should be removed via craniectomy.

EPIDURAL HEMATOMA

Epidural hematoma is an accumulation of blood between the dura mater and the inner table of the skull. These lesions most often develop after head trauma, typically as a result of bleeding from a meningeal artery (usually the middle meningeal artery located beneath the pterion) or vein or venous sinus. Spontaneous epidural hematomas are rarely documented, but have been described in association with congenital aneurysms of the meningeal artery, bleeding diatheses, sickle cell disease, pregnancy, systemic lupus erythematosus, open heart surgery, and chronic hemodialysis.[33–44]

PATHOGENESIS OF EPIDURAL HEMATOMA

Epidural hematomas are usually supratentorial. Most of them accumulate in the temporal region, where the calvarium is relatively thin and the middle meningeal artery and vein and their branches can be torn if the skull is fractured. In occasional individuals epidural hematomas collect in the frontal, parietal, or occipital region. Two or more epidural hematomas can occur, typically involving the frontal regions.[45–46]

Epidural hematomas are often associated with closed head injuries that may or may not lacerate the skin but do not perforate the skull. Their rarity in penetrating wounds is explained by the fact that blood can drain freely and hence does not dissect between the dura and the inner table of the skull. A blow forceful enough to indent the skull may loosen the dura from the inner table of the skull, so that bleeding from vessel rupture can dissect between them, creating a hematoma. At times the inner table of the skull is fractured by the displacement while the outer table remains intact. Occasionally rupture of the underlying artery or vein occurs without fracture of either table.

As the epidural hematoma increases in size, local compression of the underlying brain causes signs of focal deficit. Further enlargement pushes the brain toward the opposite side and down into the tentorial notch. In addition to causing displacement and compression of the midbrain, this impaction of the medial aspect of the homolateral temporal lobe puts pressure on the oculomotor nerve and on the homolateral posterior cerebral artery and veins.

Trauma to the occipital region may produce an epidural hematoma located in the posterior fossa, leading the compression

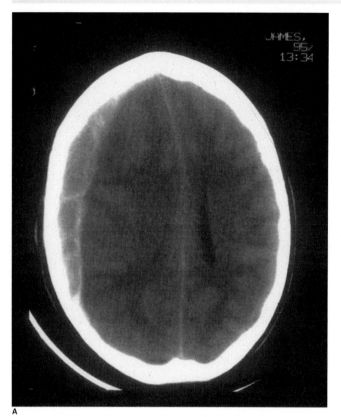
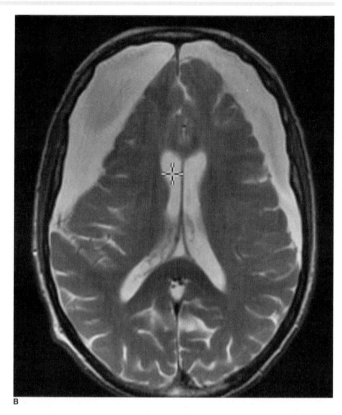

Figure 19-5. A: Cranial CT illustrates a chronic right subdural hematoma with adjacent effacement of the cortex and compression of the right lateral ventricle. Note the septations within the lesion. B: Cranial MRI from another elderly man taking warfarin who had sustained frequent falls and presented with headaches and memory loss. There are bilateral chronic subdural hematomas, slightly larger on the right than on the left with approximately 2 mm of right-to-left subfalcine shift.

of the lower cranial nerves, cerebellum, and brainstem.[39,47] Posterior fossa epidural hematomas have also been described after the evacuation of supratentorial hematomas.[48]

CLINICAL FEATURES OF EPIDURAL HEMATOMA

The clinical features of epidural hematomas depend on three variables: (1) the site of the initial injury, (2) the presence or absence of concussion and coma caused by the original blow, and (3) the rate at which the hematoma accumulates. Arterial bleeding can produce a hematoma large enough to cause compression of the brain within the hour of injury. If the initial blow caused a severe concussion, consciousness may not return during this interval. With bleeding from a small artery or a vein, the clot may accumulate more slowly, so that a lucid interval is common. In rare cases venous hemorrhages cease spontaneously, and the presence of a chronic extradural hematoma may not be suspected for weeks after the injury.

Because of these variables, four general patterns may occur: (1) initial unconsciousness from the injury with return of consciousness and the development of focal neurologic abnormalities, (2) initial coma from the injury followed by a variable period of lucidity before return to coma, (3) coma uninterrupted by a return of consciousness, (4) no initial unconsciousness from the blow but the gradual onset of coma as the hematoma accumulates. Of this group, initial unconsciousness followed by a lucid interval and gradual return of coma is said to be the typical pattern, but it occurs in only 30% of the cases.[40–49] Throbbing headache is frequent in those patients who recover consciousness.

The neurologic deficits most commonly produced by pressure on adjacent structures as blood accumulates are dysphasia (if the lesion overlies the dominant hemisphere), hemiparesis, and hemianopic field defects. Focal or generalized seizures are relatively unusual. Displacement of the brain and the herniation of the temporal lobe may produce signs of oculomotor nerve compression, beginning usually with dilatation of the pupil. When it occurs, the homolateral pupil is dilated in about 90% of cases and the contralateral in the remainder.

Increasing ICP, sometimes accompanied by papilledema, causes vomiting, slowing of the pulse rate, slow and torturous respiration, and elevation of the systolic blood pressure.

Many authorities believe that the site of scalp injury, often revealed by the presence of a palpable hematoma or a visible contusion or laceration, is as reliable a clue to the site of hematoma as is the location of the skull fracture. Injuries to the frontal region are most often associated with hematoma of the anterior fossa; injuries of the temporal area, with hematoma of the middle fossa; and blows to the occipital area, with hematoma of the posterior fossa.

DIFFERENTIAL DIAGNOSIS

The typical patient with an epidural hematoma poses no diagnostic problem, but atypical ones may be difficult to distinguish from subarachnoid hemorrhage, cerebral contusion, or laceration of the brain. Evidence of impact over the site of the middle meningeal artery and the history of a "lucid interval" (present in a minority of patients) following injury are features favoring epidural hematoma.[1,40,49]

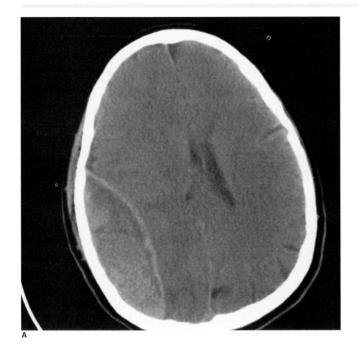
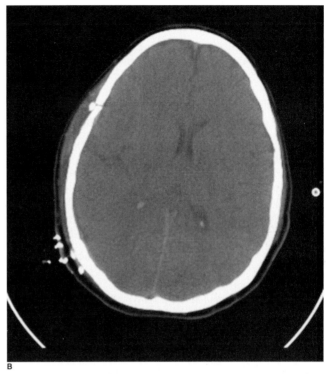

Figure 19-6. A and B: Unenhanced CT shows a large lenticular-shaped, mixed-density lesion of the right posterior convexity suggestive of an epidural hematoma along with sulcal effacement, cerebral edema, and leftward subfalcine herniation. An epidural hematoma was confirmed at surgery along with a subdural hemorrhage along the convex margin of the epidural hematoma and extending into the middle cranial fossa.

The early diagnosis of epidural hemorrhage depends to a large extent on suspicion that it may exist, and it bears well to keep in mind the possibility that extradural hematoma may follow any head injury. Many patients who die might be saved by prompt studies to identify subdural or extradural hematomas, including, in some cases, diagnostic bur holes at the site of injury.

DIAGNOSTIC EVALUATION

CT is the most common means of detecting an epidural hematoma (Figure 19-6). MRI is sometimes utilized, especially in patients with more chronic lesions. In the acute phase an epidural hematoma is isointense on T_1-weighted sequences and hyperintense or hypointense on T_2-weighted sequences.[25–26]

COURSE AND PROGNOSIS

With few exceptions, patients will die if an epidural hematoma is not removed. The degree of ultimate recovery may depend on early diagnosis and prompt operation to remove the clot and stop further bleeding. The longer the pressure remains on the brain, the more serious the sequelae. The likelihood of recovery are also related inversely to the age of the patient, degree of cerebral compression, and depth of the coma.

The overall mortality from an epidural hematoma approaches 30% to 50%. This high figure does not reflect the difficulties of surgery but indicates the rapidity with which this disorder can cause fatal compression of the brain.

TREATMENT OF EPIDURAL HEMATOMA

The management of epidural hematoma can be summarized in one sentence: Remove the clot and stop the bleeding at once.

A high index of suspicion should lead to early diagnosis, and early diagnosis to immediate surgical intervention.[50]

REFERENCES

1. Timmons SD. Extra-axial Hematomas. In: Loftus CM, ed. *Neurosurgical Emergencies*. 2nd ed. American Association of Neurological Surgeons. New York: Thieme; 2008:53–67.
2. Hoessly G. Intracranial hemorrhage in the seventeenth century. *J Neurosurg*. 1966;**24**:493–496.
3. Westermaier T, Eriskat J, Kunze E, et al. Clinical features, treatment, and prognosis of patients with acute subdural hematomas presenting in critical condition. *Neurosurgery*. 2007;**61**:482–487.
4. Bullock MR, Chesnut R, Ghajar J, et al. Surgical management of acute subdural hematomas. *Neurosurgery*. 2006;**58**:S16–24.
5. Reymond MA Marbet G, Radu EW, Gratzl O. Aspirin as a risk factor for hemorrhage in patients with head injuries. *Neurosurg Rev*. 1992;**15**:21–25.
6. Hylek EM, Singer DE. Risk factors for intracranial hemorrhage in outpatients taking warfarin. *Ann Intern Med*. 1994;**120**:897–902.
7. Gelabert-Gonzalez M, Iglesias-Pais M, Fernandez-Villa J. Acute subdural haematoma due to ruptured intracranial aneurysms. *Neurosurg Rev*. 2004;**27**:259–262.
8. Okuno S, Touho H, Ohnishi H, Karasawa J. Falx meningioma presenting as acute subdural hematoma: case report. *Surg Neurol*. 1999;**52**:180–184.
9. Bergmann M, Puskas Z, Kuchelmeister K. Subdural hematoma due to dural metastasis: case report and review of the literature. *Clin Neurol Neurosurg*. 1992;**94**:235–240.
10. Bleggi-Tores LF, Werner B, Gasparetto EL, et al. Intracranial hemorrhage following bone marrow transplantation. An autopsy study of 58 patients. *Bone Marrow Transplant*. 2002;**29**:29–32.
11. Seckin H, Kazanci A, Yigitkanli K, Simsek S, Kars HZ. Chronic subdural hematoma in patients with idiopathic thrombocytopenic

purpura: a case report and review of the literature. *Surg Neurol.* 2006;**66**:411–414.

12. Gore J, Sloan M, Price T, et al. Intracerebral hemorrhage, cerebral infarction, and subdural hematoma after acute myocardial infarction and thrombolytic therapy in Thrombolysis in Myocardial Infarction Study. Thrombolysis in Myocardial Infarction, Phase II, pilot and clinical trial. *Circulation.* 1991;**83**: 448–459.

13. Konig SA, Schick U, Dohnert J, Goldammer A, Vitzthum HE. Coagulopathy and outcome in patients with chronic subdural hematoma. *Acta Neurol Scand.* 2003;**107**:110–116.

14. Willeberger JE. Pathophysiology of the evolution and recurrence of chronic subdural hematoma. *Neurosurg Clin N Am.* 2000;**11**: 435–438.

15. Killefer JA, Killefer FA, Schochet SS. The outer membrane of chronic subdural hematoma. *Neurosurg Clin N Am.* 2000;**11**:407–412.

16. Yamashima T. The inner membrane of chronic subdural hematoma. Pathology and pathophysiology. *Neurosurg Clin N Am.* 2000;**11**:413–424.

17. Koc R, Akdemir H, Oktem I, Meral M, Menku A. Acute subdural hematoma; outcome and outcome prediction. *Neurosurg Rev.* 1997;**20**:239–244.

18. Lee KS, Bae WK, Doh JW, Bae HG, Yun IG. Origin of chronic subdural hematoma and relation to traumatic subdural lesions. *Brain Injury.* 1998;**12**:901–910.

19. Gerber P, Coffman K. Non-accidental head trauma in infants. *Childs Nerv Syst.* 2007;**23**:499–507.

20. Donohoe M. Evidence-based medicine and shaken-baby syndrome. Part I: literature review. *Am J Forensic Med Pathol.* 2003; **24**:239–242.

21. Givner A, Gurney J, O'Connor D, et al. Reimaging in pediatric neurotrauma: factors associated with progression of intracranial injury. *J Pediatr Surg.* 2002;**37**:381–385.

22. Reece RM, Sege R. Childhood head injuries: accidental or inflicted? *Arch Pediatr Adolesc Med.* 2000;**154**:11–15.

23. Kaminski HJ, Hlavin ML, Likavec MJ, Schmidley JW. Transient neurologic deficit caused by chronic subdural hematoma. *Am J Med.* 1992;**92**:698–700.

24. Gennarelli TA, Champion HR, Copes WS, Sacco WJ. Companion of mortality and morbidity, and severity of 59,713 head injured patients with 114,447 patients with extracranial injuries. *J Trauma.* 1994;**37**:962–968.

25. Besenski, N. Traumatic injuries: imaging of head injuries. *Eur Radiol.* 2002;**12**:1237–1252.

26. Gentry L, Godersky J, Thompson B, Dunn V. Prospective comparative study of intermediate-field MR and CT in the evaluation of closed head trauma. *AJR Am J Roentgenol.* 1988;**150**:673–682.

27. Moon HG, Shin HS, Kim TH, Hwang YS, Park SK. Ossified chronic subdural hematoma. *Yonsei Med J.* 2003;**44**:915–918.

28. Maxeiner H, Wolff M. Pure subdural hematomas: a postmortem analysis of their form and bleeding points. *Neurosurgery.* 2002; **50**:503–508.

29. Lee JY, Ebel H, Ernestus RI, Klug N. Various surgical treatments of chronic subdural hematoma and outcome in 172 patients. Is membranectomy necessary? *Surg Neurol.* 2004;**61**: 523–527.

30. Cartmill M, Dolan G, Byrne JL, Byrne PO. Prothrombin complex concentrate for oral anticoagulant reversal in neurosurgical emergencies. *Br J Neurosurg.* 2000;**14**:458–461.

31. Vigue B, Ract C, Tremey B, et al. Ultra-rapid management of oral anticoagulant therapy-related surgical intracranial hemorrhage. *Intensive Care Med.* 2007;**33**:721–725.

32. Siddiq F, Jalil A, McDaniel C, et al. Effectiveness of factor IX complex concentrate in reversing warfarin associated coagulopathy for intracerebral hemorrhage. *Neurocrit Care.* 2008;**8**:36–41.

33. Ng WH, Yeo TT, Seow WT. Non-traumatic spontaneous acute epidural haematoma – report of two cases and review of the literature. *J Clin Neurosci.* 2004;**11**:791–793.

34. Moonis G, Granados A, Simon SL. Epidural hematoma as a complication of sphenoid sinusitis and epidural abscess: a case report and literature review. *Clin Imaging.* 2002;**26**:382–385.

35. Szkup P, Stoneham G. Spontaneous spinal epidural haematoma during pregnancy: case report and review of the literature. *Br J Radiol.* 2004;**77**:881–884.

36. Jea A, Moza K, Levi AD, Vanni S. Spontaneous spinal epidural hematoma during pregnancy: case report and literature review. *Neurosurgery.* 2005;**56**:E1156.

37. Shahlaie K, Fox A, Butani L, Boggan JE. Spontaneous epidural hemorrhage in chronic renal failure. A case report and review. *Pediatr Nephrol.* 2004;**19**:1168–1172.

38. Ciurea A, Kapsalaki E, Coman TC, et al. Supratentorial epidural hematoma of traumatic etiology in infants. *Childs Nerv Syst.* 2007;**23**:335–341.

39. Bozbuja M, Izgy N, Polat G, Gurel I. Posterior fossa epidural hematomas: observations on a series of 73 cases. *Neurology Rev.* 1999;**22**:34–40.

40. Lee EJ, Hung YC, Wang LC, Chung KC, Chen HH. Factors influencing the functional outcome of patients with acute epidural hematomas: analysis of 200 patients undergoing surgery. *J Trauma.* 1998;**45**:946–952.

41. Cohen JE, Montero A, Israel ZH. Prognosis and clinical relevance of anisocoria-craniotomy latency for epidural hematoma in comatose patients. *J Trauma.* 1996;**41**:120–122.

42. Lobato RD, Rivas JJ, Cordobes F, et al. Acute epidural hematoma: an analysis of factors influencing the outcome of patients undergoing surgery in coma. *J Neurosurg.* 1988;**68**:48–57.

43. Bezircioglu H, Ersahin Y, Demircivi F, et al. Nonoperative treatment of acute extradural hematomas: analysis of 80 cases. *J Trauma.* 1996;**41**:696–698.

44. Chen TY, Wong CW, Chang CN, et al. The expectant treatment of "asymptomatic" supratentorial epidural hematomas. *Neurosurgery.* 1993;**32**:176–179.

45. Gupta S, Tandon S, Mohanty S, Asthana S, Sharma S. Bilateral traumatic extradural hematomas: report of 12 cases with a review of the literature. *Clin Neurol Neurosurg.* 1992;**94**:127–131.

46. Huda MF, Mohanty S, Sharma V, et al. Double extradural hematoma: an analysis of 46 cases. *Neurol India.* 2004;**52**:450–452.

47. Bor-Seng-Shu E, Aguiar PH, de Almeida Leme RJ, et al. Epidural hematomas of the posterior cranial fossa. *Neurosurg Focus.* 2004;16(2):ECP1.

48. Lui TN, Lee ST, Chang CN, Cheng W-C. Epidural hematomas in the posterior cranial fossa. *J. Trauma.* 1993;**34**:211–215.

49. Jamjoom AB. The difference in the outcome of surgery for traumatic extradural hematomas between patients who are admitted directly to the neuro hospital unit and those referred from another hospital. *Neurosurg Rev.* 1997;**20**:227–230.

50. Bullock MR, Chestnut R, Ghajar J, et al. Surgical management of acute epidural hematomas. *Neurosurgery.* 2006;**58**:S7–15.

20

Sinovenous Occlusion

No part of the body is so full of veins as the brain.

William Harvey

Before the era of cranial computerized tomography (CT) and magnetic resonance imaging (MRI), intracranial venous thrombosis was seldom diagnosed. With the introduction of these studies and MR venography, cerebral venous thrombosis is more frequently diagnosed, and an increasing number of mild clinical cases are identified.[1] Nevertheless, cerebral venous sinus thrombosis (CVST) remains relatively uncommon compared to arterial ischemic stroke and intracerebral hemorrhage, with an incidence rate of less than 0.5/100,000 cases per year, accounting for only about 1% of all strokes. However, CVST is much more common in neonates and in women of child-bearing age.[2]

CVST has multiple risk factors. The clinical presentation is highly variable and depends on the number of unaffected venous collaterals, the presence of parenchymal lesions, the widespread extension of thrombus formation, and the thrombus location.[3] Noninvasive imaging techniques allow the identification of patients with less severe manifestations, and it has become apparent that the overall prognosis is substantially better than once thought.[4–6] Knowledge of the cerebral venous anatomy and its variations is helpful in interpreting the clinical presentation and assessing prognosis.

VENOUS ANATOMY

Cerebral veins have thin walls and no valves, which allows reversal of blood flow toward the head and brain if there is an occlusion.[7] Normally, blood is drained from the brain by superficial (external) and deep (internal) veins to the heart. The former group collects blood from the cortex and the adjacent white matter, whereas the latter drains the central structures. Both systems are connected by extensive collaterals and drain principally into the dural sinuses, which empty into the internal jugular veins. Joining the subclavian veins in the superior mediastinum, they form the right and left innominate veins, which drain the blood into the superior vena cava and into the right atrium.[8]

Superficial Venous System

The superficial veins drain blood from the cortex and the underlying white matter. They are divided into superior, middle (Sylvian), and inferior cerebral groups that lie on the surface of the hemispheres and receive blood from pial branches. Attached to the underside of this network are veins that emerge from the Virchow-Robin spaces, transporting blood from the depth to the surface of the brain. The dorsal, dorsolateral, and medial aspects of each hemisphere above the corpus callosum are drained by 10 to 20 veins, through which blood flows upward into the superior sagittal sinus. These veins join to form four or five large trunks traversing into large venous lacunae adjacent to the superior sagittal sinus.

Superior Sagittal Sinus

The superior sagittal sinus, triangular in cross section, lies within the line of attachment of the falx cerebri to the calvaria. It commences at the foramen caecum and crista galli and runs to the internal occipital protuberance, where it empties into the confluens of sinuses. Anterior to the coronal suture it carries only small quantities of blood, but posteriorly it enlarges rapidly to accommodate a greatly increased blood volume. Lateral to the sinus, in the adjacent dura, are many large venous lakes. Arachnoid villi project into these sinuses to facilitate the resorption of cerebral spinal fluid. The superior sagittal sinus receives blood from the superior cerebral veins, the diploe, dura mater, the scalp, and the pericranial and nasal veins. Thrombosis of the superior sagittal sinus often causes motor deficits, bilateral neurological signs and symptoms, and seizures.[9,10] Frequently intracranial pressure is increased.[11]

Deep Venous System

The deep venous system, which drains the periventricular white matter, the basal ganglia, and other centrally placed structures, consists of the Galenic system and the paired basal veins of Rosenthal. This group collects blood from the territory perfused by the two carotid arteries and by a portion of the vertebral-basilar system. Occlusion of the deep venous system generally causes a severe clinical picture characterized by altered mental status, coma, bilateral motor deficits, and poor prognosis.[12,13]

Galenic System

The septal vein of each side joins the thalamo-striate vein and receives blood from tributaries that drain the white matter adjacent to the lateral ventricles. The choroid vein drains blood from the choroid plexus of the lateral ventricle. The internal cerebral vein of each side arises from the confluence of the septal, thalamo-striate, and choroid veins. The two internal cerebral veins run posteriorly in the roof of the third ventricle. They unite with each other to form the great vein of Galen just beneath the splenium of the corpus callosum and above the pineal gland. The great cerebral vein of Galen, after curving upward around the splenium of the corpus callosum, empties into the straight sinus at an acute angle (Figure 20-1). It receives the two basal cerebral veins of Rosenthal, the posterior cerebral veins, and small tributaries from the pineal gland and the tectum.

Basal Cerebral Veins

The basal veins are formed by the union of the anterior cerebral veins, the inferior striate veins, and the deep middle cerebral vein. The basal vein terminates in the great vein of Galen. Occasionally, however, it ends in the internal cerebral vein or the straight sinus itself. The basal veins drain the medial pallidum, the preoptic region, the hypothalamus, the subthalamus, and areas of the upper part of the brainstem. They also receive the inferior choroidal veins from the temporal lobes.

Inferior Sagittal Sinus

The inferior sagittal sinus receives blood from the corpus callosum and the cerebellum, before it becomes continuous with the straight sinus. The straight sinus has a triangular lumen and is formed by the union of the inferior sagittal sinus and the great vein of Galen. It runs caudally in the junction between the falx cerebri and the tentorium cerebelli and joins the confluens of sinuses at the internal occipital protuberance. The occipital sinus, the smallest of all intradural sinuses, is situated in the fixed margin of the falx cerebelli and runs upward from the foramen magnum to the confluence sinus. Along the way it receives veins from the tentorium cerebelli and the medial aspect of the cerebellum and communicates with the vertebral venous plexus.

Confluens of Sinuses

The superior sagittal and the straight and the occipital sinuses usually join together within the dura at the internal occipital protuberance to form the confluence of sinuses, or torcula Herophili (Figure 20-1). The majority of blood drained from the cerebrum, cerebellum, and upper part of the brainstem therefore must traverse this critical junction. In the confluence the superior sagittal sinus can turn sharply to one side, and the inferior sagittal and straight sinuses to the other, so that at times there is little or no mixing of blood within it. The transverse sinus begins at the confluence and runs to the base of the petrous pyramid. Below this point it is called the sigmoid sinus. As it descends in its groove in the mastoid portion of the temporal bone, the sigmoid sinus lies adjacent to the mastoid air cells of the middle ear. The sigmoid sinus leaves the skull at the jugular foramen, where it becomes known as the internal

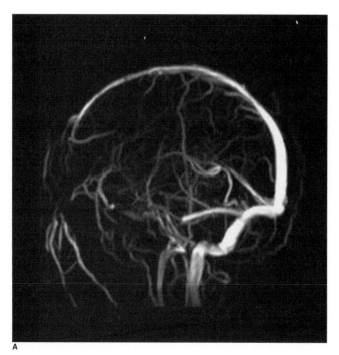

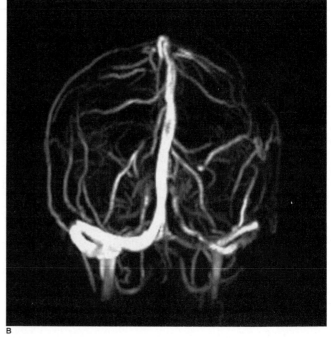

A   B

Figure 20-1. Normal venous anatomy as demonstrated by MRV in the sagittal (A) and coronal planes (B). As is often the case, there is one dominant transverse sinus.

jugular vein. The transverse sinus receives blood from the inferior group of superficial cerebral veins and the superior and the inferior petrosal sinuses, which in turn partially drain the cavernous sinus. The transverse sinuses communicate with scalp veins through emissary veins and with veins from the mastoid area.

Cavernous Sinuses

The cavernous sinuses are paired plexuses of veins situated on either side of the sella turcica, supero-lateral to the sphenoid sinus from the mucous membrane, which is separated by thin and, at times, incomplete bone. Passing through each, but separated from the bloodstream by an endothelial wall, is the internal carotid artery, the first two divisions of the trigeminal nerve, and the three nerves that control eye movements. Thrombosis of the cavernous sinus can cause orbital pain, chemosis, proptosis, and oculomotor palsies.

Superior and Inferior Petrosal Sinuses

The superior petrosal sinus is small and narrow, connecting the cavernous with the transverse sinus. It courses downward, posteriorly, and laterally, in the attachment of the tentorium cerebelli on the petrous portion of the temporal bone. It receives a few of the inferior occipital and cerebellar veins and interconnects with veins in the middle ear. The inferior petrosal sinus connects the cavernous sinus with the superior bulb of the internal jugular vein. It receives veins from the inner ear, the pons, the medulla, and the undersurface of the cerebellum.

Veins of the Cerebellum and Brainstem

Near the midline, on the superior surface of the cerebellum, lie two to four superior cerebellar veins that drain blood from the parenchyma of the cerebellum into the great vein of Galen. The posterior cerebellar veins drain the vermis and the posterior surface of the cerebellar hemisphere and empty into the straight or transverse sinuses. The central and lateral veins of the midbrain drain into the basal cerebral veins of Rosenthal.

The veins of the pons consist of a rich anastomotic network communicating with the petrosal veins on either side, and the medullary veins inferiorly. Veins of the medulla connect with cerebellar veins above and with veins of spinal cord and vertebral plexus below. They empty into the occipital sinus and, to a variable degree, into emissary veins. The basilar plexus is a network of sinusoidal veins lying in the dura that cover the clivus. It communicates with the anterior vertebral venous plexus and with the inferior petrosal sinuses.

Jugular Veins

The jugular veins are the continuation of the sigmoid sinus. They begin at the base of the skull from the posterior compartment of the jugular foramen and course through the neck within the carotid sheath. Behind the sternal end of the clavicle the jugular vein is joined by the subclavian vein to form the brachio-cephalic vein. They drain blood from the brain and parts of the face and neck and have valves that prevent blood going upwards during episodes of increase in intrathoracic pressure.

Jugular vein thrombosis can present with unilateral pulsating tinnitus or multiple cranial nerve palsies resembling occlusion of the lateral sinus.

PATHOPHYSIOLOGY

Because pressure within the jugular veins is subatmospheric during diastole, venous blood is drawn from the cranium to the superior vena cava. The cortical veins act as a capacitance system that can expand or reduce their blood volume. The rigid dural sinuses cannot do this, so that the response of the brain blood pool to changes in intracranial pressure and to compression of the jugular vein depends on changes in the quantity of blood in the cortical veins. Impairment of venous outflow expands the blood pool in distensible veins by 10% to 15%, increasing intracranial pressure accordingly. If the cerebral veins are obstructed, the resultant increase in venous pressure is transmitted back into the capillaries of the brain, causing an increase in cerebral blood volume, disruption of the blood-brain barrier, transudation of fluid, vasogenic cerebral edema, and increased intracranial pressure.[14] This results in decreased cerebral blood flow, energy failure, and impairment of the ion channel pumps with subsequent development of cytotoxic edema. Capillaries can rupture because of venous congestion causing intracerebral hemorrhage.[15]

Additionally, venous thrombosis can disrupt the resorption of cerebral spinal fluid in the arachnoid granulations that drain into the superior sagittal sinus. As a consequence intracranial pressure rises further, and patients may develop papilledema, vision loss, hydrocephalus, and possible transtentorial herniation. Elevated intracranial pressure most commonly develops after occlusion of the superior sagittal sinus, the lateral sinus, or the jugular veins.

PATHOLOGY

The thrombosed sinuses and veins are filled with thrombus of varying degrees of organization. The vessel wall is usually normal. In transverse section dural sinuses appear rounded instead of triangular and are filled with thrombus. Thrombosed veins appear bluish and stand out like cords.[16] The brain is severely edematous with flattened gyri, obliterated sulci, compressed ventricles, and, in some instances, herniation of the uncus or cerebellar tonsils. Thrombus sometimes propagates from the sinus into the smaller venous tributaries, contributing to perivenous hemorrhagic necrosis.

Hemorrhagic softening of brain tissue and patchy subarachnoid hemorrhage are other important findings. Multiple petechial hemorrhages are seen in the cortex and subcortical white matter, and these can become confluent hemorrhagic masses (Figure 20-2) with mechanical obliteration of tissue. The distribution of these lesions depends on the tributaries involved in the thrombotic process.[17] In cases of deep venous system thrombosis, hemorrhagic softening occurs in the septum pellucidum, corpus striatum, and thalamus, part of the corpus callosum, medial aspects of the occipital lobe, and medial and superior surface of the cerebellum.

Histological examination shows a variable number of shrunken nerve cells with dark staining nuclei and swollen capillary endothelial cells in the periphery. Occasional polymorphonuclear leukocytes and reactive astrocytes also occur.

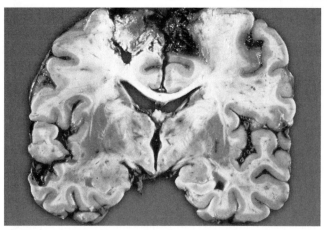

Figure 20-2. Coronal brain specimen shows bilateral hemispheric hemorrhagic infarctions due to a thrombosed sagittal sinus.

ETIOLOGY OF VENOUS THROMBOSIS

Many conditions increase the risk of cerebral venous or sinus thrombosis (Table 20-1). Frequent causes are hypercoagulable state (see Chapter 11), pregnancy and the puerperium (see Chapter 23), oral contraceptive use, and underlying malignancy.[18–20] Although infection was the predominant etiologic factor in the past, it has become less common, especially in developed countries. Cavernous sinus thrombosis is probably one of the few conditions in which infection continues to play an important causative role. Similarly children with chronic otitis media or mastoiditis may develop transverse sinus thrombosis. Precipitating factors such as dehydration, congenital heart disease, or thyroid dysfunction can contribute to the development of cerebral venous thrombosis.[21] Despite a thorough diagnostic workup, no cause can be identified in 25% of all cases.[22]

In developing countries puerperal cerebral venous thrombosis probably remains the common cause of cerebral venous thrombosis in women. Factors underlying puerperal cerebral venous thrombosis have been extensively studied. Single case studies described cerebral venous thrombosis following thrombo-phlebitis of leg veins and resulted in the hypothesis of retrograde embolization from femoral or pelvic veins via vertebral venous plexus of Batson to the cerebral veins and sinuses. This was attributed to the raised intra-abdominal pressure during labor, which was later confirmed by cadaveric and experimental studies. However, simultaneous involvement of cerebral pelvic and leg veins can be caused by a hypercoagulable state, which is probably responsible for most of these cases.

In the vast majority of patients with cerebral venous thrombosis at least one risk factor can be identified.[23] In young women the use of oral contraceptives is one of the main causes for venous thrombosis. Acquired or inherited hypercoagulable states are now the leading causes of CVST.[24,25] However, about 50% of all adult CVST patients have more than one risk factor, mandating a thorough laboratory workup and screening for conditions such as thrombophilia or an underlying malignancy even if one risk factor has already been identified. Inherited thrombophilias, for instance, can become clinically apparent in the setting of head trauma, pregnancy, infection, or dehydration leading to venous sinus thrombosis. At times the underlying etiology remains obscure, and vasculitis, inflammatory disease, or malignancy may be diagnosed long after the acute phase of cerebral venous thrombosis.[26,27]

Table 20-1: Etiology of Cerebral Venous Thrombosis

Infection
- Paranasal sinus and ear
- Systemic infections
- Meningitis (bacterial, fungal, viral)

Inflammatory disease
- Sarcoidosis
- Behçet disease
- Systemic lupus erythematosus
- Wegener granulomatosis
- Inflammatory bowel disease
- Cogan syndrome
- Polyarteritis nodosa

Thrombophilic disorders
- Antithrombin deficiency
- Protein C deficiency
- Protein S deficiency
- Factor V Leiden mutation
- Prothrombin gene *G20210A* mutation
- Hyperhomocysteinemia
- Antiphospholipid antibody syndrome

Malignancy
- Leptomeningeal carcinomatosis
- Primary or metastatic brain tumors
- Systemic tumor with hypercoagulable state

Pregnancy and puerperium

Hematological disorders
- Polycythemia vera
- Sickle cell disease
- Disseminated intravascular coagulation
- Cryofibrinogenemia
- Thrombocytosis
- Thrombocytopenia
- Paroxysmal nocturnal hemoglobinuria
- Severe anemia

Sturge-Weber syndrome

Arteriovenous malformations

Dural fistula

Mechanical injury

Pharmacological
- Oral contraceptives
- Androgens
- Tamoxifen
- L-Asparaginase
- Steroids

Idiopathic

CLINICAL PRESENTATION

The clinical features depend on the site and number of thrombosed sinuses and veins, the speed with which they are occluded, the nature of anastomotic channels, and whether the cortical veins are involved. The presentation can be acute, subacute, or chronic. Parenchymal lesions due to edema, hemorrhage (see Chapter 16), or venous infarction produce more severe neurological deficits and are more likely to be epileptogenic than isolated venous obstruction unassociated with structural brain lesions. Clinical manifestations include signs of increased intracranial pressure characterized by headaches, papilledema, nausea and visual disturbances, or focal deficits and seizures with or without altered mental status.[28]

Altered mental status in conjunction with focal neurological deficits, seizures, and headaches is highly suggestive of dural sinus thrombosis and should prompt immediate diagnostic evaluation. In the elderly, however, altered mental status tends to be more prominent than the increased intracranial pressure that dominates the clinical picture in younger individuals. Similarly, the clinical manifestations in neonates tend to be less specific than those of older children and adults.

Occasionally the presentation is atypical, making the clinical diagnosis difficult.[29] Isolated symptoms such as headache, a single seizure, or behavioral symptoms may be the only indication of cerebral venous disease. As thrombosis and fibrinolysis can occur simultaneously, symptoms can fluctuate for a time before the diagnosis becomes apparent. In patients presenting with only subacute encephalopathy, isolated seizures, or fluctuating mental status, the diagnosis can be easily missed.

Headache is the most common symptom, occurring in 75% to 95% of cases. It is typically gradual in onset, severe in intensity, and progressive. Headache is often bilateral and associated with vomiting. Any persisting headache in the first month after delivery should arouse the suspicion of cerebral vein thrombosis and should be investigated. At times the headache resembles migraine with aura, delaying the diagnosis.[30]

Next most common are seizures, which occur in about 50% to 70% of the patients. Generalized seizures are more common than focal seizures with or without secondary generalization (30%). Seizures often recur and can progress to status epilepticus that is sometimes difficult to control. Psychotic symptoms are relatively uncommon (6%), whereas alteration in consciousness is seen in over half of cases. Decreased mental status is often present in patients with thrombosis of the deep cerebral venous system and, when severe, is an indicator for poor clinical outcome.

Papilledema (Figure 20-3) occurs in individuals with occlusion of dural sinuses that impair venous drainage sufficiently to raise the intracranial pressure. Increased intracranial pressure can develop acutely (e.g., because of hemorrhage, venous infarction, or hydrocephalus) or insidiously because of impaired venous drainage or decreased cerebrospinal fluid resorption. Visual loss is the most feared complication of increased intracranial pressure.

Focal neurological deficits occur in about 40% to 60% of patients with CVST. Motor paralysis is the most frequent

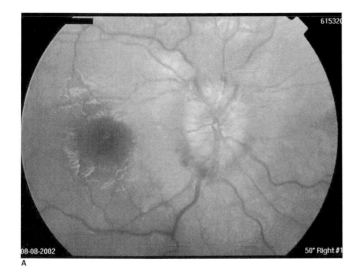

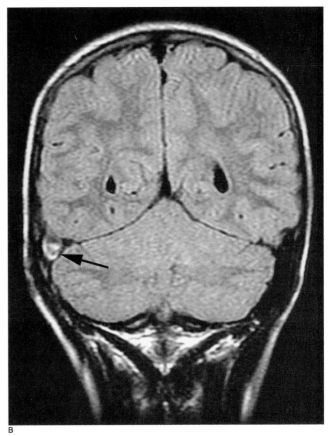

Figure 20-3. Papilledema (A) caused by thrombosis (*arrow*) of the transverse sagittal sinus (B). Reprinted with permission from Bari et al.[71]

focal neurological deficit following cerebral venous thrombosis. Weakness, when present, typically presents as mono- or hemiparesis. When the superior sagittal sinus is occluded, however, weakness is often bilateral. Exaggerated muscle stretch reflexes and extensor plantar responses can often be elicited. Aphasia, sensory deficits, and cranial nerve palsies can develop depending on the site of venous occlusion. Unilateral or bilateral CN VI palsies are nonspecific indicators of increased intracranial pressure; they usually occur in conjunction with headache, papilledema, and decreasing visual acuity.

Cavernous sinus thrombosis produces a distinctive clinical syndrome, but it is becoming increasingly rare because of the widespread use of antibiotics for paranasal sinus infections. It is often due to infection in the face and paranasal sinuses. Symptoms generally start in one eye with the development of pain, chemosis, conjunctival edema, and proptosis. This is followed by oculomotor disturbances. Within a few days the other eye is usually involved. Papilledema is common and often associated with hemorrhages of the retina. When the infection spreads to the meninges, symptoms of meningeal irritation appear. When the occlusion extends to other sinuses and cortical veins, seizures and motor weakness may develop.

Chronic otitis media and mastoiditis is often complicated by lateral sinus thrombosis, resulting in isolated intracranial hypertension (Figure 20-3). Atypical presentation is not unusual, and a high level of suspicion is necessary to make the diagnosis. Deep venous system occlusion may present with long tract signs, coma, involuntary movements, and eye motility abnormalities. Neuroimaging studies in these individuals are crucial to make the diagnosis and should include an MR-venogram (MRV).

DIAGNOSIS

Diagnostic imaging of the brain and cerebrovascular system is considered in more detail in Chapter 5. Here we will review the imaging studies only as they relate to occlusion of the venous system.

Magnetic Resonance Imaging

Brain magnetic resonance imaging (MRI) in combination with MRV has become the most sensitive diagnostic test to diagnose cerebral sinus or venous occlusion (Figure 20-4).[31,32] Typically the MRI signal changes with the age of cerebral venous thrombosis. Isolated cortical vein thrombosis remains difficult to establish even with MRV, but special MR sequences such as T_2^* can be helpful in visualizing a clot that presents as hypointense signal abnormality.[33–35] MRI also depicts associated cerebral edema, mass effect, venous infarct, and intracranial hemorrhage.[36] Like all studies, MRV has limitations. For instance, in the presence of nondominant venous flow in one of the transverse sinuses, MRV may show artifactual venous flow gaps, suggesting an occlusion.[37]

Cranial Computed Tomography

Various direct and indirect cranial computed tomography (CT) abnormalities have been documented in individuals with CVST, but cranial CT is often negative in these patients.[38] Direct signs of a sagittal sinus thrombosis include the *dense triangle sign* and the *empty delta* or *empty triangle* sign.[39,40] On a noncontrast infused scan a fresh clot in a cerebral vein or sinus appears hyperdense and is referred to as a *cord sign*. The dense triangle sign, seen on noncontrast CT scans, refers to a triangular or

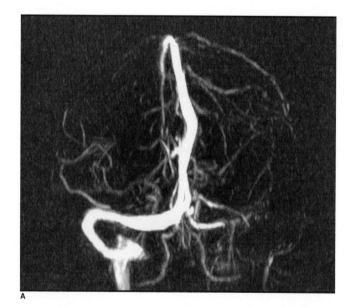

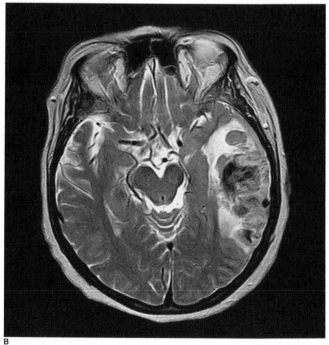

Figure 20-4. A: MRV in the coronal plane shows a normally patent sagittal sinus and right transverse sinus and a narrowed stump of the left transverse sinus. An occluded transverse sinus can be difficult to distinguish from a congenitally absent sinus (as in Figure 20-1). B: Axial view MRI shows a hemorrhagic infarction adjacent to this patient's thrombosed left transverse sinus.

rounded hyperintensity in the lumen of the sinus; it is also called the delta sign because of its shape. The empty delta sign refers to the triangular area of hypodensity resulting from displacement of contrast material by the clot. It is best seen in the posterior part of superior sagittal sinus and is the most frequent CT sign of cerebral sinus thrombosis. Computed tomography can also identify nonspecific secondary abnormalities such as cerebral edema, infarction, or hemorrhage. Intense enhancement of the falx and tentorial fissure can occur in some patients with cerebral sinus thrombosis. The enhancement is secondary to venous stasis and hyperemia caused by occlusion of the straight sinus, or rarely the superior sagittal sinus. Similarly, intense gyral enhancement can be seen, indicating venous stasis in the cortex.

Catheter Angiography

Angiography used to be the gold standard for diagnosis of cerebral venous thrombosis but has now been largely supplanted by MRI and MRV. Angiography remains indicated when the diagnosis remains uncertain. Important angiographic signs suggestive of cerebral venous thrombosis are the nonfilling of cortical veins or dural sinuses and the slowing or the stagnation of contrast medium during the capillary and venous phases. Corkscrew vessels, which are abnormally dilated anastomotic veins, and avascular mass effect are other important features. The characteristic appearance of "corkscrew" vessels is due to dilation of anastomotic veins over the cortex.

Cerebral catheter angiography is invasive, has potential complications, and can have technical limitations, such as a poor image quality of the venous phase due to anatomical variations of cerebral veins and sinuses or due to the effect of raised intracranial pressure, which causes slowing of the capillary and venous circulation and nonfilling of veins, making it impossible to localize a venous obstruction.

Ultrasound

Transcranial power or color imaging with and without contrast may have potential as noninvasive imaging modalities for the diagnosis and follow-up of patients with cerebral sinus thrombosis but require further validation before routine diagnostic use can be recommended.[41–44]

Cerebrospinal Fluid

Cerebrospinal fluid abnormalities are nonspecific in CVST and are generally not helpful in making the diagnosis. However, examination of the cerebrospinal fluid can be useful to exclude an infection, confirm the presence of subarachnoid hemorrhage, and measure the intracranial pressure. A lumbar puncture should be performed only after a neuroimaging study has been completed because it may be hazardous in the presence of increased intracranial pressure due to a mass lesion. Mild lymphocytic pleocytosis, increased protein, and red blood cells are sometimes observed. Removal of CSF can temporarily reduce pressure in patients presenting with isolated intracranial hypertension and acute vision impairment until more definitive treatment is available.

Additional Diagnostic Studies

As cerebral venous thrombosis can have multiple causes, a thorough workup is crucial to avoid recurrence. Patients should be screened for a hypercoagulable state (see Chapter 11), underlying malignancy, infection, or other medical conditions that may contribute to the development of cerebral venous thrombosis such as polycythemia vera. Medications and family history need to be reviewed in detail, and screening for acquired and inherited thrombophilia with measurement of anticardiolipin antibodies, phospholipid antibodies, lupus anticoagulant, serum homocysteine, antithrombin, protein C and S levels, factor V Leiden, and prothrombin gene *G20210A* mutation should be performed. Suspected connective tissue or other inflammatory diseases such as Behçet disease, sarcoidosis, inflammatory bowel diseases, or systemic lupus erythematosus should be systematically eliminated.

TREATMENT OF CEREBRAL VENOUS THROMBOSIS

Treatment of acute and subacute cerebral venous thrombosis focuses on anticoagulation, control of seizures, and management of increased intracranial pressure. Any underlying risk factors should be managed appropriately. The goal of anticoagulation is to prevent thrombus propagation into other veins and sinuses and to treat a potential underlying hypercoagulable state. Systemic anticoagulation may reduce mortality and risk of severe disability. Anticoagulants were first used by Stansfield in 1942.[45] However, initial conflicting reports appeared regarding the usefulness and safety of heparin, and some early investigators feared hemorrhage into the already hemorrhagic infarction. Krayenbuhl and others then observed beneficial results and advocated heparin therapy in cerebral venous thrombosis.[46] Two recent randomized trials, although based on small sample sizes, showed a positive trend for improved morbidity and mortality using systemic anticoagulation but failed to reach levels of statistical significance.[47,48]

The risk of systemic or intracerebral hemorrhage in anticoagulated patients is relatively low.[49] Patients with intraparenchymal or subarachnoid hemorrhage due to venous congestion did not have any increase in intracranial bleeding events following treatment with intravenous heparin or subcutaneous low-molecular-weight heparin. Although high-quality evidence-based data are not available, study results suggest improved clinical outcome.[50,51] Systemic anticoagulation with unfractionated or low-molecular-weight heparin is therefore the recommended treatment of cerebral sinus thrombosis, including patients who have intracranial hemorrhages due to venous congestion.[52] No data are available allowing head-to-head comparison between intravenous heparin and low-molecular-weight heparin. The choice depends on cost, patient preference, and clinical situation.

Patients with idiopathic cerebral venous thrombosis should be anticoagulated for 3 to 6 months, followed by long-term treatment with antiplatelet agents.[53,54] Some physicians advocate use of anticoagulants for 12 months because most recurrences occur within the first year. Anticoagulation is continued for at least 3 to 6 months to prevent clot extension, recurrence of cerebral thrombosis, and deep venous thrombosis of the extremities and pulmonary embolism, which occurs in 5% of untreated patients with cerebral venous thrombosis. Long-term anticoagulation beyond 12 months is recommended only for patients who are at risk for recurrent thrombotic disease because of a hypercoagulable state. Oral contraceptive use and hormonal replacement therapy need to be discontinued. It remains unclear whether antiplatelet agents have any benefits in patients with acute or subacute cerebral venous thrombosis who do not tolerate anticoagulation.[55]

Mechanical and/or pharmacological endovascular thrombolysis is currently indicated only for patients who deteriorate despite systemic anticoagulation.[56] Only data from small observational studies and case reports are available; these suggest that local thrombolysis may be safe and beneficial, potentially reducing morbidity and mortality.[57–59] In these studies patients with intracranial hemorrhage before endovascular intervention did not show an increased bleeding risk compared to those without hemorrhagic lesions before intervention.[60] However, there are valid concerns that the published data may be overly optimistic because of publication bias, resulting in reports of predominantly positive results. In observational studies the risk of intracranial hemorrhage has been reported to be about 17% following endovascular thrombolysis.[61] Clinical deterioration in earlier studies was seen in about 5% of cases, a rate that is comparable to conservatively managed patient. However, poor outcome rates were significantly higher in the recent ISCVT study. Type and dose of agents used for local pharmacological thrombolysis varied significantly between trials, indicating the need for future randomized dose response trials before general guidelines on the use of local thrombolysis become available.[53]

Secondary Complications of Venous Thrombosis

Seizures can occur in the setting of isolated cerebral venous thrombosis. However, they are more likely to develop in patients who have parenchymal lesions due to edema, venous infarcts, or intracranial hemorrhage. There is a relatively high risk of seizure recurrence in patients who have a seizure at the time of symptom onset. Although there is no clear consensus regarding seizure prophylaxis, those with supratentorial structural lesions and those with seizures at time of symptom onset should probably receive prophylactic treatment with anticonvulsants to prevent seizure recurrence and status epilepticus. Guidelines from the European Neurological Society suggest continuing treatment for 1 year in patients with early seizure onset and in those with intracranial hemorrhage.

Increased intracranial pressure may result initially from cerebral edema, venous infarct, or intracranial hemorrhage causing mass effect and potentially transtentorial herniation. Impairment in the resorption of CSF, especially when the superior sagittal sinus is thrombosed, can contribute to the development of hydrocephalus. Rarely, increased intracranial pressure can threaten vision. If there is sudden decrease in visual acuity, removal of CSF with serial lumbar punctures, ventricular-peritoneal shunt, or fenestration of the optic nerve sheath may be indicated to prevent optic nerve atrophy and permanent vision loss.[62] Measures to control increased intracranial pressure include mechanical hyperventilation aiming for a $PaCO_2$ of 30–35 mm Hg, administration of mannitol or hypertonic saline, elevation of the head to 30–40 degrees, sedation, and continuous intracranial pressure monitoring. Steroids have not proven to be of benefit, and data using hypertonic saline infusions or alternative osmotic agents are scant. For patients with a unilateral lesion that causes mass effect and midline shift with impeding herniation, hemicraniectomy can be lifesaving.[63]

Headaches usually persist for several weeks or months. In severe cases that do not respond to conservative management with analgesics, repeated lumbar punctures can help to reduce elevated intracranial pressure and pain. Acetazolamide or topiramate might help patients with milder pressure elevation. If severe disabling headaches persist that are refractory to the above measures, CSF shunting procedures should be considered.

PROGNOSIS

Before the development of modern neuroimaging modalities cerebral venous thrombosis was mainly diagnosed at autopsy, and hence the prognosis was considered poor in the majority of cases. After the introduction of angiography and before the introduction of cranial CT the mortality rate varied from 20% to 50%. With the availability of CT and MRI as routine investigative tools, milder cases are being recognized. In addition, efforts to treat CVST and its complications have improved. Together, these developments have improved the outlook of CVST considerably.

Recent mortality rates of 3% to 15% have been reported. About 3% to 4% of patients die during the acute phase of the illness. A common cause of death is the development of increased intracranial pressure with subsequent diffuse cerebral edema and transtentorial herniation. Status epilepticus can become refractory to treatment. Almost a quarter of the individuals with cerebral sinus thrombosis deteriorate after their initial presentation, developing seizures, coma, worsening focal deficits, increased headaches, and vision loss. Unexpected sudden death can result from pulmonary embolism and other medical complications.[64]

Various factors predict poor outcome.[65,66] A high mortality rate within the first months is associated with decreased mental status and coma, thrombosis of the deep cerebral venous system, rapidly progressive clinical course, large hemispheric hemorrhage, and posterior fossa lesions. Poor long-term prognosis is more common in patients with central nervous system infection, malignancy, thrombosis of the deep cerebral venous system, early intracranial hemorrhage, poor mental status, age greater than 37 years, and male gender. Intracranial hemorrhages occur in 30% to 50% of patients and can include intraparenchymal, or less commonly subdural or subarachnoid bleedings. Septic cerebral venous thrombosis, which is now rare in developed countries, has reported mortality rates between 50% and 80%. Treatment includes broad spectrum antibiotics, surgical decompression, and systemic anticoagulation.

There are few data on the recanalization rate following CVST. It has been estimated that recanalization occurs about 50% to 85% of the time, usually within the first 4 months.[67] The deep venous system and the cavernous sinus have a higher rate of recanalization. Although the data are limited, there seems to be no clear association between clinical outcome and recanalization rate.[68]

Recurrence of CVST is not common. Rethrombosis occurs in 3% to 7% of patients, typically within the first year.[69] However, the risk is greatly increased in individuals with one or more conditions causing a hypercoagulable state.[70] The recurrence risks for women with pregnancy-associated cerebral venous thrombosis and for patients with inherited or acquired thrombophilia are discussed in Chapter 23.

REFERENCES

1. Dormont D, Anxionnat R, Evrard S, Louaille C, Chiras J, Marsault C. MRI in cerebral venous thrombosis. *J Neuroradiol.* 1994;**21**:81–99.
2. deVeber G, Andrew M. Cerebral sinovenous thrombosis in children. *N Engl J Med.* 2001;**345**:417–423.

3. van den Bergh WM, van der Schaaf I, van Gijn J. The spectrum of presentations of venous infarction caused by deep cerebral vein thrombosis. *Neurology.* 2005;**65**:192–196.

4. Rother J, Waggie K, van Bruggen N, de Crespigny AJ, Moseley ME. Experimental cerebral venous thrombosis: evaluation using magnetic resonance imaging. *J Cereb Blood Flow Metab.* 1996; **16**:1353–1361.

5. Ferro JM, Canhao P, Stam J, Bousser MG, Barinagarrementeria F. Prognosis of cerebral vein and dural sinus thrombosis: results of the International Study on Cerebral Vein and Dural Sinus Thrombosis (ISCVT). *Stroke.* 2004;**35**:664–670.

6. Ferro JM, Lopes MG, Rosas MJ, Ferro MA, Fontes J. Long-term prognosis of cerebral vein and dural sinus thrombosis. results of the VENOPORT study. *Cerebrovasc Dis.* 2002;**13**:272–278.

7. Padget DH. The cranial venous system in man in reference to development, adult configuration and relation to the arteries. *Am J Anat.* 1956;**98**:307.

8. Schmidek HH, Auer LM, Kapp JP. The cerebral venous system. *Neurosurgery.* 1985;**17**:663–678.

9. Ferro JM, Correia M, Rosas MJ, Pinto AN, Neves G. Seizures in cerebral vein and dural sinus thrombosis. *Cerebrovasc Dis.* 2003; **15**:78–83.

10. Agostoni E. Headache in cerebral venous thrombosis. *Neurol Sci.* 2004;**25**(Suppl 3):S206–S210.

11. Biousse V, Ameri A, Bousser MG. Isolated intracranial hypertension as the only sign of cerebral venous thrombosis. *Neurology.* 1999;**53**:1537–1542.

12. Crawford SC, Digre KB, Palmer CA, Bell DA, Osborn AG. Thrombosis of the deep venous drainage of the brain in adults. Analysis of seven cases with review of the literature. *Arch Neurol.* 1995; **52**:1101–1108.

13. Canhao P, Ferro JM, Lindgren AG, Bousser MG, Stam J, Barinagarrementeria F. Causes and predictors of death in cerebral venous thrombosis. *Stroke.* 2005;**36**:1720–1725.

14. Gotoh M, Ohmoto T, Kuyama H. Experimental study of venous circulatory disturbance by dural sinus occlusion. *Acta Neurochir (Wien).* 1993;**124**:120–126.

15. Shinohara Y, Takagi S, Kobatake K, Gotoh F. Influence of cerebral venous obstruction on cerebral circulation in humans. *Arch Neurol.* 1982;**39**:479–481.

16. Kalbag R, Woolf A. Thrombosis and thrombophlebitis of cerebral veins and dural sinuses. In: Vinken P, Bruyn G, eds. *Handbook of Clinical Neurology.* Vol. 12. Amsterdam: Elsevier; 1972:422–446.

17. Ata M. Cerebral infarction due to intracranial sinus thrombosis. *J Clin Pathol.* 1965;**18**:636–640.

18. Weih M, Junge-Hulsing J, Mehraein S, Ziemer S, Einhaupl KM. [Hereditary thrombophilia with ischemic stroke and sinus thrombosis. Diagnosis, therapy and meta-analysis]. *Nervenarzt.* 2000; **71**:936–945.

19. Reuner KH, Ruf A, Grau A, et al. Prothrombin gene G20210->A transition is a risk factor for cerebral venous thrombosis. *Stroke.* 1998;**29**:1765–1769.

20. Cantu C, Alonso E, Jara A, et al. Hyperhomocysteinemia, low folate and vitamin B12 concentrations, and methylene tetrahydrofolate reductase mutation in cerebral venous thrombosis. *Stroke.* 2004;**35**:1790–1794.

21. Stam J. Thrombosis of the cerebral veins and sinuses. *N Engl J Med.* 2005;**352**:1791–1798.

22. Schaller B, Graf R. Cerebral venous infarction: the pathophysiological concept. *Cerebrovasc Dis.* 2004;**18**:179–188.

23. Masuhr F, Mehraein S, Einhaupl K. Cerebral venous and sinus thrombosis. *J Neurol.* 2004;**251**:11–23.

24. Hillier CE, Collins PW, Bowen DJ, Bowley S, Wiles CM. Inherited prothrombotic risk factors and cerebral venous thrombosis. *Quart J Med.* 1998;**91**:677–680.

25. Dentali F, Crowther M, Ageno W. Thrombophilic abnormalities, oral contraceptives, and risk of cerebral vein thrombosis: a meta-analysis. *Blood.* 2006;**107**:2766–2773.

26. Ferro JM, Canhao P, Bousser MG, Stam J, Barinagarrementeria F. Cerebral vein and dural sinus thrombosis in elderly patients. *Stroke.* 2005;**36**:1927–1932.

27. Enevoldson TP, Russell RW. Cerebral venous thrombosis: new causes for an old syndrome? *Q J Med.* 1990;**77**:1255–1275.

28. Bousser MG, Chiras J, Bories J, Castaigne P. Cerebral venous thrombosis: a review of 38 cases. *Stroke.* 1985;**16**:199–213.

29. Ferro JM, Lopes MG, Rosas MJ, Fontes J. Delay in hospital admission of patients with cerebral vein and dural sinus thrombosis. *Cerebrovasc Dis.* 2005;**19**:152–156.

30. Newman DS, Levine SR, Curtis VL, Welch KM. Migraine-like visual phenomena associated with cerebral venous thrombosis. *Headache.* 1989;**29**:82–85.

31. Isensee C, Reul J, Thron A. Magnetic resonance imaging of thrombosed dural sinuses. *Stroke.* 1994;**25**:29–34.

32. Ayanzen RH, Bird CR, Keller PJ, McCully FJ, Theobald MR, Heiserman JE. Cerebral MR venography: normal anatomy and potential diagnostic pitfalls. *AJNR Am J Neuroradiol.* 2000;**21**: 74–78.

33. Cakmak S, Hermier M, Montavont A, et al. T_2*-weighted MRI in cortical venous thrombosis. *Neurology.* 2004;**63**:1698.

34. Selim M, Fink J, Linfante I, Kumar S, Schlaug G, Caplan LR. Diagnosis of cerebral venous thrombosis with echo-planar T_2*-weighted magnetic resonance imaging. *Arch Neurol.* 2002;**59**: 1021–1026.

35. Fellner FA, Fellner C, Aichner FT, Molzer G. Importance of T_2*-weighted gradient-echo MRI for diagnosis of cortical vein thrombosis. *Eur J Radiol.* 2005;**56**:235–239.

36. Favrole P, Guichard JP, Crassard I, Bousser MG, Chabriat H. Diffusion-weighted imaging of intravascular clots in cerebral venous thrombosis. *Stroke.* 2004;**35**:99–103.

37. Surendrababu NR, Subathira, Livingstone RS. Variations in the cerebral venous anatomy and pitfalls in the diagnosis of cerebral venous sinus thrombosis: low field MR experience. *Indian J Med Sci.* 2006;**60**:135–142.

38. Rao KCVG, Knipp HC, Wagner EJ. Computed tomographic findings in cerebral sinus and venous thrombosis. *Radiology.* 1981; **140**:391–398.

39. Ahn TB, Roh JK. A case of cortical vein thrombosis with the cord sign. *Arch Neurol.* 2003;**60**:1314–1316.

40. Lee EJ. The empty delta sign. *Radiology.* 2002;**224**:788–789.

41. Canhao P, Batista P, Ferro JM. Venous transcranial Doppler in acute dural sinus thrombosis. *J Neurol.* 1998;**245**:276–279.

42. Valdueza JM, Hoffmann O, Weih M, Mehraein S, Einhaupl KM. Monitoring of venous hemodynamics in patients with cerebral venous thrombosis by transcranial Doppler ultrasound. *Arch Neurol.* 1999;**56**:229–234.

43. Becker G, Bogdahn U, Gehlberg C, Frohlich T, Hofmann E, Schlief MD. Transcranial color-coded real-time sonography of intracranial veins. Normal values of blood flow velocities and findings in superior sagittal sinus thrombosis. *J Neuroimaging.* 1995; **5**:87–94.

44. Ries S, Steinke W, Neff KW, Hennerici M. Echocontrast-enhanced transcranial color-coded sonography for the diagnosis of transverse sinus venous thrombosis. *Stroke.* 1997;**28**:696–700.

45. Stansfield FR. Puerperal cerebral thrombophletis treated by heparin. *Br Med J.* 1942;**1**(4239):436–438.

46. Krayenbuhl HL. Cerebral venous and sinus thrombosis. *Clin Neurosurg.* 1967;**14**:1–24.

47. de Bruijn SF, Stam J. Randomized, placebo-controlled trial of anticoagulant treatment with low-molecular-weight heparin for cerebral sinus thrombosis. *Stroke.* 1999;**30**:484–488.

48. Benamer HT, Bone I. Cerebral venous thrombosis: anticoagulants or thrombolyic therapy? *J Neurol Neurosurg Psychiatry*. 2000;**69**: 427–430.

49. Bousser MG. Cerebral venous thrombosis: nothing, heparin, or local thrombolysis? *Stroke*. 1999;**30**:481–483.

50. Bousser MG, Russell RR. Cerebral venous thrombosis. In: Warlow CP, van Gijn J, eds. *Major Problems in Neurology*. London: W. B. Saunders Company; 1997:1–175.

51. Einhaupl KW, Villringer A, Meister W, et al. Heparin treatment in sinus venous thrombosis. *Lancet*. 1991;**338**:597–600.

52. Stam J, de Bruijn SF, deVeber G. Anticoagulation for cerebral sinus thrombosis. *Cochrane Database Syst Rev*. 2002; CD002005.

53. Einhaupl K, Bousser MG, de Bruijn SF, et al. EFNS guideline on the treatment of cerebral venous and sinus thrombosis. *Eur J Neurol*. 2006;**13**:553–559.

54. Sacco RL, Adams R, Albers G, et al. Guidelines for prevention of stroke in patients with ischemic stroke or transient ischemic attack: a statement for healthcare professionals from the American Heart Association/American Stroke Association Council on Stroke: co-sponsored by the Council on Cardiovascular Radiology and Intervention: the American Academy of Neurology affirms the value of this guideline. *Stroke*. 2006;**37**:577–617.

55. Buller HR, Agnelli G, Hull RD, Hyers TM, Prins MH, Raskob GE. Antithrombotic therapy for venous thromboembolic disease: the Seventh ACCP Conference on Antithrombotic and Thrombolytic Therapy. *Chest*. 2004;**126**:401S–428S.

56. Canhao P, Falcao F, Ferro JM. Thrombolytics for cerebral sinus thrombosis: a systematic review. *Cerebrovasc Dis*. 2003;**15**: 159–166.

57. Horowitz M, Purdy P, Unwin H, et al. Treatment of dural sinus thrombosis using selective catheterization and urokinase. *Ann Neurol*. 1995;**38**:58–67.

58. Frey JL, Muro GJ, McDougall CG, Dean BL, Jahnke HK. Cerebral venous thrombosis: combined intrathrombus rtPA and intravenous heparin. *Stroke*. 1999;**30**:489–494.

59. Kim SY, Suh JH. Direct endovascular thrombolytic therapy for dural sinus thrombosis: infusion of alteplase. *AJNR Am J Neuroradiol*. 1997;**18**:639–645.

60. Wasay M, Bakshi R, Kojan S, Bobustuc G, Dubey N, Unwin DH. Nonrandomized comparison of local urokinase thrombolysis versus systemic heparin anticoagulation for superior sagittal sinus thrombosis. *Stroke*. 2001;**32**:2310–2317.

61. Wingerchuk DM, Wijdicks EF, Fulghum JR. Cerebral venous thrombosis complicated by hemorrhagic infarction factors affecting the initiation and safety of anticoagulation. *Cerebrovasc Dis*. 1998;**8**:25–30.

62. Acheson JF. Optic nerve disorders: role of canal and nerve sheath decompression surgery. *Eye*. 2004;**18**:1169–1174.

63. Keller E, Pangalu A, Fandino J, Konu D, Yonekawa Y. Decompressive craniectomy in severe cerebral venous and dural sinus thrombosis. *Acta Neurochir* 2005;**94**(Suppl):177–183.

64. Dentali F, Gianni M, Crowther MA, Ageno W. Natural history of cerebral vein thrombosis: a systematic review. *Blood*. 2006;**108**: 1129–1134.

65. Breteau G, Mounier-Vehier F, Godefroy O, et al. Cerebral venous thrombosis 3-year clinical outcome in 55 consecutive patients. *J Neurol*. 2003;**250**:29–35.

66. Girot M, Ferro JM, Canhao P, et al. Predictors of outcome in patients with cerebral venous thrombosis and intracerebral hemorrhage. *Stroke*. 2007;**38**:337–342.

67. Baumgartner RW, Studer A, Arnold M, Georgiadis D. Recanalisation of cerebral venous thrombosis. *J Neurol Neurosurg Psychiatry*. 2003;**74**:459–461.

68. Strupp M, Covi M, Seelos K, Dichgans M, Brandt T. Cerebral venous thrombosis: correlation between recanalization and clinical outcome – a long-term follow-up of 40 patients. *J Neurol*. 2002;**249**:1123–1124.

69. Kenet G, Kirkham F, Niederstadt T, et al. Risk factors for recurrent venous thromboembolism in the European collaborative paediatric database on cerebral venous thrombosis: a multicentre cohort study. *Lancet Neurol*. 2007;**6**:595–603.

70. Cakmak S, Derex L, Berruyer M, et al. Cerebral venous thrombosis: clinical outcome and systematic screening of prothrombotic factors. *Neurology*. 2003;**60**:1175–1178.

71. Bari L, Choksi R, Roach ES. Otitic hydrocephalus revisited. *Arch Neurol*. 2005;**62**:824–825.

21

Genetics of Cerebrovascular Disease

Alas, our frailty is the cause, not we!
For such as we are made of, such we be.

William Shakespeare

Cerebrovascular complications result from several monogenetic disorders (Table 21-1), but these uncommon conditions collectively account for a only small percentage of all stroke patients.[1-3] There is also a familial stroke risk that is not monogenetic. In the Framingham study, for example, a history of stroke in either parent significantly increased the likelihood of a stroke in an offspring.[4] Another large prospective study concluded that a stroke in any first-degree relative increased the odds of coronary artery disease among men and of stroke among women.[5] Family members typically share environmental risk factors as well as genes, but in twin studies the concordance rate for stroke in monozygotic twins was 17.7% whereas that of dizygotic twins was only 3.6%.[6]

Identification of single genetic disorders that cause stroke is important because some of these conditions are treatable and because family members could also be at risk. However, most of the traditional stroke risk factors – atherosclerosis, hypertension, coagulation disorders, and abnormal lipid metabolism – are ultimately controlled by genetically mediated metabolic pathways. The polygenetic traits that modulate these basic stroke risk factors account for far more patients with stroke than all of the monogenetic diseases that cause stroke risk.

In this chapter we will review several monogenetic diseases that promote cerebrovascular dysfunction. For convenience, several genetic conditions such as sickle cell disease, coagulopathies, and familial aneurysms are presented in other chapters. We will also touch on some of the vast literature on modifying genes and summarize the genetic underpinning for a few of the traditional stroke risk factors. Alberts has more thoroughly reviewed the genetics of stroke risk factors.[7]

MODIFIER GENES

The story is still unfolding, but hereditary influences on the pathophysiology of stroke are far more pervasive and complex than once imaginable. We have long appreciated that one's genetic make-up plays a major role in the occurrence and severity of stroke risk factors such as atherosclerosis, hypertension, lipid metabolism, diabetes, and coagulation. In most instances, however, it is not the presence of a single abnormal gene that alters the stroke risk but rather the interplay between numerous genes and multiple environmental factors. Additionally, genes influence the brain's ability to withstand ischemia, a person's response to stroke therapy, and the individual's capacity to recover following an injury. It is now technically possible to establish that the presence of a specific gene polymorphism or a particular combination of genes alters the stroke risk even before we fully understand their physiologic effects.

Genetic influences are potentially important even for individuals who have a well-recognized stroke risk factor, because a stroke may result from the interplay between multiple genes and environmental factors. Why, for example, do relatively few people with well-recognized risk factors such as atrial fibrillation, oral contraceptive use, or sickle cell disease have a stroke? Although everyone would agree that a 5% annual stroke risk among people with atrial fibrillation is much higher than that of an individual without atrial fibrillation, why do so many of these individuals *not* have a stroke? Clearly some individuals have additional factors that increase or decrease the stroke risk.

In one study of 1,398 individuals with sickle cell disease (92 of whom subsequently had a stroke), 12 of 39 candidate genes studied modulated the stroke risk due to sickle cell disease, primarily via an interaction with fetal hemoglobin.[8] These 12 modifier genes included three genes in the TGF-β signaling pathway and the *SELP* gene that also increase the stroke risk in individuals without sickle cell disease. Given the hundreds of genes with the potential to influence the risk of stroke, the number of possible interactions is virtually endless. To add yet another layer of complexity, some modifier genes may exert a protective effect in a given situation and a deleterious effect in another.

GENETICS OF HYPERTENSION

We have long appreciated that hypertension increases the risk of stroke and that genetic factors play a significant role in the pathogenesis of hypertension. Shared genetic traits, for example,

Table 21-1: Selected Monogenetic Stroke Risk Factors

Autosomal dominant disorders

- Antithrombin deficiency
- CADASIL
- Familial cavernous malformation
- Familial hypercholesterolemia[a]
- Hereditary hemorrhagic telangiectasia (Osler-Weber-Rendu disease)
- HERNS and related disorders
- Ehlers-Danlos syndrome (vascular type)
- Marfan syndrome
- Moyamoya disease[a,b]
- Neurofibromatosis type 1
- Arterial tortuosity syndrome
- Polycystic renal disease
- Progeria[c]
- Protein C deficiency
- Protein S deficiency

Autosomal recessive disorders

- Afibrinogenemia
- Factor XIII deficiency
- Factor X deficiency
- Factor XI deficiency
- Factor XII deficiency (Hageman factor deficiency)
- Familial hypercholesterolemia[a]
- Fanconi anemia
- Homocystinuria

- Isovaleric acidemia
- Methylmalonic acidemia
- Propionic acidemia
- Pseudoxanthoma elasticum
- Sickle cell disease
- Sickle cell–hemoglobin C disease
- Werner syndrome
- Williams syndrome

X-linked disorders

- Hemophilia A (factor VIII deficiency)
- Hemophilia B (factor IX deficiency)
- Fabry disease
- Menkes disease
- Ornithine transcarbamylase deficiency

Mitochondrial disorders

- Subacute necrotizing encephalomyelopathy (Leigh disease)
- MELAS (mitochondrial encephalomyopathy, lactic acidosis, and stroke-like episodes)
- MERRF (myoclonic epilepsy with ragged-red fibers)
- Kearns-Sayre syndrome
- NADH-CoQ reductase deficiency

Chromosomal disorders

- Turner syndrome
- Down syndrome

[a] Multiple or indeterminate inheritance patterns for similar phenotypes.
[b] Most cases are sporadic but dominant pattern seems likely in familial cases.
[c] Projected inheritance pattern (early lethal mutation).

no doubt account for the excess risk of hypertension in blacks. By some estimates, the risk of stroke is more than four times higher in an individual with hypertension than in a person with normal blood pressure, and the stroke risk is doubled even among people with intermittent or milder blood pressure elevation.[9] Hypertension is such a strong stroke risk factor, in fact, that it accounts for a substantial portion of the genetic predisposition to stroke in many families. The fact that hypertension is so easily treated enhances its importance as a stroke risk factor, and much of the well-documented recent decline in the incidence of stroke is attributable to widespread therapy of hypertension.

The interplay between environmental factors and genetic traits is complex and still largely uncharted, but there is no doubt that genetic traits strongly influence the risk of hypertension. If one parent has hypertension, over a quarter of their offspring have hypertension, and if both parents have hypertension, almost half of the offspring will also have hypertension.[9] The fact that family members typically share both environmental

risks and genetic traits makes it more difficult to segregate the influences of genes and environment. Adoption studies show that biological siblings are far more likely to be concordant for hypertension than adoptive siblings raised in the same household.[10] Blood pressures tend to be more similar in monozygotic twins than in dizygotic twins, whose genetic makeup is like that of ordinary siblings.[11]

Blood pressure is controlled via an intricate series of interrelated pathways, each of which is genetically mediated. There are acquired causes of hypertension as well as monogenetic disorders that feature high blood pressure, such as Liddle disease, familial hyperaldosteronism, and pseudohypoaldosteronism. However, the majority of people with elevated blood pressure have no single cause and have essential hypertension.

Numerous susceptibility loci contribute to essential hypertension. A partial list of candidate genes include angiotensinogen on chromosome 1q42, angiotensin receptor-1 on chromosome 3q, the endothelin-converting enzyme-1 on chromosome 1p36, the beta-3 subunit of guanine nucleotide-binding protein on chromosome 12p13, and the prostaglandin I2 synthase on chromosome 20q. There is also evidence that genetic factors help to determine which individuals respond well to therapy for hypertension. A complete review of this voluminous work is beyond the scope of the present discussion, but for additional details see Online Mendelian Inheritance in Man (OMIN) at http://www.ncbi.nlm.nih.gov/entrez/dispomim.cgi?id=145500.

GENETICS OF ATHEROSCLEROSIS

Familial hyperlipidemia and other monogenetic conditions can accelerate atherosclerosis (see Chapter 7), but numerous genetic traits influence the development of atherosclerosis even in individuals without these specific diseases. Atherosclerosis develops after an arterial injury, as occurs from hypertension, tobacco exposure, hyperlipidemia, ionizing radiation, or excess homocysteine.[12] After the vascular injury, a local inflammatory response is initiated by the cytokines tumor necrosis factor alpha and interleukin-1. Expression of intercellular adhesion molecules by the endothelial cells promotes migration of circulating monocytes into the subendothelial region, triggering the accelerated lipid uptake that represents the initial stages of atherosclerosis.[12–14] Even from this admittedly simple overview, the complexity of atheroma formation and the potential for genetic modulation becomes apparent.

One indication of genetic influence on atherosclerosis is the different location of cerebral atherosclerosis among different peoples. Among the Chinese, intracranial atherosclerosis is more severe and extracranial carotid atherosclerosis is less severe than in Caucasians.[15] Similarly, blacks are more likely to develop intracranial atherosclerosis.[16] Although these differences may be partly explainable by group differences in traditional vascular risk factors, even after accounting for variations in smoking habits, diabetes, and hypertension, race was an independent predictor of the location of cerebrovascular lesions.[17]

Several monogenetic disorders promote abnormal lipid metabolism and premature atherosclerosis, and these are summarized in Table 21-1. There are vast numbers of people with symptomatic atherosclerosis but relatively few individuals with a Mendelian gene disorder. In most individuals atherosclerosis results from the interaction between environmental factors and many different genes, each of which exerts a small effect, either alone or in tandem with other genes.

Diet, diabetes, tobacco consumption, and exercise play a well-known role in the generation of atherosclerosis, but numerous genetic susceptibility traits determine the body's response to these risk factors. Dozens of polymorphisms have been linked to the development of atherosclerosis, although the exact contribution of most genes is not clear. Even in individuals with a single gene mutation that is known to promote atherosclerosis, other genes still influence the clinical manifestations of the disease. Individuals with familial combined hyperlipidemia who become obese or hypertensive, for example, are more likely to develop symptomatic atherosclerosis, and the occurrence of genetic variations in the rennin-angiotensin-aldosterone system correlate with the likelihood of developing coronary artery disease.[18,19]

COAGULATION DISORDERS

For a discussion of hereditary coagulation disorders, see Chapter 11 and Tables 11-1 and 11-2.

Table 21-2: Clinical Features of 102 Patients with CADASIL

	Percentage Affected	Percentage as Initial Sign
Ischemic deficits	71	46
Recurrent attacks	53	NA
Cognitive deficits	48	6
Dementia	28	ND
Epileptic seizures	10	0
Psychiatric symptoms	30	1
Recurrent headache	47	ND
Migraine	38	47
Migraine with aura	33	ND

Adapted with permission from Dichgans et al.[26]
NA = not applicable; ND = not determined.

CADASIL

In 1977 Sourander and Walinder described a three-generation family in which multiple members had progressive deterioration of neurological function.[20] Typically, symptoms began between 29 and 38 years of age in individuals without systemic hypertension. They had various focal neurological deficits and a relapsing course that gradually evolved into clinical dementia. One family member suffered an intraparenchymal hemorrhage, but three siblings who underwent an autopsy had multiple small subcortical cystic infarctions and cortical atrophy. The authors postulated that this family had a new autosomal dominant condition.[20]

In 1993 Tournier-Lasserve and colleagues linked cerebral autosomal dominant arteriopathy with subcortical infarcts and leukoencephalopathy to chromosome 19q12 and coined the acronym CADASIL (cerebral autosomal dominant arteriopathy with subcortical infarcts and leukoencephalopathy).[21] CADASIL is caused by a mutation in the NOTCH3 gene, a mutation that alters the epidermal growth factor-like domain of the Notch3 receptor in vascular smooth muscle.[22–24] The prevalence of the NOTCH3 mutation is at least 4.14 per 100,000 adults, although this estimate is almost certainly low.[25]

Clinical Features of CADASIL

The clinical features of CADASIL are highly variable and age related. Recurrent ischemic episodes occurred in 71% of the 102 individuals with well-established CADASIL in one series.[26] Almost half of these individuals had cognitive deficits, a quarter had frank dementia, and 38% had migraine (Table 21-2). Most of the CADASIL patients who have headache have migraine with aura; some of these individuals present with recurrent bouts of migraine with aura or episodic hemiplegia long before there are other signs of the disease.[26–28] Although ischemic lesions are usually emphasized, intraparenchymal hemorrhage occurs as well.[29,30] The likelihood of symptoms due to CADISIL may increase during pregnancy.[31]

Most individuals with CADASIL eventually develop multiple magnetic resonance imaging (MRI) abnormalities in the white matter, basal ganglia, and brainstem (Figure 21-1).[32] The

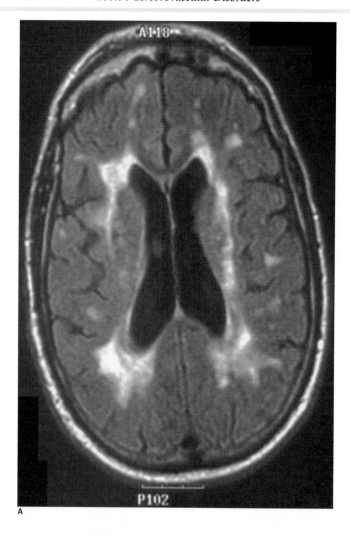

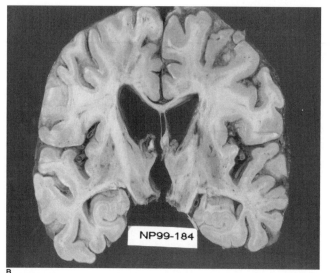

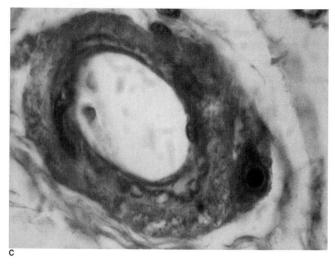

Figure 21-1. A: Brain MRI from an individual with CADASIL shows numerous small white matter infarctions especially adjacent to the ventricles. B: The brain of an individual with CADASIL has numerous small lesions in the white matter and confluent lesions in the periventricular region. C: Microscopic sections reveal the characteristic perivascular osmophilic changes of CADASIL.

lesions include both small infarctions and hemorrhages, and over time they tend to become more numerous and even confluent.[33] Later the MRI also shows cortical atrophy. Proton MR spectroscopy suggests axonal injury, myelin loss, and gliosis.[34]

Pathology of CADASIL

The brain abnormalities are more pronounced in older individuals with CADASIL. Long penetrating arterioles are most often affected.[35] These vessels have a thick wall and a narrow lumen, and some arterioles have PAS-positive granules in the media (Figure 21-1).[32] Electron microscopy reveals characteristic osmophilic granules in the basal lamina of the arterioles.[33]

Multiple small ischemic infarctions and diffuse changes with demyelination and axonal loss have been described.[33] Additionally, hemosiderin-containing macrophages occur adjacent to some of the small blood vessels. Individuals with CADASIL and findings of isolated cerebral angiitis have been described.[36]

The pathogenesis of CADASIL is still obscure, but impaired vasomotor reactivity and autoregulation in response to blood pressure changes was demonstrated in NOTCH3 mutant mice.[37]

Diagnosis of CADASIL

Although CADASIL was once considered a rare disorder, increased recognition of isolated cases and individuals with less obvious features suggests that it is still underrecognized.[38] CADASIL should be suspected in individuals with early stroke, especially those with a family history of early stroke, a strong history of migraine with aura or complicated migraine, or a history of familial dementia. DNA testing for a NOTCH3 mutation is commercially available. A few patients have a NOTCH3 mutation outside the commonly affected exons, so if CADASIL is strongly suspected, the diagnosis can be confirmed by finding typical vascular abnormalities on skin or muscle biopsy.[39]

Treatment of CADASIL

Specific treatment for CADASIL is not available. Some individuals with frequent or complicated migraine sometimes benefit from headache prophylaxis; daily calcium channel blockers may be the most effective headache prophylactic. Likewise, individuals with psychiatric symptoms may also benefit from appropriate medication. It seems intuitive to reduce other stroke risk factors (smoking, systemic hypertension, hypercholesterolemia, etc.) in individuals with CADASIL. Some patients take L-arginie, but there is limited evidence of effectiveness.

CARASIL

Cerebral autosomal recessive arteriopathy with subcortical infarcts and leukoencephalopathy (CARASIL) is an autosomal recessive arteriopathy with clinical features that overlap those of CADASIL.[40,41] CARASIL is characterized by young adult onset of nonhypertensive encephalopathy accompanied by alopecia.[41] Only a few CARASIL patients have been described in detail, and its molecular biology has not been well characterized.

Individuals with CARASIL have focal areas of demyelination and severe atherosclerosis of the small arteries, along with intimal fibrosis and hyaline degeneration and splitting of the internal elastic membrane.[41,42] CARASIL arteriopathy lacks the granular osmophilic deposits that occur in CADASIL.[43,44]

HERNS

Hereditary endotheliopathy with retinopathy, nephropathy, and stroke (HERNS) is an autosomal-dominant occlusive microangiopathy that results from a mutation of the TREX1 gene on chromosome 3p21.1-p21.3.[45–47] Cerebroretinal vasculopathy and hereditary vascular retinopathy were once considered distinct entities with features overlapping those of HERNS, but recent studies have shown that these two conditions, like HERNS, also result from a TREX1 mutation.[48] Consequently Kavanagh and colleagues suggested the new term retinal vasculopathy and cerebral leukodystrophy to describe all of the cerebral vasculopathies arising from this mutation.[48] The autosomal dominant vasculopathy disease described by Vahedi and colleagues, however, is evidently a distinct entity despite somewhat similar clinical features.[49]

Clinical manifestations of HERNS include progressive visual impairment, migraine-like headaches, focal neurologic deficits, depression or other psychiatric disturbances, seizures, and dementia.[46,50] The retinal vessels are tortuous and variable in caliber, and retinal microaneurysms and parafoveal telangiectatic capillaries are apparent.[51] Renal insufficiency and Raynaud's phenomenon are common.[52] Neurologic deficits in HERNS typically occur in the second to fourth decades of life.

MRI demonstrates diffuse, multiple, deep, white matter infarcts, although contrast-enhancing brain mass lesions may occur. Electron microscopy often reveals multilayered vascular basement membranes of the capillary and arteriolar endothelial cells in the brain and other tissues, including the kidneys, skin, stomach, appendix, and omentum.[46]

AMYLOID ANGIOPATHY

See the discussion of amyloid angiopathy in Chapter 16.

FABRY DISEASE

Fabry disease (angiokeratoma corporis diffusum or Anderson-Fabry disease) is an X-linked lysosomal defect resulting from deficiency of alpha-galactosidase A.[53,54] Mutations of the Fabry disease gene occurs in about one in 117,000 individuals.[55] Fabry disease has been documented in most ethnic groups but occurs principally in Caucasians.

Clinical Features of Fabry Disease

Fabry disease is completely penetrant in males, whereas symptoms in females are variable and generally mild.[56,57] Symptoms typically begin toward the end of the first decade with intense, painful paresthesias of the feet, but diagnosis is often delayed for several years.[58] Heterozygous females sometimes develop intermittent paresthesias, especially when febrile. Most affected males develop distinctive skin lesions (angiokeratoma corporis diffusum), especially around the umbilicus or on the buttocks, scrotum, hips, or thighs (Figure 21-2 A). However, the skin lesions become more obvious with increasing age and may be subtle or nonexistent at the time of presentation.[59,60] Whorled corneal opacities (Figure 21-2 B) occur in males and females.[61,62]

Renal failure is the most common cause of death due to Fabry disease.[59] Almost a third of the adults in a Fabry disease registry had end-stage renal disease.[60] Renal failure occasionally develops in individuals without any of the typical early signs

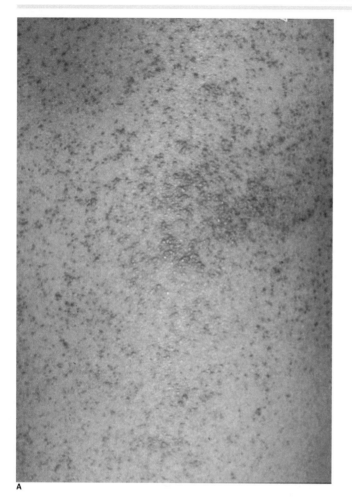

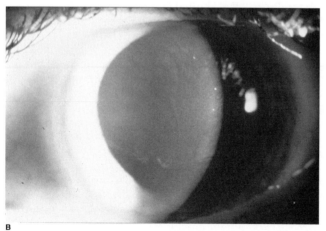

Figure 21-2. A: Cutaneous angiokeratomas of Fabry disease. B: Whorled corneal deposits of Fabry disease. Reprinted with permission from Miller and Roach.[255]

age, and individuals who have one cerebral infarction have a 76% risk of having one or more additional strokes.[71] Ischemic infarction occurs more often than cerebral hemorrhage.[70,72] Stroke or transient ischemic attacks occurred in about a quarter of the adult men in one cohort.[60] However, two-thirds of the 129 adults with Fabry disease in one series had one or more ischemic MRI lesions, whereas only one-third had previous stroke symptoms. All of the patients over 54 years of age had brain lesions.[73]

Pathophysiology of Fabry Disease

There is loss of small myelinated and unmyelinated peripheral nerve fibers and small cell bodies of the spinal ganglia.[74–76] Glycolipid granules are deposited within the cytoplasm of the vascular endothelial cells.[74–76] Accumulation of glycolipid in the vascular endothelium and smooth muscle cells causes gradual narrowing and occlusion of the lumen.[77] Cerebral infarctions result from multifocal small vessel occlusions.

Individuals with Fabry disease have markedly low enzyme activity in plasma, serum, leukocytes, or cultured fibroblasts. DNA analysis is useful for female heterozygotes whose enzyme activity is relatively normal. Prenatal diagnosis is available.[78]

Males with greater residual enzyme activity have milder symptoms.[79] Females develop symptoms more often than is generally appreciated but infrequently develop stroke, cardiac disease, or renal failure.[56] Women who are more symptomatic or have severe complications may have disproportionate inactivation of their normal X chromosome.

Treatment of Fabry Disease

Periodic infusions of recombinant human alpha-galactosidase A reduce the plasma globotriaosylceramide level and reduce the endothelial deposits in a dose-dependent fashion.[80,81] Moreover, treated patients report less pain, increased ability to sweat, and improved measures of renal function.[80,82] Sometimes dramatic improvement in cardiac function has been observed following enzyme infusions.[83]

Renal transplantation alleviates renal failure and, in some individuals, provides enough enzyme activity to alleviate the paresthesias and delay the systemic complications.[84] Carbamazepine or phenytoin may offer symptomatic relief from the paresthesias but does not reduce the vascular complications.[59]

HOMOCYSTINURIA

Homocystinuria is an autosomal recessive disorder of methionine metabolism most often caused by cystathionine β-synthetase deficiency (a few patients have a deficiency of 5,10-methylenetetrahydrofolate reductase deficiency or homocysteine methyltransferase).[85,86] Affected individuals excrete homocystine in the urine and have high levels of homocysteine in the plasma and tissue.[87]

Clinical Manifestations of Homocystinuria

The phenotype of homocystinuria varies, but skeletal and cutaneous abnormalities, lens dislocation, mental retardation, and vascular lesions are common. Many individuals have fair skin, and some have livedo reticularis or malar flushing. Dislocation of the lens is a frequent finding.[88,89] About half of the individuals with homocystinuria are mentally retarded. Homocystinuria

and symptoms of Fabry disease.[63] Similarly, isolated cardiac dysfunction has been documented in otherwise asymptomatic individuals.[64,65] Hypertrophic cardiomyopathy, angina, and arrhythmia have all been described.[66–68]

Stroke due to Fabry disease typically occurs during the third or fourth decade; it is rarely the first manifestation of Fabry disease.[69,70] The risk of stroke due to Fabry disease increases with and Marfan syndrome share enough skeletal and ocular abnormalities that the two disorders are sometimes confused.

Vascular complications include pulmonary embolism, myocardial infarction, renovascular hypertension, and thrombosis of intracranial veins or arteries. Thromboembolism was a major contributing factor in the majority of deaths in the large series of Mudd and colleagues.[90] Cerebrovascular disease may be further complicated by coexistent renovascular hypertension or heart failure. Patients who develop one thromboembolic complication have an increased likelihood of developing additional vascular complications compared to patients with no vascular complications.[90]

Elderly patients with low intake of folate and vitamin B_6 have higher serum levels of homocysteine, and hyperhomocysteinemia causes a modest increase in stroke risk.[91–93] Similarly, heterozygous cystathionine synthase deficiency may increase the risk of premature atherosclerosis and stroke in young adults.[94–97] Boers and associates documented an abnormal response to methionine loading and heterozygosity for cystathionine synthase in 14 of 50 patients with premature cerebrovascular or peripheral vascular disease.[95] In another report heterozygous cystathionine synthase deficiency was confirmed in 18 of 23 patients with both elevated homocysteine and vascular disease, whereas none of the 27 control subjects had high homocysteine levels.[91] Mudd and colleagues failed to confirm an increased risk of stroke or myocardial infarction among likely heterozygous individuals (the parents and grandparents of homocystinuria patients), but this study was limited by its reliance on questionnaires.[98]

Pathophysiology of Homocystinuria

Acute or organized thrombus may be found within the intracranial arteries, veins, or dural sinuses, and some occluded vessels show signs of recanalization. Irregular intimal proliferation and fibrosis form padlike elevations of the intimal surface.[99] Concentric proliferation slowly shrinks the lumen diameter.[100] The media may be thin and the elastica alternately attenuated or thickened and split.[99] Thrombus formation has been documented adjacent to these vascular abnormalities. Proliferative lesions of the venous system are also seen, although not with the same frequency as in the arteries.

Individuals with hyperhomocysteinemia have increased platelet aggregation, a finding that is mimicked by adding homocystine in vitro to the platelets of normal individuals.[101] There is evidence that elevated levels of homocystine are directly toxic to endothelial cells. Harker and colleagues demonstrated in baboons that a high level of homocystine provokes desquamation of the vascular endothelium, which in turn leads to platelet activation.[87,102] Continuous infusion of homocystine resulted in patchy loss of vascular endothelium, and endothelial cells could be demonstrated circulating in the peripheral blood. Platelet destruction was secondary to the endothelial abnormalities and not homocystine toxicity, and the platelet dysfunction was prevented by dipyridamole. Injecting rabbits on a high cholesterol diet with homocysteine thiolactone resulted in vascular changes resembling atherosclerosis.[103,104]

Treatment of Homocystinuria

Early diagnosis of homocystinuria is important because there is effective treatment for many individuals. About half of the patients normalize their homocysteine level in response to pharmacologic doses of vitamin B_6, a coenzyme for cystathionine synthase.[90] There is little risk to vitamin B_6 administration, and Pyeritz recommended starting 500 mg/day of vitamin B_6 (pyridoxine), then increasing the dose to 1000 mg/day if the homocysteine level does not fall.[105] Folate also reduces the homocysteine level in a few patients, perhaps by promoting the remethylation of methionine.[106–108] Folate supplementation (1–10 mg/day) is also reasonable.[105,109]

Based on the available animal studies, aspirin or other antiplatelet agents may lower the risk of thrombosis due to homocystinuria, especially in individuals who are unresponsive to vitamin B_6. It also seems reasonable to eliminate other modifiable risk factors for cerebrovascular disease.

Although vitamin supplementation may lower the risk of vascular disease due to homozygous and heterozygous homocystinuria, a multicenter trial of vitamin supplementation aimed at secondary prevention of ischemic stroke failed to demonstrate a lower recurrent stroke risk despite a reduction in the serum homocysteine levels in the individuals receiving vitamins.[110] Given the time that it takes atherosclerosis to accumulate, however, secondary prevention in a largely elderly cohort may not be the optimal test.

VASCULAR EHLERS-DANLOS

Ehlers-Danlos syndrome (EDS) is not a single entity but rather a group of connective tissue diseases with overlapping clinical manifestations that include hyperextensible joints, hyperelastic skin, vascular lesions, easy bruising, and excessive scarring after an injury.[111,112] Cerebrovascular complications are uncommon except in individuals with EDS type IV, recently dubbed vascular EDS.[113]

Vascular EDS is transmitted as an autosomal dominant trait.[111,114] It results from a mutation of the COL3A1 gene on chromosome 2, which encodes type III procollagen.[114,115] Type III collagen is the predominant collagen type in blood vessels, bowel, and the uterus.[114–116] Numerous COL3A1 mutations have been documented.[112,117,118] However, mutations of the COL3A1 gene rarely occur in unselected patients with cerebral aneurysms.[119,120]

Clinical Features of Vascular EDS

Neither hyperelastic skin (see Figure 21-3) nor hyperextensible joints are a prominent feature of vascular EDS, and consequently the diagnosis is often overlooked until after a vascular complication occurs. Cerebrovascular complications include arterial dissection, intracranial aneurysm (Figure 17-7), and carotid-cavernous fistula.[121] The probability of vascular complications increases with increasing age.[117,121] In one report of 220 individuals with vascular EDS, for example, one or more vascular complications had occurred in a quarter of the patients by age 25, but by age 40 over three-quarters of the patients had developed a vascular complication.[117]

Intracranial aneurysms due to vascular EDS (see Chapter 18) most often develop in the internal carotid artery within the cavernous sinus or just as it emerges from the cavernous sinus (Figure 17-7).[116,122,123] Rupture of an intracavernous aneurysm within the cavernous sinus creates a carotid-cavernous fistula.[124–127] Occasional individuals with bilateral carotid-cavernous fistulae due to vascular EDS have been documented. At autopsy portions of the carotid wall were fibrotic and the internal elastic membrane was fragmented.[128]

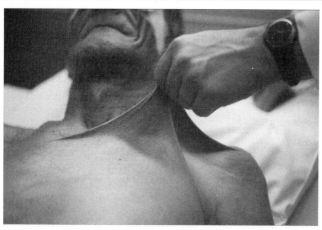

Figure 21-3. Hyperelastic skin is not characteristic of the vascular subtype (type IV) of Ehlers-Danlos syndrome, the only subtype that frequently causes vascular complications. Reprinted with permission from Roach and Riela.[256]

Arterial dissection (see Chapter 14) due to vascular EDS can affect any of the intracranial or extracranial arteries. Aortic dissection can secondarily occlude cervical vessels, and cerebral infarction distal to carotid dissection has been documented.[129,130] One patient with a vertebral dissection developed a painful, pulsatile mass of the neck.[131]

The complication rate for catheter angiography or endovascular procedures is 47% to 67% with an associated mortality rate of 6% to 17%.[121,125,132–134] Consequently, magnetic resonance angiography or CT angiography is preferable to catheter angiography in these patients.

Management of Vascular EDS

Treatment of the vascular lesions of EDS is problematic. The arteries do not hold sutures well, and tissue manipulation during either surgery or endovascular procedures often results in tears or separation of the arterial layers.[118,135,136] Despite these concerns, endovascular procedures are probably the best way to treat both arterial aneurysms and carotid-cavernous fistulae due to EDS.[125,137–141] A transvenous approach may be preferable in some patients with a carotid-cavernous fistula,[127,142] and others may require "trapping" of the fistula by occlusion of the carotid artery proximal and distal to the fistula.

MARFAN SYNDROME

Marfan syndrome is inherited as an autosomal dominant trait and results from a mutation of the fibrillin-1 (*FBN1*) gene on chromosome 15q21.1.[143–145] Fibrillin is a large extracellular matrix glycoprotein that is found in microfibrils, which, in turn, are abnormal in individuals with Marfan syndrome. New mutations are responsible for about a fourth of the patients.

Phenotypic variability is typical even among affected members of the same family. Marfan syndrome primarily affects the cardiovascular system, the skeletal system (e.g., scoliosis, anterior chest deformity, increased height, long digits and limbs, and joint laxity), and the eye (e.g., lens dislocation, myopia, and corneal anomalies). Vascular abnormalities include mitral valve prolapse, dilatation of the aortic root, and mitral or aortic

regurgitation. The most serious vascular complication is rupture of an aortic aneurysm. The life expectancy of individuals with Marfan syndrome has increased in recent years because of improved surgical and medical therapy of cardiovascular disease and the increased diagnosis of milder cases.[146]

Although intracranial aneurysms have been documented in Marfan syndrome patients, a survey of 135 individuals with Marfan syndrome identified no one with an intracranial aneurysm.[147] When intracranial aneurysms occur in individuals with Marfan syndrome, they tend to affect the intracranial internal carotid artery more often than its distal branches.[148–150]

Ischemia occurs more often than intracranial aneurysm or hemorrhage in people with Marfan syndrome. In one summary of 513 Marfan patients, 18 individuals (3.5%) developed neurovascular complications.[151] Three of these 18 individuals had an intracranial hemorrhage, but in two cases the bleeding was attributed to chronic anticoagulation. In contrast, 11 patients had TIAs, two had a cerebral infarction, and another had a cord infarction. Cardiac emboli were responsible for most instances of brain ischemia.[152]

PSEUDOXANTHOMA ELASTICUM

Pseudoxanthoma elasticum (PXE) is a disorder characterized by deterioration and calcification of elastic fibers resulting in dermatologic, ophthalmologic, and vascular dysfunction.[153–155] PXE is an autosomal recessive condition, although heterozygotes can manifest some features of the disorder.[155] It results from a mutation of the *ABCC6* gene on chromosome 16p13.1 that codes for a transmembrane transporter protein of the ATP-binding ABC family.[156,157]

Clinical Features of PXE

Yellowish plaques or papules of the lateral neck, antecubital fossae, axillae, groin, and or popliteal areas are characteristic of PXE (Figure 21-4).[158] Angioid streaks in the ocular fundus result from ruptures of Bruch's membrane, and retinal hemorrhages are common (Figure 21-5).[159] Although angioid streaks occur in about 85% of patients with PXE, they also occur with Paget disease of bone, sickle cell anemia, and Marfan syndrome.[158,160] Retinal hemorrhages are common after the fourth decade and can arise spontaneously or in response to minor trauma. Gradual occlusion of the large peripheral arteries may cause intermittent claudication, especially in the extremities.[158] Affected arteries are at times palpably rigid and can become calcified.[161] Gastrointestinal hemorrhage is relatively common in individuals with PXE.

Cerebrovascular complications due to PXE become more common with increasing age. Vascular compromise can result directly from progressive occlusion or acute rupture of a cervicocephalic artery or indirectly from systemic hypertension or cardiovascular disease.[162] The angiographic pattern of PXE mimics that of severe atherosclerosis, with vascular stenosis, occlusion, and tortuosity especially in the internal carotid or vertebral arteries.[163,164] Carotid occlusion with extensive collateral circulation is angiographically similar to moyamoya syndrome.[165]

Intracranial aneurysms are not common in individuals with PXE but usually affect the intracranial portion of the carotid artery.[162,166] Arterial aneurysms are suspected to arise because of the abnormal elastic lamina in PXE.[167]

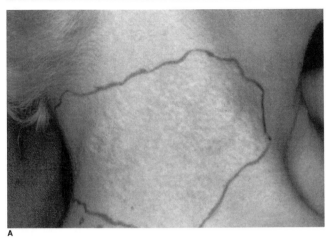
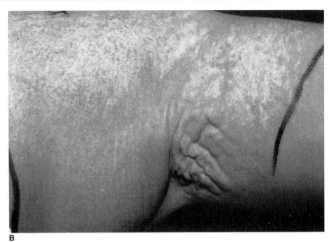

Figure 21-4. A: Characteristic cutaneous appearance of PXE on the neck of an individual with PXE (outlined in red). B: Redundant skin folds in the axilla due to PXE. Reprinted with permission from Neldner and Roach.[257]

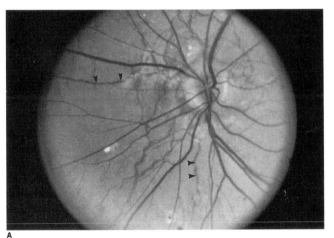
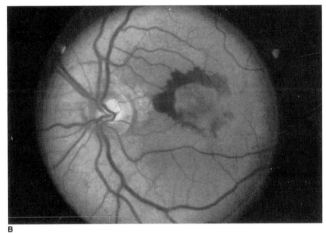

Figure 21-5. A: Angioid retinal streaks (*arrowheads*) due to PXE. B: Acute macular hemorrhage in another patient with PXE. Reprinted with permission from Neldner and Roach.[257]

Management of PXE

There is no fully effective treatment for PXE. Genetic counseling helps the patients and their families to make a more informed choice during family planning. A diet high in calcium may promote vascular dysfunction due to PXE, leading some to recommend restriction of dietary calcium in these individuals.[158] The patient should also avoid the use of tobacco, optimize the diet, and maintain a lifelong fitness regimen. Given the high risk of retinal hemorrhage, the patient should make every effort to avoid activities that might result in normally minor eye trauma. Aspirin and the nonsteroidal anti-inflammatory agents should be avoided if possible these agents could increase the likelihood of retinal and gastric hemorrhages. Surgery or endovascular procedures may be useful for some individuals with vascular complications.

NEUROFIBROMATOSIS

Various cerebrovascular lesions have been described in individuals with neurofibromatosis (NF) type 1, an autosomal dominant disorder caused by a mutation of the neurofibromin gene on chromosome 17.q11.2.[168] The most commonly mentioned cerebrovascular abnormality is moyamoya syndrome (see Chapter 13), but arterial stenosis, aneurysm, and arteriovenous malformations have been described.[169–172] Based on the number of reported patients, their age, and distribution of their vascular lesions, it seems likely that arterial stenosis, with or without the occurrence of moyamoya collateral vessels, occurs with greater than expected frequency in individuals with NF type 1.[169] In one series of 143 largely Caucasian individuals who underwent surgery for moyamoya, 16 (11%) had NF, but the incidence of cerebrovascular lesions in unselected individuals with NF has not been established.[173]

Why patients with NF develop vascular lesions is not well understood. Some individuals have added risk factors, most notably the earlier use of radiotherapy for a NF-related neoplasm.[174–176] Young age at the time of radiotherapy increases the risk of subsequent vasculopathy.[174] Hypertension due to pheochromocytoma or renal artery stenosis can add to the risk of stroke due to NF.[177,178] The genotype may influence the likelihood of vascular disease due to NF.[179,180]

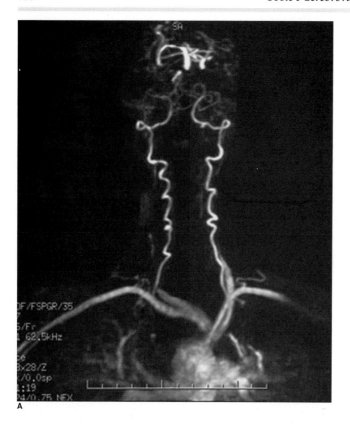

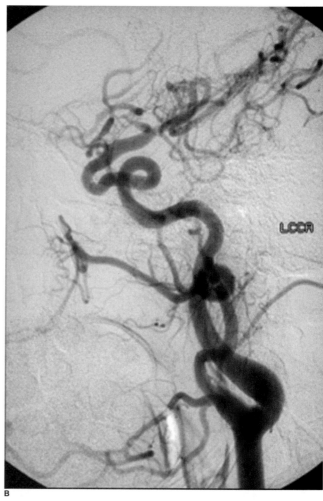

Figure 21-6. A: MRA shows severe tortuosity of both vertebral arteries in an individual with arterial tortuosity syndrome. B: Catheter angiography shows marked tortuosity of the left carotid artery in this same individual. Reprinted with permission from Cartwright et al.[183]

ARTERIAL TORTUOSITY SYNDROME

Treatment of vascular lesions in individuals with NF is identical to that offered to other patients with a similar lesion.[173]

Arterial tortuosity syndrome is a rare condition characterized by elongation, stenosis, and especially tortuosity (Figure 21-6) of the major arteries. Some patients also have joint and skin laxity, hernias, and arachnodactyly.[181] Several affected individuals are from the Mediterranean region.

Individuals with arterial tortuosity syndrome have disrupted arterial elastic fibers and fragmentation of the internal elastic membrane.[182] These histological findings, along with the arterial tortuosity and tissue laxity, suggest an as yet uncharacterized connective tissue disorder.[181]

Despite the striking arterial tortuosity and the elongation of their arteries, few individuals with this syndrome have a stroke.[183] Intuitively, disruption and fragmentation of the internal elastic membrane might promote either thrombosis or arterial dissection, but the process leading to the stroke is unknown.

The disorder is transmitted as an autosomal recessive trait, and recent studies have mapped the gene to chromosome 20q13.[184,185] The gene has not yet been cloned, and DNA testing is not available.

PROGERIA

The term *progeria* is derived from *pro*, before, and *geras*, old age. Progeria is sometimes called Hutchinson-Gilford syndrome in honor of Jonathan Hutchinson, who described this condition in 1886, and Hastings Gilford restudied Hutchinson's two patients and named the disorder progeria in 1904. Progeria is characterized by signs of premature aging and the early development of age-related complications.[186,187] By one estimate, 1 in 4 million to 8 million individuals develop progeria.[188]

Signs of aging typically begin in the first year or two of life, and invariably a premature death ensues.[189] Early features include impaired joint mobility, short stature, sparse subcutaneous fat, and alopecia (Figure 21-7). Later patients with progeria develop premature atherosclerosis, leading to angina, myocardial infarction, or stroke at an early age.[186] The cervical carotid and vertebral arteries are the first to become stenotic, but the large intracranial arteries may also be affected.[186,190–192] As with elderly patients, coronary artery disease, cardiac valvular dysfunction, congestive heart failure, arrhythmia, and systemic hypertension increase the stroke risk.[191,193–195] Survival into middle age has been documented but is rare.[196]

Progeria is caused by a mutation of the *LMNA* gene on chromosome 1q, resulting in truncation of the protein lamin A.[197,198]

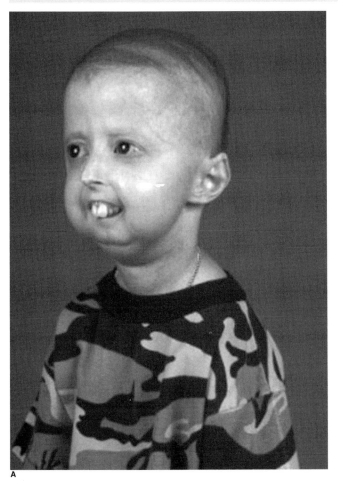
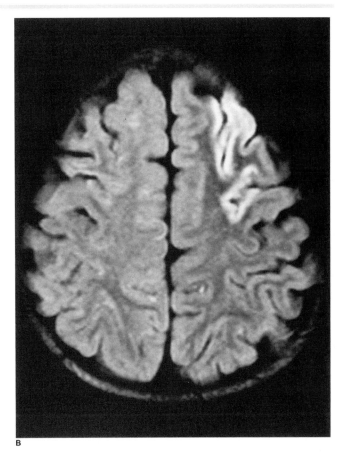

Figure 21-7. A: Physical characteristics of an individual with progeria at about 9 years of age. Note the aged appearance due to stooped shoulders, skin laxity, and alopecia. B: MRI shows a left frontal lobe infarction in this boy.

Few individuals with progeria reproduce, and consequently it usually results from a spontaneous mutation.[197] Milder phenotypes could result from somatic mosaicism. The *LMNA* mutation more often affects the paternally derived allele.[199,200] Occasional siblings who are homozygous for a *LMNA* mutation suggest the existence of an autosomal recessive form of progeria,[201] and other affected siblings result from germline mosaicism.[200]

WERNER SYNDROME

Werner syndrome is an autosomal recessive disorder that is sometimes called adult progeria, although it is now known that the two conditions result from two entirely different gene mutations. Individuals with Werner syndrome appear 20 to 30 years older than their actual age. Among other findings, they develop cataracts, early loss of hair color, senile macular degeneration, osteoporosis, diabetes, malignancies, and premature atherosclerosis.[202,203] Most patients develop a high-pitched voice because of various vocal cord abnormalities, adding further to the aura of senescence.

Unlike individuals with progeria, people with Werner syndrome often live well into adulthood, and death from cardiac disease and stroke occur less commonly than in individuals with progeria. Individuals with Werner syndrome have a higher frequency of various malignancies than patients with progeria.

The Werner syndrome gene (*WRN*) on the short arm of chromosome 8 encodes a DNA helicase.[204,205] The DNA helicase family unwinds double-stranded DNA, an important part of DNA replication, repair, and transcription.[204,206] A mutation of the Werner syndrome gene results in genomic instability, accounting for the frequency of neoplasia in this condition.

HEREDITARY HEMORRHAGIC TELANGIECTASIA

Hereditary hemorrhagic telangiectasia (HHT), or Osler-Weber-Rendu disease, is an autosomal dominant trait that occurs in one of 10,000 individuals. Four different HHT genes have been found: *HHT1* on chromosome 9q34.1, *HHT2* on chromosome 12q12-14, *HHT3* on chromosome 5q31, and *HHT4* on chromosome 7p14.[207–209] The gene products for *HHT1* and *HHT2*, endoglin and activin receptor-like kinase-1, are both transmembrane proteins of endothelial cells.

Clinical Features of HHT

The exceedingly variable phenotype of HHT includes telangiectasias of the skin and mucous membranes (Figure 21-8) along

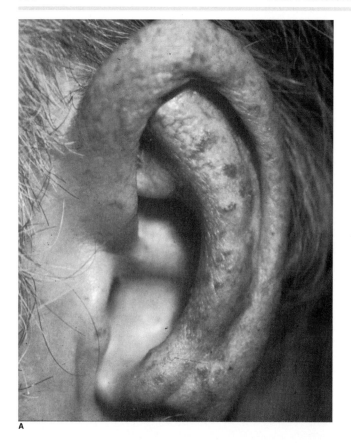

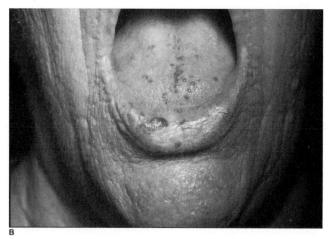

Figure 21-8. Cutaneous telangiectasias of the ear (A) and lips and tongue (B) due to hereditary hemorrhagic telangiectasia. Reprinted with permission from Dowling.[258]

with vascular malformations in various internal organs.[210–212] Based on the established clinical diagnostic criteria for HHT, a definite diagnosis requires three of four features: spontaneous recurrent epistaxis, telangiectasias in the typical locations for HHT, a visceral manifestation, and one or more affected first-degree relatives. Two of these four features are sufficient to justify a "suspected HHT" designation.[213]

Although HHT is highly penetrant, its findings may be subtle and sometimes do not become apparent until middle age.[214,215] Cutaneous telangiectasias most often occur on the face, lips, and hands. Intermittent epistaxis, due to telangiectasias of the nasal mucosa, occurs in 90% of HHT patients. Conjunctival telangiectasias occur in about a third of the individuals with HHT. One in 10 have retinal vascular malformations, although visual loss from these lesions is uncommon.[216] Vascular lesions of the lungs, intestines, or urinary system produce hemoptysis, hematemesis, melena, or hematuria, sometimes sufficiently severe to provoke anemia from iron deficiency.

In one literature review of 90 HHT patients with various neurologic complications, there were 17 arteriovenous malformations and 36 telangiectasias or angiomas.[217] However, when individuals with HHT are systematically studied with angiography, the number of people with an AVM increases substantially, although some of these remain symptom free.[218,219] Vascular lesions may occur anywhere in the brain or spinal cord and are sometimes multiple. Intracranial aneurysms have been documented in a few individuals with HHT, although their number is small enough to perhaps represent a chance occurrence.[217,220,221]

Ischemic stroke and transient ischemic attacks result from paradoxical embolism through pulmonary arteriovenous fistulae.[222] Ischemic lesions may occur more often than has been appreciated. About a third of the individuals with a large pulmonary arteriovenous malformation (AVM) have radiological evidence of stroke.[223,224] A transient neurological deficit during an episode of coughing and hemoptysis may be due to air embolism through a bleeding pulmonary arteriovenous fistula. An estimated 1% of the patients develop a brain abscess or meningitis after an infectious embolism bypasses the pulmonary circulation via a pulmonary arteriovenous fistula.[225,226] Up to half of the individuals with HHT have migraine with aura.[227]

Management of HHT

Individuals with chronic blood loss may require periodic transfusions or chronic iron therapy. Before undergoing dental procedures, HHT patients should be treated with prophylactic antibiotics to reduce the risk of brain abscess due to a pulmonary AVM.[228] Some physicians advocate prophylactic closure of pulmonary arteriovenous fistulae.

Given the risk of neurological and other complications, at-risk relatives should be screened for an HHT mutation.[229] Once a diagnosis of HHT has been established, it is reasonable also to screen for cerebral and pulmonary arteriovenous malformations. Screening studies need to be repeated at 5-year intervals or in response to specific clinical concerns. Catheter angiography may be helpful in individuals whose MRI is abnormal or those who have unexplained symptoms. Treatment of intracranial AVMs is reviewed in Chapter 19.

MELAS SYNDROME

Mitochondrial myopathy, encephalopathy, lactic acidosis, and stroke-like episodes (MELAS) is one of several multisystem disorders caused by mutations of mitochondrial DNA.[230] Mitochondrial disorders have overlapping clinical features, but the recognition of specific mutations has made classification easier.[231]

Clinical Features of MELAS

Clinical manifestations vary considerably from patient to patient, but the first signs and symptoms usually develop before adulthood.[232–235] Episodic vomiting, headache, seizures, proximal

Table 21-3: MELAS: Initial Clinical Features in 110 Patients

Initial Symptom or Sign[a]	Number	Percentage
Seizures	17	28
Recurrent headaches	17	28
Gastrointestinal symptoms (recurrent vomiting, anorexia)	15	25
Limb weakness	11	18
Short stature/stopped growth	11	18
Stroke	10	17
Altered consciousness	7	12
Impaired mentation	7	12
Hearing loss	6	10
Exercise intolerance	6	10
Visual symptom	5	8
Developmental delay	3	5
Fever	3	5
Abnormal gait	1	1

Adapted with permission from Hirano and Pavlakis.[236]

[a] Patients sometimes presented with more than one manifestation, and data were not available for all patients in every category.

muscle weakness, and recurrent episodes of focal neurological deficits are characteristic (Tables 21-3 and 21-4).[236] Recurrent neurologic deficits coincide with increasing dementia and worsening seizures, and death usually occurs in early to middle adulthood. Hirano and colleagues developed clinical diagnostic criteria for MELAS.[237]

Radiographic studies typically show multifocal infarctions of the cortex and subcortical regions with relative sparing of the deep white matter in a pattern that does not conform to the territory of a large named artery.[238] Some individuals also have calcifications in the basal ganglia. Catheter angiography is usually normal. Lactic acidosis occurs in most MELAS patients but may be intermittent, and myopathy with ragged-red fibers is variably present.[233,239,240]

Pathophysiology of MELAS

Cerebral atrophy, focal necrosis, and gliosis are present, and calcification is often noted in the vessels of the basal ganglia.[241–243] The mitochondria of the brain and other organs are increased in number and structurally abnormal. Abnormal mitochondria are also found within the smooth muscle and endothelium of small arteries and arterioles.[234,244–246]

The most common mutation in individuals with MELAS syndrome is a mitochondrial tRNA LEU(UUR) mutation. Ciafaloni and colleagues found this mutation in 21 of 23 MELAS patients.[247]

How MELAS causes stroke is not completely understood. Not all mitochondria have the MELAS mutation, and the proportion of abnormal mitochondria varies in different cells. Thus, areas of the brain with a higher proportion of abnormal

Table 21-4: Clinical Features of 110 Cases of MELAS

Sign/Symptom	Number Recorded[a]	Percentage Affected
Cardinal Manifestations		
Exercise intolerance	32/32	100
Onset before age 40	79/80	99
Stroke	106/107	99
Seizures	97/102	96
Ragged red fibers	92/98	95
Lactic acidosis	94/101	94
Frequent Manifestations		
Normal early development	56/62	90
Dementia	54/60	90
Limb weakness	58/65	89
Hemiparesis	57/69	83
Short stature	58/71	82
Hemianopsia	42/53	79
Headache	41/53	77
Nausea or vomiting	49/64	77
Onset before age 20	61/80	76
Hearing loss	46/61	75
Learning disability	28/47	60
CSF protein elevation	17/36	52
Other Manifestations		
Basal ganglia calcification	24/53	45
Family history	37/84	44
Myoclonus	27/72	38
Cerebellar signs	23/70	33
Episodic coma	9/44	20
Optic atrophy	8/41	20
Congestive heart failure	9/51	18
Pigmentary retinopathy	10/64	16
Wolff-Parkinson-White	6/43	14
PEO	9/68	13
Cardiac conduction block	3/47	6
Diabetes mellitus	2/27	8

Adapted with permission from Hirano and Pavlakis.[236]

[a] Data were not available for all patients in every category.
PEO = progressive external ophthalmoplegia.

mitochondria would have a greater risk of focal metabolic failure than other areas. A second hypothesis suggests that intermittent vasospasm caused by abnormal mitochondria within the arterial smooth muscle cells could explain the intermittent nature of the deficits and the generally normal arteriogram.

Management of MELAS

There is no effective therapy for MELAS. Seizures should be treated. One report suggested a benefit from riboflavin and nicotinamide, and others promoted coenzyme Q10 and with coenzyme Q10 plus idebenone.[243,248] However, the effectiveness of therapy is hard to gauge in part because of the variable and intermittent nature of the manifestations of MELAS.

MISCELLANEOUS CONDITIONS

Leigh syndrome (subacute necrotizing encephalomyelopathy) is a genetically heterogeneous condition that can accompany numerous different metabolic defects and be transmitted as an autosomal recessive, X-linked, or mitochondrial trait.[249,250] It typically presents in infancy or early childhood with loss of motor function, hypotonia, vomiting, irritability, seizures, apnea or hyperpnoea, external ophthalmoplegia, and stroke or stroke-like episodes. Neuroimaging studies show bilateral infarction and degeneration in the basal ganglia and brainstem.

Methylmalonic acidemia, propionic acidemia and isovaleric acidemia, and glutaric aciduria type I are autosomal recessive disorders of organic acid metabolism that cause "metabolic stroke." These conditions often develop lesions of the basal ganglia and present with acute extrapyramidal signs.[251–253] Strokes often take place during periods of dehydration or ketoacidosis. Cerebellar hemorrhage has rarely been described with methylmalonic, propionic, and isovaleric acidemia.[254]

Fanconi anemia, Down syndrome, and Turner syndrome may be risk factors for moyamoya syndrome (see Chapter 13).

REFERENCES

1. Ballabio E, Bersano A, Bresolin N, Candelise L. Monogenic vessel diseases related to ischemic stroke: a clinical approach. *J Cereb Blood Flow Metab*. 2007;**27**:1649–1662.
2. Dichgans M. Monogenic causes of stroke. *Int Psychogeriatr*. 2003;**15**(Suppl 1):15–22.
3. Razvi SS, Bone I. Single gene disorders causing ischaemic stroke. *J Neurol*. 2006;**253**:685–700.
4. Kiely DK, Wolf PA, Cupples LA, Beiser AS, Myers RH. Familial aggregation of stroke. The Framingham Study. *Stroke*. 1993;**24**:1366–1371.
5. Khaw KT, Barrett-Connor E. Family history of stroke as an independent predictor of ischemic heart disease in men and stroke in women. *Am J Epidemiol*. 1986;**123**:59–66.
6. Brass LM, Isaacsohn JL, Merikangas KR, Robinette CD. A study of twins and stroke. *Stroke*. 1992;**23**:221–223.
7. Alberts, MJ, ed. *Genetics of Cerebrovascular Disease*. New York: Futura; 2008.
8. Sebastiani P, Ramoni MF, Nolan V, Baldwin CTSMH. Genetic dissection and prognosis modeling of overt stroke in sickle cell. *Nat Genet*. 2005;**37**:435–440.
9. Svetkey LP, O'Riordan E, Conlon PJ, Emovon O. Genetics of hypertension. In: Alpers MJ, ed. *Genetics of Cerebrovascular Disease*. Armonk, NY: Futura; 2008:57–80.
10. Annest JL, Sing CF, Biron P, Mongeau JG. Familial aggregation of blood pressure and weight in adoptive families. II. Estimation of the relative contributions of genetic and common environmental factors to blood pressure correlations between family members. *Am J Epidemiol*. 1979;**110**:492–503.
11. McIlhany ML, Shaffer JW, Hines EA Jr. The heritability of blood pressure: an investigation of 200 pairs of twins using the cold pressor test. *Johns Hopkins Med J*. 1975;**136**:57–64.
12. DeGraba TJ. Genetics of atherosclerosis. In: Alpers MJ, ed. *Genetics of Cerebrovascular Disease*. Armonk, NY: Futura; 1999: 117–128.
13. van der Wal AC, Das PK, Tigges AJ, Becker AE. Adhesion molecules on the endothelium and mononuclear cells in human atherosclerotic lesions. *Am J Pathol*. 1992;**141**:1427–1433.
14. Poston RN, Haskard DO, Coucher JR, Gall NP, Johnson-Tidey RR. Expression of intercellular adhesion molecule-1 in atherosclerotic plaques. *Am J Pathol*. 1992;**140**:665–673.
15. Leung SY, Ng THK, Yuen ST, Lauder IJ, Ho FCS. Pattern of cerebral atherosclerosis in Hong Kong Chinese: severity in intracranial and extracranial vessels. *Stroke*. 1993;**24**:779–786.
16. Gorelick PB. Distribution of atherosclerotic cerebrovascular lesions. Effects of age, race, and sex. *Stroke*. 1993;**24**:I16–I19.
17. Inzitari D, Hachinski VC, Taylor DW, Barnett HJ. Racial differences in the anterior circulation in cerebrovascular disease. How much can be explained by risk factors? *Arch Neurol*. 1990; **47**:1080–1084.
18. van der Net JB, van Etten J, Yazdanpanah M, et al. Gene-load score of the renin-angiotensin-aldosterone system is associated with coronary heart disease in familial hypercholesterolaemia. *Eur Heart J*. 2008;**29**:1370–1376.
19. van der Net JB, Isaacs A, Dallinga-Thie GM, et al. Haplotype of the angiotensinogen gene is associated with coronary heart disease in familial hypercholesterolemia. *J Hypertens*. 2008;**26**: 462–467.
20. Sourander P, Walinder J. Hereditary multi-infarct dementia. Morphological and clinical studies of a new disease. *Acta Neuropathol (Berl)*. 1977;**39**:247–254.
21. Tournier-Lasserve E, Joutel A, Melki J, et al. Cerebral autosomal dominant arteriopathy with subcortical infarcts and leukoencephalopathy maps to chromosome 19q12. *Nat Genet*. 1993;**3**:256–259.
22. Arboleda-Velasquez JF, Rampal R, Fung E, et al. CADASIL mutations impair Notch3 glycosylation by Fringe. *Hum Mol Genet*. 2005;**14**:1631–1639.
23. Joutel A, Vahedi K, Corpechot C, et al. Strong clustering and stereotyped nature of Notch3 mutations in CADASIL patients. *Lancet*. 1997;**350**:1511–1515.
24. Nakamura T, Watanabe H, Hirayama M, et al. CADASIL with NOTCH3 S180C presenting anticipation of onset age and hallucinations. *J Neurol Sci*. 2005;**238**:87–91.
25. Razvi SS, Davidson R, Bone I, Muir KW. The prevalence of cerebral autosomal dominant arteriopathy with subcortical infarcts and leucoencephalopathy (CADASIL) in the west of Scotland. *J Neurol Neurosurg Psychiatry*. 2005;**76**:739–741.
26. Dichgans M, Mayer M, Uttner I, et al. The phenotypic spectrum of CASASIL: clinical findings in 102 cases. *Ann Neurol*. 1998; **44**:731–739.
27. Oberstein SAJL, van den Boom R, Middelkoop HAM, et al. Incipient CASASIL. *Arch Neurol*. 2003;**60**:707–712.
28. Golomb MR, Sokol DK, Walsh LE, Christensen CK, Garg BP. Recurrent hemiplegia, normal MRI, and NOTCH3 mutation in a 14-year-old: is this early CADASIL? *Neurology*. 2004;**62**: 2331–2332.
29. Ragoschke-Schumm A, Axer H, Fitzek C, et al. Intracerebral haemorrhage in CADASIL. *J Neurol Neurosurg Psychiatry*. 2005;**76**:1606–1607.
30. Maclean AV, Woods R, Alderson LM, et al. Spontaneous lobar haemorrhage in CADASIL. *J Neurol Neurosurg Psychiatry*. 2005; **76**:456–457.
31. Roine S, Poyhonen M, Timonen S, et al. Neurologic symptoms are common during gestation and puerperium in CADASIL. *Neurology*. 2005;**64**:1441–1443.
32. Santa Y, Uyama E, Chui DH, et al. Genetic, clinical and pathological studies of CADASIL in Japan: a partial contribution of

Notch3 mutations and implications of smooth muscle cell degeneration for the pathogenesis. *J Neurol Sci.* 2003;**212**: 79–84.

33. Dichgans M, Holtmannspotter M, Herzog J, Peters N, Bergmann M, Yousry TA. Cerebral microbleeds in CADASIL. A gradient-echo magnetic resonance imaging and autopsy study. *Stroke.* 2002;**33**:67–71.

34. Auer DP, Schirmer T, Heidenreich JO, Herzog J, Putz B, Dichgans M. Altered white and gray matter metabolism in CADASIL. A proton MR spectroscopy and 1H-MRSI study. *Neurology.* 2001;**56**:635–642.

35. Miao Q, Paloneva T, Tuominen S, et al. Fibrosis and stenosis of the long penetrating cerebral arteries: the cause of the white matter pathology in cerebral autosomal dominant arteriopathy with subcortical infarcts and leukoencephalopathy. *Brain Pathol.* 2004;**14**:358–364.

36. Schmidley JW, Beadle BA, Trigg L. Co-occurrence of CADASIL and isolated CNS angiitis. *Cerebrovasc Dis.* 2005;**19**:352–354.

37. Lacombe P, Oligo C, Domenga V, Tournier-Lasserve E, Joutel A. Impaired cerebral vasoreactivity in a transgenic mouse model of cerebral autosomal dominant arteriopathy with subcortical infarcts and leukoencephalopathy arteriopathy. *Stroke.* 2005;**36**: 1053–1058.

38. Gladstone JP, Dodick DW. Migraine and cerebral white matter lesions: when to suspect cerebral autosomal dominant arteriopathy with subcortical infarcts and leukoencephalopathy (CADASIL). *Neurologist.* 2005;**11**:19–29.

39. Peters N, Opherk C, Bergmann T, Castro M, Herzog J, Dichgans M. Spectrum of mutations in biopsy-proven CADASIL: implications for diagnostic strategies. *Arch Neurol.* 2005;**62**:1091–1094.

40. Bowler JV, Hachinski V. Progress in the genetics of cerebrovascular disease: inherited subcortical arteriopathies. *Stroke.* 1994; **25**:1696–1698.

41. Maeda S, Nakayama H, Isaka K, Aihara Y, Nemoto S. Familial unusual encephalopathy of Binswanger's type without hypertension. *Folia Psychiatr Neurol Jpn.* 1976;**30**:165–177.

42. Yokoi S, Nakayama H. Chronic progressive leukoencephalopathy with systemic arteriosclerosis in young adults. *Clin Neuropathol.* 1985;**4**:165–173.

43. Oide T, Nakayama H, Yanagawa S, Ito N, Ikeda S, Arima K. Extensive loss of arterial medial smooth muscle cells and mural extracellular matrix in cerebral autosomal recessive arteriopathy with subcortical infarcts and leukoencephalopathy (CARASIL). *Neuropathology.* 2008;**28**:132–142.

44. Yanagawa S, Ito N, Arima K, Ikeda S. Cerebral autosomal recessive arteriopathy with subcortical infarcts and leukoencephalopathy. *Neurology.* 2002;**58**:817–820.

45. Richards A, van den Maagdenberg AM, Jen JC, et al. C-terminal truncations in human 3′-5′ DNA exonuclease TREX1 cause autosomal dominant retinal vasculopathy with cerebral leukodystrophy. *Nat Genet.* 2007;**39**:1068–1070.

46. Jen J, Cohen AH, Yue Q, et al. Hereditary endotheliopathy with retinopathy, nephropathy, and stroke (HERNS). *Neurology.* 1997;**49**:1322–1330.

47. Ophoff RA, DeYoung J, Service SK, et al. Hereditary vascular retinopathy, cerebroretinal vasculopathy, and hereditary endotheliopathy with retinopathy, nephropathy, and stroke map to a single locus on chromosome 3p21.1-p21.3. *Am J Hum Genet.* 2001;**69**:447–453.

48. Kavanagh D, Spitzer D, Kothari PH, et al. New roles for the major human 3′-5′ exonuclease TREX1 in human disease. *Cell Cycle.* 2008;**7**:1718–1725.

49. Vahedi K, Massin P, Guichard JP, et al. Hereditary infantile hemiparesis, retinal arteriolar tortuosity, and leukoencephalopathy. *Neurology.* 2003;**60**:57–63.

50. Gutmann DH, Fischbeck KH, Sergott RC. Hereditary retinal vasculopathy with cerebral white matter lesions. *Am J Med Genet.* 1989;**34**:217–220.

51. Cohn AC, Kotschet K, Veitch A, Delatycki MB, McCombe MF. Novel ophthalmological features in hereditary endotheliopathy with retinopathy, nephropathy and stroke syndrome. *Clin Experiment Ophthalmol.* 2005;**33**:181–183.

52. Hottenga JJ, Vanmolkot KR, Kors EE, et al. The 3p21.1-p21.3 hereditary vascular retinopathy locus increases the risk for Raynaud's phenomenon and migraine. *Cephalalgia.* 2005;**25**: 1168–1172.

53. Brady RO, Gal AE, Bradley RM, Martensson E, Warshaw AL, Laster L. Enzymatic defect in Fabry's disease – ceramidetrihexosidase deficiency. *N Engl J Med.* 1967;**276**:1163–1167.

54. Kint JA. Fabry's disease: alpha-galactosidase deficiency. *Science.* 1970;**167**:1268–1269.

55. Meikle PJ, Hopwood JJ, Clague AE, Carey WF. Prevalence of lysosomal storage disorders. *J Am Med Assoc.* 1999;**281**: 249–254.

56. MacDermot KD, Holmes A, Minders AH. Anderson-Fabry disease: clinical manifestations and impact of disease in a cohort of 60 obligate carrier females. *J Med Genet.* 2001;**24**(Suppl 2):769–775.

57. Wilcox WR, Oliveira JP, Hopkin RJ, et al. Females with Fabry disease frequently have major organ involvement: lessons from the Fabry Registry. *Mol Genet Metab.* 2008;**93**:112–128.

58. Eng CM, Fletcher J, Wilcox WR, et al. Fabry disease: baseline medical characteristics of a cohort of 1765 males and females in the Fabry Registry. *J Inherit Metab Dis.* 2007;**30**:184–192.

59. Wallace HJ. Angiokeratoma corporis diffusum. *Br J Dermatol.* 1958;**70**:354–360.

60. MacDermot KD, Holmes A, Miners AH. Anderson-Fabry disease: clinical manifestations and impact of disease in a cohort of 98 hemizygous males. *J Med Genet.* 2001;**38**:750–760.

61. Weingeist TA, Blodi FC. Fabry's disease: ocular findings in a female carrier. *Archiv Ophthalmol.* 1971;**85**:169–176.

62. Hirano K, Murata K, Miyagawa A, et al. Histopathologic findings of cornea verticillata in a woman heterozygous for Fabry's disease. *Cornea.* 2001;**20**:233–236.

63. Nakao S, Kodama C, Takenaka T, et al. Fabry disease: detection of undiagnosed hemodialysis patients and identification of a "renal variant" phenotype. *Kidney Int.* 2003;**64**:801–807.

64. von Scheidt W, Eng CM, Fitzmaurice TF, et al. An atypical variant of Fabry's disease with manifestations confined to the myocardium. *N Engl J Med.* 1991;**324**:395–399.

65. Fisher EA, Desnick RJ, Gordon RE, Eng CM, Griepp R, Goldman ME. Fabry disease: an unusual cause of severe coronary disease in a young man. *Ann Intern Med.* 1992;**117**:221–223.

66. Ferrans VJ, Hibbs RG, Burda CD. The heart in Fabry's disease. *Am J Cardiol.* 1969;**24**:95–110.

67. Colucci WS, Lorell BH, Schoen FJ, Warhol MJ, Grossman W. Hypertrophic obstructive cardiomyopathy due to Fabry's disease. *N Engl J Med.* 1982;**307**:926–928.

68. Yoshitama T, Nakao S, Takenaka T, et al. Molecular, genetic, biochemical, and clinical studies in three families with cardiac Fabry's disease. *Am J Cardiol.* 2001;**87**:71–75.

69. Grewal RP. Stroke in Fabry's disease. *J Neurol.* 1994;**241**:153–156.

70. Wise D, Wallace HJ, Jellinek EH. Angiokeratoma corporis diffusum – a clinical study of eight affected families. *Quart J Med.* 1962;**31**:177–205.

71. Mitsias P, Levine SR. Cerebrovascular complications of Fabry's disease. *Ann Neurol.* 1996;**40**:8–17.

72. Morgan SH, Rudge P, Smith SJ, et al. The neurological manifestations of Anderson-Fabry disease (alpha-galactosidase deficiency): investigation of symptomatic and presymptomatic patients. *Q J Med.* 1990;**75**:491–507.

73. Crutchfield KE, Patronis NJ, Dambrosis JM, Banerjee TK, Barton NW, Schiffmann R. Quantitative analysis of cerebral vasculopathy in patients with Fabry disease. *Neurology*. 1998;**50**: 1746–1749.

74. Ohnishi A, Dyck PJ. Loss of small peripheral sensory neurons in Fabry disease. *Arch Neurol*. 1974;**31**:120–127.

75. Kocen RS, Thomas PK. Peripheral nerve involvement in Fabry's disease. *Arch Neurol*. 1970;**22**:81–88.

76. Kahn P. Anderson-Fabry disease: a histopathological study of three cases with observations on the mechanism of production of pain. *J Neurol Neurosurg Psychiatry*. 1973;**36**:1053–1062.

77. Rahman AN, Lindenberg R. The neuropathology of hereditary dystopic lipidosis. *Arch Neurol*. 1963;**9**:373–385.

78. Kleijer WJ, Hussaarts-Odijk LM, Sachs ES, Jahoda MJG, Niermeijer MF. Prenatal diagnosis of Fabry's disease by direct analysis of chorionic villi. *Prenat Diagn*. 1987;**7**:283–287.

79. Altarescu GM, Goldfarb LG, Park K-Y, et al. Identification of fifteen novel mutations and genotype-phenotype relationship in Fabry disease. *Clin Genet*. 2001;**60**:46–51.

80. Eng CM, Banikazemi M, Gordon RE, et al. A phase 1/2 clinical trial of enzyme replacement in Fabry disease: pharmacologic, substrate clearance, and safety studies. *Am J Human Genet*. 2001;**68**:711–722.

81. Eng CM, Guffon N, Wilcox WR. Safety and efficacy of recombinant human alpha-galactosidase A replacement therapy in Fabry's disease. *N Engl J Med*. 2001;**345**:9–16.

82. Schiffmann R, Kopp JB, Austin HA, et al. Enzyme replacement therapy in Fabry disease. A randomized controlled trial. *J Am Med Assoc*. 2001;**285**:2743–2749.

83. Frustaci A, Chimenti C, Ricci R, et al. Improvement in cardiac function in the cardiac variant of Fabry's disease with galactose-infusion therapy. *N Engl J Med*. 2001;**345**:25–32.

84. Taaffe A. Angiokeratoma corporis diffusum: the evolution of a disease entity. *Postgrad Med J*. 1977;**53**:78–81.

85. Visy JM, Le Coz P, Chadefaux B, et al. Homocystinuria due to 5,10-methylenetrahydrofolate reductase deficiency revealed by stroke in adult siblings. *Neurology*. 1991;**41**:1313–1315.

86. Schuh S, Rosenblatt DS, Cooper BA, et al. Homocystinuria and megaloblastic anemia responsive to vitamin B12 therapy. *N Engl J Med*. 1984;**310**:686–690.

87. Harker LA, Slichter SJ, Scott CR, Ross R. Homocystinemia – vascular injury and arterial thrombosis. *N Engl J Med*. 1974; **291**:537–543.

88. Schoonderwaldt HC, Boers GHJ, Cruysberg JRM, Schulte BPM, Slooff JL, Thijssen HOM. Neurologic manifestations of homocystinuria. *Clin Neurol Neurosurg*. 1981;**83**:153–162.

89. Cross HE, Jensen AD. Ocular manifestations in the Marfan syndrome and homocystinuria. *Am J Ophthalmol*. 1973;**75**:405–420.

90. Mudd SH, Skovby F, Levy HL, et al. The natural history of homocystinuria due to cystathionine B- synthase deficiency. *Am J Human Genet*. 1985;**37**:1–31.

91. Clarke R, Daley L, Robinson K, et al. Hyperhomocysteinemia: an independent risk factor for vascular disease. *N Engl J Med*. 1991;**324**:1149–1155.

92. Homocysteine and risk of ischemic heart disease and stroke: a meta-analysis. *JAMA*. 2002;**288**:2015–2022.

93. Selhub J, Jacques PF, Bostom AG, et al. Association between plasma homocysteine concentrations and extracranial carotid-artery stenosis. *N Engl J Med*. 1995;**332**:286–291.

94. Dudman NPB, Wilcken DEL, Wang J, Lynch JF, Macey D, Lundberg P. Disordered methionine/homocysteine metabolism in premature vascular disease. *Arterioscler Thromb*. 1993;**13**:1253–1260.

95. Boers GHJ, Smals AGH, Trijbels FJM, et al. Heterozygosity for homocystinuria in premature peripheral and cerebral occlusive arterial disease. *N Engl J Med*. 1985;**313**:709–715.

96. Brattstrom LE, Hardebo JE, Hultberg BL. Moderate homocysteinemia – a possible risk factor for arteriosclerotic cerebrovascular disease. *Stroke*. 1984;**15**:1012–1016.

97. Mereau-Richard C, Muller JP, Faivre E, Ardouin P, Rousseaux J. Total plasma homocysteine determination in subjects with premature cerebral vascular disease. *Clin Chem*. 1991;**37**:126.

98. Mudd SH, Havlik R, Levy HL, McKusick VA, Feinleib M. A study of cardiovascular risk in heterozygotes for homocystinuria. *Am J Human Genet*. 1981;**33**:883–893.

99. Gibson JB, Carson NAJ, Neill DW. Pathological findings in homocystinuria. *J Clin Pathol*. 1964;**17**:427–437.

100. Schimke RN, McKusich VA, Huang T, Pollack AD. Homocystinuria. *JAMA*. 1965;**193**:711–719.

101. McDonald L, Bray C, Field C, Love F, Davies B. Homocystinuria, thrombosis, and the blood-platelets. *Lancet*. 1964;**1**:745–746.

102. Harker LA, Ross R, Slichter SJ, Scott CR. Homocystine-induced arteriosclerosis. *J Clin Invest*. 1976;**58**:731–741.

103. McCully KS, Ragsdale BD. Production of arteriosclerosis by homocysteinemia. *Am J Pathol*. 1970;**61**:1–8.

104. McCully KS, Wilson RB. Homocysteine theory of atherosclerosis. *Atherosclerosis*. 1975;**22**:215–227.

105. Pyeritz RE. Homocystinuria. In: Beighton P, ed. *McKusick's Heritable Disorders of Connective Tissue*. 5th ed. St. Louis: Mosby Year Book; 1993:137–178.

106. Carey MC, Fennelly JJ, Fitzgerald O. Homocystinuria. II. Subnormal serum folate levels, increased folate clearance and effects of folic acid therapy. *Am J Med*. 1968;**45**:26–31.

107. Morrow G, Barnes LA. Combined vitamin responsiveness in homocystinuria. *J Pediatr*. 1972;**81**:945–954.

108. Ueland PM, Refsum H. Plasma homocysteine, a risk factor for vascular disease: plasma levels in health, disease, and drug therapy. *J Lab Clin Med*. 1989;**114**:473–501.

109. Jacques PF, Selhub J, Bostom AG, Wilson PW, Rosenberg IH. The effect of folic acid fortification on plasma folate and total homocysteine concentrations. *N Engl J Med*. 1999;**340**:1449–1454.

110. Toole JF, Malinow MR, Chambless LE, et al. Lowering homocysteine in patients with ischemic stroke to prevent recurrent stroke, myocardial infarction, and death: the Vitamin Intervention for Stroke Prevention (VISP) randomized controlled trial. *JAMA*. 2004;**291**:565–575.

111. Beighton P. The Ehlers-Danlos syndromes. In: Beighton P, ed. *Heritable Disorders of Connective Tissue*. 5th ed. St Louis: Mosby Year Book; 1993:189–251.

112. Byers PH. Ehlers-Danlos syndrome: recent advances and current understanding of the clinical and genetic heterogeneity. *J Invest Dermatol*. 1994;**103S**:47–52.

113. Watanabe A, Kosho T, Wada T, et al. Genetic aspects of the vascular type of Ehlers-Danlos syndrome (vEDS, EDSIV) in Japan. *Circ J*. 2007;**71**:261–265.

114. Germain DP, Herrera-Guzman Y. Vascular Ehlers-Danlos syndrome. *Ann Genet*. 2004;**47**:1–9.

115. Gilchrist D, Schwarze U, Shields K, MacLaren L, Bridge PJ, Byers PH. Large kindred with Ehlers-Danlos syndrome type IV due to a point mutation (G571S) in the COLA1 gene of type III procollagen: low risk of pregnancy complications and unexpected longevity in some affected relatives. *Am J Med Genet*. 1999;**82**:305–311.

116. North KN, Whiteman DAH, Pepin MG, Byers PH. Cerebrovascular complications in Ehlers-Danlos syndrome type IV. *Ann Neurol*. 1995;**38**(6):960–964.

117. Pepin M, Schwartze U, Superti-Furga A, Byers PH. Clinical and genetic features of Ehlers-Danlos syndrome type IV, the vascular type. *N Engl J Med*. 2000;**342**:673–680.

118. Cikrit DF, Glover JR, Dalsing MC, Silver D. The Ehlers-Danlos specter revisited. *Vasc Endovasc Surg*. 2002;**36**:213–217.

119. Kuivaniemi H, Prokop DJ, Wu Y, et al. Exclusion of mutations in the gene for type III collagen (COL3A1) as a common cause of intracranial aneurysms or cervical artery dissections: results from sequence analysis of the coding sequences of type III collagen from 55 unrelated patients. *Neurology*. 1993;**43**: 2652–2658.

120. Hamano K, Kuga T, Takahashi M, et al. The lack of type III collagen in a patient with aneurysms and an aortic dissection. *J Vasc Surg*. 1998;**28**:1104–1106.

121. Oderich GS, Panneton JM, Bower TC, et al. The spectrum of management and clinical outcome of Ehlers-Danlos syndrome type IV: a 30-year experience. *J Vasc Surg*. 2005;**42**:98–106.

122. Rubinstein MK, Cohen NH. Ehlers-Danlos syndrome associated with multiple intracranial aneurysms. *Neurology*. 1964;**14**: 125–132.

123. Schievink WI, Limburg M, Oorthuys JW, Fleury P, Pope FM. Cerebrovascular disease in Ehlers-Danlos syndrome type IV. *Stroke*. 1990;**21**:626–632.

124. Graf CJ. Spontaneous carotid-cavernous fistula. *Arch Neurol*. 1965;**13**:662–672.

125. Schievink WI, Piepgras DG, Earnest FIV, Gordon H. Spontaneous carotid-cavernous fistulae in Ehlers-Danlos syndrome type IV. *J Neurosurg*. 1991;**74**:991–998.

126. Pollock JS, Custer PL, Hart WM, Smith ME, Fitzpatrick MM. Ocular complications in Ehlers-Danlos syndrome type IV. *Arch Ophthalmol*. 1997;**115**:416–419.

127. Chuman H, Trobe JD, Petty EM, et al. Spontaneous direct carotid-cavernous fistula in Ehlers-Danlos syndrome type IV: two case reports and a review of the literature. *J Neuroophthalmol*. 2002;**22**:75–81.

128. Schoolman A, Kepes JJ. Bilateral spontaneous carotid-cavernous fistulae in Ehlers-Danlos syndrome. *J Neurosurg*. 1967;**26**: 82–86.

129. Hunter GC, Malone JM, Moore WS, Misiorowski DL, Chvapil M. Vascular manifestations in patients with Ehlers-Danlos syndrome. *Arch Surg*. 1982;**117**:495–498.

130. Pope FM, Narcisi P, Nicholls AC, Liberman M, Oorthuys JW. Clinical presentations of Ehlers-Danlos syndrome type IV. *Arch Dis Child*. 1988;**63**:1016–1025.

131. Edwards A, Taylor GW. Ehlers-Danlos syndrome with vertebral artery aneurysm. *Proc Roy Soc Med*. 1969;**62**:734–735.

132. Freeman RK, Swegle J, Sise MJ. The surgical complications of Ehlers-Danlos syndrome. *Am Surg*. 1996;**62**(10):869–873.

133. Cikrit DF, Miles JH, Silver D. Spontaneous arterial perforation: the Ehlers-Danlos specter. *J Vasc Surg*. 1987;**5**:248–255.

134. Horowitz MB, Purdy P, Valentine RJ, Morrill K. Remote vascular catastrophes after neurovascular interventional therapy for type 4 Ehlers-Danlos syndrome. *AJNR Am J Neuroradiol*. 2000;**21**: 974–976.

135. Sheiner NM, Miller N, Lachance C. Arterial complications of Ehlers-Danlos syndrome. *J Cardiovasc Surg*. 1985;**26**:291–296.

136. Driscoll SHM, Gomes AS, Machleder HI. Perforation of the superior vena cava: a complication of digital angiography in Ehlers-Danlos syndrome. *Am J Roentgenol*. 1984;**142**:1021–1022.

137. Halbach VV, Higashida RT, Dowd CF, Barnwell SL, Hieshima GB. Treatment of carotid-cavernous fistulas associated with Ehlers-Danlos syndrome. *Neurosurgery*. 1990;**26**:1021–1027.

138. Kashiwagi S, Tsuchida E, Goto K, et al. Balloon occlusion of a spontaneous carotid-cavernous fistula in Ehlers-Danlos syndrome type IV. *Surg Neurol*. 1993;**39**:187–190.

139. Foulodou P, de Kersaint-Gilly A, Pizzanelli J, Viarouge MP, Auffray-Calvier E. Ehlers-Danlos syndrome with a spontaneous caroticocavernous fistula occluded by detachable balloon: case report and review of literature. *Neurorad*. 1996;**38**:595–597.

140. Kanner AA, Maimin S, Rappaport ZH. Treatment of spontaneous carotid-cavernous fistula in Ehlers-Danlos syndrome by transvenous occlusion with Guglielmi detachable coils. Case report and review of the literature. *J Neurosurg*. 2000;**93**:689–692.

141. Desal HA, Toulgoat F, Raoul S, et al. Ehlers-Danlos syndrome type IV and recurrent carotid-cavernous fistula: review of the literature, endovascular approach, technique and difficulties. *Neuroradiology*. 2005;**47**:300–304.

142. Zimmerman CF, Batjer HH, Purdy P, Samson D, Kopitnik T, Carstens GJ. Ehlers-Danlos syndrome type IV: neuro-ophthalmic manifestations and management. *Ophthalmology*. 1994;**101S**:133.

143. Lee B, Godfrey M, Vitale E, et al. Linkage of Marfan syndrome and a phenotypically related disorder to two different fibrillin genes. *Nature*. 1991;**352**:330–334.

144. Magenis RE, Maslen CL, Smith L, Allen L, Sakai LY. Localization of the fibrillin (FBN) gene to chromosome 15, band q21.1. *Genomics*. 1991;**11**:346–351.

145. Dietz HC, Pyeritz RE, Hall BD, et al. The Marfan syndrome locus: confirmation of assignment to chromosome 15 and identification of tightly linked markers at 15q15-q21.3. *Genomics*. 1991;**9**:355–361.

146. Silverman DI, Burton KJ, Gray J, et al. Life expectancy in the Marfan syndrome. *Am J Cardiol*. 1995;**75**:157–160.

147. van den Berg JS, Limburg M, Hennekam RC. Is Marfan syndrome associated with symptomatic intracranial aneurysms? *Stroke*. 1996;**27**:10–12.

148. Hainsworth PJ, Mendelow AD. Giant intracranial aneurysm associated with Marfan's syndrome: a case report. *J Neurol Neurosurg Psychiatry*. 1991;**54**:471–472.

149. Matsuda M, Matsuda I, Handa H, Okamoto K. Intracavernous giant aneurysm associated with Marfan's syndrome. *Surg Neurol*. 1979;**12**:119–121.

150. Finney LH, Roberts TS, Anderson RE. Giant intracranial aneurysm associated with Marfan's syndrome. Case report. *J Neurosurg*. 1976;**45**:342–347.

151. Wityk RJ, Zanferrari C, Oppenheimer S. Neurovascular complications of Marfan syndrome. A retrospective, hospital-based study. *Stroke*. 2002;**33**:680–684.

152. Hypertension, hyperuricemia and iatrogenic disease. *Am J Med*. 1970;**49**:242–249.

153. Carlborg U, Ejrup B, Gronblad E, Lund F. Vascular studies in pseudoxanthoma elasticum and angioid streaks. *Acta Med Scand*. 1959;**166**(Suppl):1–68.

154. Viljoen D. Pseudoxanthoma elasticum. In: Beighton P, ed. *McKusick's Heritable Disorders of Connective Tissue*. 5th ed. St. Louis: Mosby Year Book; 1993:335–365.

155. Ringpfeil F, McGuigan K, Fuchsel L, et al. Pseudoxanthoma elasticum is a recessive disease characterized by compound heterozygosity. *J Invest Dermatol*. 2006;**126**:782–786.

156. Struk B, Cai L, Zach S, et al. Mutations of the gene encoding the transmembrane transporter protein ABC-C6 cause pseudoxanthoma elasticum. *J Mol Med*. 2000;**78**:282–286.

157. Ringpfeil F, Lebwohl MG, Christiano AM, Uitto J. Pseudoxanthoma elasticum: mutations in the MRP6 gene encoding a transmembrane ATP-binding cassette (ABC) transporter. *Proc Natl Acad Sci USA*. 2000;**97**:6001–6006.

158. Neldner KH. Pseudoxanthoma elasticum. *Clin Dermatol*. 1988; **6**:1–159.

159. Scheie HG, Hogan TF. Angioid streaks and generalized arterial disease. *Arch Ophthalmol*. 1957;**57**:855–868.

160. Lebwohl M, Halperin J, Phelps RG. Occult pseudoxanthoma elasticum in patients with premature cardiovascular disease. *N Engl J Med*. 1993;**329**:1237–1239.

161. Wahlqvist ML, Fox RM, Beech AM, Favilla I. Peripheral vascular disease as a mode of presentation of pseudoxanthoma elasticum. *Aust NZ J Med*. 1977;**7**:523–525.

162. Munyer TP, Margulis AR. Pseudoxanthoma elasticum with internal carotid artery aneurysm. *Am J Roentgenol*. 1981;**136**:1023–1029.

163. Prick JJG, Thijssen HOM. Radiodiagnostic signs in pseudoxanthoma elasticum generalisatum (dysgenesis elastofibrillaris mineralisans). *Clin Radiol*. 1977;**28**:549–554.

164. Rios-Montenegro EN, Behrens MM, Hoyt WF. Pseudoxanthoma elasticum. *Arch Neurol*. 1972;**26**:151–155.

165. Yasuhara T, Sugiu K, Kakishita M, Date I. Pseudoxanthoma elasticum with carotid rete mirabile. *Clin Neurol Neurosurg*. 2004;**106**:114–117.

166. Goto K. Involvement of central nervous system in pseudoxanthoma elasticum. *Folia Psychiatr Neurol Jpn*. 1975;**29**:263–277.

167. Iqbal A, Alter M, Lee SH. Pseudoxanthoma elasticum: a review of neurological complications. *Ann Neurol*. 1978;**4**:18–20.

168. Marchuk DA, Saulino AM, Tavakkol R, et al. cDNA cloning of the type 1 neurofibromatosis gene: complete sequence of the NF1 gene product. *Genomics*. 1991;**11**:931–940.

169. Oderich GS, Sullivan TM, Bower TC, et al. Vascular abnormalities in patients with neurofibromatosis syndrome type I: clinical spectrum, management, and results. *J Vasc Surg*. 2007;**46**: 475–484.

170. Rizzo JF, Lessell S. Cerebrovascular abnormalities in neurofibromatosis type 1. *Neurology*. 1994;**44**:1000–1002.

171. Tomsick BA, Lukin RR, Chambers AA, Benton C. Neurofibromatosis and intracranial arterial occlusive disease. *Neurorad*. 1976;**11**:229–234.

172. Woody RC, Perrot LJ, Beck SA. Neurofibromatosis cerebral vasculopathy in an infant: clinical, neuroradiographic, and neuropathic studies. *Pediatr Pathol*. 1992;**12**:613–619.

173. Scott RM, Smith JL, Robertson RL, Madsen JR, Soriano SG, Rockoff MA. Long-term outcome in children with moyamoya syndrome after cranial revascularization by pial synangiosis. *J Neurosurg*. 2004;**100**:142–149.

174. Grill J, Couanet D, Cappelli C, et al. Radiation-induced cerebral vasculopathy in children with neurofibromatosis and optic pathway glioma. *Ann Neurol*. 1999;**45**:393–396.

175. Kestle JRW, Hoffman HJ, Mock AR. Moyamoya phenomenon after radiation for optic glioma. *J Neurosurg*. 1993;**79**:32–35.

176. Edwards-Brown MK, Quets JP. Midwest experience with moyamoya disease. *Clin Neurol Neurosurg*. 1997;**99**(Suppl 2): S36–S38.

177. Pellock JM, Kleinman PK, McDonald BM, Wixson D. Childhood hypertensive stroke with neurofibromatosis. *Neurology*. 1980;**30**:656–659.

178. Holt JF. Neurofibromatosis in children. *Am J Roentgenol*. 1978;**130**:615–639.

179. Tang SC, Lee MJ, Jeng JS, Yip PK. Novel mutation of neurofibromatosis type 1 in a patient with cerebral vasculopathy and fatal ischemic stroke. *J Neurol Sci*. 2006;**243**:53–55.

180. Yamauchi T, Tada M, Houkin K, et al. Linkage of familial moyamoya disease (spontaneous occlusion of teh circle of Willis) to chromosome 17q25. *Stroke*. 2000;**31**:930–935.

181. Wessels MW, Catsman-Berrevoets CE, Mancini GM, et al. Three new families with arterial tortuosity syndrome. *Am J Med Genet A*. 2004;**131**:134–143.

182. Pletcher BA, Fox JE, Boxer RA, et al. Four sibs with arterial tortuosity: description and review of the literature. *Am J Med Genet*. 1996;**66**:121–128.

183. Cartwright MS, Hickling WH, Roach ES. Ischemic stroke in an adolescent with arterial tortuosity syndrome. *Neurology*. 2006; **67**:360–361.

184. Engel DG, Gospe SM Jr, Tracy KA, Ellis WG, Lie JT. Fatal infantile polyarteritis nodosa with predominant central nervous system involvement. *Stroke*. 1995;**26**:699–701.

185. Zaidi SH, Peltekova V, Meyer S, et al. A family exhibiting arterial tortuosity syndrome displays homozygosity for markers in the arterial tortuosity locus at chromosome 20q13. *Clin Genet*. 2005;**67**:183–188.

186. Wagle WA, Haller JS, Cousins JP. Cerebral infarction in progeria. *Pediatr Neurol*. 1992;**8**:476–477.

187. Hofer AC, Tran RT, Aziz OZ, et al. Shared phenotypes among segmental progeroid syndromes suggest underlying pathways of aging. *J Gerontol A Biol Sci Med Sci*. 2005;**60**:10–20.

188. DeBusk FL. The Hutchinson-Gilford progeria syndrome. Report of 4 cases and review of the literature. *J Pediatr*. 1972;**80**: 697–724.

189. Sarkar, PK, Shinton, RA. Hutchinson-Gilford progeria syndrome. *Postgrad Med J*. 2001;**77**:312–317.

190. Rosman PN, Anslem I. Progressive intracranial vascular disease with strokes and seizures in a boy with progeria. *J Child Neurol*. 2000;**16**:212–215.

191. Dyck JD, David TE, Burke B, Webb GD, Henderson MA, Fowler RS. Management of coronary artery disease in Hutchinson-Gilford syndrome. *J Pediatr*. 1987;**111**:407–410.

192. Smith AS, Wiznitzer M, Karaman BA, Horwitz SJ, Lanzieri CF. MRA detection of vascular occlusion in a child with progeria. *AJNR Am J Neuroradiol*. 1993;**14**:441–443.

193. Gabr M, Hashem N, Hashem M, Fahmi A, Safouh M. Progeria, a pathologic study. *J Pediatr*. 1960;**57**:70–77.

194. Nair K, Ramachandran P, Krishnamoorthy KM, Dora S, Achuthan TJ. Hutchinson-Gilford progeria syndrome with severe calcific aortic valve stenosis and calcific mitral valve. *J Heart Valve Dis*. 2004;**13**:866–869.

195. Matsuo S, Takeuchi Y, Hayashi S, Kinugasa A, Sawada T. Patient with unusual Hutchinson-Gilford syndrome (progeria). *Pediatr Neurol*. 1994;**10**:237–240.

196. Ogihara T, Hata T, Tanaka K, Fukuchi K, Tabuchi Y, Kamahara Y. Hutchinson-Gilford progeria syndrome in a 45 year-old man. *Am J Med*. 1986;**81**:135–138.

197. Eriksson M, Brown WT, Gordon LB, et al. Recurrent de novo point mutations in human lamin A cause Hutchinson-Gilford progeria syndrome. *Nature*. 2003;**423**:293–298.

198. Csoka AB, Cao H, Sammak PJ, Constantinescu D, Schatten GP, Hegele RA. Novel lamin A/C gene (LMNA) mutations in atypical progeroid syndromes. *J Med Genet*. 2004;**41**:304–308.

199. D'Apice MR, Tenconi R, Mammi I, van den Ende, J, Novelli G. Paternal origin of LMNA mutations in Hutchinson-Gilford progeria. *Clin Genet*. 2004;**65**:52–54.

200. Wuyts W, Biervliet M, Reyniers E, D'Apice MR, Novelli G, Storm K. Somatic and gonadal mosaicism in Hutchinson-Gilford progeria. *Am J Med Genet A*. 2005;**135**:66–68.

201. Plasilova M, Chattopadhyay C, Pal P, et al. Homozygous missense mutation in the lamin A/C gene causes autosomal recessive Hutchinson-Gilford progeria syndrome. *J Med Genet*. 2004; **41**:609–614.

202. Epstein CJ, Martin GM, Schultz AL, Motulsky AG. Werner syndrome. A review of its symptomatology, pathologic features, genetics and relationship to the natural aging process. *Medicine*. 1966;**45**:177–221.

203. Perloff JK, Phelps ET. A review of Werner's syndrome with a report of the second autopsied case. *Ann Intern Med*. 1958;**48**: 1205–1220.

204. Gray MD, Shen J-C, Kamath-Loeb AS, et al. The Werner syndrome protein is a DNA helicase. *Nat Genet*. 1997;**17**: 100–103.

205. Ichikawa K, Yamabe Y, Imamura O, et al. Cloning and characterization of a novel gene, WS-3, in human chromosome 8p11-p12. *Gene*. 1997;**189**:277–287.

206. Huang S, Baomin L, Gray MD, Oshima J, Saira M, Campisi J. The premature ageing syndrome protein, WRN, is a 3′–> 5′ exonuclease. *Nat Genet.* 1998;**20**:114–116.

207. McAllister KA, Grogg KM, Johnson DW. Endoglin, a TFG-B binding protein for endothelial cells, is the gene for hereditary hemorrhagic telangiectasia type 1. *Nat Genet.* 1994;**8**:345–351.

208. Johnson DW, Berg JN, Baldwin MA, et al. Mutations in the activin receptor-like kinase 1 gene in hereditary haemorrhagic telangiectasia type 2. *Nat Genet.* 1996;**13**:189–195.

209. Bayrak-Toydemir P, McDonald J, Akarsu N, et al. A fourth locus for hereditary hemorrhagic telangiectasia maps to chromosome 7. *Am J Med Genet A.* 2006;**140**:2155–2162.

210. Reilly PJ, Nostrant TT. Clinical manifestations of hereditary hemorrhagic telangiectasia. *Am J Gastroenterol.* 1984;**79**:363–367.

211. McCue CM, Hartenberg M, Nance WE. Pulmonary arteriovenous malformations related to Rendu-Osler-Weber syndrome. *Am J Med Genet.* 1984;**19**:19–27.

212. Bean WB. Congenital and hereditary lesions and birthmarks. In: *Vascular Spiders and Related Lesions of the Skin.* Springfield, IL: Charles C. Thomas; 1958:132–194.

213. Shovlin CL, Guttmacher AE, Buscarini E, et al. Diagnostic criteria for hereditary hemorrhagic telangiectasia (Rendu-Osler-Weber syndrome). *Am J Med Genet.* 2000;**91**:66–67.

214. Bird RM, Hammarsten JF, Marshall RA, Robinson RR. A family reunion: a study of hereditary hemorrhagic telangiectasia. *N Engl J Med.* 1957;**257**:105–109.

215. Plauchu H, de Chadarevian JP, Bideau A, Robert JM. Age-related clinical profile of hereditary hemorrhagic telangiectasia in an epidemiologically recruited population. *Am J Med Genet.* 1989;**32**:291–297.

216. Brant AM, Schachat AP, White RI. Ocular manifestations in hereditary hemorrhagic telangiectasia (Rendu-Osler-Weber disease). *Am J Ophthalmol.* 1989;**107**:642–646.

217. Roman G, Fisher M, Perl DP, Poser CM. Neurological manifestations of hereditary hemorrhagic telangiectasia (Rendu-Osler-Weber disease): report of 2 cases and review of the literature. *Ann Neurol.* 1978;**4**:130–144.

218. Fulbright RK, Chaloupka JC, Putman CM, et al. MR of hereditary hemorrhagic telangiectasia: prevalence and spectrum of cerebrovascular malformations. *AJNR Am J Neuroradiol.* 1998; **19**:477–484.

219. Sobel D, Norman D. CNS manifestations of hereditary hemorrhagic telangiectasia. *AJNR Am J Neuroradiol.* 1984;**5**:569–573.

220. Grollmus J, Hoff J. Multiple aneurysms associated with Osler-Weber-Rendu disease. *Surg Neurol.* 1973;**1**:91–93.

221. Fisher M, Zito JL. Focal cerebral ischemia distal to a cerebral aneurysm in hereditary hemorrhagic telangiectasia. *Stroke.* 1983;**14**:419–421.

222. Sisel RJ, Parker BM, Bahl OP. Cerebral symptoms in pulmonary arteriovenous fistula: a result of paradoxical emboli? *Circulation.* 1970;**41**:123–128.

223. White RI Jr, Lynch-Nyhan A, Terry P, et al. Pulmonary arteriovenous malformations: techniques and long-term outcome of embolotherapy. *Radiology.* 1988;**169**:663–669.

224. Lee DW, White RI Jr, Egglin TK, et al. Embolotherapy of large pulmonary arteriovenous malformations: long-term results. *Ann Thorac Surg.* 1997;**64**:930–939.

225. Berg JN, Guttmacher AE, Marchuk DA, Porteous MEM. Clinical heterogeneity in hereditary hemorrhagic telangiectasia: are pulmonary arteriovenous malformations more common in families linked to endoglin? *J Med Genet.* 1996;**33**:256–257.

226. Press OW, Ramsey PG. Central nervous system infections associated with hereditary hemorrhagic telangiectasia. *Am J Med.* 1984;**77**:86–92.

227. Steele JG, Nath PU, Burn J, Porteous ME. An association between migrainous aura and hereditary haemorrhagic telangiectasia. *Headache.* 1993;**33**:145–148.

228. Dajani AS, Taubert KA, Wilson W, et al. Prevention of bacterial endocarditis. Recommendations by the American Heart Association. *JAMA.* 1997;**277**:1794–1801.

229. Bayrak-Toydemir P, Mao R, Lewin S, McDonald J. Hereditary hemorrhagic telangiectasia: an overview of diagnosis and management in the molecular era for clinicians. *Genet Med.* 2004; **6**:175–191.

230. Pavlakis SG, Phillips PC, DiMauro S, DeVivo DC, Rowland LP. Mitochondrial myopathy, encephalopathy, lactic acidosis, and stroke-like episodes: a distinctive clinical syndrome. *Ann Neurol.* 1984;**16**:481–488.

231. DiMauro S, Moraes CT, Schon EA. Mitochondrial encephalopathies: problems of classification. In: Sato T, DiMauro S, eds. *Mitochondrial Encephalopathies.* New York: Raven Press; 1991: 113–127.

232. Inui K, Fukushima H, Tsukamoto H, et al. Mitochondrial encephalomyopathies with the mutation of the mitochondrial tRNA(Leu(UUR)) gene. *J Pediatr.* 1992;**120**:62–66.

233. Nicoll JA, Moss TH, Love S, Campbell MJ, Schutt WH. Clinical and autopsy findings in two cases of MELAS presenting with stroke-like episodes but without clinical myopathy. *Clin Neuropath.* 1993;**12**:38–43.

234. Forster C, Hubner G, Muller-Hocker J, et al. Mitochondrial angiopathy in a family with MELAS. *Neuropediatrics.* 1992;**23**: 165–168.

235. Fujii T, Okuno T, Ito M, et al. MELAS of infantile onset: mitochondrial angiopathy or cytopathy? *J Neurolog Sci.* 1991;**103**:37–41.

236. Hirano M, Pavlakis SG. Mitochondrial myopathy, encephalopathy, lactic acidosis, and strokelike episodes (MELAS): current concepts. *J Child Neurol.* 1994;**9**:4–13.

237. Hirano M, Ricci E, Koenigsberger MR, et al. MELAS: An original case and clinical criteria for diagnosis. *Neuromusc Disord.* 1992; **2**:125–135.

238. Matthews PM, Tampieri D, Berkovic SF, et al. Magnetic resonance imaging shows specific abnormalities in the MELAS syndrome. *Neurology.* 1991;**41**:1043–1046.

239. Shapira Y, Cederbaum SD, Cancilla PA, Nielsen D, Lippe BM. Familial poliodystrophy, mitochondrial myopathy, and lactate acidemia. *Neurology.* 1975;**25**:614–621.

240. Hart ZH, Chang CH, Perrin EVD, Neerunjun JS, Ayyar R. Familial poliodystrophy, mitochondrial myopathy, and lactate acidemia. *Arch Neurol.* 1977;**34**:180–185.

241. Fujii T, Okuno T, Ito M, et al. CT, MRI, and autopsy findings in brain of a patient with MELAS. *Pediatr Neurol.* 1990;**6**:253–256.

242. Ban S, Mori N, Saito K, Mizukami K, Suzuki T, Shiraishi H. An autopsy case of mitochondrial encephalopathy (MELAS) with special reference to extra-neuromuscular abnormalities. *Acta Pathol Jpn.* 1992;**42**:818–825.

243. Ihara Y, Namba R, Kuroda S, Sato T, Shirabe T. Mitochondrial encephalomyopathy (MELAS): pathological study and successful therapy with coenzyme Q10 and idebenone. *J Neurolog Sci.* 1989;**90**:263–271.

244. Yoneda M, Tanaka M, Nishikimi M, et al. Pleiotropic molecular defects in energy-transducing complexes in mitochondrial encephalomyopathy (MELAS). *J Neurolog Sci.* 1989;**92**:143–158.

245. Mizukami K, Sasaki M, Suzuki T, et al. Central nervous system changes in mitochondrial encephalopathy: light and electron microscopic study. *Acta Neuropathol.* 1992;**83**:449–452.

246. Ohama E, Ohara S, Ikuta F, Tanaka K, Nishizawa M. Mitochondrial angiopathy in cerebral blood vessels of mitochondrial encephalomyopathy. *Acta Neuropathol.* 1987;**74**:226–233.

247. Ciafaloni E, Ricci E, Shanske S, et al. MELAS: Clinical features, biochemistry, and molecular genetics. *Ann Neurol.* 1992;**31**:391–398.

248. Penn AMW, Lee JWK, Thuillier P, et al. MELAS syndrome with mitochondrial tRNA Leu(UUR) mutation: correlation of clinical state, nerve conduction, and muscle 31P magnetic resonance spectroscopy during treatment with nicotinamide and riboflavin. *Neurology.* 1992;**42**:2147–2152.

249. Yamashita S, Nishino I, Nonaka I, Goto Y. Genotype and phenotype analyses in 136 patients with single large-scale mitochondrial DNA deletions. *J Hum Genet.* 2008;**53**:598–606.

250. DiMauro S, Schon EA. Mitochondrial respiratory-chain diseases. *N Engl J Med.* 2003;**348**:2656–2668.

251. Korf B, Wallman JK, Levy HL. Bilateral lucency of the globus pallidus complicating methylmalonic acidemia. *Ann Neurol.* 1986;**20**:364–366.

252. Heidenreich R, Natowicz M, Hainline BE, et al. Acute extrapyramidal syndrome in methylmalonic acidemia: "metabolic stroke" involving the globus pallidus. *J Pediatr.* 1988;**113**:1022–1027.

253. Santos CC, Roach ES. Glutaric aciduria type I: a neuroimaging diagnosis? *J Child Neurol.* 2005;**20**:588–590.

254. Fischer AQ, Challa VR, Burton BK, McLean WT. Cerebellar hemorrhage complicating isovaleric acidemia: a case report. *Neurology.* 1981;**31**:746–748.

255. Miller VS, Roach ES. Neurocutaneous syndromes. In: Bradley WG, Daroff RB, Fenichel GM, Marsden CD, eds. *Neurology in Clinical Practice.* 3rd ed. Boston: Butterworth-Heinemann; 2000:1666–1700.

256. Roach ES, Riela AR. *Pediatric Cerebrovascular Disorders.* 2nd ed. New York: Futura; 1995.

257. Neldner KH, Roach ES. Pseudoxanthoma elasticum. In: Roach ES, Miller VS, eds. *Neurocutaneous Disorders.* Cambridge, England: Cambridge University Press; 2004:138–143.

258. Dowling MM. Hereditary hemorrhagic telangectasia (Osler-Weber-Rendu syndrome). In: Roach ES, Miler VS, eds. *Neurocutaneous Disorders.* Cambridge, England: Cambridge University Press; 2004:159–165.

22

Stroke in Children

Hemiplegia of sudden onset is not uncommon in children, especially in young children. There is considerable difference of opinion as to the exact pathological condition on which it usually depends, and it is probable that the cause is not always the same. Hence it is convenient to give a brief account of the condition as a clinical variety of disease. It is probably not a distinct pathological variety.

William R. Gowers

Cerebrovascular disorders are recognized more often in children now than in previous years, in part because of increased awareness of childhood stroke by clinicians and also because of widespread use of noninvasive neuroradiological techniques. Children have a different array of stroke risk factors than adults, although the stroke risk factors of children overlap those of young adults to a considerable degree.[1] Congenital heart disease and sickle cell disease, for example, are common causes of ischemic stroke in children, whereas stroke related to atherosclerosis and arterial hypertension is rare in children. The most common cause of nontraumatic intraparenchymal brain hemorrhage in children is arteriovenous malformation (AVM), whereas hemorrhage due to hypertension is uncommon in children.[2,3]

The stroke type and clinical presentation also vary with age. In adults, about 85% of strokes are ischemic and the remaining 15% are hemorrhagic. The proportion of hemorrhagic strokes increases in younger patients, so that spontaneous intracerebral hemorrhage (ICH) accounts for almost half of stroke cases in young adults and up to two thirds of the cases in children.

The clinical manifestations of stroke in children are often similar to those seen in adults, but children have distinctive features. The exact presentation in children depends on the patient's age, the nature of any underlying condition, the location of the lesion, and the type of lesion. Many of the acquired and genetic conditions that cause stroke in children also occur in adults and are considered in other chapters. This chapter focuses on the clinical manifestations and stroke risk factors that are unique to children.[4]

INCIDENCE OF STROKE IN CHILDREN

Schoenberg and colleagues tabulated the incidence of childhood cerebrovascular disease in Rochester, Minnesota, from 1965 through 1974. Excluding strokes related to birth, intracranial infection, and trauma, they identified three hemorrhagic strokes and one ischemic stroke in an at-risk population of 15,834, for an estimated annual incidence rate of 2.52/100,000 children/year for children 14 years of age or younger (1.89/100,000/year for hemorrhagic stroke and 0.63/100,000/year for ischemic stroke). In this population, hemorrhage occurred more often than infarction, whereas in the Mayo Clinic referral population, ischemic strokes were more common.[5] Several years later, Broderick and colleagues found a similar 2.7 pediatric stroke cases/100,000/year.[6] Stroke occurs more often in boys and in African American children, even after adjusting for trauma and for sickle cell disease.[7,8]

These figures may underestimate the stroke risk among children. One more recent report, for example, found a stroke risk of 13.0/100,000 children/year.[9] In addition, the risk of stroke is higher among neonates, who were not considered in most of the earlier surveys. Cerebral ischemic infarction is recognized in 12% to 14% of neonates with seizures, and neonates comprise a fourth of all childhood strokes. Data from the National Hospital Discharge Survey conducted from 1980 through 1998 indicate a stroke rate during the first month of life of 26.4/100,000; hemorrhagic stroke occurred in 6.7/100,000 and ischemic stroke occurred in 17.8/100,000. Based on these numbers, strokes in neonates occur in approximately 1 per 4,000 live births per year.[10]

INTRACEREBRAL HEMORRHAGE

Clinical Features of Brain Hemorrhage

Like adults, children with ICH often present with focal neurological deficits or symptoms of increased intracranial pressure. The common presenting signs and symptoms of ICH in children include headaches, emesis, irritability, seizures, and focal neurological deficits. In one series, for example, 40 of the 68 children with spontaneous ICH presented with the dominant symptoms of headache or vomiting and six others presented with irritability.[2] More than a third of the children in this series developed focal or generalized epileptic seizures acutely after the hemorrhage, a number that is higher than usually reported in adults. Alteration of mental status occurred in about half of the 85 children with an intracranial hemorrhage in another report.[3] Younger children and infants can have nonspecific or subtle manifestations even in the face of a relatively large hemorrhage.

Risk Factors for Hemorrhage in Children

Structural vascular anomalies collectively account for the largest share of nontraumatic ICH in children. In a series of 68 children with nontraumatic hemorrhage, 26 children (41.2%) had some type of congenital vascular anomaly, with AVM and arteriovenous fistula together accounting for about a third of the patients.[2] In sharp contrast to adults, arterial hypertension is not a common cause of ICH in children.[2,3] A variety of less frequent causes (e.g., bleeding diatheses, cerebral venous thrombosis, brain tumors, vasculitis, moyamoya disease, and infections) account for the remaining cases (Table 22-1).

Vascular Malformations

Cerebral AVMs are the most common vascular anomalies in clinical series of pediatric ICH patients, accounting for about 30% to 40% of children with hemorrhagic stroke.[2,3] In older children and adolescents, an AVM typically presents with an ICH or subarachnoid hemorrhage (SAH) or with seizures, much as they do in adults (see Chapter 18). Bleeding risk is increased with a central location of the AVM, small nidus size, the presence of an associated intracranial aneurysm, deep venous drainage, and venous outflow obstruction.

Symptomatic neonates may present with unexplained high-output cardiac failure or with hydrocephalus. The proportion of the total blood volume shunted through a large AVM is higher in neonates than in infants. Consequently, newborns are more likely to have congestive heart failure than infants or older children.[11,12]

Infants sometimes develop hydrocephalus, particularly when they have a posterior fossa AVM with secondary aneurysmal dilatation of the vein of Galen (Figure 22-1). A vein of Galen aneurysm is actually a choroidal type of AVM with secondary aneurysmal dilatation of the vein of Galen. It develops as a persistent embryonic prosencephalic vein of Markowski, which drains into the vein of Galen. Hydrocephalus often results when the dilated vein of Galen compresses the cerebral aqueduct or because increased intravenous pressure impedes the adsorption of the cerebrospinal fluid.

Cavernous malformations (see Chapter 18) are usually sporadic and characterized by single lesions, but less commonly, multiple cavernous malformations (see Figure 18-6) result from an autosomal dominant genetic disorder. Intracranial cavernous malformations commonly manifest as seizures, focal neurological deficits, or intracranial hemorrhage.

Intracranial Aneurysms

Symptomatic intracranial aneurysms are not as common in children as in adults, but they do occur. In one report, about 2% of 3,000 individuals with aneurysms were younger than 19 years of age.[13] The location pattern of intracranial aneurysms in children differs from that seen in adults. Children tend to develop

Table 22-1: Risk Factors for Intraparenchymal Hemorrhage in Children

AVM/AVF

Cavernous malformation

Aneurysm

Cerebral vasculitis

Brain tumor (primary or metastatic)

Hematologic/coagulopathy

Afibrinogenemia

Disseminated intravascular coagulation

Leukemia

Sickle cell disease

Thrombocytopenia

Bone marrow transplantation

Hemophilia (factor VIII or factor IX deficiency)

Factor VII (proconvertin) deficiency

Factor XIII (fibrin-stabilizing factor) deficiency

Liver failure

Liver transplantation

Warfarin therapy

Vitamin K deficiency

Anticoagulants/thrombolytics/antiplatelet agents

Hemorrhagic infarction

Venous sinus thrombosis

Intracranial arterial dissection

Moyamoya disease or syndrome

HIV infection

Systemic lupus erythematosus

Herpes simplex encephalitis

Angiophilic fungal organisms

Drug related (amphetamines, cocaine, PCP, others)

Systemic hypertension

AVF = arteriovenous fistula; AVM = arteriovenous malformation; PCP = phencyclidine.

more aneurysms of the posterior circulation and of the internal carotid artery bifurcation than do adults, who have more aneurysms of the anterior communicating artery and posterior communicating artery. Giant aneurysms are more common in children than in adults.[14]

The presentation of saccular aneurysms during the first two decades of life is biphasic, with the onset of symptoms most commonly occurring before age 2 or after age 10.[15] Approximately 5% of the children with an intracranial aneurysm have additional aneurysms, a much lower multiple aneurysm rate

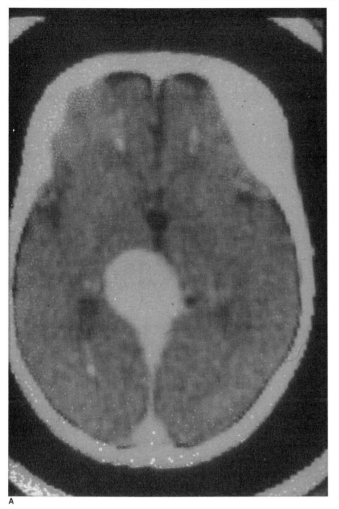
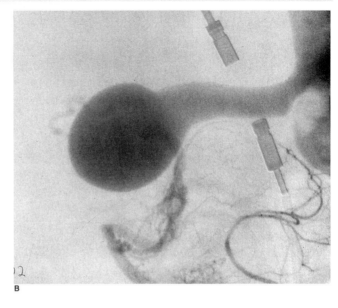

Figure 22-1. A: Cranial CT (in an infant with progressive macrocephaly and a cranial bruit) reveals a large contrast-enhancing lesion compressing the posterior III ventricle. B: Catheter angiography confirmed that the lesion was a vein of Galen aneurysm that received blood from branches of the basilar and posterior cerebral arteries.

than the 20% recorded in adults.[16] However, the likelihood of developing an additional aneurysm later in life is probably at least equivalent to the 20% risk of adult aneurysm patients.

Several disorders increase the risk of intracranial aneurysms, notably coarctation of the aorta, adult polycystic renal disease, and fibromuscular dysplasia. Despite the congenital nature of these disorders, few people with one of these conditions develop symptoms from an intracranial aneurysm before adulthood. Vascular Ehlers-Danlos syndrome, an autosomal dominant disorder of type III collagen synthesis, increases the risk of both intracranial aneurysm and arterial dissection for both children and adults. Additional information about intracranial aneurysms is provided in Chapter 17.

Thrombocytopenia

Thrombocytopenia in children most commonly results from either chemotherapeutic drugs or isoimmune thrombocytopenic purpura (ITP). In the absence of trauma, brain hemorrhage due to reduced platelets does not usually occur with platelet counts above 20,000/mm³, and even with very low platelet counts, spontaneous intracranial hemorrhage is uncommon.[17] In our series of 68 children and adolescents with non-traumatic intraparenchymal brain hemorrhage, thrombocytopenia was the most common hematological risk factor for brain hemorrhage but still accounted for only 11.8% of the patients.[2] Brain hemorrhage later in the course of ITP frequently coincides with a systemic viral infection, when production of antiplatelet antibodies increases and the number of platelets drops. Additional information about ICH due to platelet disorders is provided in Chapter 11.

Hemorrhage Due to Coagulation Disorders

Factor VIII and factor IX deficiencies (hemophilia A and B) are the two most common hereditary bleeding disorders that cause intracranial hemorrhage, but other coagulopathies (e.g., factor XIII deficiency, factor V deficiency, and congenital afibrinogenemia) occasionally cause ICH. As a rule, it is the severity of the bleeding tendency rather than the specific coagulation defect that determines the child's risk of hemorrhage.

Patients with suspected central nervous system (CNS) hemorrhage due to hemophilia should receive immediate factor replacement to achieve a factor level of 100% of normal. Patients with CNS bleeding should continue to receive factor replacement for at least 2 weeks. If available, recombinant human factor

VIII is preferred; for every 1 international unit per kilogram body weight of recombinant human factor VIII administered, the factor VIII level should increase by about 2%.

Severe acquired coagulation defects can occur with hepatic disease, malabsorption syndromes, and various other disorders that promote vitamin K deficiency. The routine use of vitamin K injections in newborns has all but eliminated brain hemorrhage due to vitamin K deficiency in developed countries, but hemorrhagic disease of the newborn still occurs in babies who are born at home and/or in regions of the world where vitamin K supplementation is not the standard practice. Infants born to mothers taking anticonvulsants sometimes bleed excessively due to loss of vitamin K–dependent coagulation factors.[18–20] These neonates require a higher dose of vitamin K after birth, and vitamins during the last trimester of pregnancy may be of value.

More than half of patients with fulminant hepatic failure have a coagulopathy. Cerebral edema and raised intracranial pressure with herniation are a common cause of death among patients with acute hepatic failure. Intracranial bleeding may complicate liver transplantation. Opportunistic infections with *Aspergillus* is sometimes responsible for this complication, which may occur either early or later in the posttransplant period.[21]

For additional information on hereditary and acquired coagulation defects, see Chapter 11.

Intracranial Tumors

Hemorrhage sometimes occurs within primary or metastatic brain tumors, sometimes as the first indication that a tumor is present. In these instances, the onset of symptoms is acute and the hemorrhage may be more obvious on initial cranial computed tomography (CT) than the surrounding neoplasm, creating a clinical picture that closely resembles that of ICH from other causes. The nature of the lesion usually becomes apparent on magnetic resonance imaging (MRI; Figure 22-2). As a general rule, highly vascular malignant tumors of the brain have a propensity to bleed, whereas less aggressive tumors do not. Reports of children with ICH document a fairly consistent 12% to 15% frequency of intracranial tumor as the cause of the hemorrhage.[2,3] Pituitary apoplexy (see Figure 23-3) occasionally occurs in children and adolescents.

Treatment of ICH in Children

Management of children with nontraumatic ICH is not entirely different from the approach used in adult patients (see Chapter 16). Supportive measures include optimizing the respiratory effort, controlling arterial hypertension, preventing seizures, and managing increased intracranial pressure. Roach and colleagues have developed recommendations (Table 22-2) for the treatment of ICH in children.[22]

Correction of treatable risk factors should reduce the likelihood of additional hemorrhages. As in older patients, vascular malformations and aneurysms should be controlled whenever possible via surgical repair or endovascular embolization, although these techniques sometimes pose special challenges in small children.[22] Several retrospective studies suggest that radiosurgery is safe and evidently effective for the treatment of children with an AVM.[23,24] Thrombocytopenia and coagulation defects should be managed.

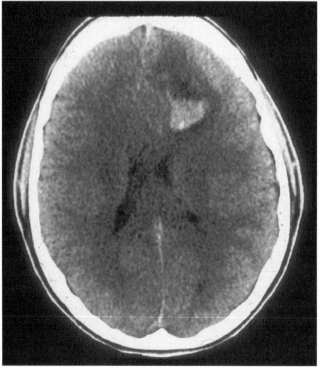

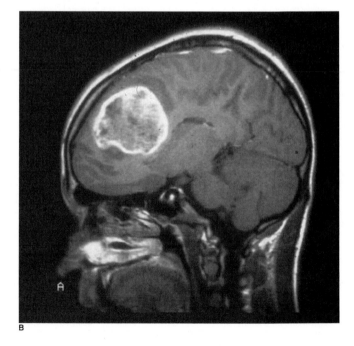

Figure 22-2. A: Cranial CT from a boy with acute headache reveals a hemorrhagic lesion in the left frontal lobe surrounded by edema. Note the blood-fluid level, an unusual finding in an acute ICH. B: Cranial MRI confirmed the presence of a brain tumor, in this instance an anaplastic oligodendroglioma.

Table 22-2: Recommendations for Evaluation and Treatment of Intracerebral Hemorrhage in Children

Class I

1. Children with nontraumatic brain hemorrhage should undergo a thorough risk factor evaluation, including catheter cerebral angiography if noninvasive tests fail to establish an etiology, in an effort to identify treatable risk factors before another hemorrhage occurs.

2. Children with severe coagulation factor deficiency should receive appropriate factor replacement therapy, and children with less severe factor deficiency should receive factor replacement after trauma.

3. Given the risk of repeat hemorrhage from congenital vascular anomalies, these lesions should be identified and corrected whenever it is clinically feasible. Similarly, other treatable hemorrhage risk factors should be corrected.

4. Stabilizing measures in patients with brain hemorrhage should include optimizing the respiratory effort, controlling systemic hypertension, controlling epileptic seizures, and managing increased intracranial pressure.

Class II

1. It is reasonable to follow asymptomatic individuals who have a condition that predisposes them to intracranial aneurysms with a cranial MRA every 1–5 years depending on the perceived level of risk posed by an underlying condition. Should the individual develop symptoms that could be explained by an aneurysm, CTA or CA may be considered even if the patient's MRA fails to show evidence of an aneurysm. Given the possible need for repeated studies over a period of years, CTA may be preferable to CA for screening individuals at risk for aneurysm.

2. Individuals with SAH may benefit from measures to control cerebral vasospasm.

Class III

1. Surgical evacuation of a supratentorial intracerebral hematoma is not recommended for most patients. However, information from small numbers of patients suggests that surgery may help selected individuals with developing brain herniation or extremely elevated intracranial pressure.

2. Although there is strong evidence to support the use of periodic blood transfusions in individuals with SCD who are at high risk for ischemic infarction, there are no data to indicate that periodic transfusions reduce the risk of intracranial hemorrhage due to SCD.

Adapted with permission from Roach et al.[22]
Class I: Should be pursued because the benefits clearly exceed the risks. Class II: Reasonable to consider because benefits probably exceed the risks, but additional studies with focused or age-specific objectives are needed. Class III: Should not be pursued because the benefits are insufficient to justify the risks.
CA = catheter angiography; CTA = computed tomography angiography; MRA = magnetic resonance angiography; SAH = subarachnoid hemorrhage; SCD = sickle cell disease.

Surgical evacuation of an ICH is of questionable value except in a few situations. Surgery can be life-saving for children with impending uncal herniation or for those with a cerebellar hemorrhage. On the other hand, surgery does not alter the dismal outcome of children with a large ICH who are deeply comatose with impaired or absent brainstem function at the time they are seen. Children with a small ICH who are fully conscious usually recover with only supportive care. Whether patients with a medium-sized ICH benefit from surgery is debatable. Hematoma evacuation in adult patients is generally unrewarding,[25,26] and there is no compelling reason to think that surgery is beneficial in children.

ISCHEMIC INFARCTION

Clinical Profile of Ischemic Stroke

The diagnosis of ischemic stroke is often missed or delayed in children. In one retrospective study of children with stroke, the average time from onset of symptoms until diagnosis was 22.7 hours.[27] This delay appears to be multifactorial; some families delay seeking medical attention for children with an acute neurological deficit, some physicians still fail to recognize or properly attribute the signs of stroke in children, and the variable clinical features that occur in some children make it harder to be confident of a stroke diagnosis.

Unique Clinical Features

Although children may have many of the same signs and symptoms of cerebrovascular disease as occur in adults (see Chapter 3), their history is often not straightforward and they are sometimes uncooperative with the examination. Stroke in younger children can present very differently than in older individuals. Infants and children, for example, are more likely to develop seizures or fever after a stroke than an adult.[28] The young stroke patient is also a diagnostic challenge because the list of stroke risk factors for children and young adults is extensive and constantly expanding. Nevertheless, the likely cause of a stroke can be identified in about three fourths of children with ischemic lesions provided a full diagnostic evaluation is performed.[1,29]

The most common sites for an ischemic stroke in children are the basal ganglia and thalamus. However, many of the children with an infarction in this region have primary occlusion of the distal carotid artery or of the middle cerebral artery, secondarily occluding the branch arteries that penetrate into this region.[30]

Neonatal Infarction

Although less common than the germinal matrix hemorrhage of premature infants, ischemic infarction in term neonates is the most common ischemic stroke syndrome in children. The infarction typically occurs in a term infant after an uneventful pregnancy and a routine delivery. The ischemic lesion is often

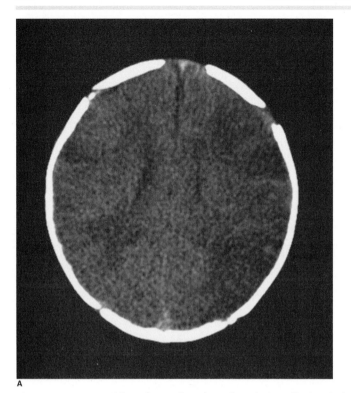
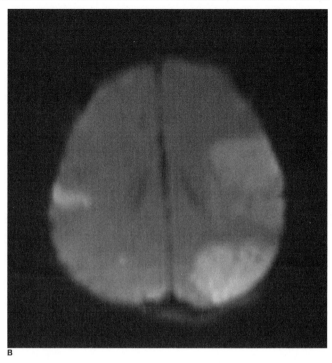

Figure 22-3. A: Cranial CT shows a large hypodense lesion affecting the left hemisphere of a neonate who presented with right-sided focal seizures one day after birth. B: Diffusion-weighted MRI suggests that these lesions are infarctions.

identified after the onset of focal seizures triggers cranial CT or a cranial ultrasound study. Typically, the physical findings are nonspecific: lethargy, irritability, hypotonia, but not hemiparesis. Focal motor seizures more often involve the right body because about three fourths of the single infarcts involve the left cerebral hemisphere (Figure 22-3). The radiographic characteristics of the lesion sometimes date the infarction to before the infant was born. The diagnosis of neonatal infarction can be missed because the findings are often subtle and not all infants develop seizures. Hence, similar lesions of long-standing duration are sometimes discovered in older children who are being evaluated for epilepsy or developmental delay.

Most neonatal infarctions probably result from emboli. The source of the emboli is not known with certainty, but they may arise from the placental vessels. Systemic emboli can sometimes be demonstrated in neonates, and the left hemisphere stroke predominance is more easily explainable by an embolus. Interruption of aortic laminar flow by blood from the still patent ductus arteriosus might explain how an embolus could be preferentially directed to the left hemisphere. Risk factors for neonatal infarction include maternal or neonatal prothrombotic disorders as well as acquired conditions such as amnionitis, pre-eclampsia, and maternal drug use.[10,31,32] The presence of two or more risk factors increases the likelihood of stroke exponentially.

Etiology of Childhood Ischemic Stroke

The list of potential risk factors for childhood stroke is long and the relative importance of each is not always certain.[29,33] The presence of multiple risk factors in the same child increases the likelihood of stroke recurrence, which in turn parallels the long-

term outcome.[34] Therefore, even when the cause of a child's stroke seems readily apparent from the start, a systematic assessment for additional risk factors is worthwhile. A list of risk factors for ischemic stroke in children is provided in Table 22-3, and several of the more common conditions are considered individually.

Cardiac Embolism

Whereas atrial fibrillation and ischemic heart disease are the most common causes of cardioembolic stroke in older individuals, congenital heart lesions predominate in children. In most series, congenital heart disease is the single most common cause of ischemic stroke in children and is sometimes also an issue in young adults, although the number of strokes due to congenital heart disease has probably decreased in tandem with the tendency to perform corrective surgery at an earlier age. In the Canadian Pediatric Ischemic Stroke Registry, cardiac disease was present in 24% of children with arterial ischemic stroke. Complex cardiac anomalies are by far the greatest problem, but particularly concerning are the cyanotic cardiac lesions with polycythemia, which increase the risk of both thrombosis and embolism.[22]

Individual genetic syndromes predispose to very specific congenital heart lesions, affecting the likelihood as well as the type of cerebrovascular complication. Individuals with Down syndrome have an increased risk of embolic stroke due to congenital cardiac disease as well as an increased risk of stroke due to moyamoya syndrome. Williams syndrome and Alagille syndrome predispose to pulmonary stenosis as well as to carotid vasculopathy.[35–39] Patients with tetralogy of Fallot and moyamoya syndrome have also been reported.[40] Patients with Turner

Table 22-3: Risk Factors for Pediatric Ischemic Stroke

Congenital heart disease
- Ventricular septal defect
- Atrial septal defect
- Patent ductus arteriosus
- Aortic stenosis
- Mitral stenosis
- Coarctation of the aorta
- Cardiac rhabdomyoma
- Complex congenital heart defects

Acquired heart disease
- Rheumatic heart disease
- Prosthetic heart valve
- Libman-Sacks endocarditis
- Infective endocarditis
- Cardiomyopathy
- Myocarditis
- Atrial myxoma
- Arrhythmia

Systemic vascular disease
- Systemic hypertension
- Superior vena cava syndrome
- Diabetes
- Vasculitis
- Meningitis
- Systemic infection
- Systemic lupus erythematosus
- Polyarteritis nodosa
- Granulomatous angiitis
- Takayasu's arteritis
- Rheumatoid arthritis
- Dermatomyositis
- Inflammatory bowel disease
- Drug abuse (cocaine, amphetamines)
- Hemolytic-uremic syndrome

Vasculopathies
- Ehlers-Danlos syndrome
- Homocystinuria
- Moyamoya disease/syndrome
- Fabry disease
- Malignant atrophic papulosis
- Pseudoxanthoma elasticum
- NADH-Coenzyme Q reductase deficiency
- Williams syndrome
- Fibromuscular dysplasia

Vasospastic disorders
- Migraine
- Ergot poisoning
- Vasospasm and subarachnoid bleed

Hematologic disorders/coagulopathies
- Hemoglobinopathy
- Thrombotic thrombocytopenic purpura
- Thrombocytosis
- Polycythemia
- Disseminated intravascular coagulation
- Leukemia or other neoplasm
- Oral contraceptive use
- Pregnancy/postpartum period
- Antithrombin deficiency
- Factor V Leiden mutation
- Protein S deficiency
- Protein C deficiency
- Prothrombin gene mutation (G20210A)
- Antiphospholipid antibodies

Trauma/iatrogenic
- Fat or air embolism
- Foreign body embolism
- Extracorporeal membrane oxygenation (ECMO) with carotid ligation
- Vertebral occlusion after abrupt cervical rotation
- Posttraumatic arterial dissection
- Blunt cervical arterial trauma
- Catheter angiography
- Amniotic fluid/placental embolism

Modified with permission from Roach and Riela.[1]

syndrome have an increased risk of coarctation of the aorta and thus of intracranial aneurysm formation. Patients with bicuspid aortic valve have an increased risk of aortic dissection compared to the general population.

Similarly, specific repair procedures for congenital heart lesions may promote specific complications. The classic Blalock-Taussig procedure may be complicated by subclavian steal syndrome and also carries the risk of damaging the recurrent laryngeal nerve. Patients with a univentricular heart (e.g., hypoplastic left heart syndrome, tricuspid atresia, double-inlet ventricle) require the Fontan procedure, which may be complicated (late sequelae) by atrial arrhythmias and thromboemboli, thus requiring long-term anticoagulation.[41–43]

Rheumatic heart disease has become less common with the extensive use of antibiotics to treat streptococcal infections, but it is still a relatively common cause of ischemic stroke in young patients worldwide. The lifetime risk of systemic thromboembolism in an individual with rheumatic mitral stenosis is 20%. The risk of thromboembolic complications is greater if there is associated atrial fibrillation. Despite the high prevalence of mitral valve prolapse, it is a rare cause of embolic stroke, and most young patients with mitral valve prolapse and cerebral infarction have another cause for their cerebral infarction. Embolic stroke also occurs in individuals with surgically replaced heart valves.

Embolic stroke attributed to cardiac arrhythmia is unusual in young patients. Atrial fibrillation is uncommon but it may occur with hyperthyroidism or rheumatic valvular heart disease, after cardiac surgery, or in isolation. Sick sinus syndrome is rare in young patients, but they may develop systemic emboli, even after pacemaker insertion. Heart block is common in patients with Kearns-Sayre syndrome.

Both myocardial infarction and cardiomyopathy increase the risk of embolic stroke in children and adolescents, but neither condition is common among children.[44] When myocardial infarction does occur in this age group, there is often a specific risk factor such as a high lipoprotein(a) or apolipoprotein A-1 level, calcific coronary arteriopathy of infancy, anomalous origin of the left coronary artery from the pulmonary artery, coronary artery emboli from an atrial myxoma, coronary artery spasm, accelerated atherosclerosis among orthotopic cardiac transplant patients, childhood polyarteritis nodosa, Kawasaki syndrome, or Behçet's disease.[45,46] Cardiomyopathy occurs in patients with Friedreich ataxia, Duchenne muscular dystrophy, Becker muscular dystrophy, limb-girdle muscular dystrophy, facioscapulohumeral muscular dystrophy, Emery-Dreyfuss muscular dystrophy, myotonic dystrophy, and a variety of congenital myopathies.

Cardiac rhabdomyomas are more common in children than atrial myxomas. However, embolism occurs relatively often in children with myxomas but rarely in those with cardiac rhabdomyomas.[47–52] Patients with myxomas are also at risk for cerebral aneurysm formation.

Right-to-left shunts can occur at the atrial level (e.g., atrial septal defect with pulmonary hypertension), ventricular level (e.g., ventricular septal defect with pulmonary hypertension), or at the arterial level (e.g., pulmonary arteriovenous fistula). Atrial septal defects (ASDs) are classified according to their location relative to the fossa ovalis into secundum ASD, primum ASD, and sinus venosus defect. During right-to-left shunting, there is an opportunity for a thrombus to pass through the defect and enter the systemic circulation, leading to paradoxical embolism. Pulmonary arteriovenous fistulas can lead to paradoxical embolism in patients with hereditary hemorrhagic telangiectasia (Osler-Weber-Rendu disease).

Patent foramen ovale (PFO) occurs in up to a third of children, making it difficult to ascertain its role, if any, in the pathogenesis of childhood stroke. Individuals with a PFO are less likely to have another identifiable risk factor, suggesting that the PFO per se increases the likelihood of ischemic stroke. Even so, PFO does not seem to be a strong risk factor for stroke in most children.

Diagnosis of infective endocarditis is based on the modified Duke's criteria.[53] A high index of suspicion is necessary, particularly whenever a stroke occurs in an individual with an unexplained fever, a new heart murmur, or peripheral manifestations of embolism. Fever may be low grade, often intermittent, and may be lacking among debilitated patients. A diligent search for Janeway lesions or Osler nodes is required. Heart valves (native or prosthetic) are most commonly involved, although infective endocarditis can also occur at ventricular septal defects or atrial septal defects. Various organisms (bacterial, fungal, etc.) cause infective endocarditis, but among the most common are *Streptococcus, Staphylococcus,* and *Enterococcus.* Culture-negative endocarditis has been reported in 5% to 10% of cases. Transesophageal echocardiography is the preferred imaging modality for suspected cases of either native or prosthetic valve endocarditis.[54]

Additional information about the general aspects of the diagnosis and treatment of embolic stroke is provided in Chapter 8. In addition, Roach and colleagues have developed management guidelines for children with stroke related to cardiac disease (Table 22-4).[22]

Atherosclerosis

Atherosclerosis is a complex multifactorial disease (see Chapter 7) that seldom becomes symptomatic before age 40 years. However, autopsies have shown that it often begins in early childhood and progresses slowly into adulthood.[55,56] Symptomatic atherosclerosis may occasionally be a concern in obese children, in children with familial hyperlipidemias, and in early aging syndromes such as progeria or Werner syndrome. One of the earliest manifestations of subclinical atherosclerosis is endothelial dysfunction, sometimes present for many decades before the onset of clinical manifestations. Impaired endothelial-dependent vasodilatation (due mainly to decreased bioavailability of nitric oxide) is a key step in the development of atherosclerosis before plaque formation.[57] Endothelial dysfunction has been associated with diabetes mellitus, hyperlipidemia, and cigarette smoking in teenagers and young adults. Although infection has been implicated in endothelial dysfunction and atherogenesis, the impact of acute common childhood infections on the vascular endothelium is unknown.

Cervicocephalic Arterial Dissection

Cervicocephalic arterial dissection (see Chapter 12) is probably an underrecognized cause of stroke in children. Neurological deficits can either begin immediately due to ischemia distal to the lesion or occur later due to an embolism arising from the dissection site. Cervicocephalic arterial dissections tend to occur in the more mobile segments of the carotid arteries or the vertebral arteries.[58] Dissection is more common in the extracranial internal carotid arteries (see Figure 12-1) than in the vertebrobasilar and intracranial carotid arteries. Extracranial vertebral artery dissections may extend intracranially in 10% of

Table 22-4: Recommendations for Children with Stroke and Heart Disease

Class I

1. Therapy for congestive heart failure is indicated and may reduce the likelihood of cardiogenic embolism.

2. When feasible, congenital heart lesions, especially complex heart lesions with a high stroke risk, should be repaired, both to improve cardiac function and to reduce the subsequent risk of stroke. This recommendation does not yet apply to PFOs.

3. Resection of an atrial myxoma is indicated given its ongoing risk of cerebrovascular complications.

Class II

1. For children with a cardiac embolism unrelated to a PFO who are judged to have a high risk of recurrent embolism, it is reasonable to initially introduce UFH or LMWH while warfarin therapy is initiated and adjusted. Alternatively, it is reasonable to use LMWH initially in this situation and to continue it instead of warfarin.

2. In children with a risk of cardiac embolism, it is reasonable to continue either LMWH or warfarin for at least 1 year or until the lesion responsible for the risk has been corrected. If the risk of recurrent embolism is judged to be high, it is reasonable to continue anticoagulation indefinitely as long as it is well tolerated.

3. For children with a suspected cardiac embolism unrelated to a PFO with a lower or unknown risk of stroke, it is reasonable to begin aspirin and continue it for at least 1 year.

4. Surgical repair or transcatheter closure is reasonable in individuals with a major atrial septal defect both to reduce the stroke risk and to prevent long-term cardiac complications. This recommendation does not apply to individuals with a PFO pending additional data.

5. There are few data to govern our management of patients with prosthetic valve endocarditis, but it may be reasonable to continue maintenance anticoagulation in individuals who are already taking it.

Class III

1. Anticoagulant therapy is not recommended for individuals with native valve endocarditis.

2. Surgical removal of a cardiac rhabdomyoma is not necessary in asymptomatic individuals with no stroke history.

Adapted with permission from Roach et al.[22]
Class I: Should be pursued because the benefits clearly exceed the risks. Class II: Reasonable to consider because benefits probably exceed the risks, but additional studies with focused or age-specific objectives are needed. Class III: Should not be pursued because the benefits are insufficient to justify the risks.
LMWH = low molecular weight heparin; PFO = patent foramen ovale; UFH = unfractionated heparin.

cases.[59] Fullerton and colleagues identified 118 dissections in individuals younger than 18 years in the English literature; they found that 74% had an anterior circulation dissection and that all patients had evidence of cerebral ischemia at the time of presentation.[60]

Cervicocephalic arterial dissections occur most often after blunt or penetrating trauma.[61] The preceding injury can be seemingly trivial, however, and spontaneous dissection is well described, suggesting that the dissecting artery may have been congenitally defective. Vertebral artery dissection occurs in children with anomalies of the cervical spine.[62] Dissection has also been described in individuals with fibromuscular dysplasia, vascular Ehlers-Danlos syndrome, coarctation of the aorta, extreme arterial tortuosity, moyamoya syndrome, pharyngeal infections, and alpha-1 antitrypsin deficiency.[63–65]

Aortic dissection occurs with increased frequency due to cystic medial necrosis, which occurs in individuals with Marfan syndrome, bicuspid aortic valves, or vascular Ehlers-Danlos syndrome but also occurs as an isolated familial disorder.[66,67] Aortic dissection can secondarily occlude the cervicocephalic arteries and cause stroke.

Vertebral artery dissections are more common among boys than girls, probably because of increased exposure to trauma.[65] Traumatic carotid dissection after peritonsillar trauma is well documented in children.[68–70] This injury typically results from a fall onto an ice cream stick, toothbrush, pen, or similar object inside the mouth. Intimal damage from blunt trauma initiates the dissection, usually without penetrating the artery.

The recurrence risk of cervicocephalic dissection is approximately 1% per year, but this risk is greater in younger patients and in individuals with an affected family member. In Fullerton's review, none of the children with posterior circulation dissection had a recurrent dissection (versus 10% when the anterior circulation was involved), and 87% of the patients with posterior circulation dissection were male.[60] The most common level of vertebral artery dissection is at the V3 segment; exaggerated rotation and or flexion-extension at the atlanto-axial joint increases the risk.

Fibromuscular Dysplasia

Fibromuscular dysplasia (FMD) is a segmental, noninflammatory angiopathy affecting medium and small-sized arteries. FMD is most often described in young and middle-aged women, but it occurs in individuals of all ages and familial cases have been described. Cervicocephalic arterial dissection is a complication of FMD based on the frequency of FMD among individuals with spontaneous dissection. However, the incidence of asymptomatic FMD is hard to pinpoint, making it difficult in turn to determine the precise contribution of FMD to the stroke risk. It is likely that most individuals with FMD remain asymptomatic. For additional information about the diagnosis and management of FMD, see Chapter 13.

Moyamoya Disease

Moyamoya disease is a chronic noninflammatory vasculopathy affecting primarily the internal carotid arteries. It is characterized by progressive occlusion of the arteries with the development of a distal telangiectatic network of collateral vessels (see Figure 13-1). The term *moyamoya disease* is used when there is no apparent cause of the vasculopathy, whereas *moyamoya syndrome* is used to describe individuals with a known risk factor for the condition. Moyamoya is more common in individuals of Asian heritage but occurs in all populations. The diagnosis and treatment of moyamoya disease are presented in more detail in Chapter 13.

The clinical picture of moyamoya varies with age, the rapidity of vascular occlusion, the availability of collateral flow, and the anatomical site of the infarction. Some children remain asymptomatic for long intervals. Moyamoya may cause transient ischemic attacks, alternating hemiparesis, headaches, seizures, and chorea. Mental retardation is common among children whose symptoms begin early; children with the onset of cerebral ischemia before the age of 4 years often develop progressive cognitive impairment. Hyperventilation or vigorous crying can provoke either ischemic symptoms or seizures. The electroencephalogram shows slowing of the background rhythm that begins just after cessation of hyperventilation (known as the "rebuild-up" phenomenon).[71]

Children with moyamoya usually present with symptoms of cerebral ischemia, whereas adults with moyamoya often present with an ICH or SAH. In general, the prognosis is worse in patients whose symptoms begin in the first 3 or 4 years of life.[72] Rapid initial progression of symptoms suggests rapid vessel occlusion, perhaps resulting in less ability to develop distal collateral branches that could maintain perfusion. The disease is not always progressive or the prognosis unfavorable. Individuals who maintain an adequate blood flow reserve distal to the occluded arteries tend to do well even without surgery, although the occurrence of a large infarction at the time of presentation does not bode well for the chances of full recovery even if surgery is performed.[72,73] Other causes of cerebral vasculopathy are summarized in Table 22-5.

Vasculitis

Numerous infectious and multisystem noninfectious inflammatory diseases promote cerebral vasculitis and stroke. Children are sometimes affected by primary cerebral arteritis, Takayasu arteritis, and polyarteritis nodosa, although they seem to be largely spared from giant cell arteritis. Additional information about cerebral vasculitis and stroke is provided in Chapter 10.

Children seem particularly prone to develop arteritis associated with infectious diseases. Up to a fourth of the children with bacterial meningitis in some series have developed radiographic evidence of a cerebral infarction.[74] Fortunately, the incidence of bacterial meningitis has diminished in developed countries because of the advent of effective vaccines. Tuberculosis continues to be a major health problem, especially in developing countries, and ischemic stroke is a relatively common complication in children with tuberculous meningitis. Stroke can even be the mode of presentation of tuberculous meningitis.[75]

Stroke occurs with increased frequency after varicella infection.[76] Herpes zoster may cause a virus-induced necrotizing arteritis similar to granulomatous angiitis. Numerous other

Table 22-5: Cerebral Vasculopathies in Children

Cervicocephalic arterial dissections

Moyamoya disease and moyamoya syndrome

Fibromuscular dysplasia

Vasculitis

Transient cerebral arteriopathy

Post-varicella angiopathy

Ergotism

Traumatic cerebrovascular disease

Radiation-induced arteriopathy

Tumor encasement of cervicocephalic vessels

Hypoplasia and agenesis of cervicocephalic vessel

Congenital arterial fenestration

Adapted with permission from Biller.[4]

infectious agents have been reported in patients with cerebral infarctions, although only a few patients have been documented with some of these infections, making it difficult to be certain of a relationship. The list of reported infections include *Mycoplasma pneumoniae,* coxsackie-9 virus, California encephalitis virus, mumps paramyxovirus, *Borrelia burgdorferi,* cat-scratch disease, and the larval stage (cysticercus) of *Taenia solium.* Internal carotid artery occlusion can complicate necrotizing fasciitis of the parapharyngeal space. Other infectious agents reported to promote systemic angiitis or cerebral infarctions include rickettsial infections (Q fever, Rocky Mountain spotted fever, Mediterranean spotted fever, epidemic typhus, murine typhus, acute febrile cerebrovasculitis), leptospirosis (*Leptospira interrogans*), brucellosis, and coenurosis (*Coenurus cerebralis*).[77] Gnasthosmiasis, endemic in Southeast Asia, and caused by the nematode *Gnasthoma spinigerum,* is also an important cause of intracranial hemorrhage among children in Thailand.[78]

Cerebral infarction is a complication of the acquired immune deficiency syndrome (AIDS) and may result from vasculitis, meningovascular syphilis, infective endocarditis, aneurysmal dilation of major cerebral arteries, nonbacterial thrombotic endocarditis, anticardiolipin antibodies, or hypercoagulable states. Another concern is the potential for antiretroviral therapy, including protease inhibitors, to induce dyslipidemia that could accelerate the atherosclerotic process.[79] In addition, some reports suggest that HIV-infected individuals are at increased risk for hemorrhagic cerebrovascular complications.[80]

Ischemic stroke can also occur as a complication of illicit drug use, glue sniffing, and a variety of multisystem vasculitides. Stroke in patients with systemic lupus erythematosus may be attributable to cardiogenic embolism (Libman-Sacks endocarditis), antiphospholipid antibodies, underlying vasculopathy, or less often to an immune-mediated vasculitis.

Migraine

Migraine alone seldom causes stroke, and migraine is so common that the likelihood of an individual stroke patient coincidentally having migraine is substantial. Cerebral infarctions complicating migraine most often involve the posterior cerebral (posterior circulation) regions. This contrasts with the predominantly anterior circulation strokes seen with emboli.

A young patient with cerebral infarction who has a history of migraines should not be assumed to have a migrainous stroke until other possible causes have been systematically eliminated. Symptoms identical to those of migraine can arise from vasculitis, AVM, and other conditions, so migraineurs who have a stroke should usually undergo a complete diagnostic evaluation to identify other stroke risk factors. Migraine and other cerebrovascular causes of headache are described in Chapter 14.

Migraine is strongly familial but in most instances polygenetic. Some people with migraine may be intrinsically at greater risk of developing a stroke than others. One gene for familial hemiplegic migraine is located on chromosome 19 adjacent to the gene for cerebral autosomal dominant arteriopathy with subcortical infarcts and leukoencephalopathy (CADASIL).[81,82] It seems intuitive that individuals with a specific tendency to develop complicated migraine would also be more likely to develop permanent deficits, and at least one report documents prolonged neurological deficits in three children with a mutation of the *FHM2* gene.[83]

Although used by many physicians, selective 5-hydroxy-tryptamine-1 (5-HT$_1$) agonists (triptans) have not been widely studied in children younger than age 12 years, nor have these agents been approved by the U.S. Food and Drug Administration. Triptan medications are usually avoided in adult patients with complicated migraine and it seems prudent to adopt the same approach for children. Similarly, it is probably best to avoid beta blocking agents in patients who developed a possible migrainous infarct while taking these medications for prophylaxis. We often use a combination of daily verapamil and aspirin if no contraindications exist to these agents.[84]

Hemoglobinopathy

Although stroke is occasionally linked to other hemoglobinopathies, sickle cell disease (SCD) is by far the most common cause of stroke due to hemoglobinopathy (see Chapter 11). The cumulative risk of stroke due to SCD is estimated to be about 25% by age 45 years. Moreover, after the first SCD-related stroke, that individual's risk of having a second stroke soars to greater than 50%, and stroke accounts for 12% of deaths in individuals with SCD. Most SCD-related strokes are ischemic infarctions, but intraparenchymal and subarachnoid hemorrhages occur.

Both large and small cerebral arteries are affected by SCD, but the intracranial internal carotid arteries and their immediate branches are affected most consistently (see Figure 11-2). Elevated cerebral blood flow velocity measured by transcranial Doppler (TCD) predicts a much higher stroke risk due to SCD.[85,86] A randomized multicenter controlled study (the STOP trial) compared prophylactic blood transfusion to standard medical care in individuals at high risk for stroke based on TCD measurements, and showed that the time averaged mean blood flow velocity measured by TCD predicts a much higher stroke risk due to SCD and that periodic blood transfusions dramatically lower the stroke risk in these individuals.[87]

The STOP trial demonstrated conclusively that prophylactic blood transfusion reduces the occurrence of first stroke by more than 90%. A 1.5 or 2 volume exchange transfusion should begin as soon as possible to reduce the hemoglobin S below 30% of the total hemoglobin. However, repeated transfusions inevitably lead to iron overload that, without effective iron chelation, leads to fatal cardiac and hepatic dysfunction. Iron chelation effectively reduces this risk, but not all patients are compliant. Halting the monthly transfusions allows the stroke risk to increase again. Hydroxyurea reduces the number of pain crises and may also lower the stroke risk, although probably not as much as blood transfusions.[88,89]

Hypercoagulable Disorders

A more detailed discussion of hypercoagulable disorders is provided in Chapter 11. Hypercoagulable disorders account for 2% to 7% of young patients with ischemic stroke. A hypercoagulable state should be suspected in patients with recurrent episodes of deep venous thrombosis, recurrent pulmonary emboli, a family history of thrombotic events, or unusual sites of venous or arterial thromboses.

Conditions that promote hypercoagulability include antithrombin deficiency, protein C or protein S deficiency, activated protein C resistance, and antiphospholipid antibodies. Strokes often complicate the clinical course of malignancies, and in rare instances a stroke may be the initial manifestation of cancer. These conditions tend to induce venous thrombosis more than arterial thrombosis.

Miscellaneous Causes of Stroke

A number of uncommon genetic and congenital conditions promote stroke or influence its course and, because of their rarity, these conditions are sometimes overlooked. Several rare metabolic derangements cause stroke by their inability to produce as much energy as the tissue needs, creating a mismatch of energy needs that results in infarction even in the face of continued blood perfusion to the area. Additional information about several of these conditions is provided in Chapter 21.

Leigh's disease (subacute necrotizing encephalomyelopathy) is an autosomal recessive or X-linked recessive disorder that typically presents in infancy or early childhood. It is characterized clinically by loss of motor control, hypotonia, vomiting, irritability, seizures, respiratory difficulties, ataxia, external ophthalmoplegia, and stroke or stroke-like episodes. Neuroimaging studies may show bilateral lesions in the basal ganglia and brainstem. Several biochemical abnormalities have been described with Leigh's disease, including abnormalities of pyruvate metabolism, cytochrome *c* oxidase deficiency, and abnormalities of thiamine metabolism.

Methylmalonic acidemia, propionic acidemia, and isovaleric acidemia are autosomal recessive conditions resulting from inborn errors of branched chain amino acid catabolism. Strokes may be seen in these conditions with dehydration and ketoacidosis. Patients typically present during an intercurrent illness with acute extrapyramidal signs due to lesions of the basal ganglia. Cerebellar hemorrhage has been described with methylmalonic, propionic, and isovaleric acidemia.[90] Glutaric aciduria is another disorder of amino acid metabolism that may cause stroke. It is an autosomal recessive condition characterized by athetosis, dystonia, and severe mental retardation. Similar to methylmalonic acidemia, there is a tendency for destructive lesions of the basal ganglia leading to extrapyramidal movement disorders.[91]

Patients with homocystinuria may display a Marfanoid habitus, malar flush, ectopia lentis, optic atrophy, psychiatric abnormalities, mental retardation, and seizures. Raised levels of plasma homocysteine may be an independent risk factor for cerebrovascular, coronary, and peripheral arterial occlusive disease. Moderate hyperhomocysteinemia also increases the risk of ischemic stroke among individuals without homozygous homocystinuria.

About half of the patients with homocystinuria have complete or partial reversal of their biochemical abnormalities if given pharmacological doses (500 mg/day initially) of pyridoxine, which normally acts as a coenzyme of cystathionine synthase. Folate (1–10 mg/day) also reduces the homocysteine level in some patients, perhaps by promoting the remethylation of methionine. Pyridoxine-responsive patients have fewer thromboembolic episodes and lower overall mortality.[92] Homocystinuria is presented in more detail in Chapter 21.

Cerebral infarction occurs in individuals with mitochondrial encephalomyopathies, such as MELAS (mitochondrial encephalomyopathy, lactic acidosis, and stroke-like episodes), mitochondrial encephalomyopathy and ragged-red fibers (MERRF), and Kearns-Sayre syndrome. Mitochondrial encephalomyopathies should be suspected in patients with intractable seizures, recurrent strokes, lactic acidosis, or episodic respiratory failure. Migraine-like headache and frequent bouts of vomiting are common. Hirano and Pavlakis distinguished six cardinal features of the syndrome.[93] These cardinal manifestations include exercise intolerance, onset before age 40 years, seizures, ragged-red fibers, lactic acidosis, and stroke-like manifestations. Symptoms of stroke are acute in onset but often superimposed on a more chronic picture of exercise intolerance, chronic headache, unexplained vomiting, and failure to thrive. MELAS is presented in more detail in Chapter 21.

Fabry disease is a rare sex-linked disorder resulting from α-galactosidase deficiency and characterized by corneal and lenticular opacities, angiokeratomas involving predominantly the thighs, periumbilical area, and scrotum, acroparesthesias, and renal failure (see also Chapter 21). Arterial hypertension and myocardial and cerebral ischemia are frequent complications. Periodic infusion of synthesized α-galactosidase relieves some of the more serious manifestations of Fabry disease and is likely to reduce the risk of stroke in these individuals.

Diffuse meningocerebral angiomatosis and leukoencephalopathy (Divry-Van Bogaert syndrome) may present with livedo reticularis, seizures, dementia, upper motor neuron signs, brain infarcts, and cerebro-meningeal angiomatosis.[94]

Vascular dysplasia, and less commonly fusiform dilatations of the cavernous segment of the carotid artery, occasionally occurs with the epidermal nevus syndrome.[95]

Carotid artery aplasia or hypoplasia is rare. Although the congenital absence of an artery per se does not usually cause a stroke, absence of a major vessel could be catastrophic should the patient occlude another major artery. Diagnosis of carotid artery hypoplasia can be more challenging than total absence of the vessel. The diagnosis of carotid artery hypoplasia can be suspected with ultrasound and confirmed by the CT demonstration of a small or absent carotid canal in the skull base.[96]

CEREBRAL VENOUS SINUS THROMBOSIS IN CHILDREN

Cerebral venous sinus thrombosis (CVST) may occur at any time from infancy to old age, although women of childbearing age are disproportionately affected during pregnancy and puerperium (see Chapter 23) or while taking oral contraceptives. In the pediatric age group, the most likely time to develop CVST is the neonatal period, when there is a relative hypercoagulable state. Neonates account for more than half of the pediatric patients with CVST.

Clinical Manifestations of CSVT in Children

Cortical vein and dural sinus thrombosis can be difficult to recognize because the clinical findings are often less dramatic than those of arterial occlusion or intraparenchymal hemorrhage. The clinical manifestations of CVST vary with the location of the occlusion and the configuration of an individual's venous anatomy. In addition, the findings are often subtle or nonspecific in neonates.

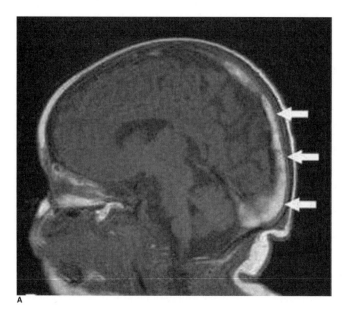
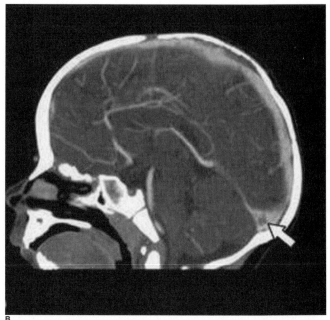

Figure 22-4. A: T_1-weighted MRI at 17 days of age shows extensive thrombus (*arrows*) in the sagittal sinus. B: CT venography at 10 months of age shows clearing of the thrombosis at the torcula (*arrow*). These abnormalities were incidental findings in an infant who was completely asymptomatic. Reprinted with permission from Golomb.[97]

Table 22-6: Disorders Reported with Cerebral Venous Sinus Thrombosis in Children

Systemic conditions
- Dehydration
- Hypoxia, e.g., post-strangulation
- Inflammatory bowel diseases
- Nephrotic syndrome
- Systemic lupus erythematosus
- Thyrotoxicosis
- Behçet's disease
- Severe malnutrition

Hematologic disorders
- Iron deficiency anemia
- Sickle cell disease
- Thalassemia
- Autoimmune hemolytic anemia
- Paroxysmal nocturnal hemoglobinuria

Prothrombotic disorders
- Antithrombin deficiency
- Protein C or S deficiency
- Factor V Leiden mutation
- Prothrombin G20210A mutation
- Elevated plasminogen activator inhibitor
- Antiphospholipid antibody syndrome
- Tissue plasminogen activator deficiency
- Dysfibrinogenemia
- Plasminogen gene mutations
- Heparin cofactor II deficiency
- Platelet glycoprotein IIIa mutation

- Disseminated intravascular coagulation
- Pregnancy and puerperium
- Increased factors VIII, IX, X or von Willebrand
- Thrombotic microangiopathies
- Homocystinuria
- Cancer (leukemia, lymphoma, other)
- Post-operative state

Cardiac disease
- Cyanotic congenital heart disease
- Postoperative or post-catheterization
- Jugular and subclavian vein catheterization
- Congestive heart disease

Head and neck infections
- Bacterial meningitis
- Mastoiditis or otitis
- Tonsillitis
- Sinusitis

Other head and neck disorders
- Head injury
- Hydrocephalus (± with or without a shunt)
- Post-lumbar puncture

Drugs
- L-Asparaginase
- Oral contraceptives
- Corticosteroids
- Intravenous immunoglobulin (IVIG)
- Epoetin-alpha

Adapted with permission from Biller.[4]

Table 22-7: Cerebral Infarction in Children: Initial Tests

Complete blood count with differential and platelet count

Prothrombin time, activated partial thromboplastin time

Blood glucose, serum electrolytes, blood chemistries

Serologic test for syphilis[a]

Erythrocyte sedimentation rate

Pregnancy test[a]

Chest roentgenogram

Electrocardiogram

M-mode and two-dimensional echocardiogram

Cranial computed tomography (CCT)

MRI of brain and MRA, in most instances

Cerebral angiography[a]

Adapted with permission from Biller.[4]
[a] Test as appropriate for age and clinical situation.
MRA = magnetic resonance angiography; MRI = magnetic resonance imaging.

Occlusion of larger dural sinuses tend to generate signs of increased intracranial pressure, while thrombosis of the cortical veins more often lead to focal neurological dysfunction or seizures. Symptoms include headaches, vomiting, and lethargy. Papilledema is common. Depending on the location of the occluded venous structure, there may be hemiparesis, paraparesis, or other focal neurological manifestations. In an individual with seizures, focal neurological dysfunction due to CVST is easily mistaken for postictal deficit. Occasional neonates remain asymptomatic despite the incidental demonstration of a thrombosed dural sinus (Figure 22-4).[97]

Sinovenous thrombosis should be included in the differential diagnosis of intracranial hemorrhage and hemorrhagic infarction. Bleeding due to CVST may be intraparenchymal, subarachnoid, or subdural. Hemorrhages involve the white matter to a greater extent than the cortex, and are often bilateral and parasagittal. Additional information about the clinical manifestations resulting from occlusion of specific dural sinuses is provided in Chapter 20.

Risk Factors for CVST in Children

Cerebral venous thrombosis in children can be divided into two broad categories: septic and aseptic. Venous occlusion is often associated with a nearby infection such as chronic otitis, mastoiditis, sinusitis, or orbital cellulitis. In the post-antibiotic area, septic dural sinus thrombosis has diminished but it is not rare.[98] An array of disorders predispose to aseptic CVST. Most of these conditions facilitate clotting in some way. The risk of venous thrombosis increases dramatically in individuals with multiple risk factors.[98–100]

Septic dural sinus thrombosis now most often involves the transverse sinus as a complication of chronic otitis media or mastoiditis (see Figure 20-3). Thrombosis of the cavernous sinus can complicate sinusitis or facial infections. Dural sinus thrombosis occasionally occurs in the setting of acute bacterial meningitis, but this too has become more and more uncommon since the advent of vaccines has lowered the incidence of meningitis.

Approximately two thirds of children with aseptic CVST have an underlying prothrombotic disorder or else a condition that results in sluggish venous blood flow.[99–101] Numerous coagulation disorders have been documented in individuals with CVST of all ages, including deficiencies of antithrombin, protein C, protein S, and activated protein C resistance. In young women, CVST occurs more frequently in the puerperium than during pregnancy. Oral contraceptive use may also predispose to this condition. Some patients have underlying malignancies and the use of l-asparaginase also promotes venous thrombosis. Several children with inflammatory bowel disease have developed CVST.[102]

Hematological disorders that have been linked to CVST include thrombocytosis, polycythemia, sickle cell disease, heparin-induced thrombocytopenia, disseminated intravascular coagulation, and paroxysmal nocturnal hemoglobinuria. Occasional individuals with congestive heart failure or dehydration develop CVST, but increasingly these individuals are found to also have a coagulopathy or another risk factor. The risk factors for cerebral venous thrombosis are summarized in Table 22-6 and additional information about the individual risk factors, diagnosis, and therapy for CVST is presented in Chapter 20.

DIAGNOSTIC EVALUATION

Finding the cause of a child's stroke is important because the recurrence risk, one major component of the long-term prognosis, is often determined by the reason for the stroke and whether it is treatable. Because a variety of conditions can cause cerebral infarction in children, no single evaluation protocol works well for every individual. The diagnostic evaluation should ideally proceed in logical steps as outlined in Tables 22-7 and 22-8.

The availability of noninvasive neuroimaging techniques has made the confirmation of stroke more accurate and expeditious. The performance and interpretation of these studies in children is similar to the techniques used for adults (see Chapter 5). One exception is neonatal cranial ultrasound, which is made possible by the acoustic window provided by the anterior fontanel during the first few months of life. With neonatal ultrasound it is possible to visualize subependymal or intraventricular hemorrhages, AVMs, cerebral infarctions, and the hydrocephalus that sometimes accompany subarachnoid hemorrhage. Cranial ultrasound can be performed at the bedside and without sedation, significant advantages for infants who are too ill to be easily transported to an imaging suite. However, the resolution afforded by cranial ultrasound is not as good it is with other neuroimaging techniques, and it is often necessary to perform one or more of these other studies to obtain more precise information.

TREATMENT CONSIDERATIONS

Less is known about treatment of stroke in children than about its etiology. Any modifiable risk factors should be eliminated in an effort to prevent recurrences. Drug therapy is largely untested in children, so treatment regimens are often adapted from experience in adults. Moreover, some stroke treatments are innately more difficult in children. Infants, for example, require a substantially higher dose of heparin and their response to warfarin fluctuates widely. Chronic anticoagulation in a toddler is riskier due to frequent falls. Because the causes of stroke are numerous in these individuals, treatment should be individualized based on the age and stroke etiology.

Anticoagulation

Anticoagulation is recommended for children with a major risk of recurrent emboli, for children with cervicocephalic arterial dissection, for patients with CVST, and for individuals with a severe hypercoagulable state. A common approach is to initiate anticoagulation with intravenous heparin and while adjusting the warfarin dose to achieve the desired international normalized ratio (INR), an approach that is not unlike the one used in adult patients. Anticoagulation is not recommended for children who have emboli and infective endocarditis.[22] The recently published pediatric stroke management recommendations also allow the use of unfractionated or low molecular weight heparin (LMWH) for up to a week after presentation during the diagnostic evaluation.[22] Anticoagulation during the initial evaluation is not usually recommended in adults, but this approach is allowed in children because they are more likely than adults to have stroke risk factors that might benefit from anticoagulation. Anticoagulation with LMWH may be used in lieu of long-term warfarin therapy.[103]

Anticoagulation for high-risk embolism patients should continue indefinitely or until the risk has been lowered by correction of the cardiac source of the emboli. Although surgery for complex congenital heart defects does not usually eliminate the risk of embolic stroke completely, surgery can greatly diminish the stroke risk for some lesions. In these patients, anticoagulation until the corrective surgery may be a reasonable option. As is the case in adults, children with artificial cardiac valves need to continue anticoagulation indefinitely.

Medical therapy of cervicocephalic arterial dissection typically involves initial anticoagulation with intravenous heparin followed by a 3- to 6-month course of warfarin adjusted to maintain an INR of 2.0 to 3.0. Antiplatelet agents are used less often for dissection, but these drugs are a reasonable option considering that neither approach has been demonstrated to be superior. Surgical correction has been proposed for selected individuals who have failed to respond to medical therapy. Surgical techniques used for cervicocephalic arterial dissections include proximal ligation, trapping procedures, and extracranial–intracranial bypass procedures.

Like adults, children with CVST may benefit from anticoagulation, even in the face of an intracranial hemorrhage (see Chapter 20). Although there are no controlled clinical trials proving the effectiveness of anticoagulation in children with CVST, several series suggest that anticoagulation is reasonably safe in these children, and one small prospective cohort study of 30 children with CVST suggested some beneficial effect from anticoagulation.[104,105] Roach and colleagues have made detailed recommendations for the evaluation and management of CVST in children.[22]

Table 22-8: More Selective Tests, Depending on Clinical Findings

If cause undetermined and suspect vasculitis:

- Drug screen
- FTA-ABS
- HIV serology (serum ELISA and Western blot)

- Antinuclear antibodies (ANA), extractable nuclear antigens (anti-S, nRNP, antibody to double-stranded DNA, only if ANA+)
- Rheumatoid factor
- Anticardiolipin antibodies
- C-reactive protein
- Antineutrophilic cytoplasmic antibody (ANCA)
- Hepatitis B surface antigen (Hbs Ag)
- Scl 70 antibody (anti-isomerase antibody)
- Anticentromere antibodies
- Serum angiotensin-converting enzyme
- Serum immunoglobulin levels
- Cryoglobulins
- Coomb's test
- Anti-SS-A antibody
- Anti-SS-B antibody
- Shirmer's test
- CSF examination
- Pulmonary function tests (spirometry, lung volumes, diffusing capacity)
- Paranasal sinus radiographs
- Gallium 647 scanning
- Visceral angiography (renal, hepatic, mesenteric circulation)
- Tissue biopsy

If cause undetermined and suspect cardiac source:

- Blood cultures
- Contrast echocardiography
- Transesophageal echocardiography
- Doppler echocardiography
- Holter monitoring
- Ultrafast (cine) cardiac CT
- Magnetic resonance imaging of the heart
- Cardiac catheterization

If cause undetermined and suspect hypercoagulable cause:

- Functional assay of antithrombin
- Immunological and functional assays of protein C
- Immunological assay of total and free protein S and functional assay of protein S
- Anticoagulant response to APC in aPTT assay
- Factor V Leiden mutation by polymerase chain reaction (PCR)
- Immunologic and functional assays of fibrinogen
- Thrombin time
- Euglobulin clot lysis time
- Plasminogen levels
- Plasmin functional activity
- Inhibitors of plasminogen activation
- Factors V, VII, VIII, IX, X, XI, and XIII assay
- Lupus anticoagulant
- Anticardiolipin antibodies (IgG and IgM)
- Circulating platelet aggregates and spontaneous platelet aggregation
- Fibrin monomers
- Fibrin degradation products
- Fibrinolytic activity
- Sucrose hemolysis test (if +, acidified serum lysis test)
- Plasma homocysteine
- Heparin-associated platelet antibodies
- Cystathionine β synthase activity in biopsy tissue
- Sickle cell testing and hemoglobin electrophoresis
- β_2 glycoprotein 1 antibodies (IgG and IgM)
- Prothrombin gene mutation (*G20210A*)

If cause undetermined & suspect miscellaneous causes:

- Apolipoprotein quantification (apolipoprotein B and E levels)
- Plasma lactate and pyruvate levels
- Leukocyte α-galactosidase activity
- Urinary sulfite or thiosulfate quantification
- Ophthalmological examination

Adapted with permission from Biller.[4]
APC = activated protein C; aPTT = activated partial thromboplastin time; ELISA = enzyme-linked immunosorbent assay; FTA-ABS = florescent treponemal antibody absorption; PCR = polymerase chain reaction; nRNP = nuclear ribonucleoprotein; anti-S = anti-Smith proteins.

Table 22-9: Protocol for Systemic Heparin Administration and Adjustment in Children

Stage		aPTT	Dose, Units/kg	Hold, min	Rate Change, %	Repeat aPTT
Loading dose[a]			75 IV over 10 min			
Initial maintenance dose	Infants < 1 yr		28/hr			
	Children > 1 yr		20/hr			
Adjustment[b]		< 50	50	0	10	4 hr
		50–59	0	0	10	4 hr
		60–85	0	0	0	Next day
		86–95	0	0	−10	4 hr
		96–120	0	30	−10	4 hr
		> 120	0	60	−15	4 hr

Obtain blood for aPTT 4 hr after heparin load and 4 hr after every infusion rate change

When aPTT values are in therapeutic range, perform daily CBC and aPTT measurement

Adapted with permission from Michelson et al.[116]
[a] Some physicians omit this step.
[b] Heparin was adjusted to maintain aPTT at 60–85 seconds, assuming that this reflects an anti–factor Xa level of 0.35–0.70.
aPTT = activated partial thromboplastin time; CBC = complete blood count.

Table 22-10: Protocol for Using LMWH in Children

Preparation		Initial Treatment Dose	Initial Prophylactic Dose
Reviparin, body weight–dependent dose, units/kg per 12 hr	< 5 kg	150	50
	> 5 kg	100	30
Enoxaparin, age-dependent dose, mg/kg per 12 hr	< 2 mo	1.5	0.75
	> 2 mo	1.0	0.5
Dalteparin, all-age pediatric dose, units/kg per 24 hr		129 + 43	92 + 52
Tinzaparin, age-dependent dose, units/kg	0–2 mo		275
	2–12 mo		250
	1–5 yr		240
	5–10 yr		200
	10–16 yr		275

Adapted with permission from Monagle et al.[117]

Table 22-9 and Table 22-10 provide a systematic method for initiating and maintaining therapy with heparin and LMWH in children. Table 22-11 offers a standardized method of initiating warfarin therapy in children.

Antiplatelet Agents

Aspirin, clopidogrel, or the combination of extended-release dipyridamole and low-dose aspirin are the mainstays of therapy in the secondary prevention of stroke from arterial thromboembolic disease. The use of these agents in children, however, is hindered by the paucity of efficacy and safety data. Nevertheless, aspirin, especially, is used extensively in children with ischemic stroke. Roach and colleagues suggest that aspirin is a reasonable option for the secondary prevention of ischemic stroke in children who do not have SCD, a severe hypercoagulable disorder, or a high risk of recurrent embolism.[22]

For children, a weight-based aspirin dose of 3 mg/kg/day is sufficient to alter platelet function, so this amount is the recommended dose.[22] Children who develop dose-related side effects on this amount can try a lower dose of 1 to 3 mg/kg/day.[22]

Reye syndrome does not seem to be a major risk for children taking this recommended dose. Nevertheless, given the

Table 22-11: Warfarin Anticoagulation Protocol for Children[a]

Stage	INR	Action
I. Day 1	1.0–1.3	0.2 mg/kg orally
II. Days 2–4	1.1–1.3	Repeat day 1 loading dose
	1.4–1.9	50% of day 1 loading dose
	2.0–3.0	50% of day 1 loading dose
	3.1–3.5	25% of day 1 loading dose
	> 3.5	Hold dosing until INR is < 3.5 then restart according to stage III maintenance guidelines
III. Maintenance	1.1–1.4	Increase by 20% of dose
	1.4–1.9	Increase by 10% of dose
	2.0–3.0	No change
	3.1–3.5	Decrease by 10% of dose
	> 3.5	Hold dosing until INR is < 3.5 then restart at 20% less than last dose

Adapted with permission from Michelson et al.[116]
[a] The protocol is designed to maintain an INR between 2 and 3 with warfarin.
INR = international normalized ratio.

propensity for Reye syndrome to develop in the aftermath of influenza or chicken pox, it is reasonable to vaccinate against these infections and to withhold aspirin during either of these two infections.[22]

Thrombolysis in Children

Safety and efficacy data for the administration of intravenous or intra-arterial tissue plasminogen activator (tPA) in children with acute arterial stroke are generally unavailable aside from several case reports documenting its use.[106–108] The reported major complication rate for tPA in children treated for systemic thrombosis is 40%, but the drug dose and the duration of therapy are typically higher in these individuals than in patients treated for stroke.[109] Janjua and colleagues analyzed 46 individuals younger than 18 years of age with arterial stroke who received tPA under diverse circumstances; they concluded that neither the safety nor the efficacy of thrombolytic therapy for these individuals could be determined.[110]

Even if tPA proves to be useful in children, it is likely that delayed tPA treatment will lead to an unacceptable rate of intracerebral hemorrhage, much as it does in adult patients. Thus, if tPA is to be administered intravenously, it should be given within 3 to 4.5 hours of symptom onset and within 6 hours for intra-arterial use.[111,112] Of course, this limitation is a serious one given the frequent delay in presentation of children with stroke.

Roach and colleagues concluded that tPA may be considered for CVST and in older children who meet the established criteria for tPA use.[22] An optimal tPA dose for children has not been determined, although most of the clinical reports describing the use of tPA in children or adolescents used the same per kilogram dose that is typically utilized in adult patients (0.9 mg/kg).[108,113–115] This seems like a reasonable approach because the tPA dose is also determined by weight even in adults.

REFERENCES

1. Roach ES, Riela AR. *Pediatric Cerebrovascular Disorders.* 2nd ed. New York: Futura; 1995.
2. Al-Jarallah A, Al-Rifai MT, Riela AR, Roach ES. Nontraumatic brain hemorrhage in children: etiology and presentation. *J Child Neurol.* 2000;**15**:284–289.
3. Lo WD, Lee J, Rusin J, Perkins E, Roach ES. Intracranial hemorrhage in children: an evolving spectrum. *Arch Neurol.* 2008; **65**:1629–1633.
4. Biller J, ed. *Stroke in Children and Young Adults.* 2nd ed. Philadelphia: Elsevier Saunders; 2009.
5. Schoenberg BS, Mellinger JF, Schoenberg DG. Cerebrovascular disease in infants and children: a study of incidence, clinical features, and survival. *Neurology.* 1978;**28**:763–768.
6. Broderick J, Talbot T, Prenger E, Leach A, Brott T. Stroke in children within a major metropolitan area: the surprising importance of intracerebral hemorrhage. *J Child Neurol.* 1993;**8**:250–255.
7. Fullerton HJ, Wu YW, Zhao S, Johnston SC. Risk of stroke in children: ethnic and gender disparities. *Neurology.* 2003;**61**:189–194.
8. Golomb MR, Fullerton HJ, Nowak-Gottl U, deVeber G. Male Predominance in childhood ischemic stroke. Findings from the International Pediatric Stroke Study. *Stroke.* 2009;**40**:52–57.
9. Giroud M, Lemesle M, Madinier G, Manceau E, Osseby GV, Dumas R. Stroke in children under 16 years of age. Clinical and etiological difference with adults. *Acta Neurol Scand.* 1997;**96**:401–406.
10. Raju TN, Nelson KB, Ferriero D, Lynch JK. Ischemic perinatal stroke: summary of a workshop sponsored by the National Institute of Child Health and Human Development and the National Institute of Neurological Disorders and Stroke. *Pediatrics.* 2007;**120**:609–616.
11. Long DM, Seljeskog EL, Chou SN, French LA. Giant arteriovenous malformations of infancy and childhood. *J Neurosurg.* 1974;**40**:304–312.

12. Amacher AL, Shillito J. The syndromes and surgical treatment of aneurysms of the great vein of Galen. *J Neurosurg.* 1973;**39**:89–98.

13. Patel AN, Richardson AE. Ruptured intracranial aneurysms in the first two decades of life – a study of 58 patients. *J Neurosurg.* 1971;**35**:571–576.

14. Huang J, McGirt MJ, Gailloud P, Tamargo RJ. Intracranial aneurysms in the pediatric population: case series and literature review. *Surg Neurol.* 2005;**63**:424–432.

15. Orozco M, Trigueros F, Quintana F, Dierssen G. Intracranial aneurysms in early childhood. *Surg Neurol.* 1978;**9**:247–252.

16. Shucart WA, Wolpert SM. Intracranial arterial aneurysms in childhood. *Am J Dis Child.* 1974;**127**:288–293.

17. Woerner SJ, Abildgaard CF, French BN. Intracranial hemorrhage in children with idiopathic thrombocytopenic purpura. *Pediatrics.* 1981;**67**:453–460.

18. Renzulli P, Tuchschmid P, Eich G, Fanconi S, Schwobel MG. Early vitamin K deficiency bleeding after maternal phenobarbital intake: management of massive intracranial haemorrhage by minimal surgical intervention. *Eur J Pediatr.* 1998;**157**:663–665.

19. Kuban KCK, Leviton A, Krishnamoorthy KS, et al. Neonatal intracranial hemorrhage and phenobarbital. *Pediatrics.* 1986;**77**:443–450.

20. Kohler HG. Haemorrhage in the newborn of epileptic mothers. *Lancet.* 1966;**1**:267.

21. Wijdicks EF, de Groen PC, Wiesner RH, Krom RA. Intracerebral hemorrhage in liver transplant recipients. *Mayo Clin Proc.* 1995;**70**:443–446.

22. Roach ES, Golomb MR, Adams RJ, et al. Management of stroke in infants and children. A scientific statement for healthcare professionals from a special writing group of the Stroke Council, American Heart Association. *Stroke.* 2008;**39**:2644–2691.

23. Shin M, Kawamoto S, Kurita H, et al. Retrospective analysis of a 10-year experience of stereotactic radiosurgery for arteriovenous malformations in children and adolescents. *J Neurosurg.* 2002;**97**:779–784.

24. Levy EI, Niranjan A, Thompson TP, et al. Radiosurgery for childhood intracranial arteriovenous malformations. *Neurosurgery.* 2000;**47**:834–841.

25. Mendelow AD, Gregson BA, Fernandes HM, et al. Early surgery versus initial conservative treatment in patients with spontaneous supratentorial intracerebral haematomas in the International Surgical Trial in Intracerebral Haemorrhage (STICH): a randomised trial. *Lancet.* 2005;**365**:387–397.

26. Batjer HH, Reisch JS, Allen BC, Plaizier LJ, Su CJ. Failure of surgery to improve outcome in hypertensive putaminal hemorrhage: a prospective randomized trial. *Arch Neurol.* 1990;**47**:1103–1106.

27. Rafay MF, Pontigon AM, Chiang J, et al. Delay to diagnosis in acute pediatric arterial ischemic stroke. *Stroke.* 2009;**40**:58–64.

28. Zimmer JA, Garg BP, Williams LS, Golomb MR. Age-related variation in presenting signs of childhood arterial ischemic stroke. *Pediatr Neurol.* 2007;**37**:171–175.

29. Roach ES. Stroke in children. *Curr Treat Options Neurol.* 2000;**2**:295–304.

30. Brower MC, Rollins N, Roach ES. Basal ganglia and thalamic infarction in children. Etiology and clinical features. *Arch Neurol.* 1996;**53**:1252–1256.

31. Curry CJ, Bhullar S, Holmes J, Delozier CD, Roeder ER, Hutchison HT. Risk factors for perinatal arterial stroke: a study of 60 mother-child pairs. *Pediatr Neurol.* 2007;**37**:99–107.

32. Golomb MR. The contribution of prothrombotic disorders to peri- and neonatal ischemic stroke. *Semin Thromb Hemost.* 2003;**29**:415–424.

33. Roach ES. Etiology of stroke in children. *Semin Pediatr Neurol.* 2000;**7**:244–260.

34. Lanthier S, Carmant L, David M, Larbrisseau A, deVeber GA. Stroke in children: the coexistence of multiple risk factors predicts poor outcome. *Neurology.* 2000;**54**:371–378.

35. Kaplan P, Levinson M, Kaplan BS. Cerebral artery stenoses in Williams syndrome cause strokes in childhood. *J Pediatr.* 1995;**126**:943–945.

36. Kawai M, Nishikawa T, Tanaka M, et al. An autopsied case of Williams syndrome complicated by moyamoya disease. *Acta Paediatr Jpn.* 1993;**35**:63–67.

37. Soper R, Chaloupka JC, Fayad PB, et al. Ischemic stroke and intracranial multifocal cerebral arteriopathy in Williams syndrome. *J Pediatr.* 1995;**126**:945–948.

38. Woolfenden AR, Albers GW, Steinberg GK, Hahn JS, Johnston DC, Farrell K. Moyamoya syndrome in children with Alagille syndrome: additional evidence of a vasculopathy. *Pediatrics.* 1999;**103**:505–508.

39. Rachmel A, Zeharia A, Neuman-Levin M, Weitz R, Shamir R, Dinari G. Alagille syndrome associated with moyamoya disease. *Am J Med Genet.* 1989;**33**:89–91.

40. Lutterman J, Scott M, Nass R, Geva T. Moyamoya syndrome associated with congenital heart disease. *Pediatrics.* 1998;**101**:57–60.

41. Oski JA, Canter CE, Spray TL, Kan JS, Cameron DE, Murphy AM. Embolic stroke after ligation of the pulmonary artery in patients with functional single ventricle. *Am Heart J.* 1996;**132**:836–840.

42. du Plessis AJ, Chang AC, Wessel DL, et al. Cerebrovascular accidents following the Fontan operation. *Pediatr Neurol.* 1995;**12**:230–236.

43. Day RW, Boyer RS, Tait VF, Ruttenberg HD. Factors associated with stroke following the Fontan procedure. *Pediatr Cardiol.* 1995;**16**:270–275.

44. Lane JR, Ben-Shachar G. Myocardial infarction in healthy adolescents. *Pediatrics.* 2007;**120**:e938–e943.

45. Crea F, Gaspardone A, Tomai F, et al. Risk factors in schoolchildren associated with a family history of unheralded myocardial infarction or uncomplicated stable angina in male relatives. *J Am Coll Cardiol.* 1994;**23**:1472–1478.

46. Zhuang J, Wang S, Zhang Z, Zeng S, Shi Y, Nong S. Acute myocardial infarction and ascending aortic aneurysm in a child with Behçet's disease. *Turk J Pediatr.* 2008;**50**:81–85.

47. Bayir H, Morelli PJ, Smith TH, Biancaniello TA. A left atrial myxoma presenting as a cerebrovascular accident. *Pediatr Neurol.* 1999;**21**:569–572.

48. Knepper LE, Biller J, Adams HP, Bruno A. Neurologic manifestations of atrial myxoma. A 12-year experience and review. *Stroke.* 1988;**19**:1435–1440.

49. Al-Mateen M, Hood M, Trippel D, Insalaco SJ, Otto RK, Vitikainen KJ. Cerebral embolism from atrial myxoma in pediatric patients. *Pediatrics.* 2003;**112**:e162–e167.

50. Ergina PL, Kochamba GS, Tchervenkov CI, Gibbons JE. Atrial myxomas in young children: an alternative surgical approach. *Ann Thorac Surg.* 1993;**56**:1180–1183.

51. Kandt RS, Gebarski SS, Goetting MG. Tuberous sclerosis with cardiogenic cerebral embolism: magnetic resonance imaging. *Neurology.* 1985;**35**:1223–1225.

52. Gomez MR. Strokes in tuberous sclerosis: are rhabdomyomas a cause? *Brain Dev.* 1989;**11**:14–19.

53. Habib G. Management of infective endocarditis. *Heart.* 2006;**92**:124–130.

54. Wilson W, Taubert KA, Gewitz M, et al. Prevention of infective endocarditis: guidelines from the American Heart Association: a guideline from the American Heart Association Rheumatic Fever, Endocarditis, and Kawasaki Disease Committee, Council

on Cardiovascular Disease in the Young, and the Council on Clinical Cardiology, Council on Cardiovascular Surgery and Anesthesia, and the Quality of Care and Outcomes Research Interdisciplinary Working Group. *Circulation.* 2007;**116**:1736–1754.

55. Tsimikas S, Witztum JL. Shifting the diagnosis and treatment of atherosclerosis to children and young adults: a new paradigm for the 21st century. *J Am Coll Cardiol.* 2002;**40**:2122–2124.

56. Enos WF, Holmes RH, Beyer J. Coronary disease among United States soldiers killed in action in Korea. *JAMA.* 1953;**152**:1090–1093.

57. Woo KS, Chook P, Yu CW, et al. Overweight in children is associated with arterial endothelial dysfunction and intima-media thickening. *Int J Obes Relat Metab Disord.* 2004;**28**:852–857.

58. Caplan LR. Dissections of brain-supplying arteries. *Nat Clin Pract Neurol.* 2008;**4**:34–42.

59. Schievink WI. Spontaneous dissection of the carotid and vertebral arteries. *N Engl J Med.* 2001;**344**:898–906.

60. Fullerton HJ, Johnston SC, Smith WS. Arterial dissection and stroke in children. *Neurology.* 2001;**57**:1155–1160.

61. Schievink WI, Mokri B, Piepgras DG. Spontaneous dissections of the cervicocephalic arteries in childhood and adolescence. *Neurology.* 1994;**44**:1607–1612.

62. Hasan I, Wapnick S, Kutscher ML, Couldwell WT. Vertebral arterial dissection associated with Klippel-Feil syndrome in a child. *Childs Nerv Syst.* 2002;**18**:67–70.

63. Schievink WI, Prakash UB, Piepgras DG, Mokri B. Alpha 1-antitrypsin deficiency in intracranial aneurysms and cervical artery dissection. *Lancet.* 1994;**343**:452–453.

64. Tyler HR, Clark DB. Neurologic complications in patients with coarctation of aorta. *Neurology.* 1958;**8**:712–718.

65. Hasan I, Wapnick S, Tenner MS, Couldwell WT. Vertebral artery dissection in children: a comprehensive review. *Pediatr Neurosurg.* 2002;**37**:168–177.

66. McManus BM, Cassling RS, Soundy TJ, et al. Familial aortic dissection in absence of ascending aortic aneurysms: a lethal syndrome associated with precocious systemic hypertension. *Am J Cardiovasc Pathol.* 1987;**1**:55–67.

67. Nicod P, Bloor C, Godfrey M, et al. Familial aortic dissecting aneurysm. *J Am Coll Cardiol.* 1989;**13**:811–819.

68. Pearl PL. Childhood stroke following intraoral trauma. *J Pediatr.* 1987;**110**:574–575.

69. Woodhurst WB, Robertson WD, Thompson GB. Carotid injury due to intraoral trauma: case report and review of the literature. *Neurosurgery.* 1980;**6**:559–563.

70. Graham CJ, Schwartz JE, Stacy T. Stroke following oral trauma in children. *Ann Emergency Med.* 1991;**20**:1029–1031.

71. Kuroda S, Houkin K, Hoshi Y, Tamura M, Kazumata K, Abe H. Cerebral hypoxia after hyperventilation causes "re-build-up" phenomenon and TIA in childhood moyamoya disease. A near-infrared spectroscopy study. *Childs Nerv Syst.* 1996;**12**:448–452.

72. Kurokawa T, Tomita S, Ueda K, et al. Prognosis of occlusive disease of the circle of Willis (moyamoya disease) in children. *Pediatr Neurol.* 1985;**1**:274–277.

73. Scott RM, Smith JL, Robertson RL, Madsen JR, Soriano SG, Rockoff MA. Long-term outcome in children with moyamoya syndrome after cranial revascularization by pial synangiosis. *J Neurosurg.* 2004;**100**:142–149.

74. Snyder RD, Stovring J, Cushing AH, Davis LE, Hardy TL. Cerebral infarction in childhood bacterial meningitis. *J Neurol Neurosurg Psychiatry.* 1981;**44**:581–585.

75. Riela A, Roach ES. Choreoathetosis in an infant with tuberculosis meningitis. *Arch Neurol.* 1982;**39**:596.

76. Sebire G, Meyer L, Chabrier S. Varicella as a risk factor for cerebral infarction in childhood: a case-control study. *Ann Neurol.* 1999;**45**:679–680.

77. Bleck TP. Central nervous system involvement in Rickettsial diseases. *Neurol Clin.* 1999;**17**:801–812.

78. Visudhiphan P, Chiemchanya S, Somburanasin R, Dheandhanoo D. Causes of spontaneous subarachnoid hemorrhage in Thai infants and children – a study of 56 patients. *J Neurosurg.* 1980;**53**:185–187.

79. Malavazi I, Abrao EP, Mikawa AY, Landgraf VO, da Costa PI. Abnormalities in apolipoprotein and lipid levels in an HIV-infected Brazilian population under different treatment profiles: the relevance of apolipoprotein E genotypes and immunological status. *Clin Chem Lab Med.* 2004;**42**:525–532.

80. Mizusawa H, Hirano A, Llena JF, Shintaku M. Cerebrovascular lesions in acquired immune deficiency syndrome (AIDS). *Acta Neuropathol (Berl).* 1988;**76**:451–457.

81. Vahedi K, Chabriat H, Levy C, Joutel A, Tournier-Lasserve E, Bousser M-G. Migraine with aura and brain magnetic resonance imaging abnormalities in patients with CADASIL. *Arch Neurol.* 2004;**61**:1237–1240.

82. Desmond DW, Moroney JT, Lynch T, Chan S, Chin SS, Mohr JP. The natural history of CADASIL: a pooled analysis of previously published cases. *Stroke.* 1999;**30**:1230–1233.

83. Jen JC, Klein A, Boltshauser E, et al. Prolonged hemiplegic episodes in children due to mutations in ATP1A2. *J Neurol Neurosurg Psychiatry.* 2007;**78**:523–526.

84. Damen L, Bruijn JK, Verhagen AP, Berger MY, Passchier J, Koes BW. Symptomatic treatment of migraine in children: a systematic review of medication trials. *Pediatrics.* 2005;**116**:e295–e302.

85. Adams RJ, Aaslid R, Gammal TE, Nichols FT, McKie V. Detection of cerebral vasculopathy in sickle cell disease using transcranial Doppler ultrasonography and magnetic resonance imaging. *Stroke.* 1988;**19**:518–520.

86. Adams RJ, Brambilla DJ, Granger S, et al. Stroke and conversion to high risk in children screened with transcranial Doppler ultrasound during the STOP study. *Blood.* 2004;**103**:3689–3694.

87. Adams RJ, McKie VC, Hsu L, et al. Stroke prevention trial in sickle cell anemia ("STOP"): Study results. *N Engl J Med.* 1998;**339**:5–11.

88. Strouse JJ, Lanzkron S, Beach MC, et al. Hydroxyurea for sickle cell disease: a systematic review for efficacy and toxicity in children. *Pediatrics.* 2008;**122**:1332–1342.

89. Vichinsky EP, Lubin BH. A cautionary note regarding hydroxyurea in sickle cell disease. *Blood.* 1994;**83**:1124–1128.

90. Fischer AQ, Challa VR, Burton BK, McLean WT. Cerebellar hemorrhage complicating isovaleric acidemia: a case report. *Neurology.* 1981;**31**:746–748.

91. Santos CC, Roach ES. Glutaric aciduria type I: a neuroimaging diagnosis? *J Child Neurol.* 2005;**20**:588–590.

92. Mudd SH, Skovby F, Levy HL, et al. The natural history of homocystinuria due to cystathionine B- synthase deficiency. *Am J Human Genet.* 1985;**37**:1–31.

93. Hirano M, Pavlakis SG. Mitochondrial myopathy, encephalopathy, lactic acidosis, and strokelike episodes (MELAS): current concepts. *J Child Neurol.* 1994;**9**:4–13.

94. Van Boagert L. Sur l'angiomatose meningee avec leukodystrophie. *Wein Z Nervenheilkd Grenzgeb.* 1967;**25**:131–136.

95. Dobyns WB, Garg BP. Vascular abnormalities in epidermal nevus syndrome. *Neurology.* 1991;**41**:276–278.

96. Ide C, De CB, Mailleux P, Baudrez V, Ossemann M, Trigaux JP. Hypoplasia of the internal carotid artery: a noninvasive diagnosis. *Eur Radiol.* 2000;**10**:1865–1870.

97. Golomb MR, Edwards-Brown M, Garg BP. Asymptomatic sinovenous thrombosis in a healthy neonate. *Neurology.* 2006;**66**:1186.

98. Carvalho KS, Bodensteiner JB, Connolly PJ, Garg BP. Cerebral venous thrombosis in children. *J Child Neurol.* 2001;**16**:574–580.

99. deVeber G, Andrew M. Cerebral sinovenous thrombosis in children. *N Engl J Med.* 2001;**345**:417–423.

100. Heller C, Becker S, Scharrer I, Kreuz W. Prothrombotic risk factors in childhood stroke and venous thrombosis. *Eur J Pediatr.* 1999;**158**(Suppl 3):S117–S121.

101. Bonduel M, Sciuccati G, Hepner M, Torres AF, Pieroni G, Frontroth JP. Prethrombotic disorders in children with arterial ischemic stroke and sinovenous thrombosis. *Arch Neurol.* 1999;**56**:967–971.

102. Standridge S, de los Reyes E. Inflammatory bowel disease and cerebrovascular arterial and venous thromboembolic events in 4 pediatric patients: a case series and review of the literature. *J Child Neurol.* 2008;**23**:59–66.

103. Dix D, Andrew M, Marzinotta V, et al. The use of low molecular weight heparin in pediatric patients: a prospective cohort study. *J Pediatr.* 2000;**136**:439–445.

104. Sebire G, Tabarki B, Saunders DE, et al. Cerebral venous sinus thrombosis in children: risk factors, presentation, diagnosis and outcome. *Brain.* 2005;**128**:477–489.

105. deVeber G, Chan A, Monagle P, et al. Anticoagulation therapy in pediatric patients with sinovenous thrombosis: a cohort study. *Arch Neurol.* 1998;**55**:1533–1537.

106. Carlson MD, Leber S, Deveikis J, Silverstein FS. Successful use of rt-PA in pediatric stroke. *Neurology.* 2001;**57**:157–158.

107. Thirumalai SS, Shubin RA. Successful treatment for stroke in a child using recombinant tissue plasminogen activator. *J Child Neurol.* 2000;**15**:558.

108. Benedict SL, Ni OK, Schloesser P, White KS, Bale JF Jr. Intra-arterial thrombolysis in a 2-year-old with cardioembolic stroke. *J Child Neurol.* 2007;**22**:225–227.

109. Gupta AA, Leaker M, Andrew M, et al. Safety and outcomes of thrombolysis with tissue plasminogen activator for treatment of intravascular thrombosis in children. *J Pediatr.* 2001;**139**:682–688.

110. Janjua N, Nasar A, Lynch JK, Qureshi AI. Thrombolysis for ischemic stroke in children: data from the nationwide inpatient sample. *Stroke.* 2007;**38**:1850–1854.

111. Manco-Johnson MJ, Grabowski EF, Hellgreen M, et al. Recommendations for tPA thrombolysis in children. On behalf of the Scientific Subcommittee on Perinatal and Pediatric Thrombosis of the Scientific and Standardization Committee of the International Society of Thrombosis and Haemostasis. *Thromb Haemost.* 2002;**88**:157–158.

112. The National Institute of Neurological Disorders and Stroke rt-PA Stroke Study Group. Tissue plasminogen activator for acute ischemic stroke. *N Engl J Med.* 1995;**333**:1581–1587.

113. Noser EA, Felberg RA, Alexandrov AV. Thrombolytic therapy in an adolescent ischemic stroke. *J Child Neurol.* 2001;**16**:286–288.

114. Heil JW, Malinowski L, Rinderknecht A, Broderick JP, Franz D. Use of intravenous tissue plasminogen activator in a 16-year-old patient with basilar occlusion. *J Child Neurol.* 2008;**23**:1049–1053.

115. Ortiz GA, Koch S, Wallace DM, Lopez-Alberola R. Successful intravenous thrombolysis for acute stroke in a child. *J Child Neurol.* 2007;**22**:749–752.

116. Michelson AD, Bovill E, Andrew M. Antithrombotic therapy in children. *Chest.* 1995;**108**:506S–522S.

117. Monagle P, Chan A, Massicotte P, Chalmers E, Michelson AD. Antithrombotic therapy in children: the Seventh ACCP Conference on Antithrombotic and Thrombolytic Therapy. *Chest.* 2004;**126**:645S–687S.

23

Stroke in Pregnancy

Nothing will sustain you more potently than the power to recognize in your humdrum routine, as perhaps it may be thought, the true poetry of life – the poetry of the common-place, of the ordinary man, of the plain, toil-worn woman, with their loves and their joys, their sorrows and their griefs.

William Osler

The tremendous physiological changes that occur during pregnancy and the postpartum period can predispose women to develop ischemic stroke, sinovenous thrombosis, and intracranial hemorrhage (see Tables 23-1, 23-2, and 23-3). Although such complications are uncommon, pregnancy is a risk factor for stroke in some individuals. Normal pregnancy induces a hypercoagulable state and significant hemodynamic changes. It can lead to unique conditions such as amniotic fluid embolism and eclampsia.

PREGNANCY-ASSOCIATED STROKE RISK

About 90% of both hemorrhagic and ischemic strokes occur during or just after the last trimester, especially around time of delivery and during the first 6 weeks of the postpartum period. The relative risk of cerebral infarction during the puerperium is 8.7 compared to only 0.7 during pregnancy. The adjusted relative risk of hemorrhage is 2.5 during pregnancy but 28.3 during the puerperium.[1–5] Rapid changes in hormonal balance, plasma volume, the coagulation system and vascular function may be responsible for this relative increase in stroke risk. The pregnancy-associated stroke risk is higher in women with arterial hypertension and other traditional vascular risk factors.[6,7] It is also higher in women with coagulopathies, migraine with aura, sickle cell disease, postpartum infection, and in those undergoing Caesarean delivery.[8,9] African American race and advanced maternal age also are associated with a higher pregnancy-related stroke risk. It is important to identify and manage modifiable risk factors during pregnancy appropriately to prevent ischemic and hemorrhagic strokes, although diagnosis and treatment are somewhat limited due to pregnancy-specific safety concerns.

Table 23-1: Hemodynamic Changes in Pregnancy

Cardiac output	+ 43%
Systemic vascular resistance	− 21%
Pulmonary vascular resistance	− 34%
Heart rate	+ 17%
Stroke index	+ 17%
Mean arterial blood pressure	− 4%

Table 23-2: Changes in Blood Flow in Normal Pregnancy

Brain	↔
Liver	↔
Uterus	↑
Kidneys	↑
Extremities	↑
Skin	↑
Breast	↑
Coronary arteries	?

PHYSIOLOGICAL CHANGES DURING PREGNANCY AND THE PUERPERIUM

Pregnancy-associated physiological changes lead to alterations in endothelial cell and platelet function and affect coagulation as well as the circulatory system. Changes in hemostasis result in a hypercoagulable state that increases the risk of thromboembolic complications.[10] In addition, pregnancy places an increased demand on cardiac function and the vascular system, which can

Table 23-3: Clotting and Fibrinolytic Shifts during Pregnancy

Increased

- Fibrinogen
- Factors VII, VIII, X, XII
- High molecular weight kininogen
- vW antigen
- PAI-1, PAI-2, plasminogen, antiplasmin
- FDP, D-dimer

Decreased

- Factor XI
- Fibrinolysis, tPA release
- Protein S

Unchanged

- Factors II, V, IX, XIII
- Antithrombin, protein C

FDP = fibrin/fibrinogen degradation product; PAI-1 = plasminogen activator inhibitor-1; PAI-2 = plasminogen activator inhibitor-2; tPA = tissue plasminogen activator; vW = von Willebrand.

predispose women to develop arterial hypertension and peripartum cardiomyopathy, conditions that are associated with an increased stroke risk. Hypertension develops in up to 10% to 15% of pregnant women and requires appropriate treatment to avoid complications.[11] Pre-eclampsia, which is a major cause for maternal and fetal morbidity and mortality, develops in 5% to 10% of all pregnant hypertensive women.[1]

Activation of platelets and the coagulation cascade are necessary to counteract the hemorrhage associated with placental separation during delivery, but when unbalanced, can predispose to thrombosis. Women with an acquired or inherited hypercoagulable state secondary to factor V Leiden mutation, antithrombin, protein C or protein S deficiency, or prothrombin gene mutation are especially at risk for thromboembolic complications. The risk of venous thrombosis is about 0.7 per 1,000

pregnant women but this number increases by three- to four-fold during the postpartum period.[12]

During the second half of pregnancy there is an increase in activated protein C resistance and a decrease in protein S activity.[13] Levels of fibrinogen, factors II, VII, VIII, X, and XII and prothrombin begin to increase by the end of the first trimester.[14,15] These changes are associated with increased fibrinolytic inhibitor activity, increased platelet turnover, and platelet activation, all of which promote hypercoagulability. With the HELLP syndrome (hemolysis, elevated liver enzymes, and low platelets during pregnancy or the postpartum period), thrombocytopenia can be severe enough to facilitate intracranial hemorrhage (Figure 23-1). In addition, platelets transition into an activated state during which they express P-selectin, CD63, and PECAM-1, which causes platelet adhesion and aggregation associated with cerebral ischemic strokes.[16,17]

Cardiovascular and hemodynamic changes during pregnancy and the puerperium cause significant physiological stress on the circulatory system. The plasma volume increases by 30% to 50% at term above the nonpregnant state, which on average equals a retention of about 1,000 mEq of sodium and 6 to 9 liters of fluid.[18–20] The red blood cell mass increases by about 20% to 30%. This increased blood volume serves as a reserve for blood loss that may occur during delivery or with postpartum hemorrhage and counteracts the pregnancy-associated hypercoagulable state. Blood pressure falls slightly, but returns to prepregnancy values around term. This fall in blood pressure reaches its nadir around 20 weeks of gestation and reflects a reduction in peripheral vascular resistance. Pregnancy also increases the heart rate, stroke volume, and cardiac output.

ECLAMPSIA/PRE-ECLAMPSIA AND THE HELLP SYNDROME

Hypertensive disorders of pregnancy encompass chronic hypertension, pregnancy induced hypertension, pre-eclampsia, and eclampsia. Eclampsia and pre-eclampsia are the most common causes of pregnancy-associated stroke and can occur at any time from the second trimester to the puerperium.[21,22] However, stroke leading to significant disability and mortality in women with pre-eclampsia and eclampsia is relatively rare.[23–25]

The pathophysiological mechanisms leading to cerebral ischemia or hemorrhage are multifactorial.[26,27] Generalized endothelial dysfunction causes altered vascular tone, hypertension, coagulopathy, and blood vessel leakage with subsequent development of proteinuria.[28–30] The resulting cerebral microangiopathy

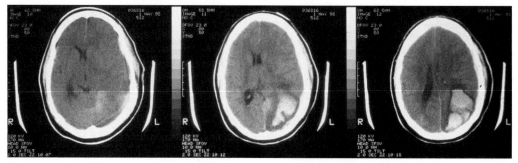

Figure 23-1. Cranial CT scan showing a lobar hemorrhage with mass effect in a hypertensive postpartum woman with hemolysis, elevated liver enzymes, and thrombocytopenia (the HELLP syndrome).

causes blood vessel leakage and increases the likelihood of both intracerebral hemorrhage and thromboembolic events.[31] Platelet aggregation and turnover are increased in pre-eclampsia, and there is a tendency for microthrombi formation. Blood vessel damage in addition causes cerebral edema which, in combination with vasospasm, can compromise cerebral blood flow, resulting in brain ischemia and infarcts.[32]

However, long before clinical symptoms of brain and systemic microangiopathy develop, changes in the placental circulation occur that result in chronic placental hypoperfusion. Normally, the trophoblast differentiates and invades the uterine vascular bed during the earliest stages of pregnancy, where it induces remodeling of the uterine spiral arteries.[33,34] The spiral arteries then transform from relatively high-resistance arterioles to low-resistance conduits, allowing exchange of oxygen and metabolites between the maternal and the fetal circulation. Several studies suggest that immunologic, hemodynamic, and genetic factors can affect normal trophoblast differentiation so that normal vascular remodeling fails. The spiral arteries remain narrow leading to placental hypoperfusion and ischemia. There is accumulating evidence that chronic placental hypoperfusion together with an increased metabolic demand during later stages of pregnancy may result in excretion of cytokines and other mediators of inflammation and oxidative stress into the maternal circulation causing generalized endothelial dysfunction and subsequent multiorgan microangiopathy.[35–38]

Clinically, pre-eclampsia is defined by new onset of arterial hypertension, that is, systolic blood pressure of $\geq$ 140 mm Hg and diastolic blood pressure $\geq$ 90 mm Hg, along with proteinuria, that is, $\geq$ 0.3 g in 24-hour urine sample, after 20 weeks of gestation in a previously normotensive woman.[39,40] Pre-eclampsia can be mild or severe. Severe pre-eclampsia frequently causes multisystem (renal, hepatic, coagulation) dysfunction.[41] Central nervous system impairment manifestations include visual changes, cortical blindness, altered cognitive function and headaches, and stroke.[42] Eclampsia is characterized by one or more generalized seizures and/or coma in an individual with pre-eclampsia and in the absence of any other medical condition that could cause these symptoms.

In women who are at moderate to high risk of developing pre-eclampsia, low-dose aspirin has shown modest, but significant, benefit in several studies and should be considered.[43–50] Relatively early treatment, within the 12th to 14th week of gestation, seems to be favorable. The safety of low dose aspirin in the second and third trimesters has been well established. The definitive treatment of pre-eclampsia is delivery, but this option must consider gestational age, maternal and fetal condition, and the overall clinical picture. In general mild cases of pre-eclampsia have good maternal and fetal outcome, but there is a predisposition to recurrent pre-eclampsia or eclampsia in subsequent pregnancies.

About 10% to 20% of women with severe pre-eclampsia develop HELLP syndrome.[51,52] Hypertension and proteinuria are common. Most cases (70%) occur between the 28th and 36th weeks of pregnancy and the rest develop during the immediate postpartum period. Thrombocytopenia and disseminated intravascular coagulation (DIC) associated with HELLP can lead to intracranial hemorrhage (Figure 23-1) or ischemic stroke which are best managed symptomatically.[53] Acute liver failure can result in increased intracranial pressure, massive cerebral edema, and death.[54] The definitive treatment of HELLP syndrome is emergent delivery.

HYPERTENSION AND PREGNANCY

Hypertension is part of the clinical picture of eclampsia/pre-eclampsia, but it also occurs in the setting of gestational hypertension or exacerbation of chronic hypertension. Gestational hypertension typically starts after the 20th week of gestation. In contrast to pre-eclampsia, which occurs at about the same time period, gestational hypertension is not associated with proteinuria. Untreated severe hypertension is associated with increased risk of hemorrhagic and ischemic stroke, acute renal and heart failure, hypertensive encephalopathy, and adverse pregnancy outcome.[39,55,56]

As there is a risk of placental hypoperfusion and fetal injury with too aggressive blood pressure management, mild hypertension should probably not be treated until after delivery. However, blood pressure needs to be closely monitored during pregnancy. Depending on preexisting blood pressure levels and concern about hypertension-related end-organ damage, systolic blood pressures should be maintained between 120 and 150 mm Hg and diastolic pressures kept between 80 and 100 mm Hg for those with severe hypertension.

Following a stroke, blood pressures must be managed to maintain cerebral and placental perfusion while avoiding complications due to severely elevated blood pressures. These patients often benefit from a multidisciplinary treatment team. Treatment options include intravenous labetalol or methyldopa.[57,58] Second-line drugs include nicardipine, nifedipine, or hydralazine.[59] Nitroprusside has a risk of cyanide exposure and should be avoided especially during the late stages of pregnancy. Angiotensin converting enzyme inhibitors and angiotensin II receptor blockers are contraindicated due to their teratogenicity. Diuretics should be avoided because of the potential risks associated with induced electrolyte abnormalities.[60,61]

CARDIOEMBOLIC STROKE DURING PREGNANCY

The risk of stroke due to cardiac disease during pregnancy and the puerperium is relatively small. About 1% to 4% of pregnancies are complicated by cardiac disease and its sequelae, and relatively few of these individuals have a stroke.[62] Most cases in developed countries are now due to congenital heart disease while rheumatic fever is becoming increasingly rare.[63,64] However, owing to increasing maternal age, which is often associated with higher incidence of traditional vascular risk factors such as hypertension or diabetes, the number of pregnant women with acquired heart disease is growing.

Poor outcome and stroke risk are high among pregnant women with New York Heart Association classes II or greater status who have obstruction of left cardiac outflow and impaired ventricular systolic dysfunction with an ejection fraction less than 40%. The frequency of cardiac events is increased in women who have a history of stroke, transient ischemic attacks (TIAs), heart failure, or cardiac arrhythmias. The fetal risk increases in parallel with maternal risk. Risk for poor fetal and maternal outcome associated with congenital or acquired untreated valvular heart disease is especially high in women with symptomatic aortic and mitral valve stenosis or regurgitation, poor cardiac output (ejection fraction < 40%), need for anticoagulation due to mechanical prosthetic valve, and in patients with Marfan syndrome and aortic regurgitation.[65]

Infective endocarditis is uncommon but can cause ischemic stroke due to dislodgement of fragments from valvular vegetations.[66]

Infective endocarditis can also lead to intracranial hemorrhages due to formation of mycotic aneurysms or other complications (see Chapter 8). Management of infectious endocarditis during pregnancy can be more challenging than in other settings because of in the use of some antibiotics.

The mortality and morbidity of hypertrophic cardiomyopathy during pregnancy is relatively low and myocardial infarctions during pregnancy are rare.[67,68] Pregnancy-associated recurrence of antepartum arrhythmias is common and can increase the risk of cardioembolic stroke and poor maternal and fetal outcome and requires close cardiac monitoring.[69]

THROMBOPHILIA

Inherited and acquired thrombophilias are an important cause of ischemic stroke and thromboembolic events during pregnancy.[70,71] Management of thrombophilia during pregnancy is somewhat different than in nonpregnant women owing to potential fetal and maternal risks associated with standard anticoagulation and antiplatelet therapy. After delivery and during the postpartum period, treatment follows the standard approach for stroke prevention in these conditions (see Chapter 25).

Inherited Thrombophilia

The factor V Leiden mutation is the most common cause of inherited activated protein C resistance and ischemic stroke during pregnancy. The prothrombin gene mutation (*G20210A*) is also common, whereas antithrombin, protein C, or protein S deficiencies are relatively rare[72–74] (see Chapter 11). Thrombosis in individuals with inherited thrombophilias tends to affect the venous system more than the arterial, and thus the primary clinical complications include pulmonary embolism, deep venous thrombosis of the legs, cerebral venous thrombosis, spontaneous abortion, and fetal loss.[75,76] Hormonal changes, generalized vasodilatation, immobility, delivery, and impairment of venous return from the lower extremities by uterine compression increase the risk of venous thrombosis and arterial events. Additional risk factors for thromboembolic events include advanced maternal age, high parity, a short interval since the last pregnancy, obesity, recent surgery, tobacco use, and presence of traditional vascular risk factors.

In women with isolated protein C or protein S deficiency and in those who are heterozygous for factor V Leiden or prothrombin gene mutation, the risk of thromboembolic events during pregnancy and the postpartum period is probably less than 1%. Women with antithrombin deficiency and those who are homozygotes or compound heterozygotes for factor V Leiden deficiency or for the prothrombin *G20210A* gene mutation are at highest risk for stroke. Their risk increases significantly if additional risk factors are present or if there is a personal or family history of previous thromboembolic complications.[77] For instance, a pregnant woman with factor V Leiden mutation who also has a history of thromboembolism increases her risk of thromboembolic complications from 0.2% to 10%. Prophylactic anticoagulation in low-risk individuals is not usually warranted unless there are additional risk factors such as other thrombophilias or a personal or family history of thrombotic complications.[78]

Women who have a pregnancy-associated ischemic stroke should be screened for antiphospholipid antibodies to detect acquired thrombophilias. Interpretation of laboratory tests for thrombophilia is complicated by the fact that protein S levels are normally reduced by 60% to 70% in healthy pregnant women and that heparin and warfarin can influence the levels of antithrombin as well as proteins S and C.

Subcutaneous heparin seems superior to low-dose aspirin for prophylaxis of recurrent thromboembolic events due to inherited thrombophilia in pregnancy.[79] Women with a history of pregnancy-associated venous or thromboembolic events require anticoagulation throughout their pregnancy and for at least 6 to 8 weeks postpartum. Women with high-risk thrombophilia and with personal or family history of unexplained previous venous thrombosis should be prophylactically anticoagulated during their pregnancy and the postpartum period.[80,81] Subcutaneous low molecular weight heparin (LMWH) is now the drug of choice for thromboembolic complications in patients with inherited thrombophilia.[82–87] Intermittent monitoring of antifactor Xa levels to evaluate therapeutic efficacy of LMWH and regular monitoring of platelet counts to detect heparin-induced thrombocytopenia are recommended.

Anticoagulation should be terminated before delivery owing to the high risk of peripartum hemorrhage. For women with antithrombin deficiency the use of antithrombin concentrate during labor and delivery can be considered. After delivery, heparin can be started after 6 to 12 hours, depending on the mode of delivery and possible complications.[88] The use of warfarin and other anticoagulants in breast-feeding women is reviewed by Clark and colleagues.[89]

Acquired Thrombophilias

Acquired thrombophilias occur in various clinical settings, including nephrotic syndrome, polycythemia vera, malignancy, acquired protein C and protein S deficiency, or the antiphospholipid antibody syndrome. Because of its unique role in pregnancy, the antiphospholipid antibody syndrome is discussed separately below. This and other thrombophilias are reviewed in more detail in Chapter 11.

Antiphospholipid Antibody Syndrome

The antiphospholipid antibody syndrome (APAS) can be responsible for recurrent fetal loss or pregnancy-associated venous or arterial thrombosis.[90,91] Ischemic stroke and TIAs are the most common arterial occlusive events.[92] The APAS can be primary or secondary. In secondary APAS antibodies develop in association with connective tissue diseases such as systemic lupus erythematosus or after the use of certain medications. Primary APAS is characterized by the presence of lupus anticoagulant, anticardiolipin (aCL) antibodies, or other antibodies such as anti-ß2-glycoprotein 1 in moderately high titers in serum or plasma on at least two occasions at least 12 weeks apart by standardized enzyme-linked immunosorbent assay (ELISA). Patients with lupus anticoagulant can develop venous thrombosis and ischemic stroke in pregnancy.[93–95] Further, antiphospholipid antibodies are associated with fetal loss, fetal growth restriction, and severe pre-eclampsia and eclampsia.[96] These antibodies can also be found in about 5% of healthy pregnant women who have no thromboembolic complications, making it at times difficult to judge their clinical relevance and need for treatment.[97,98]

The risk for ischemic stroke is highly variable and depends on the presence of other vascular risk factors or thrombophilias.

Overall, the risk of pregnancy-related thromboembolic events in women who have antiphospholipid antibodies is about 5%. Routine screening of pregnant women for antiphospholipid antibodies is usually limited to individuals with a suggestive medical or obstetrical history. High-risk individuals should be tested: women with livedo reticularis, a false-positive rapid plasma reagin (RPR) and venereal disease research laboratory (VDRL)–based syphilis serology, and prior cerebral or retinal ischemic signs during pregnancy.

Women with antiphospholipid antibodies and thromboembolic events and women with unexplained fetal loss and high titers of anticardiolipin antibodies should receive low-dose aspirin combined with LMWH during the pregnancy and for at least the first 6 to 8 weeks postpartum.[99–101] Some individuals may require lifelong anticoagulation with warfarin after delivery, but warfarin should be avoided during pregnancy owing to its potential teratogenicity. In pregnant women with lupus anticoagulant or anticardiolipin antibodies who do not meet clinical criteria for the antiphospholipid antibody syndrome, low-dose aspirin may be considered.[102] Women with stroke or TIA and anticardiolipin antibodies should at least receive antiplatelet therapy.[103] Those with cerebral ischemic events and the full antiphospholipid antibody syndrome should be anticoagulated.

In patients with a history of recurrent miscarriage associated with APAS, treatment with heparin and low-dose aspirin may improve fetal survival compared with aspirin alone.[99,104] Intravenous immune globulin therapy may reduce obstetric complications.[105]

CEREBRAL VENOUS THROMBOSIS

Cerebral venous thrombosis is more likely to occur during the postpartum period than during pregnancy and causes about 2% of pregnancy-related strokes.[106,107] However, the risk increases significantly in women with an inherited or acquired coagulopathy, those who undergo Caesarean delivery, and those who develop hypertension or a postpartum infection.[108–113]

Typical clinical manifestations (see also Chapter 20) include severe headaches, nausea, vomiting, and visual changes. Focal neurological deficits, seizures, and altered mental status are also relatively common, especially when secondary parenchymal lesions such as venous infarcts or focal edema develop. Superior sagittal sinus thrombosis often causes bilateral focal deficits due to bilateral cerebral hemorrhages (Figure 23-2). Impaired ocular motility, proptosis, chemosis, and orbital pain can be found in cavernous sinus thrombosis. Jugular vein and lateral sinus thrombosis can cause pulsating tinnitus. Isolated headaches, at times associated with papilledema, can be seen with isolated transverse sinus involvement. Stupor and coma suggest thrombosis of the deep venous system.[114,115]

The differential diagnosis includes complicated migraine. In mild cases presenting mainly with headaches, the diagnosis is frequently missed.[116] Papilledema indicates increased intracranial pressure and typically develops with chronic thrombosis. Magnetic resonance venography (MRV) confirms the diagnosis. Neuroimaging techniques are discussed in more detail in Chapter 5.

Management focuses on anticoagulation, and if present, seizure control and treatment of increased intracranial pressure. In severe cases or in the face of clinical progression, local thrombolysis, at times in combination with mechanical thrombectomy, may be useful.

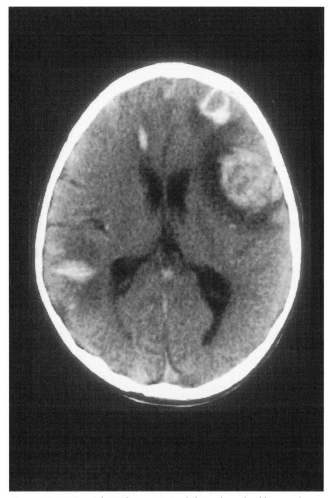

Figure 23-2. Cranial CT demonstrates bilateral cerebral hemorrhages due to sagittal sinus thrombosis.

INTRACRANIAL HEMORRHAGE

As with cerebral infarction, most pregnancy-related intracranial hemorrhages occur in the postpartum period.[117–119] However, the overall risk of pregnancy-associated intracranial hemorrhage is low, occurring in only about 6 women per 100,000 deliveries.[1,5,120] Women at highest risk include those older than 35 years of age; African American women; individuals with hypertension, pre-eclampsia, eclampsia, coagulopathy, or thrombocytopenia; and those with a history of tobacco or cocaine use.[121] The most common causes of pregnancy-associated intracerebral hemorrhages are eclampsia and rupture of an arteriovenous malformation (AVM). About 30% of hemorrhages occur in women with pre-eclampsia and eclampsia. About 40% of intraparenchymal hemorrhages are associated with poor maternal and fetal outcome.[8]

About 7% to 20% of pregnancy-associated intracranial hemorrhages are due to vascular malformations, a rate that is comparable to that of nonpregnant young women.[122] AVMs tend to bleed in the second trimester and subarachnoid aneurysms tend to bleed in the third trimester.[123] Controversy continues about whether the risk of vascular malformation rupture is substantially higher during pregnancy than at other times.

Vascular malformations and aneurysms during pregnancy are treated by aneurysm clipping or coiling in much the same way as in nonpregnant patients (see Chapters 17 and 18). Cerebral catheter angiography can be performed during pregnancy if the benefits outweigh the risks and radiation exposure is minimized by proper shielding. There are no data assessing the feasibility and safety of endovascular embolization of AVMs. Gamma knife treatment should be postponed until after delivery. After treatment of an aneurysm or AVM, spontaneous labor and delivery are reasonably safe.[124]

The safety of vaginal delivery by a woman with an untreated aneurysm or AVM remains uncertain due to concerns about hemorrhage associated with the Valsalva maneuver and pain-induced changes in cerebral hemodynamics. Some physicians advocate elective Caesarean delivery or forceps delivery during regional anesthesia in this situation, but no evidence-based data are available to help determine the best approach and aneurysm rupture during Caesarean delivery has been described.[123,125] Caesarean sections in women with untreated lesions may not afford any better maternal or fetal outcome than vaginal delivery.[124] Control of hypertension is essential for management, independent of delivery type.

AMNIOTIC FLUID EMBOLISM

Amniotic fluid embolism is an uncommon complication of pregnancy that typically occurs during labor and delivery or immediately afterwards.[126] Amniotic fluid embolism can cause severe neurological complications, including seizures in up to 50% of cases, severe headache, confusion, hypoxia, profound arterial hypotension, and cardiogenic shock, followed frequently by disseminated intravascular coagulation. Maternal mortality has been reported to be as high as 50% to 90% and the fetal mortality is estimated to be 20%. Hypoxia and disseminated intravascular coagulation can precipitate maternal and fetal intracranial hemorrhages and hypoxic ischemic brain injury. Up to 85% of women and more than 50% of children affected by amniotic fluid embolism have subsequent neurological deficits.[127]

Currently the disorder remains unpredictable and has no specific treatment, but early identification allows acute treatment of seizures, shock, and respiratory failure, measures that can significantly improve outcome.

PERIPARTUM CEREBRAL ANGIOPATHY

Peripartum cerebral angiopathy is probably the same condition as reversible multifocal segmental vasoconstriction of the cerebral arteries (Call-Fleming syndrome), which occurs with greater frequency in women of child-bearing age and may be precipitated by pregnancy or the postpartum state (see Chapter 14). The pathophysiology of this condition is not well understood, but patients develop reversible segmental vasospasm (Figure 14-1) in the absence of hypertension or arteritis.

Clinical manifestations include the sudden onset of severe headaches, visual disturbance, focal neurological deficits, and seizures. Ischemic stroke can occur with prolonged vasospasm. Rarely patients deteriorate and die. Typically the blood pressure is normal and no other pregnancy-associated complications are apparent. There is no obvious relationship with eclampsia. Women with postpartum cerebral angiopathy are not at higher risk of developing recurrent episodes of vasospasm or eclampsia in subsequent pregnancies. The differential diagnosis includes eclampsia, pre-eclampsia, thunderclap headaches, benign angiopathy of the central nervous system (CNS), isolated CNS vasculitis or vasculitis

occurring with systemic disease, migraine-associated vasospasm, reversible posterior leukoencephalopathy syndrome, and hypertensive encephalopathy.[128] More details about the evaluation and treatment of Call-Fleming syndrome are provided in Chapter 14.

GESTATIONAL TROPHOBLASTIC DISEASE

Malignant gestational trophoblastic diseases include invasive moles, placental site trophoblastic tumors, and choriocarcinoma, all of which are relatively rare conditions that can follow term, preterm, and ectopic pregnancies, or abortion. Most tumors develop from molar pregnancy.[129] The tumors metastasize to the brain in 3% to 28% of the patients and sometimes invade and erode blood vessels.[130] Choriocarcinoma is highly malignant, grows rapidly, and metastasizes early.[131,132] Brain metastases are found in up to one third of women with advanced disease and can cause single or multiple ischemic and hemorrhagic strokes. The tumor can damage blood vessels, leading to increased permeability and hemorrhage. Intracranial hemorrhage is the most common complication of cerebral metastatic disease and presents mainly as a lobar, but at times as a subdural or subarachnoid, bleed.[133,134] Neoplastic aneurysms are an extremely rare cause of subarachnoid hemorrhage.[135,136]

The diagnosis is made by measuring the ß-human gonadotropin, a selective tumor marker for choriocarcinoma and invasive mole. Confirmation by tissue biopsy is generally not required to initiate therapy.[137] Surgery should be avoided because hemorrhagic complications are common. Malignant gestational trophoblastic tumors are highly sensitive to chemotherapy, which, when followed by brain radiation, is often curative. The use of antiplatelet agents in women with arterial thrombosis most be weighed against the risk of potential hemorrhage.

PITUITARY APOPLEXY

Pituitary apoplexy results from either infarction or hemorrhage within the pituitary gland. Postpartum pituitary infarction with secondary hypopituitarism is known as Sheehan syndrome. Aside from postpartum infarction, pituitary apoplexy occurs in individuals with a pituitary macroadenoma and rarely in various other clinical settings, such as pituitary hyperplasia following adrenalectomy, intracavernous carotid artery aneurysm, or coagulopathy.[138-141]

During pregnancy the pituitary gland enlarges as a result of hyperplasia of prolactin-secreting cells. This enlargement makes it susceptible to anoxia and ischemia which causes hypopituitarism. Adrenal insufficiency can develop acutely during the postpartum period, leading to shock and hypotension or it may develop slowly over several months or even years. Therefore a high level of suspicion is key to making the diagnosis when the presentation is delayed.

Pituitary apoplexy typically presents with sudden-onset headache, visual impairment, and nausea and vomiting. Many patients have meningeal signs, confusion, and ophthalmoplegia.[142] Endocrine dysfunction is common, but given the frequency of an underlying pituitary adenoma, it is often unclear whether the endocrine dysfunction developed because of the tumor itself or because of pituitary apoplexy. Acute edema or hemorrhage is evident on CT or MRI (Figure 23-3).[143,144]

Pituitary apoplexy typically affects the anterior pituitary gland but it can also affect the posterior pituitary and can rarely present with diabetes insipidus.[145] Growth hormone deficiency

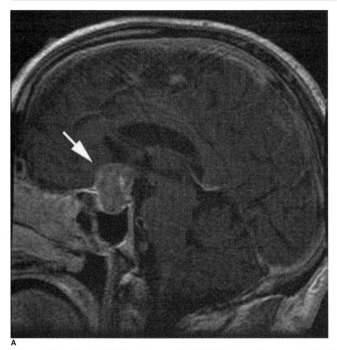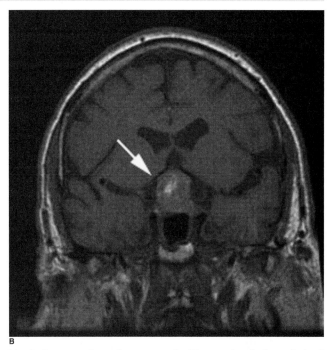

Figure 23-3. Sagittal (A) and coronal (B) MRI views from an individual with pituitary apoplexy who presented with acute headache and visual loss. The images show a large pituitary mass (*arrows*) enlarging the sella turcica and displacing the third ventricle upward.

occurs in 90%, adrenocorticotropic hormone (ACTH) deficiency in about 66%, hypogonadism in about 65%, and hypothyroidism with thyroid-stimulating hormone (TSH) deficiency in 42% of patients. Hyponatremia is often due to syndrome of inappropriate diuretic hormone (SIADH) and at times vasopressin reduction.

Treatment requires replacement of any deficient hormones. The effectiveness of surgery diminishes with longer symptom duration, and early surgery does not often prevent hormonal insufficiency. Surgical resection of the abnormal pituitary gland may be necessary in individuals with acute visual loss, but individuals whose visual symptoms are stable or improving by the time of presentation can sometimes be managed medically.[146,147] Occasional patients develop recurrent pituitary apoplexy after several years despite appropriate therapy. Individuals with a prolactin-secreting adenoma may benefit from a dopamine agonist, and steroids may be useful initially. The prognosis is generally good.[148]

NEUROIMAGING DURING PREGNANCY

In general ultrasound and MRI are the preferred imaging modalities of brain and blood vessels during pregnancy. No adverse effects on the mother or the fetus have been reported using MRI with field strengths of 1.5 Tesla or less. Potential adverse effects using higher magnetic fields are unknown in this population, and MRI studies during the first trimester should perhaps be deferred unless the potential benefits outweigh theoretical risks.[149] Gadolinium crosses the placenta, and animal studies document fetal loss, fetal growth restriction, and teratogenic effects after administration of gadolinium. The risks from gadolinium in human pregnancy are unknown, but it seems prudent to avoid it.

Despite its potential for heat- and cavitation-induced tissue damage, no harmful effects of ultrasound in pregnant women

have been observed. Ultrasound is considered to be safe and is routinely and frequently used during pregnancy. Special guidelines for use of Doppler and anatomical imaging by ultrasound for pregnant women have been developed.[150]

Cranial CT is reasonably safe if the uterus is shielded. Radiation doses from standard head CT with shielding of the abdomen typically are about 200 mrad for the mother and 10 mrad for the fetus. However, there is no lowest threshold of radiation exposure that has been determined to be biologically safe. Iodinated contrast agents cross the placenta and can cause transient biological effects on the developing fetal thyroid gland, and should therefore be avoided during pregnancy unless medically necessary for diagnosis and treatment.[151,152]

TREATMENT OF ISCHEMIC STROKE DURING PREGNANCY

Pharmacological treatment for stroke prevention is presented in other chapters, and here we only mention a few aspects of these agents that are unique to pregnancy and the postpartum period.

Antiplatelet Agents

Low-dose aspirin is generally safe for stroke prevention in pregnancy. Most experts agree that low-dose aspirin can be used during the second and third trimesters although controversy continues about its safety in the first trimester.[153,154] No safety data based on large prospective clinical trials are available for clopidogrel and dipyridamole.

Anticoagulation

Warfarin has potential teratogenic effects especially when administered between the sixth and twelfth week of pregnancy.[155] Warfarin can also cause fetal and placental hemorrhages. Cerebral hemorrhages and malformations of the CNS have been described with warfarin use during the second and third trimesters.[156] Although some controversy remains, warfarin should generally be avoided during pregnancy and should be reserved for very selected patients (i.e., women with mechanical prosthetic heart valves) due to the potential risks of warfarin-related embryopathy and CNS abnormalities.[157,158]

Use of unfractionated heparin or LMWH is safe during pregnancy.[159] Neither unfractionated heparin nor LMWH cross the placenta so they are not teratogenic. Stable blood levels are difficult to maintain as pregnancy advances. As with nonpregnant patients, there is some risk of heparin-induced thrombocytopenia (see Chapter 11), and for patients requiring more than 5 weeks of treatment, bone demineralization and associated fractures become a concern.[158,160]

Owing to its low complication rate, LMWH is often the anticoagulant of choice during pregnancy.[161] It is not recommended for the anticoagulation of pregnant women with mechanical prosthetic heart valves owing to reports of maternal deaths resulting from valve thromboses. Because of potential concerns about spinal epidural hematoma, LMWH should be changed to unfractionated heparin about 2 weeks before planned delivery, allowing reversal of the anticoagulation before spinal and epidural anesthesia or Caesarean delivery. Danaparoid can be used for systemic anticoagulation of pregnant women with heparin-induced thrombocytopenia or other heparin-associated complications.

Thrombolysis

Few data from off-label use of thrombolytic agents in pregnant women are available.[162,163] There is potential risk of placental hemorrhage, placental abruption, premature labor, and fetal death, as well as risk for significant hemorrhage if applied close to the time of labor. There are no data on the potential teratogenic effects of thrombolytics. Urokinase is FDA pregnancy category B and tissue plasminogen activator (tPA) is category C. When urokinase has been used during pregnancy for indications other than ischemic stroke, the risk of maternal hemorrhage was reported to be about 8% with a reported maternal death rate of 1.2% and a reported fetal death rate of 5.8%.[164] Reports describing the use of tPA during pregnancy have been more encouraging, but the number of treated patients remains so small that definitive recommendations are not possible. Deliveries of healthy babies and good maternal outcome after thrombolysis with tPA have been documented, but the risk/benefit ratio needs to be evaluated on a case-by-case basis and with informed patient consent.[165–167]

RISK OF RECURRENT STROKE

The risk of a recurrent ischemic stroke during a subsequent pregnancy is relatively low and comparable with recurrence rates in other pregnant women. If strokes reoccur, they tend to do so in the postpartum period.[5,8,168] In general women whose risk factors can be treated are safe to have a subsequent pregnancy.

Vascular malformations at high risk for bleeding require treatment. Subsequent pregnancies are in general not associated with a higher risk of intracranial hemorrhage in women whose vascular malformations have been treated.

The risk for recurrence of cerebral sinus venous thrombosis in pregnant women is about 6% to 12% within the first 2 years and probably higher in those with untreated thrombophilia. It is not clear whether women who had a previous cerebral sinus venous thrombosis should be prophylactically anticoagulated during a subsequent pregnancy.[80]

REFERENCES

1. Kittner SJ, Stern BJ, Feeser BR, et al. Pregnancy and the risk of stroke. *N Engl J Med*. 1996;**335**:768–774.
2. Grosset DG, Ebrahim S, Bone I, Warlow C. Stroke in pregnancy and the puerperium: what magnitude of risk? *J Neurol Neurosurg Psychiatry*. 1995;**58**:129–131.
3. Cross JN, Castro PO, Jennett WB. Cerebral strokes associated with pregnancy and the puerperium. *Br Med J*. 1968;**3**:214–218.
4. Amias AG. Cerebral vascular disease in pregnancy. I. Haemorrhage. *J Obstet Gynaecol Br Commonw*. 1970;**77**:100–120.
5. Simolke GA, Cox SM, Cunningham FG. Cerebrovascular accidents complicating pregnancy and the puerperium. *Obstet Gynecol*. 1991;**78**:37–42.
6. Wilson BJ, Watson MS, Prescott GJ, et al. Hypertensive diseases of pregnancy and risk of hypertension and stroke in later life: results from cohort study. *BMJ*. 2003;**326**:845.
7. Arnadottir GA, Geirsson RT, Arngrimsson R, Jonsdottir LS, Olafsson O. Cardiovascular death in women who had hypertension in pregnancy: a case-control study. *BJOG*. 2005;**112**:286–292.
8. Sharshar T, Lamy C, Mas JL. Incidence and causes of strokes associated with pregnancy and puerperium. A study in public hospitals of Ile de France. Stroke in Pregnancy Study Group. *Stroke*. 1995;**26**:930–936.
9. Wiebers DO, Whisnant JP. The incidence of stroke among pregnant women in Rochester, Minn, 1955 through 1979. *JAMA*. 1985;**254**:3055–3057.
10. Higgins JR, Walshe JJ, Darling MR, Norris L, Bonnar J. Hemostasis in the uteroplacental and peripheral circulations in normotensive and pre-eclamptic pregnancies. *Am J Obstet Gynecol*. 1998;**179**:520–526.
11. World Health Organization International Collaborative Study of Hypertensive Disorders of Pregnancy. Geographic variation in the incidence of hypertension in pregnancy. *Am J Obstet Gynecol*. 1988;**158**:80–83.
12. Cerneca F, Ricci G, Simeone R, Malisano M, Alberico S, Guaschino S. Coagulation and fibrinolysis changes in normal pregnancy. Increased levels of procoagulants and reduced levels of inhibitors during pregnancy induce a hypercoagulable state, combined with a reactive fibrinolysis. *Eur J Obstet Gynecol Reprod Biol*. 1997;**73**:31–36.
13. Faught W, Garner P, Jones G, Ivey B. Changes in protein C and protein S levels in normal pregnancy. *Am J Obstet Gynecol*. 1995;**172**:147–150.
14. de Moerloose P, Amiral J, Vissac AM, Reber G. Longitudinal study on activated factors XII and VII levels during normal pregnancy. *Br J Haematol*. 1998;**100**:40–44.
15. Halligan A, Bonnar J, Sheppard B, Darling M, Walshe J. Haemostatic, fibrinolytic and endothelial variables in normal pregnancies and pre-eclampsia. *Br J Obstet Gynaecol*. 1994;**101**:488–492.
16. Kjellberg U, Andersson NE, Rosen S, Tengborn L, Hellgren M. APC resistance and other haemostatic variables during pregnancy and puerperium. *Thromb Haemost*. 1999;**81**:527–531.
17. Pinto S, Abbate R, Rostagno C, Bruni V, Rosati D, Neri Serneri GG. Increased thrombin generation in normal pregnancy. *Acta Eur Fertil*. 1988;**19**:263–267.

18. Lindheimer MD, Katz AI. Sodium and diuretics in pregnancy. *N Engl J Med*. 1973;**288**:891–894.

19. Lund CJ, Donovan JC. Blood volume during pregnancy. Significance of plasma and red cell volumes. *Am J Obstet Gynecol*. 1967;**98**:394–403.

20. Pritchard JA. Changes in the blood volume during pregnancy and delivery. *Anesthesiology*. 1965;**26**:393–399.

21. Saftlas AF, Olson DR, Franks AL, Atrash HK, Pokras R. Epidemiology of preeclampsia and eclampsia in the United States, 1979–1986. *Am J Obstet Gynecol*. 1990;**163**:460–465.

22. Sibai BM, Gordon T, Thom E, et al. Risk factors for preeclampsia in healthy nulliparous women: a prospective multicenter study. The National Institute of Child Health and Human Development Network of Maternal-Fetal Medicine Units. *Am J Obstet Gynecol*. 1995;**172**:642–648.

23. Tuffnell DJ, Jankowicz D, Lindow SW, et al. Outcomes of severe pre-eclampsia/eclampsia in Yorkshire 1999/2003. *BJOG*. 2005;**112**:875–880.

24. Zeeman GG, Fleckenstein JL, Twickler DM, Cunningham FG. Cerebral infarction in eclampsia. *Am J Obstet Gynecol*. 2004;**190**:714–720.

25. Sibai BM, Spinnato JA, Watson DL, Lewis JA, Anderson GD. Eclampsia. IV. Neurological findings and future outcome. *Am J Obstet Gynecol*. 1985;**152**:184–192.

26. Sheehan HL, Lynch JB. *Pathology of toxaemia of pregnancy*. Baltimore: Williams & Wilkins; 1973.

27. Dekker GA, Sibai BM. Etiology and pathogenesis of preeclampsia: current concepts. *Am J Obstet Gynecol*. 1998;**179**:1359–1375.

28. Roberts JM, Taylor RN, Goldfien A. Clinical and biochemical evidence of endothelial cell dysfunction in the pregnancy syndrome preeclampsia. *Am J Hypertens*. 1991;**4**:700–708.

29. Agatisa PK, Ness RB, Roberts JM, Costantino JP, Kuller LH, McLaughlin MK. Impairment of endothelial function in women with a history of preeclampsia: an indicator of cardiovascular risk. *Am J Physiol Heart Circ Physiol*. 2004;**286**:H1389–H1393.

30. Lampinen KH, Ronnback M, Kaaja RJ, Groop PH. Impaired vascular dilatation in women with a history of pre-eclampsia. *J Hypertens*. 2006;**24**:751–756.

31. Okanloma KA, Moodley J. Neurological complications associated with the pre-eclampsia/eclampsia syndrome. *Int J Gynaecol Obstet*. 2000;**71**:223–225.

32. Lain KY, Roberts JM. Contemporary concepts of the pathogenesis and management of preeclampsia. *JAMA*. 2002;**287**:3183–3186.

33. Zhou Y, Damsky CH, Fisher SJ. Preeclampsia is associated with failure of human cytotrophoblasts to mimic a vascular adhesion phenotype. One cause of defective endovascular invasion in this syndrome? *J Clin Invest*. 1997;**99**:2152–2164.

34. Zhou Y, Damsky CH, Chiu K, Roberts JM, Fisher SJ. Preeclampsia is associated with abnormal expression of adhesion molecules by invasive cytotrophoblasts. *J Clin Invest*. 1993;**91**:950–960.

35. Redman CW, Sacks GP, Sargent IL. Preeclampsia: an excessive maternal inflammatory response to pregnancy. *Am J Obstet Gynecol*. 1999;**180**:499–506.

36. Levine RJ, Qian C, Maynard SE, Yu KF, Epstein FH, Karumanchi SA. Serum sFlt1 concentration during preeclampsia and mid trimester blood pressure in healthy nulliparous women. *Am J Obstet Gynecol*. 2006;**194**:1034–1041.

37. Wang X, Athayde N, Trudinger B. A proinflammatory cytokine response is present in the fetal placental vasculature in placental insufficiency. *Am J Obstet Gynecol*. 2003;**189**:1445–1451.

38. Redman CW, Sargent IL. Preeclampsia and the systemic inflammatory response. *Semin Nephrol*. 2004;**24**:565–570.

39. Report of the National High Blood Pressure Education Program Working Group on High Blood Pressure in Pregnancy. *Am J Obstet Gynecol*. 2000;**183**:S1–S22.

40. Barton JR, O'Brien JM, Bergauer NK, Jacques DL, Sibai BM. Mild gestational hypertension remote from term: progression and outcome. *Am J Obstet Gynecol*. 2001;**184**:979–983.

41. ACOG Practice Bulletin. Diagnosis and management of preeclampsia and eclampsia. *Obstet Gynecol*. 2002;**99**:159–167.

42. Cunningham FG, Fernandez CO, Hernandez C. Blindness associated with preeclampsia and eclampsia. *Am J Obstet Gynecol*. 1995;**172**:1291–1298.

43. Beaufils M, Uzan S, Donsimoni R, Colau JC. Prevention of pre-eclampsia by early antiplatelet therapy. *Lancet*. 1985;**1**:840–842.

44. Caritis S, Sibai B, Hauth J, et al. Low-dose aspirin to prevent preeclampsia in women at high risk. National Institute of Child Health and Human Development Network of Maternal-Fetal Medicine Units. *N Engl J Med*. 1998;**338**:701–705.

45. CLASP (Collaborative Low-dose Aspirin Study in Pregnancy) Collaborative Group. CLASP: a randomised trial of low-dose aspirin for the prevention and treatment of pre-eclampsia among 9364 pregnant women. *Lancet*. 1994;**343**:619–629.

46. Coomarasamy A, Honest H, Papaioannou S, Gee H, Khan KS. Aspirin for prevention of preeclampsia in women with historical risk factors: a systematic review. *Obstet Gynecol*. 2003;**101**:1319–1332.

47. Duley L, Henderson-Smart DJ, Knight M, King JF. Antiplatelet agents for preventing pre-eclampsia and its complications. *Cochrane Database Syst Rev*. 2004;CD004659.

48. Sibai BM, Caritis SN, Thom E, et al. Prevention of preeclampsia with low-dose aspirin in healthy, nulliparous pregnant women. The National Institute of Child Health and Human Development Network of Maternal-Fetal Medicine Units. *N Engl J Med*. 1993;**329**:1213–1218.

49. Kozer E, Costei AM, Boskovic R, Nulman I, Nikfar S, Koren G. Effects of aspirin consumption during pregnancy on pregnancy outcomes: meta-analysis. *Birth Defects Res B Dev Reprod Toxicol*. 2003;**68**:70–84.

50. Steyn DW, Odendaal HJ. Randomised controlled trial of ketanserin and aspirin in prevention of pre-eclampsia. *Lancet*. 1997;**350**:1267–1271.

51. Sibai BM, Ramadan MK, Usta I, Salama M, Mercer BM, Friedman SA. Maternal morbidity and mortality in 442 pregnancies with hemolysis, elevated liver enzymes, and low platelets (HELLP syndrome). *Am J Obstet Gynecol*. 1993;**169**:1000–1006.

52. Audibert F, Friedman SA, Frangieh AY, Sibai BM. Clinical utility of strict diagnostic criteria for the HELLP (hemolysis, elevated liver enzymes, and low platelets) syndrome. *Am J Obstet Gynecol*. 1996;**175**:460–464.

53. Martin JN Jr, Rinehart BK, May WL, Magann EF, Terrone DA, Blake PG. The spectrum of severe preeclampsia: comparative analysis by HELLP (hemolysis, elevated liver enzyme levels, and low platelet count) syndrome classification. *Am J Obstet Gynecol*. 1999;**180**:1373–1384.

54. Sibai BM, Ramadan MK, Chari RS, Friedman SA. Pregnancies complicated by HELLP syndrome (hemolysis, elevated liver enzymes, and low platelets): subsequent pregnancy outcome and long-term prognosis. *Am J Obstet Gynecol*. 1995;**172**:125–129.

55. Cunningham FG, Lindheimer MD. Hypertension in pregnancy. *N Engl J Med*. 1992;**326**:927–932.

56. Martin JN Jr, Thigpen BD, Moore RC, Rose CH, Cushman J, May W. Stroke and severe preeclampsia and eclampsia: a paradigm shift focusing on systolic blood pressure. *Obstet Gynecol*. 2005;**105**:246–254.

57. Abalos E, Duley L, Steyn DW, Henderson-Smart DJ. Antihypertensive drug therapy for mild to moderate hypertension during pregnancy. *Cochrane Database Syst Rev.* 2007;CD002252.

58. Duley L, Henderson-Smart DJ, Meher S. Drugs for treatment of very high blood pressure during pregnancy. *Cochrane Database Syst Rev.* 2006;**3**:CD001449.

59. Elatrous S, Nouira S, Ouanes BL, et al. Short-term treatment of severe hypertension of pregnancy: prospective comparison of nicardipine and labetalol. *Intensive Care Med.* 2002;**28**:1281–1286.

60. Walters BN, Thompson ME, Lee A, de SM. Blood pressure in the puerperium. *Clin Sci (Lond).* 1986;**71**:589–594.

61. Redman CW. Controlled trials of antihypertensive drugs in pregnancy. *Am J Kidney Dis.* 1991;**17**:149–153.

62. McFaul PB, Dornan JC, Lamki H, Boyle D. Pregnancy complicated by maternal heart disease. A review of 519 women. *Br J Obstet Gynaecol.* 1988;**95**:861–867.

63. Siu SC, Sermer M, Harrison DA, et al. Risk and predictors for pregnancy-related complications in women with heart disease. *Circulation.* 1997;**96**:2789–2794.

64. Siu SC, Sermer M, Colman JM, et al. Prospective multicenter study of pregnancy outcomes in women with heart disease. *Circulation.* 2001;**104**:515–521.

65. Hameed A, Karaalp IS, Tummala PP, et al. The effect of valvular heart disease on maternal and fetal outcome of pregnancy. *J Am Coll Cardiol.* 2001;**37**:893–899.

66. Campuzano K, Roque H, Bolnick A, Leo MV, Campbell WA. Bacterial endocarditis complicating pregnancy: case report and systematic review of the literature. *Arch Gynecol Obstet.* 2003;**268**:251–255.

67. Fett JD, Christie LG, Murphy JG. Brief communication: outcomes of subsequent pregnancy after peripartum cardiomyopathy: a case series from Haiti. *Ann Intern Med.* 2006;**145**:30–34.

68. Elkayam U, Tummala PP, Rao K, et al. Maternal and fetal outcomes of subsequent pregnancies in women with peripartum cardiomyopathy. *N Engl J Med.* 2001;**344**:1567–1571.

69. Silversides CK, Harris L, Haberer K, Sermer M, Colman JM, Siu SC. Recurrence rates of arrhythmias during pregnancy in women with previous tachyarrhythmia and impact on fetal and neonatal outcomes. *Am J Cardiol.* 2006;**97**:1206–1212.

70. Lockwood CJ. Heritable coagulopathies in pregnancy. *Obstet Gynecol Surv.* 1999;**54**:754–765.

71. Robertson L, Wu O, Langhorne P, et al. Thrombophilia in pregnancy: a systematic review. *Br J Haematol.* 2006;**132**:171–196.

72. Kupferminc MJ, Yair D, Bornstein NM, Lessing JB, Eldor A. Transient focal neurological deficits during pregnancy in carriers of inherited thrombophilia. *Stroke.* 2000;**31**:892–895.

73. Grandone E, Margaglione M, Colaizzo D, et al. Genetic susceptibility to pregnancy-related venous thromboembolism: roles of factor V Leiden, prothrombin G20210A, and methylenetetrahydrofolate reductase C677T mutations. *Am J Obstet Gynecol.* 1998;**179**:1324–1328.

74. Zotz RB, Gerhardt A, Scharf RE. Inherited thrombophilia and gestational venous thromboembolism. *Best Pract Res Clin Haematol.* 2003;**16**:243–259.

75. Friederich PW, Sanson BJ, Simioni P, et al. Frequency of pregnancy-related venous thromboembolism in anticoagulant factor-deficient women: implications for prophylaxis. *Ann Intern Med.* 1996;**125**:955–960.

76. Girling JC, de Swiet M. Thromboembolism in pregnancy: an overview. *Curr Opin Obstet Gynecol.* 1996;**8**:458–463.

77. Folkeringa N, Brouwer JL, Korteweg FJ, Veeger NJ, Erwich JJ, Van Der Meer J. High risk of pregnancy-related venous thromboembolism in women with multiple thrombophilic defects. *Br J Haematol.* 2007;**138**:110–116.

78. British Committee for Standards in Haematology. Investigation and management of heritable thrombophilia. *Br J Haematol.* 2001;**114**:512–528.

79. Gris JC, Mercier E, Quere I, et al. Low-molecular-weight heparin versus low-dose aspirin in women with one fetal loss and a constitutional thrombophilic disorder. *Blood.* 2004;**103**:3695–3699.

80. Simioni P, Tormene D, Prandoni P, Girolami A. Pregnancy-related recurrent events in thrombophilic women with previous venous thromboembolism. *Thromb Haemost.* 2001;**86**:929.

81. Lockwood CJ. Inherited thrombophilias in pregnant patients: detection and treatment paradigm. *Obstet Gynecol.* 2002;**99**:333–341.

82. Eldor A. Thrombophilia, thrombosis and pregnancy. *Thromb Haemost.* 2001;**86**:104–111.

83. Bates SM, Greer IA, Hirsh J, Ginsberg JS. Use of antithrombotic agents during pregnancy: the Seventh ACCP Conference on Antithrombotic and Thrombolytic Therapy. *Chest.* 2004;**126**:627S–644S.

84. Johnston JA, Brill-Edwards P, Ginsberg JS, Pauker SG, Eckman MH. Cost-effectiveness of prophylactic low molecular weight heparin in pregnant women with a prior history of venous thromboembolism. *Am J Med.* 2005;**118**:503–514.

85. Bowles L, Cohen H. Inherited thrombophilias and anticoagulation in pregnancy. *Best Pract Res Clin Obstet Gynaecol.* 2003;**17**:471–489.

86. ACOG Committee opinion. Anticoagulation with low-molecular-weight heparin during pregnancy. *Number 211, November 1998.* Committee on Obstetric Practice. American College of Obstetricians and Gynecologists. *Int J Gynaecol Obstet.* 1999;**65**:89–90.

87. Royal College of Obstetricians and Gynaecologists. Guideline No. 37: Thromboprophylaxis during pregnancy, labour, and after vaginal delivery. http://www.rcog.org.uk/files/rcog-corp/uploaded-files/GT37Thromboprophylaxis2004.pdf.2004. Accessed June 21, 2009.

88. Bates SM, Ginsberg JS. How we manage venous thromboembolism during pregnancy. *Blood.* 2002;**100**:3470–3478.

89. Clark SL, Porter TF, West FG. Coumarin derivatives and breast-feeding. *Obstet Gynecol.* 2000;**95**:938–940.

90. Lockshin MD. Antiphospholipid antibody. Babies, blood clots, biology. *JAMA.* 1997;**277**:1549–1551.

91. Dafer RM, Biller J. Antiphospholipid syndrome: role of antiphospholipid antibodies in neurology. *Hematol Oncol Clin North Am.* 2008;**22**:95–105.

92. Branch DW, Khamashta MA. Antiphospholipid syndrome: obstetric diagnosis, management, and controversies. *Obstet Gynecol.* 2003;**101**:1333–1344.

93. ACOG Practice Bulletin no. 68: Antiphospholipid syndrome. *Obstet Gynecol.* 2005;**106**:1113–1121.

94. Branch DW, Porter TF, Rittenhouse L, et al. Antiphospholipid antibodies in women at risk for preeclampsia. *Am J Obstet Gynecol.* 2001;**184**:825–832.

95. Lockwood CJ, Romero R, Feinberg RF, Clyne LP, Coster B, Hobbins JC. The prevalence and biologic significance of lupus anticoagulant and anticardiolipin antibodies in a general obstetric population. *Am J Obstet Gynecol.* 1989;**161**:369–373.

96. Empson M, Lassere M, Craig JC, Scott JR. Recurrent pregnancy loss with antiphospholipid antibody: a systematic review of therapeutic trials. *Obstet Gynecol.* 2002;**99**:135–144.

97. Miyakis S, Lockshin MD, Atsumi T, et al. International consensus statement on an update of the classification criteria for definite antiphospholipid syndrome (APS). *J Thromb Haemost.* 2006;**4**:295–306.

98. Galli M, Barbui T. Antiphospholipid antibodies and pregnancy. *Best Pract Res Clin Haematol.* 2003;**16**:211–225.

99. Rai R, Cohen H, Dave M, Regan L. Randomised controlled trial of aspirin and aspirin plus heparin in pregnant women with recurrent miscarriage associated with phospholipid antibodies (or antiphospholipid antibodies). *BMJ*. 1997;**314**: 253–257.

100. Kutteh WH. Antiphospholipid antibody-associated recurrent pregnancy loss: treatment with heparin and low-dose aspirin is superior to low-dose aspirin alone. *Am J Obstet Gynecol*. 1996;**174**:1584–1589.

101. Lassere M, Empson M. Treatment of antiphospholipid syndrome in pregnancy – a systematic review of randomized therapeutic trials. *Thromb Res*. 2004;**114**:419–426.

102. Erkan D, Harrison MJ, Levy R, et al. Aspirin for primary thrombosis prevention in the antiphospholipid syndrome: a randomized, double-blind, placebo-controlled trial in asymptomatic antiphospholipid antibody-positive individuals. *Arthritis Rheum*. 2007;**56**:2382–2391.

103. Tincani A, Branch W, Levy RA, et al. Treatment of pregnant patients with antiphospholipid syndrome. *Lupus*. 2003;**12**:524–529.

104. Glasnovic M, Bosnjak I, Vcev A, et al. Antibody profile of pregnant women with antiphospholipid syndrome and pregnancy outcome after treatment with low dose aspirin and low-weight-molecular heparin. *Coll Antropol*. 2007;**31**:173–177.

105. Branch DW, Peaceman AM, Druzin M, et al. A multicenter, placebo-controlled pilot study of intravenous immune globulin treatment of antiphospholipid syndrome during pregnancy. The Pregnancy Loss Study Group. *Am J Obstet Gynecol*. 2000;**182**:122–127.

106. Lanska DJ, Kryscio RJ. Risk factors for peripartum and postpartum stroke and intracranial venous thrombosis. *Stroke*. 2000;**31**:1274–1282.

107. Ferro JM, Canhao P, Stam J, Bousser MG, Barinagarrementeria F. Prognosis of cerebral vein and dural sinus thrombosis: results of the International Study on Cerebral Vein and Dural Sinus Thrombosis (ISCVT). *Stroke*. 2004;**35**:664–670.

108. Stam J. Thrombosis of the cerebral veins and sinuses. *N Engl J Med*. 2005;**352**:1791–1798.

109. Deschiens MA, Conard J, Horellou MH, et al. Coagulation studies, factor V Leiden, and anticardiolipin antibodies in 40 cases of cerebral venous thrombosis. *Stroke*. 1996;**27**:1724–1730.

110. Ludemann P, Nabavi DG, Junker R, et al. Factor V Leiden mutation is a risk factor for cerebral venous thrombosis: a case-control study of 55 patients. *Stroke*. 1998;**29**:2507–2510.

111. Martinelli I, Sacchi E, Landi G, Taioli E, Duca F, Mannucci PM. High risk of cerebral-vein thrombosis in carriers of a prothrombin-gene mutation and in users of oral contraceptives. *N Engl J Med*. 1998;**338**:1793–1797.

112. Hillier CE, Collins PW, Bowen DJ, Bowley S, Wiles CM. Inherited prothrombotic risk factors and cerebral venous thrombosis. *Q J Med*. 1998;**91**:677–680.

113. Cantu C, Alonso E, Jara A, et al. Hyperhomocysteinemia, low folate and vitamin B12 concentrations, and methylene tetrahydrofolate reductase mutation in cerebral venous thrombosis. *Stroke*. 2004;**35**:1790–1794.

114. Crawford SC, Digre KB, Palmer CA, Bell DA, Osborn AG. Thrombosis of the deep venous drainage of the brain in adults. Analysis of seven cases with review of the literature. *Arch Neurol*. 1995;**52**:1101–1108.

115. van den Bergh WM, van der Schaaf I, van Gijn J. The spectrum of presentations of venous infarction caused by deep cerebral vein thrombosis. *Neurology*. 2005;**65**:192–196.

116. Newman DS, Levine SR, Curtis VL, Welch KM. Migraine-like visual phenomena associated with cerebral venous thrombosis. *Headache*. 1989;**29**:82–85.

117. Bateman BT, Schumacher HC, Bushnell CD, et al. Intracerebral hemorrhage in pregnancy: frequency, risk factors, and outcome. *Neurology*. 2006;**67**:424–429.

118. Jaigobin C, Silver FL. Stroke secondary to post-partum coronary artery dissection. *Can J Neurol Sci*. 2003;**30**:168–170.

119. Salonen Ros H, Lichtenstein P, Bellocco R, Petersson G, Cnattingius S. Increased risks of circulatory diseases in late pregnancy and puerperium. *Epidemiology*. 2001;**12**:456–460.

120. James AH, Bushnell CD, Jamison MG, Myers ER. Incidence and risk factors for stroke in pregnancy and the puerperium. *Obstet Gynecol*. 2005;**106**:509–516.

121. Witlin AG, Mattar F, Sibai BM. Postpartum stroke: a twenty-year experience. *Am J Obstet Gynecol*. 2000;**183**:83–88.

122. Robinson JL, Hall CS, Sedzimir CB. Arteriovenous malformations, aneurysms, and pregnancy. *J Neurosurg*. 1974;**41**:63–70.

123. Horton JC, Chambers WA, Lyons SL, Adams RD, Kjellberg RN. Pregnancy and the risk of hemorrhage from cerebral arteriovenous malformations. *Neurosurgery*. 1990;**27**:867–871.

124. Dias MS, Sekhar LN. Intracranial hemorrhage from aneurysms and arteriovenous malformations during pregnancy and the puerperium. *Neurosurgery*. 1990;**27**:855–865.

125. Hunt HB, Schifrin BS, Suzuki K. Ruptured berry aneurysms and pregnancy. *Obstet Gynecol*. 1974;**43**:827–837.

126. Clark SL, Hankins GD, Dudley DA, Dildy GA, Porter TF. Amniotic fluid embolism: analysis of the national registry. *Am J Obstet Gynecol*. 1995;**172**:1158–1167.

127. O'Shea A, Eappen S. Amniotic fluid embolism. *Int Anesthesiol Clin*. 2007;**45**:17–28.

128. Singhal AB, Bernstein RA. Postpartum angiopathy and other cerebral vasoconstriction syndromes. *Neurocrit Care*. 2005;**3**:91–97.

129. Lurain JR. Gestational trophoblastic tumors. *Semin Surg Oncol*. 1990;**6**:347–353.

130. Jelincic D, Hudelist G, Singer CF, et al. Clinicopathologic profile of gestational trophoblastic disease. *Wien Klin Wochenschr*. 2003;**115**:29–35.

131. Saad N, Tang YM, Sclavos E, Stuckey SL. Metastatic choriocarcinoma: a rare cause of stroke in the young adult. *Australas Radiol*. 2006;**50**:481–483.

132. Gurwitt LJ, Long JM, Clark RE. Cerebral metastatic choriocarcinoma: a postpartum cause of "stroke." *Obstet Gynecol*. 1975;**45**: 583–588.

133. Huang CY, Chen CA, Hsieh CY, Cheng WF. Intracerebral hemorrhage as initial presentation of gestational choriocarcinoma: a case report and literature review. *Int J Gynecol Cancer*. 2007;**17**:1166–1171.

134. Weir B, MacDonald N, Mielke B. Intracranial vascular complications of choriocarcinoma. *Neurosurgery*. 1978;**2**:138–142.

135. Pullar M, Blumbergs PC, Phillips GE, Carney PG. Neoplastic cerebral aneurysm from metastatic gestational choriocarcinoma. Case report. *J Neurosurg*. 1985;**63**:644–647.

136. Ho KL. Neoplastic aneurysm and intracranial hemorrhage. *Cancer*. 1982;**50**:2935–2940.

137. Lewis JL Jr. Diagnosis and management of gestational trophoblastic disease. *Cancer*. 1993;**71**:1639–1647.

138. Biousse V, Newman NJ, Oyesiku NM. Precipitating factors in pituitary apoplexy. *J Neurol Neurosurg Psychiatry*. 2001;**71**:542–545.

139. Elsasser Imboden PN, deTribolet N, Lobrinus A, et al. Apoplexy in pituitary macroadenoma: eight patients presenting in 12 months. *Medicine (Baltimore)*. 2005;**84**:188–196.

140. Dubuisson AS, Beckers A, Stevenaert A. Classical pituitary tumour apoplexy: clinical features, management and outcomes in a series of 24 patients. *Clin Neurol Neurosurg*. 2006.

141. Lavallee G, Morcos R, Palardy J, Aube M, Gilbert D. MR of non-hemorrhagic postpartum pituitary apoplexy. *AJNR Am J Neuroradiol*. 1995;**16**:1939–1941.

142. Acikgoz B, Cagavi F, Hakki Tekkok I. Late recurrent bleeding after surgical treatment for pituitary apoplexy. *J Clin Neurosci.* 2004;**11**:555–559.

143. Piotin M, Tampieri D, Rufenacht DA, et al. The various MRI patterns of pituitary apoplexy. *Eur Radiol.* 1999;**9**:918–923.

144. Rogg JM, Tung GA, Anderson G, Cortez S. Pituitary apoplexy: early detection with diffusion-weighted MR imaging. *AJNR Am J Neuroradiol.* 2002;**23**:1240–1245.

145. Sweeney AT, Blake MA, Adelman LS, et al. Pituitary apoplexy precipitating diabetes insipidus. *Endocr Pract.* 2004;**10**:135–138.

146. Ayuk J, McGregor EJ, Mitchell RD, Gittoes NJ. Acute management of pituitary apoplexy – surgery or conservative management? *Clin Endocrinol (Oxf).* 2004;**61**:747–752.

147. Maccagnan P, Macedo CL, Kayath MJ, Nogueira RG, Abucham J. Conservative management of pituitary apoplexy: a prospective study. *J Clin Endocrinol Metab.* 1995;**80**:2190–2197.

148. Verrees M, Arafah BM, Selman WR. Pituitary tumor apoplexy: characteristics, treatment, and outcomes. *Neurosurg Focus.* 2004;**16**:E6.

149. Duncan KR. The development of magnetic resonance imaging in obstetrics. *Br J Hosp Med.* 1996;**55**:178–181.

150. ACOG Committee Opinion. No. 299, September 2004 (replaces No. 158, September 1995). Guidelines for diagnostic imaging during pregnancy. *Obstet Gynecol.* **2004**;104:647–651.

151. Ratnapalan S, Bona N, Chandra K, Koren G. Physicians' perceptions of teratogenic risk associated with radiography and CT during early pregnancy. *AJR Am J Roentgenol.* 2004;**182**:1107–1109.

152. Bentur Y, Horlatsch N, Koren G. Exposure to ionizing radiation during pregnancy: perception of teratogenic risk and outcome. *Teratology.* 1991;**43**:109–112.

153. Beeley L. Adverse effects of drugs in the first trimester of pregnancy. *Clin Obstet Gynaecol.* 1986;**13**:177–195.

154. Beeley L. Adverse effects of drugs in later pregnancy. *Clin Obstet Gynaecol.* 1986;**13**:197–214.

155. Barbour LA. Current concepts of anticoagulant therapy in pregnancy. *Obstet Gynecol Clin North Am.* 1997;**24**:499–521.

156. Ginsberg JS, Hirsh J, Turner DC, Levine MN, Burrows R. Risks to the fetus of anticoagulant therapy during pregnancy. *Thromb Haemost.* 1989;**61**:197–203.

157. Ginsberg JS, Chan WS, Bates SM, Kaatz S. Anticoagulation of pregnant women with mechanical heart valves. *Arch Intern Med.* 2003;**163**:694–698.

158. Dahlman TC. Osteoporotic fractures and the recurrence of thromboembolism during pregnancy and the puerperium in 184 women undergoing thromboprophylaxis with heparin. *Am J Obstet Gynecol.* 1993;**168**:1265–1270.

159. Melissari E, Parker CJ, Wilson NV, et al. Use of low molecular weight heparin in pregnancy. *Thromb Haemost.* 1992;**68**:652–656.

160. Pettila V, Leinonen P, Markkola A, Hiilesmaa V, Kaaja R. Postpartum bone mineral density in women treated for thromboprophylaxis with unfractionated heparin or LMW heparin. *Thromb Haemost.* 2002;**87**:182–186.

161. Ellison J, Walker ID, Greer IA. Antenatal use of enoxaparin for prevention and treatment of thromboembolism in pregnancy. *BJOG.* 2000;**107**:1116–1121.

162. Johnson DM, Kramer DC, Cohen E, Rochon M, Rosner M, Weinberger J. Thrombolytic therapy for acute stroke in late pregnancy with intra-arterial recombinant tissue plasminogen activator. *Stroke.* 2005;**36**:e53–e55.

163. Turrentine MA, Braems G, Ramirez MM. Use of thrombolytics for the treatment of thromboembolic disease during pregnancy. *Obstet Gynecol Surv.* 1995;**50**:534–541.

164. Schumacher B, Belfort MA, Card RJ. Successful treatment of acute myocardial infarction during pregnancy with tissue plasminogen activator. *Am J Obstet Gynecol.* 1997;**176**:716–719.

165. Patel RK, Fasan O, Arya R. Thrombolysis in pregnancy. *Thromb Haemost.* 2003;**90**:1216–1217.

166. Murugappan A, Coplin WM, Al-Sadat AN, et al. Thrombolytic therapy of acute ischemic stroke during pregnancy. *Neurology.* 2006;**66**:768–770.

167. Dapprich M, Boessenecker W. Fibrinolysis with alteplase in a pregnant woman with stroke. *Cerebrovasc Dis.* 2002;**13**:290.

168. van Walraven C, Mamdani M, Cohn A, Katib Y, Walker M, Rodger MA. Risk of subsequent thromboembolism for patients with pre-eclampsia. *BMJ.* 2003;**326**:791–792.

24

Vascular Diseases of the Spinal Cord

Spinal cord vascular disease is the orphan of neurology.

James F. Toole

Infarction of the spinal cord is rare compared to cerebral ischemic events, accounting for only about 1% of all strokes.[1,2] The reasons for this are not completely understood but is likely related to the characteristics of spinal cord blood supply, collateralization of blood flow, and the relative high ischemic tolerance of the spinal cord compared to the brain. Reynolds was one of the first to describe vascular occlusion as cause for spinal cord softening in his 1872 textbook,[3] and several years later the first accurate descriptions of the blood supply to the spinal cord were published by Adamkiewicz and Kadyi.[4–6]

ARTERIAL SUPPLY OF THE SPINAL CORD

Paired segmental arteries arise from the vertebral arteries, the aorta, and iliac arteries to perfuse paravertebral muscles, vertebrae, meninges, and nerve roots. Their branches travel with segmental nerves through the vertebral foramina to form the anterior and posterior radicular arteries that supply the anterior and posterior nerve roots and sensory ganglia. Unpaired medullary arteries arise from some of the segmental arteries and travel without branching to the anterior median spinal artery or the posterior pial arteriolar plexus.

All spinal cord segments receive blood from radicular arteries, but each segment is not supplied by an individual radicular artery. The largest artery is located in the lower thoracic or upper lumbar spinal cord and is named for Adamkiewicz (Figure 24-1). In about 80% of people the artery of Adamkiewicz is located on the left side, sending several ascending branches and typically one descending branch to the anterior and the posterior spinal cord. Although the anterior and posterior spinal arteries connect via a superficial arterial plexus (Figure 24-2), this network does not provide sufficient collateral blood flow at all spinal levels to stave off infarction if either system is compromised.

There are three longitudinal vascular territories: the cervicothoracic area, which includes spinal levels C1 to T2/3 and the cervical enlargement; the thoracic area encompassing levels T4 to T8; and the lower thoracolumbar territory including levels T9

to L5 and the lumbar enlargement, which are supplied by the large lumbar radicular artery. The areas between these three regions form potential watershed zones of the spinal cord.[7]

Extensive anastomoses of radicular arteries exist in the cervical and the lumbar cord, providing potential collateral blood

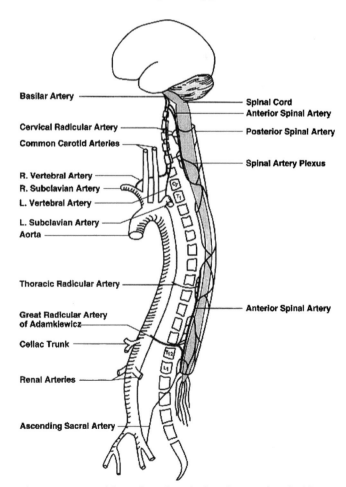

Figure 24-1. Arterial supply to the spinal cord. Reproduced with permission from Cheshire et al.[19]

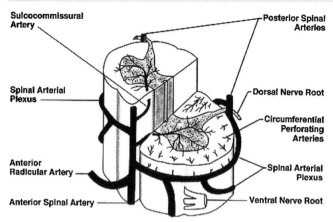

Figure 24-2. Radicular arteries from different levels contribute to the discontinuous anterior spinal artery, which connects to the vertebral arteries rostrally and to the artery of Adamkiewicz caudally. Reproduced with permission from Cheshire et al.[19]

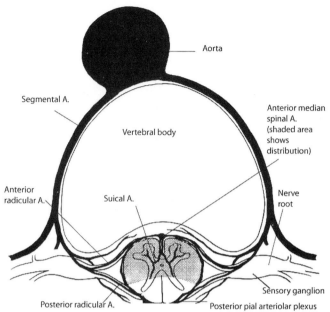

Figure 24-3. The intrinsic arterial supply to the spinal cord in cross section. The anterior spinal artery receives contributions from the radicular arteries and connects to the posterior spinal arteries via the spinal arterial plexus. Sulcocommissural branches of the anterior spinal artery penetrate to supply the anterior two thirds of the spinal cord (shaded area). Circumferential branches supply the superficial portions of the spinal cord.

supply when a radicular artery is occluded. The cervical cord receives a substantial amount of blood from the vertebral arteries, which have multiple connections with the radicular, spinal, occipital, basilar, deep cervical, ascending cervical, and inferior thyroid arteries. Comparable extensive connections exist between the radicular lumbosacral arteries and the vessels of the pelvis via internal iliac, obturator, and sacral arteries. In contrast, the thoracic cord has rather few anastomoses and is supplied by relatively small segmental arteries that travel over long distances before they reach each spinal level.

Two anterior spinal rami that arise as the first intracranial branches of the vertebral arteries descend on the anterior surface of the spinal cord to the level of the second or third cervical segment of the cord, where they unite to form a single anterior median spinal artery. One of the anterior spinal rami is small or absent 11% of the time, and in rare cases the two run parallel as far as the lower cervical region or even to the sacral cord without joining.

The posterior third of the cord receives blood from the paired posterior spinal arteries and the anterior two thirds is supplied by the anterior spinal artery via sulcocommissural branches (Figure 24-3). These penetrating arteries feed mainly the gray matter of the spinal cord except for the posterior horns and a small portion of the deep white matter. Within the cord there is a network of capillaries that is of higher density in the gray than the white matter, reflecting the higher neuronal energy demand. Peripheral branches of the posterior spinal arteries perfuse mainly the white matter.

Anterior Median Spinal Artery

The anterior median spinal artery courses along the anterior surface of the spinal cord but is frequently discontinuous in the thoracic region, adding to the relatively high ischemic vulnerability of this area. Throughout its length it varies in caliber, being largest in its cervical and lumbar enlargements. As it descends in the median fissure, the anterior median spinal artery receives sporadic contributions from the anterior medullary arteries. Although the average number of tributaries is 7 to 10, there may be as few as 5 or as many as 17. The lumbosacral portion of the cord is supplied by the unpaired anterior sacral artery, the obstruction of which may result in dysfunction of the anterior two thirds of the lumbosacral cord. Potential collateral blood supply within the spinal cord exists at two levels: in the pial arteriolar plexus and at the capillary level. This collateral circulation is sufficient to prevent neural damage only in the region of the plexus that supplies the posterior third of the cord.

Branches of the Anterior Median Spinal Artery

The anterior median spinal artery nourishes the anterior two thirds of the spinal cord through the sulcocommissural arteries and branches to the ventrolateral portion of the pial arteriolar plexus (Figure 24-2). The sulcal arteries penetrate the median fissure, turning alternately right and left into the cord parenchyma. Throughout the length of the cord their total number ranges from 250 to 300. Although there is little if any communication between the arteries of the two halves of the spinal cord, numerous capillary or precapillary anastomoses exist among those of the same side.

Penetrating branches arise from the pial arteriolar plexus and end in a capillary network with the sulcal arteries. These arteries nourish the lateral and ventral spinothalamic tracts, the corticospinal pathways, and the anterior and lateral horns of the gray matter, all of which are contained in the anterior two-thirds of the spinal cord.

Posterior Spinal Rami and Pial Arteriolar Plexus

Arising as small branches of the intracranial portion of the vertebral arteries, the paired posterior spinal rami wind around the lateral aspect of the cervicomedullary region to lie just lateral to the entrance of the posterior nerve roots on either side. They end at the second or third cervical segment of the cord by joining the lateral and ventral aspects of the pial arteriolar plexus. Throughout the length of the cord a variable number of posterior medullary branches from the segmental arteries of the cervical and thoracic regions terminate in this plexus. Below the thoracic level the great posterior medullary artery joins the network and is the only source of blood for the posterior third of the lower spinal cord. These anastomoses of the pial network are often so extensive that any one or even several of the ramifications can be occluded without producing clinical deficit.

VENOUS ANATOMY

In the cervical region the longitudinal cord veins and the internal vertebral plexus join the intracranial veins to form a continuous valveless system that may drain blood from the posterior fossa into the spinal canal or in the reverse direction from cord to the posterior fossa. The venous system of the spinal cord typically consists of one anterior and one or two posterior spinal veins draining blood from the spinal cord to radicular veins that communicate with the epidural space and empty into the vertebral, intercostal, lumbar, and sacral veins.

Whereas the vessels on the anterior aspect of the cord are chiefly arterial, those on the posterior side are primarily venous. The system is plexiform, but within the network six main channels can be distinguished: a posterior, two posterolateral, two anterolateral, and the anterior spinal veins. Most of the central veins draining the interior of the spinal cord empty into the anterior spinal vein, which runs throughout the length of the cord in the vicinity of the anterior median fissure. These six longitudinal venous channels empty into the radicular veins accompanying the ventral and dorsal nerve roots. The spinal radicular veins in the subarachnoid space penetrate the dura to join the epidural venous plexus, which in turn communicates with the internal vertebral venous plexus. The latter communicates with the inferior vena cava and the azygos system of veins through the parivertebral (Batson's) plexus.

Venous occlusions produce a highly variable clinical picture. Patients typically present with upper motor neuron paraparesis or quadriparesis, sensory dissociation, and loss of sphincter control. At its most severe, the entire cord is rendered dysfunctional. Venous infarctions have been observed in the clinical setting of ascending thrombosis, thrombophlebitis, or with mechanical obstruction.[8]

PHYSIOLOGY OF THE SPINAL CORD CIRCULATION

In many respects, the physiology of the spinal cord circulation is similar to that of the cerebral circulation. The vessels autoregulate in response to changes in systemic arterial blood pressure; they dilate when the $PaCO_2$ is increased and constrict when it is reduced. The requirement for spinal cord blood flow increases with the activity of the neurons involved. However, studies on anesthetized animals demonstrate lower unit blood flow to the spinal cord than to the brain, with an average perfusion value of about 20 ml/100 g/min in the cord that is disproportionately distributed to the cord gray matter.[9,10] It is assumed that the average arterial pressure in the spinal cord is substantially lower than that in the aorta and that tissue oxygen supply closely parallels the blood flow and systemic pressure.

Spinal cord perfusion is more directly affected by changes in systemic blood pressure than brain perfusion. Low peripheral vascular resistance with aortic hypotension diverts aortic outflow away from the spinal cord vessels. When peripheral vascular resistance in the lower extremities is high, aortic outflow is diverted toward the spinal circulation, increasing pressure and possibly cord perfusion. If the patient has hypertension and increased peripheral vascular resistance, a column of contrast medium in the aorta during aortography is diverted into the spinal cord circulation. If peripheral resistance is decreased, rapid forward flow occurs, and the aorta is virtually emptied of contrast at the end of one cardiac cycle and none is visible in the spinal arterial circulation.

The spinal cord is encased within a bony structure similar to that which protects the brain, so that any change in volume can take place only at the expense of the cerebrospinal fluid, the blood, or the spinal tissue itself. Damage to the cord typically occurs with more than 20 to 30 minutes of ischemia and during systemic hypotension with failure of the autoregulatory response. Complete interruption of aortic blood flow, as with experimental aortic ligation in cats for more than 30 minutes, causes permanent paresis, hyperreflexia, and sensory deficits.[11,12] The resulting ischemic injury to the cord first affects areas with high metabolic demand, such as the anterior horn cells and gray matter before, leading to complete cord necrosis.

CLINICAL FEATURES OF SPINAL CORD ISCHEMIA

Obstruction of the arteries supplying the spinal cord in the absence of adequate collateral blood flow results in spinal cord infarction. Cord infarction also results from prolonged hypoperfusion, as might occur with extended systemic hypotension or from chronic shunting of arterial blood away from the spinal cord by a high flow arteriovenous malformation (AVM). Hypoperfusion injuries tend to occur in watershed regions. Both infarction and transient ischemia with reversible neurological deficit have been recognized.[13–16] Table 24-1 summarizes the factors that promote spinal cord infarction for each of its major arteries.

Signs and symptoms of cord ischemia typically develop over a few minutes and rarely in stages, at times preceded by transient ischemic attacks. Sudden-onset back, neck, or radicular pain and paresthesias at the level of the involved segments are commonly followed by paresis, sensory deficits, reflex abnormalities, and sphincter disturbances depending on the location of occlusion. Table 24-2 summarizes the ischemic spinal cord syndromes.

Variations in number and caliber of radicular arteries as well as the availability of collateral vessels help to explain the striking clinical variability in individuals with spinal cord ischemia. Reduction of flow in one of the major radicular arteries can result in infarction in several cord segments, especially when flow to a watershed area is compromised. Multisegmental necrosis of the central cord affecting the vascular territory between the anterior and circumflex vessels causes signs and symptoms similar to those of the anterior spinal artery syndrome.[17]

Table 24-1: Artery-Specific Causes of Spinal Cord Infarction

Size	Causative Factors
Aorta	Dissection
	Atherosclerosis
	Aneurysm, atherosclerotic or syphilitic
	Surgery/trauma
	Hemorrhage
Vertebral arteries	Hyperextension injuries of the cervical spine
	Cervical spondylosis
	Congenital bone anomalies
	Trauma (spine fracture, dislocation)
	Vertebral artery occlusion or dissection
Intercostal Arteries	Postoperative
	Thoracoplasty
	Dorsolumbar sympathectomy
	Aortic surgery
Medullary arteries	Ligation during surgery of thoracolumbar aorta
	Occlusion by malignant tumor or tuberculosis
	Arteriography
Anterior medial spinal artery	Atherosclerosis (rare)
	Diabetes mellitus
	Syphilitic arteritis
	Mechanical compression
Sulcal arteries	Connective tissue diseases
	Endarteritis obliterans
	Air embolism
	Radiation myelopathy
	Syphilis
	Tuberculosis
	Sarcoidosis

Because infarction occurs most frequently in the midthoracic region, the pain often radiates in girdle fashion around the thorax and into the upper abdomen. An acute flaccid paralysis of the lower extremities associated with loss of pain and temperature sensations follows, perhaps with sacral sparing because of the superficial position of the sacral segments of the spinal thalamic tract which may continue to be perfused by collaterals. Sphincter control is lost immediately and there is often reflex ileus and abdominal distension secondary to the acute interruption of sympathetic enervation. Because the posterior columns are often spared, perception of vibration and joint position is preserved. This loss of spinothalamic function with preservation of posterior-column function is the distinguishing characteristic of this syndrome.

The initial flaccidity and the loss of muscle stretch reflexes result from spinal shock and are gradually replaced by spasticity in all muscles below the level of the lesion, with brisk muscle stretch reflexes and extensor plantar responses. Because of necrosis of the anterior horn cells, however, the muscles at the level of occlusion (the intercostal or abdominal muscles) remain flaccid and become atrophic.

This weakness may be intermittent with transient ischemia or permanent if spinal cord infarction occurs. The diagnosis of intermittent ischemia of the thoracic or lumbar sections of the cord should be considered when weakness of the lower limbs is precipitated by physical effort, particularly if strength is rapidly restored by rest. During this weakness the patient experiences no pain, and pedal pulses remain palpable. However, if the causative lesion is in the abdominal aorta, exercise may also lead to pain in the hips (because of ischemia of gluteal muscles) and impotence (*Leriche syndrome*). Cervical cord ischemia may also manifest as "drop attacks."

Iatrogenic damage to the vascular area of the large lumbar radicular artery is unfortunately common. The great anterior medullary artery of Adamkiewicz arises from the abdominal aorta and feeds the anterior media spinal artery. Injury usually results from surgery that involves the lumbar aorta, for example, during resection of an abdominal aortic aneurysm or renal artery reconstruction. Occlusion of this artery, which can arise at any level from T10 to L3, may cause infarction of the anterior two-thirds of the lumbosacral cord, leading to all the signs of anterior median spinal artery occlusion.

Unilateral obstruction in the intracranial portion of the anterior spinal ramus causes infarction of the homolateral pyramid, the medial lemniscus, and the hypoglossal nucleus and nerve: the ventral medullary syndrome. The results manifest as contralateral spastic paralysis of the arm and leg, with ipsilateral loss of vibration, position, and light-touch perception, and flaccid paralysis and atrophy of the tongue; perception of pain and temperature is preserved. Occlusion of both anterior spinal rami results in tetraplegia and loss of vibration and position sense in all four limbs.

ISCHEMIC MYELOPATHY SYNDROMES

Based on the spinal vascular territories affected by ischemia, there are three classic vascular syndromes of the cord:[15,18] the anterior spinal syndrome, the posterior spinal syndrome, and complete or total transverse ischemic myelopathy.

Anterior Spinal Artery Syndrome

First described by Prebaschenski in 1904, the anterior spinal artery syndrome usually results from injury or disease of the aorta or intercostal or radicular arteries, not from occlusion of the anterior spinal artery itself as the name implies. Clinical manifestations include sudden-onset radicular pain, paraplegia, or tetraplegia and dissociated sensory impairment with loss of sensation for temperature and pain but intact depth perception and vibratory sense. However, the clinical presentation is highly variable and depends on the spinal segment involved.

Table 24-2: Clinical Features of Spinal Cord Infarction

Infarcted Territory	Clinical Presentation
Anterior spinal artery	Bilateral weakness, loss of sensation for pain and temperature, hyperreflexia, sphincter and autonomic disturbances
Anterior unilateral infarct	Ipsilateral weakness with contralateral sensory loss of pain and temperature
Posterior unilateral infarct	Variable weakness with ipsilateral loss of proprioception and vibratory sense
Central cord infarct	Bilateral loss of sensation for pain and temperature with preserved motor function
Posterior spinal artery infarct	Bilateral motor deficit with loss of proprioception and vibratory sense
Transverse infarct	Bilateral complete sensory and motor deficit hyperreflexia, sphincter and autonomic disturbances

The prognosis usually is better than that of the complete transverse myelopathy but recurrent disease is not unusual.[19,20]

A vascular Brown-Séquard syndrome affecting only one side of the cord is rare but can result from occlusion of one of the two segmental sulcocommisural arteries at their bifurcation. Clinical presentations mimicking amyotrophic lateral sclerosis or primary lateral sclerosis have been observed in elderly patients with atherosclerosis following occlusion of terminal branches of sulcocommisural vessels to the anterior horn or of radicular arteries of the lower cervical/upper thoracic cord. These patients have atrophy and weakness of intrinsic hand and foot muscles, fasciculations, hyperreflexia, and often pathological reflexes.

Transverse Infarction Syndrome

Infarction of the entire transverse segment of the cord resembles the anterior spinal artery syndrome except for the loss of posterior column function with transverse infarction. Infarction is frequently preceded by signs and symptoms of intermittent claudication of the spinal cord, first described by Joseph Jules Déjerine.[16] If cord ischemia persists, there is typically a sudden onset of radicular pain followed by acute spinal shock syndrome. Depending on the spinal segment affected, patients develop paraplegia or quadriplegia, loss of all sensory modalities below the lesion, and frequently a hyperesthetic zone above the affected level. Autonomic disturbances can cause cardiac dysrhythmias, cardiovascular collapse, or pulmonary edema. Initially muscle stretch reflexes are often absent and plantar flexor responses are indifferent but will become brisk with development of pathological reflexes in the subacute to chronic stages. The clinical course varies and depends on the amount and quality of functional vascular anastomoses as well as on the duration of ischemia, among other factors. The overall prognosis is poor, but at times patients show partial or complete recovery. Not surprisingly, individuals with an incomplete loss of function tend to recover more quickly and more completely that those with complete loss of cord function.

Posterior Spinal Artery Syndrome

Vascular occlusive disease of the posterior spinal arteries results in the posterior cord syndrome, which is clinically characterized by dysfunction of the posterior columns. Depending on the segmental level involved there is sudden loss of proprioception and vibratory sense. Muscle stretch reflexes and cutaneous reflexes are decreased or absent, but neurological functions maintained by the anterior two-thirds of the cord remain intact.

DIFFERENTIAL DIAGNOSIS

Any focal lesion of the spinal cord could have clinical features that overlap those of spinal cord infarction. Other disorders to consider include inflammatory, infectious, or demyelinating conditions such as transverse myelitis, syphilis, and multiple sclerosis. Epidural abscess or hemorrhage with cord compression could be mistaken for a cord infarction, and in fact the loss of cord function in these individuals may result from cord compression with secondary infarction. A neoplasm or a syrinx could be confused with spinal cord ischemia. Infarction of the spinal cord may follow dissection or thrombosis of the aorta, trauma to the medullary arteries, or occlusion of the anterior median spinal artery or its branches. Disorders that preferentially affect the posterior columns can be confused with posterior spinal artery syndrome. These conditions could include vitamin B_{12} deficiency, copper deficiency myelopathy, vitamin E deficiency, or abetalipoproteinemia.

CAUSES OF VASCULAR MYELOPATHY

There are many risk factors for ischemic myelopathy (Table 24-3). It is caused by disease or mechanical injury of the aorta or the intercostal, vertebral, iliac, or lumbar arteries. Thrombosis of the anterior or posterior spinal arteries is relatively rare.[21,22] Aortic atheromas, dissecting aneurysm, or clamping of the aorta during surgery can result in secondary acute cord ischemia and infarction. Depending on the site of origin of the artery of Adamkiewicz, thrombosis above the renal arteries may cause ischemic myelopathy of levels T8 to L2. Vertebral artery occlusion can affect the upper spinal levels.

Spinal cord infarction is rarely attributed to embolism of cholesterol fragments, blood clots, foreign material, or herniated fragments of the nucleus pulposus. Inflammatory disorders and tumors can precipitate a cord infarction. Other causes of ischemic myelopathy include blood dyscrasias, hypercoagulable disorders, sickle cell disease, neoplastic or infectious processes such as tuberculosis or syphilis, radiation injury, vascular compromise by a disk protrusion, or severe degenerative spine disease. Air emboli during decompression sickness can

Table 24-3: Risk Factors for Arterial Spinal Cord Infarction

Atherosclerosis	Cervical spondylosis
Severe arterial hypotension or cardiac arrest	Spine fracture or dislocation
Aortic surgery	Vertebral artery occlusion or dissection
Traumatic laceration of the aorta	Rib resection for sympathectomy
Dissecting aortic aneurysm	Lumbar sympathectomy
Thrombo-occlusive aortic disease	Thoracoplasty for tuberculosis
Infection (lues, tuberculosis)	Thoracotomy
Vasculitis	Intercostal artery ligation
Carcinomatous meningitis	Celiac plexus block
Neoplastic spread to the spinal cord	Decompression sickness (Caisson disease)
Hypertensive small vessel disease	Atheromatous emboli
Subarachnoid hemorrhage	Cholesterol emboli
Sickle cell anemia	Fibrocartilaginous emboli
Systemic lupus erythematosus	Atrial myxoma
Antiphospholipid antibody syndrome	Aortic or spinal cord angiography
Disseminated intravascular coagulation	Intra-aortic balloon pump
	Lumbar artery compression

Adapted with permission from Brazis, Masdu, Biller.[64]

cause acute paralysis and sensory deficits and can be treated with emergency recompression. Venous infarctions have been observed in the setting of pelvic or abdominal phlebitis, fibrocartilaginous emboli, decompression sickness (Caisson's disease), chronic meningitis, acute myelogenous leukemia, spinal cord glioma, polycythemia rubra vera, and liver abscess.[23,24] In others infarction follows abdominal or thoracic aortic surgery, aortography, trauma, or dissecting hematoma of the aorta. Often no underlying etiology can be identified.[25,26]

Atherosclerosis

Atherosclerosis of the aorta is common in elderly individuals and often concurs with cardiovascular and peripheral arterial disease, causing vessel thickening and calcification.[14] It can result in intermittent claudication of the cord. If ischemia is unilateral, the diagnosis can be challenging. The differential diagnosis encompasses rare intermittent ischemia of paraspinal muscles, peripheral arterial disease, and spinal claudication due to a narrow spinal canal and/or disc protrusion. Transient cord ischemia can occur in isolation or can be followed by spinal cord infarction. Rare cases of chronic spinal cord ischemia due to atherosclerosis have been described that causes painless progressive

flaccid areflexic paraplegia that is unaccompanied by upper motor signs or sensory deficits.

Trauma

The spinal arteries run along a mobile structure, which makes them vulnerable for mechanic injury. Traumatic hyperextension injuries sometimes result in arterial damage and spinal cord infarction. Osteoarthritic or rheumatoid spondylosis, particularly in the cervical region where the arteries enter the spinal canal through the vertebral foramina, may impair blood supply to the cord. Protrusion of a nucleus pulposus may displace the spinal cord posteriorly, thereby stretching dentate ligaments that suspend the cord in the spinal canal. This causes venous congestion and ischemia by squeezing the cord between these ligaments and the nucleus pulposus. Flexion–extension injuries of the cervical spine (whiplash injuries), in addition to causing acute concussion of the cord, may interrupt its blood supply by compressing the arteries or by stretching them, so that vasospasm of the vertebral arteries or of their branches results. At times this constriction persists long after the acute episode and results in persistent symptoms.

Some of the effects of spinal cord injury are secondary to vascular injury which manifests as dissecting hematoma, spasm, and/or loss of autoregulation leading to tissue edema. In addition, systemic effects of cord injury can lead to further damage to the cord itself.

After injury there may be an evanescent increase in local spinal cord blood flow caused by vasoparalysis followed by a steady decline over a period of 3 or 4 hours. The resulting ischemia and edema disrupts normal signal transmission across the site of injury. When injury occurs, autonomic control is impaired and systemic arterial pressure may fall, compounding its effect. Experimentally, some of these effects can be minimized by reducing metabolic activity by cooling, glucose reduction, or the administration of naloxone, methylprednisolone, and glutamate receptor antagonists.[11]

Hypotensive–Hypoxic Myelopathy

Spinal cord blood flow and oxygenation depend on adequate systemic blood pressure regulation. In patients who suffer hypotensive shock, usually from myocardial infarction with or without cardiac arrest, paraplegia may be a sequel. This usually occurs in patients with extensive atherosclerosis, particularly of the abdominal aorta. Lesions of hypoxic myelopathy are typically symmetrical and limited to the gray matter of the cord (Figure 24-4).[27,28]

Arterial Dissection

Spontaneous or traumatic dissection of the thoracic or lumbar aorta can cause infarction of the spinal cord by occluding the ostia of the segmental arteries. Patients suffering this catastrophe have no pulse in the arteries below the abdominal aorta and require emergency surgery to correct the dissection. Unfortunately, correction of the aortic lesion seldom restores cord function.[29]

Iatrogenic Myelopathy

Contrast medium inadvertently introduced into the aorta near the ostium of a segmental artery, usually the great anterior

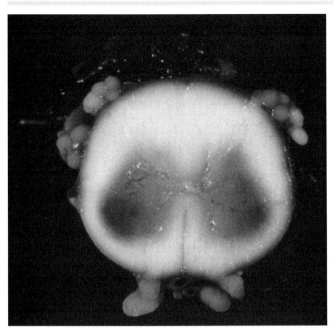

Figure 24-4. Cross section of the spinal cord shows hypoxic–ischemic myelopathy of the central portion of the cord.

medullary artery, during the performance of a lumbar or renal aortogram may promote spinal cord infarction. Ischemic spinal cord injury has been reported after sympathectomy, thoracoplasty, and particularly after aortic surgery. The prognosis of spinal cord infarction after aortic surgery, which remains one of the most frequent reasons for vascular myelopathy, is generally poor although a few patients do well. The use of magnetic resonance angiography (MRA) and computed tomography angiography (CTA) during presurgical planning, newer surgical approaches, and physiological intraoperative monitoring may help to reduce risk of myelopathy in the future.[30]

Radiation Myelopathy

After therapeutic irradiation of the thyroid, cervical lymph nodes, posterior part of the tongue, or upper part of the respiratory tract, radiation-induced damage to the small blood vessels of the spinal cord may cause infarction. Similar damage to the thoracic cord may follow irradiation for bronchogenic carcinoma. The neural deficit often becomes apparent only after a latent period of 2 or more years and is manifested by a rapidly progressive neural deficit below the level of the irradiation. This complication of radiation therapy is rare and depends on the total dose, the technique and duration of therapy, and perhaps individual sensitivity. The diagnosis should be made only after intraspinal metastasis has been excluded by appropriate neuroimaging studies.[31]

Drug-Related Vasculopathy

Spinal vascular myelopathy can be caused by heroin use, which has a predilection for damaging the thoracic cord.[32,33] Some suggest that this myelopathy is not caused by the drug itself but rather by panarteritis nodosa after hepatitis B antigen exposure that frequently occurs in this patient population.[34] Although uncommon, cocaine abuse can cause spinal cord infarction.[35] A diffuse vasculitis of the cord can be induced by amphetamines[36,37] or by the administration of toluene and buprenorphine.[38]

PROGNOSIS OF CORD ISCHEMIA

Retrospective data analysis of relatively small patient series has shown that the prognosis of ischemic myelopathy is variable but that the majority of patients have only incomplete functional recovery.[39,40] Most patients have some degree of gait impairment or are wheelchair dependent after hospital discharge. In general, motor deficits tend to have better chances of recovery than sensory, gait, or sphincter impairments. Younger patients and those with incomplete or unilateral infarction seem to have a better prognosis. It has been suggested that spinal cord infarctions due to aortic surgery have the severest clinical outcome.

VENOUS DISEASE

Subacute necrotic myelopathy (*Foix-Alajouanine Syndrome*) is uncommon but perhaps not as rare as once suspected. The subacute myelopathy of Foix-Alajouanine syndrome results from an AVM that causes congestion and increases the intravascular pressure within the cord's venous system, leading to chronic progressive dysfunction due to ischemic injury.[41] It occurs most often in middle-aged adults and typically affects the thoracic and lumbar regions. The clinical picture is that of progressive paraparesis extending over a period of a few months to several years. Both upper and lower motor neurons are involved, and there is often a sensory loss below level of the lesion. Sphincter dysfunction is also evident.

The spinal fluid may show a few cells and a moderate to marked increase in the protein level.[42] Pathological examination (Figure 24-5) reveals degeneration or necrosis of the spinal cord, with surface vessels appearing dilated and tortuous and often containing intraluminal thrombi. Some physicians believe this appearance represents a primary thrombophlebitis of the superficial veins of the spinal cord with secondary vascular dilatation. Most consider the primary lesion to be an AVM in which secondary thrombosis of veins has developed.

ARACHNOIDITIS

Arachnoiditis can follow trauma, infection, neoplasm, spinal subarachnoid hemorrhage, or the intrathecal administration of foreign substances, but often the cause remains undetermined. There is evidence of root and/or cord involvement at multiple levels. Rarely, arachnoiditis leads to secondary cavitation within the substance of the spinal cord, simulating syringomyelia. Pathological examination usually reveals an obliterative angiopathy with variable involvement of the vessels of the leptomeninges, roots, and spinal cord, accompanied by some inflammatory response.[43]

SPINAL CORD HEMORRHAGE

Spinal cord hemorrhage, like intracranial hemorrhage, may be epidural (the most common type), subdural, subarachnoid, or intramedullary and may be spontaneous or traumatic in origin. Because aneurysms of spinal arteries are very rare, the anatomic abnormality most frequently responsible for spontaneous spinal hemorrhage is spinal vascular malformation. MRI and MRA are useful initial studies for assessing spinal hemorrhage, identifying underlying vascular malformations, and planning intervention.[44]

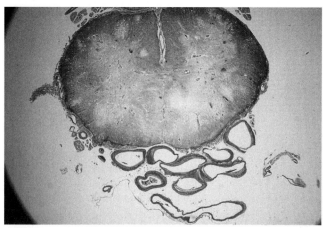

Figure 24-5. Subacute necrotic myelopathy due to an AVM (Foix-Alajouanine syndrome). Note the dilated AVM vessels anterior to the spinal cord and the widespread necrosis within the spinal cord.

Spinal Cord AVMs

Compared to those in the brain, spinal AVMs are relatively rare. They are probably underdiagnosed, but early diagnosis and treatment can in some instances prevent progressive neurological deterioration. Spinal cord AVMs can be either sporadic or hereditary. The best known genetic disorder that predisposes to spinal AVMs is hereditary hemorrhagic telangiectasia (see Chapter 21).[45–47]

Spinal vascular malformations can become acutely symptomatic when they cause intramedullary or subarachnoid hemorrhages, but they can also cause neurological deficits due to mass effect, tissue edema, subacute venous congestion, or due to a steal effect in large-volume shunts (Figure 24-5). Often these lesions produce chronic and uncharacteristic symptoms such as nonspecific back and paraspinal muscle pain, paresthesias, progressive sensorimotor deficits, weakness, impotence, or incontinence and often there is a long delay before the diagnosis is made.[48,49] The differential diagnosis of this chronic pattern typically includes degenerative spine disease, tumor, neuropathy, radiculopathy, or lumbosacral plexopathy. Timely MRI studies of the spinal cord (Figure 24-6) and surgical or endovascular intervention are key to preventing poor outcome.

AVMs of the spinal cord interconnect with the arteries and veins of the thorax and abdomen and sometimes with the pelvic vessels. They are often fed by radiculomedullary arteries and drained by the spinal venous system. In the spinal cord, AVMs may be intramedullary, meningeal, or a combination of the two. Intramedullary AVMs often have high shunt volumes leading to a circulatory steal phenomenon. AVMs represent about 3% of all spinal cord abnormalities and about 20% to 30% of all spinal vascular malformations. They usually involve the dural vessels and are most common in the lumbar and lumbosacral areas. They are rare in the cervical region. Not only do they divert blood from its normal areas of perfusion but they also compress the normal cord because the draining veins may become extremely dilated. Therefore the presentation can be subarachnoid hemorrhage or cord compression. The most common complaint is pain, usually in the lumbar area, but paresthesias occur less often.

The initial symptoms of spinal cord AVM cannot be reliably differentiated from other spinal cord lesions, but the picture at the time of presentation may suggest the diagnosis. Most patients are men with findings referable to the thoracolumbar cord and who have gradually progressive pain, weakness, and sensory and bladder disturbance. Early impairment of micturition may help suggest this lesion because it is less likely to be an early complaint in patients with disk disease or cord neoplasm.

Some patients with myelopathy caused by an AVM give a history of remissions and relapses, radicular pain made worse on standing, and aggravations during pregnancy or menstruation. Most commonly there are combined upper and lower motor neuron manifestations with nonradicular sensory deficit. The CSF is abnormal in more than 75% of cases with mild elevation of protein or presence of red blood cells and xanthochromia in cases of previous hemorrhage. Occasionally the presence of intraspinal vascular malformation is suggested by a cutaneous nevus or a bruit at the appropriate level of the spine.

Spinal MRI shows complexes of dilated vessels characterized by flow voids on T_2-weigthed imaging and tubular structures with mixed hyper- and hypointense signals on T_1-sequences (Figure 24-6 A). These lesions are most often on the posterior surface of the cord, and a small malformation may be demonstrated only after contrast application. Patients who might benefit from endovascular occlusion of a spinal cord AVM typically undergo selective arteriographic studies to demonstrate the entire extent of the lesion and to identify the feeding and draining vessels (Figure 24-6 B). Obstruction of the CSF by tumor must be excluded because dilated veins below such a tumor can mimic an AVM and serial MRI studies might be necessary.

Once the diagnosis is established and the approximate level of the malformation determined, selective arteriography is performed to plan subsequent treatment and to define the AVM type. Surgical excision is not feasible when the AVM is intramedullary, but endovascular embolization or combination of embolization and surgery is sometimes useful.[50] In other individuals, however, the AVM is not approachable either with endovascular techniques or with surgery, and the only option in most of these patients is clinical observation and supportive care.

Cavernous Malformations

Cavernous malformations (see Chapter 18) of the spinal cord are uncommon but potentially treatable lesions that constitute about 5% of all spinal vascular malformations. They occur more frequently in women and are sometimes hereditary and associated with additional cavernous malformations in the brain, retina, or spinal cord.[51,52] Cavernous malformations can be recognized on MRI by their characteristic well-defined inhomogeneous, mulberry-like hyperintensity surrounded by a hypointense rim on T_2-weighted sequences. The blood products in the hypointense rim are even better visualized by T_2^*-weighted gradient-echo images. Calcifications are sometimes evident on CT. Angiography is not helpful because of the low flow state of cavernous malformations.

Dural AV Fistulas

Dural arteriovenous fistulas are the most frequent vascular malformations in the spinal cord. They occur most often in middle-aged men. They are found predominantly within the thoracolumbar region. Shunting of blood from an intradural radiculomeningeal artery into a radicular vein significantly increases venous pressure, leading to chronic venous congestion, edema, chronic hypoxia,

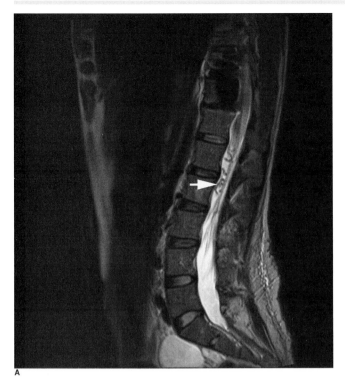

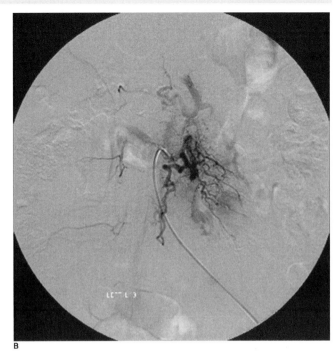

Figure 24-6. A: MRI shows the enlarged tangled vessels of an AVM (*arrow*) on the surface of the spinal cord. B: Catheter angiography confirms the serpiginous AVM vessels on the surface of the spinal cord.

and progressive cord damage (Figure 24-5). The diagnosis can be difficult to make, as symptoms often consist of nonspecific back pain and sensory disturbances radiating into the legs, impotence, and incontinence often attributed to degenerative disc and or spinal stenosis.

Spinal subarachnoid hemorrhage as presenting clinical picture is rare, but without appropriate diagnosis and therapy, functional outcome is poor.[53,54] MRI with contrast sometimes followed by MRA is the diagnostic modality of choice showing dilated and tortuous vessels on T_2-sequences presenting as flow voids. Fistulas can usually be cured by microsurgical occlusion of the draining vein or by technically often more challenging endovascular embolization of the feeding radiculomeningeal artery.

Epidural and Subdural Hemorrhage

Epidural bleeding is documented more often than subdural hemorrhage. Bleeding typically occurs after trauma but also develops in patients taking an anticoagulant medication or those with blood dyscrasias. Individuals with altered coagulation may develop an epidural hematoma after seemingly trivial trauma. Epidural hemorrhage is occasionally documented after coronary artery thrombolysis.

Clotting abnormalities in these patients should be corrected as soon as possible. At the same time, the patient should be observed carefully for signs of spinal cord involvement because emergency surgery may be required to remove a clot that compresses the cord. Hemangioma, usually involving the thoracic vertebrae, is an unusual cause of epidural hemorrhage that can be diagnosed via MRI. Any acute spinal cord syndrome is a possible neurosurgical emergency and must be investigated imme-

diately because early surgical intervention can improve functional neurological recovery.[55-57]

Subarachnoid Hemorrhage

Subarachnoid hemorrhage may be traumatic or spontaneous. If it occurs after lumbar puncture it is of no clinical consequence unless the bleeding is profuse, as it may be in rare cases in which the patient has a blood dyscrasia or has been taking anticoagulant medication. Trauma to the back sometimes causes spinal subarachnoid hemorrhage.

When a cause for spontaneous bleeding into the spinal subarachnoid space is found, it is usually rupture of an AVM or AV fistula.[58] Other causes include neoplasm of the spinal cord, blood dyscrasias (e.g., coagulopathy, thrombocytopenic purpura, or leukemia), and rarely the rupture of an atherosclerotic or inflamed artery.

Hemorrhage into the spinal subarachnoid space is usually manifested first by excruciating pain in the back, with radiation into the nerve roots. Opisthotonus followed by temporary partial paralysis of the extremities may occur. The CSF abnormalities of subarachnoid hemorrhage are described in Chapter 17. Treatment consists of bed rest and the correction of any underlying deficit in the clotting mechanism. Extramedullary angiomas may need to be excised.

Intramedullary Hemorrhage (Hematomyelia)

Like subarachnoid hemorrhage, intramedullary hemorrhage may be traumatic or spontaneous. Hematomyelia may result from rupture of a vascular malformation after Valsalva maneuver and may spread in any direction, producing a variety of clinical signs and symptoms. Sudden excruciating pain in the back, often with radicular radiation, is followed by an immediate loss of muscle tone below the level of the lesion. The results are paralysis (flaccid at first but becoming spastic after several days), retention of urine and feces, and sometimes abdominal distension caused by reflex ileus.

As the blood clot accumulates in the cord, it displaces and compresses the ascending and descending tracts. When the more laterally placed portions of the spinothalamic tracts are preserved, as is often the case, the result is preservation of sensory perception in the sacral dermatomes even though sensory perception in the thoracic and lumbar regions is lost (sacral sparing).

DIAGNOSIS OF VASCULAR MYELOPATHY

Routine laboratory evaluation might show evidence of diabetes or hypercholesterolemia and patients may have traditional stroke risk factors such as hypertension or tobacco use. Except in individuals with infectious or inflammatory disorders, the CSF is typically normal aside from the presence of a nonspecific protein elevation. A systematic assessment of the risk factors for spinal cord infarction is warranted (Table 24-3).

Whenever there is sudden paraplegia with a sensory loss on the trunk, the primary consideration is acute compression of the spinal cord by an extrinsic tumor or abscess; hence the entire length of the spine should be examined via CT or MRI as an emergency procedure. MRI of the spinal cord with sagittal and axial noncontrast T_2-weighted imaging has the highest diagnostic yield and can demonstrate hyperintense lesions associated with cord infarction. Nevertheless, up to a third of the patients with spinal cord infarction initially have no MRI abnormalities, and the likelihood of normal findings may be even higher in individuals with less severe weakness.[39] In these instances, serial imaging may be helpful. Vascular injury after aortic surgery can be visualized via serial MRI studies, and clinical deficits as well as prognosis correlate well with MRI changes.[59] Newer MRI techniques may allow more reliable diagnosis of acute spinal cord infarction.[60] If imaging studies remain negative, the diagnosis is clinically based and one of exclusion. Even intermittent spinal cord symptoms should prompt further evaluation for possible underlying spinal vascular malformations causing an intermittent circulatory steal phenomenon.[53,54]

When the pathological process is not clear initially, serial MRI studies may be required and contrast application can help to identify small vascular lesions. Blood products can be easily identified on T_2-weighted sequences or by gradient-echo imaging. Cord edema, traumatic cord transection, and cord compression can be visualized via MRI, which also is helpful to assess the prognosis of cord injury and hemorrhage.

MANAGEMENT OF SPINAL CORD VASCULAR LESIONS

Although there is no way to reverse an infarction of the spinal cord, rehabilitative measures (see Chapter 26) should be initiated immediately after diagnosis. Individuals with intermittent claudication of the spinal cord may benefit from intervention to control underlying risk factors. Selected patients at this stage may benefit from the use of anticoagulant or antiplatelet agents. Current therapy is mainly supportive and aimed at prevention and treatment of secondary complications such as skin ulcers, autonomic instability, contractures, or spasticity.

No data from large prospective clinical trials assessing the efficacy of steroids, antiplatelet agents, or anticoagulants are

available, largely because spinal cord infarction is so rare. Observational studies could not establish their clinical usefulness.[20] Animal experiments have suggested a potential therapeutic role for agents such as prostaglandins, nimodipine, riluzole, adenosine magnesium, thiopental, *N*-methyl-d-aspartate (NMDA) antagonists, or steroids, but no evidence-based data are available to support their routine clinical use.[61] Inasmuch as decreased CSF pressure may improve spinal cord perfusion pressure, temporary lumbar CSF drains have been advocated by some physicians following surgical repair of thoraco-abdominal aortic aneurysms complicated by spinal cord ischemia.[62,63]

Spinal AVMs are often amenable to intravascular embolization procedures. An epidural abscess or epidural hematoma should be surgically decompressed, although the operation may be ineffective if the cord has sustained an infarction due to the compression.

REFERENCES

1. Sandson TA, Friedman JH. Spinal cord infarction. Report of 8 cases and review of the literature. *Medicine (Baltimore)*. 1989;**68**: 282–292.
2. Weinstein M. Neurological update: ischaemic myelopathy. *Neurol Res*. 1993;**15**:212–213.
3. Reynolds JR, Bastian HC. *System of Medicine*. 2nd ed. London: Macmillan; 1872.
4. Adamkiewicz A. Die Blutgefässe des menschlichen Rückenmarks. I Die Gefässe der Rückenmarkssubstanz. *Sitzungblatt Akad Wiss Wien Math-naturw Kl.* 1881;**84**:469–502.
5. Adamkiewicz A. Die Blutgefässe des menschlichen Rückenmarks. II Die Gefässe der Rückenmarksoberfläche. *Sitzungblatt Akad Wiss Wien Math-naturw Kl.* **85**:101–130.
6. Kadyi H. Über die Blutgefässe des menschlichen Rückenmarks. *Anat Anz*. 1886;**1**:304–314.
7. Gillilan LA. The arterial blood supply of the human spinal cord. *J Comp Neurol*. 1958;**110**:75–100.
8. Gillilan LA. Veins of the spinal cord. Anastomotic details; suggested clinical applications. *Neurology*. 1970;**20**:860–868.
9. Otomo E, Van Buskirk C, Workman JB. Circulation of the spinal cord studied by autoradiography. *Neurology*. 1960;**10**:112–121.
10. Marcus ML, Heistad DD, Ehrhardt AJC, Abboud FM. Regulation of total and regional spinal cord blood flow. *Circ Res*. 1977;**41**:128–134.
11. Nystrom B, Stjernschantz J, Smedegard G. Regional spinal cord blood flow in the rabbit, cat and monkey. *Acta Neurol Scand*. 1984;**70**:307–313.
12. O'Donovan CA, Conomy JP. Neurological complications of diseases of the aorta. In: Goetz CG, Tanner CM, Aminoff MJ, eds. *Handbook of Clinical Neurology. Systemic Diseases, Part I*. Amsterdam: Elsevier; 1993:37–70.
13. Turnbull IM. Blood supply of the spinal cord. In: Vinken PJ, Bruyn GN, eds. *Handbook of Clinical Neurology*, Vol. 12. New York: Elsevier; 1972:478–491.
14. Henson RA, Parsons M. Ischaemic lesions of the spinal cord: an illustrated review. *Q J Med*. New Series 1967;**36**:205–222.
15. Garland H, Greenberg J, Harriman DGF. Infarction of the spinal cord. *Brain*. 1966;**89**:645–662.
16. Dejerine JJ. Sur la claudication intermittente de la moëlle épinière. *Rev Neurol (Paris)*. 1906;**14**:341–350.
17. Hogan EL, Romanul FCA. Spinal cord infarction occurring during insertion of aortic graft. *Neurology*. 1966;**16**:67.
18. Sliwa JA, Maclean IC. Ischemic myelopathy: a review of spinal vasculature and related clinical syndromes. *Arch Phys Med Rehabil*. 1992;**73**:365–372.

19. Cheshire WP, Santos CC, Massey EW, Howard JF. Spinal cord infarction: etiology and outcome. *Neurology*. 1996;**47**:321–330.

20. De Seze J, Stojkovie T, Breteau G, et al. Acute myelopathies: clinical, laboratory and outcome profiles in 79 cases. *Brain*. 2001;**124**:1509–1521.

21. Foo D, Rossier AB. Anterior spinal artery syndrome and its natural history. *Paraplegia*.1983;**21**:1–10.

22. Hughes JT. Thrombosis of the posterior spinal arteries. *Neurology*. 1970;**20**:6569–664.

23. Kim RC, Smith HR, Henbest ML, Choi BH. Nonhemorrhagic venous infarction of the spinal cord. *Ann Neurol*. 1984;**15**:379–385.

24. Hughes JT. Venous infarction of the spinal cord. *Neurology*. 1971;**21**:794–800.

25. Yoshizawa H. Pathomechanism of myelopathy and radiculopathy from the view-point of blood flow and cerebrospinal fluid flow including a short historical review. *Spine*. 2002;**27**:1255–1263.

26. Weidauer S, Nichtweiss M, Lanfermann H, Zanelia FE. Spinal cord infarction. MRI imaging and clinical features in 16 cases. *Neuroradiology*. 2002;**44**:851–857.

27. Azzarelli B, Roessmann U. Diffuse "anoxic" myelopathy. *Neurology*. 1977;**27**:1049–1052.

28. Imaizumi H, Ujike Y, Asai Y, Kaneko M, Chiba S. Spinal cord ischemia after cardiac arrest. *J Emerg Med*. 1994;**12**:789–793.

29. Holloway F, Fayad PB, Kalb RG, Guarnaccia JB, Waxman SG. Painless aortic dissection presenting as a progressive myelopathy. *J Neurol Sci*. 1993;**120**:141–144.

30. Yoshioka K, Niinuma H, Ehara S, Nakajima T, Nakamura M, Kawazoe K. MR angiography and CT angiography of the artery of Adamkiewicz: state of the art. *Radiographics*. 2006;**26**(Suppl 1):S63–73.

31. Komachi H, Tsuchiya K, Ikeda M, Koike R, Matsunaga T, Ikeda K. Radiation myelopathy: a clinicopathological study with special reference to correlation between MRI findings and neuropathology. *J Neurol Sci*. 1995;**132**:228–232.

32. Richter RW, Rosenberg RN. Transverse myelitis associated with heroin addiction. *JAMA*. 1968;**206**:1255–1257.

33. Pearson J, Richter RW, Baden MM, Challenor YB, Brunn B. Transverse myelopathy as an illustration of the neurologic and neuropathologic features of heroin addiction. *Hum Pathol*. 1972;**3**:107–113.

34. Gocke DJ, Christian CL. Angiitis in drug abusers (letter). *N Engl J Med*. 1971;**284**:112.

35. Schreiber AL, Formal CS. Spinal cord infarction secondary to cocaine use. *Am J Phys Med Rehabil*. 2007;**86**:158–160.

36. Citron BP, Halpern M, McCarron M, et al. Necrotizing angiitis associated with drug abuse. *N Engl J Med*. 1970;**283**:1003–1011.

37. Goldstein LH, Mordish Y, Abu-Kishak I, Toledano M, Berkovitch M. Acute paralysis following recreational MDMA (Ecstasy) use. *Clin Toxicol (Phila)*. 2006;**44**:339–341.

38. Caplan LR, Thomas C, Banks G. Central nervous system complications of addiction to "Ts and Blues." *Neurology*. 1982;**31**:623–628.

39. Novy J, Carruzzo A, Maeder P, Bogousslavsky J. Spinal cord ischemia. Clinical and imaging patterns, pathogenesis and outcomes in 27 patients. *Arch Neurol*. 2006;**63**:1113–1120.

40. de la Barrera S, Barca-Buyo A, Montoto-Marqués A, Ferreiro-Velasco ME, Cindoncha-Dans M, Rodriguez-Sotillo A. Spinal cord infarction: prognosis and recovery in a series of 36 patients. *Spinal Cord*. 2001;**39**:520–525.

41. Renowden SA, Molyneux AJ. Case report: spontaneous thrombosis of a spinal dural AVM (Foix-Alajouanine syndrome) – magnetic resonance appearance. *Clin Radiol*. 1993;**47**:134–136.

42. Mair WGP, Folkerts JF. Necrosis of spinal cord due to thrombophlebitis (subacute necrotic myelitis). *Brain*. 1953;**76**:563–575.

43. Caplan LR, Norohna AB, Amico LL. Syringomyelia and arachnoiditis. *J Neurol Neurosurg Psychiatry*. 1990;**53**:106–113.

44. White ML, El-Khoury GY. Neurovascular injuries of the spinal cord. *Eur J Radiol*. 2002;**42**:117–126.

45. Waters MF, Shields DC, Martin NA, Baloh RW, Jen JC. Novel CCM1 mutation in a patient with paraparesis and thoracic cord cavernous malformation. *Neurology*. 2005;**65**:966–967.

46. Dowling MM. Hereditary hemorrhagic telangiectasia (Osler-Weber-Rendu syndrome). In: Roach ES, Miller VS, eds. *Neurocutaneous Disorders*. Cambridge, England: Cambridge University Press; 2004:158–165.

47. Mandzia JL, terBrugge KG, Faughnan ME, Hyland RH. Spinal cord arteriovenous malformations in two patients with hereditary hemorrhagic telangiectasia. *Childs Nerv Syst*. 1999;**15**:80–83.

48. Krings T, Mull M, Gilsbach JM, Thron A. Spinal vascular malformations. *Eur Radiol*. 2005;**15**:267–278.

49. Aminoff MJ, Logue V. Clinical features of spinal vascular malformations. *Brain*. 1974;**97**:197–210.

50. Mascalchi M, Bianchi MC, Quilici N, et al. MR angiography of spinal vascular malformations. *AJNR Am J Neuroradiol*. 1995;**16**:289–297.

51. Zevgaridis D, Medele RJ, Hamburger C, Steiger HJ, Reulen HJ. Cavernous haemangiomas of the spinal caord. A review of 117 cases. *Acta Neurochir (Wien)*. 1999;**141**:237–245.

52. Weinzierl MR, Krings T, Korinth MC, Reinges MH, Gilsbach JM. MRI and intraoperative findings in cavernous haemangiomas of the spinal cord. *Neuroradiology*. 2004;**46**:238–242.

53. Jellema K, Canta LR, Tijssen CG, van Rooij WJ, Koudstaal PJ, van Gijn J. Spinal dural arteriovenous fistulas: clinical features in 80 patients. *J Neurol Neurosurg Psychiatry*. 2003;**74**:1438–1440.

54. Taylor CL, Warren RS, Ratcheson RA. Steal affecting the central nervous system. *Neurosurgery*. 2002;**50**:679–689.

55. Lawton MT, Porter RW, Heiserman JE, Jacobowitz R, Sonntag VK, Dickman CA. Surgical management of spinal epidural hematoma: relationship between surgical timing and neurological outcome. *J Neurosurg*. 1995;**83**:1–7.

56. Rodriguez Y, Baena R, Gaetani P, Tancioni F, Tartara F. Spinal epidural hematoma during anticoagulant therapy. A case report and review. *J Neurosurg Sci*. 1995;**39**:87–94.

57. Longatti PL, Freschi P, Moro M, Trincia G, Carteri A. Spontaneous spinal subdural hematoma. *J Neurosurg Sci*. 1994;**38**:197–199.

58. Shephard RH. Spinal arteriovenous malformation and subarachnoid haemorrhage. *Br J Neurosurg*. 1992;**6**:5–12.

59. Mawad ME, Rivera V, Crawford S, Ramirez A, Breitbach W. Spinal cord ischemia after resection of thoracoabdominal aortic aneurysms: MR findings in 24 patients. *AJR Am J Roentgenol*. 1990;**155**:1303–1307.

60. Lohr TJ, Bassetti CL, Lovblad KO, et al. Diffusion-weighted MRI in acute spinal cord ischaemia. *Neuroradiology*. 2003;**45**:557–561.

61. de Haan P, Kalkmman CJ, Jacobs MJ. Pharmacologic neuroprotection in experimental spinal cord ischemia: a systematic review. *J Neurosurg Anesthesiol*. 2001;**13**:3–12.

62. Crawford ES, Svensson LG, Hess KR, et al. A prospective randomized study of cerebrospinal fluid drainage to prevent paraplegia after high-risk surgery on the thoracoabdominal aorta. *J Vasc Surg*. 1991;**13**:36–45.

63. Murray MJ, Bower TC, Oliver WC Jr, Werner E, Gloviczki P. Effects of cerebrospinal fluid drainage in patients undergoing thoracic and thoracoabdominal aortic surgery. *J Cardiothorac Vasc Anesth*. 1993;**7**:266–272.

64. Brazis PW, Masdeu JC, Biller J. *Localization in Clinical Neurology*. 5th ed. Philadelphia: Lippincott Williams & Wilkins; 2007.

25

Management of Acute Ischemic Infarction

Physicians consider that, when they have discovered the cause of disease, they have also discovered the method of treating it.

Cicero

Effective specialized acute stroke management requires expertise, rigorous application of evidence-based data whenever it is available, transdisciplinary collaboration, and optimal coordination of care. Even with increased awareness of stroke by the public and improved stroke emergency infrastructure, the present 3-to-4.5-hour treatment deadline remains a major challenge for thrombolysis in stroke. Telemedicine is an important and rapidly evolving concept and discipline and represents a potential time saving means for evaluating and managing acute ischemic stroke.[1] This chapter focuses on stroke management that is applicable for most clinical care settings.

EMERGENCY STROKE EVALUATION

The clinical signs and symptoms of stroke are presented in Chapters 2 and 3. The precise diagnosis of brain ischemia must be established quickly if appropriate therapy is to be instituted, and most patients require emergency transportation to a properly equipped medical center where appropriate examinations and tests can be promptly performed. The neurological deficit resulting from a cerebral infarct usually reaches its maximum within the first 24 hours. Deterioration of clinical status after admission to hospital occurs in a third or so of stroke patients. Infarction involving the territory of the middle cerebral artery (MCA) can result in massive edema with herniation of intracranial structures across the midline and through the tentorium. The acute management of stroke patients before their arrival to the hospital is summarized in Table 25-1.

To confirm the diagnosis, an adequate history, neurovascular and cardiac examinations, electrocardiogram, cranial computed tomography (CT), or magnetic resonance imaging (MRI) must be obtained. Blood pressure and body temperature measurements and laboratory tests, including complete blood count (CBC) and platelets, prothrombin time (PT), activated partial thromboplastin time (aPTT), blood glucose, serum electrolytes, creatinine, and urinalysis, including drug screen, must be done

Table 25-1: Prehospital Management of Patients with Suspected Acute Stroke

1. Ensure airway, breathing, and circulation.

2. Assess patients for signs of trauma and provide cervical immobilization if trauma is suspected.

3. Administer oxygen.

4. Assist ventilation if necessary.

5. Monitor cardiac rhythm and blood pressure. Do not treat hypertension aggressively within the setting of an acute stroke.

6. Establish intravenous access and administer normal saline or lactated Ringer's solution at keep-open rate.

7. Assess for blood glucose concentration.

8. If hypoglycemia is strongly diagnosed, 25 g of 50% dextrose may be given intravenously.

9. Naloxone should be considered if altered mental status.

10. Notify the destination hospital of the time of arrival of the patient, the prehospital assessment (stroke), time of onset, and the patient's current condition.

11. Communicate with the patient and family and obtain contact for consent to initiate thrombolysis/thrombectomy.

12. Alert the acute stroke team to allow emergent pharmacological/endovascular intervention and enrollment into acute stroke research protocols.

emergently (Table 25-2). Pulse oximetry or arterial blood gases may be indicated. Supplemental oxygen and ventilatory assistance are added if needed. Mild hypothermia may protect the brain from ischemic injury; mild hyperthermia can worsen ischemic outcome (see Chapter 4).

The role of skilled care in stroke management is severalfold: (1) to derive accurate diagnosis, (2) to provide acute evidence-based treatment strategies, and (3) to perform specific interventions to control complications, such as treatment of

Table 25-2: Stepwise Diagnostic Evaluation for Patients with Suspected Stroke

Initial Evaluation

1. Complete blood count with platelet count
2. Chemistry profile (including glucose)
3. PT, aPTT, INR
4. Finger stick glucose
5. Pregnancy test in women of child-bearing age
6. Urine analysis (consider urinary drug screen)
7. Electrocardiogram
8. Cranial CT or brain MRI with DWI/PWI sequences
9. Noninvasive arterial imaging (ultrasound, MRA, CTA)
10. If available, consider advanced cerebral perfusion imaging

Second Step: Search for Alternative Etiology if Persistent Diagnostic Uncertainty

1. Transthoracic echocardiography with agitated saline injection
2. Transesophageal echocardiography
3. Transcranial Doppler ultrasound (emboli detection studies if indicated)
4. MRA
5. CTA
6. Cerebral arteriography
7. Antiphospholipid antibodies
8. Rheumatological screen
9. Homocysteine
10. HbA1C, fasting glucose
11. Fasting lipid profile

Other Options

1. Ambulatory ECG monitoring
2. Further screening for prothrombotic states (see Chapter 11)
3. CSF examination
4. Testing for silent myocardial ischemia (exercise ECG + thallium perfusion)
5. Cardiac troponins
6. EEG

Evaluation must be individualized to specific patient circumstances. See text for details.
aPTT = activated partial thromboplastin time; CSF = cerebrospinal fluid; CTA = computed tomography angiography; DWI = diffusion-weighted imaging; ECG = electrocardiogram; EEG = electroencephalogram; INR = international normalized ratio; MRA = magnetic resonance angiography; MRI = magnetic resonance imaging; PT = prothrombin time; PWI = perfusion-weighted imaging.

Table 25-3: Indications for Endotracheal Intubation and Initial Ventilator Setting

Intubate if:

- $PaO_2 < 50$–60 mm Hg
- $PaCO_2 > 50$–60 mm Hg
- Vital capacity < 500–800 ml
- Signs of respiratory distress
- Tachypnea > 30
- Dyspnea
- Expiratory grunting
- Use of accessory muscles
- Risk for aspiration
- Unable to maintain airway

Set ventilator at:

- IMV or CMV mode
- Tidal volume 12 ml/kg
- Respiratory rate $PCO_2 < 40$ mm Hg
- $FiO_2 = 1.0$
- I:E = 1:2–3
- Inspiratory flow 30 L/min
- PEEP: 5
- PS: 10

Used with permission from Hacke et al.[119]
CMV = controlled mandatory ventilation; FiO_2 = oxygen content; I:E = inspiration/expiration ratio; IMV = intermittent mandatory ventilation.

Table 25-4: Mimics of Acute Ischemic Stroke

Brain tumors	Hypoglycemia
Subdural hematomas	Hyperglycemia
Brain abscess	Hyponatremia
Encephalitis	Metabolic encephalopathies
Postictal state or seizure	Wernicke's encephalopathy
Migraine aura	Guillain-Barré syndrome (Fisher variant)
Hemiplegic migraine	Peripheral nerve disorders
Hypertensive encephalopathy	Myasthenia gravis
Benign paroxysmal positional vertigo	Conversion (somatoform) disorders
Ménière's disease	

Table 25-5: Acute Ischemic Stroke "Stroke Chameleons"

Movement disorders (hemiballismus, myoclonus)

Ulnar/median/radial nerve–like deficits

■ Thalamus

■ Corona radiata

■ Motor cortex

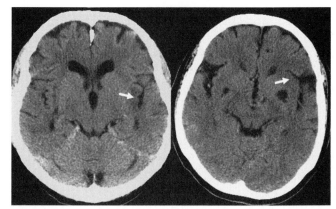

Figure 25-1. Early signs of ischemic infarct on non-contrast cranial CT. The *arrows* indicate loss of the left insular ribbon indicating cerebral ischemia.

elevated intracranial pressure (ICP), hemorrhagic transformation, or seizures that can be provided only by specialized staff. Clinical outcome can be improved if patients are managed in a dedicated stroke center.[2]

Airway evaluation and management should always take precedence over other interventions. After the stroke patient has been medically stabilized with regard to airway, breathing, and circulation (Table 25-3), a comprehensive history is taken with special emphasis on stroke risk factors and additional information that may exclude stroke-mimicking states (Table 25-4) and "stroke chameleons" (Table 25-5). Prevention of misdiagnosis is of critical importance in the thrombolytic era.

The initial physical examination (see Chapter 2) should focus on repetitive measurements of arterial blood pressure and heart rate, auscultation of the heart and cervical arteries, and neurological examination including assessment using the NIH stroke scale (see Chapter 3). Initial neurological examination focuses on level of alertness, behavioral deficits, pupillary and oculomotor signs, and severity of hemiparesis. General signs that point toward a large infarction are forced eye deviation, hemiplegia, and altered consciousness. An NIH stroke scale value of greater than 15 is another general indicator of a large infarction. Old age, coma, cardiorespiratory complications, hypoxia, hypercapnia, and neurogenic hyperventilation are adverse prognostic factors.[3–5]

In patients with acute infarction, elevation in arterial blood pressure may occur either because of the excitement of the event or secondary to the ictus itself, if it is strategically located. Such fluctuations can result in changes in perfusion pressure. In the setting of an acute stroke hypertension should not be treated aggressively due to impairment of the cerebral autoregulation.

EMERGENCY DIAGNOSTIC PROCEDURES

Emergency magnetic resonance angiography (MRA) and computed tomography angiography (CTA) can be used to identify arterial thrombi that can be treated by endovascular interventions. Diagnostic testing modalities that are used in the diagnosis of cerebrovascular disease are discussed in Chapter 5, and here we review only the aspects of these studies that are essential for acute stroke management.

Cranial CT

Cranial CT is the imaging modality of choice for the initial evaluation of stroke as it is quicker and easier to perform in critically sick patients than MRI. From the time of the initial event, CT can distinguish accurately between a brain hemorrhage and infarction in well over 95% of cases. At times, an intracranial hematoma can present symptoms and signs mimicking transient ischemic attack (TIA) or infarction and, occasionally, a brain neoplasm can do the same, so CT is of particular value. Within the first 5 hours after ischemic stroke onset, only about 50% of infarctions are visible on CT.[6] Early CT signs of infarction may include a hyperdense middle cerebral artery (MCA) sign (see Figure 5-2 D), attenuation of the lentiform nucleus, loss of the insular ribbon (Figure 25-1), and hemispheric sulcus effacement.[7] These findings also help to identify patients at greater risk for intracerebral hemorrhage after thrombolytic therapy.[8] In the hyperacute phase, early CT abnormalities tend to be subtle or absent.

Magnetic Resonance Imaging

MRI is far more sensitive and specific than CT for the detection of hyperacute stroke (Figure 25-2). Perfusion-weighted MRI

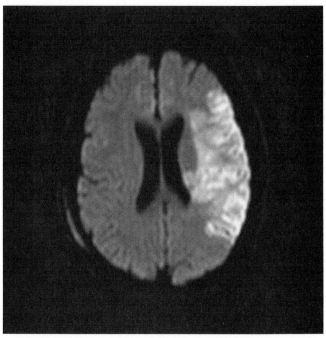

Figure 25-2. Axial diffusion-weighted imaging sequence reveals a bright area of diffusion restriction indicative of ischemic injury.

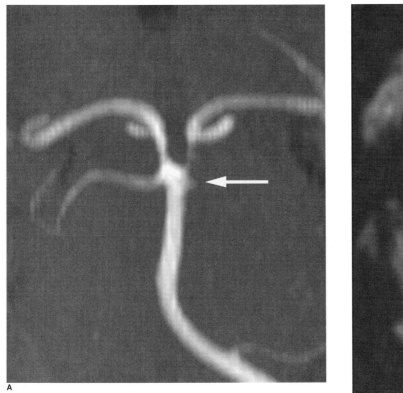

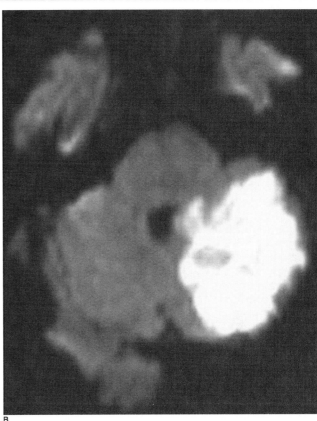

Figure 25-3. A: MRA of the posterior circulation showing occlusion of the left superior cerebellar artery (*arrow*). B: Axial DWI-weighted MRI showing a large area of restricted diffusion in the left cerebellum indicating an acute infarct.

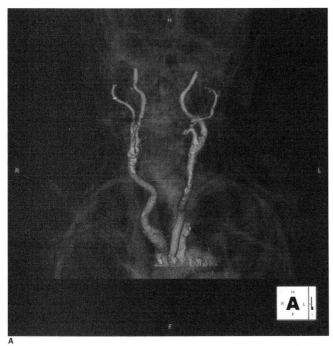

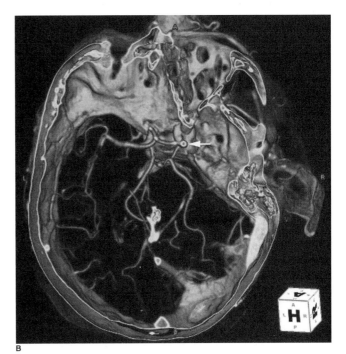

Figure 25-4. CTA is a useful diagnostic tool to rapidly assess the cerebrovascular circulation in stroke patients. A: CTA of the neck showing areas of atherosclerotic plaques in both carotid systems. There is no flow-limiting stenosis. B: CTA of the intracranial circulation showing proximal occlusion of the left M1 segment of the MCA (*arrow*).

(PW-MRI) allows imaging of hemodynamics after administration of intravenous contrast. Diffusion-weighted MRI (DW-MRI) images disturbed water diffusion in the brain. Tissue containing cells affected by cytotoxic edema are bright on DW-MRI and can already be visible within minutes after the infarction.[9] It has been postulated that brain areas with abnormal perfusion but with normal diffusion imaging, termed DW-/PW mismatch, represent the ischemic penumbra. However, acute treatment up to 6 hours after symptom onset may result in normalization of disturbed water diffusion and disappearance of signal brightness, arguing against the notion that DW-MRI changes represent an irreversibly damaged ischemic core.[10] Dynamic perfusion CT is an alternative to MRI mismatch for identifying the penumbra.[11]

In instances of cerebral infarction, MRI has several advantages over CT. MRI has better spatial resolution and shows greater contrast. Three-dimensional data acquisition by MRI makes imaging in any plane possible without image degradation. Infarctions are demonstrated more clearly and many not apparent on CT are evident on MRI. The anatomic extent and vascular distribution are distinctly demonstrated. Small cortical infarctions that are mistaken for cortical atrophy by CT are easier to recognize on MRI by virtue of associated signal changes of infarcted tissue. Lacunar infarctions are much more reliably shown by MRI than CT. MRI often helps to distinguish cortical from subcortical hemispheric infarctions during the acute phase and can, therefore, frequently influence therapeutic decisions. Many infarctions within the posterior fossa that are defined by MRI are often obscured on cranial CT by bone artifact.

In addition to imaging the penumbra and the infarction, it is important to collect information on the cerebral vascular status. Direct visualization of a clot is essential before and after intra-arterial thrombolysis. MRA and CTA are excellent methods for noninvasive evaluation of the intracranial and extracranial vessels (Figures 25-3 and 25-4). Areas of stenosis, vascular malformations, dissection, or other vascular pathology can be rapidly identified to guide further management of stroke patients.

Chest Radiography

Because cardiac decompensation, arrhythmias, myocardial ischemia, and respiratory problems are common in stroke patients, radiography of the chest may provide valuable information in the emergency evaluation of some patients with ischemic stroke.

Lumbar Puncture

Lumbar puncture is not routinely performed for evaluation of acute ischemic stroke. However, lumbar puncture occasionally confirms the diagnosis of subarachnoid hemorrhage when the CT is negative (see Chapter 17) and it may be indicated when intracranial infection is in the patient's differential diagnosis or might be the cause of the stroke. If CT suggests displacement of brain structures, a lumbar puncture is contraindicated due to the risk of cerebral herniation.

Catheter Cerebral Arteriography

Cerebral catheter arteriography remains the most precise way to assess the cerebrovascular circulation. However, it is rarely indicated in the setting of acute stroke unless endovascular thrombectomy and intra-arterial thrombolysis are contemplated. With an acute stroke, catheter angiography may reveal slow emptying of local arteries or an avascular area where arteries are obstructed.

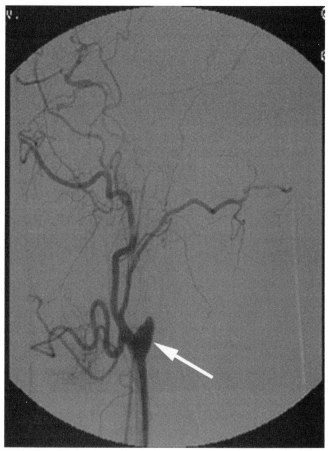

Figure 25-5. Catheter cerebral angiogram demonstrates total and abrupt occlusion of the post-bulbar left internal carotid artery (*arrow*). The right internal carotid artery injection demonstrates a normal appearing right carotid circulation (not shown). The patient was a 44-year-old woman with acute onset right hemiparesis and aphasia.

If a main stem artery is occluded, emptying of collateral arterial channels is delayed; if a peripheral artery is blocked, slow filling to the point of the obstruction occurs and transit time is delayed into the venous phase (Figure 25-5).[12,13]

Initial vasodilatation, manifested by an increase in the speed of circulation through the still perfused portion of the infarct, occurs within a few seconds after ischemia begins. Persistent vasodilatation appears in the infarct and/or the surrounding area during the first 10 days to 2 weeks after infarction and the vessels remain dilated. Early filling of the arteriolar capillary bed (luxury perfusion), which may be the only sign of vasodilatation or of shunting to the venous circulation, may be due to bypass of a blocked capillary bed. Slowing of the circulation time is common during the first week or two after the stroke and often affects the entire hemisphere. Later angiograms sometimes show recanalization. If a major vessel is occluded, a rich collateral circulation may be seen in the infarcted area.[12]

Electrocardiography

Cardiac dysrhythmias are frequent in patients with stroke, either because of coexistent cardiac disease or as a result of the infarction. Atrial fibrillation, in particular, promotes thrombus formation with cerebral embolism (see Chapter 8); at other times, the cerebral event induces cardiac irregularity, that is, dysrhythmia, S-T or Q-T segment change, or T wave abnormality.

Ultrasound

Echocardiography helps to identify cardiac sources of cerebral infarction (see Chapters 5 and 8). Carotid duplex, transcranial Doppler (TCD), and TCD-based emboli detection studies are helpful and are discussed in detail in Chapter 5.

TREATMENT OF ACUTE ISCHEMIC STROKE

Therapy to halt or reverse the progression of brain infarction requires near instant recognition that a stroke is incipient.[14] Because most people are unaware of the early warning signals for stroke, education programs for public and health care providers should be carried out to heighten awareness and knowledge about stroke symptoms.[15]

General Medical Measures

Patients with acute stroke should be admitted to the hospital for emergency evaluation and treatment, preferably to a stroke unit or intensive care unit where close medical and nursing observation is available. There is potential for death or disastrous permanent disability after a stroke, which must be prevented within a few short hours using measures that can be accomplished only in a hospital. For example, some patients develop hemorrhagic transformation of an infarction or massive brain edema with increased ICP. Other patients develop seizures or systemic complications, such as fluid or electrolyte imbalance, pneumonia, or cardiac disorders. Most particularly, the institution of thrombolytic or anticoagulant agents can be accomplished safely only in a hospital setting. Endovascular procedures and interventional treatment of stroke complications are available at specialized stroke centers and emergency identification and transfer of potential candidates for these interventions is essential.

Hyperglycemia is common in the acute phase of stroke and may reflect a stress response due to over activity in the sympathoadrenal and adrenocortical systems. Hyperglycemia evidently promotes the anaerobic metabolism of glucose to lactate. Ischemic neurons shift to anaerobic glycolysis and accumulate lactic acid, which is believed to be neurotoxic. To minimize this, blood levels of glucose should be maintained as low as practical by curtailing intravenous glucose infusions and trying to maintain normal glucose values in diabetic persons.[16–18]

Heparins and Heparinoids

Randomized studies of unfractionated heparin (UFH), low molecular weight heparins (LMWHs), or heparinoids show no benefit toward reduction of stroke-related mortality, stroke-related morbidity, early stroke recurrence, or stroke prognosis except in the case of cerebral venous thrombosis.[19,20] The lack of proven efficacy of these agents in the management of acute arterial ischemic stroke has tempered the enthusiasm for their use by most physicians.

The International Stroke Trial studied approximately 20,000 patients randomized within 48 hours of ischemic stroke onset to receive a fixed dose of 10,000 or 25,000 units of UFH subcutaneous daily (compared with no heparin). No significant difference was observed in the rate of death or recurrent ischemic or hemorrhagic stroke at 2 weeks. Patients receiving UFH had significantly fewer recurrent ischemic strokes at 2 weeks, but this benefit was negated by a similar increase in hemorrhagic strokes.[21]

Other LMWHs and heparinoids also remain unproven in acute ischemic stroke. The results of the TOAST study showed no benefit of intravenous anticoagulation with danaparoid in patients with acute ischemic stroke treated within 24 hours of symptom onset.[22]

Anecdotal evidence supports early initiation of intravenous UFH to prevent arterial ischemic stroke recurrence in several clinical situations, including cerebral infarction in the setting of inherited or acquired hypercoagulable states, intraluminal arterial thrombus, and extracranial cervicocephalic arterial dissections. Available evidence supports the use of heparin followed by warfarin in reducing mortality and dependency in patients with cerebral venous thrombosis (see Chapter 20).

When short-term heparin followed by long-term warfarin are used, both agents can be started simultaneously. A minimum of 4 days of heparin administration is generally needed to allow time to achieve a therapeutic warfarin level. The risk of immune-mediated heparin-induced thrombocytopenia (HIT), a clinicopathologic syndrome associated with thrombosis (both venous and arterial) is lower with LMWH than with UFH.

THROMBOLYSIS

Tissue plasminogen activator (tPA) is a serine protease derived from endothelial cells that activates the fibrinolytic system by converting plasminogen to plasmin. It has a high affinity for fibrin-bound and a low affinity for circulating plasminogen. Because of this, tPA is clot-specific and acts only on the clot even after intravenous administration. The selective thrombus activator of plasminogen binds with a globulin fraction of plasma and this complex activates the plasminogen permeating the thrombus mass, to an enzymatically active plasmin-globulin complex that is not inhibited by circulating antiplasmins. This enzymatically active plasmin–globulin complex digests the fibrin core of a thrombus in the presence of circulating antiplasmins. Physiological plasminogen activator, such as that released by endothelial cells or exogenous activator, such as streptokinase, converts plasminogen to an active enzyme plasmin, which can lyse fibrin. While plasmin formed in the blood may be affected by inhibiting antiplasmins, fibrin-bound plasmin is protected against such neutralization. Thus, the plasmin present in a thrombus is not only in place and ready to act during formation of thrombus but plasma plasminogen absorbed on to the fibrin/clot surface is activated by circulating activators that initiate autodigestion of thrombus.

Dissolution of a thrombus or "fibrinolysis" represents a physiological mechanism in the complex balance between hemostasis and blood flow. The fibrinolytic system is activated by factor XII, prekallikrein, high molecular weight kininogen, and vascular or tissue type plasminogen activator activation promoting the conversion of plasminogen to plasmin. Plasmin is the active fibrinolytic enzyme. On the molecular level, the activators cleave plasminogen into the two-chain plasmin compound. The plasmin heavy chain contains the "cringle structures" that include the binding site for fibrin. The light chain carries the catalytic site. When bound to fibrin, the catalytic site of plasmin becomes inaccessible to α_2-antiplasmin, its principal inhibitor, thereby providing excellent activity for local fibrin degradation. Circulating plasmin leads to a multistep degradation of fibrinogen and fibrin into specific degradation products.

Although spontaneous thrombolysis, in principle, represents a powerful mechanism mediating recanalization of an occluded cerebral vessel, it frequently occurs too late to prevent brain infarction distal to the thrombosis. Spontaneous recanalization may account for part of the nonoccluded arteries in carotid territory angiography within 6 hours of symptom onset. It has been estimated that the spontaneous recanalization rate in patients with ischemic stroke caused by large-vessel disease might be as high as 20% after 24 hours and 80% after 7 days.[23,24]

Intravenous administration of a thrombolytic agent is technically simple, comparatively time saving, and carries no additional procedural risk.[25,26] On the other hand, it requires higher doses of the thrombolytic agent to be effective which, theoretically, entails a higher risk of systemic bleeding. Local intra-arterial thrombolysis facilitates the administration of a higher local dose of the drug yet with a lower total drug dose. However, intra-arterial administration carries all the disadvantages of an additional interventional procedure.

Although early clinical trials provided fundamental data and experience on the use of thrombolytic agents, their limited sample size and patient selection methods did not allow firm conclusions about standard acute stroke patient management.[26–28] Since 1995, however, the results of five large controlled, prospective, double-blind clinical trials have become available (NINDS rt-PA Stroke Study Group, ECASS, MAST-I, MAST-E, AST trials).[36]

Three trials administering intravenous streptokinase as a thrombolytic agent[30–33] were all stopped early because of a significantly increased risk of death, largely due to intracerebral hemorrhage in the subjects receiving thrombolysis. In MAST-E, death due to intracerebral hemorrhage was 16 times more frequent in the thrombolysis group. MAST-I investigated whether intravenous streptokinase (1.5 MU) and aspirin, separately or together, showed a clinical benefit when treatment was initiated within 6 hours of symptom onset. Patients in deep coma or with signs of intracerebral hemorrhage on initial CT scan were excluded. Follow-up assessment was by telephone interview. The streptokinase group showed a significantly higher 10-day mortality; after 6 months, however, streptokinase reduced the mortality rate and the rate of severe disability. In the Australian Streptokinase Trial, streptokinase or placebo was administered intravenously to patients with anterior or posterior circulation stroke within 4 hours of symptom onset.[34] Only patients with moderate to severe stroke symptoms were included. Patients who received streptokinase within 4 hours of acute ischemic stroke had increased morbidity and mortality at 3 months. A subgroup treated within 3 hours showed better results than the 4-hour group but no significant benefit over placebo was observed. Parenchymal hemorrhage occurred in 13.2% (streptokinase group) and 3% (placebo group), respectively.

The European Cooperative Acute Stroke Study (ECASS)[35] compared the efficacy and safety of tPA (1.1 mg/kg, maximal dose 100 mg, 10% bolus) to placebo administered within 6 hours of acute hemispheric stroke onset. End points included functional (Barthel index, modified Rankin scale, combination of both) and neurological (Scandinavian Stroke Scale [SSS]) outcome measures at 90 days, 30-day mortality, as well as early neurological recovery and duration of in hospital stay. Mortality and incidence of intracranial and extracranial hemorrhage were monitored as safety parameters. The target population was defined as patients with stable, moderate to severe hemispheric stroke. Patients with mild (SSS > 50) or very severe hemispheric stroke, as well as patients with signs of intracranial bleeding or major early infarct signs, were supposed to be excluded.

Of the 620 patients randomized for the ECASS study (i.e., the intention to treat group), 17.6% were included despite major protocol violations. Of these, 52 had major early infarct signs on the initial CT scan. No statistically significant difference in functional or neurological outcome measures could be shown between the two groups in the intention to treat analysis. The target population analysis revealed a significant difference in the Rankin scale in favor of the tPA group. The mortality rate at 30 days was higher in the tPA group (22.4% vs. 15.8%), albeit not reaching statistical significance. In the intention to treat (ITT) analysis, the case fatality rate was significantly higher in the rt-PA-treated group after 90 days (ITT analysis; no difference in the target population analysis). Large parenchymal hemorrhages occurred more frequently in the tPA group (ITT-analysis: in the tPA group 6.3% died of parenchymal hematoma compared to 2.4% in the placebo group). Fatal hemorrhage was particularly frequent among patients with protocol violations.

Another large placebo-controlled clinical trial investigating thrombolysis in acute stroke was conducted by the National Institute of Neurological Disorders and Stroke (NINDS) rt-PA Stroke Study Group.[36] Similar to ECASS, t-PA was administered intravenously without prior or control angiography but the t-PA dose was smaller (0.9 mg/kg, maximal dose 90 mg, 10% bolus with the rest within 60 minutes). Patients were only included when treatment with t-PA could be started within 180 minutes post symptom onset. In contrast to ECASS, patients with symptoms indicating ischemia in the anterior or posterior cerebral circulation were included. Patients with early signs of infarction on CT were not excluded. The trial consisted of two parts. Part 1 (n = 291 patients) showed no significant difference in neurologic improvement within 24 hours after symptom onset between t-PA and placebo treated patients. Part 2 (n = 333) and Part 1 revealed a significantly better outcome of patients treated with t-PA after 90 days (Barthel index, modified Rankin scale, NIH-Stroke scale). Patients treated with t-PA were 30% more likely to have minimal or no disability at three months. Symptomatic intracerebral hemorrhage occurred in 6.4% of the t-PA treated group and in 0.6% of the placebo group. The (NINDS) rt-PA Stroke Study Group showed that treatment with intravenous t-PA within 3 hours of onset of ischemic stroke improved clinical outcome (minimal or no disability on a number of clinical assessment scales) at 3 months.[36] In the NINDS rt-PA study, intravenous administration of tPA was associated with a 12% absolute (32% relative) increase in the proportion of patients with acute ischemic stroke who were free of disability after 3 months. In other words, 1 of 8 patients given intravenous tPA had complete neurologic recovery at 90 days. Patients were considered to have attained good neurologic recovery, if at 90 days, they scored < 2 on the modified Rankin Scale (MRS).

Subsequent assessment of the NINDS tPA trial also demonstrated a sustained benefit of intravenous rt-PA at 6 and 12 months.[37] Reanalysis of the NINDS confirmed that earlier treatment of stroke patients was associated with a more favorable outcome. Based on numbers needed-to-treat (NNT) ratio, for every 8 patients treated with tPA, 1 patient had excellent or complete recovery, and for every 15 patients treated, 1 patient had a symptomatic intracranial hemorrhage. If treated within the first 90 minutes of stroke index, the NNT was 4.

Table 25-6: Intravenous tPA for Acute Ischemic Stroke: Within 3 Hours of Onset

Inclusion criteria

- Ischemic stroke onset < 3 hours (time of stroke onset is the time when patient was last known to be awake and normal)

- Diagnosis of acute ischemic stroke causing a measurable neurological deficit (NIHSS)

- Unenhanced CT does not show hemorrhage

- Neurological signs should not be rapidly improving spontaneously

- Neurological signs should not be minor or isolated (e.g., isolated INO)

Exclusion criteria

- Stroke or serious head trauma in the last 3 months

- Major surgery within 14 days

- History of intracranial hemorrhage

- SBP ≥ 185 mm Hg, or DBP ≥ 110 mm Hg

- Aggressive treatment required to reduce BP parameters to specific limits (see above)

- Symptoms suggestive of SAH

- Gastrointestinal or genitourinary bleeding in last 21 days

- Arterial puncture at noncompressible site in preceding 7 days

- Seizure at onset of symptoms

- Anticoagulant therapy or receiving heparin within preceding 48 hours and elevated aPTT or INR > 1.7

- Platelet count < 100,000/mm³

- Blood glucose level < 50 mg/dl (< 2.7 mmol)

- Myocardial infarction in previous 3 months

aPTT = activated partial thromboplastin time; DBP = diastolic blood pressure; INO = internuclear ophthalmoplegia; INR = international normalized ratio; SAH = subarachnoid hemorrhage; SBP = systolic blood pressure.

Mortality at 3 months was not statistically different; in other words, treatment did not lessen death rates or account for an excess mortality. The frequency of symptomatic intracerebral hemorrhage was 10 times greater in patients given tPA (6.4% in the treatment group compared with 0.6% in the placebo group). Most hemorrhages occurred within 36 hours of treatment. In other words, 1 of 17 patients suffered symptomatic intracerebral hemorrhage within the first 36 hours of treatment. Patients with symptomatic intracranial hemorrhage tended to have more severe deficits at baseline.

Intravenous tPA administration requires close adherence to protocol guidelines and a "no time-to-waste" approach. Patients are given 0.9 mg/kg total dose of intravenous tPA, 10% as a bolus and 90% over 60 minutes. The maximum dose is 90 milligrams. Antiplatelet and anticoagulant therapy is withheld for the first 24 hours after intravenous tPA administration (see Table 25-6).

Inclusion criteria for administration of tPA in the NINDS tPA trial were acute ischemic stroke with a clearly defined time of onset (< 3 hours), neurological deficit measurable on the NIH Stroke Scale, and CT scan without evidence of intracranial hemorrhage. Patients awakening from sleep had symptom onset defined as "when last seen awake and normal." Exclusion criteria for administration of tPA were rapidly improving or isolated minor neurological deficits, seizure at onset of stroke, prior intracranial hemorrhage, symptoms suggestive of subarachnoid hemorrhage, blood glucose level less than 50 mg/dl (2.7 mM) or greater than 400 mg/dl (22.2 mM) (currently, only the former is an exclusion), gastrointestinal or genitourinary bleeding within the 3 weeks before stroke, recent myocardial infarction (MI), current use of oral anticoagulants (PT > 15 seconds or international normalized ratio [INR] > 1.7), a prolonged aPTT or use of heparin in the previous 48 hours, platelet count less than 100,000/mm³, another stroke or serious head injury in the previous 3 months, major surgery within the previous 14 days, arterial puncture at a noncompressible site within the previous 7 days, or pretreatment systolic blood pressure ≥ 185 mm Hg or diastolic blood pressure ≥ 110 mm Hg (Table 25-6). Although the NINDS study included patients with vertebrobasilar territory stroke, data concerning this subgroup are sparse.

More recently, the use of intravenous tPA beyond the conventional 3-hour time window (3 to 4.5 hours) was found to be beneficial by the investigators of the ECASS 3 trial. This study had strict exclusion criteria such as age over 80 years, NIH Stroke Scale over 25, combination of prior stroke and diabetes mellitus, and evidence of low attenuation of more than a third of the middle cerebral artery territory on CT.[38,39] The efficacy of

Table 25-7: Thrombolytic Therapy for Individuals with Ischemic Symptoms of Longer Duration[a]

Consider intra-arterial tPA 1–5 milligram bolus followed by 0.1 to 0.2 mg/kg/h for 1–2 hours (typical dose is 20–22 mg)[b]

Consider clot retrieval (Mechanical Embolus Removal in Cerebral Ischemia [MERCI]) device in high-risk surgery patients

---

[a] For carotid territory: > 3 (or > 4.5 hours?) and < 6 hours from symptom onset. For vertebrobasilar territory: > 3–4.5 hours and < 12 hours from symptom onset.
[b] Intra-arterial tPA is not yet approved by the FDA for routine clinical use.

Table 25-8: Thrombolytic Therapy for Perioperative Acute Ischemic Stroke

Within 14 days of a surgical procedure

Less than 6 hours in carotid territory

Less than 12 to 24 hours in vertebrobasilar territory

Consider intra-arterial (IA) tPA 1–5 milligrams bolus, followed by 0.1–0.2 mg/kg/hr for 1–2 hours.[a] Typical dose is 20–22 mg.

Consider clot retrieval (Mechanical Embolus Removal in Cerebral Ischemia [MERCI]) device in high-risk surgery patients[b]

---

[a] IA tPA is not approved by the FDA for routine clinical use.
[b] MERCI is approved for clot removal and should be reserved for special cases.

combination lysis using intravenous and intra-arterial approaches is being investigated. Advanced neuroimaging studies may identify stroke patients who, although beyond the 3-hour deadline, might benefit from thrombolysis.

Because intravenous tPA can be administered only to selected patients within a 3- to 4.5-hour time window, intra-arterial thrombolysis is an alternative strategy to treat patients with a larger stroke, a longer interval since symptom onset, or individuals with perioperative strokes (see Tables 25-7 and 25-8). Intra-arterial thrombolysis within 6 hours with pro-urokinase for hemispheric stroke was studied in the PROACT trial.[38–40]

MECHANICAL INTERVENTIONS

Data on mechanical "clot" extraction show a high degree of mortality despite a high recanalization rate. The MERCI catheter has been approved for retrieval of cerebral "clots," and should be reserved for special cases.

Mechanical clot dissolving approaches such as laser-induced ablation, photoacoustic clot lysis by generation of cavitation bubbles resulting in clot liquification, or the use of high-pressure angiojets are still experimental. A major concern is arterial injury, clot dislodgement, and fragmentation with subsequent cerebral embolization of particles.

Ultrasound has been demonstrated to amplify the thrombolytic effect of tPA in acute stroke treatment in the CLOTBUST trial.[42] The use of a standard 2-MHz transcranial ultrasound

probe for continuous insonation in this study resulted in improved arterial recanalization when used in combination with intravenous thrombolysis. In vitro studies demonstrated that ultrasound insonation can increase tPA mediated thrombolysis by 20% in a static model and recanalization rate by up to 60% in a flow model. This effect might be further enhanced by use of microbubbles that adhere to the surface of a clot. When ultrasound of low frequency is applied it causes microbubbles to cavitate and burst. Jets of fluid and particles generated by the burst of microbubbles erode and then dissolve the clot. Therapeutic applications of ultrasound are limited by the bony anatomy of the skull. In patients without adequate bone windows for insonation ultrasound cannot penetrate the brain and arteries.

Future approaches will investigate the effect of adding newer neuroprotective agents or hypothermia to thrombolytic therapy.[43] Endovascular procedures such as embolectomy, angioplasty, and stenting of intracranial arteries will play an increasing role. There is urgent need for the development of safe, easily available and inexpensive acute stroke therapies.

Hemodilution

Both plasma viscosity and apparent whole blood viscosity are significantly elevated in cerebrovascular disease and in patients with established risk factors. Specifically, plasma fibrinogen is significantly elevated and serum albumin reduced. These results suggest that chronic alteration in the composition of blood, including both protein and the cellular elements, distinguishes healthy individuals from persons symptomatic or at a risk for stroke. One consequence of these alterations is an increased resistance to blood flow within the cerebral microcirculation.

Despite its appeal to logic, three major randomized prospective clinical trials in Scandinavia, Italy, and the United States reached identical conclusions that moderate hypervolemic hemodilution achieved by a combination of venisection, dextran 40, or Hetastarch administration does not have an overall beneficial effect in patients with acute ischemic stroke.[44]

Defibrinogenating and Hemorheologic Agents

Ancrod, an enzyme extracted from the venom of the Malayan pit viper, was shown to be beneficial when initiated within 3 hours of ischemic stroke onset in the multicenter Stroke Treatment with Ancrod Trial.[45] However, this early observation was not replicated in a European Trial. A follow-up study of this agent is currently underway.

Neuroprotective Therapies

Previously studied neuroprotective agents in acute stroke have not translated into improved functional outcome. Potential cerebroprotective approaches include the use of osmotherapy, magnesium, or the diversion of blood flow from the peripheral to the brain circulation by means of intra-aortic catheter devices. More debatable therapies are (1) increasing the supply of oxygen with hyperbaric oxygen, (2) decreasing the demand for oxygen and metabolic substrates by hypothermia or barbiturates, (3) increasing the supply of metabolic substrates, (4) the use of scavenger free radicals to metabolize toxic metabolites, and (5) retroperfusion through veins into the microcirculation.

Calcium ions are essential for normal cellular processes, such as endocytosis, exocytosis, mobility, and cell division. They have a preeminent role as an intracellular messenger, even though it is normally 10,000 times more concentrated extra- than intracellularly. Intracellular calcium is bound to protein, which is essential for its actions. There are at least four channels for calcium passage through the cellular membrane: leak channels, potential dependent, receptor dependent, and stretch-sensitive channels. Calcium channel blockers or antagonists, such as nimodipine, verapamil, and nifedipine, all affect different ones of these channel mechanisms, some being more active on smooth muscle cells, such as nimodipine, which, of the entire group, seems to have the most promise for neurological disorders.[46–49] It is effective for prevention of vasospasm after subarachnoid hemorrhage. Further, it has direct effects on neuron membranes by inhibiting voltage-sensitive calcium ion channels. In clinical studies, the voltage-sensitive channel blocker nimodipine has been shown to be of minor or no benefit in the treatment of ischemic stroke. Today, its value needs reevaluation concerning the treatment during the very first hours of ischemic stroke. As to receptor dependent calcium channel blockers, use of glutamate-sensitive N-methyl-d-aspartate (NMDA) and α-amino-3-hydroxy-5-methyl-4-isoxazole propionic acid (AMPA) receptor blockers may especially be indicated because during ischemia glutamate is released in excessive amounts from presynaptic nerve terminals. An interesting possibility is the prophylactic primary and secondary neuroprotection of brain ischemia with such agents as calcium and sodium channel modulators, antioxidants, growth factors, apoptosis inhibitors, and anti-inflammatory agents.

Induced hypothermia may be neuroprotective in patients with acute cerebral ischemia.[50–52] In animal studies, reduction of brain temperature has been shown to ameliorate ischemic injury. During ischemia, hypothermia seems to slow down cerebral metabolic activity and glutamate release and to protect the brain from blood-brain barrier disruption. Although the effects of mechanically or pharmaceutically induced brain temperature reduction in human stroke are unknown, experimental data suggest that special attention should be devoted on infection and temperature control in stroke patients. Aggressive management of fever should be pursued in all acute stroke patients.[53–57]

Another form of neuroprotection is protecting the brain from oxygen radicals synthesized during lipid peroxidation. During postischemic reperfusion, lipid peroxidation is very active because more arachidonic acid metabolites and oxygen are available. Aspirin and indomethacin may have therapeutic value in decreasing this peroxidation process. Compounds called the 21-aminosteroids (lazaroids) have been developed for inhibiting synthesis of oxygen radicals. However, no neuroprotective agent has been approved as yet by the FDA for acute ischemic stroke.

Miscellaneous Interventions

Pharmacologically Induced Hypertension

It has been reasoned that inducing hypertension during the early stages of infarction may increase perfusion pressure through ischemic tissue sufficiently for infarction to be minimized. While appealing, the applicability of this theory has some shortcomings, the most important of which is that the status of arterioles in ischemic zones is one of maximal dilatation no matter what the systemic arterial pressure may be. Further, they have lost their autoregulatory capacity, as well. Consequently, pharmacologically induced systemic hypertension may cause

vasoconstriction in the penumbra surrounding the ischemic zone or transmit undue pressure into vasoparalytic ischemic area, perhaps resulting in its conversion into a hemorrhagic infarction. Nevertheless, it is probably harmless and may be beneficial to raise blood pressure of normotensive patients to about 160/90 mm Hg during the acute phase. When treating relative hypotension, correction of possible hypovolemia and optimization of cardiac output are of high importance. A more common problem is the dilemma of evolving infarction in patients with sustained hypertension. Hypertension can result from stress reactions of stroke, pain, underlying hypertension, brain hypoxia, increased intracranial pressure, or even a full bladder. If repeated blood pressures are very high (> 220 mm Hg systolic or > 120 mm Hg diastolic) use of short-acting antihypertensive drugs (see Chapter 9) should be started. If possible, drugs with considerable vasodilator properties should be avoided. Hypotensive therapy for chronically hypertensive patients may be particularly hazardous because of the pre-existing disturbance in cerebral autoregulation. It should be noted that blood pressure usually normalizes spontaneously to pre-stroke levels within one week.

Blood Gas Interventions

HYPOCAPNIA

It has been suggested that prolonged hyperventilation might benefit ischemic brains by reducing pCO_2, causing vasoconstriction and shifting blood to the vasoparalytic ischemic zone, as well as by reducing intracranial pressure. There are, however, numerous reports of adverse effects produced by such therapy and no significant difference has been noted between patients with infarction treated with hypocapnic ventilation and those treated with normocapnic active ventilation.

HYPERCAPNIA

Because it is the most powerful cerebral vasodilator, carbon dioxide in varying concentrations has been administered to patients with evolving infarction. In both animals and patients with brain infarctions, an increase in regional cerebral blood flow (rCBF) has been demonstrated after the addition of 5% CO_2; however, no rigorous studies documenting its therapeutic effect on human beings are available. An objection to its use is that the nonreactive vessels in an ischemic brain are already maximally dilated and might shift blood from ischemic areas inducing a steal. Two studies, however, have shown that vasodilator response was reduced or impaired in only 25% of patients with cerebral circulatory disturbances. With recent hemispheric infarction, CBF increases in all regions after CO_2 inhalation. It is generally agreed that the steal response occurs only during the acute stages of severe and extensive cerebral infarction and then only occasionally.

HYPEROXIA

Hyperbaric oxygen therapy to increase the oxygenation of ischemic brain is an appealing idea. Patients with infarction so treated may improve during hyperbaria but the effects are not sustained when the patient leaves the chamber. Recent randomized studies by Singhal and others[58] suggest that 100% oxygen administered under normal ambient pressure, also termed normobaric oxygen (NBO), may have neuroprotective effects in acute human ischemic stroke. Although theoretically superior to NBO due to its mechanisms of action, the effect of HBOT in acute ischemic stroke is unclear. Animal studies and observational studies imply a beneficial effect of HBOT for acute stroke, but this was not validated in three applicable, small, randomized pilot trials.[59–61] These trials have not generated a clear consensus regarding either the interpretation of their results or the potential efficacy of HBOT as a treatment for acute ischemic stroke. No randomized, clinical trials with sufficient statistical power have been performed to establish a role for HBOT in acute ischemic stroke.

GENERAL MANAGEMENT AND PREVENTION OF COMPLICATIONS

Respiratory Complications

Prevention of pulmonary complications is necessary in the bedridden patient or in the patient with impaired oropharyngeal function. Pneumonia is the most common cause of fever within the first 48 hours after stroke. Pneumonia and urinary tract infections are independently associated with poor outcome after stroke. The mortality rate from pneumonia is as high as 15% to 25% in stroke patients. Risk of developing pneumonia is higher among older patients and among those with more severe infarcts. Aspiration is documented in more than one third of patients with brainstem strokes, in one fourth with bilateral hemispheric strokes, and in one tenth of patients with unilateral hemispheric strokes. Reduced level of consciousness, and mechanical devices such as nasogastric tubes and intratracheal tubes predispose patients to the development of aspiration pneumonia. Good pulmonary toilet is always needed.[56,57] Basal ganglia infarcts seem to predispose patients to pneumonia because of frequent aspiration during sleep.

Gastrointestinal Complications

Involvement of the gastrointestinal tract after stroke manifests as dysphagia and compromised bowel function. Placement of a temporary enteral feeding tube is important if there is evidence of oropharyngeal dysfunction to minimize the risk for aspiration, and reduce the risks associated with malnutrition and or dehydration. Patients with oropharyngeal dysfunction should receive nothing by mouth until appropriate swallowing studies with modified video fluoroscopy are completed by an experienced speech pathologist.

Cardiac Complications

Cardiac comorbidities are frequent after ischemic stroke. Cardiac manifestations that can occur following acute ischemic stroke include electrocardiographic (ECG) abnormalities, cardiac arrhythmias, elevation of creatine kinase-MB (CK-MB) and or cardiac troponin levels, left ventricular dysfunction, and/or MI. Strokes involving the insular cortex are more likely to be associated with ECG changes. Cardiac monitoring is recommended for the first 24 to 48 hours after stroke. An

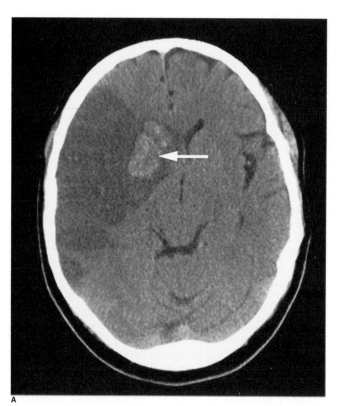
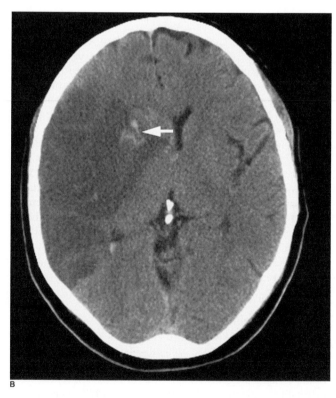

Figure 25-6. A and B: Noncontrast head CT showing hemorrhagic transformation of a large right MCA territory infarct. Blood has a hyperdense signal on CT (*arrows*). The area of stroke appears hypodense. There is a significant amount of cerebral edema and mass effect on the right lateral ventricle. The patient, a 61-year-old man with a history of atrial fibrillation, had new onset of left-sided weakness and had received IV tPA for acute ischemic stroke treatment.

immediate ECG should be obtained. Concomitant cerebral and myocardial ischemia can occur in approximately 3% to 20% of cases. Serial ECG and cardiac troponins may be needed.

Blood Pressure Instability

The blood pressure should be monitored frequently or even continuously for the first 48 to 72 hours. It is not unusual for the blood pressure to be transiently elevated after a stroke. Optimal arterial blood pressure post-stroke appears to range from 160 mm Hg to 200 mm Hg for systolic blood pressure, and 70 mm Hg to 110 mm Hg for diastolic blood pressure.[62] Blood pressure may return to pre-stroke levels within a few days. Whether transient blood pressure elevations should be treated is controversial. It is better not to over treat the blood pressure and risk arterial hypotension because cerebral autoregulation is disrupted in the setting of acute cerebral ischemia.

A key objective is to maintain adequate CBF in the presence of impaired autoregulation.[63] If urgent lowering of the blood pressure is indicated, intravenous labetalol can be given. Nicardipine may also be a reasonable alternative intravenous agent. Any blood pressure–lowering agent should be used with caution. The American Heart Association guidelines suggest lowering the blood pressure immediately post-stroke only if the patient's blood pressure is > 220/130 mm Hg,[56,57] unless the patient is a candidate for thrombolytic therapy, in which case a target goal of less than 185/110 mm Hg is appropriate before administration of intravenous thrombolysis. A systematic review by the Cochrane Study Group concluded that as yet, there is not enough evidence to reliably assess the impact of altering blood pressure (lowering or raising) in the context of acute ischemic stroke.[64]

Neurological Complications

Frequent neurological checks are essential for the early recognition of neurological changes associated with herniation, recurrent or progressive stroke, or complications.

Hemorrhagic Transformation

During the first week after stroke, neurological deterioration is observed more frequently in patients with hemorrhagic transformations than in other stroke patients (Figure 25-6). Not surprisingly, the outcome for patients with hemorrhagic transformation is also worse. Patients with petechial hemorrhagic transformation do not differ from those with parenchymal hematoma in terms of either frequency of early deterioration or poor outcome at 30 days,[65] but the administration of antiplatelet agents, heparin, or oral anticoagulants does not increase the likelihood of early deterioration or a poor 30-day poor outcome.[66,67]

Cerebral Edema

During the first week after an acute cerebral infarction, the most common cause of deterioration is development of brain edema. Brain edema occurs in up to 15% of patients with ischemic stroke and is more often a problem in individuals with large infarctions. Patients often develop drowsiness which may be accompanied by asymmetry of pupillary size and periodic breathing. Brain edema develops within the first several hours after an ischemic event, and reaches its peak approximately 72 to 120 hours after stroke.

Table 25-9: Medical Management of Raised ICP Due to Acute Ischemic Stroke

Correction of Factors Exacerbating Raised ICP

- Hypercarbia
- Hypoxia
- Hyperthermia (oral or rectal acetaminophen as needed)
- Acidosis
- Hypotension
- Hypovolemia

Positional[a]

- Avoidance of head/neck positions compressing jugular veins
- Avoidance of flat supine position
- Elevation of the head of the bed (30-degree head-up neutral position)

Medical therapy

- Rapid sequence endotracheal intubation and mechanical ventilation, if GCS ≤ 8
- Hyperventilation to a $PaCO_2$ of 35 ± 3 mm Hp (32–36 mm Hg)
- Hyperosmolar therapy (mannitol; 3% or 23.4% hypertonic saline)[b]
- High-dose barbiturates

Fluid management

- Maintenance of euvolemia with isotonic solutions (isotonic sodium chloride)
- Avoidance of glucose (D5W) containing solutions
- Replacement of urinary losses with normal saline in patients receiving mannitol

---

[a] Cerebral perfusion pressure is maximized in the supine position. Lying flat may increase intracranial pressure.
[b] As an alternative or adjunct agent to mannitol.

Ischemic edema is initially cytotoxic (cellular) and later vasogenic. Cytotoxic edema involves all the cellular elements of the brain and predominates in the gray matter. Vasogenic edema is characterized by an increase in extracellular fluid volume and involves predominantly the white matter. Those at greatest risk for development of brain edema are younger patients and those with large infarctions (malignant middle cerebral artery infarcts and large posterior fossa infarcts), often caused by large artery occlusions. Cranial CT and especially MRI are useful for diagnosis and quantification of the degree of edema. Cerebellar edema may be unapparent on cranial CT except for secondary obstructive hydrocephalus or a small fourth ventricle.

There is no completely effective pharmacological agent for ischemic cerebral edema. Corticosteroids are not helpful for acute ischemic stroke. Despite still continuing controversy and the paucity of evidence that mannitol improves survival or prevents disability after stroke, it is commonly used for the

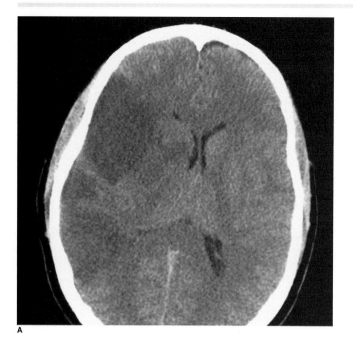

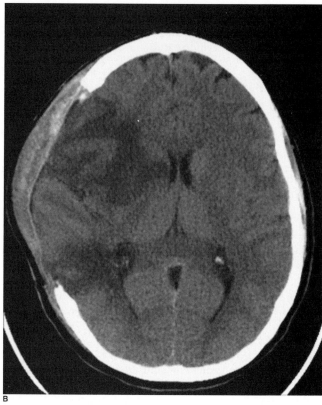

Figure 25-7. Decompressive hemicraniectomy for malignant cerebral edema in a patient with large right-sided MCA territory infarct. A: Noncontrast head CT shows a massive right hemispheric infarct resulting in significant edema and mass effect with compression of the right lateral ventricle and midline shift. B: Noncontrast head CT after decompressive right-sided hemicraniectomy. There is massive brain swelling through the hemicraniectomy site.

management of ICP.[68,69] However, it has multiple potential side effects and a short duration of action. The effects of repeated doses of mannitol are uncertain, and it requires close laboratory monitoring.

Because of these limitations hypertonic saline has been introduced as an alternative therapeutic agent. Hypertonic solution has different mechanisms of action compared to mannitol.[70] It is more effective than mannitol in lowering intracranial pressure, decreases the inflammatory response and the endothelial edema and improves immunomodulatory effects.[71–74] Hypertonic saline can significantly reduce elevated ICP that was refractory to mannitol administration. Generally continuous infusions of 3% saline are used. In cases of refractory increased ICP, boluses of 23.4% saline can be administered. The goal is to achieve a moderate degree of hypernatremia (150 mEq/L).

With increased ICP, cerebral perfusion pressure (CPP) may be impaired. CPP equals mean arterial blood pressure (MABP) minus the ICP. Guidelines for medical treatment of increased ICP associated with acute ischemic stroke are summarized in Table 25-9. In selective patients with malignant cerebral edema associated with hemispheric infarction, hemicraniectomy and durotomy may be indicated (Figure 25-7).[75] For cerebellar strokes with edema and herniation, posterior fossa decompression may be lifesaving (Figure 25-8). Ventriculostomy may also be performed, but it carries the risk for upward herniation of the cerebellum and brainstem.

Seizures

Seizures occur in 6% to 19% of patients after an ischemic stroke. Patients with cortical infarcts are at highest risk. Antiepileptic drugs should be initiated if a seizure occurs. Prophylactic therapy is usually not necessary.

Deep Venous Thrombosis and Pulmonary Embolism

Deep venous thrombosis (DVT) is a common complication in acute stroke. A lower risk has been observed among Asian patients with acute stroke, and attributed to the lower frequency of predisposing thrombophilic disorders such as the factor V Leiden mutation or the prothrombin G20210A mutation.[76] Proximal DVT is most relevant since it is associated with a high risk of thromboembolism. Pulmonary embolism (PE), the most serious complication of DVT, still carries a mortality risk between 7.5% and 17%. Lower extremity DVT in the hemiparetic limb is common if prophylaxis is not initiated. The risk for venous thromboembolism persists into the post-stroke period. If there are no contraindications, low-dose subcutaneous UFH or LMWH is used. Prophylactic doses of heparin can safely be given to patients receiving aspirin. If heparin is contraindicated, intermittent pneumatic compression of the lower extremities is recommended. Graded compression stockings may be useful for DVT prevention in stroke patients. If DVT is detected, early heparin anticoagulation is recommended. In patients with venous thromboembolism and contraindications to anticoagulation, interruption of the inferior vena cava (IVC) to prevent PE is indicated. However, IVC filters do not prevent DVT; their

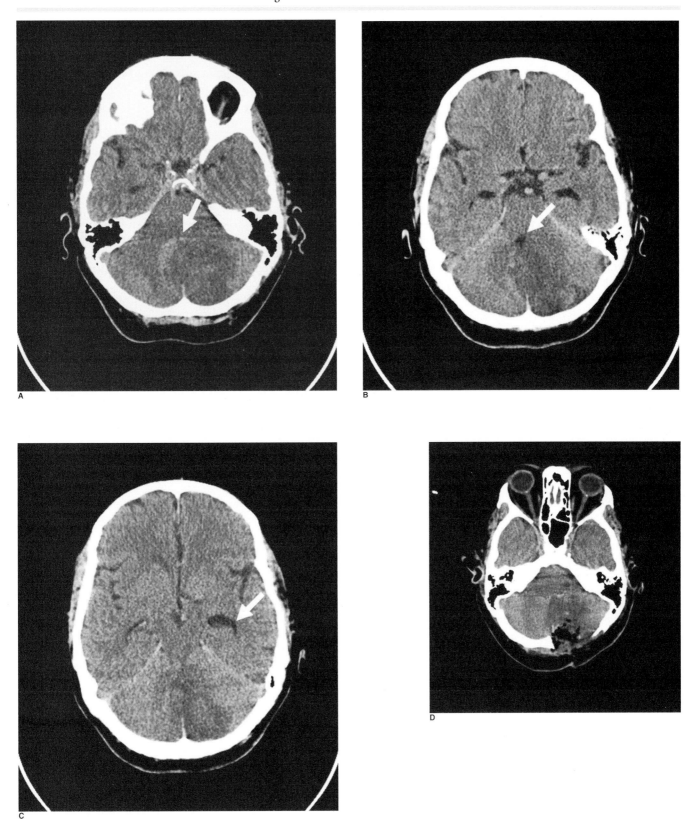

Figure 25-8. Cranial CT images from a 77 year-old woman with sudden vomiting, unsteadiness, and occipital headache. A: A hypodense lesion of the left cerebellar hemisphere and cerebellar vermis is ringed medially by faint rim of hemorrhage (*arrow*). B: The fourth ventricle is displaced anteriorly and to the right (*arrow*). C: The temporal horn is enlarged (*arrow*) due to obstruction of CSF flow. D: The postoperative cranial CT shows a left suboccipital craniectomy.

primary role is to trap and retain large fragments of venous thrombus to protect the pulmonary arterial circulation.

Urinary Incontinence

Urinary incontinence is common (40–60%) in the acute phase of stroke, with 25% of stroke patients still having problems on hospital discharge.[77] However, indwelling catheters are placed only if absolutely necessary and removed at the earliest possible time to avoid urosepsis. Chronic use of an indwelling catheter is limited to patients with incontinence or urinary retention refractory to other treatments. Treatment of asymptomatic bacteriuria is usually not indicated. However, for significant clinical infections with pyuria and fever, treatment is recommended. Catheter related urinary tract infections are usually caused by *Escherichia coli*. Polymicrobial or enterococcal infections are less common.

Fecal Incontinence and Constipation

Fecal incontinence and constipation may complicate hemiplegic stroke. Constipation may result from reduced fluid intake and body immobility. Aspirin may be a contributing factor.[78]

Decubitus

Approximately 15% of patients develop decubitus ulcers (pressure sores) after a stroke. Risk is highest in the early phases after stroke when mobility is most severely compromised. Steps to avoid decubiti include frequent inspection of the skin, skin cleansing, early mobilization, frequent turning, use of special mattresses and protective dressings (e.g., padded heel boots), maintenance of adequate nutritional status, and trying to improve the patient's mobility (see Chapter 26).

Falls

One of the most common causes of injury to the patient with a stroke is falling. Impaired gait and balance often contribute to falls. Patients with acute stroke have a propensity to hip fractures occurring on the hemiplegic side. Bone loss may be a major risk factor for post hemiplegic stroke hip fractures. Administration of folate and cobalamin has been recommended as a mean to reducing the risk of hip fractures after stroke.[79] Assessment of the risk for falling should be made at regular intervals during the acute hospitalization and also during the chronic rehabilitation phase. Reduction of postprandial systolic blood pressure has been associated with a higher incidence of falls and syncope. Strict preventative measures should be instituted to minimize the risk for falls.

Depression

Depressive symptoms (Chapter 2) are common after stroke, occurring in more than 25% of patients. Stroke patients should always be questioned and screened for depression. Whether the stroke's location affects the occurrence of depression is debated.[80–82] Treatment with antidepressants (selective serotonin reuptake inhibitors) is often successful in ameliorating symptoms.[83,84] Treatment of depression is presented in more detail in Chapter 26.

PREVENTION OF STROKE RECURRENCE

Medical Therapy

Specific measures for primary and secondary stroke prevention are provided in earlier chapters. However, the decision to imple-

ment these ongoing measures often arises at the time of the patient's first stroke, and consequently these measures are started in parallel with the acute stroke therapy. General measures, including aggressive control and modification of associated risk factors such as arterial hypertension, dyslipidemia, cigarette smoking, obesity, as well as use of antithrombotic agents (platelet antiaggregants and anticoagulants), antihypertensive agents, and lipid lowering, especially HMGCoA reductase inhibitors (statins), remain the mainstays of medical therapy for stroke prevention.

A large number of strokes should be preventable by controlling blood pressure, treating atrial fibrillation, and stopping cigarette smoking. Current cigarette smoking is more prevalent in certain regions of the world. A recent study from Asia reported a rate of 26% among 1,153 consecutive patients with acute stroke recruited from 10 Asian countries. Nicotine replacement therapy, bupropion, and varenicicline may be useful in assisting smoking cessation.

Hyperglycemia has been associated with increased mortality and worse functional outcome after stroke. Furthermore, hyperglycemia is associated with increased risk of hemorrhagic transformation in stroke patients treated with thrombolytics. Although intensive glycemic control (hemoglobin AlC < 7%) decreases microvascular complications of diabetes (retinopathy, nephropathy), such an approach has not been shown to have a significant effect on large vessel endpoints.[16,17]

Treatment with folic acid, cobalamin (vitamin B_{12}) and pyridoxine (vitamin B_6) lowers plasma homocysteine levels; however, homocysteine lowering therapy does not seem to improve cardiovascular endpoints in these patients.[85]

There are a few caveats relative to stroke-associated comorbidities. Diabetic patients taking metformin should stop this medication before performing neuroimaging procedures involving contrast administration (CT angiography, catheter cerebral angiography) and restart 2 days after. If patients have a raised serum creatinine, and these procedures are required, then *N*-acetylcysteine is given orally for 1 day preprocedure and up to 2 days postprocedure. Gadolinium administration should be avoided in patients with renal failure, as gadolinium-containing MRI contrast agents have been associated with nephrogenic systemic fibrosis (nephrogenic fibrosing dermopathy).

Platelet Antiaggregants

Antiplatelet therapy is highly effective in reducing the risk of vascular events and is recommended over oral anticoagulants for patients with noncardioembolic stroke. Evidence from several clinical studies favors the use of platelet antiaggregants as the first line of therapy in patients at high risk for stroke.[86] These agents are indicated for secondary prevention of stroke. Head-to-head comparative clinical trials versus aspirin monotherapy have shown that clopidogrel and the combination of aspirin plus extended release dipyridamole are safe and effective therapeutic options.[87–101] Practicing physicians need to synthesize the available evidence when choosing a given antiplatelet regimen for their patients.

Oral Anticoagulants

Warfarin is indicated for primary and secondary prevention of stroke in patients with nonvalvular atrial fibrillation (NVAF). NVAF patients at high risk for stroke should be treated with dose-adjusted warfarin (international normalized ratio [INR] 2.0–3.0). Anticoagulation with warfarin is also recommended for patients with atrial fibrillation (AF) and hyperthyroidism. Patients who cannot tolerate pharmacological cardioversion may benefit from electrophysiological or surgical procedures. However, cardioversion to sinus rhythm does not obviate the need for long-term anticoagulation.[102] Warfarin therapy has a protective effect against stroke following acute MI. Patients with mechanical prosthetic heart valves require lifelong therapy with oral anticoagulants to reduce the risk of thromboembolic complications. Patients undergoing elective cardioversion for AF should receive anticoagulation for 3 to 4 weeks before cardioversion unless there is documented onset of AF less than 48 hours prior to cardioversion. Use of long-term anticoagulation in patients with left ventricular aneurysms is not indicated because of a low risk for embolization. Prophylactic use of warfarin in dilated cardiomyopathy is a reasonable consideration in patients with low left ventricular ejection fractions. There are not adequate data to support anticoagulation in patients with stroke or TIA in the context of a patent foramen ovale (PFO), or complex (> 4 mm thick, or mobile, ulcerated or pedunculated) aortic arch atheroma.[103]

Likewise, there is no evidence of benefit for warfarin in preventing recurrent ischemic stroke among patients with noncardioembolic infarcts.[104] Further, warfarin has not been shown to be beneficial for symptomatic intracranial atherosclerotic vascular disease.[105] Specific guidelines for the use of warfarin are provided in Chapters 8, 11, and 20.

If used, warfarin therapy is usually initiated at a dose of 5 milligrams daily, aiming for a target INR of 2.0 to 3.0. Elderly, frail, malnourished individuals, or those with liver disease, require a lower starting dose (2–3 milligrams).

Surgical Therapy

Symptomatic Carotid Artery Stenosis

Stroke is often caused by atherosclerotic lesions of the carotid artery bifurcation. Approximately 15% of ischemic strokes are caused by extracranial internal carotid artery (ICA) stenosis. It is estimated that carotid artery stenosis > 50% is present in approximately 10% of men and in about 7% of women 65 years of age or older. Atherosclerosis, the most common cause of carotid artery disease, is most severe within 2 centimeters of the common carotid artery (CCA) bifurcation, and predominantly involves the posterior wall of the proximal ICA.

The degree of ICA stenosis remains the most important predictor of stroke among patients with extracranial carotid artery disease. Results from major prospective contemporary studies provide compelling evidence of the benefit of carotid endarterectomy (CEA) performed by experienced surgeons in improving the chance of stroke-free survival among high-risk symptomatic patients. Timely surgical intervention in selected patients with hemispheric or retinal TIAs, or completed nondisabling carotid territory strokes within the previous 6 months, and with 70% to 99% diameter-reducing carotid stenosis, can significantly reduce the risk for recurrent cerebral ischemia or death (NNT = 6).

With a low surgical risk, CEA provides modest benefit in symptomatic patients with ICA stenosis of 50% to 69%,[106] especially among men with hemispheric ischemia who are not diabetic (NNT = 15). However, CEA provides no benefit if the ICA stenosis is less than 50%.

Maximal acceptable limits of surgical risks for combined perioperative neurological morbidity and mortality are 3% for asymptomatic patients, 5% for patients with TIAs, 7% for patients with stroke, and 10% for patients with recurrent stenosis.

Options for intervention are limited when the ICA is occluded. Measurement of oxygen extraction fraction (OEF) by positron emission tomography (PET) allows clinicians to identify particular high-risk patients with ICA occlusion who might benefit from EC-IC bypass. These patients are currently being enrolled in the Carotid Occlusion Surgery Study (COSS).

Asymptomatic Carotid Artery Stenosis

Asymptomatic carotid artery atherosclerosis is prevalent in the general population, especially among elderly individuals. Carotid artery disease is a manifestation of systemic atherosclerotic disease. In fact, patients with asymptomatic carotid artery stenosis have a higher risk of cardiac ischemic events than strokes. Compared with symptomatic carotid stenosis, asymptomatic carotid artery stenosis is associated with a relatively low risk for ipsilateral cerebral infarction. The annual stroke rate of asymptomatic patients with hemodynamically consequential carotid stenosis is about 2% (range, 2–5%). Data from several randomized clinical trials concerning the efficacy of CEA in patients with asymptomatic carotid artery stenosis are now available. In the Asymptomatic Carotid Atherosclerosis Study (ACAS),[107] CEA combined with aspirin and risk factor reduction was superior to aspirin and risk factor reduction alone in preventing ipsilateral stroke in patients younger than 80 years with > 60% asymptomatic carotid artery stenosis. Based on a 5-year projection, ACAS showed that CEA reduced the absolute risk for stroke by 5.9% (ARR = 1% per year), and the relative risk for stroke and death by 53%. The surgical benefit incorporated a perioperative stroke and death rate of 2.3%, including a permanent arteriographic complication rate of 1.2%. Similar results have been reported from the MRC Asymptomatic Carotid Surgery Trial (ACST), a European trial of highly selected patients with > 70 percent carotid artery stenosis (by ultrasound) and no prior history of cerebrovascular disease.[108] In the ASCT, the 5-year stroke risk for surgery was 6.4% compared with 11.8% for medical therapy for the end points of fatal or nonfatal stroke, but the benefit was not substantiated for patients older than 75 years of age. It must be emphasized once more that these benefits require a very low perioperative stroke risk (< 3%).

Thus, controversy still exists in the selection of asymptomatic patients for CEA. Given the low risk for stroke for all deciles until 80% to 89% carotid artery stenosis is reached, some experts recommend surgery only when the degree of stenosis is > 80%, provided that the operation is performed by an experienced surgeon with a low complication rate (combined angiographic and surgical) of 3% or less.

Stenting of the Cervicocerebral Vessels

Carotid artery angioplasty and stenting (CAS) may offer an alternative treatment to CEA, particularly in patients with ICA stenosis that is in an anatomically high location in the neck (e.g., surgically inaccessible lesions above C2), carotid artery restenosis following CEA, radiation-induced carotid artery stenosis, tumor-encased carotid arteries, and among certain high-risk patients with serious medical co-morbidities who continue to have ischemic manifestations on optimal medical therapy (Figure 25-9).

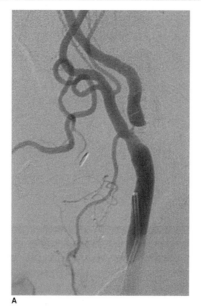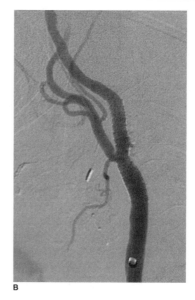

Figure 25-9. Catheter angiogram from a 75-year-old-woman with hypertension, diabetes mellitus, hyperlipidemia, congestive heart failure, and recurrent right hemisphere TIAs. A: Before stenting she has > 90% stenosis at the origin of the right internal carotid artery. B: Another injection after stenting confirms successful angioplasty and stent deployment.

An early meta-analysis of 1,154 patients suggested that the composite end point for CAS versus CEA was not different at the 1-month stroke/death end point.[109] The major difference was that the 1-month MI rate was lower for CAS (RR 0.03; 95% CI 0.1–0.9) and the cranial nerve injury rate for CAS was also lower (RR 0.05; 95% CI 0.01–0.3). At 1 year, no significant differences in the ipsilateral stroke rate were observed (RR 0.8; 95% CI 0.5–1.2). The Carotid and Vertebral Artery Transluminal Angioplasty Study (CAVATAS) was designed to evaluate the risks of endovascular therapy (percutaneous transluminal angioplasty and stenting) versus surgical intervention. Most of the patients had either a TIA or stroke within 6 months before randomization; approximately 4% were asymptomatic in both arms. CAVATAS showed no difference at 30 days in the risk of death or stroke between the groups. Cranial neuropathies were more common in the CEA group. Restenosis (> 70%) was greater for CAS versus CEA (18.5% vs. 5.2%, $p = 0.0001$).[110] However, there was a low rate of recurrent stroke in both the endovascular and CEA-treated patients, suggesting that treatment of carotid artery restenosis should be limited to patients with recurrent symptoms. Further, most of the endovascular procedures in CAVATAS were balloon angioplasties without stenting.

The Stenting and Angioplasty with Protection in Patients at High Risk for Endarterectomy (SAPPHIRE), compared stenting with deployment of a distal protection device versus CEA for patients otherwise defined as high risk for surgery.[111] The study was designed to test that carotid artery stenting (CAS) was not inferior to CEA. SAPPHIRE evaluated 747 patients of which 413 patients were treated as part of a registry, and only 334 cases were actually randomized to either CEA or CAS. The 30-day event rate showed a significant difference between CAS and CEA of 5.8% for the combined end point of stroke, MI, or death versus 12.6 ($p < 0.047$). However, these results were mainly driven by non-Q-wave MIs. At 1 year, the outcomes included a stroke rate of 6.3%, a death rate of 0.04%, and a combined end point of stroke, death, and 30-day MI rate of 12.2% for the CAS arm, and a stroke rate of 7.9%, death rate of 13.5%, and a combined end point of stroke, death at 1 year, and/or 30 day MI rate of 20.1% for the CEA arm. Major stroke was less common for CAS in the randomized arm (0.6%) compared with CEA (3.0%), but major stroke was as common in the CAS registry (3.2%) as compared with CEA, while minor stroke was less common for CEA (1.8%) as opposed to CAS in either the randomized CAS (3.6%) or registry CAS arms (3.9%). It should be noted that this analysis combined symptomatic and asymptomatic patients, and that the SAPPHIRE study was biased toward patients with asymptomatic carotid artery disease.

The Carotid Revascularization using Endarterectomy or Stenting System (CaRESS) Phase 1 also suggested that the 30-day and 1-year risk of death, stroke, or MI with CAS was equivalent to that of CEA in symptomatic and asymptomatic patients with carotid artery stenosis.[112] However, the Endarterectomy (SPACE), and Endarterectomy versus Angioplasty in Patients with Symptomatic Severe Carotid Stenosis (EVA-3S), failed to meet noninferiority criteria in patients with symptomatic stenosis of 60% or more. EVA-3S was stopped short (527 patients) of the planned enrollment of 872 patients for both reasons of safety and futility. At both 1 and 6 months after the procedure, death and stroke rates were lower with CEA.[113]

Likewise, the Stent-Supported Percutaneous Angioplasty of the Carotid Artery versus Endarterectomy (SPACE) also showed a slightly higher rate of ipsilateral ischemic stroke and death at 30 days in patents undergoing carotid stenting rather than CEA.[113] Additional randomized trials, including the Carotid Revascularization Endarterectomy versus Stent Trial (CREST) and the International Carotid Stenting Study (ICSS)–CAVATAS-2 are currently underway in the United States and Europe, for both low- and high-risk asymptomatic and symptomatic patients.[114,115]

Stenting of intracranial arteries is still a procedure under development.[116] Two small single-arm studies have been published. In the Stenting of Symptomatic Atherosclerotic Lesions in the Vertebral or Intracranial Arteries (SSYLVIA) study, restenosis occurred in 12 of 37 (32.4%) intracranial cases and 6 of 14 (42%) extracranial vertebral artery stent cases; 39.1% of the restenosis cases were symptomatic,[117] with a stroke rate of 4 in 55 (7.3%) within 6 months. In the WINGSPAN study, 45 patients had device placement for recurrent symptoms despite medical therapy.[118] Restenosis was low with this device, but the average stroke/death rate was 7.1% at 6 months.

STROKE REHABILITATION

Rehabilitation after stroke begins as soon as the diagnosis of stroke is established and as soon as any life-threatening neurological or medical complications have been stabilized. Early evaluation and referral to a rehabilitation program improve clinical outcome. A detailed description on stroke rehabilitation is provided in Chapter 26. Daily passive range of motion exercises are of critical importance. Patients are screened to evaluate whether they are candidates for further inpatient or outpatient rehabilitation. Criteria used to make this decision, including the stroke survivor's clinical and neurological status and social and environmental factors, are complex. The available evidence on the effectiveness of rehabilitation, including electrical or neuromuscular stimulation, suggests that rehabilitation is beneficial to some patients, but the superiority of one type of program or the characteristics of patients most likely to benefit are not clear.

REFERENCES

1. Levine SR. McConnochie KM. Telemedicine for acute stroke. When virtual is as good as reality. *Neurology.* 2007;**69**:819–820.
2. Jorgensen HS, Nakayama H, Raaschou HO, et al. The effect of a stroke unit: reduction in mortality, discharge rate to nursing home, length of hospital stay and cost. A community-based study. *Stroke.* 1995;**26**:1178–1182.
3. Fiorelli M, Alpérovitch A, Argentino C, et al. Prediction of death or disablement at four months based on clinical characteristics identified in the early hours of acute ischemic stroke. *Arch Neurol.* 1995;**52**:250–255.
4. Ringelstein EB, Koschorke S, Holling A, et al. Type and extent of hemispheric brain infarctions and clinical outcome in early and delayed middle cerebral artery recanalization. *Neurology.* 1992;**42**:289–298.
5. Toni D, Fiorelli M, Gentile M, et al. Progressing neurological deficit secondary to acute ischemic stroke – A study on predictability, pathogenesis and prognosis. *Arch Neurol.* 1995;**52**:670–675.
6. Horowitz SH, Zito JL, Donnarumma R, et al. Computed tomographic-angiographic findings within the first five hours of cerebral infarction. *Stroke.* 1991;**22**:1245–1253.
7. Moulin T, Cattin F, Crepin-Leblond T, et al. Early CT signs in acute middle cerebral artery infarction. Predictive value for subsequent infarct location and outcome. *Neurology.* 1996;**47**:366–375.
8. Kummer VR, Meyding-Lamade, Forsting M, et al. Sensitivity and prognostic value of early computed tomography in middle cerebral artery trunk occlusion. *AJNR Am J Neuroradiol.* 1994;**15**:9–15.
9. Warach S, Chien D, Li W, et al. Fast magnetic resonance diffusion-weighted imaging of acute human stroke. *Neurology.* 1992;**42**:1717–1723.

10. Guadagno JV, Warburton EA, Aigbirhio FI, et al. Does the acute diffusion-weighted imaging lesion represent penumbra as well as core? A combined quantitative PET/MRI voxel-based study. *J Cereb Blood Flow Metab.* 2004;**24**:1249–1254.
11. Schramm P, Schellinger PD, Klotz E, et al. Comparison of perfusion computed tomography and computed tomography angiography source images with perfusion-weighted imaging and diffusion-weighted imaging in patients with acute stroke of less than 6 hours' duration. *Stroke.* 2004;**35**:1657–1658.
12. Bozzao L, Bastianello S, Fantozzi LM, et al. Correlation of angiographic and sequential CT findings in patients with evolving cerebral infarction. *AJNR Am J Neuroradiol.* 1992;**10**:1215–1222.
13. Caplan LR, Walpert SM. Angiography with occlusive cerebrovascular disease: views of a stroke neurologist and neuroradiologists. *AJNR Am J Neuroradiol.* 1991;**12**:593–601.
14. Kothari R, Barsan W, Brott T, et al. Frequency and accuracy of pre-hospital diagnosis of stroke. *Stroke.* 1995;**26**:937–941.
15. Barsan W, Brott T, Broderick J, et al. Time of hospital presentation of patients with acute stroke. *Arch Int Med.* 1993;**153**:2558–2561.
16. Williams LS, Rotich J, Qi R, et al. Effects of admission hyperglycemia on mortality and costs in acute ischemic stroke. *Neurology.* 2002;**59**:67–71.
17. Ripley DL, Seel RT, Macciocchi SN, et al. The impact of diabetes mellitus on stroke acute rehabilitation outcomes. *Am J Phys Med Rehabil.* 2007;**86**:745–761.
18. Bethel MA, Sloan FA, Belsky D, et al. Longitudinal incidence and prevalence of adverse outcomes of diabetes mellitus in elderly patients. *Arch Intern Med.* 2007;**167**:921–927.
19. Kay R, Wong KS, Yu YL, et al. Low-molecular-weight heparin for the treatment of acute ischemic stroke. *N Engl J Med.* 1995;**333**:1588–1593.
20. Adams HP, Brott T, Crowell R, et al. Guidelines for the management of patients with acute ischemic stroke. A statement for health care professionals from a special writing group of the Stroke Council, American Heart Association. *Stroke.* 1994;**25**:1901–1914.
21. International Stroke Trial Collaborative Group. The International Stroke Trial (IST): a randomized trial of aspirin, subcutaneous heparin, both, or neither among 19435 patients with acute ischemic stroke. *Lancet.* 1997;**349**:1569–1581.
22. TOAST Investigators. Low molecular weight heparinoid, ORG 10172 (danaparoid) and outcome after ischemic stroke. A randomized controlled trial. *JAMA.* 1998;**279**:1265–1272.
23. Kassem-Moussa H, Graffagnino C. Nonocclusion and spontaneous recanalization rates in acute ischemic stroke: a review of cerebral angiography studies. *Arch Neurol.* 2002;**59**:1870–1873.
24. Kaps M, Teschendorf U, Dorndorf W. Haemodynamic studies in early stroke. *J Neurol.* 1992;**239**:138–142.
25. Hacke W, Kaste M, Fieschi C, et al. Intravenous thrombolysis with recombinant tissue plasminogen activator for acute hemispheric stroke. *JAMA.* 1995;**274**:1017–1025.
26. Hacke W, Donnan G, Fieschi C, et al. Association of outcome with early stroke treatment: pooled analysis of ATLANTIS, ECASS, and NINDS rt-PA stroke trials. *Lancet.* 2004;**363**:768–774.
27. Del Zoppo GJ, Pessin MS, Mori E, et al. Thrombolytic intervention in acute thrombotic and embolic stroke. *Sem Neurol.* 1991;**11**:368–384.
28. Wardlaw JM, Warlow CP. Thrombolysis in acute ischemic stroke: does it work? *Stroke.* 1992;**23**:1826–1839.
29. Sylaja PH, Cote R, Buchnan AM, et al. Thrombolysis in patients older than 80 years with acute ischemic stroke: Canadian

Alteplase for Stroke Effectiveness Study. *J Neurol Neurosurg Psychiatry*. 2006;**777**:826–829.

30. The Multicenter Acute Stroke Trial – Europe Study Group. Thrombolytic therapy with streptokinase in acute ischemic stroke. *N Engl J Med*. 1996;**335**:145–150.

31. Ciccone A, Motto C, Aritzu E, et al. Negative interaction of aspirin and streptokinase in acute ischemic stroke: further analysis of the Multicenter Acute Stroke Trial – Italy. *Cerebrovasc Dis*. 2000;**10**:61–64.

32. Donnan GA, Davis SM, Chambers BR, et al. Streptokinase for acute ischemic stroke with relationship to time of administration: Australian Streptokinase (ASK) Trial Study Group. *JAMA*. 1996;**276**:961–966.

33. Multicentre Acute Stroke Trial – Italy (MAST-I) Group. Randomised controlled trial of streptokinase, aspirin, and combination of both in treatment of acute ischaemic stroke. *Lancet*. 1995;**346**:1509–1514.

34. Yasaka M, O'Keefe GJ, Chambers BR, et al. Streptokinase in acute stroke: effect on reperfusion and recanalization. Australian Streptokinase Trial Study Group. *Neurology*. 1998;**50**:626–632.

35. Mouradian MS, Senthilsevan A, Jickling G, et al. Intravenous rt-PA for acute stroke: comparing its effectiveness in younger and older patients. *J Neurol Neurosurg Psychiatry*. 2005;**76**:1234–1237.

36. National Institute of Neurological Disorders and Stroke rt-PA Stroke Study Group. Tissue plasminogen activator for acute ischemic stroke. *N Eng J Med*. 1995;**333**:1581–1587.

37. Kwiatkowski TG, Libman RB, Frankel M, et al. Effects of tissue plasminogen activator for acute ischemic stroke at one year. National Institute of Neurological Disorders and Stroke Recombinant Tissue Plasminogen Activator Stroke Study Group. *N Engl J Med*. 1999;**340**:1781–1787.

38. Hacke W, Kaste M, Bluhmki E, et al. ECASS Investigators. Thrombolysis with alteplase 3 to 4.5 hours after acute ischemic stroke. *N Engl J Med*. 2008;**359**:1317–1329.

39. del Zoppo GJ, Saver JL, Jauch EC, Adams HP Jr. Expansion of the time window for treatment of acute ischemic stroke with intravenous tissue plasminogen activator: a science advisory from the American Heart Association/American Stroke Association. *Stroke*. **2009**; in press.

40. Del Zoppo GJ, Higashida RT, Furlan AJ, et al. PROACT: a phase II randomized trial of recombinant pro-urokinase by direct arterial delivery in acute middle cerebral artery stroke. PROACT Investigators. Prolyse in Acute Cerebral Thromboembolism. *Stroke*. 1998;**29**:4–11.

41. Furlan A, Higashida R, Wechsler L, et al. Intra-arterial prourokinase for acute ischemic stroke. The PROACT II study: a randomized controlled trial. Prolyse in Acute Cerebral Thromboembolism. *JAMA*. 1999;**282**:2003–2011.

42. Alexandrov AV, Moina CA, Grotta J, et al., for the CLOTBUST Investigators. Ultrasound-enhanced systemic thrombolysis for acute ischemic stroke. *N Engl J Med*. 2004;**351**;21:2170–2178.

43. Kollmar R, Henninger N, Bardutzky J, et al. Combination therapy of moderate hypothermia and thrombolysis in experimental thromboembolic stroke – an MRI study. *Exp Neurol*. 2004;**10**:204–212.

44. Lyden PD, Alving LI, Zivin JA, et al. Hemodilution with low-molecular weight hydroxyethyl starch after experimental focal cerebral ischemia in rabbits. *Stroke*. 1988;**19**:223–227.

45. Sherman DG, Atkinson RP, Chippendale T, et al. Intravenous ancrod for treatment of acute ischemic stroke, the STAT study; a randomized controlled trial. Stroke Treatment with Ancrod Trial. *JAMA*. 2000;**283**:2395–2403.

46. Tomassoni D, Lanari A, Silvestrelli G, et al. Nimodipine and its use in cerebrovascular disease: evidence from recent preclinical and controlled clinical studies. *Clin Exp Hypertens*. 2008;**30**:744–766.

47. Inzitari D, Poggesi A. Calcium channel blockers and stroke. *Aging Clin Exp Res*. 2005;**17**(4 Suppl):16–30.

48. Fogelholm R, Palomäki H, Erilä T, et al. Blood pressure, nimodipine, and outcome of ischemic stroke. *Acta Neurol Scand*. 2004;**109**:200–204.

49. Hemmen TM, Lyden PD. Multimodal neuroprotective therapy with induced hypothermia after ischemic stroke. *Stroke*. 2008; Dec 8. [Epub ahead of print].

50. Krieger DW. Stay cool in stroke. *Int J Stroke*. 2006;**1**:36–37.

51. Lyden PD, Krieger D, Yenari M, et al. Therapeutic hypothermia for acute stroke. *Int J Stroke*. 2006;9–19.

52. Gupta R, Jvin TG, Krieger DW. Therapeutic hypothermia for stroke: do new outfits change an old friend? *Exper Rev Neurotherapeutics*. 2005;**5**:235–246.

53. Hajat C, Hajat S, Sharma P. Effects of post-stroke pyrexia on stroke outcome. A meta analysis of studies in patients. *Stroke*. 2000;**31**:410–414.

54. Kammersgaard LP, Jorgensen HS, Rungby RA, et al. Admission body temperature predicts long term mortality after acute stroke: the Copenhagen Stroke Study. *Stroke*. 2002;**33**:1759–1762.

55. Krieger DW, Yenari MA. Therapeutic hypothermia for acute ischemic stroke. What do laboratory studies teach us? *Stroke*. 2004;**35**:1482–1489.

56. Adams HP Jr, Adams RJ, Brott T, et al. Guidelines for the early management of patient with ischemic stroke. *Stroke*. 2003;**34**:1056–1083.

57. Adams HP Jr, Adams RJ, Del Zoppo G, et al. Guidelines for the early management of patients with ischemic stroke. Guidelines Update. *Stroke*. 2005;**35**:916–923.

58. Singhal AB, Benner T, Roccatagliata L, et al. A pilot study of normobaric oxygen therapy in acute ischemic stroke. *Stroke*. 2005;**36**:797–802.

59. Anderson DC, Bottini AG, Jagiella WM, et al. A pilot study of hyperbaric oxygen in the treatment of human stroke. *Stroke*. **991**;22:1137–1142.

60. Nighoghossian N, Trouillas P, Adeleine P, et al. Hyperbaric oxygen in the treatment of acute ischemic stroke. A double-blind pilot study. *Stroke*. 1995;**26**:1369–1372.

61. Rusyniak DE, Kirk MA, May JD, et al. Hyperbaric Oxygen in Acute Ischemic Stroke Trial Pilot Study. Hyperbaric oxygen therapy in acute ischemic stroke: results of the hyperbaric oxygen in acute ischemic stroke trial pilot study. *Stroke*. 2003;**34**:571–574.

62. Castillo J, Leira R, Garcia MM, et al. Blood pressure decrease during the acute phase of ischemic stroke is associated with brain injury and poor stroke outcome. *Stroke*. 2004;**35**:520–526.

63. Talbert RL. The challenge of blood pressure management in neurologic emergencies. *Pharmacotherapy*. 2006;**26**:123S–130S.

64. Cochrane Study Group. Vasoactive Drugs for Acute Stroke. *Cochrane Database of Systematic Reviews*. 2003; CD002839.

65. Lapchak PA. Hemorrhagic transformation following ischemic stroke: significance, causes, and relationship to therapy and treatment. *Curr Neurol Neurosci Rep*. 2002;**2**:38–43.

66. Pessin M, Estol C, Lafranchise F, et al. Safety of anticoagulation after hemorrhagic infarction. *Neurology*. 1993;**43**:1298–1303.

67. Rosendale FR. Anticoagulation: how low can one go? *Lancet*. 1994;**343**:867–868.

68. Bereczki D, Liu M, doPrado GF, Fekete I. Mannitol for acute stroke. *Stroke*. 2008;**39**:512–513.

69. Bereckzki D, Liu M, do Prado F, Fekete I. Mannitol for acute stroke. *Cochrane Database of Systematic Reviews*, 2007, issue 3, Art No: CD00153. DOI: 10.1002/14651858. CD00153.pub2.

70. Gemma M, Cozzi S, Tommasino C, et al. 7.5% hypertonic saline versus 20% mannitol during elective neurosurgical supratentorial procedures. *J Neurosurg Anesthesiol*. 1997;**9**:329–334.

71. Ziai WC, Toung TJ, Bhardwaj A. Hypertonic saline: first-line therapy for cerebral edema? *J Neurol Sci.* 2007;**261**:157–166.

72. Horn P, Münch E, Vajkoczy P, et al. Hypertonic saline solution for control of elevated intracranial pressure in patients with exhausted response to mannitol and barbiturates. *Neurol Res.* 1999;**21**:758–764.

73. Peterson B, Khanna S, Fisher B, et al. Prolonged hypernatremia controls elevated intracranial pressure in head-injured pediatric patients. *Crit Care Med.* 2000;**28**:1136–1143.

74. Khanna S, Davis D, Peterson B, et al. Use of hypertonic saline in the treatment of severe refractory posttraumatic intracranial hypertension in pediatric traumatic brain injury. *Crit Care Med.* 2000;**28**:1144–1151.

75. Schneck MJ, Origitano TC. Hemicraniectomy and durotomy for malignant middle cerebral artery infarction. *Neurol Clin.* 2006;**24**:715–727.

76. Navarro JC, Bitanga E, Suwanwela N, et al. Complications of acute stroke: a study in ten Asian countries. *Neurology Asia.* 2008;**13**:33–39.

77. Thomas LH, Cross S, Barrett J, et al. Treatment of urinary incontinence after stroke in adults. *Cochrane Database of Systematic Reviews.* 2008; Issue 1 CD004462.

78. Bracci F, Badiali D, Pezzotti P, et al. Chronic constipation in hemiplegic patients. *World J Gastroenterol.* 2007;**13**:3967–3972.

79. Sato Y, Honda Y, Iwamoto J, et al. Effect of folate and mecobalamin on hip fractures in patients with stroke. *JAMA.* 2005;**293**:1082–1088.

80. Kim JS, Choi-Kwon S. Poststroke depression and emotional incontinence: correlation with lesion location. *Neurology.* 2000; **54**:1805–1810.

81. De Wit L, Putman K, Baert I, et al. Anxiety and depression in the first six months after stroke. A longitudinal multicenter study. *Disabil Rehabil.* 2008;**30**:1858–1866.

82. Masskulpan P, Riewthong K, Dajpratham P, et al. Anxiety and depressive symptoms after stroke in 9 rehabilitation centers. *J Med Assoc Thai.* 2008;**91**:1595–1602.

83. Hackett ML, Anderson CS, House A, et al. Interventions for treating depression after stroke. *Cochrane Database Syst Rev.* 2008 Oct 8;(4):CD003437.

84. Lenzi GL, Altieri M, Maestrini I. Post-stroke depression. *Rev Neurol (Paris).* 2008;**164**:837–840.

85. Toole JF, Malinow R, Chambless L, et al. Lowering homocysteine in patients with ischemic stroke to prevent recurrent stroke, myocardial infraction and death. The Vitamin Intervention for Stroke Prevention (VISP) Randomized Clinical Trial. *JAMA.* 2004;**291**:565–575.

86. Antithrombotic Trialists' Collaboration. Collaborative meta-analysis of randomized trials of antiplatelet therapy for prevention of death, myocardial infarction, and stroke in high risk patients. *BMJ.* 2002;**324**:71–86.

87. Adams RJ, Albers G, Alberts MJ, et al. Update to the AHA/ASA recommendations for the prevention of stroke in patients with stroke and transient ischemic attack. *Stroke* 2008;**39**:1647–1652.

88. Anderson DC, Goldstein LB. Aspirin: it's hard to beat. *Neurology.* 2004;**62**:1036–1037.

89. Sacco RL, Adams R, Albers G, et al. Guidelines for prevention of stroke in patients with ischemic stroke or transient ischemic attack: a statement for healthcare professionals from the American Heart Association/American Stroke Association Council on Stroke: co-sponsored by the Council on Cardiovascular Radiology and Intervention. *Stroke.* 2006;**37**:577–617.

90. Verro P, Gorelick PB, Nguyen D. Aspirin plus dipyridamole versus aspirin for prevention of vascular events after stroke or TIA: a meta-analysis. *Stroke.* 2008;**39**:1358–1363.

91. Sacco RL, Diener HC, Yusuf S, et al. Aspirin and extended-release dipyridamole versus clopidogrel for recurrent stroke. *N Engl J Med.* 2008;**359**:1238–1251.

92. Hass WK, Easton JD, Adams HP, et al. A randomized trial comparing ticlopidine hydrochloride with aspirin for the prevention of stroke in high-risk patients. *N Engl J Med.* 1989;**321**:501–507.

93. Gorelick PB, Richardson D, Kelly M, et al. Aspirin and ticlopidine for prevention of recurrent stroke in black patients: a randomized trial. *JAMA.* 2003;**289**:2947–2957.

94. Diener HC, Darius H, Bertrand-Hardy JM, et al. Cardiac safety in the European Stroke Prevention Study 2 (ESPS2). *Int J Clin Pract.* 2001;**55**:162–163.

95. Albers GW, Amarenco P, Easton JD, et al. Antithrombotic and thrombolytic therapy for ischemic stroke: American College of Chest Physicians Evidence-Based Clinical Practice Guidelines (Eighth Edition). *Chest.* 2008;**133**:630S–669S.

96. No authors listed. A randomised, blinded, trial of clopidogrel versus aspirin in patients at risk of ischaemic events (CAPRIE). CAPRIE Steering Committee. *Lancet.* 1996;**348**:1329–1339.

97. Diener HC, Bogousslavsky J, Brass LM, et al. Aspirin and clopidogrel compared with clopidogrel alone after recent ischaemic stroke or transient ischaemic attack in high-risk patients (MATCH): randomised, double-blind, placebo-controlled trial. *Lancet.* 2004;**364**:331–337.

98. Amarenco P, Donnan GA. Should the MATCH results be extrapolated to all stroke patients and affect ongoing trials evaluating clopidogrel plus aspirin? *Stroke.* 2004;**35**:2606–2608.

99. Liao JK. Secondary prevention of stroke and transient ischemic attack: is more platelet inhibition the answer? *Circulation.* 2007;**115**:1615–1621.

100. Bhatt DL, Fox KA, Hacke W, et al. Clopidogrel and aspirin versus aspirin alone for the prevention of atherothrombotic events. *N Engl J Med.* 2006;**354**:1706–1717.

101. Leonardi-Bee J, Bath PM, Bousser MG, et al. Dipyridamole for preventing recurrent ischemic stroke and other vascular events: a meta-analysis of individual patient data from randomized controlled trials. *Stroke.* 2005;**36**:162–168.

102. Sherman DG, Kim SG, Boop BS, et al. Occurrence and characteristics of stroke events in the atrial fibrillation follow-up investigations of sinus rhythm management (AFFIRM) study. *Arch Intern Med.* 2005;**165**:1185–1191.

103. Albers GW, Amarenco P, Easton J, et al. Antithrombotic and thrombolytic therapy for ischemic stroke: The seventh ACCP conference on antithrombotic and thrombolytic therapy. *Chest* 2004;**125**(Suppl):483–512.

104. Mohr JP, Thompson JL, Lazar RM, et al. A comparison of warfarin and aspirin for the prevention of recurrent ischemic stroke. *N Engl J Med.* 2001;**345**:1444–1451.

105. Chimowitz MI, Lynn MJ, Howlett-Smith H, et al. Comparison of warfarin and aspirin for symptomatic intracranial arterial stenosis. *N Engl J Med.* 2005;**352**:1305–1316.

106. Barnett HJM, Taylor DW, Eliasziw M, et al. Benefit of carotid endarterectomy in patients with symptomatic moderate or severe stenosis. North American Symptomatic Carotid Endarterectomy Trial Collaborators. *N Engl Med J.* 1998;**339**:1415–1425.

107. Brott T, Toole JF. Medical compared with surgical treatment of asymptomatic carotid artery stenosis. *Ann Intern Med.* 1995;Nov 1:**123**:720–722.

108. Halliday A, Mansfield A, Marco J, et al. Prevention of disabling and fatal strokes by successful carotid endarterectomy in patients without recent neurological symptoms. *Lancet.* 2004;**363**:1491–1502.

109. Qureshi AI, Kirmani JF, Divani AA, et al. Carotid angioplasty with or without stent placement versus carotid endarterectomy for treatment of carotid stenosis: a meta-analysis. *Neurosurgery.* 2005;**56**:1171–1181.

110. Dominick JH, McCabe AC, Pereira AC, et al. Restenosis after carotid angioplasty, stenting, or endarterectomy in the Carotid and Vertebral Artery Transluminal Angioplasty Study (CAVATAS). *Stroke.* 2005;**36**:281–286.

111. Yadav JS, Wholey MH, Kuntz RR, et al. Protected carotid artery stenting versus endarterectomy in high risk patients. *N Engl J Med.* 2004;**351**:1493–1501.

112. CaRESS Steering Committee. Carotid Revascularization Using Endarterectomy or Stenting Systems (CaRESS) Phase I clinical trial: 1-year results. *J Vasc Surg.* 2005;**42**:213–219.

113. Barrett KM, Brott TG. Carotid artery stenting versus carotid endarterectomy: current status. *Neurol Clin.* 2006;**26**:681–695.

114. Hacke W, Brown MM, Mas JL. Carotid endarterectomy versus stenting: an international perspective. *Stroke.* 2006;**37**:344.

115. Hobson RW II, Brott TG, Roubin GS, et al. Carotid endarterectomy versus stenting: an international perspective: reply. *Stroke.* 2006;**37**:344.

116. Chimowitz MI, Kokkhinos J, Strong J, et al. The Warfarin-Aspirin Symptomatic Intracranial Disease Study. *Stroke.* 1995;**45**:1488–1493.

117. SSYLVIA Investigators. Stenting of Symptomatic Atherosclerotic Lesions in the Vertebral or Intracranial Arteries (SSYLVIA): study results. *Stroke.* 2004;**35**:1388–1392.

118. Higashida RT, Meyers PM, Connors JJ III, et al. Intracranial angioplasty and stenting for cerebral atherosclerosis. *AJNR Am J Neurodiol.* 2005;**26**:2323–2327.

119. Hacke W, Schab S, DeGeorgia M. Intensive care of acute ischemic stroke. *Cerebrovasc Dis.* 1994;**4**:385–392.

26

Neurorehabilitation Following Stroke

David C. Good, MD, and Lumy Sawaki, MD

Perfectly exact truth is but rarely to be seen.

Hippocrates

The goal of stroke rehabilitation is to ensure that each person reaches the maximum physical, functional, and psychosocial recovery possible within the limits of his or her impairment. In theory, rehabilitation facilitates a degree of improvement greater than would occur spontaneously. In many regards, rehabilitation requires learning how to do things in new ways, a process that depends partially on the concentration and motivation of the patient. In some cases, the focus of rehabilitation is on adaptation and compensation for deficits. This may involve adaptive devices or training the family to compensate for deficits that are irreversible.

Research in the general area of stroke rehabilitation is exploding as there is increasing demand for evidence-based approaches. During the past decade there has been a dramatic increase in knowledge regarding the potential of the brain to reorganize in response to external and/or internal demands. Functional recovery has been reported for cognitive deficits, motor deficits, and sensory and perceptual deficits such as hemineglect. The potential of the brain to reorganize is due to utilization of innate reserves that lead to functional recovery. This concept has led to rapid changes in therapeutic and rehabilitative approaches using new strategies to optimize stroke rehabilitation. Still, much of day-to-day stroke rehabilitation is based on techniques that have been helpful over many years. Therefore much of this chapter is devoted to practical aspects of current stroke rehabilitation, although newer concepts and techniques are also introduced.

Stroke rehabilitation should facilitate relearning of skills and abilities that were possible before the stroke and should maximize reintegration of patients into the community. It should include:

1. Strategies that optimize improvement of neurological, psychological, and cognitive deficits
2. Strategies to assist activities of daily living
3. Prevention of secondary complications
4. Strategies to maximize independence in a home environment
5. Recreational and vocational recommendations for the best possible return to society

NATURAL HISTORY AND FUNCTIONAL RECOVERY AFTER STROKE

In most stroke patients, spontaneous improvement is usually discernible a few days after the ictus (Table 26-1). A variety of complications should be considered if there is worsening or no improvement, but there is considerable variability in the degree of restoration. Most recovery of specific impairments (motor, sensory, language) occurs during the first 6 months,[1-5] but improvements have been demonstrated in patients up to 10 to 20 years post-stroke if intensive and focused rehabilitative approaches are delivered and the patient is motivated.[6] Patients with pure motor hemiparesis usually make a good functional recovery, with most regaining independent ambulation and ability to live alone. People with hemiparesis and hemisensory loss have a more guarded prognosis, but many can ambulate and most are able to gain partial independence. Patients with hemiparesis, hemisensory loss, and homonymous hemianopsia have a worse outlook, with only a minority achieving more than assisted ambulation and most requiring long-term assistance with some activities of daily living (ADLs).[7] The Barthel Index (BI), which quantifies the ability to perform ADLs, usually shows most improvement by three months post-stroke,[3,5,8] although people with more severe initial disability may improve more slowly within the first 6 months (Figure 26-1). As with specific impairments, additional improvement in ADLs may occur in select individuals participating in an intensive program beyond 6 months.

Motor recovery almost always occurs first in the proximal muscles of the torso, hip, and leg, followed by the distal leg and proximal arm, and finally the hand. A bedside rule is that if the patient can move his hip within a week, he can learn to walk with ankle support, and if he can move his toes he will not need any bracing. Even after motor power begins to reappear, improvement may cease at any stage. Recovery may be limited by associated depression, dementia, aphasia, apraxia, sensory loss, or disturbed spatial relations. The presence of medical co-morbidities also profoundly affects stroke outcomes.[9,10]

Table 26-1: Return of Motor Function in Patients with Hemiplegia

Average time after onset of ictus	Reflex	Movement
0 hour	Loss or diminution of muscle stretch reflexes; hypotonia	No voluntary or reflex movement
4 to 48 hours	Muscle stretch reflexes more active; minimal increase in muscle tone (seen first in palmar and plantar flexors)	Reflex withdrawal to painful stimuli
3 days to 6 weeks	Finger-jerks brisk; gradual increase in muscle tone, especially adductors and flexors and flexors of the upper limb and adductors and extensors of the lower limb	Movement of proximal muscles of leg followed in 7–10 days by movement of toes
	Appearance of clonus (first seen in ankle flexors)	Movement of shoulder, "pattern" movement of upper extremity
	Clasp-knife phenomenon elicited in knee extensors or elbow flexors	

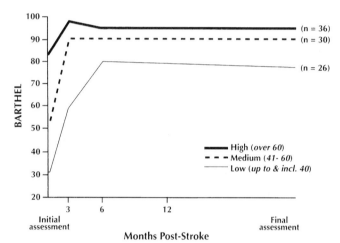

Figure 26-1. Recovery of ability to perform activities of daily living (ADLs) after stroke. The Barthel Index (B1) is a multifaceted assessment scale with a maximum score of 100. Note that patients with higher initial scores have better final outcomes than those with lower initial scores. Patients with lower initial scores (greater disability) improve more slowly. Reproduced with permission from Wade et al.[130]

EFFECTIVENESS OF REHABILITATION

There is an increasing consensus that specific stroke rehabilitation programs are effective for retraining motor skills, for preventing complications, and for teaching adaptive techniques.[11–13]

On the other hand, the degree of recovery varies greatly from patient to patient depending on the severity of deficit, side, age, and commencement of stroke rehabilitation – usually an earlier start will lead to a better outcome. In general, younger age, mild to moderate disability at admission, and absence of cognitive disturbances lead to a better outcome.[12] Another important factor affecting outcome is the availability of social and financial support.

Although there is general consensus that rehabilitation is more effective when delivered early after stroke, several studies have suggested that the therapy services provided to selected chronic stroke patients may also result in functional improvements, and this is a strong ongoing theme in stroke rehabilitation research.

Ideally stroke rehabilitation should begin within the first 24 hours of stroke, and if possible in a stroke unit. Several systematic literature reviews have reported superior stroke outcome in comprehensive multidisciplinary stroke units compared to mixed wards.[14–16] The major difference between these two groups was the interdisciplinary team approach for patients treated on stroke units rather than specific differences in acute medical management, so it seems likely that the improved outcomes may be due to in part at least to coordinated interdisciplinary rehabilitation.[17] However, it is also important to keep in mind that a comprehensive multidisciplinary stroke unit is labor intensive and expensive.

THE COMPREHENSIVE MULTIDISCIPLINARY STROKE TEAM

The comprehensive multidisciplinary stroke team should include stroke neurologists, physiatrists, internal medicine physicians, stroke specialized nursing staff, physiotherapists, occupational therapists, speech therapists, orthotists, social workers, recreation therapists, psychologists, and dietitians. Although not every patient needs all of these services, those that are required should be well coordinated. A member of the team should also ascertain the family's attitude and expectations, and their ability to care for the patient, if necessary. Education of the family or caregivers is an important role of the team.[12,13] The ultimate goal of stroke rehabilitation is to achieve the highest possible level of recovery and independence and therefore a crucial axiom of the stroke team is goal setting for an individual patient.

The comprehensive multidisciplinary stroke team should develop realistic short- and long-term goals, including plans for hospital-based care, outpatient programs, long-term care facility programs, and home-based programs according to particular profile and need of each stroke patient. Goals and care plans should be reevaluated on a regular basis and adjusted as the abilities and needs of the patient change.

THE CLINICAL SPECTRUM OF REHABILITATION SERVICES

The optimal organization of stroke services is still debated and varies across countries.[17] Rehabilitation can occur in many different settings.[12,18] Basic rehabilitation begins immediately after stroke, while the patient is still undergoing acute treatment.

More advanced rehabilitation training should progress as quickly as the patient's clinical condition allows in the acute care hospital. Further rehabilitation may occur in other settings, depending on availability and the needs of the individual patient. In most Western countries, stroke patients with functional deficits who are medically stable and have adequate cognitive function are transferred to specialized rehabilitation hospitals or units. In addition to medical stability, patients must be able to participate in 3 hours of daily therapy and have a reasonable expectation of resuming community living. The average length of stay for a stroke patient in rehabilitation units is approximately 2 weeks. Those unable to tolerate an intensive program because of the severity of deficit, concurrent illness, age, or lack of social support usually are placed in a hospital-based or skilled nursing-based subacute program, which may last several weeks to months.[19,20] Those eventually able to return home, but for whom community mobility is still a major problem, usually qualify for home-based rehabilitation services several times a week, and often for home health aides to assist with ADLs. People living in the community who are not classified as home bound are candidates for rehabilitation programs in outpatient clinics, where intensity and length of services vary considerably.

The economics of health care have resulted in shorter lengths of stay in rehabilitation hospitals and units.[21] However, there is evidence that patients are now being discharged with decreased functional gains.[22] There is also strong pressure for provision of rehabilitation in less costly settings than rehabilitation hospitals and units.[17,21] In the United States, there has been rapid growth of postacute rehabilitation programs in outpatient clinics, skilled nursing facilities, and through home health agencies.[18] These programs are less expensive and generally provide less intensive services. Nevertheless, services for stroke survivors living at home can be effective.[23,24] Decisions regarding the appropriate location for rehabilitation services should take into consideration not only the individual needs of the patient, but also the cost for such services. In the United States, guidelines provided by third-party payers, including Medicare, and rehabilitation accrediting agencies heavily influence where rehabilitation is provided.[18]

EARLY MOBILIZATION

The literature has highlighted the negative effects of prolonged immobility due to any cause, and stroke patients should be mobilized as soon as they are medically stable.[25] Prolonged immobilization results in muscle weakness and general debility. The net result is delayed recovery, a prolonged hospital stay, and increased health care costs. Despite this knowledge, there is evidence that patients with stroke spend more than 50% of their time in bed during the first 2 weeks following stroke onset.[26]

Early mobilization helps prevent secondary complications of stroke, including deep venous thrombosis, skin breakdown leading to pressure ulcer, pulmonary atelectasis, risk of aspiration, and contractures.[25] Early mobilization also has a positive psychological impact and facilitates earlier ambulation and better performance in activities of daily living.

The frequency and intensity of mobilization depend on the condition of each patient. Passive range-of-motion exercises should be initiated even in comatose patients once clinically feasible. Patients with reasonable alertness, stable vital signs, and adequate oxygenation can usually be up with assistance in a chair by 48 hours. As soon as possible, the patient should be taught to roll independently in bed and to go from supine to sitting. However, blood pressure should be monitored for orthostatic hypotension.[27] The patient should progressively advance from a sitting position, transferring from the bed to a chair and/or commode, standing, and finally walking.

A formal therapy program should begin as soon as possible, as patients who start therapy early after stroke have a better therapeutic response.[12,28,29] As active range of motion returns, it should be facilitated by therapists and the patient encouraged to engage the hemiparetic limb in functional activities. There is evidence that prolonged immobilization leads to "learned non-use" of the hemiparetic side with deleterious effects at the cortical level. Recent evidence shows that the longer it takes to engage the more affected side in relearning of skills, the longer it will take to reverse the "learned non-use."

On the other hand, use of the unaffected extremities may be necessary to assist in activities of daily living and mobility in many instances, especially at earlier stages post-stroke. For example, the patient can be taught to hook the normal foot under the affected ankle, and pull the weak leg to the side of the bed in preparation to sit or transfer. Transfers from the bed to a chair or a commode should be taught as soon as feasible. These activities should initially be practiced only with a trained therapist or nurse to prevent falls. Supervised training is especially important for patients who are impulsive or have visuospatial neglect.

Ambulation is a major goal after stroke and is eventually achieved by approximately 75% of patients.[3,30] Walking may not be possible initially, and proficiency in propelling a wheelchair is an important intermediate step. Ambulation provides a measure of independence and boosts confidence. Because hemiparetic patients must use their unaffected limbs to propel a wheelchair, the seat of the chair must be 1 to 2 inches lower than a standard wheelchair to allow the normal foot to be placed on the floor to pedal the chair. The unaffected hand is used to propel a wheel of the chair and assist in steering.

PREVENTING CONTRACTURES AND PRESSURE ULCERS

For all patients, appropriate care must be taken to prevent contractures that may delay functional recovery and restrict the potential of the patient to recover. The basic tenets of prevention are regular range of motion exercises, proper positioning in an anatomical and functional position, and preventing injury to the paretic extremities.

Active and passive range-of-motion exercises should be performed at regular intervals and initiated in bed as soon as possible. Patients should be taught to gently move their own paralyzed limbs with intact ones. Until then, nurses, physical therapists, or members of the family must move them through their full range of motion at least twice daily to prevent contractures. Hypertonicity due to spasticity increases the risk for contractions.[31] In patients with spasticity, range of motion needs to be performed more frequently.

During the flaccid stage, careful positioning of the limbs also prevents contractures and pressure ulcers. To prevent shortening of the Achilles tendon, a brace, cushioned boot, or high-top tennis shoe may be used. Care must be taken with any of these interventions to avoid undue pressure on the heels and elbows. The lateral side of the leg may be supported to prevent contracture of the hip in external rotation. A pillow may be placed in the axilla of the affected arm to maintain abduction. A resting splint can be used to maintain the fingers in a physiological position that lessens the likelihood of contracture.[32] If edema develops, the hand may be elevated on a pillow to keep it higher than the shoulder or an elastic glove may be applied.

When a fixed contracture is already present and restricts the full potential of function, a vigorous range-of-motion program should be undertaken, dynamic splinting may be applied to gradually increase range of motion, or a surgical intervention can be considered as a last resort.

Patients should be turned every 2 hours to prevent pressure ulcers. The best practice is to position the patient on the right side, then on the back, then on the left side, then back on the right side, then repeating this sequence. This minimizes the time spent lying on the back, reducing the chances of ulcers of the sacrum, heels, or occiput. Staff should examine the patient daily for any areas of nonblanching erythema of the skin over body prominences, an early sign of excessive pressure.

SHOULDER PAIN

The shoulder is a highly mobile joint that depends heavily on the rotator cuff muscles for stability (Figure 26-2), making it very vulnerable to injury, especially during the flaccid period just after a stroke. When the rotator cuff is weak, the pain-sensitive structures in and about the joint are easily injured, resulting in a variety of painful conditions, including subdeltoid bursitis, supraspinatus tendinitis, brachial plexopathy, or rotator cuff tears.[33] Inadvertent injury occurs during traction on the arm during transfers, poor positioning of the arm in the bed or chair, or forceful abduction of the shoulder. Another common problem is stretching of the joint capsule due to subluxation of the humeral head out of the glenoid fossa because of rotator cuff weakness. Although subluxation itself does not result in pain, it

is an indication of muscle weakness of the rotator cuff, which predisposes the shoulder to the conditions noted earlier.

A painful shoulder due to one or more of these factors occurs in up to 80% of stroke patients, but severe pain can often be avoided if preventive measures are undertaken.[33–35] Prevention of shoulder pain should focus on anatomically and functionally correct positioning and avoiding forceful range of motion exercises. Careful positioning of the shoulder and support of the weak arm on a wheelchair arm trough or lap tray when up in a wheelchair, or on a pillow while up in a standard chair, is advisable.[33] It is especially important to avoid traction or torsion to the shoulder when transferring the patient to a chair. A pull sheet is sometimes used to transfer the patient from the wheelchair to the bed or vice versa. When patients are able to perform self-range of motion, they should be instructed to avoid forceful movements.

Injury of the shoulder can lead to chronic pain, restriction of functional capacity and/or "frozen" shoulder. The most bothersome syndrome of shoulder pain after stroke is the shoulder-hand syndrome. It is thought to be a form of complex regional pain syndrome and may be present in as many as 25% of patients post-stroke. This syndrome includes pain in the hand and shoulder, hand swelling, stiffness, discoloration, and occasionally trophic changes. The cause is unclear, but most authorities consider it to be a sequela to one or more of other painful shoulder syndromes mentioned previously, immobilization, and possibly changes in muscle tone and decreased venous return. Shoulder-hand syndrome often occurs 1 to 2 months after the onset of stroke, and is frequently seen for the first time in the outpatient clinic.

Painful shoulder should be prevented, but once present, it should be treated with positioning, careful and progressive range-of-motion exercises, electrical stimulation, heat, anti-inflammatory agents, analgesics, and other measures.[11,33] These measures are also usually effective for shoulder-hand syndrome, but occasionally a short course of oral corticosteroid therapy or a stellate ganglion block is necessary.

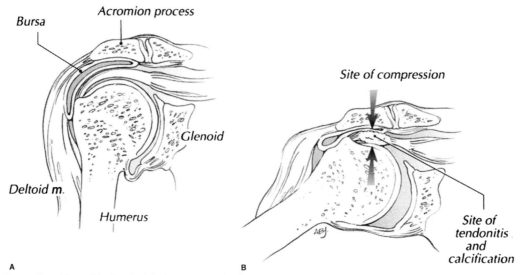

Figure 26-2. A: Normal position of the head of the humerus in the glenoid fossa. Joint stability is highly dependent on the rotator cuff, including the deltoid and supraspinatus muscles pictured here. B: When the rotator cuff is weak, there are abnormal relationships between the humeral head and pain-sensitive structures in and about the shoulder. During passive abduction, compression of the sub-deltoid bursa and supraspinatus tendon may occur.

MANAGEMENT OF SPASTICITY

Spasticity is often used to describe a constellation of findings included in the "upper motor neuron" syndrome, including hyperactive muscle stretch reflexes, increased muscle tone, muscle co-contraction, and synergistic ("pattern") motor movements.[36] It can be observed in up to 65% of patients after stroke and is occasionally debilitating. In the lower extremity, spasticity causes excessive plantar flexion and foot inversion. In the upper extremity, spasticity may increase shoulder pain, or result in functional impairments due to flexion of the elbow, wrist, or fingers. Appropriate management prevents fixed contracture and restriction of functional independence. Treatment includes a wide array of interventions such as proper positioning, stretching, splinting, and pharmacological approaches. Depending on the severity of spasticity and individual needs of the patient, *Botulinum* toxin may be used for focal spasticity. It has been shown to be effective and well tolerated to improve range of motion and prevent contractures.[37,38] Recent studies show it may result in functional improvements in selected patients.[38] Drugs such as baclofen, benzodiazepines, and tizanidine are occasionally tried for generalized spasticity;[36,39] however, because of sedative side effects and possible deleterious effects on motor recovery, these drugs should be used with caution. In occasional patients with severe generalized or segmental spasticity, intrathecal baclofen delivered by an implanted pump may be considered.[36]

AMBULATION

Ambulation is a key goal of stroke rehabilitation, and most patients and families consider independent ambulation to be an important outcome. As a general rule, household ambulation is usually possible when the preferred walking speed is 0.4 m/sec. Limited community walking is possible for patients with preferred walking speeds between 0.4 and 0.8 m/sec, while 0.8 m/sec is required for general community ambulation.

The key muscle groups necessary for standing activities are the hip and knee extensors. For the swing phase of gait, the hip flexors, knee flexors, and ankle dorsiflexors are the most important muscles. For "push off" from stance to swing phase, the ankle plantar flexors assume an important role.

When the patient is able to sit with good balance, standing practice and gait training begin.[40,41] If there is significant weakness of the hip flexors, a therapist may need to assist with advancing the leg. Patients with severe quadriceps weakness may not be able to lock the knee in stable extension during the stance phase of gait, also requiring the physical assistance of the therapist. While difficult, optimal biomechanical and neuromotor pattern of gait should be pursued, avoiding gait deviations if possible. The patient should be encouraged to place as much weight as possible on the paretic leg.

Standing and walking are especially difficult for those with nondominant parietal lobe lesions, because they tend to neglect the affected extremities. In some, neglect is much more disabling than weakness, and patients may appear to "push" toward their affected side with their unaffected leg. Feedback through verbal repetition and tactile cues is very important for all patients at this stage. Impaired proprioception or body awareness can be compensated by use of a full-length mirror showing the patient the orientation of his or her body.

As the patient improves, assisted gait may begin using a hemi-walker or wide-based quad cane. Patients with vertebrobasilar

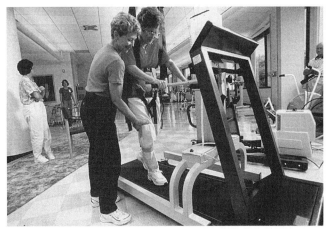

Figure 26-3. Patient with a stroke in the left anterior cerebral artery distribution with weakness in right leg undergoing gait training using treadmill with partial body weight support.

stroke and truncal ataxia rather than weakness may require a traditional walker. With additional improvement, the hemiparetic patient may progress to ambulation with a narrow-based quad cane, a straight cane, and eventually no assistive device.

Eventually, more complex gait activities, including walking over uneven ground or in crowded situations, should be practiced. Negotiating stairs is another important goal, and may be important when returning home.

The previous discussion applies to patients with moderately severe neurological deficits. People with milder stroke may begin walking immediately with supervision, although sometimes a cane is required.

Task-specific physiotherapy programs focusing on gait have been shown to promote ambulation early after stroke. Several novel techniques to enhance ambulation have been proposed. Treadmill training with partial body weight support may be useful for patients who do not have the strength or balance to do over ground therapy for ambulation.[40-43] In this technique, the body weight is partially supported over a moving treadmill, and the treadmill initially starts at slow speeds, with the therapist assisting the paretic leg in a normal gait pattern (Figure 26-3). As the person improves, the supporting harness provides less help, more of the patient's weight is borne on the treadmill, and treadmill speeds are gradually increased. Treadmill training with partial weight support has not yet been proven to be effective,[44] and this technique is currently being tested in a large multicenter randomized controlled trial.[45] In some patients, over ground training without a treadmill may be attempted using weight support. Another treatment combines body weight support and a treadmill, but uses a robotic device attached to the lower extremities to provide a normal ambulation pattern. This is currently marketed under several trade names, and although preliminary trials are encouraging, it is still not conclusively proven superior to other training techniques at this time.

ORTHOSES (BRACES)

The purposes of orthoses are to compensate for muscle weakness, joint instability, and/or deformity. While many adaptive devices are designed for a specific task or activity such as feeding or bathing, orthoses take into account the functioning of a specific body part such as the leg for standing and ambulation.

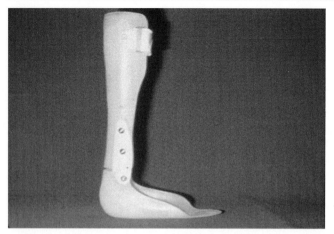

Figure 26-4. A custom-fabricated, lightweight ankle-foot orthosis with a hinged ankle joint. The joint allows free active dorsiflexion but prevents excessive plantar flexion.

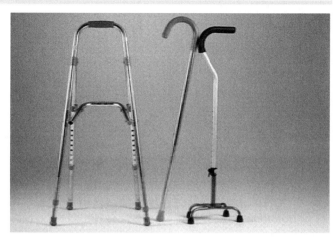

Figure 26-5. Several commonly used assistive devices for ambulation after hemiparesis, including (from right to left) a hemiwalker (walker cane), standard J-neck cane, and four-pronged quad cane.

Many patients benefit from a lower extremity orthosis. The best example is the patient who has difficulty clearing the foot during the swing phase of gait because of weakness of ankle dorsiflexion or excessive plantar flexion (Figure 26-4). In this situation, a properly designed ankle-foot orthosis (AFO) can significantly improve the biomechanics of gait.[46,47] Other patients who may benefit from an AFO are hemiparetics with mediolateral ankle instability and those with certain types of knee instability. Changing the angle of the ankle affects the force moments at the knee during ambulation. If the knee tends to buckle during weight bearing, increasing the amount of plantar flexion by a maximum of 5 to 8 degrees can bring it more quickly into extension and prevent buckling. For patients with knee hyperextension as the major problem, increasing ankle dorsiflexion in the AFO can reduce the hyperextension, although greater quadriceps strength is required to prevent the knee from collapsing in flexion. There is evidence that use of an AFO can improve walking speed in patients with hemiparesis, and may also improve balance.[47–49] The use of long leg bracing for stroke patients with severe knee weakness is controversial and seldom used.

All orthoses have their drawbacks. Custom-made orthoses are usually preferable but are expensive and need to be carefully designed to avoid pressure areas. Although orthoses can assist in the performance of some movements, they can impair others. If an orthosis does not provide a definite biomechanical advantage, the patient will usually abandon it. To ensure best results, consultation among physician, physical therapist, and an orthotist experienced in hemiparetic bracing is necessary. Cost, long-term goals, and the individual's needs should be considered when prescribing an orthosis. Because functional recovery is not a static process, the need for the orthoses should be readdressed periodically according to the level of impairment.

Upper extremity orthoses have a more limited role in stroke rehabilitation. A resting splint to maintain the hand and wrist in a neutral position in patients with plegia may help prevent contractures and prevent hand pain.[32]

ASSISTIVE DEVICES FOR AMBULATION

The two major reasons for use of these devices are to shift weight from the weak extremity and to provide improved balance while walking.[12,50,51] Most stroke patients with weakness require a cane, because hand weakness usually prevents their gripping a walker. Canes come in various styles, beginning with the standard J-shaped cane and progressing trough quad canes to walker canes, which have widely separated legs (Figure 26-5). Although they provide more stability, four-pronged (quad) canes are more difficult to maneuver on stairs and in crowded areas. All canes require some training for proper sequencing during ambulation and while ascending and descending stairs. This can be a challenge for the cognitively impaired and those with motor apraxia. The practice of merely carrying a cane without contact to the ground is potentially dangerous and should be avoided. Canes should be carried in the strong (uninvolved) hand. The proper height for any cane should be the distance from the floor to the wrist crease with the patient upright, arm extended. The handle should be at the level of the wrist crease when the cane is resting on the floor. When the cane is used, the elbow should be flexed approximately 15 degrees.

WHEELCHAIRS

Most stroke patients use a wheelchair immediately after the ictus, and some patients with restricted ability to walk will use one indefinitely. Even patients with good ability to walk may require a wheelchair for long-distance mobilization since hemiparetic gait requires high energy cost. They should be prescribed according to the individual needs of the patient, the environmental requirement, cost, and the wishes of the patient and family.[52,53]

Designs are variable but safety, comfort, and posture while seated and mobility in the community are crucial features to consider. In general, the seat should be lower than the standard wheelchair to allow propulsion with the nonaffected leg. The seat should be narrow enough to allow the patient to maneuver the wheel with the nonaffected upper extremity. The standard height of a wheelchair seat is 19 to 20 inches from the floor, but a hemiparetic patient should have a seat 17.5 to 18 inches from the floor, with a detachable footplate to allow the patient to propel the chair with the strong arm and leg. Arm and leg rests should be removable to facilitate transfers. Brake extenders may easily be added so that the patient can use the strong hand to reach across and lock the wheel on the affected side. Special devices are available on most chairs to prevent

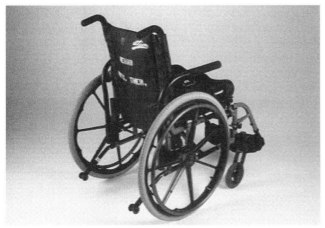

Figure 26-6. A wheelchair with standard foam cushion and commonly prescribed features, including swing-away leg rests, wheel grips to facilitate propulsion, pneumatic tires, and anti-tip bars.

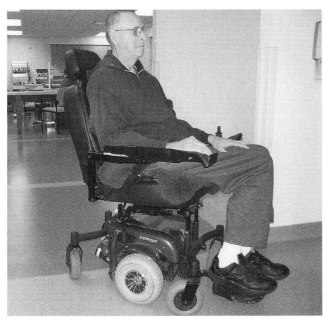

Figure 26-7. Nonambulatory patient with right hemiparesis who uses a power wheelchair. Note arm trough for support of paretic arm.

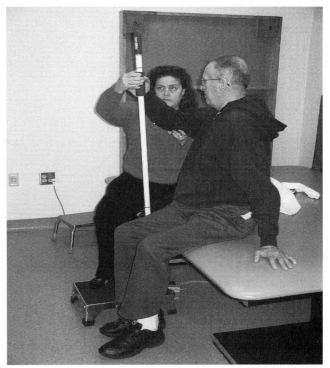

Figure 26-8. Therapist working with patient with paretic arm, spasticity, and shoulder pain. Goals are strengthening, improved active range of motion, decreased hypertonicity, and decreased shoulder pain.

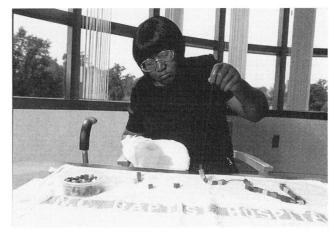

Figure 26-9. Patient with left hemiparesis receiving constraint-induced movement therapy (CIMT). She is repetitively placing beads on a string, a very difficult task for her. Note "mitt" on her right hand to prevent its involvement in this task.

backward movement while wheeling uphill. An arm trough or lap tray should be added if the arm is plegic to provide adequate support, minimize shoulder subluxation, and prevent the arm from failing off the chair or catching in the wheel (an occasional occurrence in patients with neglect). If a lap board is used, a clear plastic type allows the patient to see his or her feet and the ground ahead. If severe weakness is present, a removable or swing-away arm rest should be provided to facilitate transfers. The hammock effect of sling seats can result in asymmetric posture, which can be improved using a solid (but cushioned) seat and backboard. Care should be taken to prevent excessive ischial or sacral pressure.

Some stroke patients who are in a wheelchair for extended periods of time need a special cushion to ensure even weight distribution. Most stroke patients can use standard lightweight wheelchairs for community mobility (Figure 26-6). It should be light enough to be easily placed in an automobile. However, for nonambulatory stroke patients, a wheelchair is an invaluable means of mobility, even in the home, and must be more carefully designed.[52,53] In patients with good cognitive function, adequate balance, and ability to safely transfer on and off the seat, a motorized scooter can be considered for community mobility. These tend to be most appropriate for patients who can ambulate short distances in the home, but not in the community.

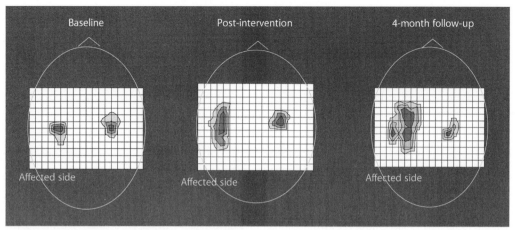

Figure 26-10. Longitudinal changes in a two-dimensional motor map obtained by using transcranial magnetic stimulation (TMS) over the motor cortex of each hemisphere in a patient receiving CIMT after stroke. The grid size is 1 cm, and motor responses at each scalp position are coded by intensity (relative to the maximal response). Note expansion of the motor map over the affected hemisphere associated with CIMT, which persists at 4 months.

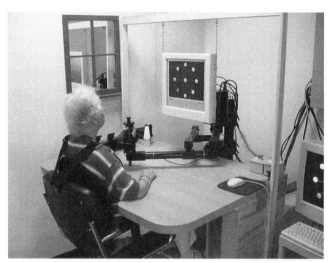

Figure 26-11. Patient undergoing robot-assisted training following stroke. The patient is presented with a visual stimulus on the computer screen and asked to move the cursor to the stimulus. Used with permission of Dr. Igo Krebs.

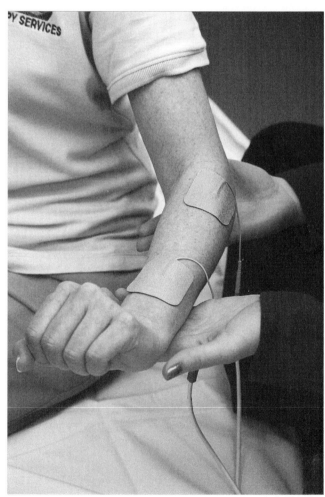

Figure 26-12. Functional electrical stimulation applied over the wrist extensors to facilitate motor movement.

Some health plans do not reimburse for these devices, requiring the patient to pay privately. Power wheelchairs are not usually required for stroke survivors except in cases of severe weakness, or co-morbid lower extremity conditions severely limiting mobility (Figure 26-7). They must be carefully prescribed, as the patient may be seated in the chair for extended periods of time.

ENHANCING MOTOR RECOVERY

The most common approach to enhance motor recovery are programs of physical and occupational therapy. A surprising number of theories of physical therapy have evolved over the years. Some carry the names of their proponents, including Bobath, Brunnstrom, and Rood, and most were based on concepts developed in the 1950s and 1960s. One of the most famous, the Bobath approach (also known as neurodevelopmental therapy), stresses the importance of normal patterns of movement, suppression of spasticity, and use of proprioceptive feedback to facilitate motor control. Despite its widespread use, it has not been proven superior to other techniques.[54] More recent approaches have stressed the practice of motor tasks in the context of specific functional skills. Because there is no compelling evidence that one method is superior to another, most modern therapists integrate components of two or more philosophies into their treatment regimens. Although the efficacy of specific therapy philosophies is unproven, most rehabilitation professionals believe that therapy accelerates and improves recovery, regardless of which specific philosophy is chosen (Figure 26-8). However, there is increasing evidence from randomized controlled trials that task-oriented training, especially when applied intensively early after stroke, is the best approach to facilitate motor recovery.[55,56]

In recent years, a number of newer techniques to enhance recovery have been studied. Constraint-induced movement therapy (CIMT) is the best example. A "mitt" (which acts as the constraint) is applied to the unaffected hand, forcing the person to use the stroke-affected hand for a series of intensive functionally related tasks (Figure 26-9). To be effective, the subject must be motivated, and have some residual motor use of the affected hand. In a large randomized controlled trial, CIMT was superior to a control group receiving no therapy when assessed 3 to 9 months after stroke.[57] This treatment is very labor intensive and not practical for all patients. Interestingly, functional MRI and transcranial magnetic stimulation (TMS) data suggest that there is cortical reorganization of motor neural networks following CIMT and other intensive training (Figure 26-10). Another new treatment is robotic enhanced recovery (Figure 26-11). A number of preliminary studies using a variety of robot designs have suggested that a properly designed training program can improve upper extremity function.[58,59] This treatment must await the results of randomized controlled trials before being widely accepted. Robotic devices have also been designed for the lower extremities, especially to assist training of ambulation. Other proposed treatments include direct cortical stimulation with repetitive TMS or direct current transcranial electrical stimulation.[60] Another strategy is to increase peripheral sensory input in the hope that this will increase cortical motor excitability, therefore promoting recovery.

Functional electrical stimulation is a term that includes several techniques to stimulate peripheral nerves and muscles in persons with hemiparesis (Figure 26-12). There is some suggestion that this may enhance recovery in some patients,[59,61,62] and

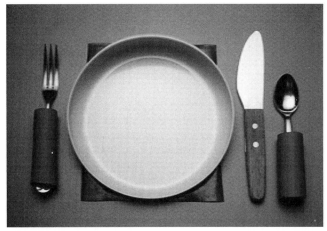

Figure 26-13. Adapted eating utensils, including built-up handles on spoon and fork, a rocker knife for one-handed cutting, a plate with raised edge, and a special surface to prevent the plate from sliding on the table.

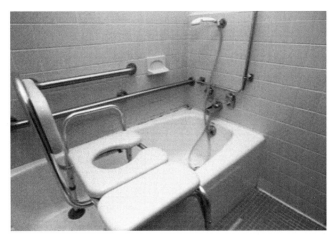

Figure 26-14. An adapted bathtub, including several types of grab-bars, a hand-held shower nozzle, and bathtub transfer bench on which the patient may safely sit.

functional electrical stimulation is now widely used in many rehabilitation facilities.

ACTIVITIES OF DAILY LIVING

One of the most important rehabilitation goals after stroke is the resumption of independence in the performance of ADLs. The ability to dress, feed, bathe, and toilet not only adds immensely to a person's sense of self-worth, but also decreases the burden on families or caregivers.[63]

Occupational therapists are skilled at teaching patients to relearn skills of daily living after stroke, but accomplishment of those activities may be difficult without modifying the strategies of the tasks.[64] For example, patients can be taught by therapists to start dressing the paretic limb first when wearing a shirt or jacket. As patients improve, they should be encouraged to resume their own ADLs, using the affected extremities as much as possible.

After returning home, some patients need adaptive equipment. Countless types of adaptive devices are available today to help the patient in becoming more functional and independent.[12]

Adaptive devices for feeding (Figure 26-13), dressing, hygiene, reading, and writing are frequently prescribed for stroke patients. Many stroke survivors need a commode or a bath tub bench for bathing (Figure 26-14). Because functional recovery may occur over months, the need for adaptive devices and equipment should be reassessed periodically. If properly selected, there is evidence that they are used long term.[65] The home may need to be adapted by building ramps, moving furniture, and widening doorways. Finally, for patients with limited functional recovery, the family or caregivers may need to be instructed in providing the ADL functions that the patient cannot perform alone.

It is important to keep in mind that adaptive devices should not circumvent the potential of the patient to relearn skills. That is to say, if the patient has the potential to improve function, he or she should be encouraged to engage in tasks with progressive complexity, limiting the use of adaptive devices.

The term instrumental ADLs (IADLs) is used to describe a higher set of activities beyond basic self-care. Examples include shopping, telephone use, preparation of simple meals, ability to do light housekeeping, and ability to manage personal finances. Because these functions are important for independent community living, they should be assessed by an occupational therapist once a patient has become proficient in basic ADLs, especially if the patient will be living alone with limited social support.

PREVENTION AND TREATMENT OF DEEP VENOUS THROMBOSIS

Deep venous thrombosis (DVT) is an important preventable cause of mortality due to subsequent pulmonary embolism and should be always addressed in stroke patients who have difficulty with walking.

Clinical signs and symptoms are not very reliable, and many patients remain asymptomatic. However, in the presence of unilateral leg swelling, leg pain that can be elicited by forceful dorsiflexion of the foot (Homans sign), low-grade fever, tenderness of the leg, or increased temperature of the leg, DVT should be strongly suspected. Diagnostic studies include Duplex ultrasonography and the D-dimer assay. Although occurring in only a small minority of patients with DVT, pulmonary embolism is the most dangerous complication. Symptoms such as chest pain, upper abdominal pain, hemoptysis, shortness of breath, or back or shoulder pain should be assessed on an emergency basis. Spiral computerized tomography (CT) of the chest is the diagnostic procedure of choice, but some patients require magnetic resonance or conventional arteriography. Stroke patients at risk for DVT should be prescribed subcutaneous unfractionated or low molecular weight heparin.[11,12,66] Physical aids, especially pneumatic compression devices, may be useful.[12,67] Prophylaxis should be continued until the patient is able to ambulate regularly. As a general guideline, DVT prophylaxis can be discontinued when a patient is able to ambulate 150 feet several times daily. Treatment of established DVT or pulmonary embolism includes anticoagulation with warfarin or high-dose low molecular weight heparin for 3 months. When anticoagulation is contraindicated, percutaneous insertion of an inferior vena cava filter is indicated.

MANAGEMENT OF DYSPHAGIA

Dysphagia involves difficulty eating due to disruption of normal swallowing mechanisms; it can lead to aspiration pneumonia,

malnutrition, and weight loss.[12] Aspiration should be suspected in stroke patients with coughing or choking when swallowing, sialorrhea, change in voice (wet or gurgly voice), oral or nasal regurgitation, impaired cough associated with absence of the gag reflex, or in the presence of recurrent pneumonia.[68,69] However, about half of patients with aspiration have no symptoms ("silent aspirators").[70] Following evaluation by a speech therapist, an X-ray swallowing study (video fluoroscopy, also called modified barium swallow) should be performed if aspiration is suspected.[12,69] An alternative diagnostic test consists of direct visualization of swallowing (fiberoptic endoscopic evaluation of swallowing-FEES). Dietary modification, head positioning, exercise and facilitatory techniques to strengthen swallowing muscles, are common treatment approaches but their effectiveness to improve swallowing remains controversial.[12,69,71] Electric stimulation has also been used to improve swallowing with mixed results.[72,73] It is often necessary to provide nutrition using a small-diameter nasogastric tube, and when no improvement is evident within 2 or 3 weeks, a percutaneous gastrostomy tube (PEG) is indicated.

MANAGEMENT OF BOWEL AND BLADDER DYSFUNCTION

Urinary and fecal incontinence are common after stroke but usually resolve spontaneously within 2 to 4 weeks.[12,74,75] Persistent cases of incontinence are often associated with severe stroke and poor prognosis. Continued incontinence has been shown to be an independent factor in predicting discharge to a long-term care facility, as this is a difficult problem for many families to deal with at home. Incontinence is more common in patients with cognitive impairment.[76] Neurogenic bladder such as hypertonic bladder with urge incontinence or hypotonic bladder leading to overflow incontinence is a common cause of urinary incontinence. However, many patients have normal bladder function but are sufficiently confused or aphasic that they simply cannot ask for assistance.[76] An individual urinary function profile should be created, listing the volume of fluid intake, frequency and volume of voiding, post-void residual urine measurements, and presence or absence of dysuria. If an indwelling catheter was used during the acute phase after stroke, every effort should be made to remove it. Urinary tract infection is the most common medical complication following stroke,[10] and the risk of UTI increases with catheterization.[11,12] A UTI may also cause bladder irritability, aggravating incontinence. A timed voiding program is effective in most cases of incontinence but intermittent catheterization may be necessary in the transitional period if post-void residual volume remains high (more than 100 ml).[12]

After the first weeks of stroke, constipation becomes more common than fecal incontinence.[12] Inactivity, insufficient fluid intake, and depression are among the common causes of constipation. Bowel training appears to be more successful when the schedule follows the routine habits of the patient before stroke.[11,12] In a majority of cases, diets with appropriate fiber, stool softeners, and fluids resolve the problem, but laxatives need to be prescribed for some patients.

MANAGEMENT OF APHASIA

Between 20% and 40% of stroke patients have impaired expression or comprehension of language.[12,77,78] The plight of a hemiplegic, globally aphasic patient is frustrating for all, as the patient can neither understand language nor speak. The individual's dependent isolation is often accentuated by the attitudes of other people. Many individuals retain some comprehension, so any discussion carried on in his or her presence should keep this in mind. Various subcategories of aphasia have been defined on the basis of the patient's fluency, ability to repeat, and language comprehension (see Table 2-1). Aphasias are often divided into fluent aphasia (with retained comprehension), nonfluent aphasia (with difficulty "expressing" themselves) and several mixed types.[79] Diagnostic evaluation includes assessment of the patient's ability to repeat, comprehend words, name objects, and follow commands. Many patients do not fit neatly into one of the classic aphasia types.

Individuals with aphasia should be encouraged to communicate by signs, sounds, and facial expressions. Aphasia is rarely an isolated disturbance; reading, writing, understanding, speaking, and calculations are all impaired, although to different degrees in different forms of aphasia. The entire process of language symbolization is disturbed, making a global approach necessary. Emotional lability, suppressed anger, frustration, and a fear of the future often compound the problem.

Fortunately, many individuals with aphasia improve over time, even without treatment.[78,79] Speech rehabilitation requires a motivated subject, a patient therapist, and an understanding family. The effectiveness of formal speech therapy in promoting actual improvement in speech and language function is hard to prove, although specific treatment techniques are useful for individual patients. Several meta-analyses have suggested that treatment is generally helpful.[12,80,81] Speech therapy requires hard work, the goal of which is not words, but communication. Several investigations have shown that intense treatment (at least 2 hours per day for at least 4 days per week) is more effective than a similar number of sessions spread out over a longer period.[3,82]

Some patients do well in a group of aphasic patients who relearn together with a speech therapist, but more often, individual therapy sessions are more successful. Usually the patient can comprehend gestures better than the spoken or written word; multilingual patients may find it simpler to comprehend his or her native tongue. Others find melodic intonations a way to circumvent their aphasia to some degree. The primary goals are to assist the patient to develop strategies to compensate for common intonations and to educate people in the patient's environment to facilitate communication.[12]

Pharmacotherapy for aphasia is an appealing concept, and many medications have been tried, including bromocriptine, amphetamine, antidepressants, and donepezil. However, there is no conclusive evidence that any of these are effective.[79,83] The evidence favoring piracetam, while not conclusive, is more encouraging.[84] Direct brain stimulation using transcranial magnetic stimulation (TMS) or transcranial direct current stimulation (tDCS) has been attempted to improve language functioning.[85] Although early results are encouraging, far more research is necessary before these techniques can be used in clinical practice.

The degree and rapidity with which patients regain use of language varies considerably. Generally, a very young child with aphasia has a better prognosis than an adult with a similar lesion, and a left-handed aphasic has a better prognosis than one who is right-handed. Recent studies of right hand dominant stroke patients using functional neuroimaging have shown that the right (nondominant) hemisphere, especially the inferior frontal cortex, also becomes active during speech, a phenomenon not seen in nonaphasic persons.[86] Whether this is compensatory or a mere consequence of damage to the left-sided homologous speech areas is still a matter of discussion.

MANAGEMENT OF NEGLECT

Neglect is a general term that refers to asymmetric inattention to stimuli (visual or sensory) or motor function on the side of the body opposite the stroke.[12] Usually, neglect occurs with right hemisphere lesions, but it also occurs with left hemisphere stroke. A syndrome that sometimes accompanies neglect is anosognosia, the inability to appreciate a neurological deficit.[87] Some patients with anosognosia can be quite adamant that they do not have weakness or other impairments that are quite obvious to everyone else. All stroke neurologists have occasionally seen patients who will even deny that their paretic arm is their own. The term spatial neglect refers to difficulty attending to one side of space. This is often accompanied by visual or sensory neglect and can be quite debilitating. Patients with this syndrome may have profound difficulty caring for the affected side of the body, including difficulty with dressing, cleaning, grooming, and feeding. Fairly common scenarios are the stroke patient who neglects the food on the left side of the plate, the person who completely misses words on the left side of the page, or the man who neglects to shave the left side of his face. Simple tests for hemispatial neglect include asking a patient to cross out all lines on a page or to draw a clock.[88,89] Another common test is to ask the patient to copy a figure drawn by the examiner. Other testing may include examination for extinction via double simultaneous stimulation in the visual or tactile domains.

No single treatment is accepted for neglect.[12,90] A novel intervention for hemispatial neglect is the use of a prism, which displaces objects in the left visual field towards the right.[91,92] Sensory stimulation on the side of neglect, eye patching, and virtual reality environments to facilitate attention to the neglected side have all been tried with varying degrees of success. Vestibular stimulation is another strategy that at least temporarily improves neglect. A variety of cognitively based rehabilitation interventions are often commonly tried by rehabilitation therapists, but studies have suggested that the immediate effect on disability is small and generally not persistent.[93]

A number of pharmacological treatments have been tried including amphetamines, amantadine, and guanfacine, a noradrenergic agonist.

A number of studies have suggested that persons with neglect following stroke have a longer hospital stay and greater long-term disability.[83,94] Fortunately, as with many other stroke-related impairments, neglect syndromes often improve over time, although when neglect persists it may become the most limiting factor in attaining a functional recovery.

DIAGNOSIS AND MANAGEMENT OF DEPRESSION

Depression is common after stroke and often is diagnosed during rehabilitation rather than immediately following the acute stroke.[3,12] Prevalence ranges from 20% to 80% depending greatly on the tools of assessment. Depression is relatively underdiagnosed and undertreated. Depressed stroke patients have greater cognitive impairments and increased mortality compared to nondepressed patients.[95] Remission of depression is associated with improved functional abilities.[96,97] Depression can be a result of the mourning of loss of function (psychosocial hypothesis) or due to alteration of brain neurotransmitter function after stroke (biological hypothesis).[98]

Depression should be suspected when a patient demonstrates apathy, constant fatigue, sleep disturbance, appetite changes, or suicidal thoughts. Crying and overt sadness have been shown to be more reliable indicators than apathy.[99] These symptoms and signs should be closely monitored. The association between depression and stroke in specific anatomical regions of the brain remains controversial.[100] Treatment regimens depend on the severity of the depression and usually involve antidepressants. A number of antidepressants have been shown to be effective in treating post-stroke depression, and the choice of agent is often determined by the side effect profile.[97,98]

PREVENTION OF FALLS

The risk of fall after stroke increases during active rehabilitation and after discharge compared to the acute phase. A major risk is hip fracture, especially in chronic stroke patients, partially due to bone loss associated with immobility.[101] Almost 40% of stroke patients experience at least one fall during rehabilitation and injuries are reported in 22% of falls.[102,103] While most fall-related injuries are contusions and abrasions, occasionally more serious injuries result. Prevention includes appropriate supervision by the staff and caregivers and management of environmental hazards. Falls are more frequent in patients with hemineglect, during transfers, in patients with cognitive impairment, in patients receiving sedative medications, and in patients with more severe functional deficits.[102,104] It should be part of the neurorehabilitation process to teach the patient and caregivers how to get up after a fall. Falls at home and/or community may be prevented if the environment is adapted with handrails, grab bars in the shower and bathtub, nonslipping mat inside the bathtub or shower room, and taller toilet seat. Patients should be also taught to push or roll objects rather than carrying them, wear nonslipping shoes, remove all electrical cords that are on the walking pathway, use a walker and/or canes with rubber tips, remove loose rugs, and rearrange chairs in different places in case the patient becomes fatigued.

ASSESSMENT OF RECOVERY

Recovery can be defined in many ways. In stroke survivors, important outcomes are return home, recovery of ambulation, and independence in ADLs.[12,105,106] A number of multifaceted scales that measure important rehabilitation outcomes have been designed. One of the earliest was the Barthel Index (BI). It has been well validated and is now a widely accepted ADL scale. The BI is an aggregate scale with a total score of 100. It consists of 15 items, 9 of which relate to self-care and 6 to mobility. It should record what a patient actually does, not what a patient could do. The BI is especially important in predicting the need for personal assistance in daily living. After a stroke, a BI score of greater than 60 correlates with ambulation and need for some assistance with ADLs. This is the point at which a spouse or caregiver can reasonably manage a patient at home. A BI score of greater than 95 correlates well with independence in ambulation and self-care activities.

A more recent comprehensive scale is the Functional Independence Measure (FIM). The FIM (Table 26-2) is basically an expanded BI, incorporating additional measures of cognitive and communication skills and social integration. The FIM is more sensitive to small changes in status, and has therefore gained favor for following the progress of individual patients during their rehabilitation. It has now largely replaced the BI in clinical settings. The FIM has also been incorporated into a large, widely used national database. It is important to realize that even though a patient has a perfect score on the BI or FIM, this does not mean that the person is neurologically normal, only that the person is independent in self-care.

Many scales have been devised to assess motor function and disability. A good example is the Fugl-Meyer Assessment[107] which is widely used as a motor outcome measure in research trials.

The Modified Rankin Scale is widely used in research studies as a simple measure of functional outcome following a stroke:

0   Asymptomatic
1   No significant disability despite symptoms; able to carry out all usual duties and activities
2   Slight disability; unable to carry out all previous activities, but able to look after own affairs without assistance
3   Moderate disability requiring some help, but able to walk without assistance
4   Moderate severe disability; unable to walk without assistance and unable to attend to own bodily needs without assistance
5   Severe disability; bedridden, incontinent, and requiring constant nursing care and attention

Successful integration into the community requires more complex skills, including ability to use private or public transportation, shop, handle finances, and engage in leisure activities. These activities may be assessed using a variety of scales. Other scales are available for assessing other facets of recovery including speech and language function, general motor abilities, and gait.

DISCHARGE PLANS

Whether and when a person can go home after stroke depends on many factors, including age, severity of neurologic deficit, cognitive impairment, presence of incontinence, and co-morbid medical conditions.[9,108] The most important variable is often the family and social situation. As is well known to every clinician, a person with considerable disability is often able to return home if a caregiver is available, whereas a person with much less disability, but without a social support system, may require placement in a nursing home. In Western societies, men are more likely than women to return home (even with similar neurological deficits), usually because of the availability of a female caregiver.

To ensure a successful return home, a number of key issues should be addressed.[109] First, the home must be accessible. If exterior access is by means of stairs, practice with stair climbing should be undertaken with a caregiver assisting as necessary. All stairs must have rails. A ramp may need to be purchased or constructed; it should have a minimum grade of one foot of ramp for each one inch of elevation attained (an 8.3% slope). If the patient is confined to a wheelchair, doors must be wide enough to accommodate the chair. Furniture may need to be rearranged to allow for maximum safety, and loose rugs should be removed.

Table 26-2: Functional Independence Measure (FIM)

Levels for scoring	No helper	7 Complete independence (timely, safely)
		6 Modified Dependence (Device)
	Helper	Modified Dependence
		5 Supervision
		4 Minimal assist (subject = 75%+)
		3 Moderate assist (subject = 50%+)
		Complete dependence
		2 Maximal assist (subject = 25%+)
		1 Total assist (subject = 0%+)
	Functional categories	Score
Self-care	A. Eating	
	B. Grooming	
	C. Bathing	
	D. Dressing: upper body	
	E. Dressing: lower body	
	F. Toileting	
Sphincter control	G. Bladder management	
	H. Bowel management	
Mobility	Transfer:	
	I. Bed, chair, wheelchair	
	J. Toilet	
	K. Tub, shower	
	Locomotion:	
	L. Walk/wheelchair	
	M. Stairs	
Communication	N. Comprehension	
	O. Expression	
Special cognition	P. Social interaction	
	Q. Problem solving	
	R. Memory	
	Total FIM (maximum 126)	

Each FIM functional category is scored from 1 (total assist) to 7 (complete independence) using the "levels for scoring" at the top of the table. The total score is obtained by adding all individual scores, with a maximum score of 126. Leave no blanks: enter 1 if patient not testable due to risk. Detailed published guidelines are available for each category to assist with proper scoring. In order to correctly score FIM categories and assure inter-rater reliability, all raters should become "FIM certified" by taking a short training course.

Grab bars may need to be placed strategically in the walls near the toilet. Safe bathing may be facilitated by providing a tub bench and arranging for a hand-held shower hose. A home visit by an occupational therapist may be very helpful in assessing the home environment and making recommendations.

Before discharge, any additional needed equipment such as canes, commodes, adaptive devices, and wheelchairs should be procured. The family or caregiver should be educated about the patient's abilities and the tasks with which the patient will need assistance. In some instances, caregivers may need to provide assistance in transferring the person in and out of the wheelchair, on and off the toilet, and in and out of bed. Car transfers must be learned for those confined to wheelchairs, to facilitate health care visits and community activities.

Caregivers often need to assist with ADLs, especially bathing and dressing. Several hands-on training sessions with the therapists facilitate learning safe, energy-efficient techniques, and greatly bolster family/caregiver confidence.[12,110] What role the stroke patient will have in other aspects of the household activities, such as meal preparation and financial management, should be discussed. For those unable to return for outpatient rehabilitation, therapy sessions can be arranged in the home, which has the advantage of providing functional training in the patient's own environment. Home health aides who can assist with personal care activities several times a week, especially bathing, can greatly relieve the family's burden. Home rehabilitation and provision of support services can permit continued functioning in the home setting for many years.[24]

For those who are able, a course of outpatient therapy helps facilitate further functional gains and has the secondary advantage of encouraging community reintegration because the patient must leave home to travel to the outpatient clinic.

DRIVING

Driving may be a very important goal, especially for younger stroke patients.[111] Most patients who have recovered sufficiently want to drive an automobile again. The decision to permit this can be particularly difficult and should be considered by the physician, patient, and family together; they must not let emotions interfere. Driving a car requires attention, concentration, good vision, intact reflex responses, and rapid decision making. If a cerebrovascular episode impairs one or more of these factors, driving should be discouraged; this is especially true for patients with homonymous hemianopsia, visual neglect, impaired judgment, or seizures. For those in whom the only deficit is hemiparesis, a specially adapted vehicle can be designed.

About 30% of stroke survivors who drove before the stroke resume driving after the stroke,[112] but almost 90% do not receive a driving evaluation. A pre-driving evaluation should include clinical and neurological evaluation, simulators or behind-the-wheel training, and car evaluation with recommendations for adaptive devices and modifications. Driving evaluation and vehicle adaptation services are available through many hospital- and community-based rehabilitation programs and should be considered for most patients. On-the-road testing with an experienced evaluator can predict safe driving with a high degree of accuracy.[113] Ultimately, the decision is the responsibility of state officials and is based not on the neurologic evaluation but on laws and road testing by appropriate licensing officials.

VOCATIONAL ASPECTS

More than 25% of stroke patients are younger than 65 years of age at the time of onset and the ability to return to work may be important for personal finances as well as for maximal quality of life. Therefore, vocational, educational and intellectual aspects need to be assessed for each patient to evaluate the possibility of resuming a previous job or seeking alternative positions. The process of returning to work is highly individual and affected by multiple factors.[114] The factors most predictive of being able to return to work include ability to walk, being a white collar worker, and having preserved cognitive ability.[115] Adequate architectural accessibility, knowledge about stroke and its consequences by the employee and employer, job coaching, appropriate seating and other environmental accommodations may be other important aspects for a successful return to work.

QUALITY OF LIFE

Quality of life is a term that is quite specific to each individual and involves many domains outside of health. Health-related quality of life (HRQOL) is more specific for illness and injury and clearly declines following stroke.[116–119] Determinants of HRQOL include depression, functional restrictions, stroke location, severity of paralysis, social support, and medical comorbidity.[120] Stroke survivors may show improvement in function, for example ADLs, but still have poor HRQOL,[116,120] even several years after stroke. Emotional well-being may remain a major concern, even in stroke survivors with high levels of social support.[120]

Therefore, maximizing quality of life often requires a multifaceted approach beyond the realm of traditional rehabilitation. At the individual level, treating depression, maximizing function, providing a safe and accessible living environment, and education of stroke survivors and their families are all important goals. At the societal level, advocating for social service support, vocational retraining programs, and accessibility in public places may benefit persons with disabilities, including those with stroke.

Quality of life also decreases for caregivers, who often must assume considerable new responsibility.[121] There is evidence that stroke caregivers have an increased risk for depression.[12] Rehabilitation professionals need to be alert to the need for counseling and education for caregivers. Stroke support groups may provide valuable assistance in this regard.

RESEARCH AND EMERGING STRATEGIES IN STROKE REHABILITATION

The adult brain can reorganize to accommodate environmental changes and to compensate for lost function, a process known as plasticity. The last few years have provided extraordinary evidence regarding the mechanisms underlying plasticity changes and spurred the development of new strategies to up-modulate these processes.[122–124] The ability of the mature brain to constantly reorganize has gained further credibility with the advances of neuroimaging techniques and the advent of transcranial magnetic stimulation.[125] Different neurophysiological techniques have demonstrated that plastic changes occur in response to pharmacological agents, in response to peripheral sensory-motor stimulation, and in association with intense motor training such as constraint-induced movement therapy. While several novel approaches seem to be promising and will someday be incorporated into standard rehabilitation programs after stroke, large-scale, well-designed, double-blind randomized trials are required to establish effectiveness.[77,126] The use of implanted stem cells or neural progenitor cells has been tried in experimental animals, but many questions remain before this technique can be used in humans. For any new therapy, a number of issues must be addressed: (1) the optimal time-window to deliver a specific intervention, (2) the detailed profile of stroke patients likely to benefit from the intervention, (3) the intensity-response of the intervention, and (4) the ultimate effect on quality of life.

In situations in which all other rehabilitation approaches fail, the emerging area of the "brain machine interface" offers hope. It is well known that brain activity, obtained from refined EEG signals,[127] from the electrical activity of neuronal ensembles, or even from the activity of single neurons,[128,129] can be used to power robots, prosthetic limbs, and other "machines." While much remains to be learned, this approach could provide a means for independence for severely disabled persons in the future.

REFERENCES

1. Jorgensen HS, Nakayama H, Raaschou HO, Olsen TS. Stroke. Neurologic and functional recovery the Copenhagen Stroke Study. *Phys Med Rehabil Clin N Am*. 1999;**104**:887–906.
2. Hendricks HT, van Limbeek J, Geurts AC, Zwarts MJ. Motor recovery after stroke: a systematic review of the literature. *Arch Phys Med Rehabil*. 2002;**8311**:1629–1637.
3. Dobkin BH. Rehabilitation after stroke. *N Engl J Med*. 2005;**352**:1677–1684.
4. Nakayama H, Jorgensen HS, Raaschou HO, Olsen TS. Recovery of upper extremity function in stroke patients: the Copenhagen Stroke Study. *Arch Phys Med Rehabil*. 1994;**754**:394–398.
5. Duncan PW, Goldstein LB, Matchar D, Divine GW, Feussner J. Measurement of motor recovery after stroke. Outcome assessment and sample size requirements. *Stroke*. 1992;**23**:1084–1089.
6. Page SJ, Gater DR, Bach-Y-Rita P. Reconsidering the motor recovery plateau in stroke rehabilitation. *Arch Phys Med Rehabil*. 2004;**858**:1377–1381.
7. Reding MJ, Potes E. Rehabilitation outcome following initial unilateral hemispheric stroke: life table analysis approach. *Stroke*. 1988;**19**:1354–1358.
8. Wade D, Langton Hewer R. Functional abilities after stroke: measurements natural history and prognosis. *J Neurol Neurosurg Psychiatry*. 1987;**50**:177–182.
9. Berlowitz DR, Hoenig H, Cowper DC, Duncan PW, Vogel WB. Impact of comorbidities on stroke rehabilitation outcomes: does the method matter? *Arch Phys Med Rehabil*. 2008;**89**:1903–1906.
10. Dromerick A, Reding M. Medical and neurological complications during inpatient stroke rehabilitation. *Stroke*. 1994;**252**:358–361.
11. Bates B, Choi JY, Duncan PW, et al. Veterans Affairs/Department of Defense clinical practice guidelines for the management of adult stroke rehabilitation care: Executive Summary. *Stroke*. 2005;**36**:2049–2056.
12. Duncan PW, Zorowitz R, Bates B, et al. Management of adult stroke rehabilitation care: A clinical practice guideline. *Stroke*. 2005;**36**:e100–e143.
13. Reddy MP, Reddy V. After a stroke: strategies to restore function and prevent complications. *Geriatrics*. 1997;**529**:59–62, 71, 75.
14. Stroke Unit Trialists' Collaboration. Organised inpatient (stroke unit) care for stroke. *Cochrane Database Syst Rev*. 2002;**1**:CD000197.
15. Langhorne P, Dennis MS. Stroke units: the next 10 years. *Lancet*. 2004;**3639412**:834–835.
16. Indredavik B, Bakke F, Slordahl SA, Rokseth R, Haheim LL. Stroke unit treatment. 10-year follow-up. *Stroke*. 1999;**308**:1524–1527.
17. Langhorne P, Cadilhac D, Feigin V, Grieve R, Liu M. How should stroke services be organised? *Lancet Neurol*. 2002;**11**:62–68.
18. Weinrich M, Good DC, Reding M, et al. Timing, intensity, and duration of rehabilitation for hip fracture and stroke: report of a workshop at the National Center for Medical Rehabilitation Research. *Neurorehabil Neural Repair*. 2004;**181**:12–28.
19. Lutz BJ. Determinants of discharge destination for stroke patients. *Rehabil Nurs*. 2004;**295**:154–163.
20. Brown RD Jr, Ransom J, Hass S, et al. Use of nursing home after stroke and dependence on stroke severity: a population-based analysis. *Stroke*. 1999;**305**:924–929.
21. Ottenbacher KJ, Smith PM, Illig SB, Linn RT, Ostir GV, Granger CV. Trends in length of stay, living setting, functional outcome, and mortality following medical rehabilitation. *JAMA*. 2004;**29214**:1687–1695.
22. Gillen R, Tennen H, McKee T. The impact of the inpatient rehabilitation facility prospective payment system on stroke program outcomes. *Am J Phys Med Rehabil*. 2007;**865**:356–363.
23. Legg L, Langhorne P; Outpatient Service Trialists. Rehabilitation therapy services for stroke patients living at home: systematic review of randomised trials. *Lancet*. 2004;**3639406**:352–356.
24. Thorsen AM, Holmqvist LW, de Pedro-Cuesta J, von Koch L. A randomized controlled trial of early supported discharge and continued rehabilitation at home after stroke: five-year follow-up of patient outcome. *Stroke*. 2005;**362**:297–303.
25. Coletta EM, Murphy JB. The complications of immobility in the elderly stroke patient. *J Am Board Fam Pract*. 1992;**54**:389–397.
26. Bernhardt J, Dewey H, Thrift A, Donnan G. Inactive and alone: physical activity within the first 14 days of acute stroke unit care. *Stroke*. 2004;**354**:1005–1009.
27. Asberg KH. Orthostatic tolerance training of stroke patients in general medical wards. An experimental study. *Scand J Rehabil Med*. 1989;**214**:179–185.
28. Cifu DX, Stewart DG. Factors affecting functional outcome after stroke: a critical review of rehabilitation interventions. *Arch Phys Med Rehabil*. 1999;**805**(Suppl 1):S35–S39.
29. Paolucci S, Antonucci G, Grasso MG, et al. Early versus delayed inpatient stroke rehabilitation: a matched comparison conducted in Italy. *Arch Phys Med Rehabil*. 2000;**81**:695–700.
30. Jorgensen HS, Nakayama H, Raaschou HO, Olsen TS. Recovery of walking function in stroke patients: the Copenhagen Stroke Study. *Arch Phys Med Rehabil*. 1995;**761**:27–32.
31. O'Dwyer NJ, Ada L, Neilson PD. Spasticity and muscle contracture following stroke. *Brain*. 1996;**119**:1737–1749.
32. Burge E, Kupper D, Finckh A, Ryerson S, Schnider A, Leemann B. Neutral functional realignment orthosis prevents hand pain in patients with subacute stroke: a randomized trial. *Arch Phys Med Rehabil*. 2008;**89**:1857–1862.
33. Turner-Stokes L, Jackson D. Shoulder pain after stroke: a review of the evidence base to inform the development of an integrated care pathway. *Clin Rehabil*. 2002;**163**:276–298.
34. Snels IA, Dekker JH, van der Lee JH, Lankhorst GJ, Beckerman H, Bouter LM. Treating patients with hemiplegic shoulder pain. *Am J Phys Med Rehabil*. 2002;**812**:150–160.
35. Dromerick AW, Edwards DF, Kumar A. Hemiplegic shoulder pain syndrome: frequency and characteristics during inpatient stroke rehabilitation. *Arch Phys Med Rehabil*. 2008;**89**:1589–1593.
36. Satkunam LE. Rehabilitation medicine: 3. Management of adult spasticity. *CMAJ*. 2003;**16911**:1173–1179.
37. Van Kuijk AA, Geurts AC, Bevaart BJ, van Limbeek J. Treatment of upper extremity spasticity in stroke patients by focal neuronal or neuromuscular blockade: a systematic review of the literature. *J Rehabil Med*. 2002;**342**:51–61.
38. Simpson DM, Gracies JM, Graham HK, et al. Assessment: *Botulinum* neurotoxin for the treatment of spasticity (an evidence-based review). *Neurology*. 2008;**70**:1691–1698.
39. Hesse S, Werner C. Poststroke motor dysfunction and spasticity: novel pharmacological and physical treatment strategies. *CNS Drugs*. 2003;**1715**:1093–1107.

40. Teasell RW, Bhogal SK, Foley NC, Speechley MR. Gait retraining post stroke. *Top Stroke Rehabil.* 2003;**102**:34–65.

41. Mauritz KH. Gait training in hemiplegia. *Eur J Neurol.* 2002; **9**(Suppl 1):23–29; discussion 53–61.

42. Barbeau H, Fung J. The role of rehabilitation in the recovery of walking in the neurological population. *Curr Opin Neurol.* 2001;**146**:735–740.

43. Hesse S. Recovery of gait and other motor functions after stroke: novel physical and pharmacological treatment strategies. *Restor Neurol Neurosci.* 2004;**223–225**:359–369.

44. Moseley AM, Stark A, Cameron ID, Pollock A. Treadmill training and body weight support for walking after stroke. *Cochrane Database Syst Rev.* 2003:CD002840.

45. Duncan PW, Sullivan KJ, Behrman AL, et al. Protocol for the locomotor experience applied post-stroke (LEAPS) trial: a randomized controlled trial. *BMC Neurol.* 2007;**7**:39.

46. Hanna D, Harvey RL. Review of preorthotic biomechanical considerations. *Top Stroke Rehabil.* 2001;**74**:29–37.

47. Teasell RW, McRae MP, Foley N, Bhardwaj A. Physical and functional correlations of ankle-foot orthosis use in the rehabilitation of stroke patients. *Arch Phys Med Rehabil.* 2001;**828**: 1047–1049.

48. Chen C-K, Hong W-H, Chu N-K, Lau Y-C, Lew HL, Tang SFT. Effects of an anterior ankle-foot orthosis on postural stability in stroke patients with hemiplegia. *Am J Phys Med Rehabil.* 2008;**87**: 815–820.

49. Wang RY, Lin PY, Lee CC, Yang YR. Gait and balance performance improvements attributable to ankle-foot orthosis in subjects with hemiparesis. *Am J Phys Med Rehabil.* 2007;**867**: 556–562.

50. Bateni H, Maki BE. Assistive devices for balance and mobility: benefits, demands, and adverse consequences. *Arch Phys Med Rehabil.* 2005;**861**:134–145.

51. Allen SM. Canes, crutches and home care services: the interplay of human and technological assistance. *Cent Home Care Policy Res Policy Briefs.* 2001;**4**:1–6.

52. Taylor SJ. An overview of evaluation for wheelchair seating for people who have had strokes. *Top Stroke Rehabil.* 2003;**101**: 95–99.

53. Trefler E, Taylor SJ. Prescription and positioning: evaluating the physically disabled individual for wheelchair seating. *Prosthet Orthot Int.* 1991;**153**:217–224.

54. Paci M. Physiotherapy based on the Bobath concept for adults with post-stroke hemiplegia: a review of effectiveness studies. *J Rehabil Med.* 2003;**351**:2–7.

55. Van Peppen RPS, Kwakkel G, Wood-Dauphinee S, Hendriks HJM, Van der Wees Ph J, Dekker J. The impact of physical therapy on functional outcomes after stroke: what's the evidence? *Clin Rehabil.* 2004;**18**:833–862.

56. Kwakkel G, van Peppen R, Wagenaar RC, et al. Effects of augmented exercise therapy time after stroke: a meta-analysis. *Stroke.* 2004;**3511**:2529–2539.

57. Wolf SL, Winstein CJ, Miller JP, et al. Effect of constraint-induced movement therapy on upper extremity function 3 to 9 months after stroke. *JAMA.* 2006;**296**:2095–2104.

58. Kwakkel G, Kollen BJ, Krebs HI. Effects of robot-assisted therapy on upper limb recovery after stroke: A systematic review. *Neurorehabil Neural Repair.* 2008;**22**:111–121.

59. Siekierka EM, Eng K, Bassetti C, et al. New technologies and concepts for rehabilitation in the acute phase of stroke: a collaborative matrix. *Neurodegenerative Dis.* 2007;**4**:57–69.

60. Webster BR, Celnik PA, Cohen LG. Noninvasive brain stimulation in stroke rehabilitation. *NeuroRx.* 2006;**3**:474–481.

61. Cauraugh J, Light K, Kim S, Thigpen M, Behrman A. Chronic motor dysfunction after stroke: recovering wrist and finger extension by electromyography-triggered neuromuscular stimulation. *Stroke.* 2000;**31**:1360–1364.

62. Chae J, Bethoux F, Bohine T, Dobos L, Davis T, Friedl A. Neuromuscular stimulation for upper extremity motor and functional recovery in acute hemiplegia. *Stroke.* 1998;**29**:975–979.

63. Lindmark B. Evaluation of functional capacity after stroke with special emphasis on motor function and activities of daily living. *Scand J Rehabil Med Suppl.* 1988;**21**:1–40.

64. Steultjens EM, Dekker J, Bouter LM, van de Nes JC, Cup EH, van den Ende CH. Occupational therapy for stroke patients: a systematic review. *Stroke.* 2003;**343**:676–687.

65. Sorensen HV, Lendal S, Schultz-Larsen K, Uhrskov T. Stroke rehabilitation: assistive technology devices and environmental modifications following primary rehabilitation in hospital – a therapeutic perspective. *Assist Technol.* 2003;**151**:39–48.

66. Hirsch J, et al. Antithrombotic and Thrombolytic Therapy. 8th ed. ACCP Guidelines. *Chest.* 2008;**133**(6 Suppl):67S-968S.

67. Mazzone C, Chiodo GF, Sandercock P, Miccio M, Salvi R. Physical methods for preventing deep vein thrombosis in stroke. *Cochrane Database Syst Rev.* 2004:CD001922.

68. Schroeder MF, Daniels SK, McCain M, Corey DM, Foundas AL. Clinical and cognitive predictors of swallowing recovery in stroke. *J Rehabil Res Dev.* 2006;**433**:301–310.

69. Finestone HM, Greene-Finestone LS. Rehabilitation medicine: 2. Diagnosis of dysphagia and its nutritional management for stroke patients. *CMAJ.* 2003;**16910**:1041–1044.

70. Horner J, Massey EW, Riski JE, Lathrop DL, Chase KN. Aspiration following stroke: clinical correlates and outcome. *Neurology.* 1988;**389**:1359–1362.

71. Bath PM, Bath FJ, Smithard DG. Interventions for dysphagia in acute stroke. *Cochrane Database Syst Rev.* 2000;**2**:CD000323.

72. Steele CM, Thrasher AT, Popovic MR. Electric stimulation approaches to the restoration and rehabilitation of swallowing; a review. *Neurol Res.* 2007;**291**:9–15.

73. Carnaby-Mann GD, Crary MA. Examining the evidence on neuromuscular electrical stimulation for swallowing: a meta-analysis. *Arch Otolaryngol Head Neck Surg.* 2007;**1336**:564–571.

74. Brocklehurst JC, Andrews K, Richards B, Laycock PJ. Incidence and correlates of incontinence in stroke patients. *J Am Geriatr Soc.* 1985;**338**:540–542.

75. Nakayama H, Jorgensen HS, Pedersen PM, Raaschou HO, Olsen TS. Prevalence and risk factors of incontinence after stroke. The Copenhagen Stroke Study. *Stroke.* 1997;**28**:58–62.

76. Gelber DA, Good DC, Laven LJ, Verhulst SJ. Causes of urinary incontinence after acute hemispheric stroke. *Stroke.* 1993;**243**: 378–382.

77. Dobkin BH. Strategies for stroke rehabilitation. *Lancet Neurol.* 2004;**39**:528–536.

78. Pedersen PM, Jorgensen HS, Nakayama H, Raaschou HO, Olsen TS. Aphasia in acute stroke: incidence, determinants, and recovery. *Ann Neurol.* 1995;**384**:659–666.

79. Hillis AE. Aphasia. Progress in the last quarter of a century. *Neurology.* 2007;**69**:200–213.

80. Robey RR. A meta-analysis of clinical outcomes in the treatment of aphasia. *J Speech Lang Hear Res.* 1998;**41**:172–187.

81. Robey RR. The efficacy of treatment for aphasia persons: a meta-analysis. *Brain Lang.* 1994;**47**:585–608.

82. Bhogal SK, Teasell R, Speechley M. Intensity of aphasia therapy, impact on recovery. *Stroke.* 2003;**34**:987–993.

83. Klein RB, Albert ML. Can drug therapies improve language functions of individuals with aphasia? A review of the evidence. *Semin Speech Lang.* 2004;**25**:193–204.

84. Liepert J. Pharmacotherapy in restorative neurology. *Cur Opin Neurol.* 2008;**21**:639–643.

85. Flöel A, Rösser N, Michka O, Knecht S, Breitenstein C. Noninvasive brain stimulation improves language learning. *J Cogn Neurosci*. 2008;**208**:1415–1422.

86. Raboyeau G, De Boissezon X, Marie N, et al. Right hemisphere activation in recovery from aphasia. Lesion effect or function recruitment? *Neurology*. 2008;**70**:290–298.

87. Jehkonen M, Laihosalo M, Kettunen J. Anosognosia after stroke: assessment, occurrence, subtypes and impact on functional outcome reviewed. *Acta Neurol Scand*. 2006;**1145**:293–306.

88. Lindell AB, Jalas MJ, Tenovuo O, Brunila T, Voeten MJ, Hämäläinen H. Clinical assessment of hemispatial neglect: evaluation of different measures and dimensions. *Clin Neuropsychol*. 2007;**213**:479–497.

89. Azouvi P, Bartolomeo P, Beis JM, Perennou D, Pradat-Diehl P, Rousseaux M. A battery of tests for the quantitative assessment of unilateral neglect. *Restor Neurol Neurosci*. 2006;**244–246**:273–285.

90. Barrett AM, Buxbaum LJ, Coslett HB, et al. Cognitive rehabilitation interventions for neglect and related disorders: moving from bench to bedside in stroke patients. *J Cogn Neurosci*. 2006;**187**:1223–1236.

91. Shiraishi H, Yamakawa Y, Itou A, Muraki T, Asada T. Long-term effects of prism adaptation on chronic neglect after stroke. *Neuro Rehabilitation*. 2008;**232**:137–151.

92. Luauté J, Halligan P, Rode G, Jacquin-Courtois S, Boisson D. Prism adaptation first among equals in alleviating left neglect: a review. *Restor Neurol Neurosci*. 2006;**244–246**:409–418.

93. Bowen A, Lincoln NB. Cognitive rehabilitation for spatial neglect following stroke. *Cochrane Database Syst Rev*. 2007;**2**: CD003586.

94. Jehkonen M, Laihosalo M, Kettunen JE. Impact of neglect on functional outcome after stroke: a review of methodological issues and recent research findings. *Restor Neurol Neurosci*. 2006; **244–246**:209–215.

95. Kauhanen M, Korpelainen JT, Hiltunen P, et al. Poststroke depression correlates with cognitive impairment and neurological deficits. *Stroke*. 1999;**309**:1875–1880.

96. Chemerinski E, Robinson RG, Kosier JT. Improved recovery in activities of daily living associated with remission of poststroke depression. *Stroke*. 2001;**321**:113–117.

97. Van de Meent H, Geurts ACH, Van Limbeek J. Pharmacologic treatment of poststroke depression: a systematic review of the literature. *Top Stroke Rehabil*. 2003;**101**:79–92.

98. Tharwani HIM, Yerramsetty P, Mannelli P, Patkar A, Masand P. Recent advances in poststroke depression. *Current Psychiatry Rep*. 2007;**9**:225–231.

99. Carota A, Berney A, Aybek S, et al. A prospective study of predictors of poststroke depression. *Neurology*. 2005;**643**:428–433.

100. Carson AJ, MacHale S, Allen K, et al. Depression after stroke and lesion location: a systematic review. *Lancet* 2000;**356**:122–126.

101. Poole KE, Reeve J, Warburton EA. Falls, fractures, and osteoporosis after stroke: time to think about protection? *Stroke*. 2002; **335**:1432–1436.

102. Teasell R, McRae M, Foley N, Bhardwaj A. The incidence and consequences of falls in stroke patients during inpatient rehabilitation: factors associated with high risk. *Arch Phys Med Rehabil*. 2002;**833**:329–333.

103. Nyberg L, Gustafson Y. Patient falls in stroke rehabilitation. A challenge to rehabilitation strategies. *Stroke*. 1995;**265**:838–842.

104. Hyndman D, Ashburn A, Stack E. Fall events among people with stroke living in the community: circumstances of falls and characteristics of fallers. *Arch Phys Med Rehabil*. 2002;**832**:165–170.

105. Dromerick AW, Edwards DF, Diringer MN. Sensitivity to changes in disability after stroke: a comparison of four scales useful in clinical trials. *J Rehabil Res Dev*. 2003;**401**:1–8.

106. Kwon S, Hartzema AG, Duncan PW, Min-Lai S. Disability measures in stroke: relationship among the Barthel Index, the Functional Independence Measure, and the Modified Rankin Scale. *Stroke*. 2004;**354**:918–923.

107. Gladstone DJ, Danells CJ, Black SE. The Fugl-Meyer assessment of motor recovery after stroke: a critical review of its measurement properties. *Neurorehabil Neural Repair*. 2002;**163**:232–240.

108. Massucci M, Perdon L, Agosti M, et al. Prognostic factors of activity limitation and discharge destination after stroke rehabilitation. *Am J Phys Med Rehabil*. 2006;**85**:963–970.

109. Reid D. Accessibility and usability of the physical housing environment of seniors with stroke. *Int J Rehabil Res*. 2004;**273**: 203–208.

110. Patel A, Knapp M, Evans A, Perez I, Kalra L. Training care givers of stroke patients: economic evaluation. *BMJ*. 20048;**3287448**:1102.

111. Legh-Smith J, Wade DT, Hewer RL. Driving after a stroke. *J R Soc Med*. 1986;**794**:200–203.

112. Fisk GD, Owsley C, Pulley LV. Driving after stroke: driving exposure, advice, and evaluations. *Arch Phys Med Rehabil*. 1997; **7812**:1338–1345.

113. Akinwuntan AE, Feys H, De Weerdt W, Baten G, Arno P, Kiekens C. Prediction of driving after stroke: a prospective study. *Neurorehabil Neural Repair*. 2006;**203**:417–423.

114. Saeki S. Disability management after stroke: its medical aspects for workplace accommodation. *Disabil Rehabil*. 2000;**10–20**; 2213–2214:578–582.

115. Vestling M, Tufvesson B, Iwarsson S. Indicators for return to work after stroke and the importance of work for subjective well-being and life satisfaction. *J Rehabil Med*. 2003;**353**:127–131.

116. Madden S, Hopman WM, Bagg S, Verner J, O'Callaghan CJ. Functional status and health-related quality of life during inpatient stroke rehabilitation. *Am J Phys Med Rehabil*. 2006;**85**:831–838.

117. Niemi ML, Laaksonen R, Kotila M, Waltimo O. Quality of life 4 years after stroke. *Stroke*. 1998;**19**:1101–1107.

118. King RB. Quality of life after stroke. *Stroke*. 1996;**27**:1467–1472.

119. Astrom M, Asplund K, Astrom T. Psychosocial function and life satisfaction after stroke. *Stroke*. 1992;**23**:527–531.

120. White JH, Alston MK, Marquez JL, et al. Community-dwelling stroke survivors: function is not the whole story with quality of life. *Arch Phys Med Rehabil*. 2007;**88**:1140–1146.

121. Adams C. Quality of life for caregivers and stroke survivors in the immediate discharge period. *Appl Nurs Res*. 2003;**162**:126–130.

122. Ward NS, Cohen LG. Mechanisms underlying recovery of motor function after stroke. *Arch Neurol*. 2004;**6112**:1844–1848.

123. Ward NS. Functional reorganization of the cerebral motor system after stroke. *Curr Opin Neurol*. 2004;**176**:725–730.

124. Sawaki L. Use-dependent plasticity of the human motor cortex in health and disease. *IEEE Engl Med Biol Mag*. 2005;**241**:36–39.

125. Baron JC, Cohen LG, Cramer SC, et al. Neuroimaging in stroke recovery: a position paper from the First International Workshop on Neuroimaging and Stroke Recovery. *Cerebrovasc Dis*. 2004;**183**:260–267.

126. Good DC. Stroke: promising neurorehabilitation interventions and steps toward testing them. *Am J Phys Med Rehabil*. 2003; **8210**(Suppl):S50–57.

127. Lenthardt EC, Miller KJ, Schalk G, Rao RPN, Ojemann JG. Electrocorticography-based brain computer interface – The Seattle experience. *IEEE Trans Neural Syst Rehab Engng*. 2008;**14**:194–198.

128. Velliste M, Perel S, Schwartz, et al. Cortical control of a prosthetic arm for self-feeling. *Nature*. 2008;**4537198**:1098–1101.

129. Kalaska JF. Neuroscience: brain control of a helping hand. *Nature*. 2008;**4537198**:994–995.

130. Wade DT, Skilbeck CF, Hewer RL. Predicting Barthel ADL score at 6 months after an acute stroke. *Arch Phys Med Rehabil*. 1983; **64**:24–28.

Index